Michael Thomas,

It was a great pleasure to meet you at the South Eastern Surgical Congress in Atlanta. I do hope that this book does not mislead you too often.

With my best wishes.

John R. Skinner.

April 28, 1980.

SURGERY OF THE ANUS, RECTUM AND COLON

To
Nancy, Susan, Jane and Michael

Surgery of the Anus Rectum and Colon

J. C. GOLIGHER

ChM(Ed), FRCS(Ed), FRCS(Eng), Hon MD(Göteborg), Hon FRCS(I), Hon FRACS, Hon FACS
Consultant in General and Colorectal Surgery, Leeds, England
Emeritus Professor of Surgery, the University of Leeds, and formerly Chairman
University Department of Surgery, the General Infirmary at Leeds
Consulting Surgeon, St Mark's Hospital for Diseases of the Rectum and Colon, London

WITH THE COLLABORATION OF

H. L. DUTHIE

MD, ChM(Glasg), FRCS(Ed), FRCS(Eng)
Professor of Surgery, University of Sheffield
Surgeon, Royal Infirmary, Sheffield, England

AND

H. H. NIXON

MA, MB, BChir(Cantab), FRCS(Eng)
Surgeon, Hospital for Sick Children, Great Ormond Street,
and Paddington Green Children's Hospital, London

Fourth Edition

BAILLIÈRE TINDALL · LONDON

A BAILLIÈRE TINDALL book published by
Cassell Ltd,
35 Red Lion Square, London WC1R 4SG
and at Sydney, Auckland, Toronto, Johannesburg
an affiliate of
Macmillan Publishing Co. Inc.
New York

First published 1961
Third edition 1975
   Reprinted 1976, 1977
Fourth edition 1980

ISBN 0 7020 0750 1

Spanish edition (Salvat Editores, Barcelona) *in preparation*
Italian edition (Precin Editore, Padua) *in preparation*

Printed in Great Britain by Spottiswoode Ballantyne Ltd.,
Colchester and London

British Library Cataloguing in Publication Data

Goligher, John Cedric
   Surgery of the anus, rectum and colon. 4th ed.
   1. Intestine, Large—Surgery
   I. Title II. Duthie, Herbert Livingstone
   III. Nixon, Harold Homewood
   617'.5547   RD541
   ISBN 0-7020-0750-1

Contents

COLOUR PLATES

Preface to the Fourth Edition

In preparing this edition, every effort has been made to bring all parts of the work fully abreast of the relevant literature at the time of completing my revision in October 1978—and even to include more recent matter subsequent to that date in the form of three appendices to the main text. I have again been most fortunate in retaining the co-authorship of Professor Herbert Duthie and Mr Harold Nixon to revise their sections on physiology and on congenital anorectal anomalies and aganglionosis respectively, and am deeply grateful to them for their valuable contributions. I myself have remained responsible for the rest of the text. In re-editing it I have drawn freely not only on the literature but also on information derived from my own practice and from recent clinical and investigative work done in conjunction with a number of former assistants and colleagues— Anthony Axon, Ali Bakran, Geoffrey Giles, Graham Hill, Peter Lee, David Lintott, John Macfie, Michael McMahon, Muriel Pollard and Keith Simpkins—to all of whom I would like to express my sincere thanks. As in previous editions, I have tried to reflect the various divergences of opinion on controversial points, but have also considered it my duty to leave the reader in no doubt as to my own views on all such issues.

Topics that have received special attention have been: Crohn's disease, the chapter on which has been largely re-written to eliminate outmoded concepts and incorporate new ideas including the results of a recent comprehensive survey of the outcome of surgical treatment on my own patients; the technique of various forms of low sphincter-saving resection of the rectum, including the use of stapling devices for construction of the anastomoses; recent innovations in the surgery and after-care of enterostomas, including the magnetic ring closing device for colostomies and the reservoir ileostomy; and the possible place of ileo-anal pull-through anastomosis with or without an ileal pouch as a treatment for ulcerative colitis. These newer technical methods have been fully illustrated and at the same time a large number of older illustrations relating to more established surgical procedures have been replaced by fresh figures to reflect more accurately my present practice. All these new illustrations have been prepared by my friend, Robert Lane, to whom I am immensely indebted for these further examples of his unsurpassed skill in surgical artwork, which, I am well aware, has contributed so much to the success of this book in the past.

In revising the text and illustrations for this new edition, the opportunity has been taken to set the type in two columns instead of one to the page, with the object of facilitating reading and economizing in precious space. One pleasing consequence is that it has been possible to accommodate a modest increase in the amount of text and number of illustrations without enlarging the book to an unwieldy size.

I have to express my grateful thanks to the editors and publishers of several journals for permission to reproduce illustrative material from articles by me, and similarly to other authors, as well as to the appropriate editors and publishers, for permission to use illustrations from their published work. The authorship and source of all such borrowed illustrations will be found separately recorded throughout the text. I must also acknowledge my heavy debt of gratitude to my secretaries, Joan Hancock and Maude Page, for their untiring efforts in preparing text, and to my publishers for their unfailing helpfulness and great expedition in the production of this edition.

I would like to think that in its present form the book will continue to be found a reliable guide to the better understanding and sound treatment of diseases of the large intestine. Nothing could afford me greater professional pleasure than the hope, however faint, that reading these pages might persuade some young surgeons that colorectal surgery is a challenging and satisfying specialty, worthy to be the main objective of their life's work.

June 1979

J. C. GOLIGHER
Glebe House, 5 Shaw Lane
Leeds LS6 4DH

1

Surgical Anatomy and Physiology of the Colon, Rectum and Anus

(With the collaboration of H. L. Duthie)

ANATOMY

By J. C. Goligher

The large intestine extends from the end of the ileum to the anus, comprises the caecum (and appendix), colon, rectum and anal canal, and is on the average about 135 cm long. Its calibre is greatest at its commencement at the caecum, and gradually diminishes as it is traced distally, but again becomes more dilated in the lowermost part of the rectum just above the contracted anal canal. In its course it describes roughly an arch which surrounds the coils of small intestine. It is readily distinguished from the small gut by its greater calibre; its sacculated appearance throughout most of its length; its possession in many parts of fatty appendages, the appendices epiploicae; the attachment to a part of it of the greater omentum; and its relatively greater fixity (Fig. 1).

The striking feature in the wall of the colon is the concentration of the outer longitudinal muscle coat into three narrow bands or taeniae, relatively shorter than the bowel itself, so that the latter is puckered with the production of the typical haustrations or sacculations. The three taeniae commence at the base of the appendix which has a complete longitudinal coat. In the distal sigmoid they eventually coalesce to provide a complete longitudinal muscle coat for the rectum, though sometimes the process of fusion is complete before the rectum is reached. Between the taeniae the colon wall is extremely thin and this accounts for the great and sometimes amazing capacity of this part of the bowel to undergo distension when obstructed, the caecum being particularly notable in this respect.

General Disposition and Relations

In the living subject there are considerable variations in the disposition of the colon, particularly of those portions equipped with a mesocolon, depending on the build of the individual. In men of sthenic type and broad build the transverse colon tends to occupy a horizontal position (Fig. 1A), while in slim women of hyposthenic type, who usually suffer from a general visceroptosis, the colon shares in this process and the transverse colon becomes very dependent, hanging down into the lower abdomen (Fig. 1B). Allowances should be made for these variations in position in reading the following rather stereotyped account of the general topography of the large intestine.

THE CAECUM

The caecum lies in the right iliac fossa above the lateral half of the inguinal ligament. Usually it is entirely enveloped by peritoneum but in some 5% of individuals the peritoneal covering is deficient posteriorly and the caecum then rests in direct contact with the fascia overlying the iliacus.

The *vermiform appendix* projects from the apex or lowermost part of the caecum. The ilium joins the large intestine on the medial and posterior aspect, and the level of this opening is accepted as an arbitrary division between caecum below and ascending colon above. The *ileocaecal* or *ileocolic* junction is guarded by a valve consisting of an upper and a lower segment or lip. These lips are semilunar in shape, run roughly horizontally and after coalescence in front and behind are prolonged

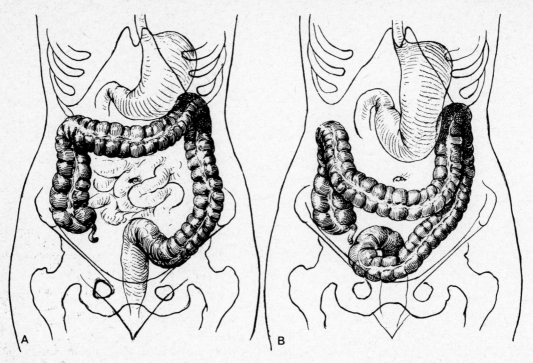

Fig. 1. General disposition of the large intestine as seen in the autopsy room: body of (A) a sthenic and (B) a hyposthenic individual. (*From Rankin et al. 1932*)

forward and backward on to the caecal wall as frenula. It is believed that when the caecum is distended the frenula and lips of the valves are rendered taut and thus brought into firm apposition, preventing regurgitation of caecal contents into the ileum.

THE ASCENDING COLON

The ascending colon is about 15 cm long. It runs upwards from the caecum to the hepatic or right colic flexure. It is invested with peritoneum on its anterior, lateral and medial surfaces, but posteriorly is devoid of peritoneal covering as a rule and lies in direct contact with the iliacus, the quadratus lumborum and the aponeurotic origin of the transversus abdominis below, and at a higher level is closely applied to the lower pole of the right kidney (Fig. 2). In front it is in relation with coils of ileum, possibly the right edge of the greater omentum and the anterior abdominal parietes.

THE HEPATIC FLEXURE

At the hepatic or right colic flexure the colon turns sharply medially, and slightly forward and downward, the site of this bend being just below the right lobe of the liver, and slightly overlapped by it, immediately in front of the lower part of the right kidney, and behind the peritoneum of the posterior abdominal wall (Fig. 2).

THE TRANSVERSE COLON

This segment of the colon is about 45 cm long in most subjects and forms a loop hanging downward across the upper and middle abdomen immediately below the greater curve of the stomach.

Its first 7·5–10 cm lie behind the posterior parietal peritoneum, closely applied to the front of the right kidney, the second part of the duodenum and the head of the pancreas to which it is connected by areolar tissue (Fig. 2). This is a most important posterior relationship for, during a right hemicolectomy, the duodenum is drawn up by its adherence to the right end of the transverse colon and may be damaged if care is not taken to separate it.

For the remainder of its course the transverse colon has a complete investment of peritoneum and is connected posterosuperiorly by the transverse mesocolon to the lower border of the pancreas. Behind, it is related to loops of small bowel including the duodenojejunal flexure. Immediately above this part of the transverse colon lies the stomach and, at its extreme left end, the lower pole of the spleen (Fig. 2). The greater omentum hanging down from the greater curve of the stomach descends in front of the transverse colon and then ascends to be attached loosely to its anterior surface and to the upper surface of the transverse mesocolon. The attachment of the omentum to the transverse colon and mesocolon is quite tenuous and can in most instances be readily divided at operation by a few touches of the scapel without severing more than a few small vessels. The entire greater omentum and upper layer of transverse mesocolon can thus be stripped off in a relatively quick and bloodless manner, this process being known as *décollement* (Fr. 'ungluing').

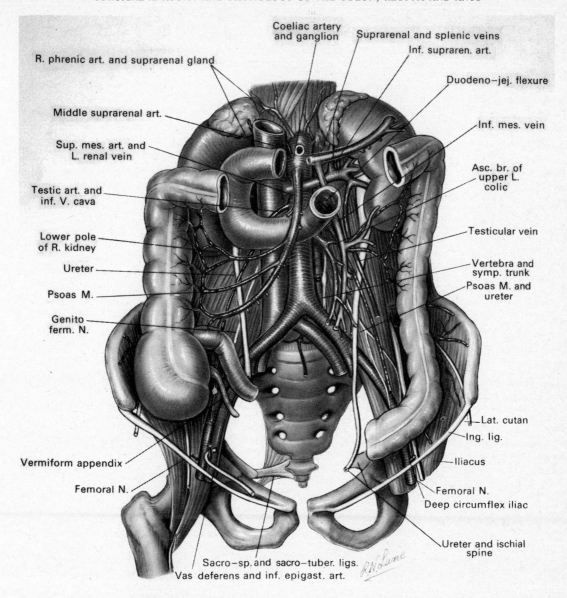

Coeliac artery and ganglion

Suprarenal and splenic veins

Inf. supraren. art.

R. phrenic art. and suprarenal gland

Middle suprarenal art.

Duodeno—jej. flexure

Inf. mes. vein

Sup. mes. art. and L. renal vein

Asc. br. of upper L. colic

Testic art. and inf. V. cava

Lower pole of R. kidney

Testicular vein

Ureter

Vertebra and symp. trunk

Psoas M.

Psoas M. and ureter

Genito ferm. N.

Lat. cutan

Ing. lig.

Iliacus

Vermiform appendix

Femoral N.

Femoral N.

Deep circumflex iliac

Ureter and ischial spine

Sacro—sp. and sacro—tuber. ligs.

Vas deferens and inf. epigast. art.

Fig. 2.   The posterior abdominal wall and large intestine demonstrating the posterior relations of the latter. (*After E. B. Jamieson*)

THE SPLENIC FLEXURE

This bend between the left end of the transverse colon and the descending colon is a much more acute angulation than the hepatic flexure. In addition, it is situated at a rather higher level than the right flexure and lies on a more posterior plane, more under the cover of the ribs and thus less accessible to surgical approach. It is covered with peritoneum in front; posteriorly it is in direct contact with the outer border of the middle of the left kidney (Fig. 2). There is a band of peritoneum extending from it laterally to the diaphragm—the *phrenicocolic ligament*—which helps to support the colon and spleen.

THE DESCENDING AND ILIAC COLON

From the splenic flexure the large intestine runs downward and slightly medially and then vertically as the descending colon as far as the iliac crest, a distance usually of about 20 cm. At this level it becomes the iliac colon, which proceeds downward and medially across the left iliac fossa to the medial border of the psoas major muscle where it becomes the sigmoid colon. [According to another anatomical terminology the descending colon extends from the splenic flexure to the sigmoid colon at the psoas major, no iliac segment being recognized (Gray 1926).] On its anterior, medial and lateral aspects the descending colon is covered by the posterior parietal peritoneum; behind, it is usually devoid of a peritoneal coat and rests directly against the left kidney, quadratus lumborum and transversus abdominis (Fig. 2). The iliac colon usually has a complete covering of peritoneum on all aspects and is provided with a short mesocolon, but almost invariably the lateral aspect of this part of the colon and its related mesocolon is adherent to the posterior parietal peritoneum of the left iliac fossa. If these adhesions are divided, however, as is regularly done by the surgeon in the initial stages of a rectal excision, the iliac mesocolon is readily re-established.

THE SIGMOID OR PELVIC COLON

The sigmoid colon extends from the lower end of the iliac colon at the margin of the psoas major muscle to the upper end of the rectum. It forms a loop which varies greatly in length, in one case being only 13–15 cm long, in another over 60 cm, but on the average is about 38 cm and normally lies within the pelvis. The actual disposition of the loop in the pelvis also varies greatly but it is convex forward and usually lies mainly in the left half of the pelvic cavity. It ends by joining the rectum in front of the third piece of the sacrum, usually slightly to the left of the midline. The sigmoid colon is completely surrounded by peritoneum which forms a mesentery, the sigmoid mesocolon; this diminishes in length from the centre toward the ends of the loop, where it disappears, so that the loop is fixed at its junctions with the iliac colon and the rectum but enjoys a considerable range of movement in its central portion. The base of the mesocolon has an attachment to the pelvic walls which forms an inverted V. The upper limb runs from the medial margin of the left psoas major upwards and medially to the midline, crossing in its course the left

ureter and iliac vessels. The lower limb extends vertically downward in front of the sacrum. The sigmoid colon itself is related to loops of small intestine, and usually also the bladder or uterus and uterine adnexa.

THE RECTUM

In cases with a fairly long loop of sigmoid colon which hangs down into the pelvis, the rectosigmoid junction is marked by a distinct flexure, as the terminal sigmoid, which is directed backward and upward, turns sharply downwards to follow the curve of the sacrum and become the rectum; but when the sigmoid colon is short such pronounced angulation may be absent. O'Beirne (1833) described a sphincter at the rectosigmoid junction and Mayo (1917) confirmed his observations. Subsequent work by Martin and Burden (1927) and others, however, has failed to substantiate their findings, and the consensus of opinion at the present day is that no such sphincter exists. At first the rectum proceeds downward, then downward and forward, closely applied to the concavity of the sacrum and coccyx for 13–15 cm. It ends 2–3 cm in front of and below the tip of the latter bone by turning abruptly downward and backward and passing through the levator muscles to become the anal canal, which has an average length of 3–4 cm and terminates at the anal orifice or anus.

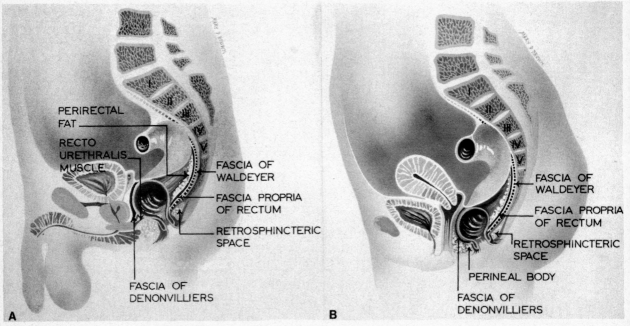

Fig. 3. Sagittal section of the male pelvis (A) and female pelvis (B) to demonstrate the anterior and posterior relations of the rectum. (*From Goligher 1959*)

RELATION OF PELVIC PERITONEUM TO
RECTUM

The relation of the pelvic peritoneum to the rectum is of considerable surgical importance. The upper third or so of the rectum has a complete peritoneal investment except for a thin strip posteriorly where the peritoneum is reflected off it as the two leaves of the thick short mesorectum (Fig. 3). As the rectum descends into the pelvis the mesorectum becomes broader and shorter and the peritoneum sweeps off, not at the back, but at the sides of the rectum, so that the uncovered portion posteriorly becomes progressively wider until only the anterior aspect has a peritoneal coat. Finally this becomes reflected forwards at the bottom of the rectovesical or recto-uterine pouch on to the back of the seminal vesicles

and bladder, or of the vagina and uterus in the female, leaving the lower third or so of the rectum without any peritoneal covering. Another difference to be detected in the peritoneal investment of the rectum as it is traced downward, is in the closeness of its attachment to the underlying muscle coat. In the upper rectum the peritoneum is closely applied, but this attachment becomes gradually looser lower down as a result of the interposition of a layer of fatty tissue, which is naturally thicker in obese subjects.

It will be seen, therefore, that it is possible to distinguish between *intraperitoneal* and *extra-peritoneal* parts of the rectum—the *rectum haut* and *rectum bas* of French surgeons—separated by the anterior and obliquely running lateral peritoneal reflections (Ewing 1952). Usually the upper one-half

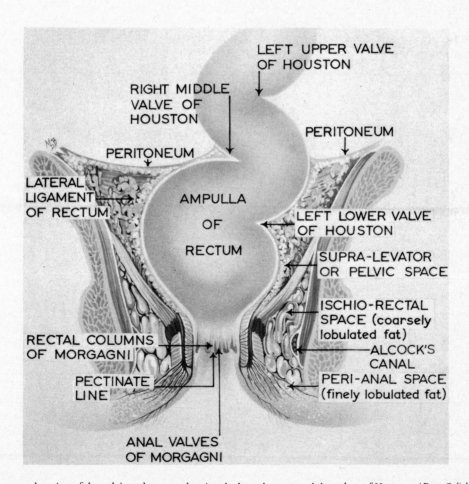

Fig. 4. A coronal section of the pelvis and rectum showing the lateral curves and the valves of Houston. (*From Goligher 1959*)

or one-third of the rectum lies in the peritoneal-covered segment, but the relative proportions of the intraperitoneal and extraperitoneal rectum vary considerably, for the peritoneal reflection is by no means a fixed landmark. On the contrary its position shows considerable individual variation and is also usually slightly lower in the female than the male. On the average the anterior peritoneal reflection lies about 8–9 cm from the perineal skin in the male and 5–8 cm in the female. In women with complete rectal prolapse the rectovaginal pouch is abnormally deep and actually protrudes into the rectum and through the anus into the prolapse (see Fig. 167).

THE FASCIAL RELATIONS OF THE RECTUM

On either side of the rectum below the pelvic peritoneum, between it and the floor of the pelvis formed by the levator ani muscles, is a space filled with fibrofatty tissue (Fig. 4). The fibrous elements in this tissue are a part of the pelvic fascia and connect the parietal pelvic fascia on the side wall of the pelvis with the rectum. They are known as the *lateral ligaments of the rectum* and seen from above, after a certain amount of definition, have a roughly triangular shape with the base on the pelvic side wall and the apex joining the side of the rectum. They may conceivably give some support to this part of the bowel. Their division is an essential step in the operation of rectal excision, and is followed by a variable amount of bleeding from the middle haemorrhoidal arteries which run in them.

The posterior aspect of the extraperitoneal rectum is loosely bound down to the front of the sacrum and coccyx by connective tissue which is easily separated by blunt dissection. When this is done it is found that there is still a thin layer of fascia covering the fat, vessels and lymph glands on the back of the rectum—this is the so-called *fascia propria* or *fascial capsule* of the rectum, and is a part of the visceral pelvic fascia (see Fig. 3A, B). The sacrum and coccyx are also still covered with a fascia; this is much stronger and tougher and is a specially thickened part of the parietal pelvic fascia which is known as the *fascia of Waldeyer* (1899). Traced inferiorly, according to Waldeyer (1899), this presacral fascia extends downwards and forwards on the upper aspect of the anococcygeal ligament to fuse with the fascia propria of the rectum at the anorectal junction, and this is the concept most surgeons have of the merging of these two fasciae. During excision of the rectum, when the coccyx is removed, or the anococcygeal raphe is

severed, the tough layer of fascia then encountered and generally known as the *fascia of Waldeyer*, has to be divided to give access to the retrorectal space. But Crapp and Cuthbertson (1974) dispute the propriety of labelling this structure with Waldeyer's name, as it had been previously described by Poirer and Charpy (1901); they prefer to call it the *recto-sacral fascia*. They also point out that in their dissections the rectosacral fascia usually lay at a slightly higher level, and extended from the fourth sacral segment to the back of the rectum, 3–5 cm above the anorectal ring. It was not to be confused with a more delicate layer of fascia immediately above the anococcygeal ligament. In carrying out the dissection from below for rectal excision it is important to sever the rectosacral fascia as it is met and not to strip the presacral fascia off the sacrum, for the middle sacral vessels, which lie between the latter fascia and the bone, are very liable to be torn if this faulty plane is struck.

Anteriorly, the extraperitoneal part of the rectum is also covered with a layer of visceral pelvic fascia which extends from the anterior peritoneal reflection above to the superior fascia of the urogenital diaphragm (triangular ligament) below, and laterally becomes continuous with the front of the lateral ligaments. It is a definite fascial layer, easily seen at operation for excision of the rectum, and known to surgeons as *Denonvillier's fascia* (see Fig. 3A, B). It intervenes between the rectum behind and the prostate and seminal vesicles or vagina anteriorly but is more closely adherent to the rectum than to these structures, so that it is more convenient to separate it from them along with the rectum in the course of a rectal excision and then to divide it transversely at a lower level. Sometimes the fascia consists of two layers.

OTHER RELATIONS OF THE RECTUM (see Fig. 3A, B)

Behind, outside the fascia of Waldeyer, the rectum is related to the sacrum and coccyx, the levator ani muscles, the left, and sometimes also the right, coccygeus muscle, the middle sacral vessels and the roots of the sacral plexus on either side.

In front, the relations of the rectum are entirely visceral and a considerable part of its surface is of course covered by peritoneum, which means that direct extension of growths forward is apt to result in implication of neighbouring organs or the peritoneal cavity. Recognition of these serious possibilities has led French surgeons to call the anterior aspect the *face dangereuse* of the rectum.

In the male, the extraperitoneal rectum is related from below upwards to the prostate, seminal vesicles, vasa deferentia, ureters and bladder wall. The intraperitoneal rectum has immediately in contact with it loops of small gut and possibly the sigmoid colon, and more remotely across the recto-vesical pouch it is related to the upper parts of the seminal vesicles and bladder.

In the female, the extraperitoneal rectum lies immediately behind the posterior vaginal wall. The intraperitoneal rectum is related across the pouch of Douglas to the upper part of the vagina and to the uterus, but occupying the pouch and separating it from these structures are frequently coils of small intestine, the ovaries, uterine tubes and the sigmoid colon.

Laterally above the peritoneal reflection are viscera, mainly loops of small gut, uterine appendages and the sigmoid colon. Below the reflection it is separated from the side wall of the pelvis, the ureter and iliac vessels by the connective tissue and fascia of the lateral ligament. At a still lower level the levator ani muscle becomes a close lateral relation, separated to some extent by the lower part of the lateral ligament.

THE CURVES OF THE RECTUM

Anteroposterior Curves. The angulations and curves of the rectum and anal canal in the sagittal plane have already been mentioned and are well shown in Fig. 3A, B.

Lateral Curves. The rectum also has lateral curves, though their prominence varies considerably. Usually there are three of them, the uppermost and lowermost being both convex to the right, the middle one convex to the left as in Fig. 4. The angulation of the bowel on the concave side of each of these curves is accentuated by infoldings of the mucosa known as *Houston's valves* (Houston 1830). There is thus an upper and lower valve on the left side and a middle valve on the right. The last-named, which is also known as *Kohlrausch's fold*, is by far the most prominent as a rule. It is situated about the same level as the anterior peritoneal reflection. The part of the rectum lying below the right valve and the peritoneal reflection has a wider lumen than has the intraperitoneal part; this dilated lower portion is known as the *ampulla* of the rectum (Fig. 4).

THE 'RECTOSIGMOID' AT OPERATION

At operation with the patient in the head-down position the sigmoid loop gravitates headwards out of the pelvis and the rectosigmoid flexure is largely undone, so that one criterion of distinction between the sigmoid and rectum is lost. No other definite criteria exist. The merging of the three separate taeniae of the lower sigmoid to provide a uniformly distributed longitudinal layer in the rectum is a gradual process which takes place over a distance of 7·5–10 cm, not always accurately centred on the precise rectosigmoid junction but sometimes a little higher or lower. The mesenteric relationships are not helpful, because the lower sigmoid and upper rectum both have short mesenteries which are quite indistinguishable. The consequence is that it is always difficult to be quite sure where the sigmoid ends and the rectum begins. That is why in surgical literature the term 'rectosigmoid' has come to have a somewhat indefinite meaning. To most surgeons it implies not one point on the bowel, but rather a segment comprising the last 5–8 cm of sigmoid and the uppermost 5 cm or so of rectum.

To provide a more precise localization of growths in this situation it has been suggested by Morgan and Lloyd-Davies (1956) that their position should always be related to the promontory of the sacrum. To do this the sigmoid loop is drawn out of the pelvis so that it and the upper rectum lie tautly along the front of the lumbosacral spine. The position of the growth is then noted relative to the sacral promontory; if it lies entirely below the promontory it should be regarded as being in the rectum, and if above in the sigmoid. If it is situated partly above and partly below the promontory it is termed a rectosigmoid growth.

Alternatively lesions of this region may be localized by reference at operation to the position of the anterior peritoneal reflection off the front of the rectum, but as previously emphasized this is a very variable landmark; or localization may be determined entirely preoperatively by sigmoidoscopic estimation of the distance of the lower edge of the growth from the anal verge—a plan that has much to commend it—the rectosigmoid junction itself being taken to be at 15 cm.

THE ANAL CANAL

This short passage, though only 3 cm long, is of the greatest surgical importance both because of its role in the mechanism of rectal continence and because it is prone to certain diseases. For that reason its anatomy and that of the closely related levator ani muscle requires to be considered in disproportionately greater detail.

In the normal living subject the anal canal is completely collapsed owing to the tonic contraction of the anal sphincters, and the anal orifice is represented by an anteroposterior slit in the anal skin. *Posteriorly*, the canal is related to the coccyx with a certain amount of fibrous, fatty and muscular tissue intervening. *Laterally*, there is the ischiorectal fossa on either side with its contained fat and the inferior haemorrhoidal vessels and nerves which cross it to enter the wall of the canal. *Anteriorly*, in the male the canal is related to the central point of the perineum, the bulb of the urethra and the posterior border of the urogenital diaphragm (triangular ligament) containing the membranous urethra (see Fig. 3A). In the female the canal is related in front to the perineal body and to the lowest part of the posterior vaginal wall (see Fig. 3B).

THE MUCOCUTANEOUS LINING

As seen in excised specimens of the rectum and anal canal and in the living anus on proctoscopy, the lining of the anal canal consists of an upper mucosal and a lower cutaneous part, the junction of the two being marked by the *line of the anal valves* about 2 cm from the anal orifice and opposite the middle or the junction of the middle and lower thirds of the internal sphincter (Figs 4, 5, 8, 9). This level is also sometimes referred to as the *pectinate* or *dentate line* because of the serrated fringe produced by the valves (pecten = cock's comb, dentate = with teeth). The pectinate line marks the junction of the postallantoic gut and the proctodeum, the valves themselves representing remnants of the proctodeal membrane. Above each anal valve is a little pit or pocket known as an *anal sinus*, or *crypt* or *sinus of Morgagni*. These sinuses may be of some surgical significance in that foreign material may lodge in them with resulting infection, or trauma may be inflicted on the related valve. It was believed by Ball (1908) that an anal fissure was due to tearing down of one of the anal valves but this theory is no longer widely accepted.

Above the pectinate line, the mucosa is thrown into 8–14 longitudinal folds, known as the rectal columns or columns of Morgagni, each adjacent two columns being connected below at the pectinate line by an anal valve. The mucosa immediately above the valves is lined by an epithelium consisting of several layers of cuboidal cells. Traced upward these give way at a variable distance, usually about 0·5–1 cm, from the valves to a single layer of columnar cells as shown in Fig. 5 (see Goligher et

al. 1955; Fowler 1957; Walls 1958). As Milligan et al. (1937) have pointed out, there are colour changes also in the living anal mucosa when followed upward from the pectinate line. For 1 cm or so above the line the mucosa is a deep purple

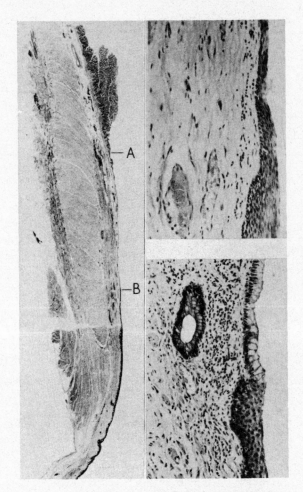

Fig. 5. Adult anal canal. Longitudinal coronal section. (A) indicates lower limit of true intestinal or columnar epithelium as determined histologically (see microphotograph). (B) indicates the level of the pectinate line as seen macroscopically; microscopical section at this point also shows that the lining of the anal canal is made up of several layers of cuboidal or slightly flattened epithelial cells. (*From Goligher et al. 1955*)

colour, but about the anorectal ring it changes to the pink colour of the rectal mucosa.

Below the pectinate line, the anal canal is lined with a modified skin devoid of hair and sebaceous and sweat glands, and closely adherent to the underlying tissues. As seen in an opened-up excised rectum and anal canal, the lining of this part of the canal for about 1 cm below the anal valves appears thin, smooth, pale and stretched. This area is sometimes known as the *pecten* (Stroud 1896). Traced further inferiorly, the lining becomes thicker and just outside the anal orifice acquires the hair follicles, glands and other histological features of normal skin.

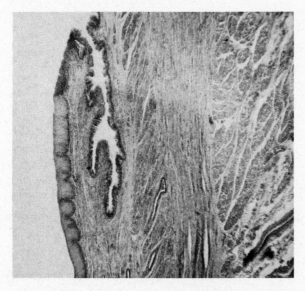

Fig. 6. Longitudinal section of anal wall showing penetration of the internal sphincter by an intramuscular gland. (*From Fowler 1957*)

ANAL INTERMUSCULAR GLANDS

It is often possible to demonstrate extensions of the anal mucosa through the substance of the wall of the anal canal—these are the *anal glands* or *ducts*, first described independently by Chiari (1878) and Herman and Desfosses (1880), and later by Harris (1929), Lockhart-Mummery (1929), Gordon-Watson and Dodd (1935), Hill et al. (1943), Kratzer and Dockerty (1947). An excellent anatomical study of these structures, with particular reference to their role in the pathogenesis of infections in the anal region, is that of Parks (1961). There are apparently four to eight of these glands in the normal anal canal as a rule. Each has a direct opening into the apex of an anal crypt and occasionally two glands open into the same crypt. About half the crypts in any anal canal have no gland communicating with them. Traced outwards from its cryptal opening,

the average gland has a short tubular portion in the submucosa which quickly branches into a racemose structure of widely ramifying ducts. Some glands appear to be confined entirely to the submucosa; but with two-thirds of them, one or more branches enter the internal sphincter (Fig. 6); and with one half, branches cross this sphincter completely to reach the intersphincteric longitudinal layer. Though some of the terminal loculi have been described as penetrating the external sphincter as well to reach the ischiorectal fossa, this is contrary to Parks' (1961) careful observations, for he found that in none of his specimens did the gland proceed beyond the longitudinal intersphincteric muscle. The general direction of extension of the glands is outwards and downwards, but *practically never upwards above the level of the anal valves.* Consequently the anal glands are always confined to the sub-mucosa, internal sphincter or longitudinal layer of the lower half of the anal canal. Branches of one gland may extend over an area about 1 cm^2. The epithelium lining the glands is of stratified colum-nar type, similar to that of the intermediate zone of the anal canal which lies between the true squamous mucosa below the anal valves and the intestinal type of epithelium of the upper anal canal. The luminal border of the cells resting on the surface stains strongly with mucin stains; they may therefore be identified even in grossly pathological material when only a remnant of epithelium remains.

It is highly doubtful whether the anal glands have any secretory function; they appear to be simply blind outgrowths of the anal crypts. Their surgical significance arises from the fact that they may provide an avenue of infection from the anal canal to the submucous and intersphincteric spaces; they may also be the site of origin of an adeno-carcinoma, as has been pointed out by Dukes and Galvin (1956).

THE MUSCULATURE

The first serious study of the anatomy of the anal musculature from the surgical point of view was made by Milligan and Morgan (Milligan and Morgan 1934; Morgan 1936; Milligan et al. 1937; Milligan 1942) whose description was widely accep-ted at one time. However, their original conception of the anatomy of this region has been shown to be incorrect in several respects by subsequent research (Eisenhammer 1951, 1953; Goligher et al. 1955; Parks 1955; Morgan and Thompson 1956), and the following account is based largely on this latter work, with reference also to some more recent research by Oh and Kark (1972) and Shafik (1975, 1976a, b).

DISPOSITION OF MUSCULATURE AS SEEN ON HISTOLOGICAL SECTION

The Internal Anal Sphincter. In longitudinal sections of the anal canal in both coronal and sagittal planes, the most striking structure is the internal sphincter (Figs 5–9). Superiorly it is continuous with the circular muscle coat of the rectum, and inferiorly it ends with a well defined rounded edge 6–8 mm above the level of the anal orifice, and 12–8 mm below the level of the anal valves. A remarkable feature of the muscle is the manner in which its constituent muscle fibres are disposed. These are grouped into discrete elliptical bundles which in the upper part of the sphincter lie obliquely with their transverse axis running internally and downward, giving them an imbricated arrangement. This obliquity becomes progressively less as the internal sphincter is traced downward so that in the lower part of the muscle the bundles lie horizontally and some of the lower ones even incline slightly upward. Sections stained by Weigert's method show that the internal sphincter consists of plain muscle fibres.

The External Anal Sphincter. On coronal and posterior sagittal section the external anal sphincter is seen to extend farther downward than the internal sphincter, and the lowermost portion curves medially to occupy a position below and slightly lateral to the lower rounded edge of the internal sphincter and close to the skin of the anal orifice (Figs 5–9). Contrary to the account of Milligan and Morgan (1934), there has been no suggestion in our histological sections of division of the external sphincter into three separate parts—the muscle is one continuous sheet. However, the lowermost or subcutaneous portion of it, which lies below the internal sphincter, does differ from the rest in that it is traversed by a fan-shaped expansion of the longitudinal muscle fibres of the anal canal which split it up into 8–12 discrete muscle bundles. At its upper end the external sphincter fuses with the puborectalis part of the levator ani muscle and it is quite impossible on histological section to say where one muscle ends and the other begins. Both muscles are, of course, made up of striped muscle fibres.

Anterior saggittal section, however, as Oh and Kark (1972) have recently pointed out, reveals a different state of affairs, which is, moreover, different in the two sexes. In the male, the lower half of the external sphincter is intersected and split up by longitudinal muscle fibres, as in coronal and posterior sagittal section; but the upper half of the muscle has longitudinal fibres not merely internal to it but also external or in front, or sometimes this part of the sphincter is bisected by such fibres into anterior and posterior halves. In the female, the

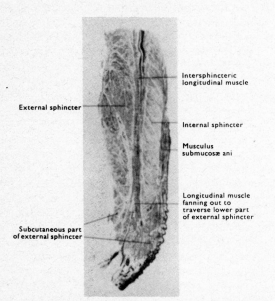

Fig. 7. Longitudinal coronal section of adult anal canal. (*From Goligher et al. 1955*)

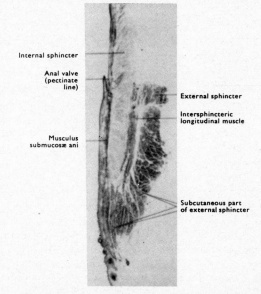

Fig. 8. Longitudinal coronal section of adult anal canal. (*From Goligher et al. 1955*)

whole external sphincter appears in anterior saggittal section as a compact rounded bundle of muscle, encased by longitudinal muscle running down anteriorly and posteriorly to it. No part of the external sphincter is traversed by longitudinal fibres in this plane of section.

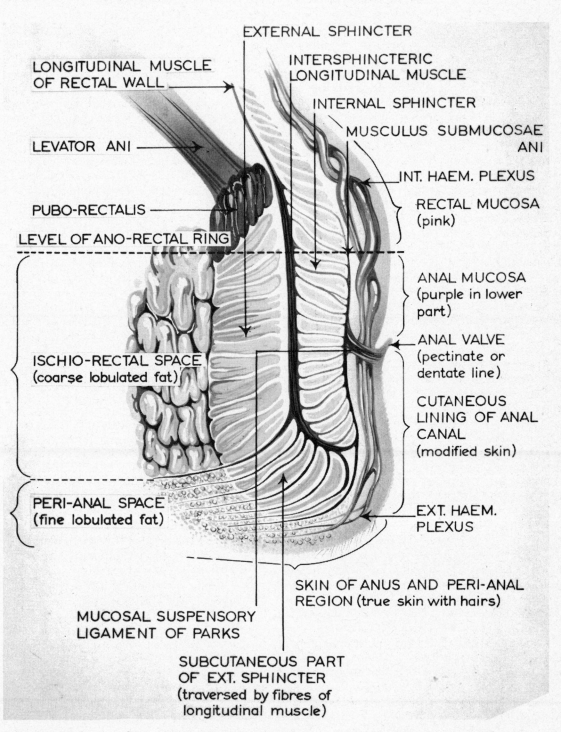

EXTERNAL SPHINCTER

INTERSPHINCTERIC LONGITUDINAL MUSCLE

INTERNAL SPHINCTER

MUSCULUS SUBMUCOSAE ANI

INT. HAEM. PLEXUS

RECTAL MUCOSA (pink)

LONGITUDINAL MUSCLE OF RECTAL WALL

LEVATOR ANI

PUBO-RECTALIS

LEVEL OF ANO-RECTAL RING

ANAL MUCOSA (purple in lower part)

ANAL VALVE (pectinate or dentate line)

ISCHIO-RECTAL SPACE (coarse lobulated fat)

CUTANEOUS LINING OF ANAL CANAL (modified skin)

PERI-ANAL SPACE (fine lobulated fat)

EXT. HAEM. PLEXUS

SKIN OF ANUS AND PERI-ANAL REGION (true skin with hairs)

MUCOSAL SUSPENSORY LIGAMENT OF PARKS

SUBCUTANEOUS PART OF EXT. SPHINCTER (traversed by fibres of longitudinal muscle)

Fig. 9. Coronal section of the anal canal to demonstrate the modern conception of anal anatomy. (*From Goligher 1959*)

The Longitudinal Muscle Fibres. In coronal and sagittal sections (Figs 5–9) the main layer of longitudinal fibres in the anal canal is seen to lie between the internal and external sphincters. Histologically, this layer consists of non-striped muscle fibres mixed with elastic tissue. Traced upward it is continuous with the outer longitudinal muscle layer of the rectal wall and is joined by some striped fibres of the levator ani. Traced downward it is seen to break up opposite the lower border of the internal sphincter into a number of septa which diverge fanwise and pass radially through the lowermost part of the external sphincter. Some of these diverging fibres are attached ultimately to the skin of the anal and perianal region from a point a little below the internal sphincter to well beyond the anal verge, while others lose themselves in the fat surrounding the lower part of the anal canal.

An additional layer of longitudinal fibres, first described by Fine and Lawes (1940), is one that lies on the inner aspect of the internal sphincter under the anal mucosa and skin (Figs 7, 8, 9). They have named it the *musculus submucosae ani*. It is composed of unstriped muscle fibres together with elastic connective tissue, and would appear to be derived chiefly from strands of the main intersphincteric longitudinal layer which make their way inward and downward between the bundles of the internal sphincter (see Fig. 7). Inferiorly, a few of the fibres of the musculus submucosae ani become continuous around the lower edge of the internal sphincter with the innermost fibres of the main intersphincteric longitudinal layer. But the majority continue downward and outward superficial to the subcutaneous part of the external sphincter, to be attached to the skin of the anus and perianal region. This extension constitutes the *corrugator cutis ani* of Ellis (1878) and Milligan (1942).

Parks (1955) has given a rather different account of the distribution of the longitudinal muscles fibres in the submucosal space. By means of a special histological technique involving distension of the submucosa with an injection of saline before fixation, he has demonstrated a strong band of longitudinal fibres passing directly from the inner aspect of the lower part of the internal sphincter to the lining of the anal canal just below the anal valves (Fig. 9). He claims that by means of this bundle, which he calls the *mucosal suspensory ligament*, the lining of the canal is firmly tethered to the underlying sphincter, and that this accounts for the well-recognized *interhaemorrhoidal groove* which appears on internal haemorrhoids when they are prolapsed or pulled down during haemorrhoidec-tomy (Fig. 15). I must confess that no trace of this suspensory ligament has been detected in any of my histological sections, but this could be due to the fact that the attachment to the anal lining is probably by serrations and my sections may not have coincided with one of the points of attachment.

Shafik (1976*a, b*) paints a more elaborate picture of the longitudinal muscle in the anal intermuscular septum, which he sees as consisting of three distinct layers of longitudinal muscle fibres with four fascial septa separating them from one another and from the internal and external sphincters respectively (Fig. 10). According to him the longitudinal muscle fibres terminate inferiorly shortly above the level of the lower margin of the internal sphincter. Below this point the fascial septa decussate to form what he terms the 'central tendon', lying between the termination of the longitudinal muscle and the subcutaneous external sphincter. Numerous fibrous bands proceed from this central tendon mainly in a downward direction, splitting the subcutaneous external sphincter into four distinct bundles of muscle and decussating below the sphincter to form the corrugator cutis ani. Incidentally, Shafik (1976*a, b*) was unable to demonstrate any structure corresponding to Parks' muscosal suspensory ligament.

ATTACHMENTS OF EXTERNAL ANAL SPHINCTER

As seen in a gross dissection of the perineal and anal region, the external sphincter is an elliptical cylinder muscle which surrounds the anal orifice and, traced upwards on the lateral sides, becomes continuous with the puborectalis and pubococcygeus muscles. *Posteriorly*, the cylinder is attached at the lowest level to the skin of the perianal region in and close to the midline. At a slightly higher level the external sphincter fibres form an anococcygeal raphe which runs backward and is attached to the dorsal aspect of the coccyx. Above this raphe the external anal musculature is devoid of posterior attachment, but forms a loop of muscle round the back of the canal. This unfixed, free-lying part of the sphincter extends up to the level at which the median raphe of the levator muscle inserts on to the front of the coccyx. Behind the anal canal, between the upper raphe of the levators and the lower one found by the external sphincter, lies a space filled with fatty tissue—the *retrosphincteric space of Courtney* (1949)—through which fistulous tracks sometimes pass (see Fig. 3A, B).

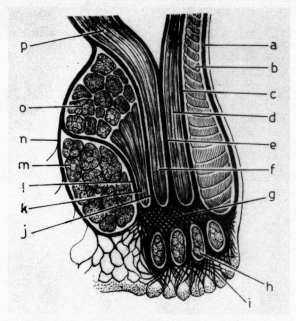

Fig. 10. The structure of the longitudinal muscle and the related fascial septa. (a) Internal anal septum. (b) Internal sphincter. (c) Inner intersphincteric septum. (d) Medial longitudinal muscle. (e) Medial longitudinal septum. (f) Intermediate longitudinal muscle. (g) Central tendon. (h) Subcutaneous external sphincter. (i) Corrugator cutis ani. (j) Lateral longitudinal septum. (k) Lateral longitudinal muscle. (l) Outer intersphincteric septum. (m) Intermediate part of external sphincter. (n) External anal septum. (o) Top part of external sphincter. (p) Puborectalis. (*From Shafik 1976*)

Anteriorly, many of the lower fibres of the external sphincter are inserted into the perianal skin in and near the midline. At a higher level corresponding roughly with the posterior attachment to the anococcygeal raphe, the external sphincter fibres merge into the transverse perineal muscles by a process of decussation at the central point of the perineum or perineal body. Above this level most of the peripheral fibres of the external anal musculature seem to proceed forward as puborectales, but some of the more centrally placed fibres are presumed to join with their fellows of the opposite side to complete the encirclement of the anal canal in front up to the level of the anorectal ring, though I have found it difficult to demonstrate these conclusively on dissection.

Shafik (1975) in his recent study has claimed that the musculature of the external sphincter is arranged essentially in a system of three loops, as shown in Fig. 11, which he believes facilitates the maintenance of continence.

THE LEVATOR ANI MUSCLES

It is important to the surgeon to understand the anatomy of the levator ani muscle because it constitutes part of the sphincter mechanism of the anal canal, and also because its accurate division is one of the key steps in the operation of rectal

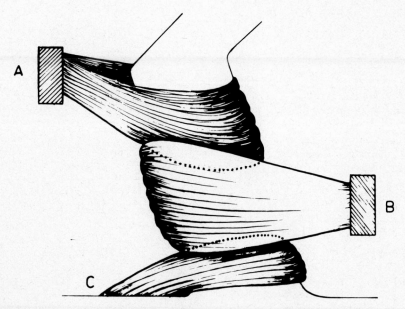

Fig. 11. The triple loop system of the external anal sphincter postulated by Shafik (1975). (A) Top loop, attached to the pubes anteriorly like the puborectalis part of the levator ani muscle. (B) Middle loop, attached to the coccyx posteriorly. (C) The lowermost loop, corresponding to the subcutaneous part of the external sphincter, attached anteriorly to the perianal skin. (*From Shafik 1975*)

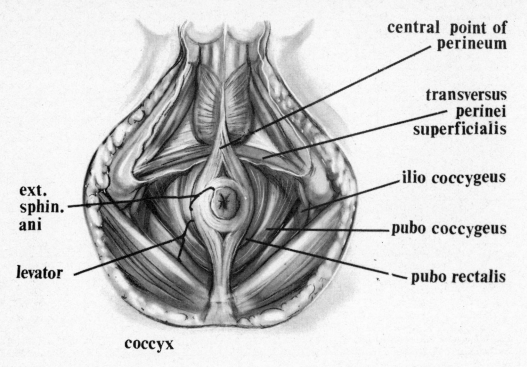

Fig. 12. The parts of the levator ani muscles as seen from the perineal aspect. (*After Naunton Morgan*)

excision. The levator ani is a broad, thin muscle, attached peripherally to the inner surface of the side of the pelvis, and united medially with its fellow of the opposite side to form the greater part of the floor of the pelvic cavity. Examined more carefully it is seen to consist of three parts as defined by Thompson (1899) (Figs 12, 13).

1. The Iliococcygeus. This is a very thin muscle which arises from the ischial spine and posterior part of the white line of the pelvic fascia covering the obturator internus. The fibres run downward, backward and medially and are inserted into the sides of the last two pieces of the sacrum and into the *anococcygeal raphe* of the levator muscles, a median fibrous band which stretches between the anus and the superior surface of the coccyx.

2. The Pubococcygeus. This arises from the back of the pubis and the anterior part of the obturator fascia, and is directed almost horizontally backward along the side of the lower part of the rectum as a flat band which lies superior to the innermost fibres of the ileococcygeus region to fuse with its fellow of the opposite side to constitute a broad fibrous band lying on the anococcygeal raphe

formed by the ileococcygeus. This band is continued up in front of the coccyx to be inserted into the anterior aspect of the first piece of the coccyx and last segment of the sacrum.

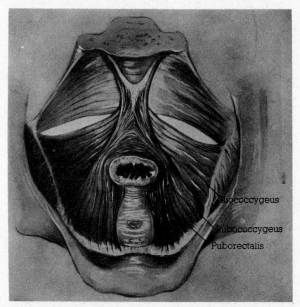

Fig. 13. The parts of the levator ani muscles as seen from the pelvic aspect. (*From Morgan 1949*)

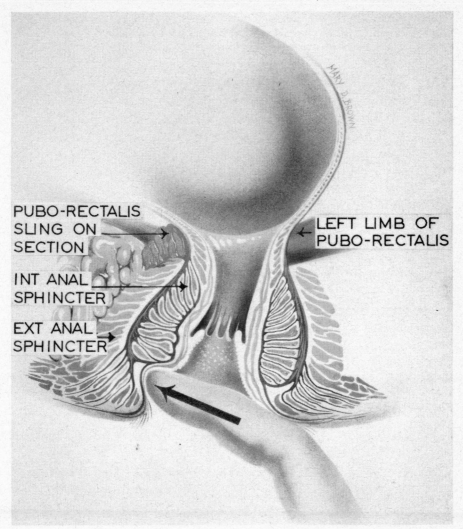

Fig. 14. Sagittal section of the anal canal to illustrate the palpation of the intersphincteric groove by the surgeon's examining finger. (*From Goligher 1959*)

3. The Puborectalis. This name is sometimes applied to those fibres of the pubococcygeus which unite with the corresponding fibres of the opposite side to form a sling behind the rectum at the anorectal junction. The puborectalis arises from the lower part of the back of the symphysis pubis and the superior fascia of the urogenital diaphragm, runs backward alongside the anorectal junction to join with its fellow immediately behind the bowel and form a strong U-shaped loop which slings the rectum to the pubes.

RECTOURETHRALIS MUSCLE OF ROUX

This consists of two slender bundles, one on either side of the midline, which are derived from the longitudinal muscle of the rectal wall and run almost horizontally forward from the front of the rectum just above the anorectal junction to the back of the urogenital diaphragm at the membranous urethra to which they are attached (see Fig. 3A). In this situation they lie sandwiched between the medial borders of the two puborectales muscles and run in roughly the same axis. During excision of the rectum the rectourethrales muscles have to be divided into the perineal dissection at the same time as the puborectales are being severed in order to open up the plane between the rectum and the prostate.

THE ANORECTAL RING

This term has been coined by Milligan and Morgan (1934) to denote the functionally important ring of muscle which surrounds the junction of the rectum and anal canal. This is composed of the upper borders of the internal and external sphincters, which completely encircle the junction, and on the posterior and lateral aspects the strong puborectales sling. As a consequence, the ring is stronger posteriorly and laterally than it is anteriorly, and its definition on the posterior aspect is accentuated by the forward angulation of the bowel at this level.

Recognition of the anorectal ring is of paramount importance in the treatment of abscesses and fistulas in the anal region, for its complete division inevitably results in rectal incontinence while its preservation, despite the sacrifice of all the rest of the sphincter musculature, at least ensures that there will be no gross lack of control, though minor degrees of incontinence may result.

DIGITAL PALPATION OF THE ANAL MUSCULATURE

As Milligan and Morgan (1934) have pointed out, the lower edges of the internal and external anal sphincters are readily recognizable on digital examination of the anus in the normal living patient. In the average individual, if the finger is inserted into the anal canal and then gradually withdrawn while pressing in a posterolateral direction, a distinct groove can be felt just inside the anal orifice (Fig. 14). The upper rim of this groove is the rounded lower border of the internal sphincter, the lower rim of the upper aspect of the subcutaneous free border of the external sphincter. On circumferential palpation the lower edge of the internal sphincter is found to form a circular ring of muscle, but the lowermost part of the external sphincter usually has a distinctly elliptical shape with the long axis running anteroposteriorly. Sometimes indeed extensions can be felt running backwards from the posterior edge of the external sphincter toward the coccyx (Fig. 15). As a consequence of the differences in shape, the anterior and posterior parts of the external sphincter are somewhat farther away from the anal verge than the lateral positions and often

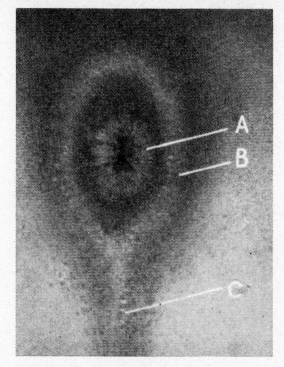

Fig. 15. Photograph of the anal region in a case where the lower edges of the internal and external sphincters were exceptionally prominent. (A) Lower edge of internal sphincter. (B) Lower edge of external sphincter. (C) Anococcygeal raphe. (*From Goligher et al. 1955*)

less easily palpated. It is possibly by firm pressure with the finger to displace the lateral portion of the external sphincter in an outward direction for 1 cm or so. Conversely, when the patient is asked to contract the anus the lower edge of the external sphincter can be felt to undergo active contraction and to provide a tight closure of the anal orifice. If the lower edge of the internal sphincter is palpated during anal contraction it is found that this muscle also contracts, presumably owing to compression by the voluntarily contracting upper two-thirds of the external sphincter which surrounds it.

The *anal intersphincteric groove*, which is often easily palpable, corresponds to the lower end of the interval between the internal and external sphincters. It is remarkable, however, that this groove should be so wide—usually 6–12 mm—for it will be remembered that in longitudinal sections of the anal canal the lower end of the external sphincter is closely applied to the inferior edge of the internal sphincter so that only a potential gap exists between them. It would appear, therefore, that in the living subject the lower part of the external sphincter lies farther downward and out-

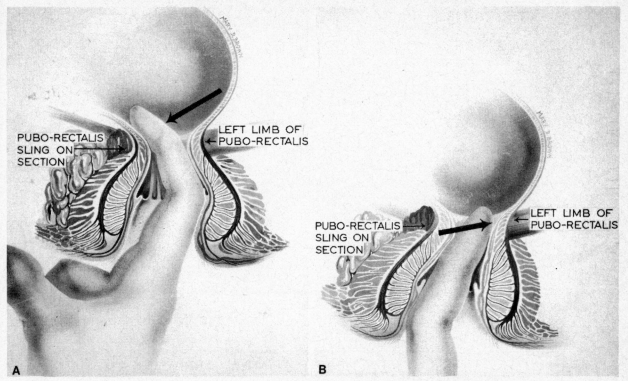

Fig. 16. Sagittal section of the anal canal to illustrate palpation of the anorectal ring during rectal examination: (A) posteriorly where it is easily felt due to the puborectalis sling and (B) anteriorly where it is virtually impalpable. (*From Goligher 1959*)

ward relative to the anal orifice than it does in fixed sections of the excised anal canal.

The foregoing remarks indicate the relative positions of the lower borders of the sphincters as usually found on clinical examination. Rarely, however, the internal sphincter may extend farther distally so that its lower edge may actually reach to the anal orifice where it may be palpable immediately internal to the external sphincter. Sometimes, indeed, the internal sphincter projects slightly beyond the external sphincter. Under either of these circumstances the intersphincteric groove lies not in the anal canal but immediately lateral to the anal verge.

If the examining finger is inserted above the intersphincteric groove it passes up along the smooth surface of the internal sphincter to the upper end of the anal canal, which terminates abruptly posteriorly in the sharply defined puborectalis sling. This indicates accurately the position of the *anorectal ring*. Above this level the finger can be passed backwards slightly and hooked on the prominent sling of muscle (Fig. 16A). The puborectales can usually be traced on to the lateral walls of the anorectal junction, but anteriorly it is impossible to palpate the anorectal ring clearly and its site has to be

gauged by reference to the posterior and lateral walls (Fig. 16B).

SPHINCTERIC DISPLACEMENTS DURING DEFAECATION AND AT OPERATION

It is important to appreciate that the two muscular tubes formed by the internal and external anal sphincters are not fixed but are capable of slight movement up and down inside one another. This probably occurs regularly during defaecation, and certainly takes place in the course of operations on the anal canal such as haemorrhoidectomy (Goligher et al. 1955). Owing to the intimate connection of the longitudinal fibres of the anal intersphincteric septum and the musculus submucosae ani with the internal sphincter, the initial traction on the haemorrhoids in the latter operation exerts a pull on this sphincter and drags it down the anal canal to the anal orifice (Fig. 17). Meanwhile owing to the effect of the anaesthetic, the external sphincter relaxes and its lower end moves laterally under the perianal skin outside the field of operation. It was failure to realize that these sphincteric displacements occur during haemorrhoidectomy and that the anatomy of this

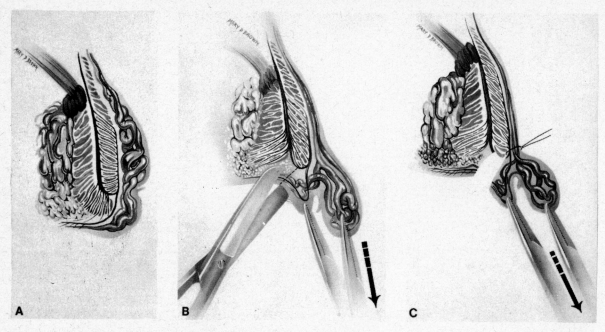

Fig. 17. Displacement of anal sphincters during haemorrhoidectomy. (A) State of anal canal in an unanaesthetized patient. (B) Patient anaesthetized and haemorrhoid drawn down. Note that traction on the pile causes the internal sphincter to descend to the anal orifice; meanwhile the lower edge of the external sphincter relaxes and moves outwards. (C) Isolation and ligature of the haemorrhoid. Note that as the skin cut is deepened it divides the longitudinal fibres which curl around the lower edge of the internal sphincter and thereby exposes this muscle and *not the external sphincter*. (*From Goligher 1959*)

region did not remain exactly as in fixed histological sections of the anal canal, that led Milligan et al. (1937) to misname the circular muscle regularly exposed during haemorrhoidectomy as the subcutaneous part of the external sphincter instead of the lower border of the internal sphincter.

THE PECTEN BAND

Miles (1919) believed that anal fissure was associated with the development of a circumferential flattened or rounded band of fibrous tissue between the skin of the lower part of the anal canal in the region of the pecten and the sphincter musculature. This he named the 'pecten band', and stated that it could always be felt on digital examination in the lower part of the anal canal in fissure cases and in many other patients as a firm ring rather like the rubber ring of an umbrella. In my experience this is exactly the sensation imparted by the lower end of the internal sphincter when it is well developed or in spasm in association with an anal fissure, and I have little doubt that what Miles called the pecten band was really the rounded inferior border of this muscle.

In treating fissures Miles stressed the necessity for dividing this pecten band, usually not through the fissure itself but posterolaterally, and considered that this was all that was required to secure inevitable healing. His second book on rectal surgery (1939) contained a drawing of the pecten band exposed at the operation of 'pectenotomy'. It is shown as lying just internal to the lowermost part of the external sphincter in exactly the same position as that occupied by the lower border of the internal sphincter in my dissections of the anal region, and it exhibits the pallor and other features of that muscle. A histological section of tissue from this 'band' would of course have immediately settled whether it was composed of fibrous tissue or plain muscle, but I have been unable to discover any report on histological findings in Miles' writings on the subject.

HILTON'S 'WHITE LINE' IN THE ANAL CANAL

Most authors of surgical textbooks dealing with the rectum apparently feel it their duty to refer to Hilton's 'white line' in the anal canal but generally manage to avoid making any clear statement about it. This is not surprising for, as Ewing (1954) has pointed out, it is quite impossible from Hilton's (1877) own account of this structure to decide exactly what or where it is. He defined it as a line with three characteristics—that it is easily recognizable, white and marks the interval between the external and internal anal sphincters. The anal intersphincteric groove is of course easily palpable, but there is absolutely nothing in the nature of a line—white or of any other colour—at this level that can be recognized on inspection through a proctoscope or on examining an excised rectum. It is to be hoped that Ewing's (1954) article will result in allusions to this 'landmark' being eliminated from surgical texts.

TISSUE SPACES IN RELATION TO THE ANAL CANAL

Certain spaces, or rather potential spaces filled with connective tissue, are of importance to the surgeon as possible sites of infection (see Figs 4, 10).

The Ischiorectal Fossa. On either side of the anal canal and lower part of the rectum, intervening between them and the side wall of the pelvis, is the ischiorectal fossa. This is a pyramid-shaped space, the apex of which is above, where the levator muscle joins the fascia on the obturator internus, the base below, formed by the perianal skin. The medial wall consists of the external anal sphincter and the obliquely lying levator ani muscle, the lateral wall of the ischium covered by the obturator internus and its overlying parietal pelvic fascia. In the obturator internus fascia on the lateral wall is Alcock's canal which contains the internal pudendal vessels and pudendal nerve. Anterior to the ischiorectal fossa is the back of the urogenital diaphragm and transversus perinei muscle. Behind, the fossa is bounded by the sacrotuberous ligament and the inferior edge of the gluteus maximus.

Milligan et al. (1937) depict the ischiorectal fossa as being subdivided by a horizontal fascia into two spaces—the perianal and ischiorectal space (see Figs 4, 8). Milligan thought that this fascia represented an outward extension of the longitudinal muscle fibres of the anal canal. My own observations do not support this conception of the formation of the fascia but confirm that there is some thin non-muscular, fascial partition.

The Perianal Space. This contains finely lobulated fat similar to that found elsewhere in the superficial fascia of the body, and laterally it becomes continuous with the subcutaneous fat of the buttocks. Medially it may be considered as extending into the lower part of the anal canal where it is lined by modified skin, probably as far proximally as the site of Parks' (1955) mucosal suspensory ligament (see Fig. 8). The space may also be said to contain the lower part of the external sphincter and the subcutaneous or external haemorrhoidal plexus. It is in the perianal space that anal haematomas and perianal abscesses form, and subcutaneous and low anal fistulas traverse this space.

The Ischiorectal Space. This comprises the upper two-thirds of the ischiorectal fossa, is filled with coarsely lobulated fat rather similar to that found in lipomas and is crossed by the inferior haemorrhoidal vessels and nerves on their way medially and forward to the anal sphincter and canal. Anteriorly, as Morgan (1949) has shown, the ischiorectal space has an important extension forward above the urogenital diaphragm, which is liable to become filled with pus in ischiorectal abscess or high anal fistula (see Fig. 129, p. 171). Posteromedially the ischiorectal space connects, under cover of the anococcygeal raphe of the external anal sphincter, through the retrosphincteric space of Courtney (1949), with the opposite ischiorectal fossa, and this is an important avenue of extension of infection from the ischiorectal space.

The Submucous Space. This space lies between the internal sphincter and the mucocutaneous lining of the upper two-thirds of the anal canal. Below, it probably extends down to the level of Parks' mucosal suspensory ligament, and above it becomes continuous with the submucous layer of the rectum. It contains the internal haemorrhoidal venous plexus and related terminal branches of the superior haemorrhoidal artery.

The Pelvirectal or Supralevator Space. This term is applied to the potential space between the pelvic peritoneal floor and the levator ani muscles, partly on either side in the area occupied by the loose connective tissue of the lateral ligaments of the rectum and partly in front and behind the rectum.

The Central Space. Attention has been drawn by Shafik (1976b) to this potential space. It is situated between the lower end of the longitudinal intersphincteric muscle and the subcutaneous external sphincter, according to his concept, and is occupied by the central tendon (see Fig. 10). It communicates externally with the ischiorectal space, inferiorly and internally with the perianal and submucous spaces and superiorly with the intersphincteric space.

The Intersphincteric Space (or Spaces). This space lying between the internal and external sphincter is considered by some surgeons to be specially important in the genesis of abscesses in the region of the anus and anal canal, because the anal intermuscular glands terminate in this space (see pp. 9, 154).

Blood Supply of the Colon, Rectum and Anal Canal

ARTERIES

The arterial supply of the *right colon*—that is, the caecum, ascending colon, hepatic flexure and right third or half of the transverse colon—is derived from the superior mesenteric artery, through its ileocolic, right colic and middle colic branches. The supply of the *left colon* is from the inferior mesenteric by means of its left colic and sigmoid branches. The *rectum and anal canal* are supplied by the lower sigmoid and terminal superior haemorrhoidal branches of the inferior mesenteric artery, by the right and left middle haemorrhoidal branches of the internal iliac arteries, and the right and left inferior haemorrhoidal arteries which come from the internal pudendal branches of the internal iliac vessels.

As the main colic arteries proceed to the colon they bifurcate and the resulting branches of neighbouring vessels unite to form arcades 2 cm or so from the mesenteric border of the bowel (Fig. 18). By means of these various arcades, some long, some short, a continuous chain of communicating

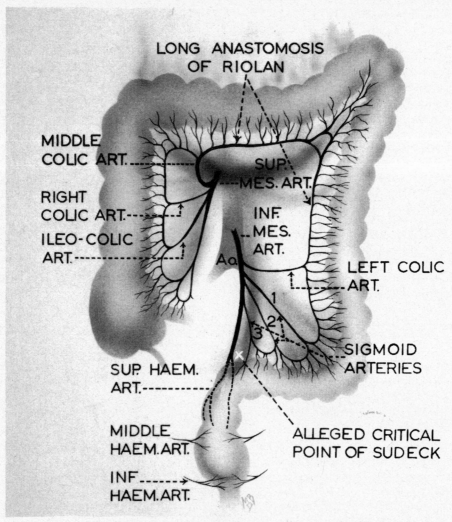

Fig. 18. The 'textbook' pattern of the arteries to the colon and rectum. (*From Goligher 1959*)

vessels is formed. This is the *marginal artery*, first so-called by Sudeck (1907). From it the ultimate branches of supply to the colon, the *vasa recti*, are distributed. The marginal artery is responsible for bringing the area of supply of the superior mesenteric artery into communication with that of the inferior mesenteric by connecting the descending branch of the middle colic with the ascending branch of the left colic by means of the long anastomosis of Riolan.

THE DETAILED ARRANGEMENT OF THE COLIC ARTERIES

The actual pattern formed by these colic vessels and their communications and the adequacy of the supply to different parts of the colon and rectum through the marginal anastomoses have been the subject of many studies in cadavers and living patients, using injection techniques and arteriography, straightforward dissections and simple observation alone or combined with selective ligations. In this connection the work of Sudeck (1907), Manasse (1907), Archibald (1908), Rubesch (1910), Drummond (1914), Pope and Judd (1929), Steward and Rankin (1933), Sunderland (1942), Bacon and Smith (1948), Goligher (1949, 1954) and Griffiths (1956) should all be mentioned.

The average arrangement of the colic vessels portrayed in standard anatomical texts is that shown in Fig. 18. *As regards the branches of the superior mesenteric artery*, Steward and Rankin (1933) and Griffiths (1956) both emphasize that in a number of individuals (25% according to the latter) the middle colic artery is absent, and is replaced by an abnormally large right colic branch. In many cases, too, the middle colic is double. *As for the inferior mesenteric system*, the typical textbook pattern of Fig. 18 was present in only 15% of the bodies studied by Griffiths (1956). The commonest disposition of the branches found by him was similar to that demonstrated by Goligher (1954) in connection with the technique of high ligation of the inferior mesenteric artery during rectal excisions (Fig. 19A, B). In this arrangement the first or highest branch of the inferior mesenteric artery, springing from the parent trunks roughly opposite the bifurcation of the abdominal aorta, runs not transversely to the left as usually described, but upward and laterally toward the splenic flexure. In the earlier part of its course this branch ascends on the surface of or just lateral to the inferior mesenteric vein; in the second part it is accompanied to the flexure by a vena comitans which enters the main vein much higher than the point of origin of the artery. This obliquely running branch might be called the accessory or ascending left colic artery, reserving the term left colic proper or descending left colic for the next branch, or alternatively it may be termed the left

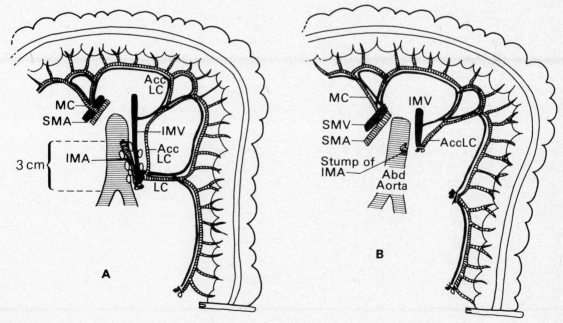

Fig. 19. Anatomy of the inferior mesenteric artery and its upper branches revealed during ligation of this vessel in the course of rectal excision. (A) Ligation at level of aortic bifurcation. (B) High ligation flush with aorta. (*From Goligher 1954*)

colic as Griffiths (1956) prefers, and all subsequent branches regarded as being sigmoid branches. The number of the sigmoid arteries varies from two to five or six and their precise arrangement is also very variable as Drummond (1914), Sunderland (1942), Goligher (1949) and Griffiths (1956) all emphasize. No useful purpose will be served in describing their detailed anatomy further except to say that they communicate freely by marginal arcades.

It should be pointed out that the main stem of the inferior mesenteric artery springs from the front of the abdominal aorta near its left margin, at least 4 cm above the level of the aortic bifurcation and 10 cm above the sacral promontory (Goligher 1949) (Figs 20, 21). At its origin it is frequently overlaid by the lower border of the third part of the duodenum, which has thus sometimes to be displaced slightly upward or to the right if a really high tie of this vessel flush with the aorta is being practised in a rectal excision. From its commencement the artery runs downward arching slightly to the left, and as it crosses the left common iliac artery close to the

aorta its name is arbitrarily changed to the superior haemorrhoidal, which continues the downward course in the base of the vertical limb of the sigmoid mesocolon to reach the back of the upper end of the rectum opposite the third piece of the sacrum. Here it divides into two main branches, the right and the left, though the level of the bifurcation shows considerable individual variation. These branches descend on the rectal wall at first posteriorly, then inclining more towards the lateral aspect, each one generally breaking up into smaller branches which penetrate the muscle coat to reach the submucosa in which they proceed downward as straight vessels which run in the columns of Morgagni and terminate usually above the anal valves as a capillary plexus. These vessels in the submucosa of the anal canal can often be clearly felt against the taut internal sphincter on digital examination of the rectum. According to Miles (1939), there is a difference in the mode of termination of the right and left main branches of the superior haemorrhoidal artery. The right branch divides into

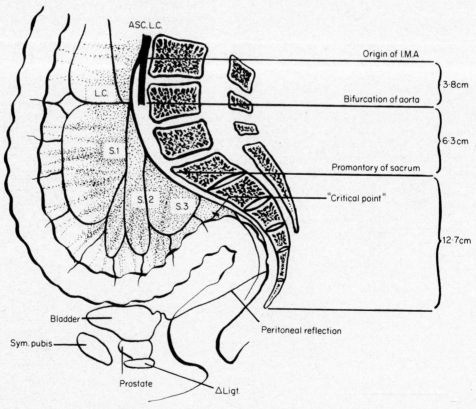

Fig. 20. Sagittal section of the pelvis and lumbar region showing the relation of the inferior mesenteric artery and its branches to the abdominal aorta and promontory of sacrum.

two major branches which run down the right anterior and right posterior aspects of the rectum, while the left branch continues undivided down the left lateral aspect. As the superior haemorrhoidal veins closely accompany the arteries, this arrangement of arterial branches is said by Miles to account for the occurrence in cases of internal haemorrhoids of two main piles on the right side, but only one on the left side.

The relationship of the ureters to the main inferior mesenteric/superior haemorrhoidal trunk is important. Owing to the deviation of the trunk to the left it passes close to the left ureter and left spermatic vessels, which are in danger during ligations of the inferior mesenteric; the right ureter is correspondingly farther distant (Fig. 21) and is not exposed to risk during this manoeuvre.

ADEQUACY OF THE MARGINAL ARTERY

Sudeck's Critical Point. There has been considerable controversy in the past as to whether a marginal anastomosis exists between the lowest sigmoid artery and the branches of the superior haemorrhoidal. Sudeck (1907) suggested that there was a failure of the marginal circulation at this point so that the role of the marginal artery had to be assumed by the last sigmoid artery itself and by the superior haemorrhoidal trunk below the original of the latter branch (see Fig. 18). He considered it important in the performance of rectal resection by the sacral route, in which for technical reasons the main vascular pedicle is inevitably tied low, that care be taken to see that the ligature is applied above the origin of the last sigmoid artery in order not to interrupt this substitute marginal circulation. According to him, necrosis of the terminal part of the colorectal stump, brought down for anastomosis or establishment of sacral colostomy in this operation, was frequently due to neglect of this precaution. At the present time, when it is generally accepted that ligation of the inferior mesenteric vessels through an abdominal approach is desirable in rectal excision, and purely sacral excisions are no longer employed, Sudeck's thesis regarding a critical point in the marginal circulation of the rectosigmoid region has ceased to be relevant. As a matter of fact, however, several subsequent workers such as Griffiths (1956) have demonstrated quite clearly by injection experiments that there are abundant anastomoses between the branches of the last sigmoid and those of the superior haemorrhoidal artery.

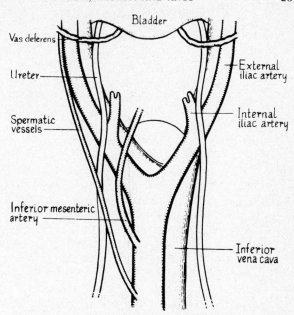

Fig. 21. The relationship of the ureters to the inferior mesenteric artery. (*From Graham and Goligher 1954*)

MARGINAL CONNECTION BETWEEN SUPERIOR AND INFERIOR MESENTERIC ARTERIES

A question that really does bear on modern surgical practice is that relating to the adequacy of the marginal communication between the middle colic (or right colic when the middle is absent) and left colic arteries. From their injection experiments and dissections, Manasse (1907), Archibald (1908), Steward and Rankin (1933), and Griffiths (1956) claimed that there is always a reliable marginal communication between these vessels. Griffiths (1956) has pointed out, moreover, that aortography in patients suffering from peripheral arterial disease occasionally shows the inferior mesenteric to be blocked (as confirmed by subsequent autopsy in many instances), and yet the sigmoid vessels fill satisfactorily, presumably through the superior mesenteric, middle colic and marginal arteries. In resection of aneurysms of the aortic bifurcation, it is the practice to ligate the inferior mesenteric artery at its origin, usually without ill effect on the colon. Finally, and most conclusively, it has been shown by Goligher (1954), Morgan (1956) and many others in actual practice that, after ligation of the inferior mesenteric artery flush with the abdominal aorta in the course of rectal excision, the blood supply through the middle colic and marginal artery is perfectly adequate to nourish the left colon in the vast majority of cases.

THE ULTIMATE ARRANGEMENT OF THE VASA RECTI IN THE COLON WALL

The vasa recti are of two types, long and short. The long branches divide into two to encircle the colon, their terminal branches running in the bowel wall, usually deep to the taeniae, to anastomose with one another on the antimesocolic border. The short branches, usually two or three to each long branch, arise from the marginal artery or from one of the long branches and supply the mesocolic two-thirds of the bowel circumference. One of them frequently penetrates the mesocolic taenia as it enters the colon wall (Fig. 22). The appendices epiploicae receive a small arterial twig from the long vasa recti. It is important in tying off these fatty appendages at operation not to draw up the long branch itself into the ligature by applying the latter too close to the bowel wall (Fig. 23).

ADDITIONAL BLOOD SUPPLY TO THE RECTUM AND ANAL CANAL

This is derived from the two internal iliac arteries via the right and left middle and inferior haemorrhoidal arteries.

The *middle haemorrhoidal arteries* spring from the anterior divisions of the internal iliacs, or rarely from their inferior vesical branches, and proceed medially and forward below the pelvic peritoneum, in the tissue of the lateral ligaments to reach the rectal wall where they anastomose with the branches of the superior and inferior haemorrhoidal vessels. However, their arrangement is very variable and the middle haemorrhoidal artery may be absent, double or treble on one or both sides.

The *inferior haemorrhoidal artery* is derived indirectly from the internal iliac through its internal pudendal branch. It leaves the latter as it is lying in Alcock's canal in the fascia of the outer walls of the ischiorectal fossa and runs medially and slightly forward breaking up into branches which penetrate the external and internal anal sphincters and reach the submucosa and subcutaneous tissues of the anal canal. They communicate with branches from the inferior haemorrhoidal artery of the opposite side and possibly from the middle haemorrhoidals of both sides.

Undoubtedly the main artery of the rectum is the superior haemorrhoidal but it is quite wrong to discount almost completely the contribution made by the middle and inferior haemorrhoidal arteries, as has been done by Steward and Rankin (1933). Experience with sphincter-saving resections for carcinomas of the upper rectum and lower sigmoid shows that after division of the inferior mesenteric/superior haemorrhoidal trunks, the middle and inferior haemorrhoidal arteries are capable of nourishing a distal rectal stump up to a point at least 8–10 cm above the peritoneal reflection. *Even when the lateral ligaments have been completely divided, sacrificing the middle haemorrhoidal supply*, a rectal stump up to just below the peritoneal reflection usually has a good blood supply, as shown by satisfactory arterial bleeding from its cut upper end. It has been suggested by Pope and Judd (1929) and by Goligher (1949) that an additional source of supply to the lower rectum may be derived from the branches of the internal pudendal artery that ramify in the puborectales, pubococcygei and transversus perinei muscles.

THE MIDDLE SACRAL ARTERY

This artery arises from the back of the aorta about 1 cm above its bifurcation and runs down in front of the last two lumbar vertebrae, the sacrum and coccyx and behind the aorta, the left common iliac vein, the presacral nerve, the superior haemorrhoidal vessels and the rectum. Some of its terminal branches may even descend along the anococcygeal raphe of the levator muscle to reach the anal canal and rectum. The significance of the middle sacral artery to the surgeon, however, is that during rectal excision it is regularly exposed as the rectum is lifted off the front of the sacrum from above and is divided when the coccyx is disarticulated from below, sometimes giving rise to troublesome bleeding.

THE ATTEMPT TO CONTROL BLEEDING DURING RECTAL EXCISION

It will be evident that the arterial bleeding encountered during the pelvic and perineal phases of the dissection in a rectal excision must come from the middle sacral artery or the branches of the internal iliac arteries, chiefly the internal pudendal. It might, therefore, be thought that preliminary ligation of these vessels would minimize or even abolish this haemorrhage. In practice, however, it is difficult to say whether such ligation makes much difference, the reason being that the gluteal branches of the internal iliacs bring blood in from the buttocks and backs of the thighs where it is derived from the external iliac and femoral artery by way of the profunda femoris, the circumflex femoral, the perforating arteries and the cruciate anastomosis. This blood is then conveyed to the other branches of the internal iliac distal to the

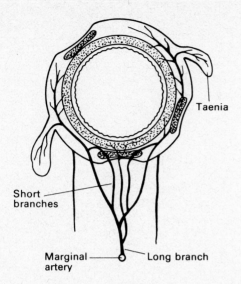

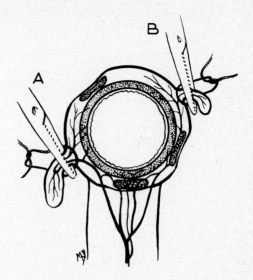

Fig. 22. Cross-section of colon and mesocolon showing the arrangement of the long and short vasa recti. (*From Goligher 1959*)

Fig. 23. The danger of damaging the long vasa recti in tying off appendices epiploicae. In (A) strong traction on the fatty appendage has drawn up a loop of the long colic branch which has been clamped by the artery forceps. In (B) by avoiding vigorous traction this danger has been averted.

ligature on that vessel, so that they are often capable of quite vigorous bleeding. Indeed, if this were not so, internal iliac ligation might frequently result in necrosis of the urinary bladder, for its blood supply is derived solely from this vessel. Fortunately this complication seldom occurs—never in my series of 70 cases so treated. To arrest all arterial haemorrhage during the pelvic or perineal operative phases of an excision of the rectum it would be necessary to control the external iliac arteries temporarily as well, as I have done occasionally in the very difficult pelvic clearance operations where a big fixed growth made accurate control of individual bleeding vessels difficult until the mass of implicated viscera had been removed.

VEINS

The veins of the colon, rectum and anal canal closely accompany the corresponding arteries and require little comment. *Those from the right colon* open into the superior mesenteric vein which lies to the right of the superior mesenteric artery and eventually joins the splenic vein to form the portal vein behind the neck of the pancreas. From *the left colon* the veins drain into the inferior mesenteric vein which lies to the left of the inferior mesenteric artery and continues upward for 5–8 cm above the origin of the latter to end by joining the splenic vein (Fig. 19A).

The veins of the *rectum* comprise the superior haemorrhoidal which drains into the inferior mesenteric and portal system, and the middle and inferior haemorrhoidal which enter the systemic venous circulation via the internal iliac veins. The superior haemorrhoidal venous plexus lies in the submucosa of the upper part of the anal canal and lower 2 cm or so of the rectum. Thence five or six collecting veins pass upwards in the wall of the rectum; at first they run in the submucosa but gradually they penetrate the muscle coat to be in the perirectal fat where they unite to form two main veins and eventually the single superior haemorrhoidal trunk. The middle haemorrhoidal vein is relatively unimportant, but the inferior haemorrhoidal vein is of more significance in that it drains the subcutaneous or external haemorrhoidal plexus of veins which lies under the skin of the anal orifice and lower part of the anal canal. Probably this plexus has communications also with the submucous or internal haemorrhoidal plexus and normally drains partly upward along the superior haemorrhoidal veins unless there is some obstruction of the portal system or distention of the internal haemorrhoidal plexus. The veins of the portal system do not have valves and are therefore specially susceptible to back-pressure.

Lymphatics of the Colon, Rectum and Anal Canal

The anatomy of the lymphatics of the large intestine was early investigated by Jamieson and Dobson (1909) and Poirier et al. (1903), using the injection technique of Gerota. They found that the lymphatics responsible for drainage of the colon could be considered as being in two closely connected groups—the intramural and the extramural lymphatics.

THE INTRAMURAL LYMPHATICS

Throughout the colon and rectum there are continuous lymphatic plexuses in the submucous and subserous layers of the bowel wall which are connected and drain into the extramural lymphatics.

THE EXTRAMURAL LYMPHATICS OF THE COLON

These consist of the lymphatic channels and lymph glands that accompany the colic blood vessels. The glands have been divided arbitrarily by Jamieson and Dobson (1909) into four groups—the epicolic, paracolic, intermediate and principal glands. The *epicolic* glands lie on the colon itself, the *paracolic* glands along the marginal artery between it and the colon, the *intermediate* glands on the main colic vessels and their branches, and the *principal* glands on the superior and inferior mesenteric vessels (see Fig. 24). The lymph usually passes through the paracolic glands in the first instance and then traverses the glands on the main colic vessels to end in glands along the superior or inferior mesenteric vessels and aorta, but sometimes lymph misses the paracolic and other more distal glands to join those on the main vessels. Poirier et al. (1903) claimed that lymph from the transverse colon instead of traversing the glands in the mesocolon could drain into the glands along the greater curvature of the stomach and in the hilum of the spleen, but this is contrary to the findings of Jamieson and Dobson (1909).

The actual course followed by lymph drainage from any part of the colon is thus determined by its blood supply, which has already been described. A knowledge of the lymphatic drainage of the various segments of the large intestine is of vital importance in the planning of radical surgical treatment and will be considered in detail in that connection in a subsequent chapter.

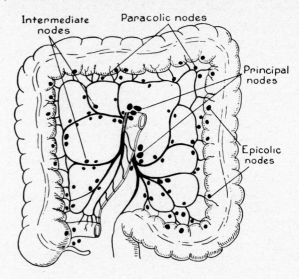

Fig. 24. The lymphatic drainage of the colon. (*From Bacon 1957*)

THE EXTRAMURAL LYMPHATICS OF THE RECTUM AND ANAL CANAL

These also follow the blood vessels supplying this part of the intestine, and there are thus three main routes of lymphatic drainage (Fig. 25):

1. Upward through the lymphatics and glands accompanying the superior haemorrhoidal and inferior mesenteric vessels essentially to the aortic glands. There may also be some drainage to the epicolic and paracolic glands along the sigmoid colon, but experience with the spread of rectal carcinoma suggests that this latter route is not ordinarily much used (p. 391).

2. Laterally along the middle haemorrhoidal vessels on either side to the internal iliac glands on the corresponding side wall of the pelvis. There may be some glands also in the course of these lymphatic channels on the upper surface of the levator ani muscles and in the substance of the lateral ligaments, but apparently the main collection is on the pelvic side wall.

3. Downward through pararectal lymph glands on the back of the rectum and along lymphatic plexuses in the anal and perianal skin, the anal sphincters and ischiorectal fat to reach eventually the inguinal lymph glands or the glands along the internal iliac vessels.

Injection experiments by Villemin et al. (1925) suggested that, while lymphatic drainage from the extraperitoneal or ampullary part of the rectum may take place along all three routes, that from the

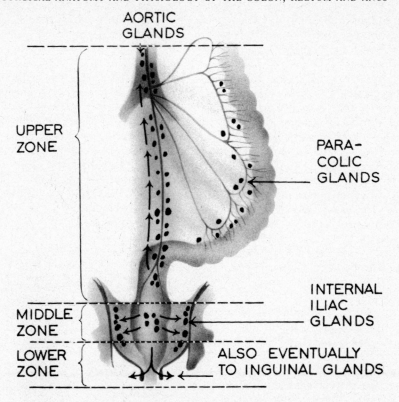

AORTIC
GLANDS

UPPER
ZONE

PARA-
COLIC
GLANDS

INTERNAL
ILIAC
GLANDS

MIDDLE
ZONE

LOWER
ZONE

ALSO EVENTUALLY
TO INGUINAL GLANDS

Fig. 25. The lymphatic drainage of the rectum and anal canal. (*From Goligher 1959*)

intraperitoneal part is exclusively upward along the superior haemorrhoidal and inferior mesenteric vessels. This is obviously a matter of great significance in regard to the spread and surgical treatment of rectal cancer. Pathological investigation of the mode of extension of this form of carcinoma shows that the main direction of spread from growths *in any part of the rectum* is upward along the superior haemorrhoidal vessels (Westhues 1934; Dukes 1940). Metastases have been demonstrated in the internal iliac glands in some cases with growths in the extraperitoneal part of the rectum, but not in cases with intraperitoneal growths (Sauer and Bacon 1952). It is well known that metastases occur in the inguinal glands in cases of rectal or anal carcinoma only when the skin of the anal canal or perianal region is involved by the growth (Gabriel 1948).

Nerve Supply to the Colon, Rectum and Anal Canal

The colon and rectum are innervated by the autonomic nervous system, with sympathetic and parasympathetic components. The nerve supply follows closely the blood supply and therefore pursues a different course to the right colon from that followed to the left colon and rectum. The account given below is based essentially on the work of Learmonth (1931), Woollard and Norrish (1933), Telford and Stopford (1934), Gask and Ross (1937), Goligher and Hughes (1951), Goligher (1951), and Smiddy and Goligher (1957).

Right Colon

Sympathetic Supply
This originates in connector cells in the right and left lateral columns of the lower six thoracic segments of the spinal cord, from which preganglionic fibres pass out in the corresponding white rami communicantes on either side to the two ganglionated sympathetic trunks. But they leave these trunks without forming synapses therein, and travel in the thoracic splanchnic nerves to the coeliac plexus and through it to the pre-aortic and superior mesenteric plexus (Fig. 26). Here they terminate in arborizations around the excitor cells

of the ganglia of this plexus, from which post-ganglionic fibres are distributed along the superior mesenteric artery and its branches to the small intestine and right colon.

Parasympathetic Supply

It is presumed that this comes from the right (posterior) vagus through its coeliac branch to the coeliac plexus (Fig. 26). Thence fibres probably pass in turn to the pre-aortic and superior mesenteric plexuses, and finally accompany the branches of the superior mesenteric artery to the small gut and right colon. There is, however, little positive evidence from dissections that vagal fibres do in fact ultimately reach the colon.

LEFT COLON AND RECTUM

Sympathetic Supply

The preganglionic fibres commence in connector cells of the right and left lateral columns of the first three lumbar segments of the spinal cord and join the lumbar ganglionated sympathetic chains on either side via the white rami communicantes. But they pass through these chains without interruption and leave them as the lumbar splanchnic nerves which join the pre-aortic plexus (Fig. 26). This plexus also contains preganglionic fibres that have descended from the thoracic splanchnic nerves through the coeliac plexus.

From the aortic plexus a prolongation extends along the inferior mesenteric artery and its branches as the *inferior mesenteric plexus*. In the course of this plexus, either close to the origin of the main artery—usually just below it—or more frequently also irregularly throughout its area of distribution, there are ganglia of various sizes. In the cells of these ganglia arise the postganglionic fibres which accompany the branches of the inferior mesenteric artery to the left colon and upper part of the rectum.

The lower rectum—and also the bladder and sexual organs in both the male and the female—receives its sympathetic supply by way of the *presacral or hypogastric nerve*. This arises from three roots: a central one, which descends over the bifurcation of the aorta from the aortic plexus which has been referred to above, and two lateral ones which are formed on each side by the junction of the lumbar splanchnic nerves, and cross the corresponding common iliac artery close to its origin. These three roots unite to form a plexus just below the bifurcation of the abdominal aorta,

known as the presacral nerve or hypogastric plexus. The presacral nerve descends into the pelvis, dividing into two branches which separate to pass to either side of the pelvis where they form plexuses of considerable size, the two *pelvic plexuses*. These plexuses also receive branches from the sacral parasympathetic nerves (nervi erigentes). From ganglion cells distributed throughout the course of the pelvic plexuses, postganglionic fibres originate which supply the lower rectum and anal canal as well as the bladder and other pelvic viscera. It will be seen that the distribution of the presacral and pelvic nerves does not follow the course of the blood vessels but proceeds directly to the walls of the organs supplied.

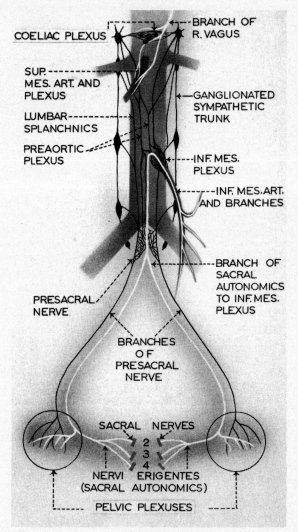

Fig. 26. The autonomic nerve supply to the rectum and colon. (*From Goligher 1959*)

The relations of the presacral nerve and pelvic plexuses are of considerable surgical significance owing to the possibility of injury to these nerves during operations such as excision of the rectum. The presacral nerve roots and nerve itself lie behind the inferior mesenteric vessels, between the two ureters, but they are very closely applied posteriorly to the abdominal aorta, the common iliac arteries, the left common iliac vein, the middle sacral artery and the fifth lumbar vertebra. Unless therefore a surgeon makes a practice of baring these structures completely during rectal excision—as perhaps he ought to—it is quite possible for him to tie the inferior mesenteric vessels either at the level of the aortic bifurcation or higher without damaging the presacral nerve or its roots. The two branches of the nerve proceed downward between the sacrum, behind, and the pelvic peritoneum, superior haemorrhoidal vessels and rectum, in front, and lower down at the back of the rectum they diverge gradually to reach either pelvic side wall below the ureter. As these two divisions separate they cling closely to the posterolateral aspects of the rectum, and unless special care is taken to brush them off the bowel they are very liable to be damaged during the posterior dissection, by either the initial scissor cut or the subsequent manual separation of the rectum from the sacral concavity. I have little doubt from dissections made in the cadaver and at operation that this is where damage to the sympathetic supply to the pelvis most frequently occurs during rectal excision. Once the divisions of the presacral nerve have reached the pelvic side wall and joined the parasympathetic nerve fibres there, they are probably less liable to injury, though they might be cut if the lateral ligament were divided unduly far laterally or a dissection of the internal lymph glands were undertaken.

Parasympathetic Supply
This is derived from small twigs, known as the nervi erigentes, or sacral autonomics, which spring from the second, third and fourth sacral nerves on either side as the latter emerge from the anterior sacral foramina (Fig. 26). They pass laterally, forward and upward to join the pelvic plexuses of sympathetic nerves on the pelvic side walls, whence fibres are distributed to the pelvic organs. Telford and Stopford (1934) have shown that the parasympathetic supply of the entire left colon is also derived from the sacral autonomics by means of fibres that travel to the pelvic plexuses and then turn up along the presacral nerve as far as the origin of the inferior mesenteric artery, where they curve downward at a sharp angle to join the inferior mesenteric plexus and to be distributed along the branches of the inferior mesenteric artery to the left colon and upper rectum (Fig. 26).

It has been stated by Ashley and Anson (1946) that the nervi erigentes pierce the fascia of Waldeyer early in their course, but this has not been confirmed by dissections made by Smiddy and Goligher (1957) which show that the nerves remain outside the parietal pelvic fascia throughout and only their ultimate branches from the pelvic plexuses to the pelvic viscera penetrate this layer. The usual mechanism of injury to the sacral autonomics during rectal excision is not quite clear, but damage probably takes places most frequently where the nerves join the pelvic plexuses and is due to the nerves being drawn inward and cut when the lateral ligament is being divided near its base. It is unlikely that the sacral autonomics are often injured by faulty stripping up of the fascia of Waldeyer during the perineal phase of the operation, as claimed by Watson (1951) and Gabriel (1948), for sacral parasympathetic injury can occur in operations such as anterior resection where there is no perineal dissection.

ANAL CANAL

Motor Innervation
The internal sphincter is supplied by the sympathetic and parasympathetic which presumably reaches the muscle by the same route as that followed to the lower rectum. The sympathetic is motor and the parasympathetic inhibitory to the sphincter.

The voluntarily contracting external sphincter has two sources of supply on either side, the inferior haemorrhoidal branch of the internal pudendal and the perineal branch of the fourth sacral nerve. The levator ani muscles which are a part of the voluntary sphincter mechanism of the anus are supplied on their pelvic aspect by twigs from the fourth sacral nerve, and on their perineal aspect by the inferior haemorrhoidal or perineal branches of the pudendal nerves.

Sensory Innervation
The normal cutaneous sensation which is felt in the skin of the perianal region and of the wall of the anal canal below the level of the anal valves is certainly conveyed by the afferent fibres in the inferior haemorrhoidal nerves and it can be abolished by an inferior haemorrhoidal nerve

block. The much less definite rather dull sensation experienced in the mucosa of the canal above the level of the valves, in response to touching or pinching with forceps or injection of haemorrhoids, is possibly mediated like rectal sensation, via the parasympathetic nerves.

PHYSIOLOGY

By H. L. Duthie

In man the large intestine receives the ileal contents, absorbs water and electrolytes and acts as a reservoir for the resultant faecal matter until it is suitable for it to be discharged from the anus. It has been calculated by Smiddy et al. (1960) that about 800–1000 ml of fluid enter the large intestine from the ileum each day; of this only about 150 ml are passed in the faeces. Complete loss of the function of the colon and rectum occurs when ileostomy and total proctocolectomy is performed, either for polyposis or for ulcerative colitis; in such cases, however, the discharge from the ileostomy is found to be less than that estimated to pass into the caecum in the normal intact individual. It has been assumed that the terminal ileum can adapt itself to take over some of the absorptive function of the colon. The exact mechanism by which this adaptation takes place is a matter for speculation, but it might be supposed that a reduced motility could allow the ileum to act a little longer on the bowel contents to reduce their volume. It is a common observation that the faeces escaping from a recently formed ileostomy are much more fluid and profuse than those discharged a week or two later which usually have a soft 'mushy' consistency. The importance of the last 30 cm of the ileum in this mechanism of compensation has been emphasized by Lillehei and Wangensteen (1955). These authors urge that the utmost conservatism should be exercised in the sacrifice of the terminal ileum when subtotal colectomy is being performed. Dilatation of the terminal ileum is also observed after total colectomy and ileostomy, and it is thought that this allows some storage of ileal contents thus imitating the reservoir function of the colon itself. On the other hand the formation of a continent ileostomy with an intra-abdominal pouch formed from the terminal ileum does not noticeably reduce the effluent after the initial period so that the capability of the ileum to concentrate its content is limited (Jagenberg et al. 1971).

When the ileocaecal valve is removed in a right hemicolectomy, bowel function is altered to give an increased stool frequency up to four times a day. This was thought, on the basis of work on animals, to be due to the loss of the valve itself (Kremen et al. 1954) but later work did not show such a change in rats and it was suggested that the findings in man were due to colonic reflux into the small bowel with resultant bacterial overgrowth (Johansson and Nylander 1969). After a left hemicolectomy only a slight increase in stool frequency occurs.

Movements of the Large Intestine

In assessing the movements of the large intestine in man, radiological examination after opaque enemas or meals has provided the most information in the past and still is the standard method of clinical assessment. In recent years measurements of pressure changes within the intestinal lumen have also received much attention.

RADIOLOGICAL OBSERVATIONS

Segmentation
The classical papers of Barclay (1933) and Alvarez (1939) give full descriptions of the activities of the normal human colon, and Alvarez (1939) emphasized their difference from movements seen in certain experimental animals. Despite this difference, the basic movements in all the alimentary canal from the stomach onwards are those of some form of segmentation; they may be looked upon as mixing movements to allow absorption of the intestinal content. In the colon, radiology has shown moulding movements at regular intervals, and these are typically seen to be small in amplitude and to occur about three to eight times in a minute. These sites of segmental constriction have been shown by cineradiography to be inconstant (Ritchie 1971). It was difficult to appreciate that such small movements could materially assist in the onward transport of colonic contents. None the less, the studies of Hurst (1909) on healthy medical students had shown that barium was transported steadily round the bowel from its entrance into the caecum about $4\frac{1}{2}$ hours after ingestion, thereafter reaching the hepatic flexure at 6 hours, the splenic flexure at 9 hours, the descending colon at 11 hours and the pelvic colon at about 18 hours. Such time intervals are too rigid and normality extends over a wide range (Brown 1959). In addition, the transport time

depends to some extent on the quantity of the opaque meal (Caldwell and Floch 1963).

Mass Peristalsis

This form of activity in the colon was first described by Holzknecht (1909) and amplified by further work of Hurst (1909), Case (1913) and Barclay (1933), and became generally accepted as the main mode of transport in the colon. It occurs most frequently immediately after a meal when all forms of motor activity in the colon are increased. The movement consists of a sudden loss of haustration in about 30–45 cm of colon, the bowel becoming extremely

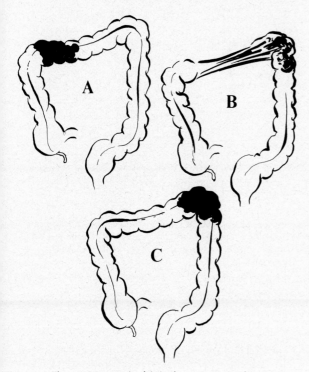

Fig. 27. Mass peristalsis in the transverse colon.

narrow and ribbon-like (Fig. 27). This state of affairs lasts for only two to three seconds and then the normal haustrated appearance returns. During this time the barium has been moved from the proximal to the distal end of the contracted areas; eventually further bursts of mass peristalsis empty some faecal matter into the rectum which can then be emptied when circumstances are suitable.

Antiperistalsis

In this movement, occasionally seen in man, waves have been shown to sweep proximally from the hepatic flexure to the caecum (Case 1913; Barclay 1933) and from pelvic to descending colon (Richie et al. 1971). This is one of the main differences between human colonic motility and that in experimental animals, for in the latter antiperistalsis is a frequent movement. Of more clinical importance is the observation by Truelove (1956) that if a small enema of say 200 ml of barium is given, a radiograph taken immediately afterwards shows all the opaque material in the rectum and sigmoid. Two or three hours later the opaque medium can often be demonstrated as far proximally as the splenic flexure and even extending into the ascending colon. This happens although the patient remains motionless in the supine position throughout this time. This evidence would suggest that a therapeutic enema, even though small in quantity, may come in contact with quite a large area of colon and would be particularly valuable in the treatment of ulcerative colitis by cortisone retention enemas.

INTRALUMINAL PRESSURE RECORDING

Initially, observations of pressure changes within the lumen of the large bowel were made by means of large balloons passed into the bowel and connected to tubes through which pressure changes were conducted to manometers or tambours. Recently smaller recording units have been used and some of the artefacts present with the larger units have been avoided. The most recent advance has been the use of the telemetering capsule which broadcasts pressure and positional changes from the inside of the gut to a special electronic receiver outside the body.

Recording Units and Fine Tubes

It is rather difficult to assign definite functions to pressure waves recorded using small balloons or fine pressure-sensitive tubes and this problem has been underlined by Connell (1961), who drew attention to the paradox of diminished wave activity in intraluminal pressure studies made on patients who had diarrhoea, with the opposite finding in patients suffering from constipation. It seems that transport through the bowel can take place rapidly with no rise in intraluminal pressure, and that when a definite rise in intraluminal pressure occurs, a segment of the bowel is temporarily closed off by the opposite sides of the bowel coming into contact. An excellent study to attempt to resolve this difficulty of interpretation was made by Ritchie et al. (1962). They measured intraluminal pressure in the human pelvic colon with a differential unit,

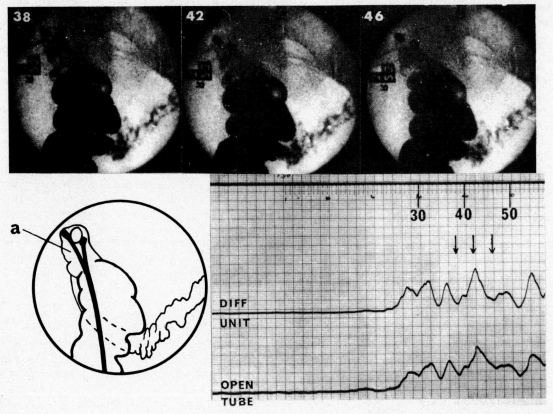

Fig. 28. Three frames from a cineradiographic record showing no movement of barium in the colon at the same time as both a differential recording unit and an open tip unit reveal active changes in the intraluminal pressure. The diagram shows the placing of the recording units and the arrows on the pressure tracing indicate the timing of the three frames. (*From Richie et al. 1962*)

consisting of a small balloon and an open-tip tube in conjunction, and at the same time made cineradiographic studies of this segment of bowel; they were able to appreciate visually the lack of correlation between a change in intraluminal pressure and the onward transport of contents of the bowel (Fig. 28). Similarly, Holdstock et al. (1970) found that physical activity of subjects increased the propulsion of radio-opaque markers in the colonic lumen, but this activity was not reflected in pressure recordings.

Telemetering Capsule

This capsule is about 1 cm in length and consists of a small electronic transmitter which is activated by a tiny dry cell, its output being altered by changes in position and by variations in intraluminal pressure. It can be swallowed and is passed along the small bowel into the colon; once the capsule is in position, the changes in pressure and position are transmitted to a recorder, and the alterations in pressure have been found to coincide with those

measured by the more conventional tube system. Radiographic studies allow the position of the capsule to be indentified accurately.

Summary

Studies of intraluminal pressure in the colon are of physiological interest but have little practical application, although they have been useful in observing the changes in diverticular disease *and the effects of colomyotomy in this condition* (Painter and Truelove 1964; Smith et al. 1971).

ELECTRICAL MEASUREMENTS FROM THE COLON AND RECTUM

Two types of electrical recordings from the colon and rectum have recently aroused interest—the electrical potential difference across the thickness of the bowel wall and the electrical waves produced in the smooth muscle cells.

Transmural Electrical Potential. A negative potential difference of around 16–28 mV exists in the normal colon and rectum. It becomes positive if the rectum is severely involved in ulcerative colitis due to a leak of potassium from the mucosal cells (Edmonds 1975). It is diminished in rectal Crohn's disease (Rudell et al. 1977).

Electrical Activity of Colonic Smooth Muscle. A rhythmic change in the electrical potential recorded from the stomach and small bowel in man has been found to form the background to the rhythmic motor activity (Bülbring et al. 1970).

Most information comes from *in vitro* studies of the taenia coli of the guinea-pig although much work has been done on the colon of the un-anaesthetized cat (Weinbeck et al. 1972). Two main types of activity are observed in man: slow waves (varying from 3 to 12/min) which provide the background for the timing of motility waves which only occur in relation to these waves. However, motor activity does not accompany each slow wave. When the muscle contracts a second form of electrical activity is seen. It consists of a burst of high frequency spikes contemporaneous with the muscle contraction and called spike activity or action potentials. In the human colon the slow waves are not present all the time, in distinction to the stomach and small bowel. Their incidence ranges from 80% in the right colon to 25% in the sigmoid colon (Duthie 1975). They also differ in that two frequencies can appear at the same site. This has been explained on the basis of the muscle fibres acting as linked relaxation oscillators and moving in and out of phase. The possible clinical significance of these waves has not been fully realized but a characteristic rhythm of around 16/min has been found in the sigmoid in diverticular disease (Taylor and Duthie 1976).

Nervous Control of Movements of Large Intestine

EXTRINSIC NERVES

It has been deduced, partly from analogy with laboratory results on animals and partly from the results of sympathetic denervation or the administration of parasympatheticomimetic drugs such as neostigmine in man, that the action of the sympathetic is to inhibit, and of the parasympathetic to stimulate peristalsis in the colon and rectum. Although total bilateral sympathectomy performed for hypertension in man had no obvious effect on bowel habit, studies in animals have shown a complex interrelation between afferent and efferent neurones at the level of the inferior mesenteric ganglion and firing patterns of post-ganglionic neurones affecting motility of the terminal colon in guinea-pigs resulted from synaptic integration inputs of preganglionic fibres of both central and peripheral origin (Weems and Szurszewski 1977).

INTRINSIC NERVES

The important role of the intramural autonomic nerve plexuses in the peristaltic activity of the colon has been dramatically revealed by the work of Swenson and Bell (1948) and Bodian et al. (1950) on the aetiology and surgical treatment of true megacolon. It is now clearly established that this condition is due to a functional obstruction of a variable part of the rectum and distal colon, caused by the inability of the normal peristaltic wave to propel itself along the relatively contracted segment of bowel distal to the lower limit of the dilated colon. Histological examination of the distal achalasic segment shows an easily recognized abnormality of its intramural nerves consisting of an absence of ganglion cells and an increase in the number of nerve fibres. These findings are further discussed on p. 279, but the correlation between achalasia and aganglionosis seems to prove the significance of the intrinsic nerve plexuses in normal colon peristalsis.

In vitro testing of strips of muscle removed from surgical specimens has shown a preponderance of adrenergic endings with noradrenaline leading to relaxation by acting on α- and β-receptors although some α-adrenergic excitatory fibres may be present (Gagnon et al. 1972). On the other hand, acetylcholine produces a contraction but probably plays a small role in resting tone since atropine results in only a slight relaxation.

Sensibility of the Colon and Rectum

It is known from the works of Lennander (1901), Hurst (1911) and others that, with the exception of the skin-lined part of the anal canal, the large gut is mainly insensitive to stimuli capable of producing pain or other sensation when applied to a cutaneous surface. It is, however, sensitive to distension by an experimental balloon introduced through the anus or through a colostomy, and it is presumed that the pain of ordinary intestinal colic is also due to natural distension (or vigorous contraction) of the gut. According to Hurst (1911) and Goligher and Hughes (1951) the sensation of fullness in the rectum that constitutes the normal call to stool or a desire to pass wind is also due to distension, and is caused by the sudden entry of faeces or flatus into this segment of the bowel.

DISTINCTION BETWEEN COLONIC AND RECTAL SENSATION

Experimental studies with balloon distension such as those of Goligher and Hughes (1951) have helped to define the characteristics of sensation in the colon and rectum respectively. Distension of the sigmoid colon in normal subjects produces a purely abdominal sensation of 'flatulent' discomfort or pain, usually referred to the suprapubic region, whereas rectal distension causes a feeling of fullness interpreted by the patient as a desire to pass wind or motion. The sensitivity of the rectum to this latter form of stimulation seems to be greater in the ampulla immediately above the anal sphincters than in the upper rectum. The distribution of the two types of sensibility in the bowel corresponds only roughly with the anatomical division into rectum and colon, and it is clear that the rectum is much more sensitive and discriminating than the colon. This is indicated experimentally by the lower pressure at which sensation can be elicited in the former and by the ability of the rectum to distinguish between flatus and faeces, which the colon cannot do. Goligher and Hughes (1951) produced some evidence that flatus normally produces a slightly lower degree of intrarectal tension than does faeces and that the rectum is able to appreciate these minor differences of pressure; but it may well be that the distinction depends, at least in part, on the recognition by the rectum and upper anal canal of other physical or chemical qualities in its contents than mere pressure (see also Sensibility of the Anal Canal, p. 35).

The difference in sensitivity of the rectum and colon is also well seen under ordinary functional conditions. During normal peristalsis considerable tension is presumably generated in the colon (pressure up to 50 cm of water), but this usually produces no sensation apart from occasional slight discomfort. It is only when peristalsis becomes greatly exaggerated as with drastic purgation that actual pain is experienced. The rectum, by contrast, is able to detect small quantities of flatus and distinguish them reliably from faeces except, perhaps, during an attack of diarrhoea.

SITE OF ORIGIN OF THE STIMULUS PRODUCING SENSATION IN THE COLON AND RECTUM

It has yet to be satisfactorily established where the nerve endings are situated which transmit sensations from the bowel. The matter cannot be decided anatomically because no recognizable organized sensory nerve endings are found in the bowel wall. Presumably the afferent nerve impulses originate from free unencapsulated nerve terminals which cannot be distinguished from the nerve endings of intramural plexuses. It was claimed by Hurst (1911) that sensation was experienced in the muscularis, while Garry (1933) tried to show, by experiments in which he painted the rectal mucosa with a cocaine solution, that afferent impulses originated in the mucous membrane. However, the anaesthetic solution might conceivably have been absorbed into the muscle coat as well, as Garry admits, and his work cannot be regarded as conclusive. The fact that a vague sensation of distension akin to the desire to defaecate is experienced during injection of irritant solutions into the submucosa of the lower rectum in the treatment of internal haemorrhoids is also in favour of the existence of some afferent nerve endings in the mucosa. Finally it should be mentioned that Lennander (1901) and more recently Lewis and Kellgren (1939) have suggested that bowel pain does not originate in the gut wall but is due to stretching of the sensitive mesentery.

In this connection it is appropriate to mention the finding of Goligher and Hughes (1951) and Goligher et al. (1965) that stumps of colon brought down into the pelvis to restore continuity after low sphincter-saving resections of abdominoanal type, sometimes acquired an imperfect sort of rectal or sacral sensation. The fact that patients with an abdominal colostomy never develop a rectal type of sensation in the piece of colon leading to the colostomy suggests that the location of the stump in the pelvis after abdominoanal excision is in some way responsible. It seemed possible that pressure on surrounding structures could contribute to rectal sensation in normal subjects. This concept has been extended since improved clinical results after coloanal anastomoses have been followed by physiological studies of continence in such patients.

In children operated upon for Hirschsprung's disease, studies of rectal sensation led to the conclusion that the urge to defaecate may arise in the puborectalis muscle (Schärli and Kiesewetter 1969). In adults after rectal excision and transanal anastomosis of the colon to the upper edge of the anal canal, pressure studies have shown a normal reflex response of both internal and external anal sphincters to balloon distension at 10 cm from the anal verge. Sensation was similar to that with an intact rectum in most cases over one year after operation (Lane and Parks 1977). It may be that surgical techniques which do not disrupt the anal canal and puborectalis permit a retention of sensory input which can give satisfactory post-operative continence in the majority without the accommodating action of the intact rectum.

NERVE PATHWAYS

It was shown by Ray and Neill (1947) that colonic pain was blocked by bilateral resection of the splanchnic nerves and sympathetic nerve chains along with the first two lumbar ganglia on both sides, and thus it can be assumed to be conveyed by the sympathetic nervous system. A pathway for the sensation of rectal fullness was investigated by Goligher and Hughes (1951). They demonstrated that rectal sensation was unaffected by bilateral and total sympathectomy or by bilateral haemor-rhoidal nerve block, but that it was abolished by a low spinal anaesthetic producing anaesthesia of the first sacral segments. This acts presumably by blocking the parasympathetic supply to the rectum from the second and third sacral nerves.

Sensibility of the Anal Canal and Anus

Skin of Perianal Region and Modified Skin below Pectinate Line. As is well known, the cutaneous covering in these parts exhibits the same sensibility to simple touch, pain and heat and cold as does the skin of the rest of the body.

Anal Mucosa above the Pectinate Line. There is a fairly widespread impression that this mucosa, like the lining of the rectum proper, is completely insensitive to ordinary tactile and painful stimuli; however experience during routine proctoscopic examination shows that this is not so. Thus the injection for haemorrhoids, which is made through this mucosa at about the level of the anorectal ring—the subsequent weal due to the injected fluid extending 6–12 mm above and below this point—usually produces a vague sensation of discomfort which is more acute the nearer the site of injection lies to the anal valves, and occasionally assumes the form of a distinct sharp and painful sensation. This accords well with the observations of Duthie and Gairns (1960) that encapsulated and free sensory nerve endings occur in abundance not only in the anal skin below the pectinate line, but also in relation to the transitional epithelium that extends for 5–10 mm or so above the valves. Encapsulated nerve endings are rarely seen beneath the rectal type of mucosa at the extreme upper end of the anal canal (Fig. 29). Anal canal dis-crimination is only preserved if at least both S_2 roots are intact and one S_3 root is undamaged (Gunterberg et al. 1976).

Anal Continence

It is difficult to formulate a generally acceptable definition of normal anal continence. The patient with total lack of control of flatus and faeces would be said by all to be incontinent. Whereas complete control is similarly easy to classify, between these two extremes the position is not so clear. Some degree of lack of control of flatus and of soiling of underclothes which might not occasion complaints from less fastidious patients could be major dis-abilities to others. Some standard form of inter-rogation must be used when this function is to be assessed especially in postoperative studies (Bennett and Goligher 1962).

Paradoxically, a patient may have a defective mechanism for anal control and yet not be inconti-nent. If colonic function is such that a firm stool is delivered into the rectum at a time suitable for defaecation, it can be passed without stressing the continence mechanism. In this way someone with a short rectal stump, after sphincter-saving resection of the rectum, may be continent when another with a longer stump but with more fluid faeces may have difficulties.

Anal continence depends on the acquired res-ponse to sensory stimuli of a complex of forces at the anorectal junction and in the anal canal. Outlines of the sensory, motor and reflex compo-nents will be presented together with some of the theories of anal continence.

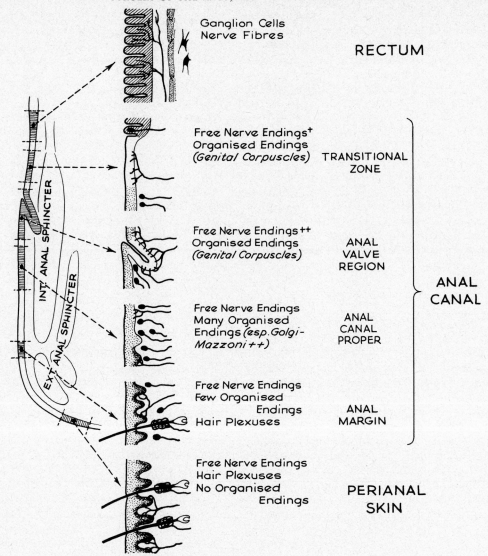

Fig. 29. Organized sensory nerve endings in the anal canal. (*From Duthie and Gairns 1960*)

SENSORY COMPONENTS

Rectal sensation (p. 34) is most important to give awareness of the arrival of material in the rectum. Anal canal sensation may contribute to the discrimination of the nature of the material (p. 35). Colonic sensation is only involved when hypermotility produces hypogastric colic.

MOTOR COMPONENTS

Numerous investigators have studied the physiology of the anus and rectum with a wide spectrum of techniques. Almost all of these methods can be said to be to some extent unphysiological as they require

the presence of a probe within the anal canal. Nevertheless, certain broad areas of agreement exist as well as several reports of conflicting findings and of differing interpretations. The exact definition of the role played by components of the continence mechanism is difficult because they overlap so much both anatomically and physiologically. Most workers have used some device to measure the pressure within the anal canal and rectum: balloons of various sizes (Denny-Brown and Robertson 1935; Hill et al. 1960; Schuster et al. 1963), open-tipped tubes (Hill et al. 1960; Duthie and Bennett 1963; Harris et al. 1966), radiopills sensitive to pressure changes (Schärli and Kiesewetter 1969), obturators with partitions to try to isolate the effect of the internal and external sphincters (Gaston 1948). At a later stage the squeeze in the anal canal has been recorded by deformation of small strain gauges placed in the canal (Collins et al. 1967; Howard and Nixon 1968).

All these methods have a fairly predictable finding, namely that there is a high-pressure zone in the anal canal. Depending on the probe used the average peak pressure found at about 2 cm from the anal verge may be from 25 to 120 mmHg in a normal adult at rest. The pressure in the anal canal relates to the viscoelastic properties of the rectum and the findings have been compared to a linear rheological model (Arhan et al. 1976). Although some relationship has been found between the

pressure recorded and the size of the balloon, this does not hold when non-compressible obturators of increasing size are used. The anal canal can quickly adapt to these and gives a resting pressure which is similar for all diameters from 5 to 21 mm (Duthie et al. 1970). Measurement of squeeze using strain gauges also gives a peak about 2 cm. This level is caudad to the puborectalis sling in the area where the internal and external anal sphincters overlap. A phasic variation in this pressure is noted by most workers. The number of these waves is increased in patients with haemorrhoids (Hancock 1977a) and in those with an anal fissure (Hancock 1977b). Electromyographic recordings show continual activity at rest in the levator ani and external anal sphincter muscles (Kawakami 1954; Floyd and Walls 1953; Taverner and Smiddy 1959; Porter

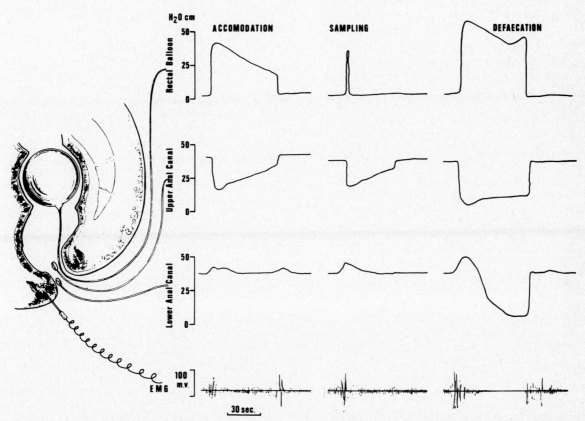

Fig. 30.   Response of upper and lower anal canal pressure and electromyogram (EMG) of the external anal sphincter to inflation of a balloon in the rectal ampulla. Accommodation (left panel) occurs when the balloon is held inflated and the rectum gradually relaxes at the same time as the upper part of the anal canal is showing a gradual return of pressure after an initial prompt relaxation. The EMG of the external anal sphincter shows a transient increase in activity on inflation and on deflation of the balloon. Sampling (centre panel): when the rectal balloon is inflated and deflated rapidly, relaxation of the upper part of the anal canal occurs. The lower part of the anal canal remains tonic with only a brief burst of action potentials on the EMG. Defaecation (right panel): with greater inflation of the balloon in the rectum, the rectal accommodation is overcome, the whole anal canal relaxes and the EMG of the external anal sphincter is inhibited and as a result the balloon is expelled.

1962; Chantraine 1966) and continuous electrical potentials have also been recorded from the internal anal sphincter at rest (Kerremans 1968; Wankling et al. 1968; Ustach et al. 1970), so that all could contribute to the resting pressure.

Agreement exists on the presence of a high-pressure zone in the anal canal but not on its importance in maintaining anal continence nor on the part played by the internal and external anal sphincters in its production. Some authors favour the internal sphincter (Duthie and Watts 1965; Katz et al. 1967; Duhamel 1969; Ustach et al. 1970) and others the external sphincter (Alva et al. 1967). In part the differing views are due to interpretation of pressures at points along the anal canal being held to be due mainly to one or other of the muscles. As has been mentioned already the overlapping of the sphincters makes this a difficult task. Even when the external sphincter is paralysed, the pressure zone is not materially altered except when a small bolus is pulled through the anal canal (Duthie and Watts 1965) so that the resting pressure would seem to be largely due to the internal anal sphincter. Although it has been demonstrated that activity is always present in the external anal sphincter and pelvic floor muscles, these muscles can only be contracted voluntarily for periods from 40 to 60 seconds. Thereafter, despite continued efforts by the subject, both the electrical activity in the muscle and pressure within the anal canal return to basal levels (Porter 1962; Taverner and Smiddy 1959; Parks et al. 1962). The striated muscles show histological changes compatible with denervation in incontinent patients (Parks et al. 1977).

RESPONSE TO ENTRY OF MATERIAL INTO RECTUM

Three patterns of response are found on the entry of material into the rectum which is usually mimicked experimentally by inflating a balloon in the rectum (Duthie 1975).

ACCOMMODATION

This occurs when the balloon is kept inflated for about a minute (Fig. 30). The rectum slowly expands to accommodate the bolus and the balloon pressure decreases. The internal sphincter shows the classical response of relaxation which remains intact in spinal man (Frenckner 1976) and the external sphincter contracts transiently when the balloon is first inflated. This reflex allows the bolus to be kept

in the rectum until a suitable time for defaecation. Sampling (see below) occurs as part of this reflex.

SAMPLING

A brief inflation of the balloon results in relaxation of the internal sphincter so that the rectal content may come in contact with the sensory epithelium of the anal canal (Duthie and Bennett 1963) (Figs 30, 31). This can be done voluntarily with a short Valsalva manoeuvre when the subject wishes to test if it is safe to pass wind.

DEFAECATION (see also p. 41)

When the balloon is inflated with increasing amounts of air, a volume (maximal tolerable volume) is reached when the urge to defaecate becomes overwhelming and the balloon is passed, with inhibition of the external sphincter electromyogram (Fig. 30). The maximal tolerable volume decreases in older subjects (Ihre 1974).

THEORIES OF ANAL CONTINENCE

PRESSURE ZONE

The most commonly accepted explanation of anal continence is that the high-pressure zone (average 25–120 mmHg) in the anal canal provides an effective barrier against pressure in the rectum (average 5–20 mmHg). Although a higher pressure is found in the anal canal than in the rectum when the subject is at rest, circumstances can arise, for example on straining or on performing a Valsalva manoeuvre, for which some investigators have made records showing a higher pressure in the rectum without any incontinence occurring. This has led to the invoking of physical factors outside the anal canal as providing additional protection (Phillips and Edwards 1965).

ANGULATION BETWEEN RECTUM AND ANAL CANAL

The angle of 80° between the axis of the rectum and that of the anal canal is maintained except when the hips are flexed more than 90° (Tagart 1966) or during defaecation (Phillips and Edwards 1965). It has long been held that this angulation, maintained by the pull of the puborectalis sling, is an important factor in anal continence.

FLUTTER VALVE

As a result of manometric and radiological studies, Phillips and Edwards (1965) suggested that ad-

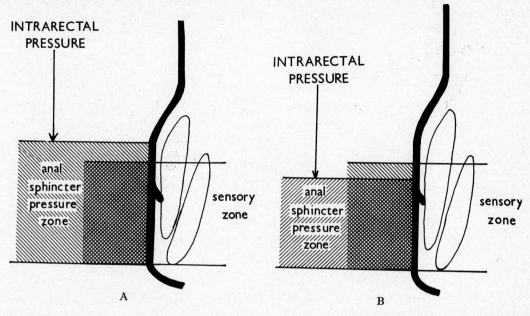

Fig. 31. Relation of the pressure zone to the sensory zone in the anal canal. A. At rest. B. When the rectum is distended. (*From Duthie, Surgical Physiology of the Gastrointestinal Tract. Symposium at Royal College of Surgeons, Edinburgh; ed. A. Smith*)

ditional protection could be afforded by intra-abdominal pressure being transmitted, at the level of the levator ani, laterally to the side of the anal canal in the region of the anorectal junction. The anal canal is an anteroposterior slit and this pressure could compress it in a way similar to the working of the simple non-return flutter valve used on some respiratory apparatus. This was proposed because when the anal canal was coated with radio-opaque material an occlusion could be seen in the region of the anorectal junction. This ingenious hypothesis is attractive but cannot exclude that the above findings are due to puborectalis activity, nor does it explain the lack of identification of a localized zone of higher pressure at the craniad part of the anal canal. While this mechanism may protect against a rise in intra-abdominal pressure it cannot provide protection against an increase in intrarectal pressure.

RESISTANCE TO OPENING

Differential pressure recording by withdrawing a probe from the rectum and re-inserting it via the anus led Harris and Pope (1964) to propose that the pressure recorded in the anal canal depended not so much on the ability of the muscles to squeeze around the anal canal but rather on their ability to resist the opening up of the canal. Various methods

have been used to assess this function. The reaction of the anal canal was measured in response to injecting microlitre amounts of water through a small tube until no further increase in pressure was observed (Harris et al. 1966). A similar technique was applied using a small balloon (Katz et al. 1967). Another procedure was to insert a special obturator which could be expanded within the anal canal and measure the resistance encountered (Inberg 1952; Yanchev 1963; Lieberman 1964). Apart from any force exerted by the muscles, the adhesion of the moist surfaces of the mucosal lining of the anal canal would have to be broken to allow the potential space to be opened. Another possible factor is a lengthening of the anal canal by the contraction of the posterior parts of the levator ani muscles, in a similar manner to the changes in the urethra when the pelvic floor is elevated.

FORCES AROUND THE ANAL CANAL

Some impression of the forces involved can be gained from Figs 32 and 33. Using a probe with numerous strain gauges set to appreciate forces in four quadrants around the anal canal (Collins et al. 1967), it was shown that the forces on the craniad portion are maximal posteriorly, less laterally and minimal anteriorly. This finding was compatible with the combined action of the puborectalis sling

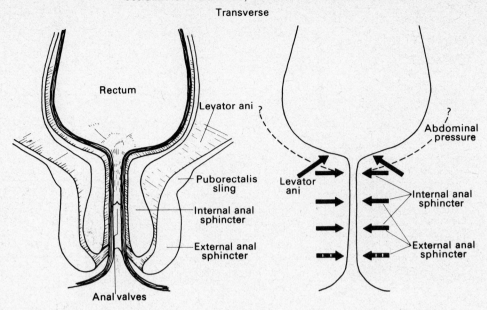

Fig. 32. Transverse section through the anal canal and lower rectum to demonstrate the factors involved in anal incontinence. The arrow represents the forces involved. (*From Duthie 1971*)

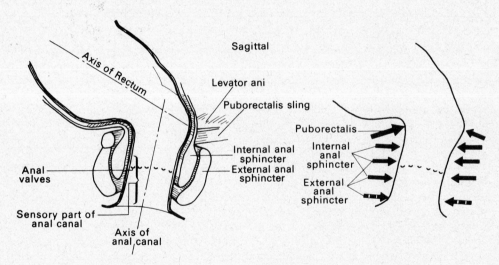

Fig. 33. Saggital section through the structures shown in Fig. 32. (*From Duthie 1971*)

and the internal anal sphincter, the latter providing the anterior component on its own. More caudad, the internal and external sphincters together provide the force which is greater laterally than anteroposteriorly. The external anal sphincter provides the final voluntary guard.

Summary

Even in 'normal' subjects a fluid stool may cause incontinence, so that anal continence is relative.

The anal canal mechanism, in combination with the suppression of the urge to defaecate, has to cope with the consistency and rate of delivery of faeces into the rectum. Sensory stimulation in the rectum and pelvic floor may reach consciousness and leads to reflex relaxation of the craniad portion of the anal canal which may allow rectal contents to be identified more accurately. Physical factors maintaining continence are the angulation between anal canal and rectum, the slit-like configuration of the anal canal and the action of the internal anal sphincter. The external anal sphincter provides additional support and acts fully as an emergency voluntary control of short (1–2 min) duration.

Defaecation

Defaecation is a complex reflex act in animals; in man, the controlling influence of the cerebral cortex makes it even more complex. The stimulus to initiation of the act is distension of the rectum. This urge may be suppressed if circumstances are not convenient for defaecation. In the adult suppression has taken place over so many years that in many cases defaecation becomes quite habitual, usually first thing on rising in the morning or immediately after breakfast. This is sometimes the only time that any urge to defaecate is felt, yet it is well known that in many people the rectum is by no means empty of faeces for the rest of the 24 hours. It is likely that a summation of impulses is necessary to achieve consciousness; a certain level of filling of the rectum, together with the conditioned reflex at the habitual time of day for that individual.

The emphasis on the cortical control of defaecation can scarcely be too great, for in the past it has received too little attention, probably because much of the information on the defaecation reflex has been obtained from animals. Apart from the cerebral control in man, there is a centre in the lumbosacral region of the spinal cord which can maintain reflex defaecation after an injury transecting the spinal cord above it. Some weak coordination of smooth muscle remains if the cauda equina is destroyed, so that automatic defaecation can occur through the already patulous anus. Obviously these lesions deprive the patients of anal continence as there is no awareness of anorectal sensation.

A factor of prime importance in beginning the act is the assumption of the squatting position. As has been already noted (p. 38) this straightens out the angulation between the rectum and anal canal and facilitates emptying of the rectum. The splinting action of the anterior surface of the thighs against the lower abdomen also assists the raising of intra-abdominal pressure. The pelvic floor descends and the physical forces in the anal canal are overcome by the intra-abdominal pressure. During defaecation the electromyogram from the pelvic floor and external anal sphincter is inhibited (Kawakami 1954). After the main mass of the faeces has passed through the anal canal the pelvic floor and anal canal muscles regain activity and finally discharge the stool.

The method of commencement of the act of defaecation varies from person to person. If one is exerting anal control during an urge, mere relinquishing of this voluntary control will allow the reflex to proceed. If, on the other hand, the urge has passed off, a voluntary straining with increase in the intra-abdominal pressure is necessary before defaecation can begin. Once begun the act can again follow either of two patterns: firstly, expulsion of the rectal contents accompanied by mass peristalsis of the distal colon clears the bowel in one continuous movement; or secondly, the stool is passed piecemeal, with several bouts of straining. The habit of the individual and the consistency of the faeces largely determine which pattern is followed.

Secretion in the Colon

Mucus

Mucus is thought to protect the mucosa and is secreted throughout the large bowel in columnar cells known as goblet cells—the collection within them of droplets of mucin appears to alter their shape into roughly that of a goblet. Mucin is synthesized in an area just above the nucleus of a cell and recent studies with the electronmicroscope have shown that the droplets appear first in the membranes of the Golgi apparatus (Bierring 1962). These cells have a life-span of about three days in experimental animals. Any irritation of the mucous membrane leads to a discharge of mucus (Florey 1962). It has been shown by autoradiography to be sulphated and to be rapidly resynthesized within the goblet cell immediately after the cell has been stimulated to discharge. No proof is available of any nervous or humoral control of its release. It has been suggested that carbachol increases the release of mucin but not its synthesis, whereas a β-adrenergic stimulus increases both release and synthesis (Smith and Butler 1974).

Absorption in the Colon and Rectum

Apart from its intrinsic interest, the absorptive function of the colon and rectum is important when considering the possible effects of proctocolectomy or of total colonic by-pass and in some cases of diarrhoea. The main substances absorbed are water and electrolytes. In addition ammonia, bile salts, urea, glucose and some drugs such as hydrocortisone and morphine are absorbed.

WATER AND ELECTROLYTES

Several methods have been used to determine the capacity of the colon and rectum to absorb water and electrolytes (Turnberg 1970). Comparing normal faecal content with ileostomy discharge in the first week after operation (Table 1) it has been estimated that 70 mmol of sodium and 400–500 ml of water are absorbed each day by the colon and rectum. Ileostomy output of water and electrolytes can be significantly reduced by giving the patient an elemental diet which also leads to a decrease in trypsin and bile acid output (Hill et al. 1976). The ileostomy discharge may not represent the state of affairs in the intact man and it has been suggested that the true volume of ileal contents reaching the caecum may be two to three times greater (Giller and Phillips 1970).

More detailed information has come from radioisotopic studies of temporarily isolated loops (Duthie and Atwell 1963) or, better, of the whole colon using perfusion methods (Levitan et al. 1962; Shields 1966; Devroede and Phillips 1969). These techniques demonstrate an active absorption of sodium with a concomitant passive movement of water. The theoretical capacity (Table 1) may be overestimated because the perfusion rate used in most studies (10 ml/min) would mean a total load of 14 litres/day and less sodium is present in colonic fluid than in isotonic saline. Potassium is secreted into the lumen of the colon against a concentration gradient of up to 15 mmol/litre. This seems to be active secretion because the transmural electrical potential difference is not great enough for the movement of potassium to be due to passive transport down an electrochemical gradient (Edmonds and Godfrey 1970). Comparisons of the right and left halves of the colon indicate that the caecum and ascending colon may have the greater absorptive capacity.

Any diminution in the amount of sodium absorbed from the colon would impair water absorption and predispose to diarrhoea. Objective measurements of such changes have been made in ulcerative colitis (Duthie et al. 1964; Harris and Shields 1970) and also following instillation of dihydroxy bile salts into the colon (Mekhjian et al. 1971) giving support for the role of bile salts in the production of some types of diarrhoea. The stimulation of cyclic AMP produced in the human colon by bile salts can be inhibited by propranolol acting as an adenyl cyclase inhibitor (Coyne et al. 1977). In contrast, presumably bran used in the conservative treatment of diverticular disease (see p. 898) has its effect by diminishing water absorption from the colonic content: an effect varying with the type of bran (Brodribb and Groves 1978).

AMMONIA

The production and absorption of ammonia in the colon is important in the aetiology of portasystemic encephalopathy in cirrhosis especially after portacaval shunting. Neomycin therapy to cut down the bacterial population and surgical by-pass of the colon are methods to reduce the severity of symptoms. After some initial debate, it now seems clear that ammonia is absorbed from the colon in proportion to its concentration in the lumen and is better absorbed at pH 7–9 than at pH 4–5. Thus non-ionic diffusion would seem to be the main method of transport (Castell and Moore 1971; Bown et al. 1972).

Physiology of the Small Bowel

The importance of the terminal ileum in absorption of fluid from ileostomy dejecta has been mentioned, but other aspects of ileal function are worthy of consideration. Despite the fact that this book is mainly concerned with colonic function, inevitably some ileum is removed in a total colectomy or right hemicolectomy and quite an extensive area may be removed or be diseased in patients with regional enteritis.

TABLE 1. *Daily Water and Electrolyte Content of Ileal Discharge, Ileostomy Discharge and Faeces*

	Volume (ml)	Sodium (mmol)	Potassium (mmol)
Normal faeces*	200–400	2–5	6–12
Ileostomy discharge within first week	up to 1000	up to 130	1–12
when established	200–500	40–60	1–12
Ileal volume passed into caecum†	1500	185	9
Faeces (mean of 4 subjects)	40	1	5
Theoretical absorptive capacity of colon in 24 hours‡	2500	400	—

* Smiddy et al. (1960); † Giller and Phillips (1970); ‡ Levitan et al. (1962).

MOTILITY

When the ileocaecal area is resected either in a right hemicolectomy or in a total colectomy the controlling effect of the ileocaecal valve is removed and the frequency of bowel actions is increased disproportionately to the length of small bowel which has been ablated. After an ileostomy is formed the discharge from the stoma changes in consistency from fluid to semi-solid over the first 10 to 12 days. This has been attributed to be an adaptation of the terminal ileum. Some objective evidence to show an adaptation in the motility pattern has been found from studies of the motility of the terminal ileum after formation of an ileostomy. The initial rate of motility in the terminal ileum is higher in the first week than when studies are made three to four weeks after the operation (Waterfall et al. 1971).

ABSORPTION

The contribution of the terminal ileum to absorption of water and electrolytes and most nutrients is small compared with that of the rest of the small intestine. Overt malabsorption does not occur if the rest of the small bowel is not diseased. However, two constituents of diet are specifically absorbed in this area and mention will be made of their importance.

VITAMIN B12

There is a highly specific mechanism for the absorption of B12 in the terminal ileum. The vitamin combines with intrinsic factor from the parietal cells of the body of the stomach, and this complex adheres to specific receptors on the microvillous membrane of the mucosal cells of the ileum. Some workers have suggested that the intrinsic factor–vitamin B12 complex may be absorbed intact (Rothenberg et al. 1972). Calcium ions seem to be essential for this attachment. The vitamin B12 is released from the complex by enzyme reaction and 95% passes via the portal system. Although most of the vitamin B12 is absorbed by the terminal ileum, large oral doses of the vitamin can be absorbed more proximally presumably by diffusion. Thus when the terminal ileum is resected or is extensively diseased, e.g. in regional enteritis, the patient is liable to develop a deficiency of vitamin B12 which will take some time to become obvious and, if the resection is not large, may remain at a subclinical level, being detected only by measurement of the serum vitamin B12.

BILE SALTS

The total pool of bile salts in the body is about 3–5 g and these are circulated through the liver several times in 24 hours, being secreted into the bile and re-absorbed by a specific mechanism in the terminal ileum. Normally about 1 g of bile salts is lost in the faeces each day, but this amount would be increased in ileostomy, especially if any substantial amount of the terminal ileum has to be removed. The liver synthesis of bile salts has then to be increased to compensate for this loss and, eventually, the bile salt pool in the body can become depleted and, as a result of this deficiency, the absorption of lipids is impaired and steatorrhoea can result. If, after resection, the small bowel is joined to the colon, the resultant increase in bile salts in the colon is acted upon by the colonic bacteria to produce free bile acids. These may irritate the colon so that as well as having a tendency to steatorrhoea the patient may have colonic diarrhoea from this factor. When less than 1 m of small bowel is resected the effect of the increased amount of bile salts in the colon predominates. When more than 1 m of the small gut is removed the steatorrhoea is the prime factor in producing diarrhoea (Hofmann and Poley 1972).

Autonomic Innervation of the Urinary Bladder and Sexual Organs in Relation to Rectal Surgery

Actually the function of the autonomic nervous system that is most important in regard to rectal surgery is not its action on the rectum or colon, but its influence on the bladder and male sexual organs, for damage to the sympathetic or parasympathetic nerves in the pelvis is liable to show itself by disorder of the function of these organs. The work of Learmonth (1931) has established that the sympathetic nerve supply is motor to the bladder neck, trigone and internal urethral sphincter, and inhibitory to the body of the bladder (the detrusor muscle), and that it also causes contractions of the seminal vesicles. Surprisingly enough, division of the presacral nerve causes no obvious alteration of bladder function apart possibly from a transient slight increase in the frequency of micturition. But it does affect sexual function, the patient being capable of normal erection and orgasm but not of ejaculation. He is therefore potent but sterile.

Stimulation of the nervi erigentes in animals is known to cause relaxation of the bladder neck and contraction of the detrusor, in addition to producing erection of the penis. Division of these nerves in animals and man results in retention of urine, possibly with paradoxical overflow incontinence, and in impotence.

REFERENCES

ALVA, J., MENDELOFF, A. I. and SCHUSTER, M. M. (1967) Reflex and electromyographic abnormalities associated with fecal incontinence. *Gastroenterology, 53*, 101.

ALVAREZ, W. C. (1939) *An Introduction to Gastro-enterology*, 3rd ed. London: Heinemann.

ARCHIBALD, E. (1908) Operative treatment of cancer of the rectum. *J. Am. med. Ass., 50*, 73.

ARHAN, P., FAVERDIN, C., PERSOZ, B., DEVROEDE, G., DUBOIS, F., DORNIC, C. and PELLERIN, D. (1976) Relationship between viscoelastic properties of the rectum and anal pressure in man. *J. appl. Physiol., 41*, 677.

ASHLEY, F. L. and ANSON, B. J. (1946) The pelvic autonomic nerves in the male. *Surgery Gynec. Obstet., 82*, 598.

BACON, H. E. (1957) Cancer of the rectum and colon: a critical analysis with recommendations to extend the rate of survival. *Surgery, St Louis, 41*, 387.

—— and SMITH, C. H. (1948) Arterial supply of distal colon. *Ann. Surg., 127*, 28.

BALL, C. B. (1908) *The Rectum: its Diseases and Developmental Defects*. London: Frowde; Hodder and Stoughton.

BARCLAY, A. E. (1933) *The Digestive Tract*. Cambridge: Cambridge University Press.

BENNETT, R. C. and GOLIGHER, J. C. (1962) Results of internal sphincterotomy for anal fissure. *Br. med. J., 2*, 1500.

BIERRING, F. (1962) Electron microscopic observations on the mucus production in human and rat intestinal goblet cells. *Acta path. microbiol. scand., 54*, 241.

BODIAN, M., STEPHENS, F. D. and WARD, B. C. H. (1950) Hirschsprung's disease. *Lancet, 1*, 19.

BOWN, R. L. SLADEN, G. E., CLARK, M. L. and DAWSON, A. M. (1972) The production and transport of ammonia in the human colon. *Biol. Gastroentérol., 5*, 644c.

BRODRIBB, A. J. M. and GROVES, C. (1978) Effect of bran particle size on stool weight. *Gut, 19*, 60.

BROWN, F. O. (1959) On routine barium examination of the small bowel. *Lancet, 2*, 530.

BÜLBRING, E., BRADING, A. F., JONES, A. W. and TOMITA, T. (1970) *Smooth Muscle*. London: Edward Arnold.

CALDWELL, W. L. and FLOCH, M. H. (1963) Evaluation of the small bowel barium motor meal with emphasis on the effect of volume of barium suspension ingested. *Radiology, 80*, 383.

CASE, J. T. (1913) X-ray observations on colonic peristalsis etc. *Proc. 17th int. Congr. Med., London* (quoted by Barclay 1933).

CASTELL, D. O. and MOORE, E. W. (1971) Ammonia absorption from the human colon. The role of nonionic diffusion. *Gastroenterology, 60*, 33.

CHANTRAINE, A. (1966) Électromyographie des sphincters striés urétral et anal humains: étude descriptive et analytique. *Revue neurol. 115*, 396.

CHIARI, H. (1878) *Med. J. Wien*, 419.

COLLINS, C. D., DUTHIE, H. L., SHELLEY, T. and WHITTAKER, G. E. (1967) Force in the anal canal and anal continence. *Gut, 8*, 354.

CONNELL, A. M. (1961) The motility of the pelvic colon. II. Paradoxical motility in diarrhoea and constipation. *Gut, 3*, 342.

COURTNEY, H. (1949) Posterior subsphincteric space; its relation to posterior horseshoe fistula. *Surgery Gynec. Obstet., 89*, 222.

COYNE, M. J., BONORRIS, G. G., CHUNG, A., CONLEY, D. and SCHOENFIELD, L. J. (1977) Propranolol inhibits bile acid and fatty acid stimulation of cyclic AMP in human colon. *Gastroenterology, 73*, 971.

CRAPP, A. R. and CUTHBERTSON, A. M. (1974) William Waldeyer and the rectosacral fascia. *Surgery Gynec. Obstet., 138*, 252.

DENNY-BROWN, D. and ROBERTSON, E. G. (1935) An investigation of the nervous control of defaecation. *Brain, 58*, 256.

DEVROEDE, G. J. and PHILLIPS, S. F. (1969) Studies of the perfusion technique for colonic absorption. *Gastroenterology, 56*, 92.

DRUMMOND, H. (1914) The arterial supply of the rectum and pelvic colon. *Br. J. Surg., 1*, 677.

DUHAMEL, B. (1969) Physio-pathology of the internal anal sphincter. *Archs Dis. Childh., 44*, 377.

DUKES, C. E. (1940) Cancer of the rectum: an analysis of 1000 cases. *J. Path. Bact., 50*, 527.

—— and GALVIN, C. (1956) Colloid carcinoma arising within fistulae in the ano-rectal region. *Ann. R. Coll. Surg. Engl., 18*, 246.

DUTHIE, H. L. (1975) Colonic motility in man. *Mayo Clin. Proc., 50*, 519.

—— and ATWELL, J. D. (1963) The absorption of water, sodium, and potassium in the large intestine with particular reference to the effects of villous papillomas. *Gut, 4*, 373.

—— and BENNETT, R. C. (1963) The relation of sensation in the anal canal to the functional anal sphincter: a possible factor in anal continence. *Gut, 4*, 179.

—— and GAIRNS, F. W. (1960). Sensory nerve endings and sensation in the anal region of man. *Br. J. Surg., 47*, 585.

—— KWONG, N. K. and BROWN, B. (1970) Adaptability of the anal canal to distension. *Br. J. Surg., 57*, 388.

—— and WATTS, J. M. (1965) Contribution of the external anal sphincter to the pressure zone in the anal canal. *Gut, 6*, 64.

—— —— DE DOMBAL, F. T. and GOLIGHER, J. C. (1964) Serum electrolytes and colonic transfer of water and electrolytes in chronic ulcerative colitis. *Gastroenterology, 47*, 525.

EDMONDS, C. J. (1975) Electrical potential difference of colonic mucosa. *Gut, 16*, 315.

—— and GODFREY, R. C. (1970) Measurement of electrical potentials of the human rectum and pelvic colon in normal and aldosterone-treated patients. *Gut, 11*, 330.

EISENHAMMER, S. (1951) Surgical correction of chronic internal anal (sphincteric) contracture. *S. Afr. med. J., 25*, 486.

—— (1953) The internal anal sphincter: its surgical importance. *S. Afr. med. J., 27*, 266.

ELLIS, G. V. (1878) *Demonstrations of Anatomy*, 8th ed., p. 420. London: Smith, Elder.

EWING, M. R. (1952) The significance of the level of the peritoneal reflection in the surgery of rectal cancer. *Br. J. Surg.*, *39*, 495.

—— (1954) The white line of Hilton. *Proc. R. Soc. Med.*, *47*, 525.

FINE, J. and LAWES, C. H. W. (1940) On the muscle-fibres of the anal submucosa, with special reference to the pecten band. *Br. J. Surg.*, *27*, 723.

FLOREY, H. W. (1962) The secretion and function of intestinal mucus. *Gastroenterology*, *43*, 326.

FLOYD, W. F. and WALLS, E. W. (1953) Electromyography of the sphincter ani externus in man. *J. Physiol., Lond.*, *122*, 599.

FOWLER, R., Jr. (1957) Landmarks and legends of the anal canal. *Aust. N.Z. J. Surg.*, *27*, 1.

FRENCKNER, B. (1976) Function of the anal sphincters in spinal man. *Gut*, *16*, 638.

GABRIEL, W. B. (1948) *The Principles and Practice of Rectal Surgery*, 4th ed. London: H. K. Lewis.

GAGNON, D. J., DEVROEDE, G. and BELISLE, S. (1972) Excitatory effects of adrenaline upon isolated preparations of human colon. *Gut*, *13*, 654.

GARRY, R. C. (1933) Responses to stimulation of the caudal end of the large bowel in the cat. *J. Physiol., Lond.*, *78*, 208.

GASK, G. E. and ROSS, J. P. (1937) *The Surgery of the Sympathetic Nervous System*, 2nd ed. London: Baillière.

GASTON, E. A. (1948) Physiology of fecal incontinence. *Surgery Gynec. Obstet.*, *87*, 280.

GILLER, J. and PHILLIPS, S. F. (1970) Colonic absorption of electrolytes and water in man: a comparison of 24 hour ileal content and feces. *Gastroenterology*, *58*, 951.

GOLIGHER, J. C. (1949) The blood-supply to the sigmoid colon and rectum. *Br. J. Surg.*, *37*, 157.

—— (1951) Discussion on urological complications of excision of rectum. *Proc. R. Soc. Med.*, *44*, 824.

—— (1954) The adequacy of the marginal blood-supply to the left colon after high ligation of the inferior mesenteric artery during excision of the rectum. *Br. J. Surg.*, *41*, 351.

—— (1959) In *Diseases of the Colon and Ano-rectum*, ed. R. Turell. Philadelphia: W. B. Saunders.

—— DUTHIE, H. L., DE DOMBAL, F. T. and WATTS, J. M. (1965) Abdomino-anal pull-through excision for tumours of the mid third of the rectum. *Br. J. Surg.*, *52*, 323.

—— and HUGHES, E. S. R. (1951) Sensibility of the rectum and colon: its role in the mechanism of anal continence. *Lancet*, *1*, 543.

—— LEACOCK, A. G. and BROSSY, J.-J. (1955) The surgical anatomy of the anal canal. *Br. J. Surg.*, *43*, 51.

GORDON-WATSON, SIR C. and DODD, H. (1935) Observations on fistula in ano in relation to peri-anal intramuscular glands, with reports on three cases. *Br. J. Surg.*, *22*, 703.

GRAHAM, J. W. and GOLIGHER, J. C. (1954) The management of accidental injuries and deliberate resections of the ureter during excision of the rectum. *Br. J. Surg.*, *42*, 151.

GRAY, H. (1926) *Anatomy, Descriptive and Applied*, 23rd ed., Fig. 718. London: Longmans.

GRIFFITHS, J. D. (1956) Surgical anatomy of the blood supply of the distal colon. *Ann. R. Coll. Surg. Engl.*, *19*, 241.

GUNTERBERG, B., KEWENTER, J., PETERSEN, I. and STENER, B. (1976) Anorectal function after major resections of the sacrum with bilateral or unilateral sacrifice of sacral nerves. *Br. J. Surg.*, *63*, 546.

HANCOCK, B. D. (1977a) The internal anal sphincter and anal fissure. *Br. J. Surg.*, *64*, 92.

—— (1977b) Internal sphincter and the nature of haemorrhoids. *Gut*, *18*, 651.

HARRIS, H. A. (1929) Some embryological aspects of the problem involved (in fistula-in-ano). *Proc. R. Soc. Med.*, *22*, 1341.

HARRIS, J. and SHIELDS, R. (1970) Absorption and secretion of water and electrolytes by the intact human colon in diffuse untreated proctocolitis. *Gut*, *11*, 27.

HARRIS, L. D. and POPE, C. E., II (1964) 'Squeeze' vs. Resistance: an evaluation of the mechanism of sphincter competence. *J. clin. Invest.*, *43*, 2272.

—— WINANS, C. S. and POPE, C. E., II (1966) Determination of yield pressures: A method for measuring anal sphincter competence. *Gastroenterology*, *50*, 754.

HERMANN, G. and DESFOSSES, L. (1880) Sur la muquese de la région cloacale du rectum. *C.r. hebd. Séanc. Acad. Sci., Paris*, *90*, 1301.

HILL, G. L., MAIR, W. S. J., EDWARDS, J. P. and GOLIGHER, J. C. (1976) Decreased trypsin and bile acids in ileal fistula drainage during the administration of a chemically defined liquid elemental diet. *Br. J. Surg.*, *63*, 133.

HILL, J. R., KELLEY, M. L., Jr., SCHLEGEL, J. F. and CODE, C. F. (1960) Pressure profile of the rectum and anus of healthy persons. *Dis. Colon Rect.*, *3*, 203.

HILL, M. R., SHRYOCK, E. H. and ReBELL, F. G. (1943) Role of the anal glands in the pathogenesis of ano-rectal disease. *J. Am. med. Ass.*, *121*, 742.

HILTON, J. (1877) In *On Rest and Pain*, 2nd ed., ed. W. H. A. Jacobson. London: Bell.

HOFMANN, A. F. and POLEY, J. R. (1972) Role of bile acid malabsorption in pathogenesis of diarrhea and steatorrhea in patients with ileal resection. *Gastroenterology*, *62*, 918.

HOLDSTOCK, D. J., MISIEWICZ, J. J., SMITH, T. and ROWLANDS, E. N. (1970) Propulsion (mass movements) in the human colon and its relationship to meals and somatic activity. *Gut*, *11*, 91.

HOLZKNECHT, G. (1909) Die normale Peristaltik des Kolons. *Münch. med. Wschr.*, *56*, 2401.

HOUSTON, J. (1830) Observations on the mucous membrane of the rectum. *Dublin Hosp. Rep.*, *5*, 158.

HOWARD, E. R. and NIXON, H. H. (1968) Internal anal sphincter observations on development and mechanism of inhibitory responses in premature infants and children with Hirschsprung's disease. *Archs Dis. Childh.*, *43*, 569.

HURST, A. F. (1909) *Constipation and Allied Disorders*. London: Henry Frowde.

—— (1911) *The Sensibility of the Alimentary Canal. Goulstonian Lectures*. London and Oxford: Frowde.

IHRE, T. (1974) Studies on anal function in continent and incontinent patients. *Scand. J. Gastroenterol.*, *9*, Suppl. 25.

INBERG, K. R. (1952) Contractile power and resting tone of the anal sphincter during intravenous tetraethylammonium chloride block. *Acta chir. scand.*, *104*, 302.

JAGENBURG, R., DOTEVALL, G., KEWENTER, J., KOCK, N. G. and PHILIPSON, B. (1971) Absorption studies in patients with intra-abdominal ileostomy reservoirs and in patients with conventional ileostomies. *Gut*, *12*, 437.

JAMIESON, J. K. and DOBSON, J. F. (1909) The lymphatics of the colon. *Proc. R. Soc. Med.*, *2*, 149.

JOHANSSON, H. and NYLANDER, G. (1969) Ileo-colic transit in rats subjected to ileo-caecal resection. *Acta chir. scand.*, *135*, 455.

KATZ, L. A., KAUFMANN, H. J. and SPIRO, H. M. (1967) Anal sphincter pressure characteristics. *Gastroenterology*, *52*, 513.

KAWAKAMI, M. (1954) Electromyographic investigation on the human external sphincter muscle of anus. *Jap. J. Physiol.*, *4*, 196.

KERREMANS, R. (1968) Electrical activity and motility of the internal anal sphincter: an *in vivo* electrophysiological study in man. *Acta gastro-ent. belg.*, *31*, 465.

KRATZER, G. L. and DOCKERTY, M. B. (1947) Histopathology of anal ducts. *Surgery Gynec. Obstet.*, *84*, 333.

KREMEN, A. J., LINNER, J. H. and NELSON, C. H. (1954) An experimental evaluation of the nutritional importance of proximal and distal small intestine. *Ann. Surg.*, *140*, 439.

LANE, R. H. S. and PARKS, A. G. (1977) Function of the anal sphincters following colo-anal anastomosis. *Br. J. Surg.*, *64*, 596.

LEARMONTH, J. R. (1931) A contribution to the neurophysiology of the urinary bladder in man. *Brain*, *54*, 147.

LENNANDER, K. G. (1901) Über die Sensibilität der Bauchhöhle und über lokale und allgemeine Anästhesie bei Bruch- und Bauchoperationen. *Zentbl. Chir.*, *28*, 209.

LEVITAN, R., FORDTRAN, J. S., BURROWS, B. A. and INGELFINGER, F. J. (1962) Water and salt absorption in the human colon. *J. clin. Invest.*, *41*, 1754.

LEWIS, T. and KELLGREN, J. H. (1939) Observations relating to referred pain, viscero-motor reflexes and other associated phenomena. *Clin. Sci.*, *4*, 47.

LIEBERMAN, W. (1964) Objective measurement of external anal sphincter tension. *Am. J. Proctol.*, *15*, 375.

LILLEHEI, R. C. and WANGENSTEEN, O. H. (1955) Bowel function after colectomy for cancer, polyps, and diverticulitis. *J. Am. med. Ass.*, *159*, 163.

LOCKHART-MUMMERY, J. P. (1929) Discussion on fistula-in-ano. *Proc. R. Soc. Med.*, *22*, 1331.

MANASSE, P. (1907) Die arterielle Gefässversorgung des S romanum in ihrer Bedeutung für die operative Verlagerung desselben; Mittheilung über eine Anastomose bei Mastdarmstenosen (Sigmoideo-rectostomia externa). *Arch. klin. Chir.*, *83*, 999.

MARTIN, E. and BURDEN, V. G. (1927) The surgical significance of the rectosigmoid sphincter. *Ann. Surg.*, *86*, 86.

MAYO, W. J. (1917) Surgery of the rectosigmoid. *Surgery Gynec. Obstet.*, *25*, 616.

MEKHJIAN, H. S., PHILLIPS, S. F. and HOFMANN, A. F. (1971) Colonic secretion of water and electrolytes induced by bile acids: Perfusion studies in man. *J. clin. Invest.*, *50*, 1569.

MILES, W. E. (1919) Observations upon internal piles. *Surgery Gynec. Obstet.*, *29*, 497.

—— (1939) *Rectal Surgery*, p. 133, Fig. 48. London: Cassell.

MILLIGAN, E. T. C. (1942) The surgical anatomy and disorders of the perianal space. *Proc. R. Soc. Med.*, *36*, 365.

—— and MORGAN, C. N. (1934) Surgical anatomy of the anal canal, with special reference to anorectal fistulae. *Lancet*, *2*, 1150, 1213.

—— —— JONES, L. E. and OFFICER, R. (1937) Surgical anatomy of the anal canal, and the operative treatment of haemorrhoids. *Lancet*, *2*, 1119.

MORGAN, C. N. (1936) The surgical anatomy of the anal canal and rectum. *Postgrad. med. J.*, *12*, 287.

—— (1949) The surgical anatomy of the ischiorectal space. *Proc. R. Soc. Med.*, *42*, 189.

—— (1956) Quoted by Griffiths.

—— and LLOYD-DAVIES, O. V. (1956) In *Modern Operative Surgery*, ed. G. Grey Turner and Lambert Charles Rogers, 4th ed., p. 1307. London: Cassell.

—— and THOMPSON, H. R. (1956) Surgical anatomy of the anal canal, with special reference to the surgical importance of the internal sphincter and conjoint longitudinal muscle. *Ann. R. Coll. Surg. Engl.*, *19*, 88.

O'BEIRNE, J. (1833) *New Views of the Process of Defaecation and their Application to the Pathology and Treatment of Diseases of the Stomach, Bowels and Other Organs*. Dublin: Hodges and Smith.

OH, C. and KARK, A. E. (1972) Anatomy of the external anal sphincter. *Br. J. Surg.*, *59*, 717.

PAINTER, N. S. and TRUELOVE, S. C. (1964) The intraluminal pressure patterns in diverticulosis of the colon. *Gut*, *5*, 201.

PARKS, A. G. (1955) The surgical treatment of haemorrhoids. *Br. J. Surg.*, *43*, 337.

—— (1961) Pathogenesis and treatment of fistula-in-ano. *Br. med. J.*, *1*, 463.

—— PORTER, N. H. and MELZAK, J. (1962) Experimental study of the reflex mechanism controlling the muscles of the pelvic floor. *Dis. Colon Rect.*, *5*, 407.

—— SWASH, M. and URICH, H. (1977) Sphincter denervation in anorectal incontinence and rectal prolapse. *Gut*, *18*, 656.

PHILLIPS, S. F. and EDWARDS, D. A. W. (1965) Some aspects of anal continence and defaecation. *Gut*, *6*, 396.

POIRIER, P. and CHARPY, A. (1901) *Traité d'Anatomie Humaine*, vol. IV, p. 372. Paris: Masson.

—— CUNEO, B. and DELAMERE, G. (1903) *The Lymphatics*. London: Constable.

POPE, C. E. and JUDD, E. S. (1929) Arterial blood supply of the sigmoid, rectosigmoid and rectum. *Surg. Clins N. Am.*, *9*, 957.

PORTER, N. H. (1962) A physiological study of the pelvic floor in rectal prolapse. *Ann. R. Coll. Surg. Engl.*, *31*, 379.

RANKIN, F. W., BARGEN, J. A. and BUIE, L. A. (1932) *The Colon, Rectum and Anus*. Philadelphia: W. B. Saunders.

RAY, B. S. and NEILL, C. L. (1947) Abdominal visceral sensation in man. *Ann. Surg.*, *126*, 709.

RITCHIE, J. A. (1971) Movements of segmental constrictions in the human colon. *Gut*, *12*, 350.

—— ARDRAN, G. M. and TRUELOVE, S. C. (1962) Motor activity of the sigmoid colon of humans. A combined study by intraluminal pressure recording and cineradiography. *Gastroenterology*, *43*, 642.

—— TRUELOVE, S. C., ARDRAN, G. M. and TUCKEY, M. S. (1971) Propulsion and retropulsion of normal colonic contents. *Am. J. dig. Dis.*, *16*, 697.

ROTHENBERG, S. P., WEISBERG, H. and FICARRA, A. (1972) Evidence for the absorption of immunoreactive intrinsic factor into the intestinal epithelial cell during vitamin B12 absorption. *J. Lab. clin. Med.*, *79*, 587.

RUBESCH, R. (1910) Uber die Vermeidung der Darmgangrän bei Rektumoperationen. *Beitr. klin. Chir.*, *67*, 480.

RUDDELL, W. S. J., BLENDIS, L. M. and LOVELL, D. (1977) Rectal potential difference and histology in Crohn's disease. *Gut*, *18*, 284.

SAUER, I. and BACON, H. E. (1952) A new approach for excision of carcinoma of the lower portion of the rectum and anal canal. *Surgery Gynec. Obstet.*, *95*, 229.

SCHÄRLI, A. F. and KIESEWETTER, W. B. (1969) Imperforate anus: anorectosigmoid pressure studies as a quantitative evaluation of post-operative continence. *J. pediat. Surg., 4*, 694.

SCHUSTER, M. M., HENDRIX, T. R. and MENDELOFF, A. I. (1963) The internal anal sphincter response: manometric studies on its normal physiology, neural pathways, and alteration in bowel disorders. *J. clin. Invest., 42*, 196.

SHAFIK, A. (1975) A new concept of the anatomy of the anal sphincter mechanism and the physiology of defaecation. *Investigative Urology, 12*, 412.

—— (1976a) The longitudinal anal muscle: anatomy and role in anal sphincter mechanism. *Investigative Urology, 13*, 271.

—— (1976b) Anatomy of the perianal spaces. *Investigative Urology, 13*, 414.

SHIELDS, R. (1966) Absorption and secretion of water and electrolytes by the human colon with special reference to benign adenoma and papilloma. *Br. J. Surg., 53*, 893.

SMIDDY, F. G. and GOLIGHER, J. C. (1957) Unpublished data.

—— GREGORY, S. D., SMITH, I. B. and GOLIGHER, J. G. (1960) Faecal losses of fluid, electrolytes, and nitrogen in colitis before and after ileostomy. *Lancet, 1*, 14.

SMITH, A. N., GIANNAKOS, V. and CLARKE, S. (1971) Late results of colomyotomy. *J. R. Coll. Surg. Edinb., 16*, 276.

SMITH, B. and BUTLER, M. (1974) The autonomic control of colonic mucin secretion in the mouse. *Br. J. exp. Path., 55*, 615.

STEWARD, J. A. and RANKIN, F. W. (1933) Blood supply of the large intestine. *Archs Surg., Chicago, 26*, 843.

STROUD, B. B. (1896) On the anatomy of the anus. *Ann. Surg., 24*, 1.

SUDECK, P. (1907) Über die Gefässversorgung des Mastdarmes in Hinsicht auf die operative Gangrän. *Münch. med. Wschr., 54*, 1314.

SUNDERLAND, S. (1942) Blood supply of the distal colon. *Aust. N.Z. J. Surg., 11*, 253.

SWENSON, O. and BELL, A. H., Jr. (1948) Resection of rectum and rectosigmoid with preservation of the sphincter for benign spastic lesions producing megacolon. *Surgery, St Louis, 24*, 212.

TAGART, R. E. B. (1966) The anal canal and rectum: their varying relationship and its effect on anal continence. *Dis. Colon Rect., 9*, 449.

TAVERNER, D. and SMIDDY, F. G. (1959) An electromyographic study of the normal function of the external anal sphincter and pelvic diaphragm. *Dis. Colon Rect., 2*, 153.

TAYLOR, I. and DUTHIE, H. L. (1976) Bran tablets and diverticular disease. *Br. med. J., 1*, 988.

TELFORD, E. D. and STOPFORD, J. S. B. (1934) Autonomic nerve supply of the distal colon; anatomical and clinical study. *Br. med. J., 1*, 572.

THOMPSON, P. (1899) *The Myology of the Pelvic Floor.* Newton, McCorquodale and Co.

TRUELOVE, S. C. (1956) Treatment of ulcerative colitis with local hydrocortisone. *Br. med. J., 2*, 1267.

TURNBERG, L. A. (1970) Electrolyte absorption from the colon. *Gut, 11*, 1049.

USTACH, T. J., TOBON, F., HAMBRECHT, T., BASS, D. D. and SCHUSTER, M. M. (1970) Electrophysiological aspects of human sphincters in function. *J. clin. Invest., 49*, 41.

VILLEMIN, F., HUARD, P. and MONTAGNÉ, M. (1925) Recherches anatomiques sur les lymphatiques du rectum et de l'anus. Leurs applications dans le traitement chirurgical du cancer. *Revue Chir., 63*, 39.

WALDEYER, W. (1899) Quoted by Thompson.

WALLS, E. W. (1958) Observations on the microscopic anatomy of the human anal canal. *Br. J. Surg., 45*, 504.

WANKLING, W. J., BROWN, B. H., COLLINS, C. D. and DUTHIE, H. L. (1968) Basal electrical activity in the anal canal in man. *Gut, 9*, 457.

WATERFALL, W. E., BROWN, B., WHITTAKER, G. and DUTHIE, H. L. (1971) Gastrointestinal hormones and electrical activity in the terminal ileum. *Br. J. Surg., 58*, 868.

WATSON, P. C. (1951) Discussion on urological complications of excision of the rectum. *Proc. R. Soc. Med., 44*, 820.

WEINBECK, M., CHRISTENSEN, J. and WEISBRODT, N. W. (1972) Differential effects of morphine and cholinergic agents on the electrical activity of the colon of the unanaesthetised cat. *Biol. Gastroentérol. 5*, 31C.

WEEMS, W. A. and SZURSZEWSKI, J. (1977) Modulation of colonic motility by peripheral neural inputs to neurons of the inferior mesenteric ganglion. *Gastroenterology, 73*, 273.

WESTHUES, H. (1934) *Die Pathologisch-anatomischen Grundlagen der Chirurgie des Rektumkarzinoms.* Leipzig: Thieme.

WOOLLARD, H. and NORRISH, R. E. (1933) The anatomy of the peripheral sympathetic nervous system. *Br. J. Surg., 21*, 83.

YANCHEV, V. G. (1963) Anal tonometry. *Fedn Proc. Fedn Am. Socs exp. Biol.*, Suppl. *22*, 110.

2

Diagnosis of Diseases of the Anus, Rectum and Colon

The diagnosis of diseases of the rectum and colon depends on a careful assessment of the information derived from one or more of the following sources:

1. A well-taken medical history.
2. A complete rectal examination, including sigmoidoscopy.
3. Abdominal and general clinical examination.
4. Radiological investigations, including plain radiographs of the abdomen or chest, and X-ray examination after a barium enema or barium progress meal.
5. Colonoscopy.
6. Rarely certain other investigations.

The extent to which these different sources are used naturally varies from patient to patient. Thus with some complaints the diagnosis is virtually evident from a consideration of the history alone or on very simple physical examination. In other cases a diagnosis may only be reached after enlisting the aid of all the available means of investigation. Rarely even after utilizing all these methods, it may be found impossible to come to a firm conclusion. Under these circumstances, re-examination when symptoms are maximal or after an interval of two or three months may sometimes prove helpful; or, very occasionally now that colonoscopy is available, an exploratory laparotomy may be required.

THE HISTORY

In his book *Diseases of the Rectum and Colon* the late Mr J. P. Lockhart-Mummery (1934), who did so much to advance rectal surgery, stated that in the diagnosis of rectal diseases the history was of little significance, and everything depended on the physical examination. This arresting remark was of course an overstatement—as it was doubtless intended to be—but it does contain a solid kernel of truth. One of the reasons why the physical findings tend to dwarf the symptomatology in the assessment of rectal complaints is the great accuracy of our methods of examination in this region. As a rule lesions of the anus, rectum or distal part of the sigmoid colon are accessible to direct approach, either with the finger or by endoscopy, and this allows a very precise and reliable appreciation of their nature, quite apart from any consideration of symptoms. With lesions in the colon beyond the reach of the sigmoidoscope, however, the physical diagnosis depends in large measure on radiological examination after a barium enema, and though this generally provides accurate information from which a tentative diagnosis can be inferred, a consideration of the patient's history often plays an important part in interpreting the significance of the radiological appearances.

The other reason why physical examination dominates in making a rectal diagnosis is the great difficulty which the average patient experiences in describing rectal complaints with delicacy and precision. To clarify his initial complaint of, say, 'piles', bleeding or a swelling may call for a great deal of questioning. To avoid much time-consuming and confusing circumlocution, particularly in a busy out-patient clinic, it is advisable to break one of the first rules of medical history-taking, and to ask the patient quite deliberately a series of leading questions about specific symptoms and their duration, as follows:

Bleeding: at defaecation or apart from it; some idea of how much (a mere streak on the motions or a considerable drip).

Prolapse: at defaecation only, or at other times as well; whether it reduces itself spontaneously or has to be replaced digitally; roughly how far it projects.

Swelling: painful or not; whether it has discharged blood or pus.

Pain: at defaecation only or at other times; character (burning, throbbing, stabbing); aggravated by constipation or not.

Discharge (Apart from Defaecation): purulent or serous; continuous or intermittent; roughly how much.

Anal Irritation: by day or night, or both; if nocturnal, whether it interferes seriously with sleep; associated with discharge or not.

Bowel Habits: normal with or without aperients (if the former, whether the dose has had to be increased recently); constipation, diarrhoea. If diarrhoea, frequency and character of motions by day and night and whether containing blood or slime.

Continence: in relevant cases, whether able to appreciate and control faeces and flatus.

Abdominal Pain and Other Symptoms: in relevant cases, a detailed interrogation about the characteristics of any abdominal complaint such as pain, vomiting, loss of appetite, flatulence.

Loss of Weight: how much and over what period.

General Health: any loss of energy or failure of general health.

Previous Illnesses: with particular reference to abdominal and rectal complaints, dysentery or diarrhoea, residence in tropical or subtropical countries.

Previous Operations: particularly abdominal, rectal and gynaecological or obstetrical operations.

RECTAL EXAMINATION

No elaborate equipment is necessary for rectal examination. A very few simple instruments and other items suffice, but it is essential that the surgeon should be thoroughly familiar with their use. The following is a description of the equipment that I personally employ and recommend for rectal work.

Examination Couch

In ordinary general clinical work it is often necessary to perform at least a partial examination of the rectum with the patient in his bed. But this is most inconvenient for endoscopic examination, mainly because the bed is too low and the patient's buttock tends to sink into the soft mattress. For a full rectal examination the patient should ideally be on a proper examination couch with a firm padded top (see Fig. 49). Many such couches are not sufficiently high for rectal work; the top should be at least 80 cm from the ground otherwise the surgeon will have to stoop unduly and this may prove exhausting during the course of a long clinic. I have no personal experience of the special examination tables used by certain American surgeons such as Buie (1932) of the Mayo Clinic. A good example of the latter is the Ritter table, which is electrically operated to give a head-down tilt whilst the patient kneels on it. This is certainly much more comfortable for the patient than the ordinary knee–shoulder position on a flat fixed couch, and is very satisfactory for the surgeon; but it is a costly piece of equipment.

Lighting

A good light is absolutely essential for efficient rectal examination, both for preliminary inspection of the anal region and possibly also for directing illumination down the proctoscope. For this purpose the Anglepoise (or a similar type) examination lamp, mounted on a special stand on wheels, is excellent (Fig. 34). Due to the flexibility of its arm this lamp can be made to assume an infinite variety of different positions and to shine light in whatever direction is required. The bulb should be of at least 100 watts; the best type is one with a reflector mechanism, such as the Phillips reflector flood-lamp, which concentrates the light on the area to be examined.

them on the hands between cases so that the same pair is used throughout the entire clinic.

Lubricant

Soft paraffin is often used for this purpose but is not really satisfactory because of the difficulty in removing it from instruments and gloves. A water-soluble lubricant of the type used for lubricating catheters, but of rather firmer consistency, is much more convenient from this point of view. For clinic use it should be supplied in large wide-necked jars into which the finger or instruments can be easily dipped, though for an isolated rectal examination it may be more convenient to have it in an ordinary collapsible metal tube. A suitable prescription for a water-soluble lubricant is as follows:

Pulv. Tragacanth	21 ml
Glycerine	125 ml
Solution Hydrarg. Perchlor. 1/200	568 ml

Wool and Gauze

For swabbing out the lumen of the bowel during proctoscopy or sigmoidoscopy small pledgets of dry cotton wool, previously prepared by being rolled into small balls, serve admirably. For swabbing or holding the perianal skin medium-sized squares of gauze are best, but ordinary toilet paper is a good cheap substitute.

Proctoscope and Long Non-Toothed Dissecting Forceps

Tubular Proctoscope. Many different patterns of tubular proctoscope exist, all derived from the original Kelly type of instrument. The variations affect the length, calibre and shape (whether cylindrical or slightly conical) of the tube, the setting of the terminal opening (whether transverse or oblique), the possession of side slits, grooves, or sliding attachments, and the method of illumination. The larger the bore of the instrument that can be passed, the better will be the view obtained, and so for ordinary purposes it is best to have a fairly large proctoscope. My preference is for the Śt Mark's Hospital pattern which is illustrated in Fig. 35. Its tubular part is 7 cm long and has a diameter of 22 mm at the tip and 32 mm at the base, the slight widening towards the base being useful in facilitating the withdrawal of the obturator and the

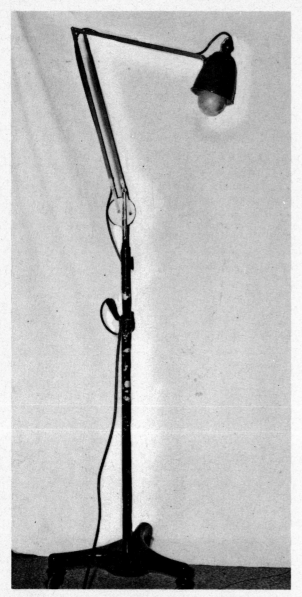

Fig. 34. Anglepoise lamp mounted on stand with wheels.

Gloves and Finger Cots

For occasional rectal examination rubber finger cots were once popular, but they have been completely replaced by rubber or plastic gloves in recent years, the plastic version being specially favoured. In using plastic gloves a pattern such as those made by Travenol, which fits closely on the hand, is preferable to more loosely fitting ones. *For work in the outpatient clinic* a convenient plan is for the surgeon (and nurses!) to wear a pair of ordinary rubber surgical gloves constantly, and to wash and dry

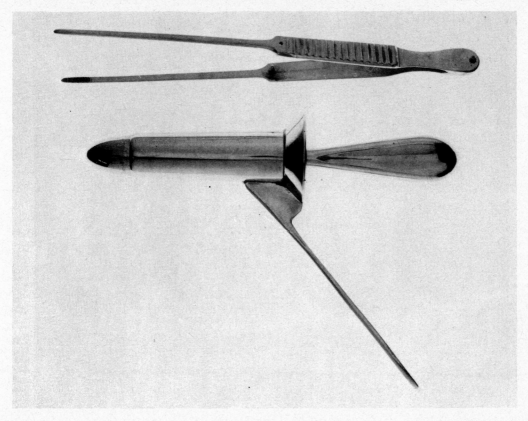

Fig. 35. St Mark's hospital pattern of proctoscope with (*above*) Emmett's 20-cm long non-toothed dissecting forceps.

manipulation of instruments within the lumen. An alternative version is available with a small obliquely placed tunnel in the handle of the instrument through which the terminal of a fibreoptic system can be passed. In actual practice, however, this is seldom used.

For patients with painful anal lesions or with some degree of anal spasm or stenosis, a narrower instrument is necessary. One possibility is the *Bensaude* proctoscope, which has a tube slightly tapered towards the tip and a minimum diameter of 16 mm; another possibility is to use the narrow Lloyd-Davies sigmoidoscope (Fig. 38) to examine the anal canal as it is withdrawn. The same plan may also be useful for very young children though as a matter of fact the anal canal of the child is remarkably distensible and is generally quite capable of admitting an adult-sized proctoscope (as it is of passing large hard motions!).

Long Non-toothed Dissecting Forceps. It is essential to have available for use with the proctoscope a pair of fairly long non-toothed dissecting forceps for swabbing out the lumen. Emmett's 20-cm forceps (Fig. 35), which were originally devised for gynaecological surgery, are absolutely ideal for proctoscopic work, and I regard them as well-nigh indispensible.

Nasal Punch Forceps. Occasionally it is necessary to take biopsies of low-lying rectal carcinomata seen through the proctoscope. For this purpose Hartmann's conchotome is very useful (Fig. 36).

Bivalve Speculum. For certain purposes a bivalve speculum is preferable to a tubular proctoscope—for example for inspecting anal crypts or removing hypertrophied anal papillae, and for carrying out internal sphincterotomy. My own speculum of this kind is illustrated in Fig. 37. It has the advantage of possessing a third blade for retracting the side of the anal canal opposite to that being examined. A version of this retractor capable of a wider separation of blades is available for transanal operations to remove benign rectal tumours or complete coloanal anastomoses. Another very popular pattern of bivalve speculum is that of Parks.

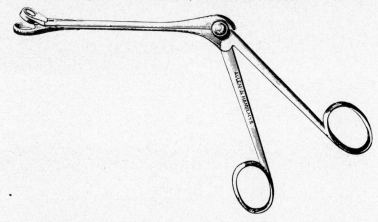

Fig. 36. Conchotome, useful for taking a biopsy of a low rectal growth.

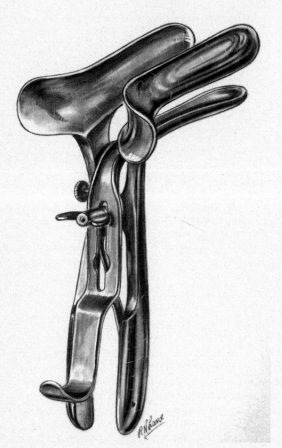

Fig. 37. Bivalve anal speculum with attachable third blade.

Sigmoidoscope

STANDARD METAL TUBULAR SIGMOIDOSCOPES

These can be divided into two main groups according to whether the lighting is situated distally or proximally. The classical example of *a sigmoidoscope with distal illumination* was the original Strauss pattern, the light being carried on the distal end of a long wire attachment which projected inside the tube. Unfortunately if liquid faeces or discharge were present in the bowel, the light quickly became submerged and had to be withdrawn for cleansing. This constituted a serious objection to this otherwise excellent type of instrument and led to its being largely supplanted by *sigmoidoscopes with proximal illumination*. An excellent pattern of sigmoidoscope of this latter type is that designed by O. V. Lloyd-Davies, which has fibreoptic illumination to its proximal end (Fig. 38). It has the merit of great simplicity and reliability. It is made in two sizes of different length and calibre, the tube in the larger size having an effective length of 30 cm and a bore of 19 mm, the dimensions of the smaller one being 25 cm and 13 mm respectively. For all ordinary purposes the narrower model is perfectly adequate and is undoubtedly more comfortable for the patient than the larger one. Its only slight defect is that sometimes it is difficult in the restricted lumen to see clearly when taking a biopsy, and often biopsy has to be carried out blindly, but with correct preliminary siting of the end of the tube against the tumour this really presents no difficulty. A magnifying lens is available for attachment to the proximal end of the instrument for examining the mucosa in greater detail. Recently there has become available a sigmoidoscope with distal illumination secured by the incorporation of fibre-optic fibres in the wall of the tube to convey light from a powerful bulb at the head end. This pattern, made by Welch–Allyn, can be obtained in two sizes (Fig. 39) corresponding to the two models of the Lloyd-Davis sigmoidoscope. (A third larger model is also available for operative sigmoidoscopy and

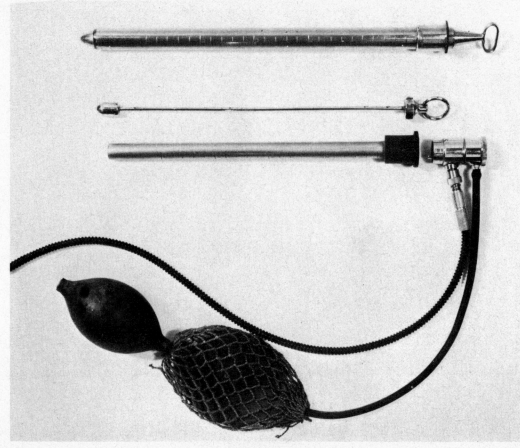

Fig. 38. Lloyd-Davies pattern of sigmoidoscope with proximal fibreoptic illumination. The tube is made in two sizes; the same eye piece fits both.

snaring of polyps, see Fig. 251.) The window at the proximal end of the Welch–Allyn sigmoidoscope magnifies two times. The tube and obturator of the narrower sizes of the Welch–Allyn sigmoidoscope are also available in disposable plastic instead of metal, but I do not find these plastic versions as comfortable for the patient.

Long Alligator Forceps for Holding Swabs. Forceps of this pattern, 35 cm or so long, with small serrated blades for gripping pledgets of wool to swab out the lumen of the bowel, are an integral part of the equipment for sigmoidoscopy, and it is seldom that they are not required at some stage of the proceedings (see Fig. 40). A very convenient alternative for this purpose is cotton-wool buds on long sticks—'scopets' (Fuller Pharmaceutical Co., Minn., U.S.A.).

Long Suction Tube. When the faeces are very liquid and profuse as in cases of severe ulcerative colitis a thin suction tube is a useful alternative to repeated swabbing to empty the lumen and afford a clear view of the mucosa. I use a tube similar to that employed in bronchoscopy and oesophagoscopy; it is connected to a mobile suction motor.

Long Alligator Forceps for Biopsy. 35-cm long alligator forceps with sharp cupped blades for taking biopsies of tumours or other lesions should also be available during sigmoidoscopy. A very good pattern is that devised by Lloyd-Davies which has very strong blades capable of taking a good bite of tissue (see Fig. 41).

Probes and Directors

For examining fistulae it is necessary to have probe-pointed directors, both rigid and malleable, and a selection of malleable probes including some fine lacrimal-duct probes (Fig. 42).

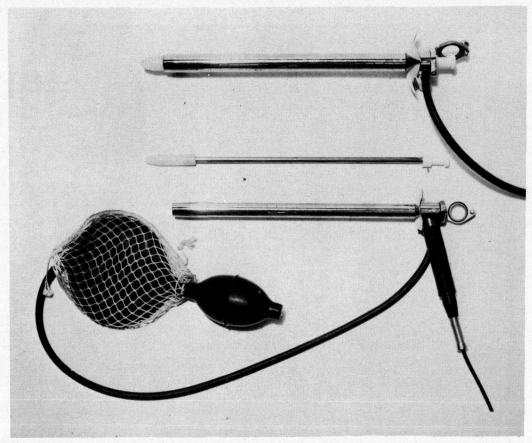

Fig. 39. The Welch–Allyn sigmoidoscope which has a light bulb at the proximal end and contains fibre-optic fibres in the wall of the shaft to convey illumination to the distal end. Two sizes are shown corresponding roughly to the two versions of the Lloyd-Davies instrument (Fig. 38).

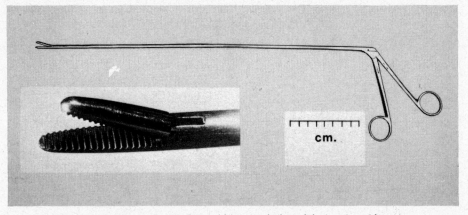

Fig. 40. Long alligator forceps for swabbing out the bowel during sigmoidoscopy.

Miscellaneous Other Instruments

Several other instruments may be required in the out-patient rectal clinic depending on the extent to which minor operations are undertaken. Thus a scalpel may be necessary for opening abscesses, and toothed dissecting forceps and fine, blunt-ended strabismus scissors, curved on the flat, for excision

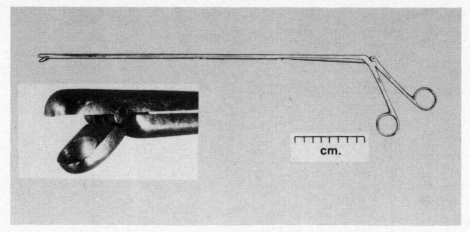

Fig. 41. Lloyd-Davies biopsy forceps for use during sigmoidoscopy.

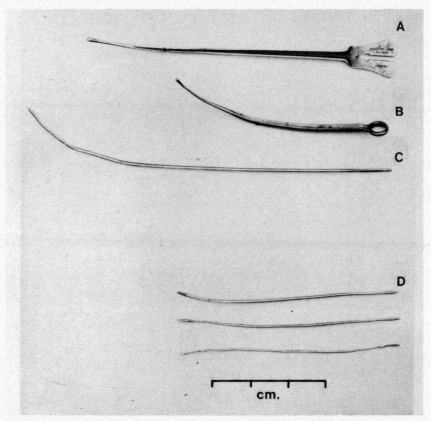

Fig. 42. Selection of probes and probe directors used in the diagnosis and treatment of rectal conditions: (A) St Mark's Hospital pattern of probe-pointed director. (B) Allingham's smaller probe-pointed director. (C) Malleable silver probe of medium size. (D) Fine lacrimal-duct probes.

of anal haematomata or skin tags; fine artery forceps and silk or catgut for ligating bleeding points may also be needed. Suitable syringes and needles will also be required for injection of local anaesthetic solutions for these operations. Special syringes and needles for injections of haemorrhoids which are in constant use in a rectal clinic will be described in detail in the section dealing

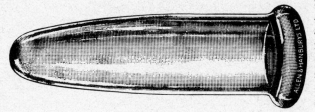

Fig. 43. St Mark's Hospital pattern of anal dilator; it is made in metal, glass or plastic material.

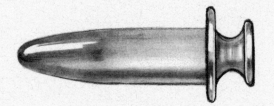

Fig. 44. Thorlakson's modification of the St Mark's Hospital pattern of anal dilator. It is made in light plastic material in three sizes, of which the version illustrated is the medium.

with this condition. For treating an anal stenosis or preventing its development after anal operations such as haemorrhoidectomy or the laying open of an anal fistula, an anal dilator such as the St Mark's Hospital pattern is very useful (Fig. 43). A more convenient version of this instrument was recently designed by R. H. Thorlakson (Fig. 44); it has a distal knob for holding it. For dilating strictures of the rectum proper the most useful instrument is the double-ended Hegar dilator in its largest sizes, from say $\frac{14}{11}$ to $\frac{26}{23}$ (Fig. 45).

Dressing Trolley, Bowls, Dishes and Bucket

Some form of table is necessary on which to place the surgeon's instruments and materials. An ordinary dressing trolley about 80 × 65 × 45 cm answers this purpose admirably, the underneath shelf and cupboards being useful for storing equip-

ment and dressings in the intervals between clinics. A certain number of bowls and kidney dishes are also required and there should be a bucket for receiving dirty swabs. The layout of equipment on the trolley in readiness for rectal examination is shown in Fig. 46. Note the use of the long holder suspended from the rail of the trolley to accommodate a sheaf of sigmoidoscopes and long alligator forceps.

TECHNIQUE OF RECTAL AND SIGMOIDOSCOPIC EXAMINATION

Position of the Patient

The *genupectoral position* (note knee–*shoulder* not knee–*elbow*) is preferred by many surgeons and I have used it myself a certain amount in the past (Fig. 47). It is certainly the best position for proctoscopy, for when the obturator of the proctoscope is withdrawn air is sucked into the bowel which becomes ballooned, and an excellent view is thus obtained of the lower rectum. But it is an uncomfortable and rather embarrassing position for patients, particularly for women.

The *left lateral or Sims's position* is the simplest and most satisfactory for all ordinary purposes and is the one I now invariably use in my rectal clinic for both male and female patients. Certain details of the position require attention if optimum conditions are to be obtained for the surgeon (Fig. 48). First of all, the patient's left hip should rest on a small firm sandbag placed immediately adjacent to the surgeon's side of the couch, so that the buttocks, slightly elevated, project beyond that edge. Secondly, his trunk should lie *obliquely* across the couch top so that the head rests on a pillow near the opposite edge. Thirdly, the position of the lower limbs should be so arranged that the hips are flexed

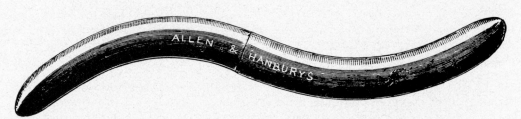

Fig. 45. Hegar's double-ended uterine dilator.

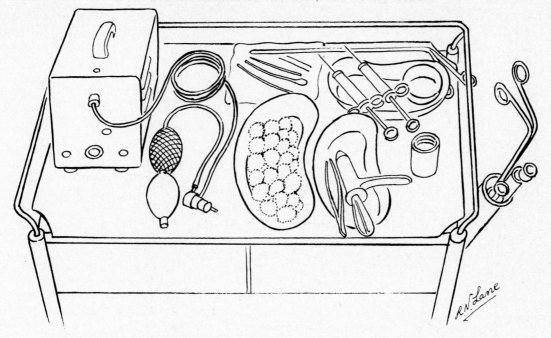

Fig. 46. Layout of equipment on instrument trolley in preparation for rectal examination.

to an angle slightly greater than 90°. The effect is to place that part of the legs between the knees and ankles parallel and close to the opposite side of the couch. Finally, the right shoulder and buttock should be displaced a trifle forwards, giving the patient a slightly prone inclination with his face directed partly into the pillow; spectacles should therefore be removed to avoid damage. It is important that this inclination of the body should be maintained throughout the examination, for there is a natural tendency for the patient to rotate his right shoulder backwards and turn his face upwards to see what is happening or to talk to the surgeon.

Position of the Light, Instrument Trolley and Surgeon

The most convenient position for the Anglepoise light is at the foot end of the examination couch, accurately in the midline. In this position it does not impede the surgeon's access to the instrument trolley which is placed immediately behind the light, symmetrically arranged in relation to the couch. The arm of the lamp is sufficiently long to extend to any position close to the anus that may be desired (Fig. 49).

The surgeon then takes up his position close to the patient's buttocks and facing slightly towards

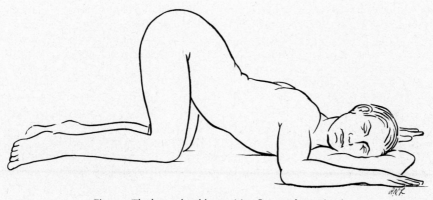

Fig. 47. The knee–shoulder position for rectal examination.

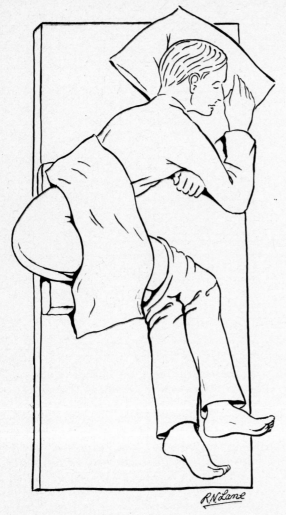

Fig. 48. The Sims's position adapted for rectal examination including sigmoidoscopy. Note that the left hip rests on a small sandbag, the buttocks project slightly beyond the edge of the table, the trunk crosses the top of the table obliquely, and the knees and legs lie along the opposite side.

the feet. With his left hand he can retract the right buttock upwards to expose the anus thoroughly for examination and hold the proctoscope or sigmoidoscope when it is in position; whilst the right hand is able to adjust the light, stretch to the trolley for equipment, or carry out digital examination or instrumentation as required.

Conduct of the Examination

It is important never to forget that rectal examination is a distinctly embarrassing experience for the patient. Allied to this discomfiture is the natural apprehension for the future which any patient who has recently noticed alarming symptoms, such as the passage of blood, is liable to feel. If, in addition, one of his symptoms has been pain in the anal region he is, needless to say, frightened lest he should be hurt by the examination, particularly if he has already suffered in this respect at the less experienced hands of his general practitioner or another surgeon.

The effect of all this is to produce a rather tense, apprehensive patient and, though he may succeed in concealing his anxieties completely, his feeling of tension is apt to reveal itself in a tight spastic condition of his anal sphincters and buttock muscles. This does not make for easy examination, and if the surgeon proceeds regardless of it and in the process does hurt the patient, his spasm increases, which in turn magnifies the surgeon's difficulties. Thus a vicious circle is quickly established, making the examination an extremely unpleasant performance for both patient and surgeon and probably preventing it from achieving its object.

The surgeon's first duty therefore is to allay any anxiety, evident or concealed, and to encourage the patient to relax his musculature and keep it relaxed throughout the examination. A *sympathetic yet confident manner* during the taking of the history is an important first step towards this end. Secondly the surgeon must exercise the *utmost gentleness* at every stage of his examination from the moment he first lays a hand on one buttock till the final withdrawal of the sigmoidoscope. If he finds that the sphincter tightens as he attempts to pass his finger or an instrument, he must not proceed at the ordinary tempo but must delay till the muscle relaxes, meanwhile maintaining a constant gentle pressure and exhorting the patient to remain 'quite loose'. Eventually after a minute or two the spasm yields and the instrument or finger can be passed without discomfort. Any attempt to overcome spasm by undue force not only hurts the patient and increases the tension of his muscles but also results in the loss of his newly won confidence, so that he begins to fear every further move by the surgeon. An essential feature of gentleness in examination is the avoidance of instruments that are badly designed and the *restriction of inflation on sigmoidoscopy to a minimum*.

The third way in which the unpleasantness of a rectal examination can be minimized is by *warning the patient in advance* as the examination proceeds of any sensations or discomforts he may experience. However gentle the examiner may be, a complete

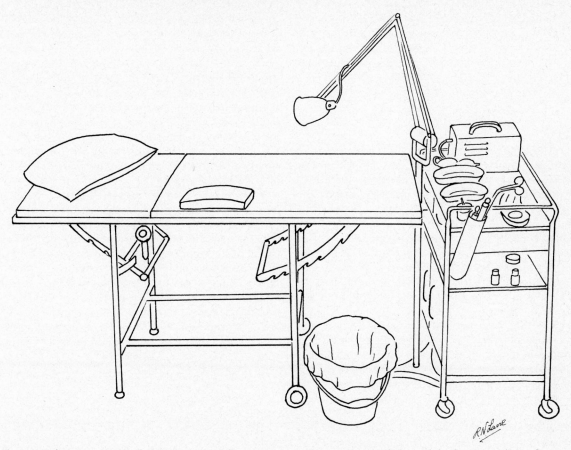

Fig. 49. Relative positions of examination couch, instrument table, Anglepoise light and bucket in readiness for rectal examination.

and thorough examination generally produces some sensations of a physiological nature due to distension or stretching of the bowel wall; these are liable to be interpreted by the patient as the prelude to actual pain, and, in aggravated form, may indeed amount to pain. Thus when the finger is being firmly pressed into the pelvis on digital palpation the patient often feels that his bowels are going to act or he is going to pass wind, and a similar but even more urgent sensation is produced by inflation of the rectum in the earlier stages of sigmoidoscopy. If the patient is assailed suddenly and quite unexpectedly by these sensations his immediate reaction is to assume that he is going to pass flatus or faeces, and to make every effort to save himself from such an embarrassment by contracting his sphincters as strongly as he can. If, however, he is warned in advance that he may have such sensations, but that they are due simply to the pressure of the finger or the instrument, as the case may be,

and that no 'accidents' will occur, he is usually able to maintain his equanimity and the relaxed state of his muscles. Similarly if, as the sigmoidoscope approaches the rectosigmoid junction, he is warned to expect a slight 'windy' sensation in the abdomen, he is less alarmed and better able to endure this temporary discomfort. A further advantage of anticipating for the patient any physiological sensations he may experience is that it impresses him with the examiner's complete mastery of his specialty. As he finds the slight discomforts or more unpleasant sensations of the examination accurately forecast in this way his confidence in his surgeon mounts and his anxieties diminish.

By attention to these points it is usually possible to carry out a complete examination. Sometimes due to the presence of a painful lesion such as an anal fissure or prolapsed thrombosed piles the examination has to be restricted, but nearly always it is possible to examine the patient sufficiently to establish a diagnosis and initiate treatment. Occasionally, however, general anaesthesia is required to permit a proper assessment of the condition, and this is also rarely necessary in the case of certain nervous uncooperative patients even without painful lesions.

INSPECTION

This is one of the most neglected parts of the rectal examination in ordinary general clinical work. Internists in their somewhat cursory palpation of the rectum generally manage to avoid seeing the anal region at all and, even in surgical practice, due to indifferent lighting and faulty positioning of the patient on a bed or low couch, inspection is often little more than an ineffectual gesture. The more is the pity for with certain lesions, such as an anal fissure or haematoma, warts, a pilonidal sinus or pruritus ani, the diagnosis rests essentially in simple inspection.

With the layout of lighting and equipment described on p. 57, inspection is carried out under ideal conditions. The surgeon draws the Anglepoise lamp fairly close to the anus and with his left hand gently lifts the uppermost buttock to expose the anus and perianal region to clear view (Fig. 50).

It will be noted at once whether there is any obvious pathological condition such as an anal haematoma, prolapsed internal piles with exposed mucosa, skin tags, the lower edge of a carcinoma, the external opening of an anal fistula, or the localized swelling with reddening of the overlying skin of an abscess. Any more generalized pruritic condition of the perianal skin, with redness and excoriation or with thickening of the normal radiating folds and a white sodden epidermis, will also be observed. The presence of any discharge at the anal orifice or on the perianal skin should be noted, as should the scars of previous operations on the anal region. Faecal soiling of the skin around the anus is an important point to note; it may signify a lack of personal fastidiousness or a defect of normal anal continence.

The state of tone of the anal sphincters can be judged more directly by observing whether the anal orifice is completely closed or patulous in the resting condition and on voluntary contraction, and whether it remains closed when the buttocks are forcibly separated. A tightly contracted anus is highly suggestive of sphincter spasm due to an anal fissure, especially if a dorsal sentinel skin tag is present as well.

To examine the anus itself more thoroughly the fingertips of the two hands should be placed on the

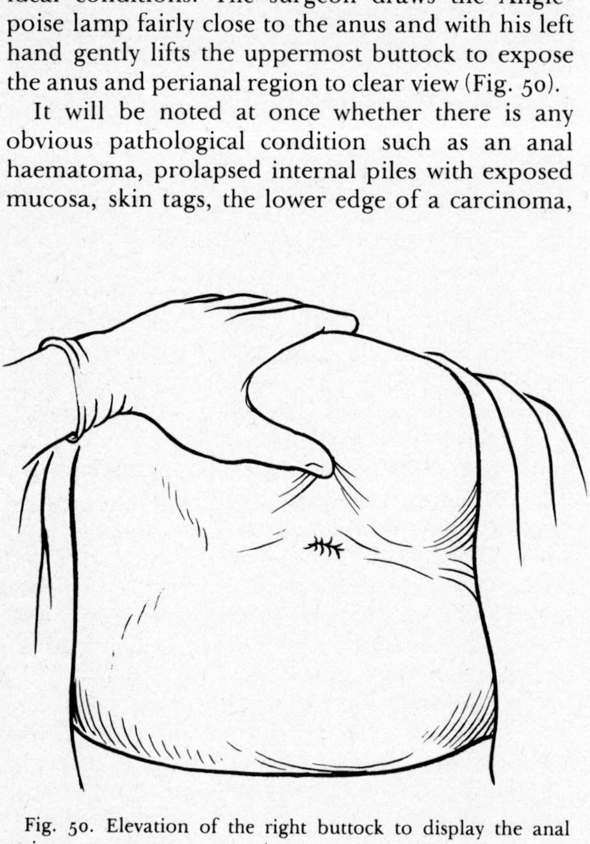

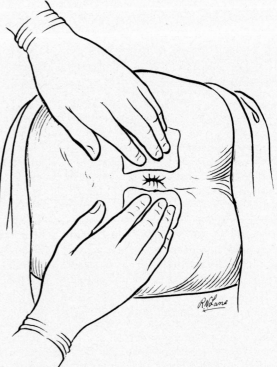

Fig. 50. Elevation of the right buttock to display the anal region.

Fig. 51. Strong retraction of the edges of the anal orifice to allow of a closer inspection as for a fissure-in-ano.

skin over gauze squares close to the anal verge on either side, and the margins of the anus gently but firmly separated (Fig. 51). This manoeuvre generally succeeds in showing at least the lower end of a fissure.

Lastly the postanal region should be examined for evidence of pilonidal sinus.

PALPATION

Of the Perianal Region

In cases with obvious lesions around the anus careful palpation of the perianal region may be informative. This is preferably done with the *unlubricated* finger. Any suspected abscess or haematoma is palpated for tenderness and, if a fistulous opening is present, palpation around it, particularly in the interval between the opening and the anus, may detect induration indicating the course of the fistulous track. It will be noted whether the pressure of the finger causes any discharge to escape from the opening. Similarly scars of previous operations should be palpated to determine if they are soft and supple or whether there are any areas of induration to suggest residual inflammation.

Of the Anal Canal and Rectum

The left buttock is retracted rather firmly upwards to draw redundant skin away from the anus and clearly expose the actual orifice. The tip of the lubricated right index finger is next stroked across the anus once or twice to smear some of the lubricant on to it and the surrounding skin, and then gently inserted into the canal. As already explained on p. 16 certain normal anatomical landmarks can be readily appreciated in most patients.

The anal intersphincteric groove. The lower borders of the external and internal sphincters and the *anal intersphincteric groove* between them can usually be palpated without difficulty. In certain individuals, generally thin middle-aged or elderly women with a prominent 'conical' anus, the muscular tube of the internal sphincter projects actually beyond the lower border of the external sphincter. The intersphincteric groove then lies not in the lowermost part of the anal canal but outside the anal orifice.

The anorectal ring. If the finger is inserted farther into the anus and directed posteriorly it reaches the sharply defined puborectalis sling at the upper end of the anal canal. The position of *the anorectal ring* having thus been located posteriorly and posterolaterally, its level can be determined by comparison on the anterior wall where there is of course no clearly palpable indication of the exact situation of this important junction.

In certain cases, notably those with complete rectal prolapse, the tone of the sphincter muscles and puborectalis sling may be distinctly subnormal. If the patient is asked voluntarily to contract the anus it may be found that the contractile power of these muscles is also much impaired or completely lost. The reverse condition of excessive tonic or fibrous contraction of the internal sphincter is encountered regularly in association with an anal fissure, and occasionally apart from this lesion in patients who have indulged in regular purgation with paraffin or salts for many years. In these cases the lower edge of the tightly contracted internal sphincter is especially prominent and the fingertip can be inserted only with difficulty and pain, if at all. If a fissure is present the maximum tenderness will be elicited when the finger presses directly on it in the lower part of the posterior or anterior wall of the canal. In very chronic cases there may be palpable thickening of the edges of the fissure due to fibrosis. An anal papilla may be felt at the upper end of a fissure; in other cases similar swellings may be palpable anywhere in the circumference of the canal along the line of the anal valves. Certain other lesions may be detected at the same level; thus foreign bodies such as bone, if impacted in the anal canal, tend to lodge in the anal crypts, and can be felt there; and the internal orifices of anal fistulae are often in this situation causing a recognizable opening or induration. But apart from such abnormalities the pectinate line is not clearly distinguishable on palpation. Induration due to anal fistulae may also be felt above the anorectal ring, a striking example being the high posterior horseshoe fistula which produces thickening palpable both above and below the puborectalis sling, which itself often becomes fibrosed, rigid and unduly prominent. An integral part of the palpation of fistulae is the use of the probe and director, which is described on p. 173.

Abscesses, if of ischiorectal type, may cause a considerable, tender bulging of one side of the anal canal, or, if of perianal variety, may produce a more localized swelling in the lower part of the canal and at the anal orifice. If the latter type is very small it is sometimes best appreciated by *bidigital palpation* with the tip of the index finger in the canal and the thumb on the perianal region.

Internal haemorrhoids are not normally palpable, but very long-standing piles associated with much fibrosis may be felt as longitudinal ridges or folds in the wall of the lower rectum and upper part of the anal canal as the finger is swept round the bowel. In cases of thrombosis in the internal haemorrhoidal plexus the firm tender cord of the thrombosed veins can be felt extending from the canal into the lower rectum. The induration following injection treatment may remain palpable just above the anorectal ring for several weeks.

The finger is now passed farther into the rectum proper and a careful palpation made of its contents and walls. It will be noted whether the bowel is completely empty and if so whether it is relatively collapsed or ballooned. More usually some semi-solid faeces are palpable. Cases with faecal impaction are immediately recognized by feeling a large hard mass of faeces distending the lower rectum. The finger is next swept systematically round the bowel to palpate its wall thoroughly for irregularities, excrescences, induration or narrowing. Normally the rectal mucosa is perfectly smooth. In cases of ulcerative colitis the granularity of the mucosa can sometimes be detected by the examining finger; at the same time any rigidity or actual narrowing of the bowel will be appreciated. A sessile adenoma is usually easily recognized if felt, but is so small as a rule that it may be missed if the palpation of the rectal wall has not been thorough. A pedunculated adenoma is usually larger but its mobility may render it elusive, or, if felt, its apparent lack of fixity may lead to it being dismissed as a piece of faeces. Further palpation, however, will demonstrate that it is tethered to the wall of the bowel and that it does not indent on firm pressure with the finger. Villous papillomas are larger than adenomas; they have a characteristic granular feel and, owing to their softness, it may be difficult to define their edges with accuracy on palpation. The feel of a carcinoma with its raised indurated edge is usually quite unmistakable, though the size of growth may vary from a relatively small malignant ulcer or projecting lesion to a massive tumour completely encircling the bowel. The exact position and extent of the growth should be noted in relation to the anorectal ring and to the cervix uteri and prostate; its mobility should also be determined.

The extent to which the finger can be inserted into the rectum depends on the length of the surgeon's finger and on the build of the patient and his willingness to relax his muscles. The average index finger is approximately 10 cm long from tip to metacarpophalangeal joint, but the effective length is to the distal edge of the interdigital web which is about 7·5 cm. In a slim patient who flexes his hips fully and relaxes his muscles well the examiner will probably be able to increase the range of his palpation by forcing the anal sphincters and perineum upwards with the knuckle and web at the base of his finger, so that he can reach about 10 cm from the normal resting position of the anus. This is generally reckoned to be at, or a little above, the anterior peritoneal reflection in the male and about 2·5 cm above the reflection in the female. In a fat patient, however, the protrusion of the obese buttocks impinging against the examiner's hand may considerably reduce the range of his digital examination, especially if in addition the patient fails to relax his muscles completely.

Various manoeuvres have been suggested for increasing the effective reach of the finger during rectal palpation:

1. By carrying out a bimanual examination, the surgeon using his left hand simultaneously to palpate the abdomen in the suprapubic and left iliac region and exert considerable downward pressure on the lower abdominal and pelvic viscera. In this way a tumour which was previously just out of reach of the finger in the rectum may, it is claimed, be depressed sufficiently to be touched by the fingertip.

2. By making the patient stand for examination leaning over the back of a chair or across an examination couch whilst the surgeon kneels to palpate the rectum. During the examination the patient is asked to bear down in the hope that this will cause a lesion to descend somewhat in the pelvis.

3. By examining the patient in the *right* lateral position. Abel (1936) has pointed out that when the patient is lying on the left side the sigmoid colon falls back into the left iliac fossa away from the examining finger. By placing the patient in the *right* lateral position (and of course using the left index finger for examination) the sigmoid drops back on to the finger, and some centimetres of bowel inaccessible to palpation in the left lateral position now become palpable by the finger in the rectum.

Actually the ready availability of sigmoidoscopy in any well-organized rectal clinic renders these efforts to extract the maximum out of simple palpation quite superfluous. A narrow bore sigmoidoscope will give all the information that can be gleaned by vigorous palpation of the upper rectum and causes much less discomfort to the patient.

Palpation of extrarectal structures. The main interest is focused on structures related to the anterior rectal wall. Opposite the lower part of the rectum in men the prostate and seminal vesicles are easily felt. Assessment of enlargement of the former may be important in relation to any operation being planned for lesions of the rectum or colon. In women, the cervix uteri and often the retroverted body of the uterus can be equally easily palpated. Sometimes the prominence of the cervix is such that it is mistaken by the inexperienced practitioner for an anterior rectal carcinoma; I have had several such 'tumours' referred to me with a confident diagnosis by the family doctor. Through the rectal wall in the rectovesical or rectouterine pouch other structures may be palpated, such as a tumour of the upper rectum or pelvic colon, hard faecal masses in that part of the bowel, or a secondary deposit of growth in the pelvic peritoneum as from a carcinoma of the stomach or transverse colon. The diagnostic significance of this 'rectal shelf' of growth was strongly emphasized by Blumer (1909) and it is therefore often known as Blumer's shelf. Buie et al. (1941) have given an interesting account of some of the causes of such deposits in a large series of cases at the Mayo Clinic.

Posteriorly the sacrum and coccyx are easily palpable through the rectal wall. Deformities of the coccyx can often be best appreciated by rectal palpation or by a combined bidigital examination; it may also be important to determine the mobility and amount of pain produced by palpating the coccyx from within the rectum. Presacral tumours such as lipomas or teratomas can be readily detected on palpation if situated low enough in the sacral hollow.

Examination of examining finger on withdrawal. An important step in the conduct of rectal palpation is inspection of the examining finger on final withdrawal. If blood, mucus or pus is observed it clearly suggests the presence of a neoplasm or a colitis.

A vaginal examination is often required to supplement rectal palpation, particularly in cases of carcinoma to determine whether the posterior vaginal wall is implicated, and in cases of suspected rectovaginal fistula.

PROCTOSCOPY

No special preparation is required for proctoscopy. From his preliminary inspection with digital palpation the examiner will have formed a pretty shrewd opinion as to whether the patient is likely to admit an ordinary sized proctoscope without discomfort or whether the smaller Bensaude instrument should be employed.

The proctoscope is smeared with lubricant and held in the right hand with the obturator thrust well home. The uppermost buttock is then raised with the left hand to display the anal orifice more clearly, and, with the handle directed backwards towards the sacrum, the point of the instrument is engaged in the anal orifice (Fig. 52/1, 2). At first it is gripped by the anal sphincters, but if gentle pressure is maintained in the long axis of the canal, which runs *from the anus towards the umbilicus*, the muscles gradually relax. In most instances this takes place in a few seconds, in other cases it may require 30–60 seconds or longer. Once relaxation occurs insertion of the instrument is rapid and its point quickly arrives at the upper end of the anal canal. When this level is adjudged to have been reached, the axis of introduction is altered to direct the instrument more backwards into the hollow of the sacrum and avoid injurious and uncomfortable pressure on the anterior rectal wall and prostate. In this new axis the proctoscope is passed to its full length, till in fact the outer flange impinges firmly against the anal verge. The surgeon now takes the handle of the instrument in his left hand, the fingertips of which can be rested on the skin of the sacral region and buttock to steady them, whilst the obturator is removed with his right (Fig. 52/3). Lastly the Anglepoise lamp is adjusted so as to shine the light into the lumen, and Emmett's forceps are taken up in the right hand ready for any swabbing that may be necessary.

It is important to note whether the end of the obturator after removal was soiled with faeces, blood or pus. A trace of blood may be due to slight trauma to the mucosa of the anterior rectal wall during introduction, but any heavy coating of blood is highly suggestive of an inflammation of the mucosa due to a proctocolitis, as a result of which it is thickened and friable and bleeds readily on minimal contact.

The lumen is now examined and the nature of any contained faeces is noted and also the presence of blood, pus or mucus. The mucous membrane is next observed, being swabbed clear of faeces or discharge if necessary to enable this to be done. Normally it is a pale pink colour and the submucous vessels forming a fine network are clearly seen through it. In proctocolitis (ulcerative colitis) it becomes thickened and granular or velvety in appearance, the vascular pattern ceases to be evident and almost invariably, when the mucosa is gently rubbed with a swab on forceps, it bleeds: this is 'contact bleeding', a most important and delicate sign of an inflamed mucosa. Occasionally low-lying rectal tumours can be seen through the proctoscope and, if required, biopsies taken by

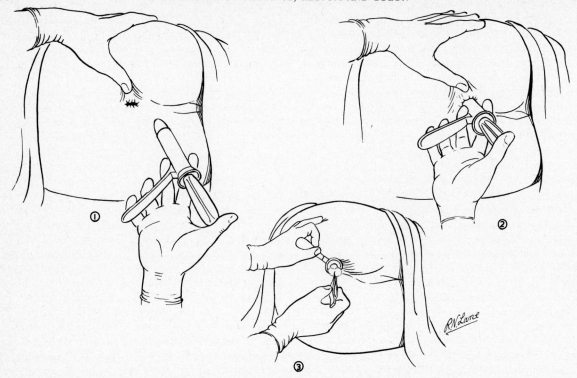

Fig. 52. Introduction of the proctoscope. (1) Note that the instrument is held in the palm of the right hand with the handle lying posteriorly. The upper buttock is raised with the left hand to expose the anal orifice clearly. (2) The point of the obturator is now engaged in the anus and directed *towards the umbilicus*. (3) The obturator has been withdrawn and the handle of the proctoscope is held in the left hand with *the left fingertips resting on the skin of the upper buttock and sacral region*. Emmett's forceps are available for swabbing as required.

means of the conchotome. In cases of threadworm infection the worms may sometimes be seen writhing in the lower rectum on proctoscopy and provide an unforgettable picture.

The proctoscope is now slowly withdrawn. As its end passes into the anal canal the mucosa closes over it at the level of the anorectal ring shutting off the spacious cavity of the rectum. If internal haemorrhoids are present they will prolapse into the lumen of the instrument as it is withdrawn. To gauge more accurately their size and degree it is helpful to ask the patient to bear down as the proctoscope is being removed. Due to the congestion caused by this manoeuvre bleeding may be produced, the actual point of haemorrhage being usually clearly visible on one of the piles when finally the instrument is completely removed; large haemorrhoids if present will probably be found to project at the anal orifice. During the passage of the proctoscope down the anal canal a special note is made of the state of the anal valves and whether any hypertrophied anal papillae are present. An anal fissure will also be looked for as a flattened raw area in the midline posteriorly or anteriorly from which

a little bleeding, or more rarely a discharge of pus, may take place. Lastly in fistula cases the internal opening. of the fistulous track may be evident on proctoscopy, usually in the vicinity of the anal crypts, and as the end of the instrument passes over it a bead of pus may be expressed.

It is often necessary to re-insert the proctoscope for a further assessment of the condition of any haemorrhoids observed, or for a more careful scrutiny of the walls of the canal for a fissure or fistulous opening. To do so, it should always be withdrawn completely and re-fitted with its obturator as at the first passage. Any attempt to replace the obturator with the tube still in the lower part of the anal canal is liable to nip the mucosa between the end of the obturator and the tube and cause pain.

SIGMOIDOSCOPY

Many surgeons have the erroneous idea that sigmoidoscopy is not likely to be worthwhile unless the bowel has been thoroughly cleared by an enema, wash-out or suppository. On the contrary, a preparatory enema is usually not only quite unnecessary, it is actually a drawback in two ways. First, the soap in the enema is excessively irritating to the mucosa and causes a discharge of mucus which may give rise to confusion in diagnosis if this explanation is not borne in mind; secondly, if the enema or wash-out has not been all returned before the patient presents for sigmoidoscopy, the surgeon may find to his annoyance that the rectum and sigmoid are full of liquid motion. The same state of affairs may also result from the incomplete action of purgatives administered the evening before the day of examination. Fluid faeces are much more difficult to cope with during sigmoidoscopy than is loading due to semi-solid faeces. In other words inefficient preparation is much worse than no preparation at all.

In actual practice I find that all but a very small minority of cases coming as out-patients without any preparation whatsoever to my rectal clinic are suitable for a complete rectal examination including sigmoidoscopy. An occasional patient is altogether too loaded and has to be requested to attend on another occasion for the administration of an enema or a glycerine or bisacodyl suppository in the out-patient department immediately before the rectal clinic.

No anaesthesia is needed as a rule for sigmoidoscopy. Even when painful anal lesions such as fissures are present it is usually possible to pass a small bore sigmoidoscope without too much discomfort. If however the anus is too tender and tight even for this, and sigmoidoscopy is urgently required it may be possible after an inferior haemorrhoidal nerve block (see p. 85); alternatively the examination will have to be conducted under general anaesthesia. Resort to a general anaesthetic is also required exceptionally in cases with a presumptive diagnosis of carcinoma of the rectosigmoid, where the end of the sigmoidoscope cannot be negotiated round the sharp rectosigmoid flexure without causing unbearable abdominal pain, and subsequent barium enema examination has not provided a good view of the distal sigmoid and upper rectum.

The patient has already been placed in the correct position at the commencement of the rectal examination, of which sigmoidoscopy is but a part, but in case he may have moved slightly during the initial stages of the examination it is verified that his position is still satisfactory. The points requiring particular attention are that the buttocks project as far as possible over the edge of the couch, that the trunk lies obliquely across the couch top, that the hips are not too strongly flexed and that the ankles rest adjacent to the edge of the couch distant from the surgeon.

The sigmoidoscope is taken in the right hand, with the obturator held firmly in position in the tube, and lubricated by dipping it in a jar of lubricant, some of the lubricating jelly thus acquired being also smeared along the more proximal part of the shaft to prevent it sticking to the skin of the buttocks during introduction. The patient's uppermost buttock is now lifted by the surgeon's left hand and the tip of the instrument inserted into the anal canal again in the classical direction 'towards the umbilicus' (Fig. 52/1, 4). The same resistance from the anal sphincters as was encountered during proctoscopy may be felt at first, but usually it is less marked during sigmoidoscopy because the instrument is narrower and the patient has recovered from some of his initial nervousness. As soon as the rectum proper is entered, the proximal end of the sigmoidoscope is swung anteriorly so that the axis of the shaft is directed more backwards towards the sacral concavity. Sometimes the instrument can be introduced blindly for several centimetres in this new axis without encountering any resistance, but it is a wise rule that once the end of the sigmoidoscope is in the rectum *further advancement should always be under direct vision*, otherwise damage may be done to tumours and other obstructing lesions.

The obturator is removed and the tube is rotated so that the calibrations are on the side facing the surgeon. The proximal end of the sigmoidoscope, carrying the glass window, light and bellows, is then firmly attached (Fig. 53/2). The shaft of the instrument is grasped close to the proximal lighted end with the left hand, whilst the left arm is steadied *by resting the elbow and upper part of the forearm on the patient's buttocks* (Fig. 53/3). The further movement of the instrument is now controlled throughout by the left hand. The bellows are taken in the right hand and with a few puffs of air the rectum is distended sufficiently to demonstrate its lumen. This is seen to be quite capacious as a rule, and in order to inspect all parts of its circumference a certain amount of rotation of the outer end of the sigmoidoscope is necessary at each level. In addition some side-to-side movement may be necessary to negotiate the point past the lower and middle valves of Houston, which are often prominent. The instrument is slowly advanced with as little inflation with air as possible for over-distension is one of the causes of pain during the examination. The general direction is at first upwards and backwards, the point of the sigmoidoscope being directed quite

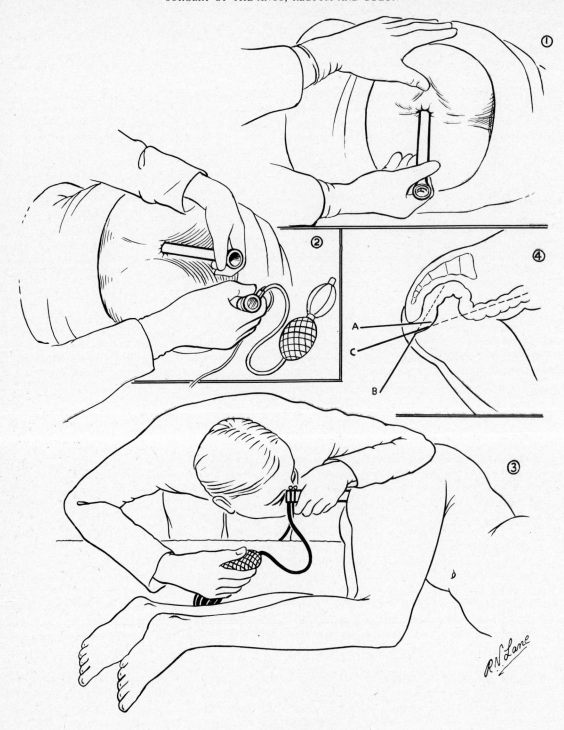

Fig. 53. Sigmoidoscopy: (1) Introduction of sigmoidoscope, the point being directed *towards the umbilicus* till the top of the anal canal is reached. (2) Attachment of light to sigmoidoscope tube after withdrawal of obturator. (3) Viewing with the sigmoidoscope. Note that the tube is held by the surgeon's left hand whilst the left forearm is steadied by resting it on the patient's buttock; bellows held by right hand, but *very little air need be inflated*. (4) Alterations in the axis of the instrument during sigmoidoscopy. (A) Axis 'through umbilicus' whilst point is in anal canal. (B) Axis towards sacral concavity when rectal ampulla being inspected. (C) Eye-piece end rotated backwards, and point forwards during negotiation of the sharp rectosigmoid angulation.

markedly posteriorly into the hollow of the sacrum.

This has the effect of carrying the outer end of the instrument well forwards and, unless the precaution was taken to place the patient with his trunk obliquely across the couch and his legs along the opposite edge, the examiner's head in following the eye-piece will impinge uncomfortably on the back of the patient's legs and heels. Correct initial positioning largely obviates any such awkwardness.

This axis of instrumentation continues till the rectosigmoid junction is reached at about 12–15 cm from the anal margin. At this level the lumen appears to end in a blind cul-de-sac, till it is appreciated that it in fact bends sharply forwards and to the left. To enable the point of the instrument to follow it round this angulation the eye-piece has to be swung backwards and slightly to the right (Fig. 53/4). Unless done with the utmost gentleness—and sometimes despite such care—this manoeuvre may cause a certain amount of discomfort in the anus from distortion of the anal sphincters by the shaft of the sigmoidoscope, or a colicky type of pain in the lower abdomen due to stretching of the wall of the distal colon by the point of the instrument. The difficulty in negotiating the rectosigmoid junction is frequently aggravated by the occurrence of spasm in this region. This spastic condition together with the sharpness of the bend, which varies greatly in different individuals, and the pain being experienced by the patient may combine to prevent further passage. In fact many sigmoidoscopies come to a stop at this level, but it is remarkable how frequently a really experienced sigmoidoscopist can surmount this obstacle by a combination of gentle but firm manipulation of the instrument and judicious inflation with the bellows. Once the sigmoid colon proper has been entered further passage is usually very rapid and easy right up to the full length of the instrument—25–30 cm. The conduct of the examination may of course be impeded at this level or elsewhere by loading with faeces. If these are solid it is quite surprising how easy it is to slip a narrow-bore sigmoidoscope, such as the small Lloyd-Davies instrument, between the faecal masses and the rectal or colonic wall, so that fair progress can still often be made. Liquid faeces or a profuse discharge of pus or blood are usually more troublesome, but, with the aid of a suction tube inserted periodically down the sigmoidoscope during the examination, a satisfactory sigmoidoscopy can sometimes be achieved.

So much for the mechanics of sigmoidoscopy. As for the findings on sigmoidoscopic examination, the following points should be observed:

The Contents of the Rectum and Colon. It should be noted whether the rectum is empty or contains normal semi-solid motion, liquid faeces, mucus, pus, blood or undigested food particles such as fruit skins.

The Lumen of the Bowel. Whether it is normal, ballooned or contracted; and whether any localized stricture or spasm is present.

The Appearance of the Mucosa. The normal rectal and colonic mucosa is smooth and glistening, has a pale pink colour with a faint orange tinge, and allows the vessels of the submucosa to be seen clearly through it giving the characteristic 'vascular pattern' (Plate IIIA). Another feature of the normal mucosa is its suppleness, so that it moves easily over the end of the sigmoidoscope, and loose mucosal folds flatten out rapidly on distension of the bowel with air. *The inflamed mucosa* (of proctocolitis or Crohn's colitis) may exhibit several different appearances, which are described on pp. 702 and 834.

The Presence of Benign Polyps Projecting from the Mucosa. The characteristics and situation of any polyps present should be carefully observed. Such tumours may be single or multiple, sessile or pedunculated, and may represent true adenomas, villous papillomas, projecting submucous connective tissue tumours, or inflammatory swellings of remnants of the mucosa in colitis—the so called pseudo-polyps. A special note should be made of evidence of ulceration or friability in polyps as a possible indication of malignant changes (Plates II and IIIF).

The Existence of a Carcinoma of the Rectum or Colon. This may take the form of projecting papilliferous mass, like a small cauliflower, but far more commonly it is seen as a typical malignant ulcer with raised everted edges and a grey sloughing base. Almost as distinctive as the appearance of a malignant lesion is the sensation of induration experienced by the examiner through the shaft of the sigmoidoscope as its distal end impinges on the hard growth (p. 412).

It is advisable to resort freely to biopsy of any doubtful lesion to confirm or refute endoscopic impressions as to its precise nature. It is an easy matter to obtain representative snippets of tissue for such histological examinations by means of the forceps shown in Fig. 41, but the taking of the biopsy should be the last step in the sigmoidoscopy for it may cause a certain amount of bleeding which obscures subsequent views.

RECORDS

The findings of a rectal examination should always be clearly recorded. For example the precise situation of any lesion observed on sigmoidoscopy should be stated in terms not only of height (i.e. distance from the anal margin) but also of the aspect of the bowel wall affected (anterior, posterior, right lateral, left lateral). The findings on inspection, palpation and proctoscopy should be similarly clearly recorded, and there is much to be said for the use of diagrams such as those shown in Figs 54 and 55, on which the position and extent of any lesion may be depicted with accuracy and great saving in verbal description. These diagrams may be printed on the case sheet or added by means of inked rubber stamps as required. They are valuable for recording not only the findings on initial examination, but also the type and scope of operations and other forms of treatment. They reach their maximum usefulness in cases with complicated fistulae, the anatomy of which it is difficult to describe accurately without recourse to diagrams of this kind.

ABDOMINAL AND GENERAL CLINICAL EXAMINATION

A general clinical examination ought perhaps ideally to be carried out prior to rectal examination in all instances, but in many cases in which the symptoms suggest particularly a lesion of the rectum it is more convenient in the running of a rectal clinic to examine the patient rectally first of all and to supplement this as required subsequently by examination of the abdomen and other parts. Such examination follows the lines of an ordinary clinical examination, special attention being paid to the presence of abdominal distension, visible peristalsis, free fluid in the peritoneal cavity, a palpable mass in the line of the colon, hepatomegaly, enlargement or induration of the inguinal glands. I may perhaps be forgiven for reminding the reader of the importance of a vigorous bimanual technique in palpating for a carcinoma of the splenic or hepatic flexure, one hand being placed behind on the loin, the other in front below the costal margin and the patient meanwhile being instructed to breathe deeply in and out during the palpation. I have known palpable carcinomas in these situations to elude clinical detection through lack of attention to these elementary practical details.

In all cases with major lesions of the colon and rectum such as carcinoma or colitis an assessment

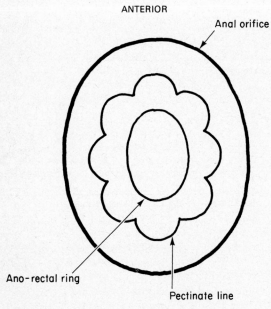

Fig. 54. Outline of the anal canal and perianal region as seen from below, showing the lower edges of the two sphincters, the pectinate (mucocutaneous) line, and the anorectal ring. This diagram is of value in depicting graphically the position of lesions encountered clinically or at operation.

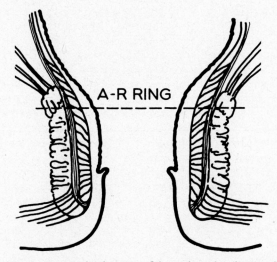

Fig. 55. Longitudinal section of the anal canal, indicating the inter-relationships of the sphincters and other anatomical landmarks; of great assistance in describing the course of anal fistulae.

of the patient's general condition is important, partly to exclude distant manifestations of the disease such as pulmonary deposits or metastatic arthritis or skin eruptions, and partly in relation to the prospects of carrying out operative treatment. In this latter connection the presence of gross malnutrition, chronic bronchitis, diabetes, anaemia, hypertension, or a cardiac or renal lesion must be specially noted and their effects corrected as far as possible in the preoperative period. The collaboration of a general physician or cardiologist may be desirable in assessing and treating the patient from this point of view.

RADIOLOGICAL INVESTIGATIONS

Radiological examination may be required in several ways. *A plain radiograph of the chest* may be necessary to help to exclude a tuberculous pulmonary focus or secondary deposits of growth in the lungs, and to show the extent of structural changes in cases with chronic bronchitis. *A plain X-ray examination of the abdomen* is particularly valuable in cases with obstructive intestinal symptoms; the presence of gaseous distension of the bowel with fluid levels confirms the diagnosis of obstruction and a careful study of the distribution of the gas shadows may be of the greatest assistance in determining the site of the obstructing lesion and its nature. Plain X-ray plates of the abdomen are also helpful in cases of suspected perforation of the colon due to carcinoma or colitis and in the diagnosis of the extent of the disease and the presence or absence of toxic megacolon in severe attacks of colitis or Crohn's disease of the large bowel. *Mesenteric arteriography* has recently emerged as an important aid in the investigation of certain cases of intestinal haemorrhage (see p. 897). *Intravenous pyelography* is advisable in any cases with an extensive fixed upper rectal growth or growth in any part of the colon where it might become adherent to the ureter. The pyelograms will show whether there is any obstruction of the ureter with the development of hydronephrosis and will also provide evidence as to the functional and anatomical state of the opposite kidney, information that will be valuable and reassuring to the surgeon embarking on a difficult rectal or colonic excision. Rarely *radiological examination of the pelvis* may be useful in deciding whether there is bony involvement by a growth, and *X-ray examination of the sacrum and coccyx* is generally required in cases of coccygeal pain to exclude old or recent bony injury or sacrococcygeal arthritis. The most important radiological investigation, however, in diseases of the rectum and colon is naturally the direct examination of the alimentary tract itself after *barium enema or barium progress meal.*

Barium Enema Examination

The barium enema is the sheet anchor of the radiological investigation of diseases of the colon. Two main types of opaque enema examinations are in regular use:

The simple barium enema technique, in which the patient is screened as the bowel is gradually filled with the barium mixture, and radiographs are taken to illustrate various stages in the process and to record obvious morbid appearances. The enema is then evacuated and further radiographs taken of the collapsed colon with only a trace of barium in it. This method suffices as a rule for the demonstration of gross lesions like obvious carcinomas, but frequently fails to display small polypoid growths.

The barium–air double contrast enema technique, originally introduced by Fischer (1925) of Frankfurt, in which radiological examination by the simple barium enema is followed by inflation of the colon with air. The distended bowel then has a thin coating of barium mixture on its mucosa, and radiological studies at this stage give a good display of the mucosal pattern, usually showing very clearly any projecting polypoid lesion arising from it. This method is specially valuable in the diagnosis of early plaque-like carcinomas or polyps and gives a beautiful demonstration of the multiple polyps in familial polyposis. These show mainly as a mosaic of 'negative' shadows, but larger polyps may retain a complete coating of barium and stand out clearly in the air-filled colonic lumen. For full details of radiological technique standard works on radiodiagnosis should be consulted, such as Shanks and Kerley (1971), and Margulis and Burhenne (1967); particularly detailed and helpful accounts of the double contrast technique are given by Welin (1958) and Welin and Welin (1976) of Malmö and by Young (1964) in this country.

A most important point to emphasize is the need for very thorough preparation of the bowel by purgation and enemas or wash-outs (perhaps using an irrigating machine such as the Henderson apparatus made by McCarthy) in order to cleanse it of its faecal content before undertaking a double contrast study. The precise details of preparation vary with the radiologist.

Barium Progress Meal Examination

Because it is less embarrassing and uncomfortable for the patient than a barium enema, or because the lesion is thought to lie in the right colon, a barium progress meal is sometimes ordered as an alternative by the clinician in investigation of patients with presumed disease of the large intestine. But, owing to the patchy distribution of barium which it gives in the large bowel and the inadequate filling that results, no reliable conclusion as a rule can be drawn from it. Further it is not without danger in cases with a constricting lesion of the colon, for the barium is liable to 'cake' and form scybala which may impact in the narrowed portion of the bowel and precipitate an 'acute on chronic' intestinal obstruction. It cannot be too strongly urged therefore that priority be given to the barium enema in the radiological investigation of diseases of the large intestine.

The progress meal, however, has a valuable supplementary role to play in the investigation of certain patients who initially appeared to be suffering from a lesion of the colon or rectum, but on whom a barium enema examination and other investigations have proved negative, and the possibility arises that the symptoms may be due to disease of the small gut such as ileitis or to idiopathic steatorrhoea. Owing to reflux of barium from the colon through the ileocaecal valve into the lower ileum, which occurs in a large proportion—possibly as many as 50%—of barium enema examinations, the terminal small bowel is often outlined fairly well and disease conditions are sometimes demonstrated in it in this way. But for more thorough radiological investigation of the jejunum and ileum a progress—or small bowel—meal study is required. In the conduct of a small bowel meal examination it is essential to use a non-flocculating preparation of barium (e.g. Raybar) otherwise the irregular flocculation of the opaque medium in the small bowel may produce an appearance similar to that seen in steatorrhoea, either idiopathic or due to some forms of ileitis (Ardran et al. 1950). Further details of radiological technique and interpretation should be sought in radiological texts (Shanks and Kerley 1971; Margulis and Burhenne 1967; Marshall and Lindner 1976).

The Small-bowel Enema

In 1943 Schatzki devised a technique for radiological examination of the small bowel, which he designated the 'small-bowel enema'. This was designed to overcome the disadvantage of pyloric control by intubating the pylorus so that the opaque medium could be introduced in a continuous flow directly into the small bowel itself. Actually it is an advantage to use a double tube for this purpose: an outer more rigid rubber tube which is passed down to the pylorus, and an inner more flexible polythene tube which is then manipulated through the pyloric sphincter into the duodenum and jejunum (Scott-Harden 1960). The opaque medium employed is 20–30 ml non-flocculating barium diluted with 60–90 ml water. The solution is injected rapidly by means of a 20 ml syringe, onward progress being achieved by the subsequent injection of tap water, the barium left behind adhering to the mucosa and serving to give a double contrast. Good accounts of the achievements of the modern small-bowel enema technique are given by Pygott et al. (1960) and Scott-Harden et al. (1961).

COLONOSCOPY

Equipment

COLONOSCOPES

The introduction of fibreoptic endoscopy in the investigation of the upper gastrointestinal tract in the mid-1960s was followed a few years later by the development by three firms—the American Cytoscope Makers Incorporated, and Olympus and Machida of Tokyo—of instruments for examination of the large bowel, which are essentially similar to fibreoptic oesophagogastroscopes but somewhat strengthened to stand up to the twisting strains involved in manoeuvring the instrument through the colon. The first pattern evolved was a 'short' colonoscope 60–70 cm long, really a fibre-sigmoidoscope, but it was soon supplanted by instruments with a greater reach, though it was recently revived to some extent as a means of conducting a more extended examination in the out-patient clinic or consulting room, the patient having taken a disposable enema beforehand (Marks 1977; Carter 1978). The two patterns of instrument now in regular use are the 'medium' and 'long' colonoscope respectively. The medium instrument, which is usually about 110 cm long, can as a rule reach the splenic flexure or distal trans-

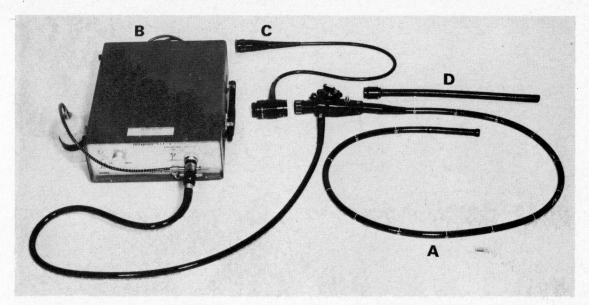

Fig. 56. The Olympus TCF two-channel colonoscope with accessories. (A) The colonoscope itself. (B) The light source. (C) The teaching attachment. (D) The sigmoid stiffener.

verse colon, the long instrument, which is 165–190 cm long, is designed to bring the right colon as far as the ileocaecal junction into view.

The general structure of a colonoscope is exemplified by the Olympus TCF 2 channel instrument, which is depicted in Fig. 56A. This colonoscope is 190 cm long, with a working length of 173 cm and a tube diameter of 16 mm. The greater part of the length of the instrument is passively flexible, the distalmost 10 cm can be actively bent to 170° upwards and downwards, and 140° to the right and to the left by turning knobs on the rigid proximal segment, which carries the eyepiece. The light source (Fig. 56B) is provided in a separate box, which contains a halogen quartz lamp, and the cold light is supplied to the proximal end of the instrument through a connecting cable. In the colonoscope itself some of the optical fibres convey this light from the proximal to the distal end, the remainder carry the visual impressions from the distal end to the eyepiece and the observer. The view from the distal end is in the long axis of the instrument, not from its side, as in some forms of gastroscope. The colonoscope has its own pump housed in the box containing the light source; by means of controls on the rigid proximal segment of the scope the pump can be operated to inflate the bowel with air or to irrigate the surface of the lens at the distal end if it gets fouled with faeces. Similarly a built-in suction line is provided for withdrawing air or liquid faecal content from the bowel. A separate channel is also available in colonoscopes for the passage of a flexible biopsy forceps or a diathermy snare, and in this particular Olympus TCF instrument two channels are provided for this purpose, allowing a biopsy or holding forceps to be passed down one and simultaneously a snare to be passed down the other, a helpful manoeuvre in polypectomy (see Fig. 344).

ADDITIONAL ITEMS

Teaching Attachment. In instructing others in the technique and findings of colonoscopy a teaching attachment is well nigh indispensible. It consists of an additional eyepiece with a fibreoptic side-arm leading to a second eyepiece, so that the colonoscopist and another can be viewing simultaneously (Fig. 56c). If, as is often the way, some of the advancement of the colonoscope is left to an assistant, it helps him to be able to see what is happening through the teaching attachment.

Sigmoid Stiffener. This is a flexible hollow tube of slightly greater width than the colonoscope. It is passed over the colonoscope before the examination commences and slid up to the proximal part of the shaft out of the way during the initial passage of the instrument (Fig. 56D). When the distal end of the colonoscope has reached the descending colon, the stiffener is passed into the rectum and sigmoid over the instrument after it has been straightened.

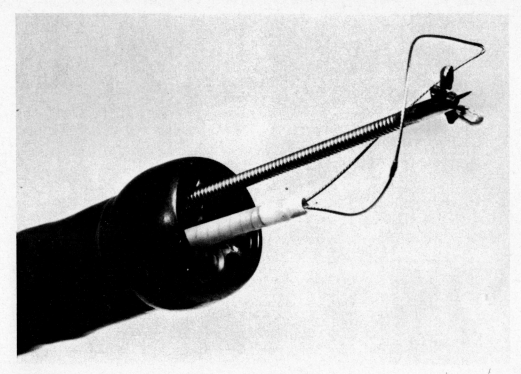

Fig. 57. The distal extremity of the Olympus TCF two-channel colonoscope with a biopsy forceps and a snare projecting from the two channels.

Biopsy Forceps and Snares. Examples of the fine biopsy forceps and snares used in connection with the colonoscope are shown in Fig. 57. An electro-surgical source of current is necessary in using snares and some of these are also capable of delivering carbon dioxide or other inert gas to the bowel to displace air during polypectomy and thereby obviate any risk of explosion.

Fluoroscope with Television Image-intensification. Though for many colonoscopic examinations X-ray control is not necessary, in some cases it proves very helpful in orientating the instrument and judging how far it has passed. It is advisable therefore to have a mobile intensifier available.

Organization

The arrangements for colonoscopy have become more stereotyped in the last four or five years. Most colonoscopies are now performed on an out-patient basis and in my practice that applies also to most patients undergoing colonoscopic poly-pectomies. It is essential to have some conveniently adjacent recovery space in which the patient can recover from the effects of sedation for a couple of hours after the colonoscopy before going home, whilst the examination of other patients is proceed-ing. For the colonscopy itself an ordinary exam-ination couch would suffice for most cases, but, as fluoroscopic control occasionally becomes neces-sary, it is preferable to be prepared for this require-ment by carrying out the examination on an X-ray table. The colonoscopist needs one nurse or techni-cian to look after the instrumentation during the examination (and to be responsible for the cleaning and maintenance of the equipment before and afterwards as well), and another nurse to care for the patient. It is also sometimes a help at various stages in the passage of the instrument to have the collaboration of an assistant, who at the same time is learning the technique of colonoscopy. But an experienced colonoscopist will often feel happier to handle the controls of the instrument entirely with one hand, keeping the other hand for advance-ment, rotation or withdrawl of the tube at the anus. Colonoscopes can be sterilized with ethylene oxide or glutaraldehyde (Cidex); the latter has the advan-tage of being quicker and better suited to use be-tween cases on a colonoscopy list (Axon et al. 1974).

BOWEL PREPARATION

It cannot be too strongly stressed that thorough preparation of the bowel is an absolute essential for successful colonoscopy. For 48 hours before the examination the patient is on essentially a liquid diet. If the day of examination is regarded as Day 3, on the evening of Day 1 he is given three tablets of Senokot, and on the morning of Day 2 45 ml of castor oil. He reports to hospital on the morning of Day 3 and is given two enemas of Veripaque, each consisting of 3 g in 1 litre of fluid, the second enema being not less than two hours before the colonoscopy.

MEDICATION

It is possible in some cases to perform colonoscopy without any form of medication at all, and this plan has the advantage of retaining the patient in a thoroughly rational and cooperative state throughout provided that he does not experience too much pain. In general, however, it is better to give sedation and analgesia in the form of an intravenous injection of diazepam 10–25 mg and pethidine 50–75 mg just before the colonoscopy commences. The antispasmodic hyoscine butylbromide may sometimes be useful in relaxing circular muscle spasm in the colon, but I have not used it much.

TECHNIQUE OF COLONOSCOPY

The examination commences with the patient lying on his left side with his knees moderately flexed. After the anal region and skin of the adjacent buttocks has been smeared with jelly, the well-lubricated end of the colonoscope is pressed gently but firmly against the ánal orifice. With continued pressure the sphincters relax and the scope passes into the rectum for a distance of 10–12 cm. A little air is now introduced and viewing starts. It is better not to withdraw to examine the lower rectum at this stage but to continue the advancement of the instrument under vision. In doing so the important principle is to keep the lumen constantly in view by a certain amount of *inflation* combined with *angulation* in the various directions possible and *rotation* of the instrument. If a so-called 'red-out' develops and a clear view of the lumen and mucosa is lost, it can always be regained by withdrawing the scope slightly. (Sometimes cautious blind onward passage of the instrument—the 'slide by' manoeuvre—will recover the lumen at a higher level, but more often it proves unavailing and, because of the risk of perforation, should be stopped immediately if the colon wall shows increasing pallor or the patient complains of pain.) By the judicious use of these manoeuvres the rectosigmoid flexure can usually be negotiated and the scope passed along the sigmoid loop into the descending colon and round the splenic flexure to the transverse and right colon and caecum. Once the scope has entered the sigmoid, it is usually an advantage to have the patient turn from the left lateral into the supine (or prone) position, and this is essential if X-ray screening is to be carried out. Such screening for a few seconds at a time can be very helpful in negotiating the sigmoid loop and other flexures, through the frequency with which it is necessary varies a good deal with the experience and policy of the colonoscopist. For example Shinya and Wolff (1975) and Sugarbaker et al. (1976) make relatively limited use of fluoroscopy and that has also been my practice.

One of the most difficult areas in colonoscopy is the sigmoid loop and particularly the angle which it makes with the descending colon. Sometimes the end of the scope fails to negotiate this bend and impacts there, so that further feeding of the instrument into the bowel through the anus merely leads to the development of a larger and larger sigmoid loop, with resulting pain but no advancement of the tip. There are two ways of dealing with this difficulty. One is to try to fix the distal end of the scope by strong angulation of it in the upper end of the sigmoid and then under X-ray control to withdraw the shaft of the instrument a certain distance through the anus so as to straighten and shorten the sigmoid loop (Fig. 58A, B). If the tip of the instrument is then unhooked, it can often be advanced with or without a certain amount of rotation of the instrument into the descending colon (Fig. 58C). The other plan for dealing with an initially impassable sigmoido-descending angle is to employ what is known as the 'alpha manoeuvre', which is also ideally conducted under X-ray control. In it the scope is withdrawn to 25 cm approximately from the anus and the distal end is angulated to the patient's left (Fig. 59A). Then, whilst the instrument is strongly rotated 180° or so in an anticlockwise direction to turn the tip to the patient's right (Fig. 59B), it is again advanced. If the manoeuvre is successful, the scope makes a loop to the patient's right and proceeds from below up the descending colon forming an elegant alpha in its course (Fig. 59C). Once the tip of the instrument has reached the upper descending colon or beyond the splenic flexure, the alpha loop in the sigmoid can be undone, if desired, by a combination of slight withdrawal and clockwise rotation under X-ray viewing.

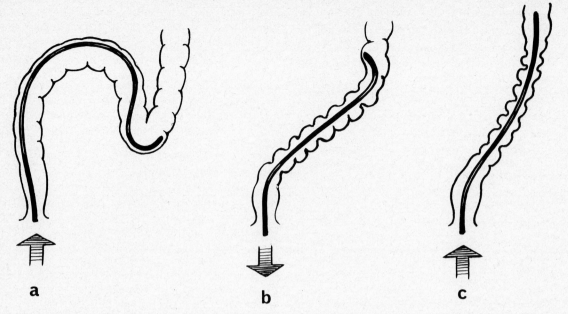

Fig. 58. The method of dealing with sharp angulation between sigmoid and descending colon by straightening the sigmoid loop. (a) Strong angulation of the distal end of the scope to fix it. (b) Withdrawal of the scope to straighten the sigmoid. (c) Unhooking of the scope and advancement into descending colon.

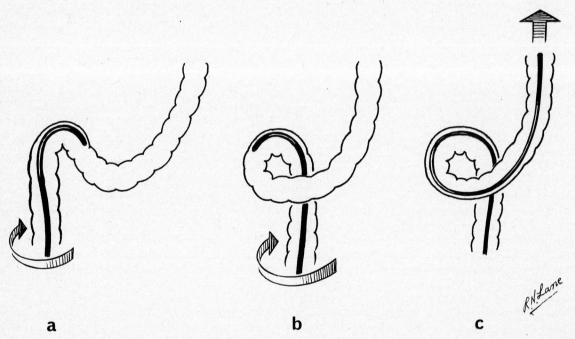

Fig. 59. The 'alpha manoeuvre'. (a) Withdrawal of the scope to 25 cm or so from the anal verge and angulation of the end to the patient's left. (b) Anti-clockwise rotation of scope through 180°. (c) Advancement of the scope which then makes a loop to the patient's right and sweeps into the descending colon.

Another way in which the sigmoid may give rise to difficulty during colonoscopy is by its forming a very large loop which 'uses up' a certain amount of

the length of the colonoscope and gives rise to considerable discomfort to the patient. The loop can be undone by fixing the distal end of the instrument in the descending colon by forcibly flexing it and then withdrawing the shaft of the scope somewhat from the anus. When the sigmoid has thus been straightened out as shown on the fluoroscopic screen, it may be possible by undoing the terminal hook to advance the instrument along the descending and transverse colon without the sigmoid loop reforming. But if troublesome loop formation recurs, the same process of straightening it should be carried out and the 'sigmoid stiffener' (see p. 71), previously placed on the upper part of the scope, is then slid down over it into the rectum and sigmoid as far as the lower descending colon.

Though the state of the mucosa and the presence of any lesions is noted *en passant* as the instrument is being advanced during the colonoscopy, the really detailed and comprehensive survey of the lining of the bowel is reserved till after the colonoscopist has reached what he considers to be the limit of his examination—be it caecum, mid-transverse or upper ascending colon. Then, during the phase of slow withdrawal, every effort is made by bending and rotating the scope, and occasionally by temporary retracing of steps, to see the mucosa of all parts of the circumference of the bowel throughout the length examined. This is often much easier said than done, for it may be quite difficult to bring some areas behind folds of the bowel wall fully into view, and lesions may lurk in these 'blind spots'. When abnormalities are observed, multiple biopsy specimens are taken as necessary. (Incidentally the pathologist needs some practice in working with these small specimens before he is able to make confident pronouncements on them.) One of the most exciting developments in colonoscopy has been the introduction of diathermy snaring of polyps (see p. 341 for further consideration of this subject).

For a more detailed account of the technical aspects of colonoscopy reference should be made to the papers by Williams and Muto (1972), Wolff et al. (1972), Morrissey (1972), Teague and Read (1974), Sakai (1972), Williams and Teague (1973) and Sugarbaker et al. (1976). It is important to emphasize, however, that in this difficult form of endoscopy a very essential quality in the examiner is a certain flair, which combined with experience enables him to judge in a semi-instinctive way the correct mixture of inflation, aspiration, angulation, rotation, advancement and withdrawal needed to negotiate the various bends and twists of the large bowel. But even the most expert colonoscopist will usually find it hard to predict with confidence how easy or difficult colonoscopy will

turn out to be in an individual patient. In some cases to reach the caecum may take but 10–15 minutes, in others nearly an hour may be required or it may prove impossible. Not that a complete colonoscopy is necessary in every case examined by this method. For example, sometimes the objective is a radiologically clearly defined lesion, such as a polyp or dubious carcinoma in the left colon, when, if the standard of radiology is good, colonoscopic examination of the right colon may not be required. But, if colonoscopy is being undertaken to investigate the occurrence of persistent diarrhoea or bleeding, for which no cause has been found on clinical or radiological examination, complete inspection of the entire large bowel round to the caecum is absolutely essential.

COMPLICATIONS

The two main complications of colonoscopy are colonic perforation and bleeding.

Perforation of the colon is extremely rare with highly skilled and experienced examiners (Wolff et al. 1972; Williams and Teague 1973), but much more common in the hands of occasional colonoscopists. When it occurs it is usually in the sigmoid and is produced during one of the special manoeuvres to negotiate this part of the bowel, but it may also arise from errors of technique during diathermy snaring of polyps in any part of the colon (Spencer et al. 1974; Greenen et al. 1975; Smith and Nivatongs 1975). Perforation may manifest itself by the early or dramatic onset of abdominal pain and appropriate signs, leading to emergency laparotomy and suture, usually with a successful outcome (Greenen et al. 1975), or it may reveal itself much more insidiously by the gradual development of a peritonitis, with considerable delay in resorting to surgical intervention and a poorer prognosis.

Bleeding is virtually exclusively a complication of polypectomy and will be considered in connection with this operation (see p. 344).

Selection of Patients

Unlike ordinary sigmoidoscopy with the rigid sigmoidoscope, which should be a routine investigation in virtually all patients with colorectal complaints and *should as a rule precede barium enema study*, fibreoptic colonoscopy is only exceptionally required, *usually after barium enema examination* in patients on whom the radiological verdict has been equivocal or negative despite the presence of strongly suggestive symptoms and signs, such as the persistent passage of blood and mucus. Clearly, the more expert the radiological service available, the less the place for colonoscopy. In my experience the main diagnostic contribution of colonoscopy has been in the detection of polyps or small carcinomas in radiologically-negative patients, in the differentiation of diverticular disease and carcinoma, and occasionally in the recognition or histological confirmation of the precise nature of inflammatory disease above the level of ordinary sigmoidoscopy. In patients known (or found at colonoscopic examination) to have a polyp, colonoscopy is of the utmost value in complementing the radiological exclusion of other polyps, and in securing biopsies or preferably removing the lesion or lesions in toto by diathermy snaring.

OTHER INVESTIGATIONS

In certain cases additional investigations may be required such as the following:

INSPECTION OF THE STOOLS

We are far removed from the days when learned physicians made their diagnosis solely from inspection of the excreta without even seeing the patient! But it may be that we have gone too far in this direction, and in certain cases it may be desirable to examine the stools to confirm the patient's statements regarding their consistency and colour, and the presence of mucus, blood or other abnormality.

DETECTION OF OCCULT BLOOD IN THE FAECES

In sigmoidoscopically and radiologically negative cases of suspected carcinoma of the large intestine a traditional supplementary diagnostic measure is examination of the stools for occult blood. Three main methods are available for the performance of this test—spectroscopic, isotopic and chemical. The first two, and especially the second employing red cells tagged with chromium-51 (see Stephens and Lawrenson 1970), are unquestionably the more reliable, but their complexity renders them unsuitable for routine examination of large numbers of specimens. For chemical testing the substance formerly used was benzidine, but its production has been discontinued because it was discovered that there was a high incidence of cancer amongst persons engaged in its manufacture. Recognized substitutes are the orthotoluidine test, the Occultest tablet, and the Hematest tablet. According to Kay (1962), the Hematest tablet is inadequately sensitive and is liable to give false negative results. The other two would seem to be good replacements for benzidine but, like the original compound, they err on the side of oversensitivity when used on the faeces of patients on unrestricted diets or those who may be suffering from slight blood-loss from the gums due to trauma whilst brushing their teeth. It is important, therefore, for patients to be on a meat-free diet and

not to brush their teeth while undergoing this test. It is customary to repeat the test on three successive days.

However, the practical value of such tests in the diagnosis of neoplasms of the colon is debatable. Like Cameron et al. (1961), I have not found them to be as reliable as the clinical history and seldom use them. More recently the guaiac test in the form of the Hemoccult test has acquired a certain popularity in the U.S.A. as a very convenient, not too sensitive, screening test for colorectal cancer in large groups of asymptomatic persons (see p. 417 for details).

BACTERIOLOGICAL AND PROTOZOAL EXAMINATION OF STOOLS

In cases thought to have a specific dysenteric infection examination of the stools for organisms is obviously required.

For *bacteriological* examination a sample of faeces is taken from the centre of a freshly passed stool on to a swab, which is then placed in a sterile test tube and sent to the bacteriological department forthwith. For *examination for protozoa* in cases of suspected amoebic dysentery even greater expedition is required in dispatching the specimen of faeces, for the amoebae lose their motility within an hour or two of leaving the intestine, though cystic forms of the parasite can still be demonstrated for two or three days.

EXAMINATION OF COLON WASHINGS FOR EXFOLIATED MALIGNANT CELLS

The application of exfoliative cytological studies to the diagnosis of carcinoma of the large intestine has lagged behind its use in the detection of growths in several other situations, partly because of the reliability of other diagnostic methods which, together with a careful assessment of the history for suspicious symptoms, seldom permit a misdiagnosis. Another drawback to cytological studies of this kind is that, in general, they are time-consuming and require much technical assistance for their execution. Oakland (1961) and Knoernschild et al. (1961) described techniques with which they have obtained a high proportion of accurate results.

Oakland (1961) used the more conventional colonic lavage method, in which a wide-bore rectal tube is introduced through a sigmoidoscope, which has been passed to as high a level as possible without causing discomfort; thereafter the instrument is withdrawn. By means of a tube and funnel 400 ml of warmed normal saline is then introduced and, if the lesion is in the sigmoid colon, the saline is washed in and out of the bowel for several minutes, while the patient lies on his left side and has the lower abdomen gently massaged. If the site of the suspected lesion is unknown a more elaborate technique of total colonic lavage is employed: the tube is spigotted off, and the patient lies first on his back and then on his right side in a slightly head-down position, while the abdomen is massaged. Finally, he turns on to his left side again and the fluid is evacuated through the tube. The saline lavage specimen is filtered and then centrifuged. Smears are made of the deposit and stained by Papanicolaou's technique.

The method used by Knoernschild et al. (1961) is simpler in that the preparation for cytological study is that used for a barium enema, and no sigmoidoscope is employed, so that it can be carried out entirely by the nurse without professional supervision. Five hours after receiving 60 ml of castor oil, the patient is given two or three saline enemas. The return from the last enema is placed in an alcohol fixative and stored in a refrigerator. An aliquot of this specimen is passed through a series of filters to remove debris or mucus. The filtrate is finally passed through a millipore filter with a 5 micropore diameter to recover the cells, and the filter is stained by a modified Papanicolaou method.

Knoernschild et al. (1961) have applied their method to the examination of 700 patients, 70 of whom were subsequently shown to have had carcinomas of the colon or rectum. They claim correct diagnoses by cytological examination in 64 (91·5%) of the latter group. There were three false-positive diagnoses. Oakland (1961) reports accurate positive diagnosis in 30 cases (70%) with proven carcinoma of the large intestine. He had five false-negative and five false-positive diagnoses.

The plain fact is that cytological examination as a supplement to radiology has never gained much popularity and in the last few years in most centres it has been supplanted in this role by colonoscopy.

SILICONE-FOAM ENEMA EXAMINATION

Cook and Margulis (1962, 1963) and Cook (1963) reported the use of a diagnostic enema that could be retrieved as a precise mould of the distal large bowel to permit of naked-eye inspection for surface irregularities suggestive of mucosal projections or indentations due to polypoid or diverticular lesions. In addition the cast could be specially examined for the presence on it of adherent exfoliated cells.

Method

After the colon has been emptied by a 112 ml sodium phosphate enema, the patient is placed in the knee–chest position and a specially designed balloon catheter (like a Foley catheter) is inserted into the rectal ampulla and inflated. Then 125 ml of liquid polysiloxanes is injected, which is polymerized to a soft resilient foam within 4 minutes of the addition of a non-toxic organometallic oxidizing agent. During polymerization the liquid expands gradually by action of an included intumescent and contacts the mucosal surface of approximately 50 cm of the distal colon. The balloon is then deflated and the catheter removed. The patient next sits on a dry bedpan and in due course evacuates the mould, which usually happens within 10 minutes. If necessary 0·5 ml of neostigmine may be given subcutaneously to assist evacuation, or the passage of the cast may be left till the colon fills with faeces and the patient has his next normal urge to defaecate.

Cook and Margulis (1963) examined silicone casts obtained in this way from 150 patients with diverse colonic diseases, including polyps, villous papillomas and carcinomas. The method has also been used in cases of diverticular disease. Fallacies in the interpretation of impressions on the surface of the mould may arise from imprints due to faecal particles or to bubbles of flatus.

This method has not gained general acceptance and is to be regarded as a research tool rather than a routine diagnostic measure.

DETERMINATION OF MALABSORPTION OF FAT

Frazer (1955), Cooke and Brooke (1955) and Cooke (1956) drew attention to the significance of impaired absorption of fat in the recognition of disease of the *small intestine*, such as Crohn's enteritis, the severity of the malabsorption being roughly proportional to the extent of small bowel implicated. Thus, with a regional ileitis confined to, say 15–20 cm of gut, there would usually be no alteration in fat absorption, but with more extensive involvement of up to half the jejuno-ileum an increased loss of fat in the faeces is invariably found. Probably disease of the jejunum or upper ileum is more prone to interfere with fat absorption than is a lesion confined to the distal part of the small gut. It has been established by Cooke (1956) that, no matter how severely diseased the large intestine may be from ulcerative colitis, fat absorption is not affected as a rule even if there is a short segment of regional 'ileitis' extending proximally from the ileocaecal junction.

Interesting though these observations are, I have to record that with the increased accuracy of small bowel radiological examination in recent years, little use is now made by me of fat absorption studies in the assessment of patients with Crohn's disease and ulcerative colitis.

BACTERIOLOGICAL EXAMINATION OF PUS OR TISSUE FROM ABSCESSES OR OTHER LESIONS

The examination of pus for pyogenic organisms and the determination of their sensitivity to antibiotics follows routine lines and needs no comment. Samples of granulation and fibrous tissue from the walls of abscess cavities and fistulous tracks are often taken for examination *for the presence of a tuberculous infection*. A simple histological technique is that generally chosen for routine use because of its convenience, the tissue being sent in a formol-saline jar and subsequently fixed and sectioned in due course. The diagnosis then rests on recognition of the typical histological features of a tuberculous infection, with tubercle formation and the presence of giant cell follicles *with central caseation*. When only non-caseating giant cell follicles are found, it is impossible for the histopathologist to diagnose tuberculosis with confidence, though not infrequently in the face of these findings he returns a report that the histological features are 'suggestive of a tuberculous infection'. Actually they are much more suggestive of Crohn's disease for, as Morson and Lockhart-Mummery (1959) have shown, the granulation tissue of abscesses and fistulae in the anal region, secondary to Crohn's lesions of the small or large intestine, frequently shows on microscopical examination appearances very like those of tuberculosis, except that the giant cell follicles are non-caseating in type. It must also be remembered that a foreign-body reaction in an ordinary pyogenic fistula may sometimes simulate this histological picture to the extent of producing giant cells. Only very rarely can actual tubercle bacilli be demonstrated by suitable staining in histological preparations even in cases known to be tuberculous.

The more reliable method of establishing the existence of a tuberculous infection is by guinea-pig inoculation. For this purpose the sample of tissue is taken with full aseptic precautions and sent in a sterile jar *without formalin*. It takes up to six weeks from the time of inoculating the guinea-pig's abdomen for the result to be assessed, which minimizes the value of the test, for unfortunately it gives no help in deciding whether to institute early postoperative chemotherapy.

DEMONSTRATION OF TREPONEMA PALLIDUM IN FLUID DERIVED FROM ANORECTAL LESIONS

In cases with lesions in the anal region suspected to be either condylomata or a primary chancre, direct bacteriological confirmation is often possible. It is provided by microscopy with dark ground illumination of fluid taken from the lesion. The fluid is obtained for this examination by being sucked up into a fine capillary tube—as non-sanguineous a sample as possible being chosen—and then extruded on to a microscopic slide and covered with a coverslip. The appearance of the spirochaetes as seen with the oil-immersion lens in a positive case is characteristic.

THE BLOOD WASSERMANN REACTION

In cases with suspected syphilitic lesions the blood Wassermann reaction may also be helpful in reaching a diagnosis.

FREI'S TEST

The antigen for performing this test was originally obtained by withdrawing pus from a softening inguinal bubo (Frei 1925), but the latest and most reliable form of antigen is that known as Lygranum ST (Squibb). It is prepared by growing the virus in the yolk sac of the developing chick embryo. The dose for the test is 0·1 ml injected intradermally on one forearm, a similar quantity of normal saline being injected at a different site as a control. A positive result is a red papule 6 mm or more in diameter surrounded by a fainter erythematous area; this reaches its maximum in 48–72 hours and then gradually fades.

THE COMPLEMENT-FIXATION TEST FOR LYMPHOGRANULOMA VENEREUM

A complement-fixation test on blood serum, using the same specific antigen as in the Frei test, is also available for lymphogranuloma. It is generally agreed that this is a more sensitive and reliable test than the intradermal reaction, and one likely to give positive results earlier in the course of the disease. The test is reported quantitatively, a positive result in dilutions of the serum to 1 in 16 or above being usually taken to indicate the presence of active or recent infection with lymphogranuloma virus. Positive results at a lower titre suggest that the patient has suffered from the disease but that it is now inactive.

HAEMATOLOGICAL EXAMINATION AND ESTIMATION OF PLASMA ELECTROLYTES AND PROTEINS

These investigations are all frequently required in the elucidation and preparation of patients with rectal and colonic lesions, but they are such an integral part of routine practice that no special comment is called for in this chapter.

REFERENCES

ABEL, A. L. (1936) Examination of the rectum. *Postgrad. med. J., 12*, 301.

ARDRAN, G. M., FRENCH, J. M. and MUCKLOW, E. H. (1950) Relationship of the nature of opaque medium to small intestine radiographic pattern. *Br. J. Radiol., 23*, 697.

AXON, A. T. R., COTTON, P. B., PHILLIPS, I. and AVERY, S. A. (1974) Disinfection of gastrointestinal fibre-endoscopes. *Lancet, 1*, 656.

BLUMER, G. (1909) The rectal shelf: a neglected rectal sign of value in the diagnosis and prognosis of obscure malignant and inflammatory disease within the abdomen. *Albany med. Ann., 30*, 361.

BUIE, L. A. (1932) In *The Colon, Rectum and Anus*, ed. F. W. Rankin, J. A. Bargen and L. A. Buie. Philadelphia: W. B. Saunders.

—— JACKMAN, R. J. and VICKERS, P. M. (1941) Extrarectal masses caused by tumors of the rectouterine or rectovesical space. *J. Am. med. Ass., 117*, 167.

CAMERON, A. B., KNOERNSCHILD, H. E. and ZOLLINGER, R. M. (1961) Detection of cancer and adenomas of the colon. *Am. J. Surg., 101*, 23.

CARTER, H. G. (1978) Routine office use of the 60-cm. flexible fiberoptic colonscope. *Dis. Colon Rectum, 21*, 101.

COOK, G. B. (1963) Silicone foam examinations in asymptomatic persons. *Am. J. Gastroent., 41*, 619.

—— and MARGULIS, A. R. (1962) Use of silicone foam for examining human sigmoid colon. *Am. J. Roentgen., 87*, 633.

—— —— (1963) Detecting small sessile colon cancers with silicone foam. *J. Am. med. Ass., 183*, 66.

COOKE, W. T. (1956) Steatorrhoea. *Med. Ann.*, 392.

—— and BROOKE, B. N. (1955) Non-specific enterocolitis. *Q. Jl Med., 24*, 1.

FISCHER, A. W. (1925) Über die Röntgenuntersuchung des Dickdarms mit Hilfe einer Kombination von Lufteinblasung und Kontrasteinlauf (Kombinierte Methode). *Arch. klin. Chir., 134*, 209.

FRAZER, A. C. (1955) Steatorrhoea. *Br. med. J., 2*, 805.

FREI, W. (1925) Eine neue Hautreaktion bei 'Lymphogranuloma inguinale'. *Klin. Wschr., 4*, 2148.

GREENEN, J. E., SCHMITT, M. G., Jr., WU, W. C. and HOGAN, W. T. (1975) Major complications of coloscopy: bleeding and perforation. *Am. J. dig. Dis., 20*, 231.

KAY, A. W. (1962) Management of obscure alimentary bleeding. *Br. med. J., 1*, 1709.

KNOERNSCHILD, H. E., CAMERON, A. B. and ZOLLINGER, R. M. (1961) Millipore filtration of colonic washings in malignant lesions of the large bowel. *Am. J. Surg., 101*, 20.

LOCKHARD-MUMMERY, J. P. (1934) *Diseases of the Rectum and Colon*, 2nd ed. London: Baillière.

MARGULIS, A. R. and BURHENNE, H. J. (1967) *Alimentary Tract Radiology*, vol. 2. St Louis: C. V. Mosby.

MARKS, G. (1977) Personal communication.

MARSHALL, R. H. and LINDNER, A. E. (1976) *Radiology of the Small Intestine*. Philadelphia and London: W. B. Saunders.

MORRISSEY, J. F. (1972) Progress in gastroenterology. Gastrointestinal endoscopy. *Gastroenterology, 62*, 1241.

MORSON, B. C. and LOCKHART-MUMMERY, H. E. (1959) Anal lesions in Crohn's disease. *Lancet, 2*, 1122.

OAKLAND, D. J. (1961) The diagnosis of carcinoma of the large bowel by exfoliative cytology. *Br. J. Surg., 48*, 353.

PYGOTT, F., STREET, D. F., SHELLSHEAR, M. F. and RHODES, C. J. (1960) Radiological investigation of the small intestine by small bowel enema technique. *Gut, 1*, 366.

SAKAI, Y. (1972) The technique of colonfiberoscopy. *Dis. Colon Rect., 5*, 404.

SCHATZKI, R. (1943) Small intestinal enema. *Am. J. Roentgen., 50*, 743.

SCOTT-HARDEN, W. G. (1960) Examination of the small bowel. In *Modern Trends in Diagnostic Radiology (Third Series)*, ed. J. W. McLaren, p. 84. London: Butterworths.

—— HAMILTON, H. A. R. and SMITH, S. W. (1961) Radiological investigation of the small intestine. *Gut, 2*, 316

SHANKS, S. C. and KERLEY, P. J. (1971) *A Textbook of X-ray Diagnosis by British Authors*, 4th ed., vol. 4. London: H. K. Lewis.

SHINYA, H. and WOLFF, W. I. (1975) Colonoscopic polypectomy: technique and safety. *Hospital Practice, 9*, 71.

SMITH, L. E. and NIVATONGS, S. (1975) Complications in colonoscopy. *Dis. Colon Rect., 18*, 214.

SPENCER, R. J., COATES, H. L. and ANDERSON, M. J., Jr. (1974) Colonoscopic polypectomies. *Mayo Clin. Proc., 49*, 40.

STEPHENS, F. O. and LAWRENSON, K. B. (1970) The pathologic significance of occult blood in faeces. *Dis. Colon Rect., 13*, 425.

SUGARBAKER, P. H., VINEYARD, G. C. and PETERSON, L. M. (1976) Anatomic localization and step-by-step advancement of the fibreoptic colonoscope. *Surgery Gynec. Obstet., 143*, 457.

TEAGUE, R. H. and READ, A. E. (1972) Use of fibreoptic colonoscopy for investigating rectal and colonic disease. *Proc. R. Soc. Med., 65*, 966.

WELIN, S. (1958) Modern trends in diagnostic roentgenology of the colon. *Br. J. Radiol., 31*, 453.

—— and WELIN, G. (1972) *The Double Contrast Examination of the Colon: Experiences with the Welin Modification*. Stuttgart: Georg Thieme.

WILLIAMS, C. and MUTO, T. (1972) Examination of the whole colon with the fibreoptic colonoscope. *Br. med. J., 3*, 278.

—— and TEAGUE, R. (1973) Progress report: colonoscopy. *Gut, 14*, 990.

WOLFF, W. I., SHINYA, H., GEFFEN, A. and OZAKTAY, S. Z. (1972) Colon fiberoscopy. A new and valuable diagnostic modality. *Am. J. Surg., 123*, 180.

YOUNG, A. C. (1964) The Malmö enema at St. Mark's Hospital: a preliminary report. *Proc. R. Soc. Med., 57*, 275.

3

Principles and General Conduct of Minor Rectal Surgery

HEALING BY GRANULATION

One of the first principles of so-called minor rectal—really anal—surgery has hitherto been that *sepsis is inevitable* in this region and that *anal wounds must be so managed that they can resist infection and proceed to satisfactory healing despite it*. This in effect has meant laying the wounds widely open at the time of operation and keeping them open subsequently by suitably applied dressings; they then fill from the depths with granulations, which eventually become covered by epithelium growing from the periphery (Fig. 60). This principle goes back several hundreds of years, indeed to antiquity, and it is clearly described in the writings of John Arderne, a fourteenth century surgeon (see Power 1910). But it would, I think, be correct to say that the modern, more radical version of this technique with free excision of the skin edges to give a wide guttered or saucerized wound has been popularized mainly by the teaching of Lockhart-Mummery (1934), Gabriel (1948) and Milligan et al. (1948).

We all know what reliable healing by second intention can be obtained by this method if carefully applied in the treatment of haemorrhoids, fissures and, above all, fistulae. There are however several obvious disadvantages in leaving anal wounds open to granulate. *First* there is the length of time required for complete healing to take place, which with a large horseshoe fistula may amount to two or three months, and even with a low fistula or anal fissure is seldom less than four or five weeks. *Secondly* there is the not inconsiderable discomfort from the large raw area, which during the initial postoperative week or two may occasion a great deal of pain, not lightly to be dismissed. And *thirdly*

the scarring that inevitably follows healing by granulation may lead to troublesome stenosis if special precautions are not observed—sometimes indeed despite such measures. In the present antibiotic era, when potent antibacterial substances, which have wrought revolutionary changes in many aspects of surgical practice, are available for systemic and enteral use, it is appropriate to ask whether sepsis and healing by granulation must still

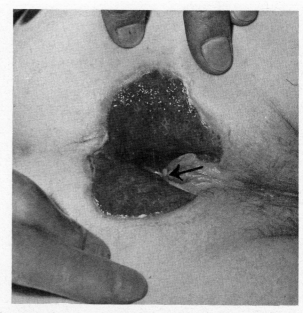

Fig. 60. Large horseshoe fistula wound three weeks after operation showing extensive area of granulation tissue and narrow rim of young epithelium growing in from the periphery (anus marked by arrow).

80

remain the hall-marks of minor rectal surgery. Is primary skin cover still an unattainable ideal in this situation?

IMMEDIATE SKIN COVER FOR ANAL WOUNDS

This has been attempted in two ways—by primary suture of the wound and by the application of split thickness (Thiersch) skin grafts.

Primary Suture

Primary suture of wounds *after excision of anal fistulae* was warmly recommended in selected cases many years ago by Tuttle (1903). In the application of this technique he emphasized that special care must be taken to remove the fistulous track completely and to bring the walls of the wound into firm apposition by buried sutures. But the method never became popular, presumably because it seemed unsound in theory or the results were found to be unsatisfactory in practice, and suture of fistula wounds was universally condemned or ignored by authorities such as Goodsall and Miles (1900), Gabriel (1948) and Milligan et al. (1948). Then Starr (1953, 1959) of Sydney attempted to revive primary suture for dealing with fistula and fissure wounds, employing sulphonamides or antibiotics for bowel antisepsis and systemic use before and after operation and claimed to have been invariably successful in securing uneventful union.

Stimulated by Starr's experiences I also practised primary suture in a few patients with what appeared to be specially suitable wounds following the laying open of low anal fistulae. Particular care was taken to excise the fistula in its entirety and leave fresh supple raw surfaces which were then opposed by two or more layers of buried fine, plain,

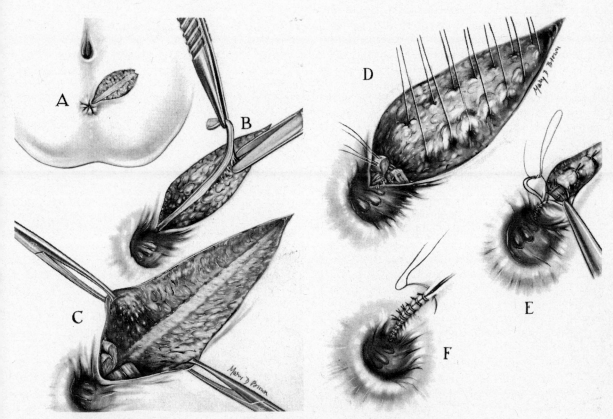

Fig. 61. Excision of fistula-in-ano with primary suture: (A) Fistulous tracks laid open. (B) Excision of the track. (C) The fresh raw surfaces, free from fibrous scar tissue, ready for suture. (D) Suture of sphincter muscles and fat with interrupted fine plain catgut stitches. (E) Apposition of lining of anal canal with chromic catgut stitches. (F) Suture of skin with serum-proof silks.

catgut sutures. Finally the skin was co-apted with Michel clips or silk sutures and any part of the anal lining implicated in the wound sutured with catgut (Fig. 61). Antibiotics were used for intestinal antisepsis and systemic chemotherapy in all instances. Of 20 cases treated in this way 12 secured uncomplicated primary healing, but in 7 the wounds became infected and had to be laid open to heal by granulation. I had no doubt from these results that, while primary union could sometimes be achieved by this technique the proportion of successes was too small to make it a practicable method for routine use, even in apparently favourable cases.

In regard to the small *external anal wounds resulting from haemorrhoidectomy*, though Lockhart-Mummery (1934) favoured closing these to some extent by suturing the skin edges to the ligatures on the main pile pedicles, the consensus of surgical opinion in this country at the present time is that they should be left widely open to granulate. American surgeons, however, such as Buie (1932), David (1949) and Ferguson and Heaton (1959) advocate partial or complete suture of these wounds, as have Starr (1959) and Failes (1966), but it is difficult to judge from their writings how successful this practice is in securing primary union. Such sutured wounds look very tidy in the theatre at the conclusion of the operation, and even more so as depicted by the medical artist, but the result five or seven days later in my experience is apt to be bitterly disappointing. For a period in 1947–8 under cover of colon antisepsis with phthalyl-sulphathiazole and systemic chemotherapy with penicillin, I employed routinely for haemorrhoidectomy the method of clamping and overstitching described by Mitchell (1903) (see Fig. 73 and p. 109), and closed the external wounds completely with catgut sutures. Most of these wounds became to some extent infected and underwent partial or complete separation. Moreover in their inflamed and oedematous condition they were, I should say, more painful than the open wounds usually left after haemorrhoidectomy. These impressions were strongly confirmed by a more careful subsequent study in my department (Watts et al. 1964), leaving me in no doubt that haemorrhoidectomy wounds are better left open to granulate than sutured.

Perhaps the most promising use of primary suture in the anal region has surprisingly been *in connection with perianal and ischiorectal abscesses*. It is clear from the work of Ellis (1959), which is referred to in greater detail on p. 160, that with the aid of systemic penicillin/streptomycin therapy, it is now possible to treat these abscesses by incision and evacuation of pus followed by curettage of the lining of the cavity and immediate suture, with a high probability of securing primary union. The fact that this method can be applied as an outpatient procedure confers considerable advantages on it which outweigh the disadvantage that about 20% of the cases so treated develop a fistula-in-ano requiring subsequent operative treatment (Wilson 1964). I imagine that one reason why these sutured wounds do relatively so well is that the incision usually lies outside the anal verge and does not extend into the anal canal itself.

Another more recent example of primary suture of the perianal skin in surgical practice is in connection with *open lateral internal sphincterotomy* for anal fissure (see p. 150). The small wound in the left lateral perianal region in this operation is closed by immediate suture and usually heals *per primam*, again possibly because it lies beyond the anal margin.

Split-Skin Grafting

The first move towards using skin grafts to expedite the healing of anal wounds was made by Gabriel in 1927 when he applied *secondary Thiersch grafts*, once the crevices and irregularity of the wound surface had evened out with granulation tissue. In only one of his 21 cases treated in this way did the grafts fail to take (Gabriel 1948). Most other surgeons, including myself, who have essayed secondary grafting, have had a very much lower percentage of 'takes'—so low in fact as to make them extremely doubtful whether it had been worthwhile.

Primary split-skin grafting was perhaps first used in this region by Rank (1944) who employed this method in the treatment of the wounds resulting from the excision of pilonidal sinuses. In 1953 Hughes, also of Melbourne, utilizing colon antisepsis and penicillin/streptomycin therapy, applied primary grafting to anal wounds proper, as after laying open fistulae or excising fissures. In certain instances, where there was too much initial oozing of serum and blood from large deep wounds to permit of the immediate use of grafts, Hughes recommended *delayed primary* grafting two or three days later, the wound meanwhile being packed with dry gauze. The grafts were taken from the medial aspect of the thigh and applied as sheets to the raw surface, having been sutured to one another and to the skin edges to provide a complete covering. They might have needed to be snicked with scissors in places to facilitate the escape of serous fluid and

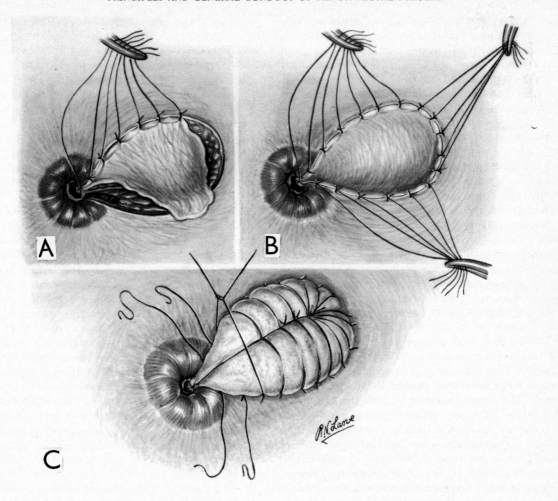

Fig. 62. Application of split skin graft to fistula wound. (A) The upper edge of the graft has been stitched in position using fine serum-proof silks on small curved cutting needles to fix it to the margin of the skin. (B) The suture of the graft completed. Note that the tails of the silk stitches are left 15 cm long. (C) The graft is covered with a layer or two of soft paraffin gauze and over this is placed a pack of cotton wool soaked in acriflavine, the silk 'tails' being tied over the wool to fix it firmly in place and exert pressure firmly against the wound surface.

prevent them being 'floated off'. Finally a pack of cotton wool soaked in acriflavine, or a pad of sponge rubber, was applied to the graft and fixed in position by tying over it the tails of the stitches uniting the graft to the skin. In this way the graft was firmly compressed against the raw surface of the wound (Fig. 62). Fixation and compression of the grafts were further enhanced by a generous pad of gauze and wool held in position by strapping extending across both buttocks. As the grafting was only carried out as the final step in a formal excision of fistula (or fissure), the area to which it was applied was roughly concave or guttered, and in the case of high posterior horseshoe fistulae, might have

been a very deep furrow indeed. Firm pressure by a moulded pack was therefore essential if good apposition was to be secured. The pack was retained in position for five or six days, at the end of which time the sutures were removed and the bowels opened by an enema or aperient. The healing of any remaining raw areas was completed under a regimen of baths, irrigations and Eusol dressings as required.

Hughes (1953) reported most impressive results—40 cases treated by grafting, with virtually complete 'takes' in 30, and substantial, though incomplete, 'takes' in most of the others. My own results with primary Thiersch grafting in 22 cases,

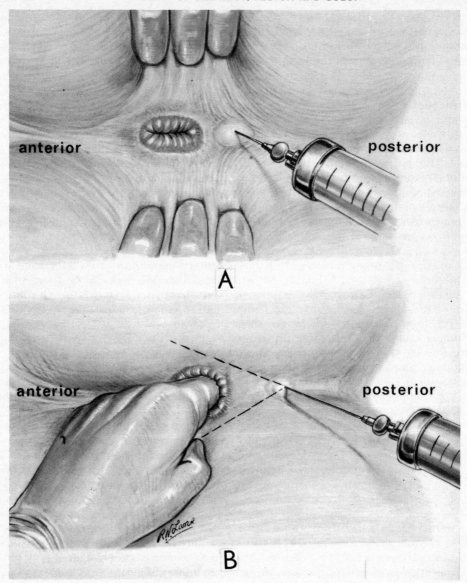

Fig. 63. Inferior haemorrhoidal nerve block. Note that the patient lies on his *right* side for the nerve block (though the subsequent minor anal operation will probably be performed with him on his left side). (A) Whilst the buttocks are gently separated, the post-anal skin is swabbed with an antiseptic solution and, using a fine needle on the syringe, an intradermal weal is raised with the anaesthetic solution in the midline 2·5 cm behind the anal verge. (B) With the index finger of the left hand in the anus as a guide and with a stouter 7·5 cm long needle on the syringe, a deep injection of 15–20 ml of 2% lignocaine or procaine with adrenaline hydrochloride is then given on either side of the anal canal. It should be stressed that the needle should be kept quite deep so that no visible swelling of the perianal tissues develops as the fluid is injected.

conscious patient. I also prefer this position for operations on postanal pilonidal sinuses for which the lithotomy position is unsuitable.

In America the *prone or jack-knife position* is popular, the patient lying face down with the buttocks elevated and the hips slightly flexed by 'breaking' the table or by using sandbags (see Fig.

89). The main advantages claimed for it are that bleeding is much reduced and that the operative field is displayed horizontally rather than vertically, which may be more convenient for arranging towelling, lighting and instruments. I have tried to evaluate this position in my own practice, but having done several thousands of minor rectal

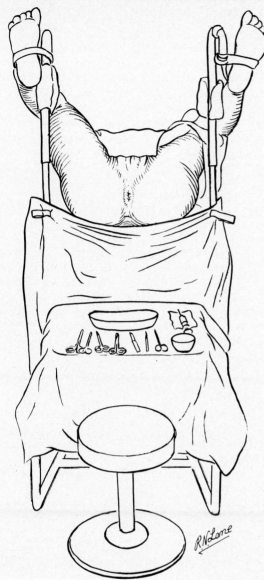

Fig. 64. The lithotomy position for anorectal operations. Note the use of pole clips to fasten the mackintosh towel to the leg supports on either side, also the instrument table immediately over the surgeon's knees.

easy one for the anaesthetist, and it was mainly for this reason that I ceased using it.

Lighting

When the lithotomy or lateral positions are being used it is usually difficult to obtain adequate illumination from the average fixed theatre light, however much it may be tilted. A theatre lamp on a mobile stand is essential, the light being lowered sufficiently to direct the beam *horizontally* at the wound. A good alternative is a head-light, such as the Welch–Allyn, if the surgeon is accustomed to it.

Rectal Toilette

As already explained, one of the governing principles of much minor rectal surgery is that asepsis in this region cannot usually be complete and some contamination is inevitable. Whether this contamination can possibly be somewhat lessened by the adoption of an antiseptic technique with the free use of weak, watery, antiseptic solutions such as cetrimide, Lysol or Dettol for swabbing purposes before and during the operation is rather dubious. My own practice is to cleanse the anal region and lower rectum briefly with swabs soaked in cetrimide immediately prior to operation. This soapy solution is then removed with dry gauze swabs and the operation is commenced. A bowl of sterile water or of a 1/5000 solution of chlorhexidine stands by the surgeon's side during the operation for cleansing the gloved hands and instruments of blood, and for soaking gauze for occasional moist swabbing of the wound and perianal skin.

Digital Stretching or Partial Division of the Anal Sphincters

In the past many surgeons, such as Gabriel (1948), have made a point of stretching the anal sphincters as a routine at the beginning of every minor rectal operation. This was done in the belief that some degree of anal spasm was common in patients with minor rectal ailments, that stretching allowed better delivery of offending piles and was followed by a more comfortable convalescence. Miles (1919) also subscribed to the theory that contraction of the anus was a common finding in cases with haemorrhoids, etc., but attributed it to the development of the 'pecten band' (see p. 18) which he recom-

operations in the lithotomy position it is difficult to avoid bias in favour of the latter. I doubt if the amount of bleeding is much affected by the use of the prone position. Certainly employing the methods which are described below, haemorrhage in the lithotomy position is not a problem. As for the convenience of the surgeon, that is a very personal matter. To my mind the chief disadvantage of the jack-knife position is that it is not an

mended should be divided in the majority of these cases at the outset of the operation. We now know that by such a 'pectenotomy' he inadvertently performed a partial internal sphincterotomy. In recent years Eisenhammer (1953) has advocated deliberate division of the internal sphincter, not merely for the treatment of anal fissure but as a sort of universal panacea in the prevention of post-operative pain in connection with other minor rectal operations such as haemorrhoidectomy.

At one stage I was distinctly sceptical of the value of this ritual stretching or dividing of the sphincter apparatus, particularly as regards the lessening of postoperative pain. However, our experiences during the conduct of trials of various forms of haemorrhoidectomy in my department over the past few years (Watts et al. 1964, 1965) suggested that sphincter stretching was probably beneficial in this connection. They also prompted us to institute a properly controlled prospective trial of this manoeuvre in association with haemorrhoidectomy. The outcome of this enquiry (Goligher et al. 1969) was that there was less pain in the patients who had had a sphincter-stretch immediately prior to haemorrhoidectomy than in the control group who had not had this manoeuvre, but the difference overall was not statistically significant, though in male patients it almost achieved significance. Unfortunately another effect of the sphincter stretching was also disclosed by this trial—namely an increased incidence of *temporary* minor imperfections of anal control, such as slight leakage of flatus or liquid faeces and some degree of anal soiling. Though the functional disturbances were minimal and practically invariably cleared up completely in a few months, they were something of an inconvenience whilst they lasted, and on balance it seemed to me that the disadvantages of stretching the anal sphincters in conjunction with haemorrhoidectomy outweighed the possible advantages. Accordingly I no longer practise sphincter stretching as a routine procedure in the conduct of minor rectal operation, but reserve it for a special indication, as in the treatment of anal fissure (see p. 144 where the technique is described in detail).

DESIGN OF OPEN ANAL WOUNDS

The design of an open anal wound is generally considered important in securing sound healing by granulation. One thing strenuously to be avoided is overhanging edges of skin and subcutaneous tissue which might fall together and unite prematurely before the main wound cavity has had a chance to become filled with granulation tissue. If this should happen exudate is liable to accumulate with the formation of an abscess or fistula. It is advisable therefore at the time of the operation to trim the skin margin and subcutaneous fat generously to produce a wide guttered or saucerized wound, the walls of which, with reasonably efficient nursing, are unlikely to come together in this way. The best instrument to use for wound trimming and indeed for much of minor rectal surgery is a 15-cm pair of blunt-pointed scissors. These cut better at their tips than do the more popular Mayo's scissors.

An additional disadvantage of leaving lax, redundant skin at the edges of an anal wound is that post-operatively this loose skin usually becomes oedematous, swollen and painful, and thus contributes greatly to the patient's discomfort. For this reason a well-shaped open wound with trimmed edges, which presents a relatively large raw area, is often paradoxically less uncomfortable than a much smaller, badly designed wound which has been left with much redundant skin and fat.

HAEMOSTASIS

For the ligation of pedicles of piles or of rectal polyps surgical opinion is divided on the relative merits of strong braided silk or chromic catgut, and whether to transfix the pedicle as well or not. My own practice is to employ silk, usually without transfixion.

Larger vessels divided in open anal wounds can be tied with fine thread or plain catgut. However, for most smaller bleeding points, diathermy coagulation is attractively convenient to the surgeon at the operation, though it causes extensive sloughs which often take a considerable time to separate.

Much of the haemorrhage liable to occur with anal wounds can be avoided or controlled by the *topical use of adrenaline*. This may be employed as a preliminary infiltration of the perianal tissues with a 1/100 000 solution in sterile water as is my routine practice before haemorrhoidectomy. The fluid is introduced through an injection in the midline 2·5 cm behind the anal verge, 15–20 ml being deposited in the subcutaneous tissues on either side of the anus (see Fig. 80). After a delay of three or four minutes, operations such as haemorrhoidectomy can be performed with virtually no bleeding from the cuts in the perianal skin. It might be anticipated that reactionary haemorrhage would be common after such an injection of adrenaline but this has not been so in my experience of many hundreds of cases treated in this way. Another method of using adrenaline is to soak gauze swabs in the BP solution of 1/1000 adrenaline hydrochloride and apply them to the oozing wound surfaces. I have found this practice most effective in checking bleeding and reducing the need for multiple ligatures or diathermy coagulation.

CONCLUSION OF OPERATION

RECTAL TUBE

It is traditional practice to insert a short length of rubber tubing, 13 mm in outside diameter, into the anal canal at the end of many minor rectal operations. The alleged object of the tube is to act as an external vent for flatus and to give warning of haemorrhage by allowing blood to escape from the rectum. Such an indwelling tube is decidedly uncomfortable for the patient, and he is usually very grateful when it is removed. For this reason most surgeons withdraw the tube after 18 or at most 36 hours. During this time there is no real risk of bleeding from pile pedicles and the only haemorrhage likely to be encountered at this stage is reactionary bleeding from one of the external wounds. The tube cannot therefore be really claimed to have any value as an indicator of haemorrhage. Nor can it be of much use as a flatus tube if, as is often done, it is removed on the morning after operation, for in that time few patients have much flatus to pass. I personally have not used a rectal tube of any kind for several years, I believe, to the additional comfort of my patients.

DRESSINGS

Open anal wounds are best dressed with flat pieces of gauze. These may be used dry but preferably are soaked in a hypochlorite solution such as Eusol or Milton (12 ml/litre of tepid water). First of all the entire raw surface is given a covering of flat gauze dressings, as many pieces of gauze as necessary being used for the purpose. Special care is taken to tuck an edge of gauze into any wound crevices, and similarly the drawn-out corner of one of the squares is inserted along any extension of the wound into the anal canal. Then further flat or bunched-up pieces of gauze are packed lightly on top of this lining to fill the hollow of the wound cavity up to the level of the surrounding skin and to maintain the shape of the wound. Finally more

gauze and wool are applied on the surface and the whole dressing is held firmly in position by a T-bandage as in Fig. 65. It is a convenience to have the transverse part of this bandage already tied in position when the patient comes into the theatre for his operation, the tails being rolled up underneath him. When the dressing has been applied the tails can be quickly drawn down and tied, fixing it in place with the minimum of delay.

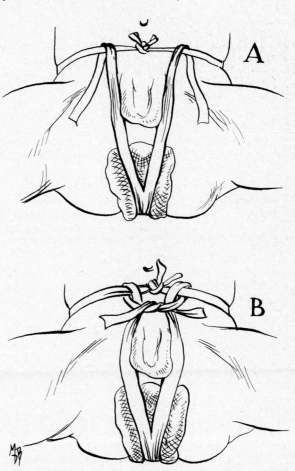

Fig. 65. The T-shaped bandage used to hold the dressings in position.

A simple gauze dressing of this kind soon becomes adherent to the wound surface. This is both a good and bad thing. It is an advantage because it provides a firm protective covering for the raw area and wound edges, and as long as it remains in position pain is much reduced. The disadvantage is that by the time the patient has his first bowel action the dressing has become quite firmly fixed in position and its separation may cause some pain. This is not usually a serious matter with smaller haemorrhoidectomy wounds, but may be troublesome in fistula cases unless the routine is adopted of separating the dressings under general anaesthesia shortly before the bowels act. Some surgeons seek to avoid this difficulty by using soft paraffin gauze or one of the non-adherent patterns of gauze. In my experience these dressings are less satisfactory than ordinary gauze because they do not remain in position and the wound surfaces are thus allowed to come together and may unite in a disorderly fashion.

Postoperative Care

MANAGEMENT OF THE WOUND DURING THE FIRST TWO DAYS AFTER OPERATION

Up to the time the bowels act the wound requires little attention. It is a good plan to change the outer dressing of wool and gauze each morning and evening, but the inner gauze dressing, which is in intimate contact with the wound surface and provides a protective covering for it, should not be disturbed. A fresh dressing of gauze squares soaked in Eusol or Milton is place over it and further wool applied.

More fastidious patients may prefer to have a bath the day after operation and to continue with this routine morning and evening even before the bowels have started acting. After each bath the entire dressing will have soaked off or will have been removed and it will need to be replaced by a new one each time.

THE FIRST BOWEL ACTION

In the eyes of the patient this is the major event of the whole postoperative period, and one which he approaches with considerable trepidation. He feels sure that it cannot fail to be a painful experience, and is moreover worried lest he should damage the anal region in the process and thereby undo the good effects of the operation. It is not surprising therefore that he should often suffer inhibition of his normal mechanism of defaecation, and should fail to achieve a satisfactory motion with a dose of aperient that would ordinarily prove thoroughly effective for him. Instead he is apt to experience a series of false alarms and to make a number of disturbing and exhausting abortive efforts to open his bowels.

To overcome these uncertainties some surgeons make it their practice to prescribe a powerful aperient, such as 30–45 ml of castor oil, but this can be very uncomfortable for the patient if it produces a short succession of motions and is better reserved as a last resort. The plan which I favour is to give 15 ml of liquid paraffin twice daily from the time of operation. In a few cases this mild laxative will suffice to produce a bowel action during the next couple of days, but if, as is usually the way, no action has occurred by *the evening of the second postoperative day*, counting the day of operation as 0, a more drastic agent, such as 3·5–5 ml of liquid extract of cascara or three tablets of Senokot, is given. The following morning the bowels usually act in an adequate manner but, if they do not, either another dose of the stronger aperient is prescribed or a soap and water enema is given. This consists of 850–1200 ml of soap and water administered through a tube and funnel attached to a No. 10 Jacques catheter. The insertion of the latter, well lubricated, through the anal canal, need not cause any real discomfort despite the anal wounds, if carefully done. The patient retains the enema as long as possible and then uses a bedside commode rather than a bed pan for the resulting motion.

In cases with small anal wounds, such as after haemorrhoidectomy, the inner gauze dressings come away without difficulty as a rule at the time of the initial bowel action. With larger wounds, as in fistula cases, such separation is not so certain and is apt to be painful. A better scheme in these cases is to *change the inner dressing under a short general anaesthetic* the evening before the bowel action or on the morning itself shortly before the enema is given. The original dressing is removed and fresh gauze squares soaked in Eusol are placed lightly in position. They are unlikely to become firmly adherent by the time defaecation occurs. The catheter for administration of the enema may conveniently be introduced whilst the patient is anaesthetized and left in position for subsequent use.

After the bowels have acted the patient has a hot bath and soaks in it for 20–30 minutes; this will relieve most of his anal pain. Thereafter he returns to his bed and the wound is dressed as described below.

SUBSEQUENT ROUTINE

After the initial defaecation a normal diet is resumed and mild aperients, such as liquid paraffin at a dose of 15 ml each evening, are given as required to secure a regular movement of the bowels each morning after breakfast; the bath and dressing then follow. Later in the day, before his evening meal, the patient has a second bath and dressing, and this routine of morning and evening bath, and dressings continues during his stay in hospital.

TECHNIQUE OF ANAL WOUND IRRIGATION AND DRESSING

The patient lies on his left side with the buttocks projecting over the edge of the bed. If it is the intention to irrigate the anal wound with hydrogen peroxide and then Milton before doing the actual dressing, a mackintosh sheet should be placed underneath the buttock, leading down into a dressing bucket. This arrangement allows of vigorous irrigation of the anal region with large quantities of fluid without any risk of wetting the bed. Another pail is available for receiving dirty dressings. An Anglepoise lamp shines on the anal region. A sterilized 1-litre douche can, fitted with 90–120 cm of rubber tubing and a glass nozzle, is filled with 5-volume strength hydrogen peroxide solution, and the anal region and wound are irrigated to remove all faeces, discharge and adherent dressings. When this fluid has run through, the can is refilled with weak Eusol or 2·5% Milton solution, and the irrigation repeated. Finally the wound area is swabbed dry and examined carefully.

Whilst such irrigations do help to clean up big septic anal wounds, especially large fistula wounds, they are certainly not essential and, provided the patient is having two baths a day with a certain amount of swishing to and fro in the bath, they can be dispensed with, at any rate so far as smaller anal wounds are concerned. In these days of shortage of nurses, it is always important to work out an order of priority for the various demands on their limited time. For some years now I have felt obliged to absolve my nursing staff from any obligation to irrigate ordinary haemorrhoidectomy wounds. Yet these wounds seem usually to have healed very satisfactorily.

For the actual dressing a flat gauze square soaked in Milton solution is then applied, being gently tucked at its inner end into the anal canal if the wound extends in this direction. Further gauze squares and then dry wool are placed on top. At a later stage of the postoperative course, the dressing lotion may with advantage be changed to lotio rubra. A change may be indicated earlier if the skin becomes irritated by the Milton. Alternatively an attempt may be made to protect the skin by applying soft paraffin gauze to it and confining the Milton or Eusol gauze to the raw area of the wound itself.

The dressings are done by the nursing staff, but the surgeon should review the wound every week till healing is well advanced. If occasionally he does the entire dressing himself, it has a very salutary effect on the ward staff and helps to maintain a high standard of attention to anal dressings.

By the time the patient comes to be discharged from hospital, a domiciliary modification of this dressing routine is usually possible with the assistance of the district nurse, one dressing only being performed each day. Alternatively if the wound is then small, it may suffice to have one or two baths daily and to apply a little dry cotton wool to the unhealed area to absorb discharge and protect the clothing; generally it stays satisfactorily in position without a bandage if tucked gently into the anal orifice.

The Use of a Silicone Foam Sponge in Granulating Anal Wounds. Wood and Hughes (1975) have reported their experiences with a silicone foam sponge to replace the gauze packs normally used in open anal wounds. Usually the switch from gauze packing to the sponge was made on the fourth or fifth day after operation. The sponge is created by mixing 10 ml of silicon elastomer No. 386 Dow Corning with 0·6 ml of the catalyst. The best plan is to draw the appropriate quantities of the two viscous fluids up into separate syringes, which are then emptied into a small bowl and stirred with a wooden spatula. The elastomer is then poured into the granulating wound whilst the skin edges are drawn slightly apart. During this period the foam expands to four times its original volume, setting to a soft pliable foam in about 2 minutes.

Immediately after setting, the sponge is removed from the wound cavity and then replaced to demonstrate to the patient how simple and painless a process this can be. It is then fixed in place with a strip or two of 2·5 cm micropore tape. The patient is instructed to have two salt baths a day and to remove the sponge in the bath. It is then washed under running water, squeezing it like an ordinary rubber sponge, and a final rinse is given in an antiseptic such as aqueous chlorhexidine solution.

The patient replaces the sponge in the wound cavity himself. He is seen at hospital weekly and either the size of the sponge is reduced at each visit as required by diminution in the dimensions of the wound by cutting off portions of it with scissors or a knife, or a new sponge is made.

Wood and Hughes (1975) employed this technique of wound management initially in connection with operations for pilonidal sinuses, but have subsequently extended it to other forms of open wound particularly in relation to the anus (Wood et al. 1976). The main advantage of the foam elastomer technique would seem to be not that the wounds heal any better, but that their care can, to a large extent, be left to the patient himself, thus economising on the need for district nursing attention. The silicon elastomer is about to become available on a commercial basis.

PASSAGE OF A FINGER OR ANAL DILATOR

It is important during the healing of anal wounds to make sure that no stenosis is developing in the anal canal by passing a finger periodically. If a tendency to stricture formation is noted it should be countered by instituting the regular passage of an anal dilator, such as the Thorlakson pattern (Fig. 44), once or twice daily as part of the ordinary dressing routine. However at the present time stenosis is a relatively rare complication of anal surgery and I find that I seldom need to prescribe anal dilatation in this way. I think that in the past routine dilatation of the anus has often been ordered as a prophylactic measure in cases that were not in any real danger of developing a stricture. The avoidance of such unnecessary instrumentation adds considerably to the comfort of the patient.

REFERENCES

BUIE, L. A. (1932) In *The Colon, Rectum and Anus*, ed. F. W. Rankin, J. A. Bargen and L. A. Bure. Philadelphia: W. B. Saunders.

DAVID, V. C. (1949) quoted by Orr, T. G.(1949) In *Operations of General Surgery*. Philadelphia: W. B. Saunders.

EISENHAMMER, S. (1953) The internal anal sphincter: its surgical importance. *S. Afr. med. J.*, *27*, 266.

ELLIS, D. (1959) In *British Surgical Practice*, ed. E. R. Carling and J. P. Ross. London: Butterworths.

FAILES, D. (1966) Primary suture of the operative wounds after haemorrhoidectomy. *Aust. N.Z.J. Surg.*, *36*, 63.

FERGUSON, J. A. and HEATON, J. R. (1959) Closed haemorrhoidectomy. *Dis. Colon Rect.*, *2*, 176.

GABRIEL, W. B. (1927) Skin grafts for fistulae. *Proc. R. Soc. Med.*, *20*, 1278.

—— (1948) *Principles and Practice of Rectal Surgery*, 4th ed. London: H. K. Lewis.

GOLIGHER, J. C., GRAHAM, N. G., CLARK, C. G., DE DOMBAL, F. T. and GILES, G. (1969) The value of stretching the anal sphincters in the relief of post-haemorrhoidectomy pain. *Br. J. Surg.*, *56*, 859.

GOODSALL, D. H. and MILES, W. E. (1900) *Diseases of the Anus and Rectum*, Part I. London: Longmans.

HUGHES, E. S. R. (1953) Primary skin grafting in proctological surgery. *Br. J. Surg.*, *41*, 639.

LOCKHART-MUMMERY, J. P. (1934) *Diseases of the Rectum and Colon*, 2nd ed. London: Baillière.

MILES, W. E. (1919) Observations on internal piles. *Surgery Gynec. Obstet.*, *29*, 497.

MILLIGAN, E. T. C., MORGAN, C. N., LLOYD-DAVIES, O. V. and THOMPSON, H. R. (1948) In *British Surgical Practice*, ed. E. R. Carling and J. P. Ross, vol. 4, p. 102. London: Butterworths.

MITCHELL, A. B. (1903) A simple method of operation on piles. *Br. med. J.*, *1*, 482.

POWER, D'ARCY (1910) *Treatise of Fistula-in-Ano, Haemorrhoids and Clysters, by John Arderne*. Oxford: Oxford University Press.

RANK, B. K. (1944) Plastic principles in common surgical procedures. *Aust. N.Z.J. Surg.*, *14*, 14.

STARR, K. W. (1953) Primary closure in proctology. *Postgrad. Med.*, *14*, 365.

—— (1959) Personal communication.

TUTTLE, J. P. (1903) *Diseases of the Anus, Rectum and Pelvic Colon*. New York: Appleton.

WATTS, J. M., BENNETT, R. C., DUTHIE, H. L. and GOLIGHER, J. C. (1964) Healing and pain after haemorrhoidectomy. *Br. J. Surg.*, *51*, 808.

—— DUTHIE, H. L. and GOLIGHER, J. C. (1965) Pain after haemorrhoidectomy. *Surgery Gynec. Obstet.*, *120*, 1037.

WILSON, D. H. (1964) The late results of anorectal abscess treated by incision, curettage and primary suture under antibiotic cover. *Br. J. Surg.*, *51*, 828.

WILSON, E. (1969) Skin grafts in surgery for anal fistula. *Dis. Colon Rect.*, *12*, 327.

WOOD, R. A. B. and HUGHES, L. E. (1975) Silicone foam sponge for pilonidal sinus: a new technique for dressing open granulating wounds. *B. med. J.*, *3*, 131

—— WILLIAMS, R. H. P. and HUGHES, L. E. (1977) Foam elastomer dressing in the management of open granulating wounds: experience with 250 patients. *Br. J. Surg.*, *64*, 554.

4

Haemorrhoids or Piles

Piles are certainly one of the commonest ailments that afflict mankind. It is difficult to obtain any accurate idea of their incidence, but clinical experience suggests that very many people of both sexes suffer from haemorrhoids, and that even more perhaps have piles in a symptomless form. It is a frequent experience to find haemorrhoids on routine rectal examination in patients who have never had any complaint referable to them. The incidence of piles apparently increases with age, and it seems likely that at least 50% of people over the age of 50 have some degree of haemorrhoid formation. However the disease is by no means confined to older individuals, and piles are encountered in people of all ages, including occasionally young children. Men seem to be affected roughly twice as frequently as women.

By common consent the terms haemorrhoids and piles are used quite interchangeably, but etymologically the words have entirely different meanings. The term haemorrhoid is derived from the Greek adjective *haimorrhoides*, meaning bleeding (*haima* = blood, *rhoos* = flowing), and emphasizes the most prominent symptom in the majority of cases. But it cannot be accurately applied to all the conditions diagnosed as haemorrhoids, for a number of them do not at any time give rise to bleeding. The term pile on the other hand, derived from the Latin word *pila*, a ball, can be aptly used for all forms of haemorrhoids or piles, for literally every such condition does produce a swelling of some kind, even though it may not show externally.

CLASSIFICATION

Piles are classified as internal and external piles, the former arising in the upper two-thirds of the anal canal which is lined by columnar-celled epithelium, the latter in the skin-covered lower one-third of the canal or at the anal orifice itself. These definitions, however, refer solely to the site of origin of the piles, for, after they have been present for some time and have enlarged sufficiently, internal haemorrhoids also appear externally at the anus.

INTERNAL PILES

Pathological Anatomy and Pathogenesis

Internal piles have traditionally been regarded as essentially varicosities of the venous plexuses in the wall of the anal canal and lower-most centimetre or so of the rectum. These form swellings covered with mucosa, which bulge into the lumen of the anal canal, especially when the portal venous pressure is raised and the sphincters are relaxed during defaecation and straining. The veins concerned are chiefly those of the submucous or internal haemorrhoidal plexus, which are mainly radicles of the superior rectal (haemorrhoidal) vein. But, except in the very earliest stages of internal haemorrhoids, the subcutaneous or external haemorrhoidal venous plexus of the corresponding segment of the anal canal also participates in the varicose process. The so-called internal haemorrhoid is therefore really often more accurately an intero-external pile, and has an upper two-thirds, above the level of the anal valves, covered with mucosa and a lower one-third below the valves, covered with the skin of the anal canal and anus. In addition to veins, the contents of the pile include a small arterial twig, which is one of the ultimate branches of the superior rectal (haemorrhoidal) artery—and can

93

sometimes be quite clearly palpated against the firm internal sphincter muscle by the examining finger in the anal canal—and also a certain amount of loose submucous and subcutaneous areolar tissue surrounding the vessels. In long-standing piles this latter is converted into denser fibrous tissue so that the piles, instead of being easily collapsible, venous swellings, become palpable on rectal examination.

So much for conventional belief regarding the pathogenesis of piles. But contrary opinions have been expressed. Thus Graham-Stewart (1963) has suggested that internal haemorrhoids could be divided into two categories: (a) *vascular* haemorrhoids, seen mainly in younger persons, in which the distended veins are the main component; and (b) *mucosal* haemorrhoids, more often encountered in older subjects, which are composed in large measure of thickened mucosa. Thomson (1975) has taken an even more iconoclastic view. In an interesting study, in which he injected the superior rectal vein in cadavers, he demonstrated that fusiform, saccular or serpiginous dilatations of the veins of the submucous plexus of the anal canal—the so-called corpus cavernosum recti of Stelzner (1963)—were a regular feature of normal anatomy. Thomson (1975) further claimed that the histological appearances of haemorrhoidectomy specimens did not differ materially from those of the normal anorectal submucosa. For these reasons he maintains that venous congestion need not be invoked to explain the development of internal haemorrhoidal swellings. Instead he favours the suggestion, originally made by Gass and Adams (1950) and supported by Hughes (1957) and Patey (1972), that internal piles are due simply to a sliding down of part of the lining of the anal canal as a result of stretching or fragmentation of the muscularis submucosae ani (see p. 12).

To my mind the serious weakness of this theory of prolapse of mucosal cushions as the primary factor in the production of piles is that it entirely fails to explain adequately the frequent occurrence of bleeding first-degree piles, detected only on proctoscopy and unassociated with descent of the mucosa to that anal orifice. Thomson (1975) meets this criticism in effect by denying the existence of such cases and claiming that the initial symptom in cases of internal haemorrhoids is always prolapse, but this is quite contrary to my experience. On clinical and operative grounds also I would seriously doubt the correctness of his contention that the corpus cavernosum recti is not often considerably more distended in patients with large haemorrhoids than in normal people, especially when the patient is bearing down and the piles are prolapsing.

FURTHER AETIOLOGICAL CONSIDERATIONS

From the aetiological point of view internal piles may be divided into two main categories:

INTERNAL HAEMORRHOIDS IN PATIENTS WITH A DEFINITE ORGANIC OBSTRUCTION IN THE PORTAL CIRCULATION, INTERFERING WITH VENOUS RETURN FROM THE SUPERIOR HAEMORRHOIDAL VEINS

Examples of such an obstruction are:
    Cirrhosis of the liver
    Thrombosis of the portal vein
    Abdominal tumours, notably pregnancy

In surgical practice it is remarkable how rarely patients present with haemorrhoids due to these causes, the explanation presumably being that these conditions are usually recognized by their other symptoms, rectal bleeding being very rare or completely overshadowed by the other manifestations.

Special mention must be made of that commonest of all abdominal tumours, pregnancy, for it leads to haemorrhoids not only by the venous obstruction which it produces, but also by the greatly increased vascularity and laxity of the tissues of the pelvis which result from it. As a consequence haemorrhoids are extrmely common during the later stages of pregnancy. The conclusion of the pregnancy of course corrects these factors and the piles usually undergo a rapid improvement after parturition, but that is not to say that the haemorrhoidal condition always returns to complete normality. Quite frequently the woman is left with small or moderate-sized haemorrhoids which become progressively worse with subsequent pregnancies or advancing age. Pregnancy may thus be considered the commonest known factor in the production of piles in women.

Another mechanical cause of internal haemorrhoids frequently quoted is carcinoma of the rectum, it being alleged that the presence of the growth in, say, the middle one-third of the rectum obstructs the tributaries of the superior rectal veins in its wall and thus leads to venous engorgment and internal piles. It is impossible to say that this very plausible sequence of events may not sometimes take place, but it is probable that the more usual relationship between rectal cancer and haemorrhoids is that they may both give rise to bleeding, and this may be wrongly attributed to long-standing, entirely coincidental piles, when it is really due to a carcinoma.

IDIOPATHIC HAEMORRHOIDS WHERE NO EVIDENT ORGANIC VENOUS OBSTRUCTION IS PRESENT

These cases represent the vast majority of patients with piles encountered by the surgeon. Usually it is impossible to ascribe the haemorrhoids to any particular cause and the most that can be done is to point to a number of factors that may have played a part in the production of the condition in any individual patient:

Heredity. Just as with varicose veins of the lower extremities, heredity seems to be an important aetiological factor in many cases of piles. Thus certain families appear to be specially predisposed to the development of haemorrhoids, so that many or all its members become affected, often at an early age, presumably as a result of some structural weakness of the wall of the haemorrhoidal veins. It is well known that haemorrhoids and varicose veins of the legs often coexist, suggesting a more widespread defect of venous structure.

Anatomical and Physiological Factors. A characteristic of the portal system of veins is that it is completely devoid of valves so that in the erect position the entire column of blood in the superior rectal, inferior mesenteric, splenic and portal veins from anal canal to liver bears directly on the internal haemorrhoidal venous plexus. In the ordinary way, however, the haemorrhoidal veins in the submucosa of the anal canal are firmly supported by the close apposition of the walls of the canal under the contraction of the anal sphincters. It is during defaecation when the anal canal is opened to atmospheric pressure, and at the same time the pressure on the portal system is greatly increased by straining, that distension of the haemorrhoidal veins is liable to occur. Additional factors promoting venous congestion during defaecation are compression of the superior haemorrhoidal veins as they lie in the submucosa in the lower rectum by the descending mass of faeces, especially if the motion is hard and constipated, or constriction of the veins by the contracting muscle of the rectal wall as they make their way through it at a higher level.

Some degree of distension of the haemorrhoidal venous plexus in the anal canal is presumably an inevitable accompaniment of every act of defaecation. It seems possible that this regularly recurring momentary haemorrhoidal engorgement in people who have perfectly normal bowel habits may be quite sufficient in the course of years to result in the development of internal piles by the time late middle age is reached. Especially will this be so if there is any inborn weakness of venous structure.

Constipation, Diarrhoea and Straining at Stool. Clearly the distending effect of normal defaecation on the haemorrhoidal plexus may be greatly magnified if the patient suffers from constipation and has to engage in prolonged and repeated straining to pass large hard motions. Diarrhoea if associated with much tenesmus and futile straining may have a similar, but slightly less injurious effect, and the same may be said of irritating aperients such as aloes, phenolphthalein and salts, which may result in some degree of tenesmus with straining. Faulty habits of defaecation can be equally bad, for some individuals instead of having a smooth, easy daily motion lasting at most a few minutes, indulge in an orgy of protracted straining at stool interspersed with reading of the morning newspaper. Such a practice may concentrate into 12 months the injurious effects on the haemorrhoidal veins of 12 years of normal defaecation.

Epidemiology and Diet. Burkitt (1972) has drawn attention to the fact that haemorrhoids are excessively rare throughout rural Africa and almost unknown in the more primitive communities. This contrasts with the not infrequent occurrence of haemorrhoids in American negroes and in the urban population of Africa where a more Western type of life and, in particular, diet obtains. Burkitt (1972) believes that the important difference between the primitive African and the African who has become or is in the process of becoming Westernized lies in the elimination of cereal fibre from the diet of the latter two groups with a resulting considerable delay in faecal transit time in the bowel and a high incidence of chronic constipation.

Deficiency of the Anal Sphincters, Alterations of Sphincter Tone. In patients who have had operations for anal fistulae involving division of a considerable part of the sphincters on one aspect of the anal canal, the venous plexus in the opposite wall, deprived of its normal support, frequently develops a haemorrhoidal swelling. In haemorrhoid patients who have not had anal operations there has been some difference of opinion as to whether the sphincter tone is normal or not. In anal pressure studies comparing patients with haemorrhoids and normal control subjects Hancock and Smith (1975) and Arabi et al. (1977a) observed significantly higher pressures in the former, though how this raised pressure might be aetiologically relevant is difficult to understand. Arabi et al. (1977a) were struck by the poor correlation between the impression of laxity of the anal sphincters on digital examination in such patients and the actual pressure recordings.

NUMBER AND POSITION OF INTERNAL PILES

It might be expected that the number and arrangement of internal haemorrhoids in the anal canal would vary greatly from patient to patient, but in fact the distribution is remarkably constant. In the great majority of patients there are three main piles which occupy well-defined positions; two are present on the right side of the anal canal and are termed the *right anterior* and *right posterior* piles respectively, and the third forms on the left side and is the *left lateral* pile (Fig. 66). Additional haemorrhoids may be present between these main piles but it is surprising how rare they are; I should estimate that some 60–70% of patients with internal piles seen by me have little other than three primary haemorrhoids.

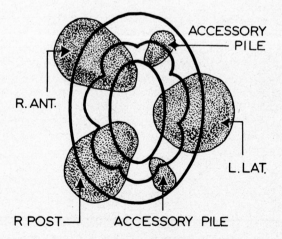

Fig. 66. Diagram of the anal region indicating the position of the three primary piles and secondary or accessory piles.

Miles (1939) postulated—without producing any evidence for his belief—that this arrangement of the piles was due to the difference in the termination of the right and left main branches of the superior rectal artery, the left branch continuing essentially as a single vessel, whilst the right branch splits into an anterior and a posterior branch; consequently when the associated radicles of the superior rectal vein become varicose, two sets of haemorrhoids form on the right side but only one on the left. But Thomson (1975) injected the superior rectal artery in cadavers and was quite unable to substantiate Miles' (1939) statement.

DEGREES OF HAEMORRHOID FORMATION

Internal haemorrhoids vary greatly in size. In their earliest stages they merely project slightly into the lumen of the anal canal when the veins are congested at defaecation. These are said to be *first-degree haemorrhoids*. In time, however, the piles tend to form larger swellings which not only protrude into the canal, but also descend towards the anal orifice so that eventually the mucosal surface corresponding to the piles may appear externally whilst the patient is straining, but return spontaneously to the anal canal when the motion has been passed and the defaecating effort has ceased. These are *haemorrhoids of the second degree*. At a still later stage the piles prolapse even more readily and not only protrude during defaecation but remain prolapsed afterwards until they are digitally replaced within the anus. Further exertion of any kind is liable to force the piles down once more, necessitating further reposition. Piles which prolapse in this way are classified as *haemorrhoids of the third degree*. Lastly some very long-standing piles in elderly subjects become so large and develop such considerable skin-covered components they they cannot be properly returned to the anal canal, but instead remain as a permanent projection of anal mucosa. These completely irreducible piles are *haemorrhoids of the fourth degree*. In the past the term *intero-external haemorrhoids* has often been reserved for this advanced state of affairs.

Symptoms

There are two cardinal symptoms of internal haemorrhoids, *bleeding* and *prolapse*, and it is on account of one or other of these that the average patient with haemorrhoids reports to his doctor. *Pain* is not usually considered to be a symptom of uncomplicated internal piles; however a history of some pain was elicited in 86% of 138 haemorrhoid patients carefully interrogated by Bennett et al. (1963), and was the main complaint in 18% of these cases. Particularly severe pain may occur if the piles become prolapsed and thrombosed. Other symptoms which may develop in certain cases are *discharge* and *anal irritation*. In patients who have been bleeding fairly severely for some time, regeneration may not keep pace with blood loss and symptoms of a *secondary anaemia* may develop. It is traditional teaching that patients with piles tend to become depressed and introspective.

BLEEDING

This is usually the first symptom and occurs initially as a slight streak of blood on the motion or toilet paper, especially when the patient is constipated. At this stage it can often be avoided by securing regular easy bowel actions. Later it takes place more readily and the patient may find that there is a steady drip of blood for a few minutes after the motion has been passed. At a still later stage, when the piles have become much larger, bleeding may occur apart from defaecation at any time when the piles prolapse and become congested. Under these circumstances the patient may find that he is apt to loose blood quite spontaneously into his clothing and may suffer several severe haemorrhages in this way.

Stelzner (1958) has emphasized that the blood that escapes from haemorrhoids is bright red in colour and therefore arterial rather than venous in character. He explains this fact by his finding of arteriovenous communications in the corpus cavernosum recti, making it a sort of erectile tissue.

PROLAPSE

Prolapse of the haemorrhoids is a later development as a rule. It occurs initially at defaecation, the pile appearing at the anal orifice at the height of the expulsive effort, and slipping back immediately afterwards. Later the piles tend to remain in a prolapsed condition after the motion has been passed and the patient finds it necessary to replace them digitally into the anal canal. At this stage they are also liable to come down on any exertion such as sneezing, coughing, lifting, walking or on passing flatus, so that the patient may find himself frequently inconvenienced by the piles prolapsing at various times during the day. Finally a stage is reached when the piles are more or less permanently prolapsed, with anal mucosa exposed and in contact with the underclothing.

DISCHARGE

A mucoid discharge from the rectum can occur in any case with prolapsing piles but is most severe in patients with piles that are in a permanently prolapsed condition. The soiling of the underclothing with mucus and sometimes faecal matter then becomes a troublesome symptom.

ANAL IRRITATION

Irritation of the perianal skin, due to its becoming moist and sodden from discharge, is an almost invariable accompaniment of large third-degree haemorrhoids, and may also occur in other cases with a less severe degree of prolapse.

SYMPTOMS OF SECONDARY ANAEMIA

It is important to remember that bleeding from internal haemorrhoids can be a cause of secondary anaemia. In addition to the local symptoms, therefore, the patient may complain of breathlessness on exertion, dizziness on standing, lethargy and pallor due to increasing anaemia. Also occasionally, from a sense of false modesty, patients may omit to mention to their doctor that they are having rectal bleeding but may describe only their general symptoms. It behoves him therefore to bear in mind this cause of an unexplained secondary anaemia.

Examination

Examination follows the routine lines adopted in any rectal case, and includes examination of the abdomen and, if necessary, haematological investigation of any suspected anaemia.

INSPECTION

Large third-degree haemorrhoids will be readily recognized as projecting masses, the outer part of which is covered with skin, the inner portion with red or purplish anal mucosa, the junction between these two areas being marked by a linear furrow. In long-standing cases of prolapsing haemorrhoids, where the mucosa has been in frequent contact with the clothing over a period of months or years, the lining epithelium often undergoes metaplasia to a squamous type, which is seen as a pale white *pannus*

extending from the mucocutaneous junction over the most dependent part of the mucosal surface and terminating in a rather irregular edge. In advanced cases of this kind the perianal skin frequently shows characteristic changes of pruritis ani.

With second-degree internal haemorrhoids there is naturally no projection of the mucosa, but the skin-covered components of the piles may be evident at the anal orifice as distinct swellings in the three main positions, and most frequently on the right anterior aspect. Gentle traction with the fingers on these loose folds or swellings often succeeds in drawing down some of the anal mucosa, again most frequently in connection with the right anterior haemorrhoid. First-degree haemorrhoids do not usually produce any abnormality of the anal region that can be detected on simple inspection.

PALPATION

Piles in their earlier stages are soft, easily collapsible, venous swellings, quite imperceptible on digital palpation. It is only after they have been present for some time and have prolapsed that the submucous connective tissue undergoes fibrosis and the pile becomes palpable. It can then be felt as a soft longitudinal fold, as the finger is swept round the lower rectum.

PROCTOSCOPY

Proctoscopy is the essential step in the examination for internal haemorrhoids. If haemorrhoids are present they tend to bulge into the end of the proctoscope like grapes, when the patient bears down slightly and the instrument is gradually withdrawn. Sometimes when this is done one of the piles starts to bleed, and the actual spot from which the haemorrhage is occurring can be clearly seen.

To assess the size and degree of the haemorrhoids the withdrawal of the proctoscope is continued till it just emerges from the anal orifice, the patient being instructed to maintain his expulsive effort. If now no red anal mucosa is evident at the anal orifice the piles are only first-degree; alternatively if mucosa does project the piles are second- or third-degree. The patient is next requested to cease straining. If the piles are of second-degree variety they immediately slip back into the anal canal out of view, and the anal orifice closes over them. But if they are third-degree piles the mucosal prolapse persists after the cessation of straining till it is reduced digitally.

SIGMOIDOSCOPY

This becomes specially important when procto-scopy fails to reveal any significant haemor-rhoids to account for the patient's bleeding, but it is a wise routine measure in all cases attending a rectal clinic with haemorrhoids or other minor rectal complaint, especially if the patients are over 40 years of age. Occasionally—admittedly very rarely—an entirely unsuspected rectal or sigmoid carcinoma is detected in this way.

ABDOMINAL EXAMINATION

This requires no comment.

Complications and Sequelae

THROMBOSIS

This is almost always a complication of large prolapsing second- or third-degree haemorrhoids and is believed to be due to their becoming nipped by the sphincter muscles whilst in the prolapsed position, so that congesion and thrombosis result. As a consequence the pile becomes hard and tender and is usually irreducible. At the same time considerable oedema develops in the adjacent peri-anal skin and subcutaneous tissues, forming a large swelling external to the pile and partly concealing it at the anal orifice. Thrombosis may occasionally occur in the external haemorrhoidal plexus as well and contribute to the swelling. Prolapse and thrombosis is a complication which may affect all the haemorrhoids present in a particular patient or may be confined to one or two. Very rarely thrombosis occurs quite spontaneously apart from prolapse and produces a tender induration of a pile in its normal position inside the anal canal and rectum.

CLINICAL FEATURES

The symptom which suggests that a patient has pro-lapsed thrombosed piles is the occurrence of a painful swelling at the anus which makes sitting on the part or having a motion extremely uncomfort-able. This state of affairs is known to the laity as 'an attack of piles'. Inspection of the part shows a very considerable oedematous swelling in the anal and perianal region (Fig. 67A). The outer and greater part of this swelling is covered with skin and is usually soft and oedematous, but sometimes tender hard areas of thrombosis of the external haemor-rhoidal plexus may be detected in it. The inner aspect of the swelling is covered with mucosa which

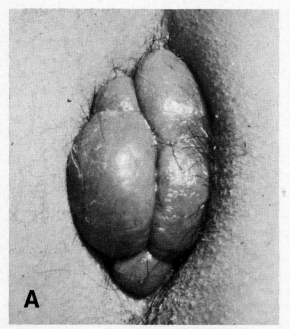

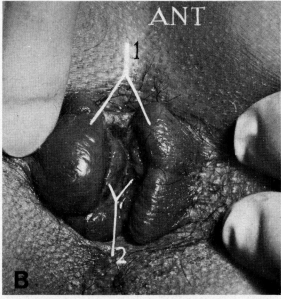

Fig. 67. Prolapsed thrombosed internal haemorrhoids. (A) The gross oedema of the skin and subcutaneous tissues at the anal orifice. (B) On retracting the larger oedematous, skin-covered perianal swelling (1), the inflamed mucosa (2) of the piles is seen.

differs from the mucosal prolapse of ordinary third-degree haemorrhoids in that it is firm and exquisitely tender due to clotting in the underlying veins. Often this prolapsed mucosa is completely overshadowed by the oedematous skin-covered part of the pile and may indeed not be evident till the latter has been retrated laterally to expose it (Fig. 67B). Digital examination of the anal canal and rectum is extremely uncomfortable in cases with thrombosis, but if it can be tolerated by the patient it confirms the extent of the process and shows whether all three piles are involved or not. Usually proctoscopy is quite impossible because of the pain.

COURSE

The natural course of events in the majority of cases with this complication is *spontaneous resolution*. After a few days the swelling and oedema diminish and the thrombosed pile gradually recedes into the anal canal. As a consequence of the episode of thrombosis the pile may eventually undergo considerable shrinkage and become reduced in size compared with its condition before the attack, and this may be attended by a corresponding symptomatic improvement with cessation of bleeding and prolapse at defaecation. Very rarely after an attack of thrombosis the pile undergoes a dense fibrosis and projects as a large fibroid mass at the anal orifice.

In certain cases the course after thrombosis is less favourable and the condition progresses to actual *sloughing and ulceration* of one or more of the piles. The necrotic process is often confined to localized areas of the mucosa, but at other times may involve a considerable part or all of the substance of the pile, and very exceptionally, due to the spread of the thrombosis, the sloughing may extend to the rectal wall with resulting serious sepsis in the pelvis (see Lockhart-Mummery and Joshi 1915). With the more usual, less extensive forms of necrosis, the devitalized portion of tissue gradually separates leaving an ulcerating area which gradually becomes retracted into the anal canal where it persists as a raw surface till epithelialization occurs.

Though thrombosis in prolapsed piles would appear to be primarily a non-infective process in the first instance, obviously when necrosis and ulceration takes place some degree of infection becomes inevitable. Sepsis may also occasionally occur apart from sloughing. *Abscess formation* may then result either in the submucosa or in the perianal or ischiorectal region and may be difficult to detect in the first instance, so that it may actually discharge spontaneously before it is diagnosed.

Another more serious, but fortunately excessively rare, septic complication is *portal pyaemia* due to infection of the clots in the internal haemorrhoidal venous plexus with discharge of septic emboli into the superior haemorrhoidal and portal veins. I have never personally encountered this complication but fatal examples of it in cases with prolapsed thrombosed piles have been recorded by Lockhart-Mummery (1934) and Gabriel (1948).

Diagnosis

The diagnosis of internal haemorrhoids is usually readily established by consideration of the history combined with careful examination, especially by proctoscopy. Minor degrees of the condition may be difficult to distinguish with confidence, for most individuals have normally a certain laxity of the anal mucosa, so that it may prolapse slightly into the proctoscope on straining. It is difficult to say when this state of affairs ceases to be normal and becomes first-degree piles. If the history is compatible with small haemorrhoids and not particularly suggestive of any other lesion such as carcinoma, and abdominal examination and sigmoidoscopy are negative, the correct policy is to carry out injection treatment as a therapeutic test. Early piles of this kind respond dramatically as a rule to such treatment and the bleeding ceases immediately. Any continuation or rapid recurrence of the bleeding therefore demands further investigation by barium enema.

If in the first instance examination shows quite definite or even large internal haemorrhoids and no other abnormality, but the patient has some symptoms such as a recent increase in constipation or looseness of the motions, he must obviously be submitted to radiological examination of the colon before a final diagnosis is made, especially if he is over middle age. Internal haemorrhoids are so common that they are frequently present coincidentally with carcinoma of the rectum or colon.

Treatment

Three forms of treatment are available for internal haemorrhoids:
   Palliative
   Injection
   Operative

PALLIATIVE TREATMENT

Small piles which are discovered during the course of a routine examination for another condition and which have caused no symptoms are usually best left without treatment of any kind. But if the patient has had any complaint referable to his piles—either directly as bleeding or prolapse, or indirectly in the form of, say, pruritus ani—then active treatment by injections or operation should be advised. Injection treatment is so safe and disturbs the patient so little whatever may be the state of his general health, that there can seldom be any justification for treating piles by medical measures alone as is sometimes recommended. (The management of piles in pregnancy admittedly represents to some extent an exception to this generalization as will be discussed later on p. 102.) Medical measures have usually consisted of aperients or advice regarding diet to overcome habitual constipation. Unquestionably the most fashionable prescription for this purpose in recent years has been unprocessed bran (see p. 898) or other preparations such as Fybogel, designed to increase the bulk of the stools. Just how successful bulk-forming agents *per se* may be in lessening the symptoms of haemorrhoids is difficult to judge. One controlled trial by Broader et al. (1974) showed only a very slight insignificant advantage for such as agent over a non-bulk-forming placebo, but Webster et al. (1978) in their trial found Fybogel to be significantly more successful than a placebo. Local medical treatment for haemorrhoids has comprised the use of ointments and suppositories of various kinds, one of the most popular of the latter being Anusol. The value of these preparations is in the highest degree doubtful, but in the eyes of the patients they have the great psychological advantage of being applied directly to the site of origin of their symptoms. If the patient should be anaemic an iron mixture should be prescribed to help to correct this state of affairs.

INJECTION TREATMENT

Graeme Anderson (1924) and Bacon (1949) have outlined for us the early history of this form of treatment. Apparently the first person to practice injection of haemorrhoids was Morgan of Dublin who in 1869 treated a case of piles with an injection of persulphate of iron. The method was used also by the well-known Dublin surgeon, Colles, in 1874, but did not find popular favour in Britain, and was allowed to lapse till it was reintroduced from America some years later. Mitchell of Clinton, Illinois, was the pioneer in that country, and, starting in 1871, treated many hundreds of cases of piles by injection with a solution consisting of one part of carbolic acid to two parts of olive oil with good results. Unfortunately Mitchell kept his method a secret and before his death sold the secret to a large number of quacks who roamed the United States and were known as travelling 'pile doctors'. For the most part they used carbolic acid solutions of strengths ranging from 27 to 95% for their injections. Eventually Andrews of Chicago discovered the secret from one of the quacks and gave it to the medical profession in 1879. At first most surgeons spurned the method, but due to the firm advocacy of Andrews and Andrews (1892), Kelsey (1883) and Martin (1904) injection treatment was slowly adopted in America.

In England the revival of the method was encouraged by Swinford Edwards (1888), who used a 10% (sometimes 20%) solution of carbolic acid in equal parts of glycerine and water, and for many years this remained the favourite preparation for injecting haemorrhoids in this country. At first the usual practice was to make the injection into the substance of the pile itself. In 1928 Blanchard described the technique, originally suggested by Albright, of placing the injection not in the pile but above it, and using for the purpose a much weaker solution of 5% phenol in almond oil in doses of 3–5 ml. This method was introduced into England by Morley (1928) and has since become the generally accepted practice. In America however it would appear from the writings of Bacon (1949) and Turell (1959) that the injection of a quinine and urea hydrochloride solution directly into the piles is still the preferred method, but injection treatment is not nearly so popular in the U.S.A. as in Britain.

RATIONALE

The object of injection treatment for haemorrhoids is quite different from that of similar treatment for varicose veins of the lower limbs. In the treatment of varicose veins by injections the aim is to damage the intima and produce intravascular thrombosis. No such effect is sought with injections for haemorrhoids. One reason for this is that it is extremely difficult to inject into the veins of a haemorrhoid, however large the latter may be. Even with a vigorous thrust of the needle into the centre of the pile, the point usually ends up between the veins, not in their lumen.

In practice then the injection is given *into the submucous aerolar tissue* in which the haemorrhoidal veins lie, and the effect of the irritant solution is to produce an inflammatory reaction. The histological features of this reaction have been studied by Dukes (1924) and Pruitt (1931), in internal piles excised at varying times after administration of a haemorrhoid injection of 10–20% phenol in glycerine and water. They found that within 24 hours of the injection there was a marked oedema of the perivenous tissues with infiltration by leucocytes, red blood cells and many large mononuclear cells, often arranged as clusters round the vessels. They observed also proliferation of fibroblasts which increased during the succeeding few days. It is specially to be noted that at this stage there was no thrombosis of the vessels, but clotting became increasingly evident after the fifth day, when also there was an increase in the fibrous elements of the submucosa. More recently Graham-Stewart (1962), using oily solutions, re-investigated the histological reaction to submucosal injections of sclerosants, and found a cellular response consisting of multi-nuclear giant cells, histiocytes, lymphocytes and eosinophils, concentrated round the globules of fat in the submucosa. Extravasation of red blood cells was minimal and there was no evidence of early changes of fibrosis or of thrombosis in any of the blood vessels. Surprisingly, he observed identical reactions after injections of 5% phenol in almond oil and after injections of pure almond oil.

Clinically the fibrous induration at the site of the injection is the outstanding feature two or three weeks after the injection and it presumably corresponds to the increase in the amount of fibrous tissue observed histologically by Dukes (1924). Actually not all patients develop a clearly palpable fibrous nodule, and this may be related to Graham-Stewart's (1962) observation that as much as half or two-thirds of a haemorrhoid injection may subsequently escape through the hole in the mucosa into the lumen of the bowel. Fortunately a good symptomatic response may often be obtained despite the absence of any demonstrable thickening. It is a matter for conjecture really as to how injections achieve their effect. Two possible modes of action may be postulated:

1. Conceivably the fibrous tissue that forms, surrounds and constricts the veins (and arteries) in the submucosa. If the injection has been given low into the pile itself this fibrous tissue may provide a supporting and encasing layer protecting the veins from the trauma associated with the passage of faeces. It also contracts on the vessels and may even obliterate their lumen or lead to thrombosis as has been shown. If the injection has been given high, above the pile, the fibrosis will constrict and possibly completely obliterate the radicles of the superior haemorrhoidal vein and accompanying branches of the superior haemorrhoidal artery in the pile pedicle. This will protect the veins of the pile itself from becoming distended by increased back-pressure in the portal system during the exertions of defaecation and straining. The consequence of these changes will be to diminish venous congestion in the pile and to reduce the tendency to bleeding. In fact this devascularization is the main effect of injection treatment.

2. The fibrosis may also increase the fixation of the pile or its pedicle to the underlying muscular coat and in that way it may reduce the amount of prolapse, but though sometimes very striking this is a much less certain effect.

INDICATIONS AND CONTRAINDICATIONS

It follows from what has been said that injection treatment is chiefly directed at the control of bleeding. Where bleeding is slight or absent but the piles are large and fibrosed and prolapse freely, injection treatment is less likely to be beneficial.

Selection of Cases for Injection Treatment

In selecting cases for injection treatment the most important consideration is undoubtedly the degree of haemorrhoid formation present (Milligan 1939), though other factors have to be taken into account as well. The indications and contraindications for injections may be listed as follows:

Indications

1. For all cases of first-degree internal haemorrhoids, unless there are special contraindications, injection treatment is the method of choice and will give an excellent prospect of complete cure or long freedom from symptoms.

2. Most second-degree internal haemorrhoids should be carefully considered for injection treatment. If they are relatively small the chances of cure or prolonged relief before further injections are required are very good. The larger they are and the more they approach third-degree cases, the poorer become the prospects with injections.

3. As a rule third-degree haemorrhoids cannot be cured by injection treatment, but sometimes injections will afford a very remarkable degree of temporary palliation. For example in patients whose extreme age, poor general condition, or domestic or business commitments make it desirable to avoid or postpone operation, injections may control bleeding temporarily and may even mitigate the amount of prolapse.

Contraindications

1. No injections for piles must ever be given through the skin but only through the mucosa of the upper two-thirds of the anal canal or lower rectum. Injection into a cutaneous covered part would be a most painful experience for the patient. *It follows from this that external piles or the lower, skin-covered components of large internal piles must never be injected.*

2. Injections may be contraindicated in patients who would otherwise be suitable for them because of some associated anal lesion. This is most fre-

quently an anal fissure. The presence of this condition may make the proctoscopy, necessary for diagnosis and injection of the haemorrhoids, too painful for this form of treatment to be commenced till the fissure has been induced to heal. Alternatively, if the piles are pretty large, the simpler plan may be to proceed to an operation at which the fissure and haemorrhoids are dealt with simultaneously. Another anal lesion frequently associated with internal haemorrhoids is skin tags or chronic external piles. Though these can be removed separately from the internal haemorrhoids leaving the latter to be treated by injections, if the external piles are large and numerous it will generally be considered more satisfactory to deal with the entire condition at operation, especially if the internal components are moderately large and therefore likely to recur in the long run after injection treatment.

3. It is generally considered unwise to give injections in the course of an attack of thrombosis of internal haemorrhoids or for some three or four weeks afterwards. Subsequently, however, injection treatment may be very useful in assisting the natural resolution of the piles.

4. After patients have had a certain number of injections the submucosa may become so fibrosed that it will not admit further injection fluid. It may be possible to inject at a lower level but eventually a time will be reached when further injections are quite impossible.

5. Some surgeons regard internal haemorrhoids in pregnant patients as unsuitable for injection treatment, because the condition will improve enormously after parturition, and because there may be a risk of disturbing the course of the pregnancy if injections are given during its later stages. I do not share this view, for many of these patients suffer severely from bleeding which can be relieved by injection and, when required, I have given such treatment to pregnant patients at all stages up to term.

Proportion of Haemorrhoid Patients Suitable for Injection Treatment

The proportion of patients suffering from haemorrhoids whom a surgeon will treat by injections will obviously depend on the way in which he interprets. the indications for this treatment. If the employs injections only for early haemorrhoids, he will probably treat not more than a third of his cases in this way. If, on the other hand, he is prepared to try injections for practically all second-degree internal haemorrhoids as well, and as a

temporary palliative measure for an occasional case of third-degree piles, he will treat a very much larger proportion, though of course he will have many recurrences necessitating further injections or eventually operation. I reckon that *85–95% of the patients with haemorrhoids seen by me receive injection treatment in the first instance.*

PRACTICAL DETAILS OF INJECTION TREATMENT

The Albright method of high injection of a weak carbolic solution into the submucosa just above the anorectal ring has been found by me to be much more satisfactory for routine use than the technique of injection into the pile itself and it alone will be described in detail.

Instruments Required

The Proctoscope. The first essential is a tubular proctoscope of fairly large size. It must be capable of reaching above the anorectal ring. Personally I use the St Mark's Hospital pattern of instrument which has a length of 7 cm (see Fig. 35).

The Syringe and Needle. It is possible to make these injections with an ordinary Record syringe with a long needle, but however carefully the syringe is filled and the needle fitted some of the oily fluid is liable to run down the exterior making it slippery and difficult to handle with confidence. For that reason it is advisable to use a syringe with lateral rings on the barrel and a ring on the end of the piston for the fingers, so that a secure grip can be obtained. An excellent pattern of syringe is that designed by Gabriel for the purpose (Fig. 68). It is made in two sizes and the one of 10 ml capacity is advised. It is fitted with a 7·5-cm long needle which may be either straight or slightly angulated. There is a shoulder on the needle 2 cm from its sharp end which serves as a marker, enabling the surgeon to judge by its distance from the surface of the mucosa how far the point of the needle has penetrated into the tissues. The calibre of the needle is adequate to allow easy passage of the viscous oily fluid along it.

The Solution. A 5% solution of phenol in almond or arachis oil is recommended. My experience (Clark et al. 1967) is that, contrary to the findings of Graham-Stewart (1962) (p. 101), injections of almond oil alone cannot be relied upon to give as good results as those of phenol in oil. The total amount of solution used on the average case having injection treatment is 12–15 ml, so that in the

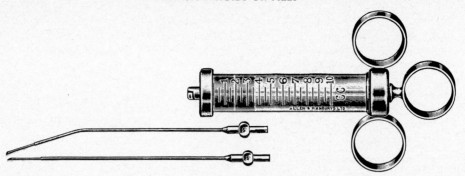

Fig. 68. Gabriel syringe for injection of haemorrhoids. Note that the needle, which fits on to the syringe with a bayonet joint, has a shoulder 2 cm from its tip to enable the surgeon to judge how deeply the point has progressed into the tissues during the injection.

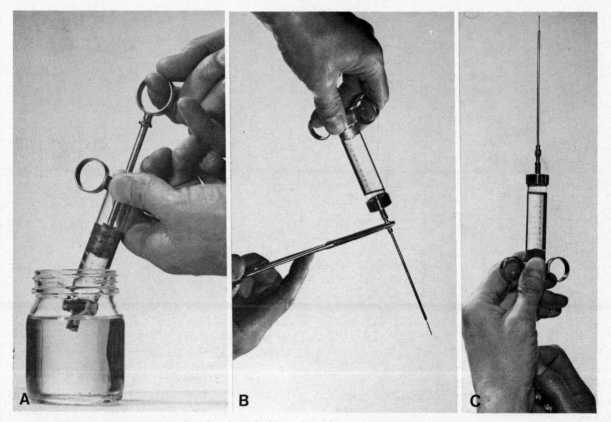

Fig. 69. Filling the syringe with 5% phenol in almond oil in readiness for use. (A) Drawing the oily solution directly into the barrel of the syringe from a wide-necked jar. (B) Fitting the needle tightly with the aid of artery forceps to avoid leaks at the joint. (C) Expelling any air from the syringe.

course of a busy rectal clinic 400–500 ml may easily be required during one session. It is therefore a great convenience in refilling syringes to have the fluid dispensed in a large wide-necked jar into which the nozzle of the sterile syringe may be dipped, rather than in small ampoules which have to be filed open for each case (Fig. 69A). The syringe having been filled, the needle is connected and firmly screwed in position, preferably with the aid of a strong pair of dissecting or artery forceps so as to avoid disconcerting leaks during the actual injection (Fig. 69B). The syringe is then held vertically with the needle point uppermost and any contained air is expelled (Fig. 69C). Finally the

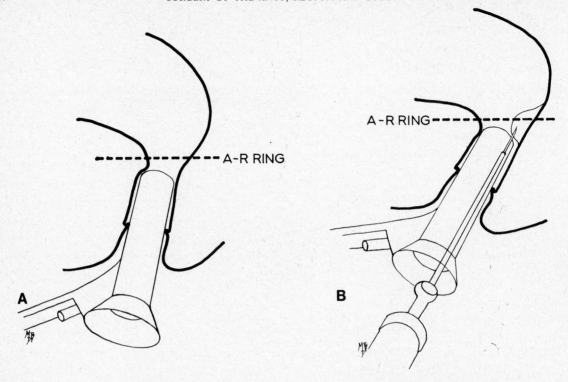

Fig. 70. Mechanics of injection for right anterior haemorrhoid. (A) Proctoscope withdrawn to just below anorectal ring. (B) Proctoscope tilted sharply forwards to bring site for injection of submucosa at or immediately below the ring, clearly into view.

exterior of the syringe and the finger rings are swabbed with a piece of gauze or cotton wool to get rid of any contaminating oily solution. The syringe is now laid down, preferably across a small round bowl or kidney dish ready for use, and it is a good plan to have two loaded syringes prepared as a routine for each rectal case (see Fig. 46).

Technique of Injection

The injection treatment of haemorrhoids is essentially an out-patient procedure which is performed in the course of routine examination in an out-patient rectal clinic or consulting room. It requires no special preparation of the patient or the bowel and can be carried out even when the rectum is rather loaded. As a rule the patient is quite unaware that any treatment has been given or that anything has been done over and above simple proctoscopy.

When a decision has been reached to treat the case by injections the proctoscope is re-introduced, the upper part of the anal canal is inspected and *the anorectal ring is identified.* This is usually easily recognized by the projection of the puborectalis posteriorly. The position of the ring can then be surmised on the anterior or lateral walls.

The next step is to bring the proposed site of injection at or just above the anorectal ring clearly into view. To do this the proctoscope is advanced almost to the ring and then sharply tilted so that its long axis is brought to bear more directly on the bowel wall in the appropriate quadrant. This manoeuvre is most easily done for the right anterior pile because the proctoscope is normally directed to some extent towards the lower anterior rectal wall as it lies in the anal canal, and the surgeon has merely to increase this forward inclination of the instrument as Fig. 70A, B shows. The most difficult injection is undoubtedly that for the right posterior pile, for the proctoscope has to be very sharply angulated backwards to give a view of the rectal mucosa just above the fold which marks the posterior segment of the anorectal junction (Fig. 71).

The Actual Injection. If necessary the mucosa at the proposed site of injection is swabbed clear with a pledget of cotton wool on Emmett's forceps. The needle is then inserted obliquely through the mucosa with a sudden jab. This usually carries it further into the bowel wall than is desirable for the injection, and it is necessary to withdraw it grad-

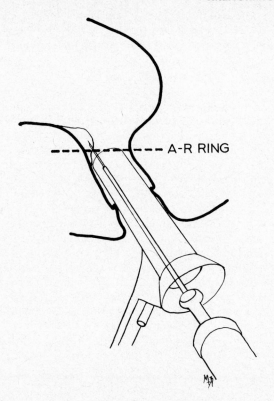

- - - - - - - - - A-R RING

Fig. 71. Mechanics of injection for right posterior haemorrhoid. Note that the proctoscope has to be angled very strongly
backwards to make the site for injection accessible.

On withdrawal of the needle there is sometimes a
little bleeding and escape of phenol solution from
the puncture in the mucosa, but this practically
invariably stops of its own accord or after pressure
with a cotton wool swab on forceps for a few
moments. Very occasionally it is necessary to touch
the bleeding spot with the end of a stick of silver
nitrate to arrest the haemorrhage.

The surgeon now turns to the next injection and
alters the axis of the proctoscope to bring the area
required into view. The swelling resulting from the
other injections may prove a slight impediment,
and this is even more likely to be so when he is
dealing with the last of three piles. But usually with
the aid of forceps and cotton wool swabs it is possible to pack these oedematous folds out of the way
and secure an uninterrupted view of the next site,
and it is practically never necessary to desist without dealing with all three haemorrhoids, where
necessary, at the one examination. However because the right posterior pile is always the most
difficult it is generally wise to inject it first, when no
additional difficulty will be presented by the presence of other previously injected haemorrhoids.

The amount of fluid to be injected at each site will
depend on the laxity of the submucosa, but will
seldom be less than 3–5 ml in a new case, except in
patients who have had previous injections, for in
them it will be found that the submucosa has
usually become so fibrosed that it will only accept a
small amount of fluid. It is because of this fibrosis
interfering with subsequent injections that the
surgeon is well advised *to seek the maximum effect with
the first set of injections and to make these as large as
reasonably possible.*

After-care Following Injections

As a rule no special treatment is required after the
injections have been given. Most patients return to
their ordinary activities on leaving the hospital out-
patient department or consulting room, but it may
be wise to advise against any strenuous exertion for
the rest of the day and to warn them that they may
have a little discomfort in the anal region or rectum
that evening. After each defaecation for a few days
the patient should take particular care to replace
any prolapsing piles. He is asked to attend for
review of his condition and a decision regarding
further treatment after an interval of three weeks.

Immediate Effects of Injections

Pain and discomfort during the injection. It is usually
stated that high injections for internal haemorrhoids are quite painless. This is not entirely true.

ually, judging the position of the point of the needle
from the gap between the shoulder of the needle
and the mucosal surface. During the withdrawal a
very small amount of fluid is injected cautiously
and the reaction in the tissues carefully noted. If the
latter immediately balloons up in an oedematous
weal with obvious vessels crossing it—the so-called
'striation sign'—the surgeon knows that the fluid is
spreading in the submucous plane and the point of
the needle must be in the submucosa as desired. If
on the other hand no weal of any kind is produced
the needle is too deep and the injection is being given
into the muscle coat of the bowel or even possibly
into extrarectal structures. The needle should
therefore be gradually withdrawn till a satisfactory
effect is achieved. If at any stage the mucosa at the
site of the injection becomes dead white this signi-
fies that the fluid is being injected into the mucosa
itself. The result of a mucosal injection is a small
area of superficial necrosis and subsequent ulceration, so that it should be avoided if possible
and the needle inserted again more deeply.

Certainly any severe pain is unusual in competent hands and generally indicates that there has been some fault in the technique and the injection has been given low down in the anal canal into a skin-covered part of the pile. But even with perfectly administered injections there is quite frequently a sense of discomfort of an aching kind experienced deep in the anal canal or rectum. This is felt particularly with large injections, presumably due to the larger amount of fluid extravasating downwards in the submucosa into the pile proper. The sensation becomes progressively more unpleasant as the injection proceeds, especially if it is given unduly rapidly. Once the injection has ceased it soon wanes and disappears altogether within 30–60 seconds, to be renewed with the commencement of the next injection.

Faintness and collapse. Very occasionally a patient feels faint after an injection, not whilst he is lying on the examination couch but when he steps off it and is dressing subsequently. This is probably an entirely non-specific effect, related more to the patient's psychological and physical make-up than to the solution or dosage used. The only treatment required as a rule is for him to lie down for a few minutes and then to resume the erect position more gradually.

Rapid cessation of symptoms. This is the most striking effect to the patient, for usually within 24–48 hours the bleeding has stopped. Improvement in the prolapse is much less marked as a rule and may take some time to show itself.

The reaction to the injection in the rectal wall. This becomes apparent on rectal examination within two or three days of the injection as areas of induration in the wall of the rectum at the sites of the injections just above the anorectal ring and extending into the upper parts of the piles. Generally these areas are about 2–2·5 cm in diameter and they become more prominent during the succeeding two or three weeks and then gradually fade. But they may still be palpable in some cases three to four months later. The mucosa over the indurated areas is closely adherent to the underlying fibrosed submucosa and this can be appreciated by the finger on palpation and seen when the mucosa is touched with forceps during proctoscopy. This fibrous reaction to injections can on occasion feel very like a malignant tumour spreading in the submucosa, and in patients who sometimes present with no clear history of previous injections, the reactionary induration may be mistaken for a growth especially if a small injection ulcer is present as well. Another objective result of the injection is a lessening in the tendency of the piles to prolapse, which, though often a negligible effect, in certain cases may be quite appreciable on proctoscopic examination.

The Need for Further Injections

The fibrous reaction in the wall of the rectum following injections renders further injections much more difficult, especially during the first few weeks. Even months or years afterwards further injections have usually to be smaller than the initial ones, so that I believe the surgeon should concentrate his efforts on the first injections, making them as large as experience has shown to be safe; subsequent injections are accorded a very subsidiary role, and are reserved essentially for patients whose symptoms continue to recur. Some patients who develop further bleeding after an interval of freedom of two or three years can be kept going for fairly long periods in comfort with further injections as required; the technical difficulties of injecting increase each time and may be the limiting factor in the long run.

In repeating injections the problem is usually to find a site that will take a further submucous injection. Points in between the three initial injections above the anorectal ring will be tried first of all, but after several treatments all this region may become quite unusable for further injections. At this stage the surgeon should consider injecting at a lower level directly into the piles themselves. It is generally recommended that when making injections into the piles only small injections should be given, preferably of a rather stronger solution than usual so as to avoid causing much swelling of the pile which might then prolapse and become strangulated. A popular solution for this purpose is 20% phenol in equal parts of glycerine and water. conveniently administered through a Graeme Anderson syringe. In administering low injections, however, I have always employed the standard 5% solution of phenol in almond oil used in the Albright technique, giving up to 4 or 5 ml if possible into each pile, the patient being warned of the necessity to reduce any prolapse after defaecation or straining.

COMPLICATIONS

Necrosis and formation of injection ulcers. In the evolutionary phase of injection treatment, when very strong solutions of carbolic and other chemicals were often used, extensive sloughing sometimes resulted. With the 5% phenol solution now employed necrosis is rare, and when it occurs it is due either to an excessively large dose having been given, or to the fact that the patient has had injections before. Most patients having initial injections can tolerate 5 ml at each site without risk of necrosis. For a period I used regularly to give 10 ml as the standard dose at first injections. Most patients stood this very well but a small proportion, about 1 in 20 or 30, developed some necrosis at one of the sites of injection. Since reducing the dose to 5 ml this risk has been virtually completely eliminated.

The effect of necrosis is to produce a so-called *injection ulcer*. This is often entirely symptomless and is discovered in the course of a routine follow-up examination three weeks after the injections. It usually takes another three to six weeks to heal completely. In other cases it does cause some symptoms, the most common of these being a recurrence of the bleeding which was initially stopped by the injections and which recurs after two or three weeks. This is a source of great disappointment to the patient who naturally assumes that the piles have recurred. Exceptionally an injection ulcer may cause other symptoms such as diarrhoea with passage of a purulent discharge per anum and sometimes a mild pyrexia. Very rarely the bleeding from an injection ulcer may be severe enough to be dignified by the description of a secondary haemorrhage. The condition is immediately diagnosed by digital and proctoscopic examination which reveals ulceration in the centre of one or more of the areas of reactive induration in the rectal wall. In the cases with constitutional disturbance and rectal discharge there may be pus in the rectum, but more usually no suppurative reaction is evident. Usually the condition heals spontaneously in a few weeks and no local treatment has any effect on the rapidity of healing.

Submucous abscess is mentioned by Gabriel (1948) as a rare complication of injections for haemorrhoids but I have never encountered it. Likewise *haematuria* or *prostatic abscess*, due to too deep an injection of the right anterior haemorrhoid with penetration of the prostatic capsule by the point of the needle, has been recorded by Dickson Wright (1950), but must be regarded as a complication of very inexpert treatment.

The inflammatory reaction to injections in the rectal wall is sometimes excessive and may almost completely surround the bowel to form a *stricture and encroach on the lumen*, but this usually subsides in the course of a few weeks without producing a permanent narrowing. The formation of a persistent fibrotic tumour around oil retained in the bowel wall—so called *paraffinoma*—has been described by Rosser (1931), but I have yet to meet this complication.

Operative Treatment
A. Formal Haemorrhoidectomy

The surgical treatment of piles was one of the earliest exercises in operative surgery and was practiced even in ancient Greece and Rome (Parks 1955). The methods used comprised excision, ligation and the use of the cautery. These very same manoeuvres have been passed down through the ages and represent in essence the three main types of operation available for the treatment of haemorrhoids at the present day:

1. LIGATION AND EXCISION

As practised by the ancients and by most surgeons in the Middle Ages down to the first part of the nineteenth century, this operation consisted in applying a ligature to the entire haemorrhoid, including skin- and mucosa-covered portions, and cutting off some of the pile distal to the tie. In those pre-anaesthetic days it must have been an incredibly painful procedure, aggravated by the fact that skin was included within the ligature. This technique continued till Frederick Salmon, the founder of St Mark's Hospital, introduced his modification, which consisted of making a cut with scissors at the mucocutaneous junction of the pile and stripping the mucosa-covered portion up to the top of the anal canal, where it was ligated and the excess excised. This operation was said by Allingham (1901), one of Salmon's successors at St Mark's Hospital, to be followed by much less pain than the older type of ligature operation. The criticism that came to be levelled at Salmon's 'stripping' operation by later surgeons who practiced it, such as Anderson (1909), Milligan (1930) and Gabriel (1948), was that extensive raw areas created by it in the anal canal frequently resulted in wide scarring and fibrous stenosis requiring anal dilatation.

To overcome this weakness of the Salmon operation Lockhart-Mummery (1934) recommended keeping the ends of the main haemorrhoidal ligatures long and suturing them to the edge of the skin wounds below, so as to draw the pile pedicles down and provide a mucosal covering to the raw areas in the canal. Miles (1919) employed a different device to obviate this drawback to the ligature operation. He suggested making the scissor-cut, not at the mucocutaneous junction, but through the perianal and anal skin up to but not beyond the mucocutaneous junction. This separated V-shaped piece of skin, together with the mucosal part of the pile, was then included in the ligature which, when tied, dragged the mucosa down to the level of the mucocutaneous junction and thus avoided extensive denudation of the anal canal of its mucous lining. This might be regarded as a *low ligation* in contrast with Salmon's operation of *high ligation*, but it was none the less a very radical method, which Miles performed over 5000 times with apparently good results. Incidentally Miles never excised any of the pile distal to the ligature because he thought that the escape of blood might reduce the size of the pile stump and predispose to slipping of the tie. The entire haemorrhoid was thus left to slough off.

In 1937 Milligan et al. described a low ligation technique similar in essentials to that of Miles (1919); they emphasized that the ligated pile pedicle in their operation was tethered in the lower part of the anal canal by the longitudinal fibres running through the internal sphincter, and so was prevented from riding up and leaving a large raw area in the wall of the anal canal. This maintenance of mucosal cover, they claimed, avoided the risks of stricture formation associated with high ligation. Their writings have been very influential and as a consequence their technique is, perhaps, the most widely used, at least in this country.

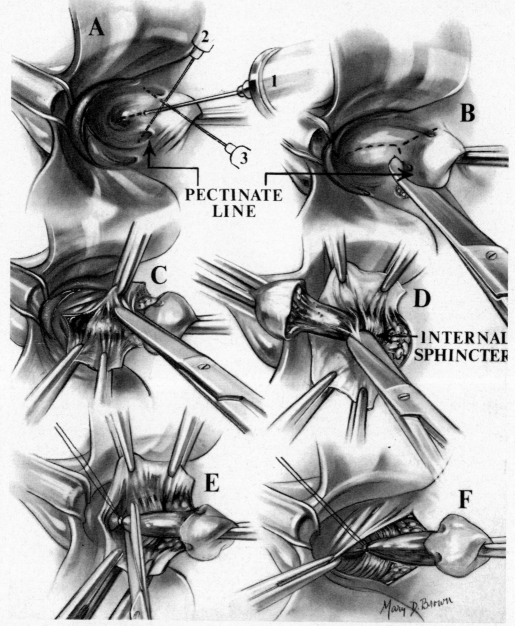

Fig. 72. Submucosal haemorrhoidectomy. (A) The left lateral pile has been drawn outwards by an artery forceps grasping its skin-covered lower pole, whilst a 1/100 000 solution of adrenaline hydrochloride is injected under the mucosa for haemostasis (1). Subsequently the needle is reinserted in different positions (2 and 3) to infiltrate the region of the pectinate line on either side; the solution is also injected under the skin of the lower part of the pile, a total of 20–30 ml being used. (B) The racket-shaped incision, with its handle in the long axis of the pile, is being made with scissors. (C) The lower flap of mucosa and skin has been elevated from the vascular substance of the pile, and the upper flap is in the process of being freed by scissor dissection. (D) The pile is drawn medially whilst its deep surface is separated from the fibres of the internal sphincter. (E) The pile has been transfixed and ligated with fine chromic catgut and is about to be excised. (F) As an alternative technique, the 'handle' of the incision may be dispensed with, and the mucosa dissected up as a cowl or hood. This is actually easier than splitting the mucosa into two flaps, and allows just as high a ligation.

2. SUBMUCOSAL HAEMORRHOIDECTOMY

More recently Parks (1956) has proposed a modification of the ligature operation, originally suggested by Petit (1774) and Cooper (1809), which may be termed a *submucosal haemorrhoidectomy with high ligation*. This operation is performed entirely within the anal canal with the aid of a bivalve speculum, such as Parks' or that shown on p. 52, which exposes the canal throughout its length. The submucous and subcutaneous tissues overlying the pile are then infiltrated with a weak solution of adrenaline (Fig. 72A), not less than 20 ml being used for each pile in turn. A longitudinal inverted racket-shaped incision is made with scissors in the covering of the haemorrhoid; the handle is placed in the mucosa and the circular portion in the skin of the anal canal and perianal region (Fig. 72B). Mucocutaneous flaps are next raised on either side (Fig. 72C), particular care being taken to divide the mucosal suspensory ligament (see p. 12). Then, starting from below, the pile is dissected off the underlying sphincter muscles (Fig. 72D) to the upper end of the anal canal, where the slender pedicle is tied off with fine catgut and the rest of the pile excised (Fig. 72E). The flaps fall back more or less accurately on to the raw area, covering most of it except for the lower portion which extends out into the perianal region where a small open wound remains. One or two catgut stitches may be used to bring the flaps together and fix them to the internal sphincter but it is easy to tear the very friable mucosal leaves by so doing. I have recently employed a modification of this technique in which the handle of the incision is omitted and the dissection is made entirely through the lower circular portion, the mucosa being separated from the pile as a cowl or hood (Fig. 72F).

The *main advantages* claimed for submucosal haemorrhoidectomy are (a) that the main ligature does not include any anal mucosa, which Parks alleges is particularly sensitive, and so pain is very much reduced, and (b) that mucosa and skin are not removed, merely incised so that they fall back into place again after the haemorrhoidectomy and no large raw areas are left to produce fibrosis and stricturing. Parks (1956) states that in 50 cases treated by this method postoperative pain was surprisingly slight, that the wounds healed remarkably rapidly, usually within a week, that spasm was notably absent and that stricture formation occurred in only two cases, but rectified itself without the need for anal dilatation. *The disadvantages* of the operation are (a) that technically it is by no means easy to dissect the mucosa off the pile because of bleeding, which may be very troublesome; (b) the operation is much more time-consuming than most other forms of haemorrhoidectomy; and (c) that recurrences have apparently been more frequent than with the Miles or Milligan–Morgan operation (see also pp. 110–13).

3. EXCISION WITH SUTURE

Excision of Individual Piles with Suture over a Clamp

This method was introduced by Mitchell (1903) of Belfast. As performed by him no attempt was made to define and narrow a pile pedicle, the pile was merely drawn down as far as possible and a large pair of straight artery forceps placed radially across its base, including skin and mucosa-covered portions. That part of the pile lying distal to the clamp was then excised. Next a catgut suture on a curved needle was passed as a continuous stitch over the clamp. Its upper or inner end was knotted, the rest of the suture being left loose after insertion till finally the forceps was released and withdrawn. The stitch was then tightened and this effectively controlled all bleeding. By this method no raw

areas were left to granulate and Mitchell claimed that the wounds were invariably soundly healed within eight to ten days, but gave no actual details of the number of cases treated. It will be noted that in this original version the skin was clamped and sutured along with the mucosa. Many other surgeons subsequently modified the technique to provide for a preliminary skin cut and the preparation of a pedicle to the pile as in the ligature operation. The pedicle was then treated by Mitchell's method of clamping and suturing (Fig. 73).

This has been a very popular method in America where it is generally associated with the name of Earle (1911). Bacon (1949) of Philadelphia has varied the technique further by passing the suture not *over* but, as a continuous mattress stich, *under* the clamp and states that this controls haemorrhage satisfactorily. Mitchell's method has never enjoyed the same popularity in this country, where the ligature operation has usually held the field.

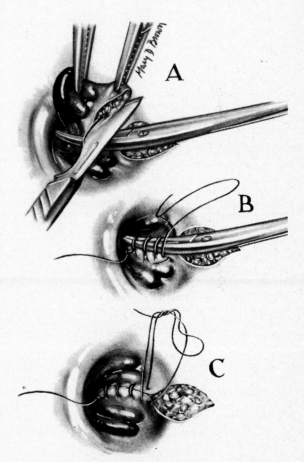

Fig. 73. Clamp and suture method of excision of haemorrhoids (Mitchell's operation). (A) After the skin-covered part of the pile has been separated from the rest of the anal skin by a wedge-shaped cut extending up to the dentate line, a strong crushing clamp or artery forceps is placed radially across the base of the pedicle and the tissue lying distal to it is excised. (B) Continuous catgut suture tied at one end has been inserted over the clamp. (C) As the clamp is removed the suture is tightened and the ends tied.

Excision of Individual Piles and Immediate Suture without a Clamp

More recently a method of haemorrhoidectomy without the use of a clamp has been strongly advocated by Ferguson (Ferguson and Heaton 1959; Ferguson et al. 1971; Ganchrow et al. 1971) and has been widely adopted in America and in some centres in Australia (Failes 1966). In this so-called 'closed haemorrhoidectomy' technique an anal retractor like a Sims vaginal speculum is inserted into the anal canal and exposes the haemorrhoid on the opposite wall. A complete haemorrhoidectomy with high ligation is then carried out and the resulting longitudinal wound in the lining of the anal canal and in the perianal skin is closed with a continuous suture of fine catgut or Dexon. The remaining two piles are then dealt with in turn in the same way leaving the patient with three sutured wounds.

4. EXCISION OF THE ENTIRE PILE-BEARING AREA WITH SUTURE

This is the operation described by Whitehead (1882) of Manchester, which provides for excision of the entire pile-bearing area of the anal canal as a tubular segment, the lower edge of the rectal mucosa then being sutured circumferentially to the skin of the anal canal. Whitehead actually performed the excision in piecemeal fashion through a circular incision in the lower part of the canal just at or above the dentate line. He then made a series of longitudinal incisions extending upwards from it, separating the anal mucosa into areas corresponding to the main piles. These areas were stripped up and ligated individually at the anorectal junction, the rectal mucosa then being drawn down and sutured to the skin of the pecten, providing the anal canal with a new mucosal lining.

In several respects the results of this operation were most unsatisfactory. Firstly, its performance was attended by quite considerable blood loss, which in pre-transfusion days sometimes involved shock and some risk to life. Secondly, the removal of the sensitive anal and lower rectal mucosa often interfered seriously with the normal mechanism of continence. These patients frequently developed a form of sensory incontinence which was further aggravated by the fact that the rectal mucosa often protruded at the anal orifice and greatly increased the tendency to leakage of mucus. Thirdly, though the idea of immediate mucocutaneous apposition by suture with the avoidance of all raw areas was theoretically attractive, in actual practice primary union was seldom achieved. As a result the patients were frequently left with a circular granulating wound which usually led to the production of a stricture at the anal orifice, as Anderson (1909) found in a follow-up survey of cases treated by this operation at St Mark's Hospital. And lastly, though this may seem a very radical method of dealing with internal piles, it could be argued, as it was by Allingham and Allingham (1901), that there is no reason why the patient should not develop further piles in the new lining of the anal canal. In fact several instances of recurrence were encountered by Lockhart-Mummery (1934).

As a result of these experiences the Whitehead operation has long since been abandoned in Britain, but it has continued to be used by some American surgeons, such as Buie (1932), Granet (1953), McMahon (1956) and White et al. (1972), either for cases with very large intero-external piles, or even routinely, apparently with satisfactory results, though how critically these have been viewed is not always clear. Another enthusiastic advocate of this technique is Starr (1959) of Sydney, who emphasizes that many of the bad results with the Whitehead operation have been due to the fact that the initial cut was made at or below the anal verge with resulting sacrifice of the anal canal skin and eventual suture of the rectal mucosa to the perianal skin. As stressed by Whitehead (1887) himself, the lower limit of the excision should be in the mucosa just above the dentate line, so that the *suture line will be in the anal canal*. With large haemorrhoids, the lower skin-covered parts of the piles are said to shrink up subsequently.

Readers who desire accounts of more recent experiences with the Whitehead operation should consult the publications of the surgeons mentioned above.

5. EXCISION WITH CLAMP AND CAUTERY

Though cauterization had been used as a treatment for haemorrhoids from antiquity, the modern clamp and cautery method probably originated with Cusack (1846) of Dublin. As in the method of excision with suture over a clamp, so in the clamp and cautery operation some surgeons place the clamp radially across the skin and mucosa of the base of the pile. Others make a cut at the mucocutaneous junction or in the anal skin and apply the clamp to the mucosal pedicle thus created. A specially heavy clamp such as Smith's (1875) or Farquharson's (Fig. 74B) is used, with ivory or plastic plates fitted to the under aspect of the blades to diminish conduction of heat to the skin. Moist packs are placed under the clamp on either side further to protect the skin. Most of the pile protruding beyond the clamp is then excised with angled scissors, leaving about 6–7 mm of tissue to be cauterized (Fig. 74D). For this purpose it is best to use the actual cautery in the form of a poker, a soldering-iron, or a special rectangular block of metal on a long handle (Fig. 74A). The cautery should be heated to a dull red heat; it is then applied firmly to the projecting remnant of pile and held in contact with the blades of the clamp for 2 minutes to heat them and thus cauterize and 'gum together' the tissue included in their grasp (Fig. 74E). Finally the clamp is released allowing the linear eschar to recede, and the other piles are dealt with in turn (Fig. 74F).

It would appear from the report of Anderson (1909) that if care is taken to exclude skin from the clamp the method is probably less painful than any other technique for haemorrhoidectomy. Cormie and McNair (1959) thought that, even if skin were included in the clamp, the method caused less discomfort than the standard low ligature operation. It is commonly believed that it is more liable to be followed by re-actionary or secondary haemorrhage than other methods, but this was not the experience of Anderson (1909). He found also that the clamp and cautery technique very seldom led to stricture formation. Yet despite these favourable results it has never been widely used in Britain, probably because it has seemed to most surgeons a cumbersome way of accomplishing what can be done more easily by a simple ligature.

COMPARATIVE ASSESSMENT OF DIFFERENT FORMS OF HAEMORRHOIDECTOMY

Though a certain amount of information is available in the literature on the outcome of various forms of haemorrhoidectomy, remarkably few papers provide any controlled comparisons of the different methods. To rectify this defect in our knowledge a number of studies were undertaken a few years ago in my department contrasting five types of haemorrhoidectomy—excision with low ligation, excision with high ligation (Milligan–Morgan operation), excision with primary suture, submucosal excision and excision with the clamp and cautery—in regard to the initial healing of the wounds and the subsequent development of fibrosis, skin tags and recurrent haemorrhoids and to the occurrence of postoperative pain:

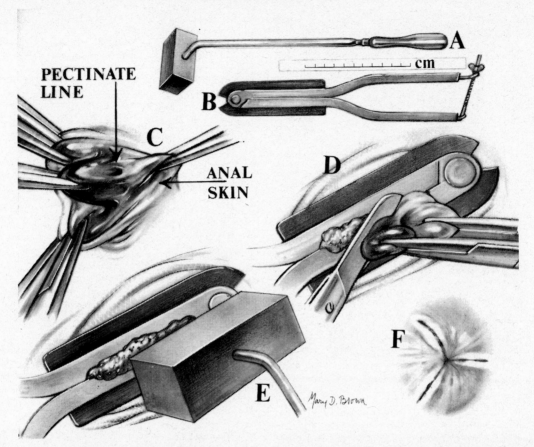

PECTINATE LINE

ANAL SKIN

Fig. 74. Haemorrhoidectomy by clamp and cautery method. (A) Farquharson's haemorrhoidectomy cautery. (B) Farquharsons' haemorrhoidectomy clamp. (C) After the anus has been stretched and the three main piles have been drawn down with artery forceps, the left lateral pile is held out for application of the clamp. (D) The clamp is placed radially across the base of the entire pile, including the skin-covered part. Dry or moist abdominal packs are tucked round the pile under the plastic blades of the clamp, to increase the insulation of the surrounding skin and mucosa from the heat of the cautery. All but 6 mm of the substance of the pile projecting beyond the clamp is excised with scissors. (E) The cautery iron, heated to just short of a dull red heat, is applied firmly to the projecting remnant of tissue and held in position for 10–20 seconds after all smoking has ceased, so as to heat the blades of the clamp as well. The clamp is then quickly released and removed. (F) The three radial linear eschars left at the end of the complete operation.

WOUND HEALING

Most ideas on the subject of healing after haemorrhoidectomy seem to have been based on observation of the external wounds together with palpation of the anal canal at varying intervals after operation, and supplemented by a good deal of conjecture. But these methods of examination provide little reliable information regarding the state of the wounds *in the anal canal itself*, except retrospectively, when, on occasion, on the examining finger, a gross fibrous stricture is detected by the examining finger. To display the *intra-anal* wounds during the phase of healing requires the passage of an anal speculum (see Fig. 37) as was done in our study (Watts et al. 1964).

Initial Raw Areas and Subsequent Epithelialization

The raw areas present in the anal canal and perianal region at the conclusion of the different operations and during the next 10 days are depicted in Figs 75–79. It will be seen that, contrary to

the claim of Milligan et al. (1937), there is actually little difference in the extent of the raw surfaces left after excision with low ligation and excision with high ligation. Excision with primary suture was disappointing too in that by 10 days after operation the intra-anal wounds had almost invariably separated, but primary healing of the skin wounds was more common and nearly 50% of these wounds united satisfactorily, though never more than one or two in any individual patient. As regards epithelial cover the most impressive method was submucosal haemorrhoidectomy, for 10 days after operation most of the intra-anal wounds had healed and the remainder were usually represented by narrow longitudinal strips of granulation tissue; the external skin wounds were usually open, but were generally rather smaller than those resulting from ordinary haemorrhoidectomy with low ligation. Unquestionably the most destructive method was that of haemorrhoidectomy with the clamp and cautery, for, when the linear eschars resulting from this operation separated, the mucosal edges usually retracted widely leaving wide open wounds. In many of the cases one or two of the mucosal strips between the piles were entirely

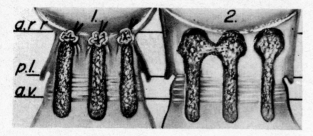

Fig. 75. The opened-up anal canal showing state of wounds after excision of haemorrhoids with *high ligation*. 1. Immediately on completion of operation. 2. Ten days later. (a.r.r. = ano-rectal ring. p.l. = pectinate line. a.v. = anal verge). (*From Watts et al. 1964*)

destroyed and in some cases there was complete circumferential loss of anal canal lining.

If the striking feature at 10 days postoperatively was the great amount of destruction of the lining of the anal canal after several of the techniques employed, the remarkable thing about the findings on later examination was the rapidity with which the mucosa regenerated. Even after the most extensive necrosis of the mucosal lining, this upper part of the anal wounds had invariably healed completely by six weeks from the time of operation. Any delay in healing always related to the skin-lined part of the canal below the pectinate line and to the perianal skin. Actually there was little difference in the incidence of delayed skin healing after the different operations, except that external healing after the clamp and cautery method sometimes took a very long time.

Development of Fibrosis and Stenosis

Of the 100 patients in our detailed study (Watts et al. 1964), none developed stenosis of such severity as to interfere with passage of

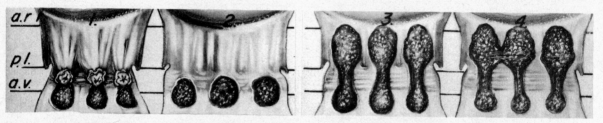

Fig. 76. The state of wounds in the anal canal following excision of haemorrhoids with *low ligation*. 1. At conclusion of operation. 2. Expected findings at 10 days. 3 and 4. Actual findings at 10 days with wounds extending up to anorectal ring and sometimes coalescing. (*From Watts et al. 1964*)

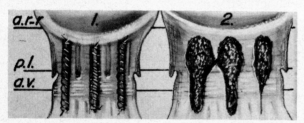

Fig. 77. The condition of the anal canal after haemorrhoidectomy with *primary suture*. 1. At completion of operation. 2. Ten days later, when it is seen that the sutured wounds have largely separated, especially above the pectinate line. (*From Watts et al. 1964*)

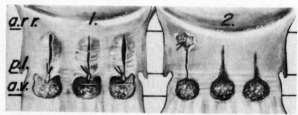

Fig. 78. Wounds in the anal canal following *submucosal* haemorrhoidectomy. 1. At completion of operation. 2. Ten days later, with only narrow linear wounds extending above the pectinate line. (*From Watts et al. 1964*)

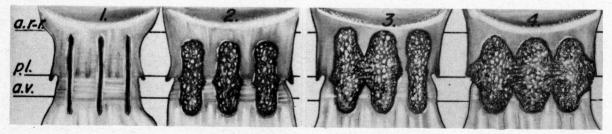

Fig. 79. The state of the anal canal after haemorrhoidectomy by *clamp and cautery*. 1. Linear eschars at completion of operation. 2, 3 and 4. Typical findings at 10 days, with wide wounds reaching up to the anorectal ring and often merging to form partial or complete circumferential raw areas. (*From Watts et al. 1964*)

a finger, but four had sufficient narrowing to prevent the passage of an average sized proctoscope and eight had easily palpable fibrosis which was unassociated with any difficulty in passing a finger or proctoscope. The impression was that fibrosis and stenosis were least common after submucosal excision and most common after the clamp and cautery operation, but the figures were too small for significant statistical analysis.

Formation of Skin Tags

Skin tags were found in 35 of the 100 patients six months after operation. They were particularly common after submucosal haemorrhoidectomy and, contrary to the experience of Cormie and McNair (1959), not specially so after the clamp and cautery operation.

Recurrence of Piles

On proctoscopic examination after any type of haemorrhoidectomy it is not uncommon to find that when the patient bears down vigorously the mucosa between the intra-anal scars and above the sites of excision bulges into the lumen. It is very difficult to evaluate this state of affairs in terms of haemorrhoidal recurrence, unless it is sufficient to result in mucosal protrusion at the anal orifice when the proctoscope is withdrawn, or is associated with recurrent symptoms. In our enquiry, therefore, we disregarded objectively demonstrated symptomless small piles and accepted as significant recurrences only sizeable haemorrhoids accompanied by symptoms for which no other cause could be found. On this basis five patients were considered to have recurrences at six months, four in the group of 28 treated by submucosal haemorrhoidectomy and one in the group of 35 submitted to standard low ligature and excision, none after any of the other three methods. These incidences are too small for proper comparison, but they would arouse some tentative misgiving about the relative efficacy of the submucosal method in avoiding recurrent haemorrhoid formation.

SEVERITY OF POSTOPERATIVE PAIN

Amongst the laity the surgical treatment of piles carries a notorious reputation for the amount of postoperative pain, and not a few patients have long deferred a much-needed haemorrhoidectomy because of their apprehension on that score. Recognition of this fact has been a powerful stimulus to surgeons in introducing various modifications of technique for this operation, yet evidence that postoperative pain is reduced thereby is often flimsy in the extreme and is usually based on rather vague, frequently retrospective, clinical impressions.

Our comparative assessment of pain after different forms of haemorrhoidectomy has been based on three separate studies (Watts et al. 1964, 1965; Goligher et al. 1969), the method of judging the amount of pain being similar in all three. Each patient was interviewed and examined before a panel of six or seven members of the departmental surgical staff on the eighth postoperative day. Initially he was questioned regarding the severity of the discomfort experienced during the first two days and nights after operation, special note being taken of how well he slept, the amount of analgesic required and the reports of the nursing staff and house surgeon. Enquiry was then made about the severity of pain caused by the first and subsequent bowel actions after operation. A careful and gentle digital examination of the anal region was next performed by a member of the panel other than the surgeon who did the operation, and a report given of the amount of discomfort and spasm elicited by this procedure. Finally, with the aid of all this information, members of the panel were asked to write down their individual opinion of the severity of the pain, using one of the following five categories:

A. Almost none
B. Less than average
C. Average
D. More than average
E. Severe

The majority opinion was accepted as the final verdict, it being notable, incidentally, that there was usually fairly close agreement between the members of the panel. By adopting a scoring system in which each patient was allotted so many points according to his category (as A = 1, B = 2, C = 3, D = 4, E = 5) it was possible to work out the total number of points for the group of patients treated by each operation. The mean score could then be calculated for each group by dividing this figure by the number of cases in the group and a comparison made between the mean scores after the different operative methods, the lower the score the less the pain.

Our first two studies (Watts et al. 1964, 1965) compared patients after submucosal haemorrhoidectomy, excision with low ligation (the Milligan–Morgan operation) with and without sphincter-stretching, excision with primary suture, excision with clamp and cautery. They showed no statistically significant difference in the amount of pain after the different methods but suggested that in a larger series of cases the addition of sphincter-stretching might be demonstrated to be of real benefit in reducing the amount of pain after haemorrhoidectomy. In our third study (Goligher et al. 1969) the value of a four-finger sphincter-stretch for four minutes immediately prior to a Milligan–Morgan haemorrhoidectomy was more carefully assessed in 100 cases. It confirmed that patients who had been given a sphincter-stretch appeared to have rather less pain, but this effect for some reason was confined largely to male patients and even in them the difference in the amount of pain just failed to reach statistical significance at the 5% level. Another point that emerged from this study was that after sphincter-stretching there was a higher incidence of minor imperfections of anal control than in patients who did not have this manoeuvre. These disturbances of function were only temporary and cleared up completely in 6 to 12 months as a rule, but whilst they lasted they were an inconvenience to the patients and certainly outweighed the marginal advantage of stretching as regards relief of pain.

CHOICE OF FORMAL HAEMORRHOIDECTOMY OPERATION

It is probably fair to say that good results can be obtained from a number of different methods of haemorrhoidectomy, and in his choice of technique a surgeon will naturally be influenced to a great extent by personal predilection based on past experience. But in the light of our own investigations I would make certain points.

First of all, a preliminary sphincter-stretch is no longer advocated because the modest benefits of this manoeuvre in the relief of postoperative pain do not compensate for its disadvantages in the form of the occurrence of minor degrees of temporary incontinence after operation in the patients on which it was done. Nor have I adopted the alternative procedure, claimed by Eisenhammer (1969, 1974) without controlled evidence, to lessen the pain of haemorrhoidectomy—namely a sphincterotomy of the distal half of the internal sphincter through one of the haemorrhoidectomy wounds.

Secondly, as between submucosal haemorrhoidectomy, the clamp and cautery operation and excision with low ligation, there appears to be little to choose as regards pain. The clamp and cautery operation is a simple procedure in principle, but the administrative and technical difficulties enountered in putting it into practice in a modern operating theatre make it a rather cumbersome way of removing piles at present. Furthermore, it is not readily adaptable to varying patterns of haemorrhoids. In my opinion the ordinary ligature and excision operation is the most generally serviceable procedure, as it is quick and simple to perform, requires no special equipment and is easily within the compass of the average surgeon and surgical trainee. For these reasons it remains my standard form of haemorrhoidectomy and will be described in detail below.

Thirdly, as for excision with primary suture, contrary to expectation, this method was found in our studies to be slightly more, rather than less, painful than other methods. Admittedly the prospect that it offers of avoiding open external wounds is attractive, but even in this respect it is only partly successful, for in most patients at least one of the three sutured anal skin wounds breaks down during the early postoperative period. For these reasons I have not myself felt inclined to adopt 'closed haemorrhoidectomy' as a routine procedure, but because it is so popular in America a full description of its technique will be given (see below).

Fourthly, as the Whitehead operation was not included in our enquiries, I am unable to offer any personal assessment of it in comparison with other methods.

DETAILED TECHNIQUE OF LIGATURE AND EXCISION OPERATION

The ligature and excision operation I use is virtually identical with that described by Milligan et al. (1937).

The patient is placed in the lithotomy position with the buttocks projecting well beyond the end of the table, the anal region is cleansed and sterile towels and instrument table arranged as in Fig. 46.

An invariable routine is the infiltration of the subcutaneous tissues of the immediate perianal region with a

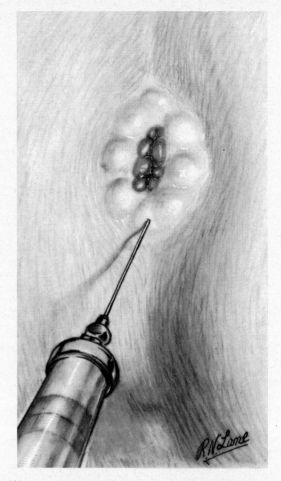

Fig. 80. Ligature and excision operation. Infiltration of perianal tissues with 1/100 000 solution of adrenaline hydrochloride for haemostatic purposes.

1/100 000 solution of adrenaline hydrochloride for haemostatic purposes (*Fig. 80*). This greatly reduces the amount of bleeding during the initial skin cuts and the subsequent steps in the isolation of the piles.

Application of 'skin forceps'. The skin-covered components of each of the main piles are now seized in artery forceps and retracted outwards (Fig. 81). This has the effect of causing the lower poles of the mucosal-covered parts of the piles to protrude to a varying extent depending on the degree of haemorrhoid formation present.

Application of 'mucosa forceps'. The purple anal mucosa of each pile is now taken in another forceps and drawn downwards and outwards. This pulls the pile well out of the anus and brings into view pink rectal mucosa at its upper pole (Fig. 82).

Demonstration of triangle of exposure of Milligan. The traction of the three piles is maintained till pink

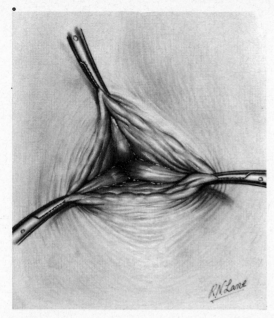

Fig. 81. Ligature and excision operation. Applications of artery forceps to the skin-covered components of each of the three primary piles.

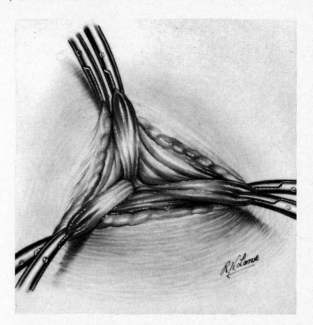

Fig. 82. Ligature and excision operation. Forceps have been applied also to the mucosal-covered parts of the three main piles which are drawn down to produce the 'triangle of exposure'.

rectal mucosa shows not only at the upper part of the piles, but also on the mucosal folds running between the piles (Fig. 82). This indicates that the piles have been drawn down to their maximum extent so that the ligatures will be applied at their upper poles and not about their middle.

Isolation of pedicle of left lateral pile. The two forceps attached to the left lateral pile are taken in the palm of the operator's left hand and drawn downwards and to the opposite side, whilst the operator's index finger rests in the anal canal and exerts pressure outwards and downwards on the upper pole of this pile. With blunt-pointed scissors in his right hand he now makes a V-shaped cut in the anal and perianal skin corresponding to this pile, the limbs of the V abutting on the muco-cutaneous junction but not extending into the mucosa, the point of the V lying 2·5–3 cm distal to the junction (Fig. 83). It will be found that if the tip of the surgeon's index finger is pressed firmly against the end of the scissors as the two parts of this cut are made, the lower edge of the internal sphincter is laid bare, and holding the edge of the skin wound aside exposes it quite clearly (Fig. 84). If the 'skin forceps' is drawn well medially to expose the outer raw surface of the pile, it will be seen that longitudinal strands of fascia and muscle descend into it from the region immediately internal to the inferior margin of the internal sphincter. These

represent the musculus submucosae ani on its way to be attached to the anal skin. In the classical low ligation technique they are not divided, and the only further dissection of the pile consists of making a slight nick in the mucosa above and below to narrow the mucosal pedicle somewhat before applying the ligature. But sometimes recently I have freed the pile further by dissecting it off the internal sphincter for 13–20 mm. This involves division of the longitudinal fibres as they proceed from between the imbricated bundles of the internal sphincter into the substance of the pile. As each set of fibres is severed with the scissors just medial to the edge of the pale internal sphincter muscle bundle pulled down from a higher level, the latter slips laterally and its place is then taken by a still higher bundle. Finally the mucosa is cut upwards for about 6 mm on either side of the pedicle, care being taken to make these cuts parallel or slightly converging as they ascend, otherwise a very broad mucosal pedicle may result. One of the reasons for restricting the incision of the mucosa is that it may bleed in an embarrassing manner.

Application of ligature to left lateral pile. A 30-cm strand of No. 16 braided silk is used for this purpose, applied as a simple ligature usually without transfixion of the pedicle (Fig. 84). The strength of the material allows it to be tied with great force which makes for a very secure ligature

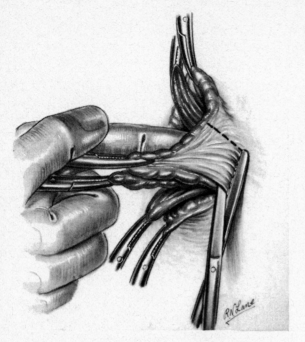

despite the fact that it does not transfix the tissues. There is no reason, however, why it should not be inserted on a needle. If catgut (No. 3, 21-day chromic) is used instead, as some surgeons prefer, it is better to apply it as a transfixion ligature for catgut is more likely to slip. As the ligature is tied the 'mucosa forceps' is removed and applied to the ends of the ligature, so that the left lateral pile is now held by a skin forceps and a ligature with forceps on its tails (Fig. 85). The surgeon hands these forceps to the assistant to hold outwards to the left whilst he turns to the right posterior pile.

Isolation and ligature of pedicle of right posterior pile. This follows the same lines as the isolation of the left lateral pile but the pile forceps are held in the surgeon's right hand and retracted to the right, whilst the *scissor cuts are made with the left hand* (and scissors have to be very sharp and tight at the joint for it to be possible to wield them with the left hand!). Also in making the skin cut it is important to note carefully the position of the skin wound of

Fig. 83. Ligature and excision operation. Making the skin cuts in connection with the left lateral pile.

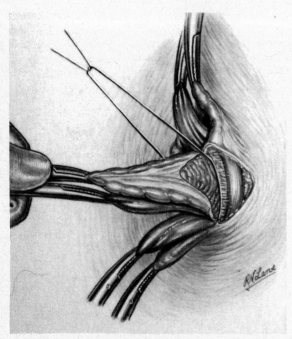

Fig. 84. Ligature and excision operation. After snicking the mucocutaneous junction with scissors at the neck of the pile, the ligature of stout braided silk is applied.

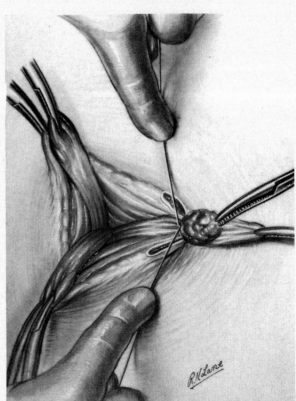

Fig. 85. Ligature and excision operation. Strong traction is exerted on the forceps as the ligature is tied, and finally the 'mucosa forceps' are released allowing the silk to sink into the tissues.

the left lateral pile, and to preserve an intact bridge of skin and mucosa running into the anal canal between it and the right posterior pile.

Isolation and ligature of right anterior pile. Lastly the pedicle of the right anterior pile is prepared and tied along the same lines, care being taken to preserve the skin mucosa on either side of it.

Excisions of piles and cutting of tails of ligatures. It will have been noted that as each pile was isolated and ligated it was not excised but, on the contrary, was retracted in position outside the anus till all the piles had been similarly prepared. Now all three piles are excised leaving at least 1–2 cm of tissue beyond the ligatures, and as the tails are cut short the stump of the piles recede within the anus (Fig. 86).

Passage of finger to assess size of lumen of anal canal. A finger is passed to determine the size of the passage at the site of the ligatures for it is possible to narrow the lumen unduly (Fig. 87). Usually any tightness can be stretched adequately with the finger.

Insertion of dry gauze into anal canal and trimming of anal wounds. To reduce the pile pedicles completely a dry gauze swab is inserted into the anal canal, and the three anal skin wounds examined in turn. Any loose edges are trimmed with scissors to leave three pear-shaped raw areas, which experience has shown heal more satisfactorily as a rule than do smaller haemorrhoid wounds.

Application of Milton gauze dressing, wool and bandage. My practice is to use no indwelling rectal tube or dressings in the anal canal itself. The only dressing applied is a gauze swab soaked in Milton, bunched up and placed on the anal orifice and external wounds (Fig. 87). This is covered with further swabs soaked in Milton, and with dry gauze and wool maintained in position by means of a firm T-bandage.

Recording of operative details. The operative details are recorded most simply and effectively in diagrammatic form as in Fig. 88.

Management of associated accessory piles and anal fissure. Accessory piles can generally be taken along with one of the main piles so that even when several accessory piles are present only three skin wounds are left, but occasionally this is impossible and the inclusion of a large accessory pile necessitates throwing two skin wounds together. This leaves the patient with only two skin and mucosa bridges instead of three and exposes him to a slightly greater risk of developing stenosis, which requires to be watched carefully during the postoperative period. Alternatively one or more of the bridges may be 'filletted' of their vascular elements by

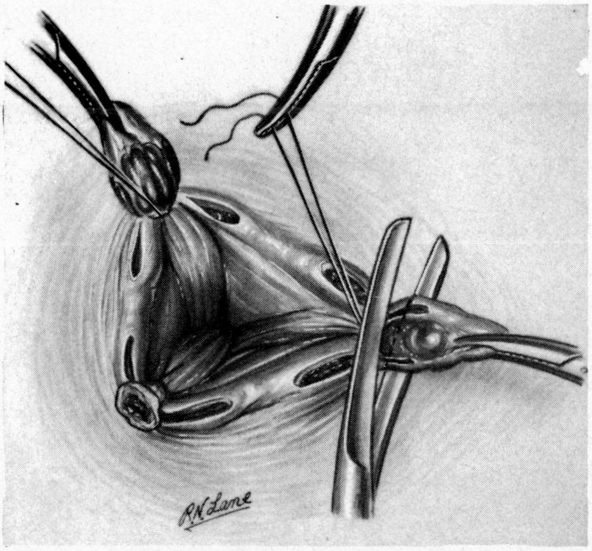

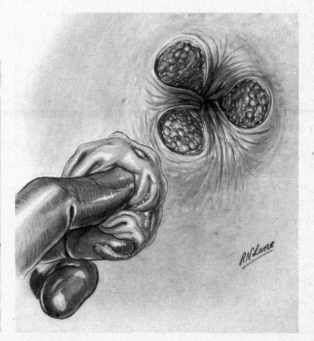

Fig. 86. Ligature and excision operation. All three main piles have now been isolated and ligated. The tissue beyond the ligatures is then excised with scissors leaving an adequate stump to avoid slipping of the thread. Finally the silk tails are cut off.

Fig. 87. Ligature and excision operation. The skin wounds have been trimmed to remove loose edges and leave oval or pear-shaped raw areas. No tube or pack is left in the anal canal. A dressing of gauze soaked in Eusol is simply applied to the external wounds.

ANT.

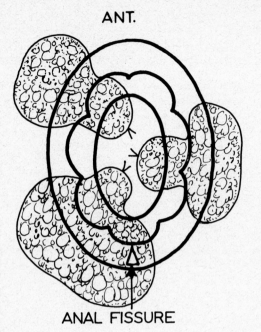

ANAL FISSURE

Fig. 88. Diagrammatic record of straight-forward haemorrhoidectomy.

scissor dissection from either side, keeping the skin and mucosa intact, or the skin may be temporarily divided and subsequently reconstituted by suture.

An associated anal fissure is dealt with essentially by internal sphincterotomy or digital stretching of the sphincters, but it is possibly as well to excise the actual fissure by throwing it into the wound of the right posterior pile.

CLOSED HAEMORRHOIDECTOMY

Position of patient. Though this operation can be done quite conveniently in the standard lithotomy or left lateral position (see p. 85), most American surgeons who use it prefer the prone 'jack-knife' position with the buttocks retracted laterally by means of broad strips of adhesive plaster attached to the lateral edges of the operating table (Fig. 89). I must admit that this prone posture always seems to be a very comfortable one for the surgeon practising this particular technique of haemorrhoidectomy.

Anaesthesia. Many surgeons who choose this form of haemorrhoidectomy find that they can usually do the whole operation under local infiltration anaesthesia, injecting up to 50 ml of 0·5% xylocaine together with 1/100 000 adrenaline circumferentially in the perianal subcutaneous tissues and in the wall of the anal canal. It is wise to supplement the local analgesia with an intravenous injection of diazepam 10–20 mg or of pentothal. Even if a full general or caudal anaesthetic is preferred, a local infiltration of the anal tissues with a weak adrenaline solution in saline is highly desirable for its haemostatic properties during the operation.

Insertion of a Hill–Ferguson anal retractor. Once relaxation of the sphincters has been obtained by local or general anaesthesia, a Hill–Ferguson retractor (which is not unlike a Sims vaginal retractor and comes in three sizes) is inserted into the anal canal to open it up and expose fully the haemorrhoid arising from the opposite anal wall. It is a good plan to start with the pile that seems to be the main offender and to use the largest size of retractor for it.

Incising around the haemorrhoid. The extent of the proposed haemorrhoidectomy on this first pile is outlined by a light elliptical incision with the scalpel, extending from the level of the anorectal ring above to the perianal region below (Fig. 90).

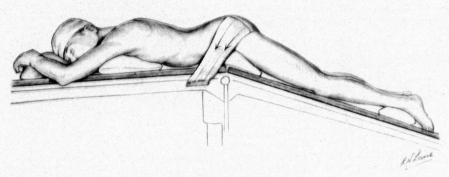

Fig. 89. The prone jack-knife position.

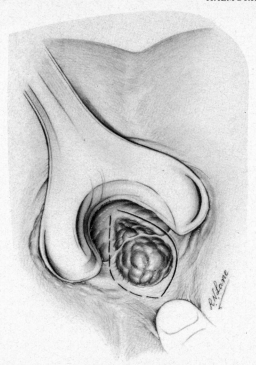

Fig. 90. Anal haemorrhoidectomy. The Hill–Ferguson retractor in position exposing the right anterior haemorrhoid. The dotted line indicates the proposed extent of the haemorrhoidectomy.

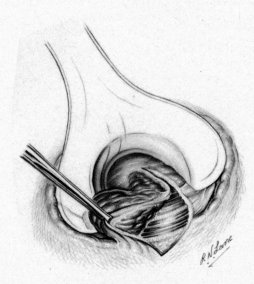

Fig. 91. Anal haemorrhoidectomy. The incision is being extended down to the sphincter musculature.

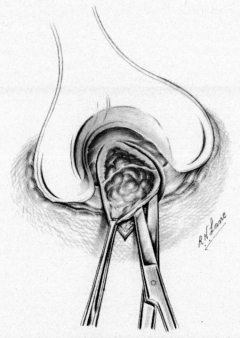

Fig. 92. Anal haemorrhoidectomy. Further dissection with scissors to free the main part of the pile from the underlying structure, up to the inferior pedicle.

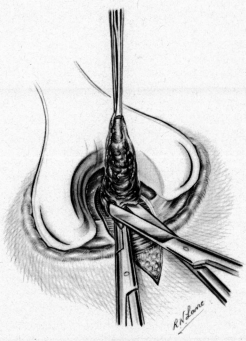

Fig. 93. Anal haemorrhoidectomy. Superior pedicle clamped with artery forceps and about to be divided with scissors.

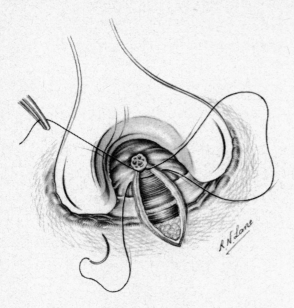

Fig. 94. Anal haemorrhoidectomy. The superior pedicle has been tied off and the wound is being closed with a running suture of 3/0 Dexon.

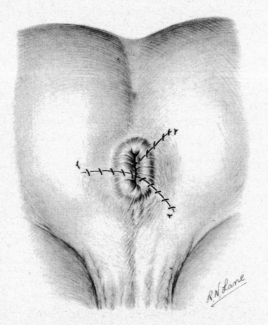

Fig. 95. Anal haemorrhoidectomy. All three haemorrhoids have been dealt with in the same way, leaving three sutured radiating wounds.

This incision is deepened either with the scalpel or scissors down to the underlying sphincter musculature and the haemorrhoid is dissected off these structures from either side and from the perianal

end (Figs 91, 92). Haemorrhage is controlled temporarily by suction or gauze swabbing till individual bleeding points can be coagulated with the diathermy.

Mobilizing the haemorrhoid and tying off the superior pedicle. The pile is freed up to its superior pedicle, which is then clamped (Fig. 93) and tied off. Actually in this technique of haemorrhoidectomy there frequently appears to be very little in the way of a major vascular stalk superiorly and one can often simply cut across the upper end of the mucosa without causing any significant bleeding.

Closing the haemorrhoidectomy wound. It only remains to suture the gap in the lining of the anal canal caused by the excision of the haemorrhoid. This is accomplished by a running suture of 3/0 Dexon or chromic catgut (Fig. 94), if necessary preceding this step by slight freeing of the cut edges of the mucosa by undermining scissor or scalpel dissection.

Dealing with the remaining haemorrhoids. The remaining two haemorrhoids are dealt with in like fashion, the anal retractor being re-positioned to expose each in turn. Obviously the lumen of the anal canal becomes progressively narrower as tissue is excised from its wall and the gap closed by suture, so that a medium or small sized retractor will be more convenient for the second and certainly for the third pile. When all three piles have been removed the patient is left with three sutured wounds extending out into the perianal region (Fig. 95). No dressing is required in the anal canal, but the anal orifice and perianal region is covered with a piece of dry gauze and a pad of cotton wool, held in position by a T-shaped bandage.

POSTOPERATIVE MANAGEMENT AFTER HAEMORRHOIDECTOMY

This is described on p. 90. I would merely refer to the traditional practice of passing a finger on the seventh or eighth day after haemorrhoidectomy ostensibly to detect any undue narrowing and, if necessary, to order the daily passage of an anal dilator to guard against the development of stenosis. I doubt if much good comes from this practice and have long since abandoned it. Any tightness of the anus at this stage is due to spasm, which in turn is caused by discomfort in the wounds, and usually subsides spontaneously as healing takes place. In any event, my patients are usually discharged from hospital on the fourth or fifth day. When the patient reports to the out-patient department two to three weeks after opera-

PLATE I

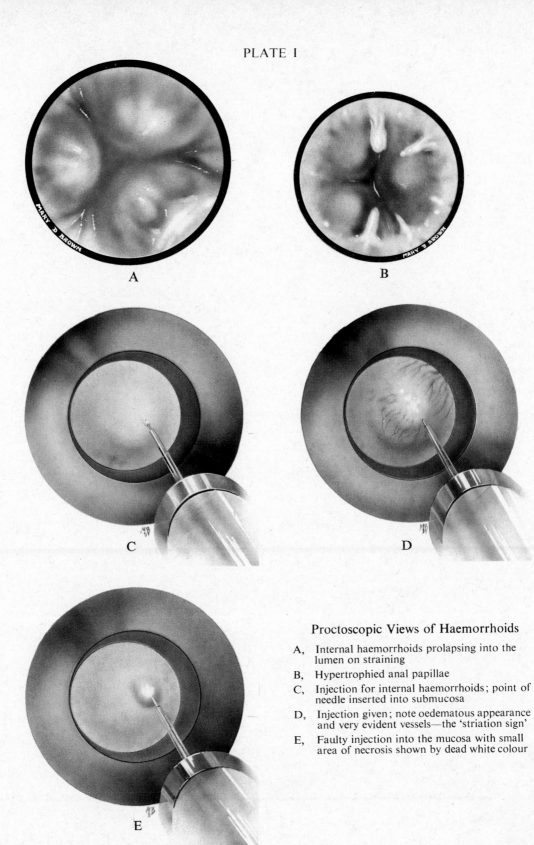

Proctoscopic Views of Haemorrhoids

A, Internal haemorrhoids prolapsing into the lumen on straining

B, Hypertrophied anal papillae

C, Injection for internal haemorrhoids; point of needle inserted into submucosa

D, Injection given; note oedematous appearance and very evident vessels—the 'striation sign'

E, Faulty injection into the mucosa with small area of necrosis shown by dead white colour

tion, the raw areas are usually very small, if not yet completely healed. A finger is invariably passed at this stage into the anal canal, which should be smooth and without stricture; if any narrowing is found, regular use of an anal dilator should be prescribed. The patient is advised that no further formal dressing is required but that he should have a bath or wash the anal region after defaecation and again in the evening, and should tuck a little wisp of dry cotton wool into the anal orifice to absorb any slight discharge for the next week or so. Thereafter he can lead an entirely normal existence, but should preferably be seen again in one month's time for a final examination, at which the anal wounds will usually be found completely healed and the patient can be finally discharged from specialist care.

POSTOPERATIVE COMPLICATIONS

Pain
It is the general impression that haemorrhoidectomy is one of the more painful operations of surgery, certainly as a rule more uncomfortable than the average minor abdominal operation, such as appendicectomy or inguinal herniotomy. Our enquiries into post-haemorrhoidectomy pain (Watts et al. 1965) have provided some interesting and reliable data on the subject (see p. 113). They confirm that there is a very considerable personal factor in the amount of discomfort—which ranges from virtually nil to very severe, following an identical operative technique—suffered by different patients. But, on the average, pain is distinctly less than I personally had previously imagined. It is rare for a patient to require more than one injection of morphine postoperatively, and a few patients decline all opiates. Indeed discomfort during the first 24–48 hours after operation is usually tolerable or relatively insignificant and severe pain is experienced mainly at the time of defaecation, especially the first motion, but in this respect also there is a considerable variation from patient to patient. In a few cases the act is surprisingly easy and hardly painful. Other patients complain of a stinging sensation in the anal region during the motion and for some time afterwards, and others say that it was an agonizing experience which felt 'like passing bits of broken glass' or 'having a red hot poker inserted'. Subsequent motions rapidly became less painful.

In the management of postoperative pain it is important to recognize that occasionally it may be quite severe and to prescribe sedatives in a generous and humane manner as required. For the pain of defaecation itself the most effective measure is an immediate hot bath, which the patient invariably finds most soothing.

The influence of operative technique on the amount of postoperative pain has already been discussed on p. 113. It has been my impression that haemorrhoidectomy with primary suture of the raw areas, including the skin wounds is more painful than methods leaving the external wounds open. It also appears that the latter heal better if they are oval or pear-shaped than if they are left as slits with loose edges. Postoperatively these redundant edges tend to become oedematous and swollen and form painful skin tags.

The use of long-acting anaesthetic solutions as a perianal injection immediately before haemorrhoidectomy to minimize postoperative discomfort was at one stage strongly recommended by Morgan (1935) and others (see p. 143), but the complications and disadvantages of this practice have led to it being dropped.

Retention of Urine
Difficulty in passing urine is another allegedly common complication after haemorrhoidectomy. It was certainly more frequent when a low spinal anaesthetic was used, but at the present time, when general anaesthesia or a caudal block is the rule, serious retention occurs in only about 3% of my haemorrhoidectomy cases. Obviously, if the patient is an elderly prostatic type, the risk of urinary difficulties is increased, and in certain patients of this kind preliminary surgical treatment directed to the prostate may be a wise precaution before proceeding to deal with the rectal condition. In male cases a great help in passing urine postoperatively is to stand the patient up at the edge of the bed to use the bottle. The next step is the administration of a parasympatheticomimetic drug such as prostigmine 1 ml by subcutaneous injection. This has its maximum effect within 15–20 minutes and often helps the patient to overcome his or her retention. Unfortunately it may rarely produce a sufficient increase of intestinal peristalsis to necessitate a bowel action which may be inconvenient at this stage of the convalescence, but this drawback can usually be ignored. Lastly if one or two such injections are ineffective the patient will have to be catheterized, but this should be avoided as long as reasonably possible, for it always introduces a small risk of infecting the urinary tract, especially as there is a very distinct tendency for these patients, once catheterized, to require a repetition of this procedure. Actually less than 0·7% of my patients have

needed to be catheterized after haemorrhoidectomy.

Formation of Skin Tags

The occurrence of oedema in the perianal skin adjacent to haemorrhoidectomy wounds with the formation of painful skin tags has already been referred to above as a cause of discomfort in the postoperative period. To avoid these as far as possible it is recommended that all lax wound edges should be trimmed to leave flat open wounds. However, there is a limit to the application of this technique, and sometimes the whole skin–mucosa bridge between two adjacent haemorrhoidectomy wounds is slack and redundant and becomes oedematous subsequently. A firm dressing pad of wool and T-shaped bandage also helps to restrain this oedematous swelling. The oedema eventually subsides and the prominent skin remnant either settles down to a normal appearance or fibroses and forms a permanent skin tag which may be readily palpated by the patient and considered by him a blemish on the result of his operation.

Reactionary or Secondary Haemorrhage

This is an important complication, not because of its frequency but because it may cause considerable alarm. *Reactionary bleeding* occurred in 1·7% of cases after the ligature and excision operation, but was rather more common after submucosal haemorrhoidectomy in my experience. It occurs soon after the patient's return to the ward or later that evening. It is usually due to opening up of a small bleeding point in one of the external anal wounds. With proper operative technique it is impossible for any displacement of the main pile ligatures to occur at this stage. The bleeding takes place externally into the dressings and is soon detected by the nursing staff as an excessive ooze. Removal of the dressings reveals the bleeding vessel. It may be possible to secure haemostasis with an artery forceps and ligature in the ward, or a return to the theatre and a general anaesthetic may be necessary for this purpose.

Secondary haemorrhage is more serious, for the bleeding from it may be considerable and the blood may accumulate in the rectum and escape detection for some time. It is due to the occurrence of sepsis in the pile pedicles with resulting softening of the wall of the main artery to the pile and its eventual disintegration. Secondary haemorrhage, like reactionary bleeding, occurred in 1·2% of my patients after ligature and excision. It usually takes place between the seventh and tenth postoperative days and, now that patients are discharged four or five days after operation, the complication is apt to occur at home. The bleeding follows defaecation; some evidence of it may have been observed at the time with the motion. Subsequently the bleeding continues into the rectum and colon without escaping externally unless the patient has a desire to have another motion, when he finds that he is passing mainly fluid and clotted blood. Meanwhile if the condition is undetected the signs of continuing internal haemorrhage become evident; the patient develops an increasing pallor, the pulse rate rises and the blood pressure falls. The condition should be readily thought of and quickly investigated. On examination of the anal region a trickle of dark blood may be seen to be escaping from the anus. A finger passed into the rectum usually detects large soft clots in the bowel, and on withdrawal some blood may come away at the same time. The diagnosis is confirmed by the passage of a proctoscope, which allows blood to escape from the bowel and shows that much clotted blood remains in the rectum. Needless to say proctoscopy in a patient one week after a haemorrhoidectomy may be an uncomfortable and rather difficult proceeding, so that a small-bore instrument should be used. A general anaesthetic may be required.

Treatment of secondary haemorrhage. If the blood loss seems relatively small, conservative management with bed-rest and sedation may suffice. However, if bleeding continues or is initially very severe the patient should be examined in the theatre under general anaesthetic. The important item of equipment for dealing with this complication is a bivalve speculum for it permits of insertion of sutures in the anal canal or rectum—something which is not readily possible through a tubular proctoscope, however large. The speculum having been passed and opened up, the rectum is emptied of blood and clots by swabbing and irrigation with hot saline. It will then usually be possible to see the bleeding point which can be under-run with a catgut stitch using a small half circle or 5/8 needle on a needle holder. If direct haemostasis proves impossible or the surgeon is not quite satisfied that it will suffice, a large Foley catheter may be passed, so that when the balloon is inflated and traction is exerted on the catheter it may press on the bleeding site. During and after the operation a blood transfusion is required, and the condition of the patient is assessed by half-hourly pulse and blood pressure recordings. If a tube or catheter has been used it is retained for three days. Thereafter the motions are kept soft and regulated by liquid paraffin, and there is usually no recurrence of the haemorrhage.

Fissure Formation

Considering the frequency of haemorrhoidectomy, this is a very rare complication which occurred in none of a series of my patients. It may occur in the midline posteriorly or anteriorly, in connection with the right posterior or right anterior haemorrhoid wounds, especially when the latter have included accessory piles in the median plane itself. If it is found that either of these wounds is failing to heal completely and developing into a fissure despite proper attention to baths, irrigations and dressings, the best plan is to give the patient a short general anaesthetic and perform a sphincter stretch or internal sphincterotomy.

Development of an Abscess or Fistula

With the technique of operation here recommended providing for large wide external wounds, it is almost impossible for abscesses or fistulae to form if the postoperative care is adequate. But if the patient is left with narrow external wounds the redundant skin edges may become adherent and lead to pocketing of pus with resulting abscess or fistula formation. It may be possible to separate the edges by manipulation or, more usually, the wound requires to be reshaped under general or local anaesthesia.

Stricture Formation

As pointed out on p. 112 this is, in my experience, a comparatively rare complication of the ligature and excision operation, even though I do not use anal dilatation as part of the postoperative care. Moreover if some degree of narrowing is found at follow-up examination, it is seldom that it causes any symptoms. When there is a tendency to stenosis it is probably wise to use a dilator (see Figs 43, 44) regularly for a time; sometimes it is necessary to make the first dilatation under general anaesthetic.

Recurrence

This is discussed on p. 113.

OPERATIVE TREATMENT:
B. ALTERNATIVE FORMS

In the last few years three alternative forms of treatment to formal haemorrhoidectomy have been evolved. They are rubber band ligations, manual dilatation of the anus and cryosurgery. One of the major advantages claimed for all these methods is that they can be performed in the out-patient department or consulting room and thus obviate the necessity for finding a bed in hospital—an important logistical consideration, at any rate in Britain, where in competition with patients suffering from more serious ailments a patient requiring haemorrhoidectomy (or an operation for hernia or varicose veins) may wait a considerable time for in-patient facilities to become available. Indeed, on this score it could be argued that, even if these new procedures should prove to be less effective than a formal haemorrhoidectomy, their readier availability should make them serious contenders for surgical favour.

RUBBER BAND LIGATION

This operation has been developed by Barron (1963, 1964) as a modification of an out-patient ligature method originally proposed and practised by Blaisdell (1958). The principle of the method is to apply a rubber ring ligature through a proctoscope to the mucosal-covered part of the internal pile. Over a period of seven to ten days this elastic band gradually cuts through the tissues and the pile sloughs off spontaneously. The special instrument devised by Barron for this operation is illustrated in Fig. 96A; a slight modification of it, the McGivney ligator, is obtainable in this country from Down Bros. of Mitcham, Surrey.* It consists of a small metal cylinder or drum on a long handle into which the pile can be drawn by special seizing forceps (Fig. 96B). A rubber ring ligature has to be placed round the end of the drum, and to get it in this position a special conical metal tip is used. The latter is stood upright on a hard flat surface and the ring is threaded on to it from its apex to its more cylindrical base (Fig. 96C). It is customary to apply two rings in this way. The metal cone is then fitted to the end of the drum on the ligator and the rings are rolled from the loader to the drum (Fig. 96D). When the ligator has been thus charged, the cone is removed and the instrument is ready for use (Fig. 96E). A proctoscope is passed, the patient is asked to strain gently to display the piles. The ligator is then inserted through the proctoscope and brought to bear on the mucosal part of the most prominent pile. The long alligator forceps (or, alternatively, a long pair of Allis' tissue forceps) are next passed through the proctoscope and through the drum on the end of the ligator. With it the pile is seized and drawn well into the drum, whilst the distal end of

---

* A new Belgian combined proctoscope and ligator may have some advantages (see p. 935).

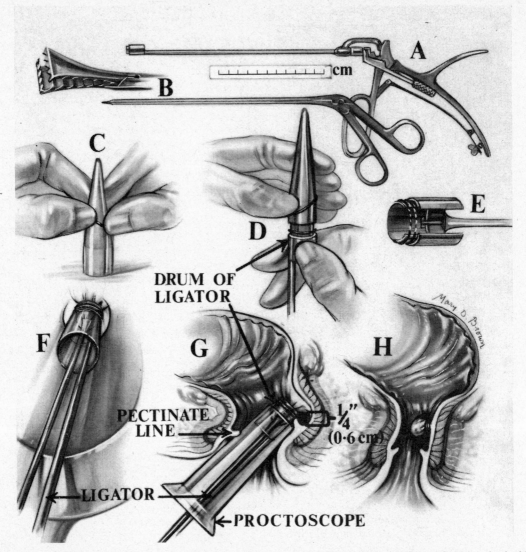

Fig. 96. Barron technique for rubber ring ligation of haemorrhoids. (A) The *ligator*, the essential part of which is the double drum at the distal end, which bears the rubber rings. (B) The *seizing forceps* for pulling the pile into the drum of the ligator. (C) Method of rolling rubber rings on to conical metal loader, whilst the latter is stood on a firm flat surface. (D) The loader, bearing two rings on its basal more cylindrical part, is fitted on to the drum of the ligator, and the rings are transferred from one to the other; thereafter the conical tip is removed. (E) The drum of the ligator, charged with two rubber rings and ready for use. (F, G) A tubular proctoscope has been passed and the ligator is inserted through it, to bear on the mucosal aspect of the pile, the substance of which is drawn into the drum by the seizing forceps. Note that the inferior edge of the drum lies *at least 6 mm above the pectinate line*. The two rubber rings are then pushed off the drum by closing the handles of the ligator. (H) The state of affairs when the proctoscope and ligator are withdrawn, a small nub of tissue about the size of a cherry being strangulated by the rings.

the latter is firmly pressed against the anal canal wall, special care being taken to see that *its inferior edge is at least 6 mm above the pectinate line* (Fig. 96F, G). By closing the handles of the ligator the rubber rings are pushed off the drum and instantly close on the base of the pile; the resulting nub of strangulated tissue is usually about the size of a small cherry (Fig. 96H).

No anaesthetic is required for ligation by the Barron technique, which is claimed by him to be virtually painless as a rule—or at least to cause no more discomfort than does an injection for haemorrhoids. It is usual to ligate only one pile at a time and to carry out further ligations on the remaining piles at intervals of three weeks or so, as required.

The obvious criticism of this method is that it does nothing to remove the skin-covered component of the pile or an associated skin tag, which, in patients with large piles, may be of considerable size and troublesome. It is clear, therefore, that the operation is unsuited as a curative measure for cases in this latter category. However, Barron (1964) claims that the lower remaining portion of the pile may undergo some shrinkage once the mucosal-covered part has been dealt with, and if the skin tags continue to bother the patient, they can subsequently be removed under local anaesthesia in the out-patient department. Another objection that might be levelled at this method is that it might be followed by secondary haemorrhage, which could be alarming and specially dangerous when occurring in a patient at home. In over 600 cases treated by this technique Barron (1964) has had two instances of fairly severe secondary haemorrhage, requiring a return of the patient to hospital. It must be admitted, however, that it is the practice of many surgeons to discharge their cases on the fifth or sixth day following ordinary haemorrhoidectomy, so that if these patients were to develop secondary bleeding, it also would occur whilst they were at home.

My own initial experience of Barron's technique (Clark et al. 1967) was encouraging and enabled me to confirm its easy practicability, though I was disappointed that it caused rather more pain that I had anticipated and I found it necessary to prescribe pethidine for the first night or two. Moreover, continued practice with the method, taking particular care not to place the rubber rings too close to the pectinate line, has not succeeded in regularly eliminating this discomfort. It seems to me, too, that rubber ring ligation is best suited to moderately big second-degree piles, and perhaps preferably to patients with one main pile. With piles smaller than that, there is insufficient tissue to pull into the ligature drum to make the method worthwhile, and in any event such piles can very successfully be managed by injections. For really large second- or third-degree piles, particularly if multiple, my experience is that rubber ring ligations are of very limited and temporary value and are certainly no substitute for a formal haemorrhoidectomy.

MANUAL DILATATION OF THE ANUS AND LOWER RECTUM

Lord (1968, 1969) has suggested that internal haemorrhoids are caused by circular constricting fibrous bands in the wall of the lower rectum or of the anal canal, which interfere in some way with normal defaecation, leading to abnormal raising of the intrarectal pressure during the act and to consequent venous congestion. He admits that these bands are not usually discernible when the anorectum is palpated with one finger clinically, but maintains that they can be felt regularly when one or two fingers of both hands are inserted simultaneously into the lower rectum under a general anaesthetic. He claims, moreover, that, if these bands are broken down under anaesthesia by a very vigorous stretching of the anal canal and lower rectum with the four fingers of both hands inserted as far as they can reach into the bowel and dilating in all directions, the haemorrhoidal state can be corrected in the great majority of patients.

As soon as the dilatation has been completed, a moistened plastic sponge, $12 \cdot 5 \times 10 \times 5$ cm, is immediately packed into the lower rectum and anus to prevent the development of a submucous and perianal haematoma. It is left *in situ* whilst the patient returns to the ward or recovery room, and is removed an hour later. After full recovery from the anaesthetic the patient is allowed to go home, but takes with him a supply of Normacol (sterculia) and a very large Perspex anal dilator (made by Vann Bros. of London), 4 cm in diameter at its widest part. He is instructed to take a suitable dose of the Normacol to ensure a soft, bulky motion daily and to pass the anal dilator regularly to its fullest extent for at least one minute, at first daily and then less frequently, but to continue using it occasionally for several months.

Lord (1969) and his colleagues have used this method on several hundred patients and he claims very satisfactory results in the great majority, so much so, indeed, that he himself has almost completely given up doing haemorrhoidectomy. Three complications have been encountered, though only in a small proportion of the cases. (*a*) *Splitting of the anal and perianal skin*, but usually this heals quite quickly of its own accord. (*b*) *Mucosal prolapse* in some patients who have had third-degree piles. Lord (1969) claims that the venous element in these cases has shrivelled up, so that what is prolapsing is not haemorrhoid so much as mucosa. Where the protrusion has been troublesome he has removed it under a short general anaesthetic, by clamping it across its base with a special forceps of his own design and shaving off the tissue beyond the clamp, which is left in position for an hour. (*c*) *Anal incontinence*, though how often it has occurred is difficult to deduce from Lord's (1968, 1969) writings.

However, manual dilatation has now been used in many centres in Britain and a number of reports have appeared on its results. Macintyre and Balfour (1972), on a one-year follow-up assessment of 55 patients treated by the Lord procedure, found that 80% were symptom-free or greatly improved, but on proctoscopic examination 75% still had significant haemorrhoids and 43·6% had anal skin tags. In addition 21·8% of the cases complained of incontinence for flatus and 36% for faeces, but the majority of the patients so affected apparently did not regard this lack of control as a serious inconvenience. Sames (1972) also reported that in 149 cases of haemorrhoids treated by manual dilatation the objective state on proctoscopy postoperatively was largely unchanged but the symptomatic results were mostly very satisfactory with only a few instances of temporary incontinence and none of permanent incontinence. Fussell (1972), on the other hand, encountered incontinence in four patients of 11 treated by dilatation, and Bates (1972) reported the development of complete rectal prolapse after Lord's operation in two elderly patients. Walls and Ruckley (1976) reported a five-year follow-up on 100 patients who had had manual dilatation for haemorrhoids. Two patients could not be traced and one had died. Seventy-five patients were symptom-free or greatly improved, but in 22 cases the treatment was unsuccessful and 19 of these have since undergone formal haemorrhoidectomy.

Chant et al. (1972) conducted a controlled trial of manual dilatation versus haemorrhoidectomy in 51 patients. In assessing the results they paid attention to the persistence, disappearance or aggravation of preoperative symptoms following either procedure. Apart from minor complaints, such as anal irritation, there were no failures in the 24 patients who had haemorrhoidectomy, but in the 27 who had anal stretching, five complained of continued bleeding, 11 of continued or aggravated prolapse, and three of aggravation of soiling or irritation. Altogether five of the cases treated by stretching were deemed to be failures and four of these subsequently came to haemorrhoidectomy. As a result of their experience Chant et al. (1972) considered that, whilst vigorous stretching may continue to have a role in the treatment of haemorrhoids, it should not be used for patients whose chief complaints are prolapse and soiling but should be reserved for those with painful bleeding piles. Ortiz et al. (1978) was also unfavourably impressed by the frequency of prolapse and incontinence after manual dilatation compared with a standard haemor-

rhoidectomy. In another controlled comparison of manual dilatation and haemorrhoidectomy in 100 patients Anscombe et al. (1974) had rather similar findings to those of Chant et al. (1972). Six months postoperatively the overall success rate of dilatation was put at 84% as against 98% for haemorrhoidectomy, and 24% of patients had prolapse after dilatation but only 2% after haemorrhoidectomy. Incontinence was present in 3% of patients after dilatation and minimally in 1% after haemorrhoidectomy. But the shorter time in hospital and the more rapid return to work after dilatation than after haemorrhoidectomy convinced Anscombe et al. (1974) that in general the Lord procedure was preferable to haemorrhoidectomy.

My own personal experience of manual dilatation for haemorrhoids is relatively small. It has not convinced me of the reality of the constricting bands described by Lord (1968, 1969) in the rectal wall (and even if they were present, I must say, I find the mechanism whereby they are alleged to produce internal haemorrhoids rather implausible). In the 26 patients with large haemorrhoids treated by me by dilatation some years ago I was impressed by the occurrence of incontinence and prolapse in four, which dampened my enthusiasm for the method.

(As a postscript to this account of manual dilatation it may be mentioned that Notaras (1977) and Arabi et al. (1977b) have suggested the use of lateral subcutaneous internal sphincterotomy instead of forcible dilatation in the treatment of haemorrhoids—see p. 187.)

CRYOSURGERY

Recent advances in cryogenic techniques have made it easily possible to freeze limited areas of living human tissue in many parts of the body. Such tissue, after being frozen solid, undergoes a gradual necrosis, due partly to thrombosis of the microcirculation (Fraser and Gill 1967). The method of cryodestruction has in the last few years been applied by many surgeons to the treatment of haemorrhoids (Lewis et al. 1969; Lewis 1973; Lloyd-Williams et al. 1973; O'Connor 1976). One of the great advantages claimed for this method is that it is painless, rendering it specially suitable for application to out-patients without anaesthesia. In the following account of cryosurgery in the treatment of haemorrhoids I am reflecting mainly my personal experience in the management of 68 patients by this technique (Goligher 1976).

Equipment
The essential item is the cryoprobe (Fig. 97), which

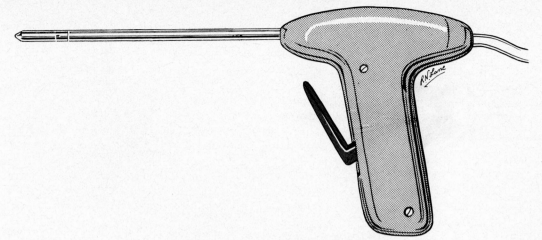

Fig. 97. The cryoprobe (*From Goligher 1976*)

has an active end 3–4 cm long, capable of being cooled by circulation through it of liquid nitrogen or nitrous oxide gas. Liquid nitrogen can produce a reduction of temperature to −180°C as compared with −70°C with nitrous oxide gas, but a cryoprobe apparatus using liquid nitrogen costs roughly £2000 as against about £500 for a nitrous oxide cryoprobe. Such equipment is manufactured or marketed in Britain by Spembly Ltd of Andover, Hants, and by Key-Med of Southend.

Anaesthesia

Though the freezing process itself is indeed painless, the sensitivity of the anal region is such that the pressure of the cryoprobe alone tends to cause some discomfort and excite alarm, which in turn usually leads to anal spasm, rendering it impossible to secure adequate access to the haemorrhoids. Even a sedative such as diazepam, as recommended by Lloyd-Williams et al. (1973), did not in my experience afford sufficient anal relaxation. In order to keep cryosurgery as an out-patient or office procedure, general anaesthesia was avoided and instead local anaesthesia in the form of an inferior haemorrhoidal block was employed, as described on p. 85. Generally this produced satisfactory sphincteric relaxation.

Exposure of Haemorrhoids

To give good access to the full length of the haemorrhoids, including both mucosa-covered and skin-covered portions, a bivalve speculum was used (see Fig. 37) and was rotated around the circumference of the anal canal to expose each haemorrhoid in turn.

Application of Cryoprobe

One method was that of simple application of a single probe in the long axis of the pile whilst the nitrous oxide was circulated (Fig. 98). Almost immediately the active portion of the probe would develop a white frost on its surface and become adherent to the part of the haemorrhoid with which it was in contact. Then gradually an increasing margin of tissue around the probe would turn white, reaching a maximum width of about 6–7 mm after two minutes. Generally the freezing was continued for three minutes in all. What is not known for certain is how deeply into the tissues the freezing extends; presumably it varies depending on the vascularity of the part. Probably the maximum penetration of freezing that one could reasonably expect into a moderately vascular pile would be 6–7 mm. When the flow of nitrous oxide was stopped, it usually took 10–20 seconds, and sometimes rather longer, before the frost on the surface of the active end of the instrument thawed and the tissues ceased to be adherent to it. Until the probe became freed in this way, it was important not to attempt to withdraw it for fear of tearing the pile and causing haemorrhage.

The alternative method of application, which was employed in the majority of my cases and was especially suitable for patients with large second- and third-degree haemorrhoids projecting well into the lumen of the anal canal when the bivalve speculum was in position, was that of compression of the attachment of the haemorrhoid to the anal wall between two simultaneously applied probes (Fig. 99). The object of this manoeuvre was to narrow the base of the haemorrhoid to a width of

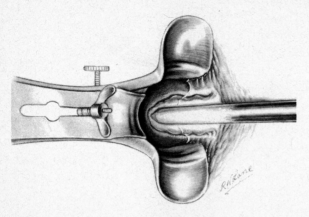

Fig. 98. Application of a single cryoprobe to the long axis of an anterior haemorrhoid. Note the frosting of the active end of the cryoprobe and adjacent tissues during freezing. (*From Goligher 1976*)

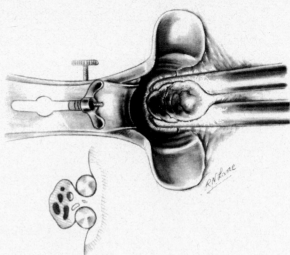

Fig. 99. The two-cryoprobe technique in which the base of the haemorrhoid is constricted by two cryoprobes placed in parallel and firmly approximated. *Inset:* probable extent of freezing of tissues. (*From Goligher 1976*)

tissue of 6 or 7 mm, which the freezing process extending from either side might confidently be expected to bridge (Fig. 100), thus destroying the pile without having to freeze its entire substance.

Usually two or three haemorrhoids could be dealt with in sequence at one session, but occasionally only one was treated either because there were no other significant haemorrhoids or because the patient had not reacted well to the treatment.

After-care

Patients were allowed home within 20–30 minutes of completion of the treatment. They were given pentazocine, 50 mg tablets, for use eight-hourly as required for pain. In addition they were advised of the possibility of an anal discharge and the necessity for frequent hot baths and the wearing of an external anal pad of wool. As regards bowel actions, they were told to use mild aperients as necessary to secure soft easy motions. Patients attended for review after an interval of a week and thereafter periodically till healing was complete.

Results

One patient had to be admitted to hospital because of bleeding which soon ceased with bed-rest and without the necessity for blood transfusion. There were no other major postoperative complications in the 68 patients.

When patients reported a few days or a week after treatment there was usually evident *necrosis* of some part of the tissues comparable to that resulting from the application of diathermy or the cautery. In some of the initial cases the area of necrosis was

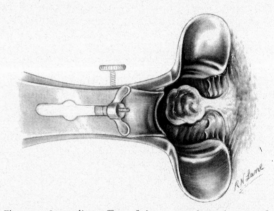

Fig. 100. Immediate effect of the two-probe technique after removal of the probes. Note that the constricted base of the haemorrhoid is frozen but much of the haemorrhoid itself is unaffected. (*From Goligher 1976*)

much less than the superficial extent of the freezing at the time of treatment, but with more prolonged freezing for at least three minutes for each haemorrhoid, and particularly with the use of the double-cryoprobe technique (Fig. 99), underfreezing appeared to be much less common. The slough would usually take two or three weeks to separate; complete healing of the resulting granulating areas would often require another two weeks or so.

Pain during the first few days, and sometimes lasting a week or more, was a prominent symptom in many of the patients after cryosurgery. It was described as very severe in 11, quite bad in 29, mild in 20 and insignificant in 8. A *discharge* of serous or brown offensive fluid from the anal canal occurred in most patients and was quite profuse in about half of them. Because of the pain and to a lesser extent the anal discharge, most patients were *unable to return to work for a period* varying from a few days to more usually at least a week.

Review of our 68 patients after three months revealed that there had been good destruction of the piles in 50, but that in 18 residual haemorrhoids were present and were causing symptoms in 12, on whom further treatment was necessary—re-freezing in two, injections in five and formal haemorrhoidectomy in five. Persistent anal skin tags were a feature in 17 patients. As for the patients' own verdict on the outcome, 38 were very pleased, 18 on balance were reasonably satisfied, and 12 were disappointed because of continued symptoms.

Comparison with Other Authors' Experience

Some other writers such as Lewis (1973), Lloyd-Williams et al. (1973) and O'Connor (1976) have reported very favourably on cryosurgery for haemorrhoids, particularly in regard to the avoidance of discomfort and the rapid return to work, often the day after treatment. By comparison my experience can only be described as bitterly disappointing, for to very many of my patients the postoperative course for a week or so after this form of treatment was decidedly unpleasant. It could be that some of these other authors have confined their freezing to the suprapectinate parts of the piles. If so, this would certainly greatly lessen the amount of postoperative discomfort, but it would also greatly reduce the efficiency of the method in dealing with third-degree haemorrhoids, which would otherwise really need formal haemorrhoidectomy.

AUTHOR'S PRESENT PRACTICE REGARDING CHOICE OF TREATMENT

In view of the multiplicity of methods now available for the elective treatment of internal haemorrhoids and the competing claims of efficacy, it may be helpful for me to state my own current practice regarding choice of therapy. First of all, amongst the welter of information about newer methods of management it is, I think, important not to lose sight of the fact that injection treatment is easily the most comfortable for the patient and the most convenient and expeditious for the surgeon. It is, moreover, remarkably effective, at any rate for a

time, in the great majority of patients, and repeat injections will often secure relief for another considerable period. Accordingly I use injection treatment in the first instance in most of my cases, and the other methods are reserved for the 20% or so of patients who either have very large prolapsing piles when they first present or soon develop recurrent symptoms after injections and possibly re-injections. For these primarily more severe cases or failed-injection cases my own preference is for formal haemorrhoidectomy, which I still regard as a very good operation. However, for some of these patients, preferably those with one particularly large haemorrhoid, I have used rubber band ligations as a substitute. I no longer offer cryosurgical treatment (either alone or in combination with rubber banding) and in this type of patient with large mainly prolapsing piles I am unattracted to forcible manual dilatation because of the risk of persisting prolapse or incontinence.

MANAGEMENT OF PROLAPSED THROMBOSED INTERNAL HAEMORRHOIDS

If, in the very earliest stages of an attack of prolapse and thrombosis, the prolapsed piles were to be released from the grip of the sphincter muscles by being reduced under a short general anaesthetic, it is just conceivable that the whole process of thrombosis might be aborted as claimed by Bailey (1936) and Gabriel (1948). But, by the time the average case reaches hospital, the thrombosis is well established and the swollen piles are quite irreducible. The choice of treatment then rests between strictly conservative management and immediate haemorrhoidectomy. Opinion on this issue has been sharply divided with, perhaps, the majority of surgeons, such as Gabriel (1948) and Aird (1957), favouring a conservative approach on the grounds that removal of haemorrhoids at this stage is considerably more difficult, may lead to extensive loss of tissue because of the large size of the inflamed piles with a risk of subsequent stricture formation, and exposes the patient to the risk of developing suppurative pylephlebitis. My own practice for 17 years now has been to advise immediate haemorrhoidectomy to the majority of these cases. I find that usually there is no special difficulty in the conduct of the operation, but I agree that, if care is not taken, one may end up with negligible skin bridges between the haemorrhoid wounds which might predispose to stricture formation. It is to be noted that Tinckler and Baratham (1964) had three strictures in 39 cases submitted to emergency haemorrhoidectomy for prolapsed thrombosed piles. As for the risk of portal pyaemia, this seems to be largely a myth. Certainly my experience of immediate operation would encourage me to continue with this practice as a rule, for it carries the great advantages that it immediately relieves the patient's discomfort and also cures his underlying haemorrhoids with the greatest of time-saving for him and hospital alike. What appears to be a useful aid in reducing the amount of oedema and facilitating the performance of emergency haemorrhoidectomy, in these cases, is the injection of hyaluronidase (3000 units in 40 ml of a freshly prepared solution of 1:200 000 adrenaline/saline) into the perianal tissues immediately before operation and the subsequent massage of the part for five minutes, as suggested by Raynham (1970).

The alternative of conservative management entails bed-rest, sedatives, possibly antibiotics, hot baths, soothing compresses, as with evaporating lead lotion, and mild aperients. Usually the pain and tenderness gradually settle over a period of a week or so, and the swelling subsides more slowly, but the patient is generally off work for at least 10–14 days—and at the end of it all he still has his haemorrhoids and may well eventually come to elective haemorrhoidectomy. Occasionally, too, the attack proceeds to actual necrosis of the piles, with considerable prolongation of the period of incapacity.

EXTERNAL PILES

External piles form at or just outside the anal orifice. They are invariably covered with skin, not mucosa, and as this is endowed with ordinary cutaneous sensation they may be extremely painful. External piles may be divided into two groups—acute thrombosed external piles or anal haematomas, and chronic anal skin tags.

Thrombosed External Piles or Anal Haematomas

The term thrombosed external piles implies a thrombosis of blood in the veins of the external or subcutaneous haemorrhoidal plexus, in the same way as clotting occurs in the veins of the internal or submucous plexus in thrombosed internal haemorrhoids. This may conceivably occur, but the more usual course of events appears to be a rupture of one of the external veins during straining at defaecation with the escape of blood into the subcutaneous tissues, where it clots and forms a tense painful swelling. The term anal haematoma is thus a more accurate description of the condition present.

Symptoms and Signs

The patient complains of the sudden development of a painful lump at the anus and often relates its onset to a bout of constipation which necessitated undue straining at stool. The pain is continuous but is aggravated by defaecation and by sitting. If the condition began some days previously there may already have been some mitigation of the pain and swelling, or alternatively, the symptoms may not have waned or may even have been accompanied more recently by bleeding due to rupture of the haematoma.

On examination an anal haematoma usually shows as a rounded swelling at the anal orifice, covered with tense stretched skin, through which the bluish colour of the contained clot can generally be appreciated. In the early stages the swelling is exquisitely tender, but after a few days the tenderness as a rule diminishes markedly, and after a week or so the swelling may be quite painless. Sometimes multiple haematomas are present, and occasionally these are conglomerate and form a swelling which occupies the greater part or all of the anal circumference.

Subsequent Course

In most cases spontaneous resolution occurs with gradual subsidence of the pain and diminution of the swelling. Eventually after several weeks the swelling may be completely absorbed, but often a residual loose tag of skin remains. *Rupture of the haematoma* sometimes occurs. This may be followed by complete extrusion of the clot, but more often this sticks in a partially extruded condition and has to be digitally expressed. If the clot remains exposed or sometimes even if completely evacuated, *infection* is liable to occur with resulting *abscess* or *fistula formation*.

Treatment

This may be expectant or by operation.

Expectant treatment is based on the experience that the majority of anal haematomas soon become painless and are usually absorbed without incident. Conservative treatment is designed to assist this process. It is an advantage if the patient can be confined to bed or be laid up for the greater part of the day for two or three days when the pain is severe, but this is sometimes not practicable for economic reasons. Frequent hot baths will be found very soothing, and sedatives, such as codeine or pethidine, may be prescribed as required. The motions should be kept soft by mild aperients. Within three or four days the more severe pain usually subsides, and the patient may then be able to return to non-strenuous work which does not involve prolonged sitting. Rarely the discomfort may persist unabated or may be so severe when the patient first presents that he is unwilling to accept conservative treatment. In either event operation will be required.

Operative treatment consists of evacuation of the clot either under a short general anaesthetic or with the aid of local anaesthesia. All that is required is a very short incision, say 1 cm long, radially placed over the clot, which can then be squeezed out between finger and thumb. Postoperative care comprises frequent baths and a dry cotton wool pad over the anal region for a few days.

ANAL SKIN TAGS

These are exceedingly common, and it is impossible to examine more than a few rectal patients without encountering a varied assortment of anal skin tags. In any individual case they may be single or multiple, and may vary from a slight excrescence of the skin to grossly projecting tags. An important practical distinction is between idiopathic skin tags, which are not associated with any obvious causal condition, and secondary skin tags, occurring in connection with an anal fissure, or pruritis ani. *Idiopathic skin tags* may possibly represent a legacy of resolved haematomas, but in many instances there is nothing in the patient's history to suggest that such thrombotic events had ever occurred. Usually idiopathic tags are soft and pliable and are covered by normal skin. *A secondary skin tag* found in relation to a fissure-in-ano is normally stiff with oedema when the fissure is open, but, after healing has taken place it becomes more flaccid like any ordinary skin tag. Some of the grossest examples of skin tags are found in association with pruritus ani; they are to be regarded as simply oedematous, infected skin rugae, and the anal and perianal skin in these cases shows the typical changes of pruritus ani.

Diagnosis

A careful examination will quickly differentiate anal skin tags from other lesions at the anus such as anal warts, condylomata or a carcinoma, and will indicate whether they are part of a pruritus ani, are associated with an anal fissure or are occurring quite idiopathically.

Treatment

Idiopathic anal skin tags require no treatment as a rule. Exceptionally they may be so large as to become something of a nuisance to the patient in cleansing the anal region after defaecation, or he may complain of discomfort in one or more of them and ask for its removal. This is a simple operation which can if necessary be performed under local anaesthesia, care being taken to leave a flat pear-shaped or triangular open wound which cannot fail to heal satisfactorily by granulation. Often, however, it is necessary to remove associated internal haemorrhoids by a formal ligature and excision operation, the skin cut being made sufficiently wide to embrace as many of the skin tags as possible; it may be worth sacrificing one of the skin bridges if required to facilitate wider excision of the cutaneous swellings.

The treatment of secondary skin tags is bound up with the treatment of the causal fissure or pruritus (see pp. 222–3). In particular it should be stressed that the skin tags in the latter condition are an effect and not a cause of pruritus, so that it is futile to undertake their excision in the hope of relieving the patient's condition. (To undertake complete excision of the pruritic anal and perianal skin in stages, with immediate grafting, is a different and more extensive procedure, which, as explained on p. 222, may be of value in the cure of the pruritus.)

HYPERTROPHIED ANAL PAPILLAE

These may be conveniently considered here. Anal papillae are the fine points of projection of the extreme upper end of the anal canal skin at the mucocutaneous junction, seen in 50 or 60% of cases examined. Usually they are small and just sufficiently prominent to give the pectinate line its characteristic serrated appearance on proctoscopy; they cause no symptoms and are to be regarded as normal structures. In certain patients, however, one or more of the papillae becomes hypertrophied and elongated, possibly to a length of 1 cm or more. Such a papilla is liable to undergo considerable fibrous thickening and to acquire a rounded expanded tip; at this stage it is usually termed a fibrous polyp. An hypertrophied papilla or fibrous polyp may give rise to symptoms by projecting at

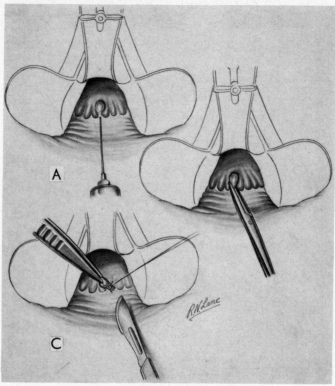

Fig. 101. Excision of hypertrophied anal papilla. (A) Exposure of papilla by means of bivalve speculum and injection of 0·5 to 1 ml of 0·5% lignocaine solution into its base. (B) Crushing the base of the papilla. (C) Ligation and excision of papilla.

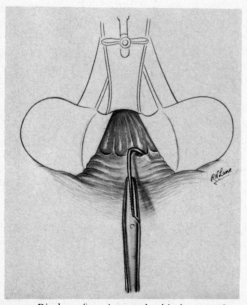

Fig. 102. Display of anal crypt by bivalve speculum and exploration by means of a hooked probe. The probe shown here is an ordinary fine malleable silver probe bent back at the tip and held in artery forceps to give better control.

the anal orifice during defaecation and requiring to be replaced digitally, the patient then complaining that he has prolapsing piles. A fibrosed hypertrophied papilla is also frequently found at the upper end of a chronic anal fissure, but the symptoms of the latter then completely dominate the clinical picture.

Diagnosis

If hypertrophied to any size, anal papillae can be easily palpated by the examining finger either as minute nodules of thickening at the mucocutaneous junction or as a definite fibrous polyp. They are, however, best appreciated on proctoscopy (Plate Iʙ).

Treatment

Formerly it was believed by Wallis (1911) and a number of other surgeons that hypertrophied anal papillae were a frequent cause of pruritus ani, and their removal was often advised on that account. At the present time this view is not widely held, and it seems unlikely that anal papillae play any part in the production of anal irritation, unless they actually project at the anus, when they may be responsible for a mucous leak with resulting increased anal moisture. If papillae are causing definite symptoms they may be very simply removed under local anaesthesia or a short general anaesthetic, a bivalve speculum being the ideal instrument for displaying the part (Fig. 101).

ACUTE CRYPTITIS AND PAPILLITIS

This is described particularly by American surgeons such as Buie (1937), Whitney (1948), Nesselrod (1949), Bacon (1949) and Granet (1954), but seems to be rarely diagnosed in this country. In this condition the anal valve or papilla affected becomes swollen, reddened and tender, and sometimes a drop of pus can be expressed from the adjacent crypt. As emphasized by Buie (1937) and Nesselrod (1949) this state of affairs may progress to produce an abscess in the connective tissues of the anal canal and perianal and ischiorectal spaces (see p. 154). It is well in cases of anal cryptitis to explore the affected crypt gently with a hooked probe to determine whether a fistulous track has already formed (Fig. 102). In the latter event operative treatment will be required to lay the track open, but in the earlier stages before the occurrence of definite fistulation, the only treatment required is mild aperients to soften the motions and lessen the pain of defaecation, frequent hot baths, and systemic penicillin 600 000 units and streptomycin 1 g twice daily.

Chronic anal cryptitis and papillitis is described at some length by Buie (1937), Whitney (1948) and Bacon (1949), and remote symptoms have been attributed to it in the belief that it acts as a focus of infection and reflex disturbance of the gastrointestinal tract. I must confess that I am completely unconvinced that there is such a disease.

REFERENCES

AIRD, I. (1957) *A Companion in Surgical Studies*, 2nd ed. Edinburgh and London: Livingstone.
ALLINGHAM, W. and ALLINGHAM, H. W. (1901) *The Diagnosis and Treatment of Diseases of the Rectum*, 7th ed. London: Baillière.
ANDERSON, H. G. (1909) The after-results of the operative treatment of haemorrhoids. *Br. med. J., 2*, 1276.
—— (1924) The injection treatment of haemorrhoids. *Practitioner, 113*, 399.
—— and DUKES, C. (1924) The treatment of haemorrhoids by submucous injection of chemicals. *Br. med. J., 2*, 100.
ANDREWS, E. (1879) The treatment of haemorrhoids by injection. *Med. Rec., 15*, 451.
—— and ANDREWS, E. W. (1892) *Rectal and Anal Surgery*. Chicago: W. T. Keener.
ANSCOMBE, A. R., HANCOCK, B. D. and HUMPHREYS, W. V. (1974) A clinical trial of the treatment of haemorrhoids by operation and the Lord procedure. *Lancet, 2*, 250.
ARABI, Y., ALEXANDER-WILLIAMS, J. and KEIGHLEY, M. R. B. (1977a) Anal pressures in haemorrhoids and anal fissure. *Am. J. Surg., 134*, 608.
—— GATEHOUSE, D., ALEXANDER-WILLIAMS, J. and KEIGHLEY, M. R. B. (1977b) Rubber band ligation or lateral subcutaneous sphincterotomy for treatment of haemorrhoids. *Br. J. Surg., 64*, 737.
BACON, H. E. (1949) *The Anus, Rectum and Sigmoid Colon*, 3rd ed. Philadelphia: Lippincott.
BAILEY, H. (1936) *Emergency Surgery*, 2nd ed. Bristol: John Wright.
BARRON, J. (1963) Office ligation of internal haemorrhoids. *Am. J. Surg., 105*, 563.
—— (1964) Personal communication.
BATES, T. (1972) Rectal prolapse after anorectal dilatation in the elderly. *Br. med. J., 2*, 505.
BENNETT, R. C., FRIEDMAN, M. H. W. and GOLIGHER, J. C. (1963) The late results of haemorrhoidectomy by ligature and excision. *Br. med. J., 2*, 216.
BLAISDELL, P. C. (1958) Prevention of massive haemorrhage secondary to haemorrhoidectomy. *Surgery Gynec. Obstet., 106*, 485.
BLANCHARD, C. E. (1928) *Text-book of Ambulant Proctology*, p. 134. Youngstown, Ohio: Medical Success Press.
BROADER, J. H., GUNN, I. F. and ALEXANDER-WILLIAMS, J. (1974) Evaluation of a bulk forming evacuant in the management of haemorrhoids. *Br. J. Surg., 61*, 142.
BUIE, L. A. (1932) In *The Colon, Rectum and Anus*, ed. F. W. Rankin, J. A. Bargen and L. A. Buie. Philadelphia and London: Saunders.
—— (1937) *Practical Proctology*. Philadelphia and London: Saunders.
BURKITT, D. (1972) Varicose veins, deep vein thrombosis and haemorrhoids. Epidemiology and suggested aetiology. *Br. med. J., 2*, 556.
CHANT, A. D. B., MAY, A. and WILKEN, B. J. (1972) Haemorrhoidectomy versus manual dilatation of the anus. *Lancet, 2*, 398.
CLARK, C. G., GILES, G. and GOLIGHER, J. C. (1967) Results of conservative treatment of internal haemorrhoids. *Br. med. J., 2*, 12.
COOPER, S. (1809) *A Dictionary of Practical Surgery*. London: Longmans.
CORMIE, J. and McNAIR, R. J. (1959) The results of haemorrhoidectomy. *Scot. med. J., 4*, 571.
CUSACK, J. W. (1846) *Dublin Q. J. med. Sci., 2*, 562.
DUKES, C. E. (1924) In Anderson and Dukes (1924).
EARLE, S. T. (1911) *Diseases of the Anus, Rectum and Sigmoid*. Philadelphia: Lippincott.
EDWARDS, F. S. (1888) The treatment of piles by injection. *Br. med. J., 2*, 815.
EISENHAMMER, S. (1969) Proper principles and practices in the surgical management of haemorrhoids. *Dis. Colon Rect., 12*, 288.
—— (1974) Internal anal sphincterotomy plus free dilatation versus anal stretch, with special criticism of the anal stretch procedure for haemorrhoids: the recommended modern approach to haemorrhoid treatment. *Dis. Colon Rect., 17*, 493.
FAILES, D. (1966) Primary suture of the operative wounds after haemorrhoidectomy. *Aust. N.Z. J. Surg., 36*, 63.
FERGUSON, J. A. and HEATON, J. R. (1959) Closed haemorrhoidectomy. *Dis. Colon Rect., 2*, 176.
—— MAZIER, W. P., GANCHROW, M. I. and FRIEND, W. G. (1971) The closed technique of haemorrhoidectomy. *Surgery, St Louis, 70*, 480.

FRASER, J. and GILL, W. (1967) Observations on ultrafrozen tissue. *Br. J. Surg., 54*, 770.

FUSSELL, K. (1972) Personal communication.

GABRIEL, W. B. (1948) *The Principles and Practice of Rectal Surgery*, 4th ed. London: H. K. Lewis.

GANCHROW, M. I., MAZIER, W. P., FRIEND, W. G. and FERGUSON, J. A. (1971) Haemorrhoidectomy revisited: a computer analysis of 2038 patients. *Dis. Colon Rect., 14*, 128.

GASS, O. C. and ADAMS, J. (1950) Hemorrhoids: etiology and pathology. *Am. J. Surg., 79*, 40.

GOLIGHER, J. C. (1960) Cryosurgery for hemorrhoids. *Dis. Colon Rect., 19*, 223.

—— GRAHAM, N. G., CLARK, C. G., DE DOMBAL, F. T. and GILES, G. (1969) The value of stretching the anal sphincters in the relief of post-haemorrhoidectomy pain. *Br. J. Surg., 56*, 859.

GRAHAM-STEWART, C. W. (1962) Injection treatment of haemorrhoids. *Br. med. J., 1*, 213.

—— (1963) What causes haemorrhoids? A new theory of etiology. *Dis. Colon Rect., 6*, 333.

GRANET, E. (1953) An anorectoplasty for extensive and complicated hemorrhoids. *Surgery, St Louis, 34*, 72.

—— (1954) *Manual of Proctology*. Chicago: Year Book Publishers.

HANCOCK, B. D. and SMITH. K. (1975) The internal anal sphincter and Lord's procedure for haemorrhoids. *Br. J. Surg., 62*, 833.

HUGHES, E. S. R. (1957) *Surgery of the Anus, Anal Canal and Rectum*, pp. 2, 129. Edinburgh: Livingstone.

KELSEY, C. B. (1883) *The Pathology, Diagnosis and Treatment of Diseases of the Rectum and Anus*. London: Sampson, Low [etc.].

LEWIS, M. I. (1973) Diverse methods of managing haemorrhoids: cryohaemorrhoidectomy. *Dis. Colon Rect., 16*, 175.

—— DE LA CRUZ, T., GAZZANGA, D. A. and BALL, T. L. (1969) Cryosurgical haemorrhoidectomy: preliminary report. *Dis. Colon Rect., 12*, 37.

LLOYD-WILLIAMS, K., HAQ, I. U. and ELEM, B. (1973) Cryodestruction of haemorrhoids. *Br. med. J., 1*, 666.

LOCKHART-MUMMERY, J. P. (1934) *Diseases of the Rectum and Colon*, 2nd ed. London: Baillière.

—— and JOSHI, M. K. (1915) Death from strangulated internal haemorrhoids. *Lancet, 1*, 332.

LORD, P. H. (1968) A new regime for the treatment of haemorrhoids. *Proc. R. Soc. Med., 61*, 935.

—— (1969) A day-case procedure for the cure of third-degree haemorrhoids. *Br. J. Surg., 56*, 747.

MACINTYRE, I. M. C. and BALFOUR, T. W. (1972) Results of the Lord non-operative treatment for haemorrhoids. *Lancet, 1*, 1094.

McMAHON, W. A. (1956) Anoplasty: complications and final results. *Am. J. Surg., 92*, 739.

MARTIN, C. F. (1904) The injection treatment of internal hemorrhoids. *Am. Med., 8*, 365.

MILES, W. E. (1919) Observations upon internal piles. *Surgery Gynec. Obstet., 29*, 496.

—— (1939) *Rectal Surgery*. London: Cassell.

MILLIGAN, E. T. C. (1930) In discussion on the complications of operations for piles. *Proc. R. Soc. Med., 23*, 706.

—— (1939) Haemorrhoids. *Br. med. J., 2*, 412.

—— MORGAN, C., NAUNTON JONES, L. E. and OFFICER, R. (1937) Surgical anatomy of the anal canal, and the operative treatment of haemorrhoids. *Lancet, 2*, 1119.

MITCHELL, A. B. (1903) A simple method of operating on piles. *Br. med. J., 1*, 482.

MORGAN, C. N. (1935) Oil-soluble anaesthetics in rectal surgery. *Br. med. J., 2*, 938.

MORLEY, A. S. (1928) An improved technique for the treatment of internal haemorrhoids by injection. *Lancet, 1*, 543.

NESSELROD, J. P. (1949) In *A Textbook of Surgery*, ed. F. Christopher, 5th ed., p. 1092. Philadelphia and London: Saunders.

NOTARAS, M. J. (1977) Personal communication.

O'CONNOR, J. J. (1976) Cryohaemorrhoidectomy: indications and complications. *Dis. Colon Rect., 19*, 41.

ORTIZ, H., MARTI, J., JAURRIETA, E., MASDEVALL, C., FERRER, J. and SITGES, A. (1978) Lord's procedure: a critical study of its basic principle. *Br. J. Surg., 65*, 281.

PARKS, A. G. (1955) De haemorrhois. *Guy's Hosp. Rep., 104*, 135.

—— (1956) Surgical treatment of haemorrhoids. *Br. J. Surg., 43*, 337.

PATEY, D. H. (1972) Aetiology of varicosity (letter to the editor). *Br. med. J., 2*, 712.

PETIT, J. L. (1774) *Traité des Maladies chirurgicales et des Opérations qui leur conviennent*, Vol. 2, p. 137. Paris: T.-F. Didot.

PRUITT, M. (1931) *Modern Proctology*. St Louis: Mosby.

RAYNHAM, W. H. (1970) Strangulated prolapsed piles. *S. Afr. J. Surg., 8*, 29.

ROSSER, C. (1931) Chemical rectal stricture *J. Am. med. Ass., 96*, 1762.

SAMES, C. P. (1972) Experiences of Lord's procedure for the treatment of haemorrhoids. *Proc. R. Soc. Med., 65*, 782.

SMITH, H. (1875) A second series of cases illustrating the treatment of haemorrhoids and prolapse by the clamp and cautery. *Lancet, 2*, 89.

STARR, K. W. (1959) Personal communication.

STELZNER, F. (1958) Über die Haemorrhoiden. *Dt. med. Wschr., 83*, 569.

—— (1963) Die Hämorrhoiden und andere Krankheiten des Corpus cavernosum recti und des Analkanals. *Dt. med. Wschr., 88*, 689.

THOMPSON, W. H. F. (1975) The nature of haemorrhoids. *Br. J. Surg., 62*, 542.

TINCKLER, L. F. and BARATHAM, G. (1964) Immediate haemorrhoidectomy for prolapsed piles. *Lancet, 2*, 1145.

TURELL, R. (1959) In *Diseases of the Colon and Anorectum*, p. 888. Philadelphia and London: Saunders.

WALLIS, SIR F. (1911) Pruritus ani. *Practitioner, 87*, 417.

WALLS, A. D. F. and RUCKLEY, C. V. (1976) A five-year follow-up of Lord's dilatation for haemorrhoids. *Lancet, 1*, 1212.

WATTS, J. M., BENNETT, R. C., DUTHIE, H. L. and GOLIGHER, J. C. (1964) Healing and pain after different forms of haemorrhoidectomy. *Br. J. Surg., 51*, 88.

—— DUTHIE, H. L. and GOLIGHER, J. C. (1965) A controlled study of pain after different forms of haemorrhoidectomy. *Surgery Gynec. Obstet., 120*, 1037.

WEBSTER, D. J. T., GOUGH, D. C. S. and CRAVEN, J. L. (1978) The use of bulky evacuant in patients with haemorrhoids. *Br. J. Surg., 65*, 291.

WHITE, J. E., SYPHAX, B. and FUNDERBURK, W. W. (1972) A modification of the Whitehead haemorrhoidectomy. *Surgery Gynec. Obstet.,* *134,* 103.

WHITEHEAD, W. (1882) Surgical treatment of haemorrhoids. *Br. med. J., 1,* 149.

—— (1887) Three hundred consecutive cases of haemorrhoids cured by excision. *Br. med. J., 1,* 449.

WHITNEY, E. T. (1948) Infection of the anal glands. *Gastroenterology, 15,* 451.

WRIGHT, A. D. (1950) Complications of rectal injections. *Proc. R. Soc. Med., 43,* 263.

5

Anal Fissure

This is a common disease of the anus which causes an amount of suffering out of all proportion to the size of the lesion. A fissure consists essentially of a crack in the skin-lined part of the anal canal, which often shows a considerable reluctance to heal. It is usually encountered in young or middle-aged adults, but is sometimes seen at other ages, including infancy and early childhood, and is equally common in the two sexes (Bennett and Goligher 1962).

PATHOLOGY

One of the remarkable features of this condition is the constancy of its situation, which is nearly always in the midline of the posterior wall of the anal canal or immediately to one or other side of it. Occasionally it occurs in the middle of the anterior anal wall, and exceptionally it is found elsewhere on the circumference of the anus. Anterior fissures are more common in women than in men, and account for some 10% of all fissures in that sex as contrasted with only 1% in men. Fissures are nearly always single but rarely two or more fissures co-exist.

The situation of the fissure in the vertical axis of the anal canal is also very constant. It lies in the cutaneous portion of the anal lining between the level of the anal valves and the anal orifice. In this position it is situated superficial to the lowermost quarter or third of the internal sphincter muscle. Initially it is separated from the sphincter by the thin layer of longitudinal muscle spread on the inner surface of the latter, but eventually it may deepen down to the sphincter so as to expose its circular fibres in its floor (Fig. 103). It is particularly to be noted that it bears no direct relationship to the external sphincter, for it was formerly held by some authorities that anal fissures invariably lay on the lowermost or subcutaneous part of the external sphincter and that it was external sphincter fibres that were usually revealed in the base of the fissure (Milligan and Morgan 1934; Blaisdell 1937; Milligan 1943; Gabriel 1948). An alternative view advanced by Miles (1919, 1939) was that the pale tissue exposed by a chronic fissure was not sphincter muscle at all but instead a condensation of fibrous tissue in the submucous plane of the anal canal, forming a ring of fibrosis which he termed the 'pecten band', and which he believed played an important part in the aetiology of anal fissure. The work of Eisenhammer (1953), Goligher et al. (1955) and Morgan and Thompson (1956), however, leaves no doubt that the tissue underlying a fissure-in-ano is the internal sphincter, that the structure identified by Miles as the pecten band is simply the prominent lower edge of this sphincter, and that at no stage is the external sphincter in direct contact with an anal fissure.

Secondary Changes

In its early stages a fissure is a simple split in the skin of the anal canal, but there soon develop in connection with it certain secondary changes. One of the most striking of these is a swelling of the skin at the lower end of the fissure, actually at the level of the anal orifice, so that it forms a tag-like swelling—the so-called 'sentinel pile' (Fig. 103). This is presumably due to low-grade infection and lymphatic oedema, and often the tag has a very inflamed, tense and oedematous appearance; later it may undergo fibrosis and persist as a permanent fibrous skin tag even after the fissure has healed.

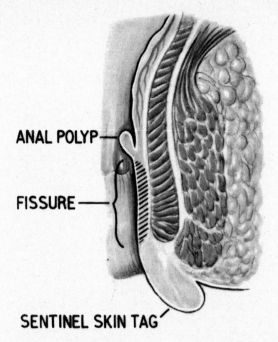

ANAL POLYP

FISSURE

SENTINEL SKIN TAG

Fig. 103. Sagittal section of the posterior wall of the anal canal showing the relation of a chronic fissure in the usual situation to the sphincters. Note that it overlies the lower third of the internal sphincter.

Quite frequently the anal valve immediately above the fissure also becomes swollen due to oedema and fibrosis, and forms *an hypertrophied anal papilla or polyp*, which does not usually reach anything like the same size as the sentinel pile. Another feature in a long-standing case is the development of *fibrous induration in the lateral edges* of the fissure. At any stage frank suppuration may occur and extend into the surrounding tissues to form a *perianal abscess*, which may discharge through the fissure into the anal canal or may burst externally to produce a *low anal fistula.* Usually the external opening of this fistula lies in or close to the midline a short distance behind the anus, and an anal fissure should always be thought of as the commonest cause of such a median low dorsal anal fistula (see Fig. 133).

Special mention must be made of the changes in the internal sphincter muscle in the presence of an anal fissure, for they have an important bearing on the treatment of the condition. Even when the fissure is relatively superficial the sphincter usually undergoes a tight spasm, but when the fissure deepens and bares the sphincter fibres this becomes even more pronounced. Eventually after several months the muscle may become fibrosed in its spastic condition so that a *rather fibrotic, tightly*

contracted, internal sphincter may result. It is easy to understand how the prominent, rigid, lower edge of this stenosed muscle could have been mistaken by Miles for a ring of fibrous tissue. The external sphincter may also share to some extent in the contraction of the anal musculature associated with the pain of the fissure, but it does not undergo the intense persistent contraction and eventual fibrosis seen so often in the internal sphincter.

Rather surprisingly attempts to demonstrate an increase of sphincter tone in association with fissure-in-ano by recording the pressure in the anal canal have resulted in somewhat discordant findings. In controlled studies comparing patients with anal fissures with normal subjects Graham-Stewart et al. (1961) found no difference, but Hancock (1977) and Arabi et al. (1977) demonstrated significantly higher pressures on average in the fissure patients.

AETIOLOGY

It must be admitted that our conception of the aetiology of anal fissure is to a large extent speculative. However it would seem that trauma to the anal canal during the passage of a large hard motion is generally responsible for initiating the condition. A majority of patients certainly relate the onset of their symptoms to the passage of such a constipated motion. Frequently also they will describe with some pride how they had hitherto been most regular in their bowel habits with the invariable use of mild aperients such as liquid paraffin or a saline purgative. In fact as a result of this regular medication many of these patients have had only liquid motions for months or years, and their anal canal has undergone some contraction so that the sudden passage of a hard scybalous mass could be particularly difficult and traumatizing to it. The occurrence of constipation is also frequently incriminated by patients as the factor responsible for producing a recurrence of their fissure symptoms after healing had taken place.

Why the fissure should be so prone to occur in the median plane and posteriorly is difficult to explain. Owing to the elliptical shape of the inferior edge of the external sphincter the lower part of the internal sphincter is perhaps less well supported posteriorly and anteriorly and the skin more liable to split behind or in front. But this leaves the much greater predilection to dorsal fissures still unexplained.

We know that superficial fissures may heal spontaneously in a week or two, especially if the motions are kept soft and constipation avoided. It is a matter for conjecture as to why others become chronic and refuse to heal. *Infection* may be a factor, but in many cases at any rate there is no more florid sepsis in long-standing chronic fissures than in very recent ones. *Spasm of the sphincter* has been freely indicted as the factor responsible for chronicity, it being alleged that the spasm of the anus brings the lateral edges of the fissure together so that discharge from the crack is dammed back or pocketed, and healing by granulation from the depths cannot take place. Certainly painful sphincter spasm is a notable feature in all cases of chronic fissure. One of the strongest arguments in favour of the view that sphincter spasm is aetiologically important is that division of the internal sphincter in part or in whole is usually followed by rapid relief of the pain and healing of the fissure. The evaluation of this step is often confused by other manoeuvres carried out at the same time, such as excision of the chronic fissure, but an equally good result is generally achieved if the internal sphincter is merely divided at a point remote from the fissure itself, or if a simple stretching of the sphincters is carried out under general anaesthesia.

No account of the aetiology of anal fissure would be complete without mentioning the ingenious theory of the late Sir Charles Ball of Dublin (1908). He believed that anal fissures resulted from tearing down of an anal valve by a faecal mass, leaving a linear wound extending from the pectinate line to the anal orifice, where the coiled-up strip of separated skin formed the sentinel pile. However, this explanation can seldom be the correct one, for usually in cases of anal fissure the anal valve is seen to be intact at the upper end of the fissure, and sometimes indeed it is hypertrophied to form an anal papilla.

So far we have been considering what might be termed *primary or idiopathic* fissure-in-ano. It should be added that a *secondary* form of fissure sometimes develops in patients who have undergone anal operations, such as haemorrhoidectomy (p. 123) or laying open of a low anal fistula, where the resulting wound is situated in the midline posteriorly or anteriorly. Presumably the aetiological factors responsible are similar to those leading to the establishment of a chronic fissure from a superficial anal crack. Considering the large number of minor anal operations regularly performed it is surprising that secondary anal fissures are not more common.

Other conditions to which fissures may be secondary are non-specific proctocolitis and Crohn's disease. Such fissures have certain characteristic features which are described on pp. 719 and 833.

SYMPTOMS

Pain. The chief symptom of anal fissure is pain in the anus during and after defaecation. It is usually described as a sharp, cutting, or tearing sensation during the actual passage of the motion; subsequently it may continue as a less severe burning or gnawing discomfort for three or four hours after defaecation. To some patients with an anal fissure the pain is so agonizing that they are frightened to have a motion and may remain in a constipated condition for several days on end. In less severe cases the patient may have become to some extent accustomed to the condition and may have discovered that by using mild aperients to avoid constipation and hard motions, the pain can be greatly lessened or completely obviated.

Bleeding. This is by no means an invariable symptom of fissure, but is very common. Usually the bleeding is quite slight and amounts to little more than a streaking of the motion, but occasionally the loss is more profuse and may cause anaemia.

Swelling. Some patients with a large sentinel tag may become aware of this as a lump at the anus and may complain of having a painful external pile.

Discharge and Pruritus. If there is much discharge this may lead to soiling of the underclothes, and to increased moisture of the perianal skin with resulting pruritus ani.

Urinary Symptoms. Sometimes patients with a painful anal fissure develop disturbances of micturition, either dysuria and retention or increased frequency.

EXAMINATION

Fissure-in-ano is an extremely painful condition and the patient suffering from it is usually very apprehensive of rectal examination. It is necessary

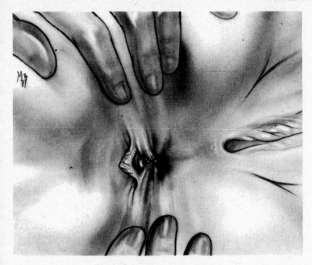

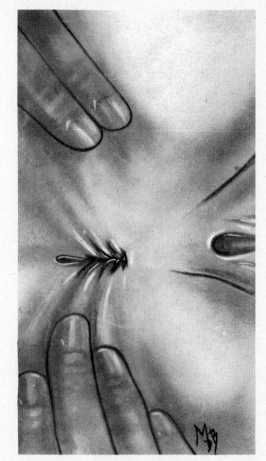

Fig. 104. Dorsal anal fissure with well marked sentinel pile seen on simple inspection of the anal region.

therefore to display particular gentleness in examining him.

INSPECTION

This is by far the most important step in examination, for anal fissures can always be seen if properly sought. The difficulty in demonstrating them arises from the associated anal spasm which closes the anal orifice tightly and conceals the fissure from view. Indeed the finding of marked spasm of the sphincters in a patient with a suggestive history is strong presumptive evidence of the existence of a fissure. The spasm can usually be overcome by gentle but determined lateral separation of the edges of the anal orifice, by traction with the fingers placed close to either side of the anus. If this causes too much pain it may be helpful to try the local effect of a 10% amethocaine ointment, applied on a wiped wooden probe inserted into the anal orifice for 5–10 minutes.

The first thing that will probably be noted is a sentinel skin tag posteriorly or anteriorly. This may be as big as a small grape but is usually less than half or a third that size. The fissure itself appears as a triangular or pear-shaped slit in the skin of the anal canal just above the base of the sentinel pile (Fig. 104). The floor of the fissure may consist either of connective tissue or, in really chronic lesions, of the internal sphincter, the pale transversely running fibres of which can often be clearly distinguished. In

Fig. 105. A more superficial anal fissure without sentinel tag.

cases with a very superficial fissure, this may present as the merest crack in the anal wall unassociated with any sentinel tag (Fig. 105), or the anal skin may be found to tear as it is stretched, leading to bleeding and suggesting that the symptoms are due to recurrent splits of this kind when a particularly constipated motion is passed. Occasionally, in patients whose symptoms have recently abated, a sentinel tag and depression corresponding to a fissure are observed, but the fissure is covered with epithelium, and in these cases there is no anal spasm. On the other hand, with deep chronic lesions there may be a considerable amount of acute inflammation with frank pus exuding from the fissure. There may in addition be an inflammatory swelling behind the fissure due to an intersphincteric or perianal abscess, and even an external fistulous opening, through which a probe can be passed to emerge through the fissure.

Palpation

This confirms the presence of sphincter spasm, the rounded lower edge of the internal sphincter being usually easily palpable just distal to the fissure itself. The passage of the finger is uncomfortable but the maximum tenderness is elicited when the finger is placed on the fissure itself. Pressure on other parts of the circumference of the anal canal does not produce the same exquisite pain. Induration of the lateral edges of the fissure, indicating fibrosis, is specially to be noted. At the upper end of the fissure an hypertrophied anal papilla may be palpable. The digital examination is, of course, important as a means of excluding other lesions in the lower rectum, such as a carcinoma or polyp, which might be present in addition to the fissure.

Proctoscopy

This is often impossible owing to pain, or has to be performed with a smaller proctoscope than usual, for the final withdrawal of the end of the open instrument over a tender fissure may be very uncomfortable indeed. In doubtful cases, however, it may show the fissure more clearly than was possible on simple inspection. Protoscopy may also demonstrate other lesions such as internal haemorrhoids or a proctitis which may have a bearing on the patient's complaint.

Sigmoidoscopy

This is best performed with a narrow-bore instrument, its main value being to exclude proctitis or a Crohn's lesion of the distal large bowel; but it may also rarely reveal an unsuspected carcinoma.

DIAGNOSIS

The history of pain on defaecation is, of course, very suggestive of an anal fissure and examination of the anal region usually demonstrates the characteristic anal spasm and fissure and excludes other possible causes for the complaint. As emphasized, the essence of the physical examination is simple inspection and it is important to detect the fissure at the outset of the examination so that unnecessary use of instruments may be avoided. In some patients, despite the utmost gentleness by the surgeon, pain and spasm are severe enough to prevent the proper demonstration of a suspected fissure. Final diagnosis then depends on a more thorough examination under general anaesthesia, made as the initial step in operative treatment.

DIFFERENTIAL DIAGNOSIS

Most other conditions presenting with anal pain, and possibly swelling or bleeding, are usually easily distinguished on examination. Thus anal haematoma, prolapsed thrombosed internal haemorrhoids, and various forms of abscess in the anal region are generally quickly recognized for what they are. A few other lesions, however, produce an ulcer or crack in the anal region and obviously require more careful discrimination:

PRURITUS ANI WITH SUPERFICIAL CRACKS OF OF THE ANAL SKIN

This is sometimes a source of difficulty in diagnosis. Many cases of anal fissure develop pruritus ani due to irritation of the perianal skin by the discharge, and it would be possible on cursory examination to overlook the fissure and diagnose the condition as being due entirely to idiopathic pruritus. On the other hand, the skin in a case of primary pruritus frequently shows superficial cracks extending radially from the anus. One of these may on occasion simulate a dorsal anal fissure and lead to a faulty diagnosis of fissure-in-ano with secondary pruritus. Careful examination of the suspected lesion in these cases, however, will show that it does not present the characteristic features of a true anal fissure, that there is no true anal spasm or tenderness and that other less obvious cracks are present in the anal skin elsewhere.

ULCERATIVE COLITIS OR PROCTOCOLITIS WITH ASSOCIATED ANAL FISSURE (see also p. 719)

Septic complications, including fissures, are not at all uncommon in the anal region in cases of colitis. Usually the anal fissures are extremely painful and soon become broad, deep, and very septic, so that they readily lead to abscess and fistula formation. In addition they are often situated off the midline, and may be multiple. If the patient has a frank ulcerative colitis involving the greater part or all of the large bowel he will, of course, have severe diarrhoea and constitutional symptoms so that he will be admitted primarily on account of these and the fissure will be recognized as a complication of this condition. But patients with a distal form of proctocolitis, confined to the rectum and lower part of the sigmoid, who may have only mild diarrhoea and little general disturbance, may also develop these large painful fissures, unlike those seen in ordinary individuals. It is possible for such a patient to report with his complaint of pain in the anal region on defaecation and to say nothing about the slight diarrhoea which he has had for some months or years previously, and it is also possible for the surgeon to overlook the proctocolitis on examination because of the difficulty of instrumentation owing to pain. These fissures, however, are, as mentioned, usually broad and the surrounding skin is inflamed, and this should put the surgeon on the alert for the associated proctocolitis, which can be easily diagnosed if a view of the rectal mucosa can be obtained by endoscopy. It is important to recognize that the fissure is but a complication of the colon condition.

CROHN'S DISEASE WITH ANAL ULCERATION
(see also p. 833)

Equally important in the differential diagnosis of anal fissure is Crohn's disease of the large or small intestine, for this condition may be associated with ulceration in the anal region. Again, the fissuring is usually much grosser than an idiopathic fissure and more akin to that seen in ulcerative colitis, though often much more extensive than in that condition. Even when the ulcer is relatively restricted in size its appearances should arouse suspicion that it is no ordinary fissure and lead to investigation by sigmoidoscopy and barium studies; yet I have seen several cases where a Crohn's anal ulcer had been excised elsewhere in the mistaken impression that it was a simple fissure-in-ano. The histological examination of tissue secured by biopsy or excision may be helpful by showing characteristic appearances of Crohn's disease. Sigmoidoscopy may reveal disease in the rectum, but very rarely the rectal mucosa appears normal and the intestinal lesion is situated at a higher level in the bowel.

SQUAMOUS-CELL CARCINOMA OF THE ANUS,
OR ADENOCARCINOMA OF THE RECTUM
INVADING THE ANAL CANAL OR ANUS

Either of these carcinomata involving the anal skin will cause severe pain on defaecation and on inspection may occasionally be found to produce an appearance not unlike that of a very chronic and indurated simple fissure and in the correct position for a fissure. But digital palpation will usually detect more induration than could be reasonably accounted for by a simple fissure, however long-standing, and may reveal further that the anal ulcer is but the lowermost edge of a more extensive lesion of the anal canal or rectum. The inguinal glands may also be hard and enlarged. Any doubt about the diagnosis can be resolved by biopsy.

SYPHILITIC FISSURES

Anal fissures due to syphilis may be either primary chancres or condylomas (secondary lesions). *A chancre* in its initial stages may closely resemble an ordinary anal fissure, but it soon acquires a good deal of induration at its margins and base and the inguinal glands become enlarged. A highly characteristic feature is the presence of a symmetrical lesion on the opposite wall of the anal canal. If suspicion is aroused the diagnosis is quickly established by microscopic examination by the method of dark ground illumination of a sample of the discharge from the ulcer for the presence of spirochaetes. The Wassermann reaction may also be positive by the time the patient attends hospital. *Anal condylomas* may occur at the anal orifice as well as in the perianal region and may there cause multiple anal fissures. The whole anal region is usually moist and pruritic in these cases. This finding, together with the presence of several superficial, rather septic fissures, should suggest the possibility of syphilis. Secondary skin lesions and mucous patches in the mouth are usually present, and the Wassermann reaction is strongly positive. Contrary to popular belief, *syphilitic lesions in the anal region are not by any means painless.*

TUBERCULOUS ULCER

Very rarely a tuberculous ulcer occurs in the anal canal and may closely resemble a simple anal fissure at first. Later it tends to enlarge and to develop an undermined edge. Unless there are other manifestations of tuberculosis in the anal region or in the lungs it may be very difficult to differentiate from an ordinary anal fissure till a biopsy and guinea-pig inoculation are done. The diagnosis from anal ulceration in association with Crohn's disease may be very difficult unless the latter test has been done. It seems probable, indeed, that some cases diagnosed as tuberculous on histological and clinical examination alone may have really been manifestations of Crohn's enteritis.

IDIOPATHIC STENOSIS OF INTERNAL SPHINCTER

This seems to be a definite clinical entity. It occurs in certain older patients, usually women, who have been accustomed to taking aperients over many years so that the anal canal has for a long time been spared the regular dilating action of a normal solid motion. As a consequence the internal sphincter undergoes contraction and may become fixed in this contracted condition by fibrosis, as in a case of chronic anal fissure. There may be no symptoms, or when the contraction becomes extreme, the patient may find difficulty in passing motions. The condition is easily recognized by finding a tightly contracted internal sphincter on palpation, without any evidence of a past or present fissure. If required it can be treated by internal sphincterotomy exactly as for chronic anal fissure.

MISCELLANEOUS CONDITIONS

Lastly in a certain number of cases with anal pain there may be on examination no evidence of an anal lesion of any kind. The surgeon will then have to consider carefully whether the patient might not have had an anal fissure which has recently healed. A superficial fissure may heal without leaving any traces, but in a case of a chronic fissure, even after healing, there is nearly always some evidence of a previous chronic fissure, in the form of a sentinel tag or a deep radial furrow in the midline covered with thin skin tightly applied to the lower part of the internal sphincter muscle. Only when all possibility of a fissure or other local organic anal cause for the patient's pain has been firmly excluded should less definite conditions be considered, such as proctalgia fugax, coccygodynia, rectal crisis of tabes, or frank psychoneurosis.

TREATMENT

Many fissures heal spontaneously, often in two or three weeks. These are usually superficial lesions which have been attended by a relatively short history of pain. By contrast really chronic fissures are most resistant to any form of conservative treatment, and though there may be temporary abatements of symptoms, the trouble tends to recur frequently. To save the patient unnecessary discom-

fort and uncertainty it is therefore desirable to make an early decision as to whether a fissure is likely to heal under an expectant regimen or whether an operation will be required.

FEATURES INDICATING CHRONICITY AND THE NEED FOR OPERATION

A long, continuous, or intermittent history of pain obviously suggests that a very fibrosed chronic lesion is present. On examination the findings that indicate chronicity are *a large sentinel tag of skin, induration in the edges of the fissure,* and, most important of all, *the exposure of the fibres of the internal sphincter in the floor of the fissure.* When these signs are present, and especially the last-mentioned, a lasting cure is unlikely to be achieved without operation. It will be appreciated, too, that with relatively recent fissures of a more superficial character operative measures may sometimes be required because of the severity of the pain which the patient is unwilling to tolerate any longer, or because of abscess or fistula formation.

Conservative Treatment

Avoidance of Constipation
This is probably the most important item of conservative treatment, and if the repeated anal trauma occasioned by passage of hard faeces can be avoided many fissures heal rapidly without any other treatment. To achieve this state of affairs mild aperients are usually required, of which oily preparations such as liquid paraffin, Petrolagar, Agarol or Milpar are especially suitable for they tend to produce soft easily passed motions. The patient may, however, be accustomed to some other purgative and may prefer to take it in slightly increased doses. When the fissure has finally healed care should be taken that the patient does not discard the regular bowel habits that have by then been acquired, for a bout of constipation will often result in a recurrence of the fissure. Only gradually should the dosage of the aperient be reduced till the patient finds that he can dispense with it entirely without becoming constipated. Alternatively he may have to continue with it indefinitely, but only sufficient should be taken to keep the motions soft and easy and not to produce liquid actions which may result, over a period of months or years, in a gradually increasing anal stenosis.

Use of Anaesthetic Ointment
To lessen the pain of the fissure and relieve anal

spasm ointments containing anaesthetic agents may be applied locally. Popular preparations are 3% amethocaine ointment or lignocaine 5%, though the regular use of amethocaine may cause dermatitis and it should not be repeatedly applied in any concentration greater than 3%. They should be inserted on the finger into the anal canal and not merely smeared on the perianal skin. Another convenient way of applying them so that they reach the fissure is to use them as a lubricant for an anal dilator which is passed into the anus. The best times to use the ointment are probably in the morning before defaecation and again after the motion has been passed, but it may be employed at other times as required.

Use of an Anal Dilator

This is warmly recommended by Gabriel (1948) but it is difficult to see any convincing rationale for its use; in fact it seems rather illogical to advise dilatation of the anus in this condition. It is, however, a simpler and more reliable way of applying an anaesthetic ointment which is regularly used in conjunction with it, than is a digital insertion, and that is the only reason why I sometimes prescribe it. A suitable dilator is the St Mark's Hospital pattern (see Fig. 43) or Thorlakson's (see Fig. 44), which are manufactured in three sizes. A small or medium size is usually preferable.

Injection of Long-acting Local Anaesthetics

The sensory nerve supply to the skin in the region of an anal fissure is derived from the inferior rectal (haemorrhoidal) nerves, and blocking of these nerves by injection of a long-acting anaesthetic solution would seem an eminently rational step in the conservative treatment of fissure-in-ano. Several solutions are available for this purpose; they are mostly put up in sterile oil, the object of which is to delay the absorption of the anaesthetic agent and prolong its local action. Two well-known preparations of this kind contain cinchocaine.

An important practical point in handling these oily solutions is that they are more easily drawn into the syringe and injected into the tissues if the ampoules in which they are supplied are *heated by immersion in hot water immediately before use*. The fluid should be *sucked directly into the syringe* through its nozzle, and then the needle attached. The latter should be of sufficient calibre, say No. 19 or 20, to transmit the warm oil fairly freely, and at least 5 cm long. The technique of injection of the fluid follows closely the account given on p. 86, a small weal of 0·5% lignocaine being raised in the skin 2·5 cm

behind the anal verge and the needle injected at this spot, 5–10 ml of solution being placed on either side of the anal canal. In addition 2–3 ml may be injected immediately behind the anus deep to the fissure. The strictest asepsis should be maintained throughout and on withdrawal of the needle the skin puncture should be sealed with collodion on a wisp of cotton wool or with a plastic spray. Under no circumstances should a second injection be given in less than three months, and it is probably unwise for the treatment to be repeated within a period of a year.

Long-acting local anaesthetics enjoyed a considerable vogue in the 1920s and 30s, being strongly recommended by Gabriel (1929) and Morgan (1935) in this country and by Yeomans et al. (1927) and Gorsch (1934) in America, and used not only in the treatment of fissure but also the prevention of pain after haemorrhoidectomy. However, they are irritating solutions to the tissues and with the slightest contamination during the injection are liable to be followed by sepsis, so that abscesses and fistulae have been not infrequently encountered after their use. Further, their anaesthetic action has not always been very effective or prolonged unless the amount given is increased to a total of over 20–25 ml. With dosage of this order temporary incontinence may result from paralysis of the external sphincter, and the risks of infective complications seem to be increased. In cases of really chronic fissure ultimate resort to operation is seldom avoided by cinchocaine injection, whilst the relief and healing or more superficial fissures seems to take place just as effectively under treatment with aperients and simple anaesthetic ointments as with such injections. As a result of these considerations, the popularity of these preparations has waned dramatically in recent years. Personally, I no longer use them and in the management of an extremely painful anal fissure, for which immediate relief is urgently required, I now prefer to carry out a sphincter-stretch or an internal sphincterotomy (see pp. 144, 150).

Operative Treatment

There is considerable divergence of opinion as to the essential step in the operative treatment of anal fissure—whether it is correction of spasm and contraction of the internal sphincter muscle by stretching or by partial or complete division, or excision of the fissure so as to provide a wide external wound in which discharge cannot pocket.

STRETCHING OF THE ANAL SPHINCTERS

This operation, which is associated with the name of Récamier (1829), has long been a favourite method of treating anal fissure with many surgeons, perhaps more especially general surgeons without any particular interest in rectal work. The great attractions of the procedure have been its extreme simplicity, so that it can be easily performed by relatively junior staff without special equipment, and the fact that it requires virtually no aftercare other than a daily bath.

TECHNIQUE

A local anaesthetic, however carefully injected, does not usually provide satisfactory conditions for a thorough stretching of the sphincters, and deep general anaesthesia is required, preferably with a relaxant. With the patient in the lithotomy or lateral position, the anus is forcibly stretched by introducing first both index fingers and then the index and middle fingers of both hands, which maintain a firm distraction for three or four minutes (Fig. 106). During this manoeuvre the forearms are fully

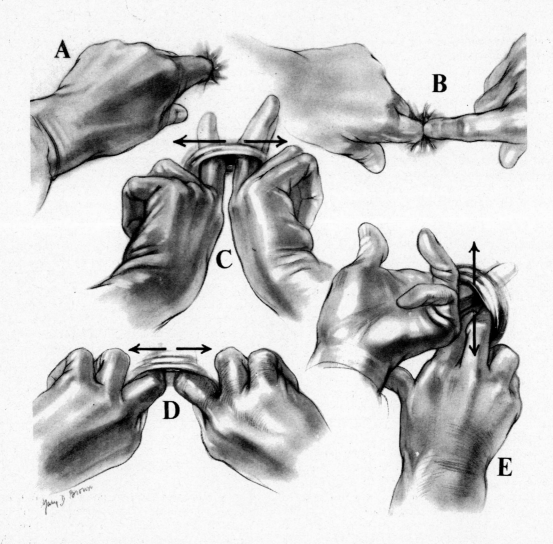

Fig. 106. Anal sphincter stretching. At first one and then two fingers are inserted (A, B) and a certain amount of distraction is exerted to stretch the anus sufficiently to allow three and finally four fingers to be passed (C, D). The anal canal is then stretched in a transverse axis with gradually increasing force over a period of three or four minutes. In male patients a better stretch is often obtained in the vertical or anteroposterior axis (E), because the more closely placed ischia tend to impede lateral distraction.

pronated so as to stretch particularly the posterior wall of the anal canal. Often a better stretch is obtained in male patients by using the sagittal rather than the transverse plane as this avoids the fingers coming in contact with the ischial tuberosities. The problem does not arise in women owing to their wider pelves. The effect on the internal—and external—sphincter is to produce a temporary paralysis usually lasting several days or a week, and there may be some incontinence during this time. Usually some sphincter fibres are torn in the process and as a consequence there is often some extravasation of blood leading to perianal bruising and discoloration which may be quite extensive. As a result of the stretching, moreover, the fissure itself is often torn more widely open, but the pain is completely relieved as a rule, and the condition heals generally with great rapidity.

RESULTS

For a time I employed stretching of the anal sphincters as the routine surgical treatment for fissure-in-ano, as part of a deliberate policy to evaluate this operation, and was thus able to report the results obtained in 99 patients (Watts et al. 1965). They were as follows.

Relief of Pain. In 94 of the 99 patients early and complete relief of pain was achieved by the treatment and was usually apparent within a day or two of operation.

Time off Work. Though a few patients returned to their jobs almost immediately, it was more usual for them to remain off work for a few days.

Complications. Two patients developed painful perianal oedema within a few hours of stretching. One of these patients also had prolapsed, thrombosed haemorrhoids. It would seem that this is a method to be avoided in cases with concomitant large internal piles.

Recurrence. Of the 94 patients initially relieved, 11 subsequently complained of further pain although a second fissure was not found in all of them. If the five patients whose original pain was not relieved by stretching are added to those, there is a total of 16 cases (16%) in which the treatment did not prove completely successful. Presumably additional recurrences may appear on more prolonged follow-up, but it is perhaps significant that all but two of our patients who have developed recurrence so far did so within six months of the stretching. (Incidentally,

Fries and Rietz (1964) of Stockholm reported nine recurrences on a 1–10-year follow-up of 59 patients after sphincter-stretching for anal fissure, and Moore (1964) of Exeter had two recurrences only in 41 cases traced for 1–9 years.)

Results of Further Treatment. Some form of further treatment was necessary in nine of our 16 patients with an unsatisfactory response to the initial operation. Six patients were submitted to internal sphincterotomy, with satisfactory results in five; the other patient required yet further treatment by triangular excision of the fissure. Three patients were treated by a repeat sphincter-stretch, which was ineffective in all cases, even in one patient when repeated on two occasions. Two of these three patients have had a subsequent internal sphincterotomy with satisfactory results to date.

Functional Results. When questioned about anal continence since operation, slightly imperfect control for flatus was mentioned by 12% of our patients and for faeces by 2%, whilst 20% had noticed unaccustomed soiling of the underclothes (see also Defects of Anal Function after internal sphincterotomy, p. 148).

EXCISION OF ANAL FISSURE

This operation was popularized chiefly by Gabriel (1948), who believed that in excising a fissure it was important to remove a broad triangle of perianal skin along with the lesion itself. The advantage of so doing, according to him, was that the apical part of the wound corresponding to the site of the former fissure was given a chance to epithelialize before the basal portion could close, so that there was little prospect of being left within an unhealed area of granulation in the posterior wall of the anal canal. Also, the triangular shape of the wound was said to promote freer external drainage and avoid any accumulation of discharge which might impair healing. However, Gabriel also took two additional steps of considerable therapeutic significance. He divided the edge of sphincter muscle exposed in the area of the wound, which he stated was the subcutaneous or lowermost part of the external sphincter, but was really the rounded inferior margin of the internal sphincter, as demonstrated by Goligher et al. (1955). He also usually stretched the anal sphincters. But he attached particular importance to the triangular excision of skin and advised that it should be of a precisely triangular shape and of a size not less than 4 cm from apex to middle of base. It would probably be correct to regard this operation as essentially an internal sphincterotomy done through a large triangular wound. Its popularity has waned considerably in recent years in favour of simpler ways of doing a sphincterotomy.

The technique of excision of an anal fissure by Gabriel's method is shown in Fig. 107. The postoperative care is similar to that after haemorrhoidectomy. It usually takes the wound about four to six weeks to heal completely.

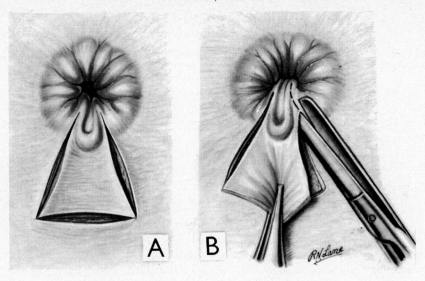

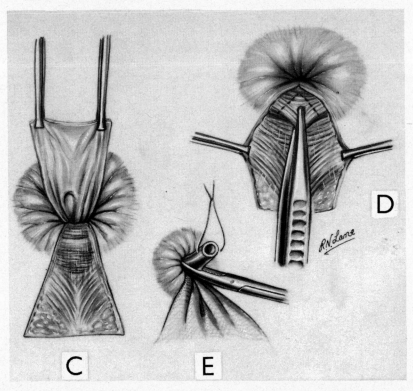

Fig. 107. Excision of anal fissure by Gabriel's method. (A) Triangular incision. (B) Dissecting up the skin flap. (C) Freeing the apical part of the triangular flap of skin from the lower border of the internal sphincter. (D) Division of the lower third of the latter muscle. (E) A corner of gauze dressing is tucked into the anal canal in relation to the wound. The use of an indwelling tube is optional.

RESULTS

Though Gabriel (1963) reported excellent results for the operation, this statement does not appear to be based on any detailed follow-up study. I myself have performed very many Gabriel fissurectomies in the past, but never subjected the outcome to careful analysis. I can only say that my clinical impression is that this is a very good and reliable operation. The main criticism levelled at it is that it leaves the patient with a large, rather uncomfortable, external wound, which by design takes a long while to heal.

EXCISION OF ANAL FISSURE WITH IMMEDIATE SKIN GRAFTING

A modification of the operation, suggested by Hughes (1953) to expedite healing and shorten the convalescence, is to apply an immediate split-thickness skin graft to the wound after excision of the fissure (see p. 82). Hughes has claimed a high percentage of complete 'takes' with this method, and years ago I used it myself in some cases with success. The main objections to the technique are that it is a rather finicky procedure and the bowels must be confined for five to six days, which may be uncomfortable for the patient. A further practical disadvantage is that, although grafting does reduce the period required in hospital, the patient has still to remain at least a week in hospital, which compares unfavourably with the three or four hours required after sphincter-stretching or sphincterotomy.

DIVISION OF THE INTERNAL ANAL SPHINCTER—INTERNAL SPHINCTEROTOMY

Internal sphincterotomy was originally performed for the surgical treatment of anal fissure under a complete misapprehension. Miles (1939) stated that he had been treating idiopathic fissure-in-ano for many years by 'pectenotomy', or division of what he called the 'pecten band' in the lower part of the anal canal, access being obtained through a short longitudinal incision in the lining of the posterolateral part of the canal. This apparent fibrous band was eventually shown by Eisenhammer (1951) and Goligher et al. (1955) to be the spastic prominent lower edge of the internal sphincter. Milligan and Morgan (1934) and Gabriel (1948), in the course of excising anal fissures, made a practice of dividing what they maintained was the spastic, subcutaneous part of the external sphincter. But again this band of muscle was demonstrated beyond doubt to be the wrongly identified inferior margin of the internal anal sphincter (Eisenhammer 1951; Goligher et al. 1955).

Credit for suggesting the treatment of anal fissure by internal sphincterotomy alone under its correct designation must rest with Eisenhammer (1951, 1953). Morgan and Thompson (1956) also helped greatly to popularize this operation. The method favoured by Eisenhammer (1953) and Morgan and Thompson (1956) for this procedure was to divide the lower half of the internal sphincter through an incision in the midline of the posterior wall of the anal canal—usually through the fissure itself—the resulting wound being left open to heal by granulation.

1. TECHNIQUE OF OPEN POSTERIOR INTERNAL SPHINCTEROTOMY

Internal sphincterotomy can be performed under a local anaesthetic block of the inferior rectal nerves, as described on p. 83 (see Fig. 63). After the block has been given with the patient on his *right* side, he is turned on his *left* side for the actual operation. However, my experience is that patients with anal fissures are specially sensitive about rectal examination and instrumentation, and much prefer to have their operation for this condition conducted under general anaesthesia. With suitable recovery space available, it is possible to do the operation on an out-patient basis and for the patient to go home two or three hours later. If the patient is having a general anaesthetic it is more convenient to do the operation in the lithotomy position as for haemorrhoids, rather than in the side position.

For the easy execution of this operation two special instruments are essential—a bivalve type of anal speculum and a long No. 7 Bard Parker scalpel handle carrying a small No. 10 blade (Fig. 108). A convenient pattern of speculum is my own model which is illustrated in Fig. 37. The detachable third blade, which provides for forward retraction, is useful for controlling any bulging of a coexistent anterior haemorrhoid into the operation field. During the operation it is also an advantage to have some 1/1000 solution of adrenaline hydrochloride solution (BP) in which to soak small gauze pledgets for application to the cut surface of the mucosa and muscle to control haemorrhage and permit of a better view of the progress of the sphincterotomy.

The steps of the operation are depicted in Fig. 109, the legend to which gives an adequate description of the operative procedure. If there is still some bleeding at the end of the operation it is usually checked by the application of a piece of adrenaline gauze or a strip of absorbable haemostatic such as oxycellulose to the cut surface, and over this a piece of ordinary gauze soaked in Milton. For anterior fissures the sphincterotomy is best carried out at a separate point posteriorly or posterolaterally.

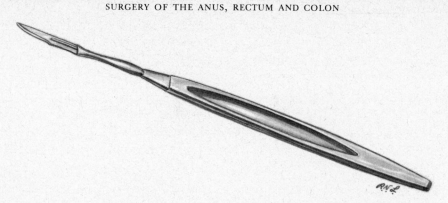

Fig. 108. No. 7 long Bard-Parker scalpel handle with No. 10 blade, used for internal anal sphincterotomy.

POSTOPERATIVE MANAGEMENT

This is usually very simple and can easily be carried out in the patient's home. He is supplied with two or three doses of 100 mg of pethidine to take during the first two nights if necessary, and tablets of aspirin or codeine to use as required during the first two or three days. He is advised to take a mild aperient, such as liquid paraffin 15–30 ml daily, for a few days, and to have a hot bath twice a day, the anal region subsequently being covered with a Milton gauze or dry cotton wool dressing. He is seen by the surgeon twice in the first week and thereafter at weekly intervals till the wound is completely healed.

RESULTS

Eisenhammer (1959) and Morgan and Thompson (1956) claimed excellent results for open posterior internal sphincterotomy, as did Lockhart-Mummery (1957). But a more critical appraisal by Bennett and Goligher (1962) of the results obtained by them in 127 patients treated by this operation, whilst confirming the great efficacy of the procedure in curing anal fissure, disclosed some less satisfactory features. The following facts were ascertained in their study.

Immediate Relief of Pain

The great majority of cases were immediately relieved of their pain. This relief was noted by nearly all patients at the time of the first bowel action which, despite the operation wound, was much more comfortable than defaecation had been for a long time. The few who denied having had immediate relief stated that their discomfort gradually subsided over a period of 5–6 weeks, *pari passu* with the healing of their wounds.

Period Off Work and Time Required for Complete Wound Healing

The period during which patients were off work ranged from a few days to six weeks, depending on the nature of their employment and their psychological make-up, the average time being 17 days. The length of time taken for the wound to heal was seldom less than four weeks, more usually about seven weeks, and this was so even in patients who had experienced immediate and lasting relief of pain. It was difficult to account for this delay in healing, but it was certainly regarded as something of a nuisance by many of the patients.

Recurrence

In nine of the 137 patients (7%) symptoms of anal fissure recurred, but in only four cases was there objective evidence of a recurrent fissure. Seven of these patients were satisfied with the result despite the further symptoms, but two underwent a second operation with complete relief in one but with further pain in the other.

Defects of Anal Function

The other disappointing aspect of the results of open posterior internal sphincterotomy was the disturbingly high incidence of minor imperfections of anal continence after it. During the first few weeks after operation control for flatus was said to be impaired by 34% of the patients, and for faeces by 15%. These impairments of function tended to improve in time, so that in the cases that had been followed up for three years the incidence of incontinence for flatus had declined to 13% and for faeces to 9%. Another functional defect, which quite frequently occasioned a good deal of embarrassment, was anal discharge with resulting faecal staining of the underclothes. This was present in

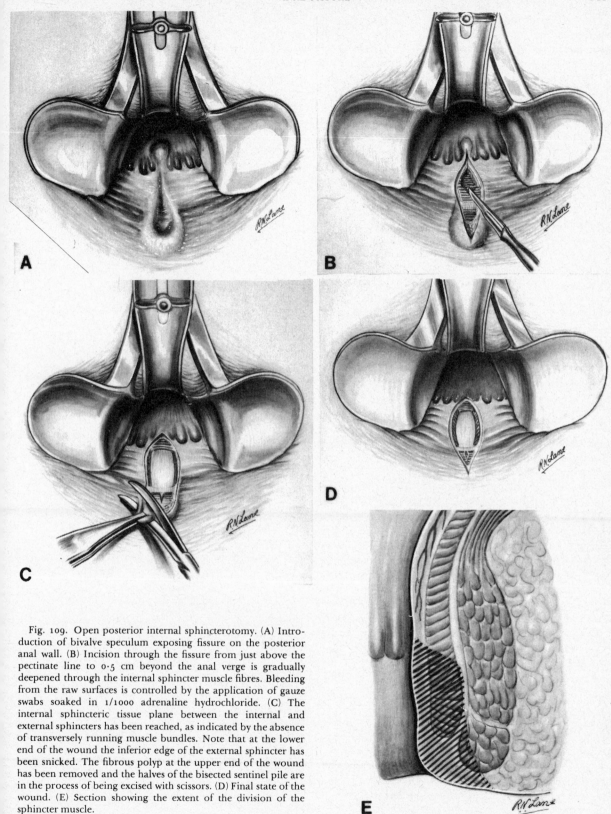

Fig. 109. Open posterior internal sphincterotomy. (A) Introduction of bivalve speculum exposing fissure on the posterior
anal wall. (B) Incision through the fissure from just above the
pectinate line to 0·5 cm beyond the anal verge is gradually
deepened through the internal sphincter muscle fibres. Bleeding
from the raw surfaces is controlled by the application of gauze
swabs soaked in 1/1000 adrenaline hydrochloride. (C) The
internal sphincteric tissue plane between the internal and
external sphincters has been reached, as indicated by the absence
of transversely running muscle bundles. Note that at the lower
end of the wound the inferior edge of the external sphincter has
been snicked. The fibrous polyp at the upper end of the wound
has been removed and the halves of the bisected sentinel pile are
in the process of being excised with scissors. (D) Final state of the
wound. (E) Section showing the extent of the division of the
sphincter muscle.

28% of the patients and showed no trend towards spontaneous improvement. In the majority of cases the operation involved division of the distal half of the internal sphincter, but in a number of cases the extent of the sphincterotomy varied from the lower third to the entire muscle. Contrary to what might reasonably have been expected, there was no clear correlation between the quality of the functional result and the height of the sphincterotomy. Therefore it did not seem possible to prevent interference with continence, with any degree of certainty, by restricting the operation to the distal half or third of the muscle.

Our impression, which was borne out by a more detailed study by Bennett and Duthie (1964) of the physiology of the internal anal sphincter and its disturbance by internal sphincterotomy, was that an important factor in the production of these imperfections of control was the longitudinal furrow that developed in the scar of the sphincterotomy wound in the posterior wall of the anal canal. It seemed that faecal matter and flatus could leak down this groove despite the action of the sphincter musculatore. The possibility that a lateral sphincterotomy might cause a less prominent furrow on the wall of the anal canal than a posterior sphincterotomy and be followed by fewer functional disturbances was suggested by Eisenhammer (1959), and Bennett and Goligher (1962). More recently Parks (1967) strongly recommended lateral sphincterotomy through a short circumferential incision in the skin outside the lateral anal verge, which is subsequently closed by suture. The great advantage of this method, which is also favoured by Hawley (1969), is that it avoids an open wound in the anal canal itself. Even simpler and more expeditious, however, is the technique of *lateral subcutaneous internal sphincterotomy*, described by Notaras (1968, 1969, 1971), in which the lower part of the internal sphincter is divided as in a subcutaneous tenotomy, which leaves virtually no wound at all. This is the method which I have been using exclusively for the treatment of anal fissure during the past ten years (Hoffmann and Goligher 1970).

2. TECHNIQUE OF LATERAL SUBCUTANEOUS INTERNAL SPHINCTEROTOMY

As for open posterior internal sphincterotomy, this operation can be done under local anaesthesia, but I prefer to do it under a short general anaesthetic with the patient in the lithotomy position. A bivalve speculum is introduced into the anal canal and rotated so that the handles lie to the patient's right and the blades are situated in front and behind. The instrument is then gently opened to a diameter approximating two fingerbreadths. This manoeuvre has the effect of exposing the left lateral wall of the anal canal and of rendering the lower margin of the internal sphincter in that sector taut and easily palpable, sometimes even visible—especially if the speculum is pulled slightly downwards in the long axis of the anal canal, dragging the internal sphincter tube with it—as a definite curvilinear prominence (Fig. 110). For the myotomy a von Graefe cataract knife is used.

Unlike Notaras (1968, 1969, 1971), who divides the internal sphincter from within outwards, I have preferred usually to introduce the knife on the outer side of this muscle and to cut medially. Accordingly, the point of the blade is inserted through the perianal skin, immediately lateral to the lower edge of the internal sphincter (Fig. 110) and passed vertically upwards in the intersphincteric plane till it is adjusted to lie at or just above the level of the pectinate line (Fig. 111). By means of delicate strokes of the blade in the direction of the anal canal, the lower half of the

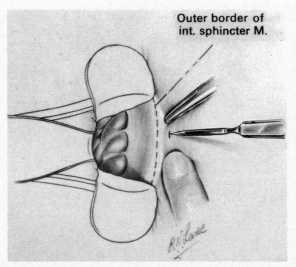

Outer border of int. sphincter M.

Fig. 110. Lateral subcutaneous internal sphincterotomy. A bivalve anal speculum has been inserted and opened in the sagittal plane so as to expose the left lateral wall of the anal canal. If slight traction is exerted on the retractor, as if to withdraw it from the canal, the lower edge of the internal sphincter is brought into relief, so that it may be felt by the finger or demonstrated by the end of an artery forceps and a point chosen just lateral to it for insertion of the cataract knife.

internal sphincter is then divided, care being exercised not to penetrate the lining of the canal. A useful precaution to avoid such penetration is to leave a few of the innermost fibres of the muscle undivided (Fig. 111) and, after the knife has been withdrawn, to rupture them by firm lateral pressure with the finger (Fig. 112). The pressure is maintained for a few moments. Then the bivalve speculum is removed and the finger is replaced by a small pad of wool or a plastic sponge which is kept in place by a firm T-bandage. If there is a large associated sentinel skin tag or fibrous polyp it can be excised at the same time, preferably just before the sphincterotomy.

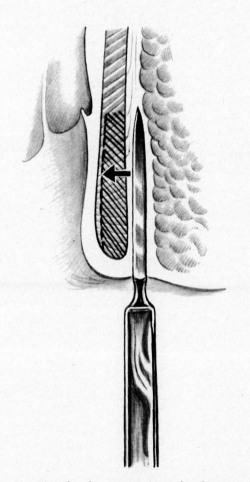

Fig. 111. Lateral subcutaneous internal sphincterotomy. Transverse section of the wall of anal canal showing how the blade of the knife is passed upwards in the intersphincteric plane till its tip is level with the pectinate line, the cutting edge being directed internally. By to-and-fro movement of the blade the lower half of the internal sphincter is then divided completely or nearly so, possibly a few of the most internal muscle fibres being preserved to protect the skin of the anal canal from damage.

AFTERCARE

The patient is allowed home within a few hours, armed with codeine and pethidine for use as required. He takes liquid paraffin or another mild aperient for a few days and has a daily bath, preferably after defaecation. A dry dressing is worn if there is any discharge.

RESULTS

My results in 99 patients treated by lateral subcutaneous internal sphincterotomy have recently been analysed (Hoffmann and Goligher 1970):

Immediate Relief of Pain and Healing of Fissure. Satisfactory relief of pain was achieved in all patients but one, and the fissure was found to heal completely in all but two patients, usually within a week or two of operation. The persistence or recurrence rate is thus reckoned to be 3%, which compares favourably with that of 7% in our hands for open posterior sphincterotomy and 17% for sphincter-stretching.

Time Off Work. The length of time off work averaged about a week for men and two or three days for women.

Surgical Complications. One patient had a brisk *reactionary haemorrhage* from the sphincterotomy stab wound two hours after operation. The bleeding was controlled by firm pressure and the patient was able to leave hospital after one day. Another patient developed a *perianal abscess and subsequent fistula* at the site of the sphincterotomy, which required to be laid open eventually. It is remarkable that significant haematoma formation requiring further surgical intervention did not occur in any case, but minor *ecchymoses* were observed postoperatively in 22 cases. Two patients complained that following sphincterotomy they had troublesome *prolapse of internal haemorrhoids*, in one case requiring emergency haemorrhoidectomy.

Alterations of Anal Sphincter Function. This is perhaps best indicated by reference to Table 2 which records the frequency of such disturbances after lateral subcutaneous internal sphincterotomy, by comparison with their incidence after open posterior internal sphincterotomy and after sphincter stretching. It will be seen that continence is less impaired after lateral subcutaneous internal sphincterotomy.

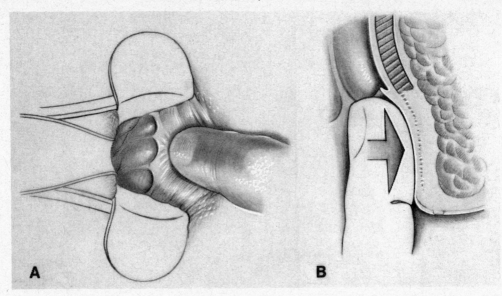

Fig. 112. Lateral subcutaneous internal sphincterotomy. After withdrawal of the knife, the tip of the finger is pressed firmly against the wall of the anal canal at the site of the sphincterotomy for a moment or two (A), the object being to rupture any residual fibres of the lower half of the internal sphincter (B). As soon as the finger is removed a pad of wool or plastic sponge is applied to the lower anal canal to control any tendency to haematoma formation.

AUTHOR'S PREFERENCE IN OPERATIVE TREATMENT

Lateral subcutaneous internal sphincterotomy is now my preferred operation for the treatment of idiopathic anal fissure, though I recognize that some surgeons, lacking the equipment or interest, may still favour simple sphincter-stretching. I think that open posterior internal sphincterotomy should be strenuously avoided because of its complications, and the operation of triangular excision of the fissure, with or without skin grafting, should never now be necessary, except perhaps for a very occasional recalcitrant fissure which has failed to heal with other operations.

If haemorrhoids are associated with the fissure and are of first- or moderate second-degree size, they need not contraindicate treatment of the fissure by lateral subcutaneous internal sphincterotomy in the first instance; they themselves can be treated by injections two or three weeks later when the fissure has healed and a proctoscope can be passed without discomfort. But if there are very large second- or third-degree haemorrhoids, sphincterotomy as a separate manoeuvre should be avoided, for it may be followed by prolapse and thrombosis of the piles. What is required is a formal haemorrhoidectomy, at which an internal sphincterotomy is performed through one of the haemorrhoid wounds, preferably the left lateral one, or alternatively a four-finger sphincter-stretch is performed as an immediate preliminary to the haemorrhoidectomy.

TABLE 2. *Incidence (%) of Minor Disturbances of Anal Continence following Various Operations for Anal Fissure*

Type of operation	No. of patients reviewed	Impaired control for		Faecal soiling of underwear	One or more defects
		Flatus	Faeces		
Open posterior internal sphincterotomy (Bennett & Goligher 1962)	127	24	11	28	43
Sphincter-stretching (Watts et al. 1964)	90	12	2	20	28
Lateral subcutaneous internal sphincterotomy (Hoffmann & Goligher 1970)	99	6	1	7	12

REFERENCES

ARABI, Y., ALEXANDER-WILLIAMS, J. and KEIGHLEY, M. R. B. (1977) Anal pressures in hemorrhoids and anal fissure. *Am. J. Surg., 134*, 608.

BALL, C. (1908) *The Rectum: its Diseases and Developmental Defects.* London: Frowde; Hodder and Stoughton.

BENNETT, R. C. and DUTHIE, H. L. (1964) The functional importance of the internal anal sphincter. *Br. J. Surg., 51*, 753.

—— and GOLIGHER, J. C. (1962) Results of internal sphincterotomy for anal fissure. *Br. med. J., 2*, 1500.

BLAISDELL, P. C. (1937) Pathogenesis of anal fissure and implications as to treatment. *Surgery Gynec. Obstet., 65*, 672.

EISENHAMMER, S. (1951) Surgical correction of chronic internal anal (sphincteric) contracture. *S. Afr. med. J., 25*, 486.

—— (1953) The internal anal sphincter: its surgical importance. *S. Afr. med. J., 27*, 266.

—— (1959) The evaluation of the internal anal sphincterotomy operation with special reference to an anal fissure. *Surgery Gynec. Obstet., 109*, 583.

FRIES, B. and RIETZ, K. (1964) Treatment of fissure-in-ano. *Acta chir. scand., 128*, 312.

GABRIEL, W. B. (1929) Treatment of pruritus ani and anal fissure: the use of anaesthetic solutions in oil. *Br. med. J., 1*, 1070.

—— (1948) *Principles and Practice of Rectal Surgery*, 4th ed. London: H. K. Lewis.

—— (1963) *Principles and Practice of Rectal Surgery*, 5th ed. London: H. K. Lewis.

GOLIGHER, J. C., LEACOCK, A. G. and BROSSY, J.-J. (1955) Surgical anatomy of the anal canal. *Br. J. Surg., 43*, 51.

GORSCH, R. V. (1934) Oil soluble anaesthetics in proctology. *Med. Rec., 139*, 35.

GRAHAM-STEWART, C. W., GREENWOOD, R. K. and LLOYD-DAVIES, R. W. (1961) A review of 50 patients with fistula-in-ano. *Surgery Gynec. Obstet., 113*, 445.

HANCOCK, B. D. (1977) The internal sphincter and anal fissure. *Br. J. Surg., 64*, 92.

HAWLEY, P. R. (1969) The treatment of chronic fissure-in-ano. *Br. J. surg., 56*, 519.

HOFFMANN, D. C. and GOLIGHER, J. C. (1970) Lateral subcutaneous internal sphincterotomy in treatment of anal fissure. *Br. med. J., 3*, 673.

HUGHES, E. S. R. (1953) Anal fissure. *Br. med. J., 2*, 803.

LOCKHART-MUMMERY, H. E. (1957) In *Operative Surgery*, ed. C. Rob and R. Smith, Vol. 3, p. 11. London: Butterworths.

MILES, W. E. (1919) Observations upon internal piles. *Surgery Gynec. Obstet., 29*, 497.

—— (1939) *Rectal Surgery.* London: Cassell.

MILLIGAN, E. T. C. (1943) The surgical anatomy and disorders of the peri-anal space. *Proc. R. Soc. Med., 36*, 365.

—— and MORGAN, C. N. (1934) Surgical anatomy of the anal canal, with special reference to ano-rectal fistulae. *Lancet, 2*, 1213.

MOORE, H. D. (1964) Treatment of fissure-in-ano. *Lancet, 1*, 909.

MORGAN, C. N. (1935) Oil-soluble anaesthetics in rectal surgery. *Br. med. J., 2*, 938.

—— (1954) Personal communication.

—— and THOMPSON, H. R. (1956) Surgical anatomy of the anal canal with special reference to the surgical importance of the internal sphincter and conjoint longitudinal muscles. *Ann. R. Coll. Surg. Engl., 19*, 88.

NOTARAS, M. J. (1968) Personal communication.

—— (1969) Lateral subcutaneous sphincterotomy for anal fissure—a new technique. *Proc. R. Soc. Med., 62*, 713.

—— (1971) The treatment of anal fissure by lateral subcutaneous internal sphincterotomy—a technique and results. *Br. J. Surg., 58*, 96.

PARKS, A. G. (1967) The management of fissure-in-ano. *Hosp. Med., 1*, 737.

RÉCAMIER, N. (1829) Quoted by Maisonneuve, J. G. (1849) Du traitement de la fissure à l'anus par la dilatation forcée. *Gaz. d'Hôp., 1*, 220.

WATTS, J. M. BENNETT, R. C. and GOLIGHER, J. C. (1965) Stretching of the anal sphincters in the treatment of fissure-in-ano. *Br. med. J., 2*, 342.

YEOMANS, F. C., GORSCH, R. V. and MATHESHEIMER, J. L. (1927) Benacol in the treatment of pruritus ani (preliminary report). *Trans. Am. proct. Soc., 28*, 24.

6

Anorectal Abscess

Cellulitis leading to abscess formation is relatively common in the tissues surrounding the anal canal and lower rectum. According to Ellis (1958) it is usually due to staphylococci, more rarely to streptococci, *E. coli*, or *Proteus* spp. In recent years with the more regular use of anaerobic culture it has become evident that anaerobes, such as *Clostridium welchii* and particularly *Bacteroides*, are frequently responsible for these abscesses. Sometimes the tubercle bacillus is found, though usually in association with a mixed pyogenic infection.

AETIOLOGY

Cause Obvious

In a minority—perhaps 20%—of the cases the portal of entry of the infection is obvious as for example when a posterior perianal abscess arises secondary to a dorsal anal fissure, or an abscess forms in a ruptured anal haematoma. Other instances are the infection that sometimes occurs in the submucous, perianal or ischiorectal spaces in relation to prolapsed thrombosed internal haemorrhoids, and the severe infections with extensive necrosis that may follow injection of oily anaesthetic solutions or alcohol into the ischiorectal or perianal spaces in the treatment of anal fissure or pruritus. Injections for internal haemorrhoids are much less frequently complicated in this way—in fact surprisingly rarely in view of the very large number of haemorrhoid patients treated by injections. Lastly, abscesses in this region are sometimes clearly attributable to injuries of the anal skin or mucosa by the nozzle of an enema syringe or are sequels to anal operations such as haemorrhoidectomy.

The rare pelvirectal type of anorectal abscess, which forms in the loose connective tissue between the pelvic peritoneum and the levator muscles as complication or sequel of septic lesions in the pelvis, has also usually a definite cause. Perhaps the commonest antecedent is acute appendicitis or acute salpingitis, but it may also arise from acute suppuration in connection with a diverticulitis, growth, or stricture of the sigmoid colon, or rectum, or infections of the prostate, seminal vesicles, pelvic bones or sacrum.

No Cause Immediately Evident

In the majority of cases of anorectal abscess there is no evident pre-existing lesion to provide an entry for micro-organisms into the tissue spaces and there has been much discussion as to how infection usually occurs under these circumstances. Some of the mechanisms suggested are the following:

ABRASION OR TEARING OF THE LINING OF THE ANAL CANAL OR OF THE PERIANAL SKIN

It is probable that minute, almost imperceptible, abrasions or tears of the lining of the anal canal are not infrequently produced by hard faeces, especially by hard objects in the faeces such as fish or rabbit bones, or particles of egg shell. These breaches of the epithelium might allow bacteria to effect an entry into the tissue spaces and subsequently close or remain as an internal fistulous opening. In the same way any abrasion of the perianal skin caused by the friction of rough underclothes or trousers may provide an avenue for entrance of organisms into the subcutaneous tissues with resulting cellulitis and abscess formation.

INFECTION FROM AN ANAL CRYPT VIA AN ANAL GLAND

The anatomy of the so-called anal 'glands', first described by Hermann and Desfosses (1880), has been outlined on p. 9. The possible significance of these epithelium-lined tracks, which extend from the anal crypts through the lower half of the internal sphincter, in the aetiology of anorectal infection was long ago pointed out by Lockhart-Mummery (1929), Gordon-Watson and Dodd (1935), Hill et al. (1943), Kratzer and Dockerty (1947) and Kratzer (1950). It has been widely accepted in America that practically all anorectal abscesses or fistulae originate in anal cryptitis and anal glandular infections (Buie 1937; Bacon 1949; Nesselrod 1949; Granet 1954). In Britain acceptance of this concept has been much less general and most surgeons in this country long inclined to the view that the majority of these abscesses were due to some other cause. However, work by Eisenhammer (1956, 1958, 1961) and Parks (1961) has again

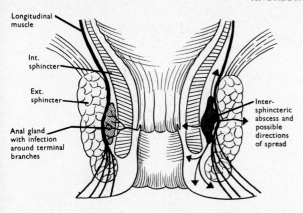

Fig. 113. The genesis of intersphincteric abscess from anal glandular infection, and the possible avenues of extension.

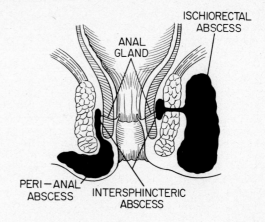

Fig. 114. The concept of perianal and ischiorectal abscesses as further extensions of an intersphincteric abscess.

emphasized the role of the anal glands in the production of abscesses and fistulae in this region.

Parks (1961) has demonstrated characteristic stratified, mucus-secreting, columnar epithelium of anal glandular type in biopsy material from 21 of 30 cases of fistula-in-ano, in 13 of which it formed part of the lining of the inner end of the fistulous track or of an intersphincteric abscess. He has convincingly argued the case for regarding the anal glands as the essential aetiological factor in most fistulae-in-ano. He gives his support to Eisenhammer's (1956, 1958, 1961) suggestion that the first step in the pathogenesis of an anal abscess or fistula is the formation of an *intersphincteric abscess* in relation to the termination of an anal gland lying between the internal sphincter and the longitudinal intersphincteric muscle fibres (Fig. 113). Subsequently the pus may force its way downwards along the longitudinal fibres to emerge at the anal orifice as a *perianal abscess* (Figs 113, 114), laterally through the longitudinal muscle and external sphincter to enter the ischiorectal space and give rise to an *ischiorectal abscess* (Figs 113, 114), or upwards in the intersphincteric space to produce what Eisenhammer (1961) terms a *high intermuscular abscess* (Fig. 113), which he believes has usually been wrongly regarded in the past as a submucous abscess.

The theory of anal glandular infection and the formation of an intersphincteric abscess as the initial event in the development of most anorectal abscesses is attractive, in so far as the internal opening in many cases of anal fistulae that open internally is at an anal crypt. On the other hand, on this hypothesis one might expect virtually all abscesses in this region to have an internal opening at the level of the anal valves when, in fact, the majority do not in my experience. Admittedly, in examining and treating acute anorectal abscesses, one does not always scrutinize and palpate the anal canal very searchingly in the first instance for an internal opening. But certainly the majority of these cases, treated solely by an adequate external incision, heal without ever developing a fistula into the anal canal (see p. 160). If infection along an anal gland is accepted as the primary lesion in anorectal abscess, it must be allowed that the fine track of the gland itself does not invariably, or even usually, drain pus back into the anal canal, which is somewhat surprising.

A more careful study of the incidence of internal openings and of intersphincteric abscess formation in association with anorectal abscesses and fistulae has been conducted at the General Infirmary in Leeds (Goligher et al. 1967). In a series of 29 cases

with acute abscesses in the anal region (20 perianal, eight ischiorectal and one pelvirectal) coming to emergency operation, the following manoeuvres were employed. First of all, the lining of the anal canal was examined with the aid of a bivalve speculum, particular attention being directed to the region of the anal valves in the corresponding sector of the canal and also posteriorly. Firm pressure was exerted on the abscess to see if pus could be expressed from any of the anal crypts. The crypts were also gently probed in search of an internal opening. Of the 29 cases, five had a demonstrable communication with the crypt region (five with perianal and none with ischiorectal abscesses).

Next, after infiltration of the subcutaneous and submucous tissues of the relevant quadrant of the anal canal, and using a bivalve speculum, a broad flap of anal canal lining was dissected up to 6 mm above the pectinate line (see Fig. 149). The lower edge of the internal sphincter was defined and the plane between the two sphincters opened up sufficiently to allow passage of the blades of two pairs of straight artery forceps to grasp a rectangle of the lower half of the internal sphincter (see Fig. 149). This portion of the muscle was excised by cutting on the outer side of each forceps, and horizontally above the points of the forceps, thus opening up the intersphincteric space to inspection. Adrenaline gauze swabs and diathermy were used freely to give a bloodless field. Of the 29 cases dissected in this way eight had intersphincteric abscesses (seven with perianal and one with an ischiorectal abscess). Actually in three of the patients with perianal abscesses the internal sphincter was semi-necrotic and pus already lay directly under the lining of the anal canal.

These experiences would seem to show that whilst some anorectal abscesses are probably caused by anal glandular infections operating through the medium of an intersphincteric abscess, in some two-thirds of the cases this aetiological mechanism does not apply.

BLOOD-BORNE INFECTION

In septicaemic conditions abscesses may arise in the perianal and perirectal region as elsewhere due to blood-borne infection; but this state of affairs, with a very ill patient showing other mani-.

festations of sepsis, bears no relationship to ordinary cases of anorectal abscess.

ADDITIONAL AETIOLOGICAL FACTORS

It is most important for the surgeon to bear in mind *three additional aetiological factors*, which are not infrequently found in cases of anorectal abscess, and which, if present, require special consideration in planning treatment. They are *Crohn's disease, ulcerative colitis* and *tuberculosis*. Abscesses associated with these conditions usually terminate in the formation of fistulae and will be considered in more detail in the section dealing with fistulae (see p. 195).

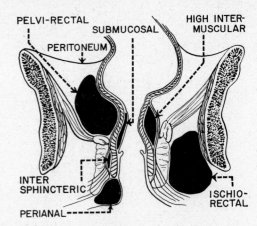

Fig. 115. The sites of abscess formation in the region of the anus and rectum.

INCIDENCE

Anorectal abscesses are much commoner in men than in women. Of 200 cases of anorectal abscess treated in the casualty department of the Leeds General Infirmary during an 18-month period, 143 were males and 77 females (Ellis 1958). The difference in the incidence in the two sexes may be explained by the less fastidious attitude of men in general towards anal cleanliness, by their rougher type of underclothing, causing greater friction on the perianal skin, and by their often more arduous work causing more sweating in the anal region.

CLASSIFICATION

Anorectal abscesses are generally classified according to their site of origin in the different tissue spaces as perianal, ischiorectal, submucous (or high intermuscular) and pelvirectal (Fig. 115). But in time the inflammatory process tends to spread, and may do so widely in neglected cases. Thus an abscess originating in the perianal space may extend into the ischiorectal space, or *vice versa*, and a supralevator abscess may eventually burst through the levator muscle and present as an ischiorectal abscess. The frequency of the different types of abscess in the series mentioned above (Ellis 1958) was as follows:

Perianal	109
Ischiorectal	78
Submucous (or high intermuscular)	0
Pelvirectal	0
Atypical	13

These figures perhaps slightly underrate the incidence of submucous (or high intermuscular) and pelvirectal abscesses, in so far as some patients with these lesions may possibly have been referred not to the casualty department but to individual surgical clinics. But they are certainly very infrequent as compared with the other varieties of abscess. Similarly, the absence of intersphincteric abscesses in this list is misleading, for this form of abscess is not ordinarily evident clinically and has to be sought for by special dissection (see pp. 188 and 189), which was not employed on these cases. It will be noted that perianal abscess is slightly more common than ischiorectal abscess.

CLINICAL FEATURES

PERIANAL AND ISCHIORECTAL ABSCESSES

The initial symptom with these abscesses is acute pain in the anal region, which is throbbing in character, and aggravated by sitting, coughing, sneezing and defaecation. Usually by the time the patient presents at hospital he has noticed an actual swelling in the vicinity of the anus, and found that it is exquisitely tender on touching. Occasionally the abscess has burst and the patient reports that following the discharge of pus his pain was much relieved. Small perianal abscesses are not as a rule attended by much constitutional upset, but larger

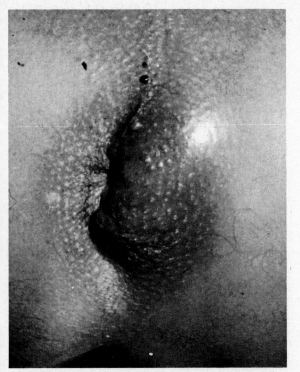

Fig. 116. Perianal abscess producing diffuse swelling of the perianal region of the left side of the anus (Mr M. Ellis' case).

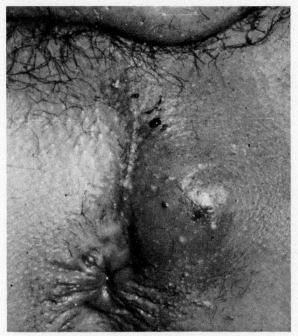

Fig. 117. Perianal abscess showing as a localized, ovoid swelling to the left and in front of the anus (Mr M. Ellis' case).

abscesses, especially those of ischiorectal type, generally produce a moderate fever up to say 39°C, and the usual pyrexial accompaniments.

On examination a perianal abscess usually shows itself as a red, tender, localized rounded or ovoid swelling close to the anus. It stands out above the surrounding skin (Figs 116, 117), which is not tender on palpation. At a later stage obvious fluctuation may be elicited in the swelling and the skin may become purple or necrotic or actually give way allowing pus to escape. Digital examination of the rectum reveals no tenderness, induration or bulging of the corresponding aspect of the anal canal above the visible swelling at the anal orifice.

An *ischiorectal abscess* causes a more diffuse brawny swelling of the entire perianal region on one side of the anus, which is tender but not usually fluctuant till a late stage is reached. Rectal examination with the finger elicits a similar tender induration bulging into the anal canal on that side. Sometimes an ischiorectal abscess is bilateral with these signs evident on both sides and usually posteriorly as well. Also some ischiorectal abscesses arising high in the ischiorectal fossa may produce no obvious external signs, and the only manifestation of inflammation may be a little tenderness and indura-

tion or firm palpation of the apical part of the fossa between index finger and thumb. Such cases may present with a pyrexia of obscure origin without spontaneous pain of any kind.

In other cases with gross inflammatory swelling of one or both sides of the anus, considerable areas of necrosis of the overlying skin may develop. These extensive abscesses are often due to gas-forming organisms which may be further indicated by the elicitation of frank crepitation and the presence of intense toxaemia.

SUBMUCOUS OR HIGH INTERMUSCULAR ABSCESS

This type of abscess is usually most insidious in its onset. It may cause a dull aching pain in the rectum rather than the anus. Not infrequently the patient does not present till the abscess has burst, discharging its contents into the rectum, so that one of the symptoms is passage of pus per anum.

There are no external signs with a submucous abscess unless it is complicated by an associated perianal or ischiorectal abscess. Digital examination reveals a smooth swelling on one aspect of the upper part of the anal canal and of the lower rectum. This is tender and may be indurated, or there may be an area of central softening. If the abscess has already burst the opening through which it ruptured may be palpable, or may sometimes to be seen on proctoscopy, pus being observed to escape from it as pressure is exerted with forceps on the surrounding mucosa.

PELVIRECTAL ABSCESS

A pelvirectal abscess also usually has an insidious onset with pyrexia and a certain amount of constitutional upset, but no local anal or rectal pain or external signs. Digital examination of the rectum, however, may reveal a tender mass high up in the pelvis, and this is confirmed on vaginal examination. Later the mass may extend downwards into one or other ischiorectal fossa, where it may be palpable on rectal examination or may even produce an external swelling. There may be a clear history of some recent pelvic infection, but not infrequently this is lacking.

DIAGNOSIS

In the great majority of cases of anorectal abscess, the diagnosis is very obvious, but sometimes the clinical distinction between different types of abscess is not so easy, especially in late cases when the suppurative process has spread and the features of more than one classical type may be present. Thus it may be difficult to distinguish before operation between a pelvirectal abscess with a downward extension into the ischiorectal fossa, and a large primary ischiorectal abscess. At operation, however, in the former case an opening will be found in the corresponding levator ani muscle connecting the supralevator abscess with its ischiorectal prolongation.

With abscesses situated anterior to the anus in men the possibility of confusion with a *periurethral abscess* may arise if the lesion extends forwards towards the urethral bulb. Enquiries as to a previous urethritis, urethral stricture or urethral instrumentation are important, and it may be necessary to investigate the state of the urethra by passage of sounds. In the female anteriorly situated abscesses may be mistaken for *infective conditions of Bartholin's glands*.

Very occasionally a patient may present with an exceptionally early perianal or ischiorectal abscess which is causing anal pain, but on examination the only physical sign that can be elicited is tenderness on palpation in the appropriate region. It is easy to fall into the error of diagnosing this state of affairs as being psychogenic, and the possibility of anal pain and tenderness with no signs being due to an incipient anorectal abscess must always be kept in mind.

A *tuberculous anorectal abscess*, which is usually of perianal or ischiorectal type, may present acutely like an ordinary pyogenic abscess—for the infection is often a mixed one. More often, however, it manifests itself as a swelling which is only slightly tender, gradually increases in size, and may eventually burst before the patient seeks advice. The discharge is usually thinner and more watery than in an ordinary pyogenic abscess, and the skin around the opening may be undermined and unhealthy, but often there are no special features to suggest a tuberculous infection. The patient may have a known pulmonary tuberculous lesion or this may be disclosed on radiological examination and examination of the sputum.

TREATMENT

It has generally been held in the past that a cellulitis in the tissues around the anus and rectum will never resolve spontaneously, but always proceeds to suppuration. Since the advent of antibiotics this is no longer entirely true, for I have seen a very few cases with incipient inflammatory changes in the perianal region which subsided on antibiotic therapy. However I have seen far more patients whose development of a perianal or ischiorectal abscess has continued despite the administration of penicillin and streptomycin by their general practitioners. I would say therefore that *as a rule operation will be required and that the sooner it is carried out the better*.

INTRA- OR EXTRA-ANAL INCISION?

On the basis of his claim that anorectal abscesses usually originate in cryptoglandular infections of the intersphincteric space, Eisenhammer (1956, 1958, 1961) has advocated that most of these abscesses should be opened into the anal canal through their site of origin. To do so he uses an internal sphincterotomy, similar to that employed in the treatment of anal fissure, but situated in the appropriate sector of the canal to drain the intersphincteric abscess. It would seem that sometimes he extends his incision well outwards into the perianal skin to deal more adequately with abscesses lying wide of the anus, but if

DETAILS OF USUAL OPERATIVE TREATMENT

so subsequently sutures most of the external part of the wound. He acknowledges that this is a complete reversal of the usual practice in operating on anorectal abscesses and fistulae, of having the wounds widely open externally so that their inner portions have a chance to heal before the outer part closes. Though a generally favourable impression is conveyed of the outcome of his method, no details are given of the number of cases so treated or of the results obtained.

It will be appreciated that an internal sphincter*otomy* of this kind merely drains the abscess, it does not remove the epithelium-lined anal glandular track, which is presumed to provide the avenue for entrance of infection into the intersphincteric space. An even more logical operation would be to unroof the intersphincteric abscess by an internal sphincter*ectomy*, consisting of removal of a flap of anal canal lining and a piece of the

These patients are usually suffering considerable discomfort and it is best to omit all bowel preparation in the form of enemas. Shaving of the perianal skin should be postponed till the anaesthetic has been given.

To open and explore an abscess of the anal region properly a general anaesthetic is essential. With the patient in the lithotomy position, a linear incision is made over the swelling (Fig. 118), usually

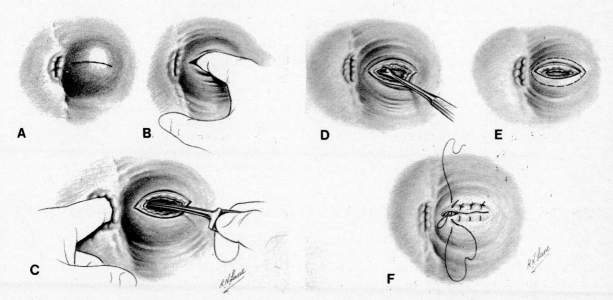

Fig. 118. The steps in the operative treatment of perianal and ischiorectal abscesses: Incision; exploration of abscess cavity with finger; seeking an internal fistulous opening with probe or director; cruciate enlargement of the wound and some trimming of the skin edges preparatory to leaving wound open, if *Gabriel's method* is being adopted; or curetting of the abscess cavity with a sharp spoon and complete closure of the skin wound with deep vertical mattress sutures, if *Ellis' technique* is being followed.

lower half of the internal sphincter. This procedure would eliminate the glandular epithelium of that part of the anal canal, and ought to provide better insurance against recurrent abscesses or fistula formation at that site. But, as already mentioned on p. 155, I have used this operation on 29 patients with anorectal abscesses and succeeded in demonstrating intersphincteric abscesses in only eight (in seven of 20 cases with perianal abscesses, and in one of eight cases with ischiorectal abscesses). These experiences would not encourage one to treat anorectal abscesses by routine internal sphincterotomy or sphincterectomy. It would seem, indeed, that any attempt to do so would inevitably result in a fair proportion of patients having quite unnecessary damage done to their sphincteric musculature, and one can readily see that in the hands of relatively junior staff, to whom these cases often fall, there could be many disastrous consequences.

4 cm long in the first instance, and certainly of sufficient length to allow the finger to be inserted freely into the abscess cavity. After the main gush of pus has escaped and a specimen has been taken for bacteriological examination, the wound is thoroughly explored with the index finger, dividing septa being gently broken down and subsidiary abscess cavities brought into communication with the main cavity. Attention is now directed to determining whether an internal fistulous opening is present or not, any suggestive depression detected on the inner wall of the wound with the finger being *very gently* tested with a medium-sized probe or

probe-pointed director. This manoeuvre calls for the utmost delicacy for, in the oedematous state of the tissues in the presence of an acute abscess, a false passage is all too easily produced. Assistance in the search for a fistulous opening may be obtained by examining with the aid of a bivalve anal speculum the lining of the anal canal in the sector corresponding to the abscess, especially at the level of the anal valves. The manner of completion of the operation is determined by the presence or absence of a fistula.

NO OBVIOUS FISTULA DEMONSTRATED

This is the state of affairs in the great majority of abscess cases in my experience. Under these circumstances the management of the wound may follow either of two courses:

Further Incision or Excision of Skin to Lay the Abscess Cavity Widely Open
This is the classical method, the skin being further incised or excised to give a wide cruciate or saucer- or bowl-shaped wound. The practice of excision has been particularly strongly advocated by Lockhart-Mummery (1934) and Gabriel (1948), who recommend removing with scissors all the skin and subcutaneous fat overlying the abscess cavity so as to 'unroof' it (Fig. 118). After careful haemostasis the raw surfaces are dressed with gauze soaked in Milton and a firm external dressing with plenty of wool is applied. The subsequent management is similar to that of any open fistula wound, with baths, irrigations and changes of dressings twice daily, starting after the bowels act on the second or third postoperative day. Complete healing usually takes four or five weeks or longer depending of the size of the abscess, and that is the main objection to this technique. However, unless an internal fistulous opening has been overlooked it is generally considered to be a very reliable method, though good information on this point has been lacking till the recent paper by Buchan and Grace (1973) (see p. 161). Actually in recent years I have generally compromised in my application of this technique and have excised only a limited amount of skin from the edges of the initial incision, sufficient to prevent them coming together and adhering. This shortens the period of convalescence apparently without seriously impairing the reliability of the method.

Primary Suture Under Systemic Antibiotic Therapy
Since the introduction of antibiotics a new fashion has grown up in several casualty departments in British hospitals of treating cellulitic abscesses, not by the traditional method of incision and drainage, but, *under systemic antibiotic cover*, by incision, curettage and primary suture. The rationale of the curettage is that it is alleged to destroy the layer of granulations lining the abscess wall thereby allowing the antibiotic to penetrate freely from the blood stream into the abscess cavity and keep it sterile. My colleague Ellis (1959) at the Leeds General Infirmary stated that the vast majority of abscesses so treated heal by first intention. He has extended this method also to the treatment of perianal and ischiorectal abscesses. Primary suture for such lesions has struck many as revolutionary and the method has not been widely accepted, but Ellis has treated over 1000 such abscesses along these lines in out-patients in the last ten years and his results command attention. His detailed management is as follows:

Half an hour before operation 500 mg of each of ampicillin and cloxacillin (or 600 mg of lincomycin) are given by injection. Under general anaesthesia the abscess is then incised and explored as described above. *Cases with a fistulous opening into the anal canal are unsuitable for this method.* The wall of the cavity is well curetted with a sharp spoon or rubbed with a gauze swab (Fig. 118). Finally the skin edges and as much of the wall of the cavity as possible are approximated accurately with three or four deep vertical mattress sutures of silk-worm gut or nylon (Fig. 118), and a dry dressing is applied and kept firmly in place with a T-shaped bandage and adhesive strapping. The patient *is allowed home that day* and is given a four-day supply of ampicillin and cloxacillin for oral administration (500 mg of each six-hourly) or, more recently, of clindamycin (150 mg six-hourly by mouth). He re-attends on the fourth and sixth days for inspection of his wound and re-dressing, the sutures being removed on the latter occasion. During this time his bowels are not confined but act as required with the assistance of a mild aperient if necessary. He is able to return to work usually within a week of the operation unless fistulation occurs.

Follow-up by Ellis and myself in 1955 of 100 consecutive cases of perianal or ischiorectal abscess treated by this method or primary suture in the receiving room of the Leeds General Infirmary during 1953 revealed that 86 had healed by first intention and remained well subsequently, but that 14 either failed to heal, or healed and subsequently broke down to form a fistula-in-ano. Many of these fistulae were quite symptomless and were only brought to light by our enquiry. They have all been dealt with satisfactorily since by a further operation. In a similar follow-up study by Wilson (1964) of 100 cases of anorectal abscess treated by Ellis' method and traced for an average of just over two years, 15 patients developed recurrent abscesses and seven anal fistulae—an overall rate of recurrent infection of 22%. The incidence of recurrence was 15·6% in cases with perianal abscesses initially, but 33·3% in those with ischiorectal abscesses.

These results with primary suture are perhaps not very impressive, but the results of classical unroofing operations, as reported by Buchan and Grace (1973), with 25% of recurrences on a two-year follow-up, also leave a great deal to be desired. In terms of the time taken for complete healing and the period lost from work postoperatively, the method of primary suture under antibiotic cover certainly has advantages over the conventional type of operation, as a recent controlled comparison by us—with unfortunately a rather brief follow-up period—has confirmed (Leaper et al. 1976).

AN ASSOCIATED INTERNAL FISTULOUS OPENING HAS BEEN FOUND

The discovery of an internal fistulous opening in association with a perianal or ischiorectal abscess alters the plan of operation, for whatever is done to the external wound, satisfactory healing will not be obtained till the fistulous track into the anal canal has been dealt with. The question is whether the latter should be laid open right away or whether the surgeon should be content to drain the abscess externally in the first instance and tackle the fistulous track at a later stage when the acute inflammation has subsided—and possibly a more experienced operator is available. It is usually advised that the latter course should be adopted. If this is done, no extensive 'unroofing' or further incision should be carried out in the first instance, but the wound should be sufficiently enlarged to provide free external drainage. An attack on the fistula is best deferred for seven to ten days, but if necessary can be delayed indefinitely, the wound being allowed to close round the fistulous track, and the patient discharged and then re-admitted to suit his convenience at a later date.

If the fistulous opening is low down in the anal canal at the level of the anal valves my own practice is to lay it open at the time of the original abscess operation. The resulting wound is then shaped and managed as described for a low anal fistula on p. 180. A high fistula, on the other hand, is better not dealt with at this stage unless the surgeon is specially experienced in the management of anal fistulae, and then only if he feels absolutely confident that it lies below the anorectal ring. Usually the wiser plan will be to leave it, possibly marking its position by means of a silk ligature threaded through the opening on a probe and tied *loosely* round the sphincter musculature. Subsequently in the ward with the patient conscious and able to contract his sphincter and puborectalis muscles, it may be possible to determine more accurately its relationship to the anorectal ring, and if this is satisfactory to lay it open at a second operation one week later (see Fig. 138).

HIGH INTERMUSCULAR (SO-CALLED SUBMUCOUS) ABSCESS

This form of abscess presents special problems in treatment. By the time it is diagnosed, it has already frequently ruptured into the rectum, sometimes with considerable sloughing of the overlying mucosa. It may thus be found on examination that a large internal opening is present which freely admits the tip of the finger, and which may be assumed to provide adequate drainage. Alternatively any existing opening may be small so that the abscess shows a tendency to refill. Under these circumstances enlargement of the opening will be required. Also, in cases where the abscess is still intact, it will of course need to be opened.

Under general anaesthesia and with the patient in the lithotomy position the lesion is further palpated, and then inspected. For this latter purpose a bivalve speculum is ideal. It is inserted so as to bring the appropriate sector of the anal canal and lower rectum into view. If the tissue overlying the abscess is incised with a scalpel or even cutting diathermy there is apt to be troublesome haemorrhage. A better plan therefore is to find the internal opening with a probe-pointed director, which is then passed upward for 2–2·5 cm and made to emerge again into the lumen through the mucosa (see Fig. 147A). A strong silk ligature is then threaded on a malleable silver probe with an eye, passed from the original internal opening to the newly created one and tied very tightly round the isolated bridge of mucosa—and round the circular muscle as well if the abscess is intermuscular rather than submucosal (see Fig. 147B). A second ligature may be passed and tied in a similar manner alongside the first (see Fig. 147C). These ligatures slowly strangulate the tissue, eventually cutting through after four or five days and in the process laying the abscess widely open. If no internal opening already exists the abscess is opened by a small stab incision through the mucosa with a pair of artery or sinus forceps. This in turn is enlarged by the method of strangulating ligatures just outlined or by cutting diathermy.

Sometimes a submucous or intermuscular abscess coexists with a perianal or ischiorectal abscess. A more elaborate operation will then be required, consisting of adequate incision of the latter abscess together with laying open of the submucous extension along the lines already indicated.

PELVIRECTAL ABSCESS

It may only be at the opening of an ischiorectal abscess that the existence of a pelvirectal abscess is discovered by finding that pus is coming down from above the levator muscle. The opening in the latter muscle should be found and enlarged with forceps or scalpel till it will admit two fingers. A rubber drainage tube of at least 1 cm diameter is then passed through it and secured with a plain catgut stitch to the muscle edge. The ischiorectal abscess, if not already opened, is dealt with by further incisions and removal of skin especially posteriorly to provide for wide unroofing.

The underlying cause of the pelvic infection resulting in the formation of the pelvirectal abscess also needs to be considered, and may require to be dealt with by a later operation through the abdomen.

CROHN'S OR TUBERCULOUS ABSCESS

A Crohn's abscess or tuberculous infection may sometimes be suspected clinically by the indolent character of the condition, or at operation by the pale greyish appearance of the granulations lining the abscess cavity. In all suspicious cases samples of the granulation tissue should certainly be sent to the laboratory for histological examination and if necessary guinea-pig inoculation. It is indeed a wise precaution to send such specimens in all cases even when the clinical and operative features have not particularly suggested a tuberculous aetiology.

REFERENCES

BACON, H. E. (1949) *The Anus, Rectum and Sigmoid Colon*, 3rd ed. Philadelphia: Lippincott.

BUCHAN, R. and GRACE, R. H. (1973) Anorectal suppuration: the results of treatment and the factors influencing the recurrence rate. *Br. J. Surg.*, *60*, 537.

BUIE, L. A. (1937) *Practical Proctology*. Philadelphia and London: Saunders.

EISENHAMMER, S. (1956) The internal anal sphincter and the anorectal abscess. *Surgery Gynec. Obstet.*, *103*, 501.

—— (1958) A new approach to the anorectal fistulous abscess based on the high intermuscular lesion. *Surgery Gynec. Obstet.*, *106*, 595.

—— (1961) The anorectal and anovulval fistulous abscess. *Surgery Gynec. Obstet.*, *113*, 519.

ELLIS, M. (1958) Personal communication.

—— (1959) Progress in the casualty department. In *British Surgical Practice*, ed. E. R. Carling and J. P. Ross, p. 379. London: Butterworth.

GABRIEL, W. B. (1948) *Principles and Practice of Rectal Surgery*, 4th ed. London: H. K. Lewis.

GOLIGHER, J. C., ELLIS, M. and PISSIDES, A. (1967) A critique of anal glandular infection in the aetiology and treatment of idiopathic anorectal abscesses and fistulas. *Br. J. Surg.*, *54*, 977.

GORDON-WATSON, C. and DODD, H. (1935) Observation on fistula-in-ano in relation to intramuscular perianal glands. *Br. J. Surg.*, *22*, 303.

GRANET, E. (1954) *Manual of Proctology*. Chicago: Year-Book Publishers.

HERMANN, G. and DESFOSSES, L. (1880) Sur la muqueuse de la région cloacale du rectum. *C.r. hebd. Séanc. Acad. Sci., Paris*, *90*, 1301.

HILL, M. R., SHYROCK, E. H. and REBELL, F. G. (1943) Role of anal glands in the pathogenesis of anorectal disease. *J. Am. med. Ass.*, *121*, 742.

KRATZER, G. L. (1950) Anal ducts and their clinical significance. *Am. J. Surg.*, *79*, 34.

—— and DOCKERTY, M. B. (1947) Histopathology of the anal ducts. *Surgery Gynec. Obstet.*, *84*, 333.

LEAPER, D., PAGE, R. E., ROSENBERG, I. L., WILSON, D. H. and GOLIGHER, J. C. (1976) A controlled study comparing the conventional treatment of idiopathic anorectal abscess with that of incision, curettage and primary suture under systemic antibiotic cover. *Dis. Colon Rect.*, *19*, 46.

LOCKHART-MUMMERY, J. P. (1929) Discussion on fistula-in-ano. *Proc. R. Soc. Med.*, *22*, 1331.

—— (1934) *Diseases of the Rectum and Colon*, 2nd ed. London: Baillière.

NESSELROD, J. P. (1949) In *A Textbook of Surgery*, ed. F. Christopher, 5th ed., p. 1092. Philadelphia and London: Saunders.

PARKS, A. G. (1961) Pathogenesis and treatment of fistula-in-ano. *Br. med. J.*, *1*, 463.

WILSON, D. H. (1964) The late results of anorectal abscess treated by incision, curettage and primary suture under antibiotic cover. *Br. J. Surg.*, *51*, 828.

7

Fistula-in-Ano

Fistula is the Latin word for a reed, pipe, or flute. In surgery it implies a chronic granulating track connecting two epithelial-lined surfaces. These surfaces may be cutaneous or mucosal. In its simplest form an *anal fistula* is a single track with an *external* opening in the skin of the perianal region, and an *internal* opening in the modified skin or mucosa of the anal canal or rectum. However, the fistulous track is often more complicated in its course and has several external openings; multiple internal openings are very rare. The *wall* of the track is composed of a thick tough layer of fibrous tissue which, in the intact fistula, forms a fibrous tube lined on its inner aspect by a layer of granulation tissue. Its structure is seen to best advantage when the fistula is laid open at operation and the thick velvety inner coat of granulations is scraped off the white fibrous base (see Fig. 139c).

The term *sinus* (L. = bay or recess) is taken to mean a granulating track which is open at only one end. However such culs-de-sac are often referred to loosely as *blind fistulae*, and in this chapter it is not proposed to differentiate rigidly between true fistulae and sinuses, but to include both lesions under the comprehensive term fistula-in-ano.

AETIOLOGY

The following aetiological factors require to be considered:

PREVIOUS PYOGENIC ABSCESS

Fistula-in-ano most commonly develops as a legacy of an ano-rectal abscess, particularly if the latter has been allowed to burst spontaneously or has been inadequately opened at operation.

The tendency for suppurative lesions in this region to become chronic, if neglected, is notorious, though just why they should behave in this way has not always been clear. The liability to chronicity has been attributed to several circumstances, some of them of a rather hypothetical nature:

(a) *If an internal opening into the anal canal is clearly present*, as in abscess associated with anal fissure, or in many other idiopathic anorectal abscesses, it is readily understandable that repeated re-infection of the abscess cavity from the bowel may occur, with establishment of a fistula. Occasionally a foreign body, such as a rabbit- or fish-bone or particle of egg-shell, may be lodged in the abscess cavity helping to maintain the chronic infective process.

(b) *If there is no obvious opening into the anal canal*, the development of a chronic discharging fistula has always appeared particularly mysterious. Surgeons have then often fallen back on such dissatisfying explanations as that the fatty tissues around the anus have a poor resistance to infection, or that repeated retrograde infection has occurred from the external opening in the highly contaminated perianal skin. However it would seem, particularly from the work of Eisenhammer (1958, 1961) and Parks (1961), that the solution of this mystery may lie with contamination from the bowel along the minute anal glands. As described on p. 154, this may result in the formation of an intersphincteric abscess, which is believed to be responsible for the initial ano-rectal abscess and also to act as a reservoir of infection, leading to the development of a chronic discharging fistula. This theory affords a plausible explanation for the occurrence of fistulae in the absence of a macroscopic communication with the bowel. It could provide an equally valid basis for the development of fistulae with a clearly demonstrable internal opening, for Parks (1961) has frequently found anal glandular epithelium lining the inner end of the track connecting with the anal canal, and claims that, if it were not for this epithelial continuity, such openings would usually close spontaneously. Detrimental to this theory of anal glandular infection with resulting intersphincteric abscess formation is our finding, mentioned on p. 155, that in 29 specially dissected cases of perianal or ischiorectal abscess an intersphincteric abscess was present in only eight. In this connection it may be added that similar dissections in 34 cases of anal fistulae disclosed the existence of a definite intersphincteric abscess in only nine. If, therefore, anal glandular infection is responsible for the development of most anal fistulae, it does so by the mechanism of intersphincteric abscess formation in only a minority. Alternatively some other aetiological factor may be the important agent in most cases (see Goligher et al. 1967).

TUBERCULOSIS

It has long been known that anorectal abscesses and fistulae may sometimes be due to a tuberculous infection. This occurs as a well-recognized complication in patients with known pulmonary tuberculous lesions. Thus Granet (1954) reported a 6% incidence of anorectal tuberculous abscesses and fistulae in patients undergoing treatment for pulmonary tuberculosis at the Sea View Sanatorium, New York City. The method of infection of the anal region in these cases is presumably that tubercle bacilli are swallowed in the sputum and enter the perianal tissue through

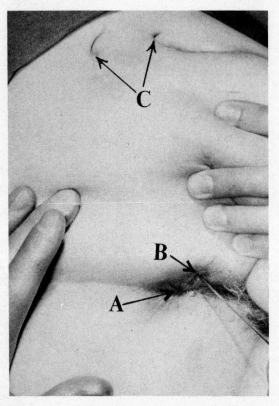

Fig. 119. Tuberculous fistula-in-ano secondary to tuberculous arthritis of the hip. (A) Anal orifice. (B) External opening of fistula marked by probe. (C) Scars in trochanteric region representing old sinuses from tuberculous hip.

minute abrasions of the lining of the anal canal. The alternative of a blood-borne infection from the pulmonary lesion is theoretically possible, though it seems much less plausible. It is also conceivable, though again unlikely, that infection might occur as a direct inoculation of tubercle bacilli during anal toilet on to excoriations or cracks in the perianal skin from the patient's fingers, contaminated by contact with his own infected sputum.

What was perhaps not so widely appreciated, till Gabriel (1921) emphasized this fact, was that a proportion of fistulae-in-ano in patients presenting in apparently good health at ordinary

surgical out-patients clinics could in fact be tuberculous. He examined histologically and by guinea-pig inoculation samples of granulation tissue from 75 consecutive cases of fistulae-in-ano operated on at St Mark's Hospital and found clear evidence of tubercle in 12 (16%). In a subsequent series of over 1500 fistulae treated at St Mark's Hospital he found the incidence of tuberculosis as determined mainly by histological examination to be 11·7% (Gabriel 1948).

Jackman and Buie (1946) surveyed 600 cases of fistula-in-ano at the Mayo Clinic, and from a consideration of the clinical and histological features combined with guinea-pig inoculation concluded that between 7 and 8% were tuberculous. The great majority of their cases with tuberculous fistulae had a coexistent focus also in the lung, and usually this was in an active condition. Under these circumstances it is easy to understand how the tuberculous anal infection might have arisen by the mechanism of swallowed sputum.

In my experience of 28 proven tuberculous fistulae, however, an active pulmonary focus was present in only 15. Of the remaining cases nine had a well-healed pulmonary lesion which had either been unsuspected prior to the development of the fistula, or had been known to be quiescent for several years. In these cases we must presumably postulate that the inoculation of the perianal region with tubercle bacilli took place some considerable time previously, and that they remained inactive or encapsulated in the tissues till some lowering of general or local resistance occurred or till there some super-added pyogenic infection, leading to the production of an abscess and fistula. In the four cases with no evidence whatsoever of an old or recent pulmonary lesion, it is difficult to account for the tuberculous anal infection. Blood spread from some other unspecified tuberculous focus in the cervical, mediastinal or mesenteric lymph glands is another possibility, as is infection with the bovine type of tubercle bacillus ingested in infected milk. At the present time, with the widespread, almost universal use of pasteurized milk or milk from tuberculin tested herds in this country, the opportunities for infection with bovine tubercle bacilli must be rare. Another way in which a tuberculous fistula-in-ano may arise is by direct extension from a tuberculous lesion of the hip, sacrum, prostate or seminal vesicles, as was the case in one of my patients (Fig. 119).

The incidence of tuberculosis in anal fistulae at the present time is probably much less than these earlier estimates suggest. In my experience about 8–10% of fistulae show a suggestive histological picture on biopsy, but in half of these it is probably due to a foreign body reaction rather than tuberculosis or to a Crohn's lesion (see below).

ULCERATIVE COLITIS

Another condition that undoubtedly predisposes to the development of anorectal abscess and fistula is ulcerative colitis, and any large series of cases of frank ulcerative colitis includes a number of patients whose condition has been complicated by the development of abscesses and fistulae. Thus in a series of 465 of my patients with ulcerative colitis analysed (see p.718), there were 63 with anorectal abscesses or fistulae. The usual course of events in the development of these fistulae seemed to be that first of all small septic cracks or fissures appeared and provided an avenue of infection. In a proportion of these cases an abscess then formed and developed into a fistula.

It must be remembered that this predisposition to abscess and fistula exists also in the cases of mild distal proctocolitis or proctitis. As the bowel symptoms in these patients may be relatively slight, the underlying inflammatory condition of the rectal mucosa may easily be overlooked if a complete rectal examination with proctoscopy and sigmoidoscopy is not performed. Anal abscess and fistula may also be complications of segmental forms of colitis in which the rectum itself remains normal.

CROHN'S DISEASE

Unquestionably the most important predisposing cause, at the present time, for anal abscesses and fistulae is Crohn's disease (see also p. 833). In a series of 332 cases of Crohn's disease treated at the Leeds General Infirmary, 16% had anorectal abscesses and 20% anal fistulae. The site of the primary disease in the intestinal tract had an important bearing on the likelihood of these complications occurring, for, when the enteritis was confined to the small intestine, the incidence of abscess was 9% and of fistula 10%, but, when the large bowel was involved, the incidence of abscess rose to 21% and of fistula to 25%. When the rectum itself was implicated, the figures rose to 23% and 35% respectively.

In view of the absence of any direct continuity between small bowel lesions and anal abscesses it must be assumed that the infection is conveyed along the lumen of the colon and enters the tissues of the anal region through minute breaches of the lining of the anal canal, or along an anal gland. As Morson and Lockhart-Mummery (1959) have pointed out, the characteristic histological appearances of Crohn's disease, with non-caseating giant cell follicles, are often seen in the granulation tissue of secondary anal abscesses and fistulae.

CARCINOMA OF THE RECTUM AND ANAL CANAL, ESPECIALLY COLLOID CARCINOMA

Carcinomata of the colon or rectum are occasionally complicated by the occurrence of pericolonic or perirectal abscesses. Indeed, bearing in mind the high bacterial content of the faeces in the large intestine and the ulcerated condition of these growths, it is perhaps remarkable that septic complications of this kind do not take place more frequently. If the growth lies in the lower rectum or in the anal canal and such an abscess should develop, it will be situated in one of the tissue spaces around the anal canal, and when it ruptures it will give rise to a fistula-in-ano. Undoubtedly the carcinoma most likely to be so complicated is a colloid carcinoma of the anorectal region. Moreover, the causal carcinoma is sometimes relatively inconspicuous and may be overlooked on cursory rectal examination. As Dukes and Galvin (1956) point out, some of these colloid carcinomata of the anorectal region may arise, not in the mucosa of the rectum or anal canal, but in the epithelial lining of anal intramuscular glands, when there may be no growth evident in the rectal or anal lumen but only in the fistulous track.

LYMPHOGRANULOMA VENEREUM

Strictures due to lymphogranuloma inguinale are quite frequently accompanied by abscesses and fistulae in the anal region (see p. 868).

ACTINOMYCOSIS OF THE ANORECTAL REGION

Actinomycosis of the rectum is excessively rare but when it occurs it is often associated with the development of anal fistulae discharging typical actinomycotic pus (see p. 865).

PREVIOUS RECTAL, OBSTETRICAL, OR GYNAECOLOGICAL OPERATIONS

Sometimes—though very rarely—a fistula develops following an operation such as haemorrhoidectomy or evacuation of an anal haematoma, due to skin edges falling together and uniting to form a bridge. In female patients anterior fistulae-in-ano quite frequently arise after complete perineal tears during parturition, or after perineorrhaphy. What happens is that the wound becomes infected and the resulting abscess bursts into the anal canal or rectum and on to the perineum or posterior vaginal wall. The consequence is often a rectovaginal fistula.

CLASSIFICATION

Anal fistulae are best thought of in relation to the vertical and horizontal axes respectively of the anal canal.

Vertical Disposition

The most important point to be determined in this axis is the position of the fistulous track in regard to the anal musculature. Milligan and Morgan (1934) classified fistulae according to their relationship to the anal sphincters and in particular to the *anorectal ring* (see p. 16). Their classification has been the guide for most surgeons for many years, though it suffered slightly from some, now exploded, misconceptions on the part of its originators regarding the anatomy of the anal musculature (see p. 9) and from a lack of precision in the definition of the course of some of the higher fistulae relative to the levator muscles. It was, therefore, modified in a few minor respects in previous editions of this book to correct these criticisms. Recently Parks et al. (1976) have formulated a new classification which takes into account the important work of Eisenhammer (1958, 1961), Stelzner (1976) and Parks (1961) on the pathogenesis and course of anal fistulae. It emphasizes especially the relationship of fistulae to the *external sphincter* and is a good deal more detailed and probably more accurate than that of Milligan and Morgan (1934). However, though the terms used in this new classification are

TABLE 3. *Comparison of Classifications of Fistulae in Anal Region*

Milligan and Morgan (1934) and Goligher (1975)	Parks et al. (1976)
Subcutaneous (5%)	Scarcely recognized
Low anal (75%)	Low intersphincteric
High anal (8%)	Transsphincteric
Anorectal (7%)	
Ischiorectal or infralevator	Trans- or suprasphincteric with high blind infralevator extension
Pelvirectal or supralevator	Trans- or suprasphincteric with blind supralevator extension
	Extrasphincteric
Submucous (or high intermuscular) (5%)	High intersphincteric

quite different from those in the older classification, for the most part the categories of fistula recognized are substantially the same—at least as regards therapeutic implications—as those described in the modification of the Milligan–Morgan classification used previously by us (Goligher 1975). The two classifications are compared in Table 3, which also gives some indication of the frequency of the different types of fistula.

It is worth remembering that it is sometimes difficult to determine the precise course of a complex fistula at operation and even more difficult to record the findings in such a way that they will be intelligible to subsequent readers. Conse-

quently classifications based on a survey of the operative notes of fistula cases inevitably depend on a certain amount of imaginative interpretation. To simplify description of different types of fistulae they will be portrayed on a standard diagram of a coronal section of the anorectal region (Fig. 120).

SUBCUTANEOUS FISTULAE

These fistulae have tracks that lie just deep to the perianal skin or cutaneous lining of the lower part of the anal canal below the pectinate line (Fig. 121). They may be true fistulae or sinuses. Parks et al.

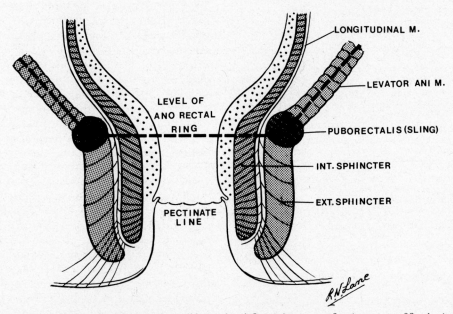

Fig. 120. Standard diagram of a coronal section that will be used in defining the course of various types of fistulae in relation to the anorectal musculature. Note particularly the position of the anorectal ring and the levators.

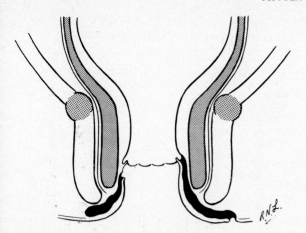

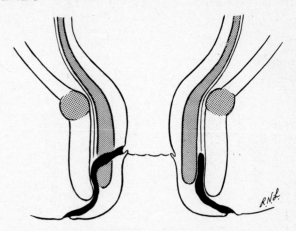

Fig. 121. Section of the anal canal showing the course of a *subcutaneous* fistula.

Fig. 122. Section of the anal canal showing the course of a *low anal* fistula (low intersphincteric fistula of Parks et al. 1976).

(1976) rather belittle the purely subcutaneous fistula, but I have no doubt from my experience that this type of fistula does occasionally occur.

LOW ANAL (LOW INTERSPHINCTERIC) FISTULAE

They may be defined as fistulae with tracks that do not extend above the level of the anal crypts, and indeed usually open at this level into the anal canal (Fig. 122). Milligan and Morgan (1934) believed that such fistulae, when traced inwards, would pass through the external sphincter just above its subcutaneous portion and would skirt the lower border of the internal sphincter. We now know, however, that these fistulae usually run below the subcutaneous external sphincter, enter the intersphincteric plane and then pass through the lowermost part of the internal sphincter to open on the lining of the anal canal at the level of the pectinate line (Fig. 122). Included under the heading of low anal (low intersphincteric) fistulae are also sinuses with an external opening and a blind track that extends up in the anal intermuscular septum usually to the level of the pectinate line.

As will be seen in Table 3, low anal (or low intersphincteric) fistulae constitute the bulk of the fistulae in the anal region.

HIGH ANAL (TRANSSPHINCTERIC) FISTULAE

In these fistulae the track rises to a higher level and is in relation to the upper parts of the anal sphincters, but does not extend above the anorectal ring, though it may reach close to it. It may be either a true fistula, with an internal opening anywhere from the pectinate line to just below the anorectal ring but usually at the pectinate line (Fig. 123), or a blind external fistula with the closed end of the track reaching to a point anywhere up to the anorectal ring, but usually with an additional blind side track extending through the external sphincter to end in the intersphincteric septum at the level of the anal valves.

ANORECTAL FISTULAE

These are the very much rarer fistulae with tracks that extend *above the level of the anorectal ring* and thus lie opposite both the anal canal and the lower part of the rectum (Fig. 124). There may exceptionally be an internal opening in the rectum above the ring. By far the commoner arrangement, fortunately, is for that part of the track which lies above the ring to be a closed cul-de-sac; the fistula then either has an external opening alone or, more usually, there is a subsidiary internal opening into the anal canal anywhere between the anorectal ring and the anal orifice and commonly at the pectinate line posteriorly, though it may be quite difficult to demonstrate at operation. In the extremely rare instances where the alternative arrangement exists of an internal opening in the rectum above the anorectal ring, it is highly probable that this opening has been 'man-made'—due to injudicious probing of the upper blind end of an anorectal or high anal fistula, or to faulty exploration of a pelvirectal or high ischiorectal abscess.

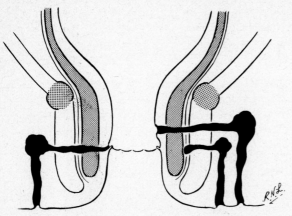

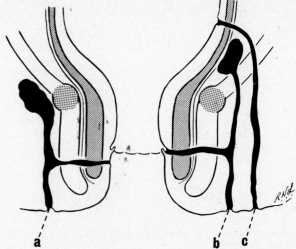

Fig. 123. Section of the anal canal showing the position of *high anal* fistulae (mostly transsphincteric fistulae of Parks et al. 1976).

Fig. 124. Section of the anal canal showing the pattern of *anorectal* fistulae. (*a*) Ischiorectal or infralevator type (transsphincteric of Parks et al. 1976*c* with high blind extralevator track. (*b*, *c*) Pelvirectal or supralevator types (transsphincteric of Parks et al. 1976*c* with high blind supralevator extension or extrasphincteric).

RELATIONSHIP TO THE LEVATOR MUSCLE

Unfortunately the Milligan–Morgan description of anorectal fistulae did not clearly define their relationship to the levator ani muscle, and it is important to rectify this omission as Parks et al. (1976) have done. With reference to the levator, anorectal fistulae are of two main types:

1. A very few of them extend upwards through the muscle. For example, if the fistula is complete with an opening into the rectum above the sphincters, it must traverse the levator in order to reach the rectum. Also certain fistulae originating in a pelvirectal or supralevator abscess will clearly

have a blind extension above the levator muscle without an opening into the rectum. To such extremely rare fistulae, which lie partly above the levator musculature in the pelvis proper, the term *pelvirectal* or *supralevator anorectal fistula* may conveniently be applied (Fig. 124*b*, *c*). The extremely rare *suprasphincteric* type of fistula of Parks et al. (1976) (Fig. 125) will also be included in this category.

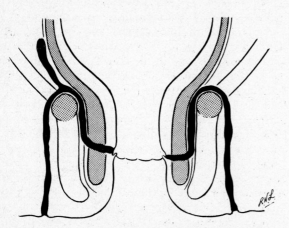

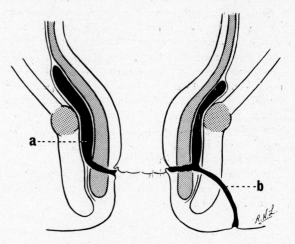

Fig. 125. The rare *suprasphincteric* fistula of Parks et al. (1976), which extends upwards from the pectinate line in the intersphincteric plane to just above the anorectal ring and then turns outwards over the top of the puborectalis sling and external sphincter and downwards through the levator and the ischiorectal fossa to reach the perianal skin.

Fig. 126. Section of the anal canal showing the position of so-called *submucous*, really high intermuscular fistulae (high intersphincteric fistulae of Parks et al. 1976). They may exist alone (A) or may occur as an extension of an ordinary low anal canal fistula (B).

2. Owing to the obliquity of the levator muscle, however, it is quite possible for a fistulous track to rise above the level of the anorectal ring and yet be entirely within the ischiorectal fossa, separated from the lower rectum by the levator muscle and its overlying fascia. This is in fact the state of affairs in the vast majority of anorectal fistulae and, because of their situation in the ischiorectal fossa and of the fact that most of them originate in ischiorectal abscesses, it is appropriate to call them *ischiorectal* or *infralevator anorectal fistulae* (Fig. 124*a*).

SUBMUCOUS OR INTERMUSCULAR (HIGH INTERSPHINCTERIC) FISTULAE

These usually take the form of blind sinuses extending upwards from an opening at the level of the pectinate line and lie not in the submucosa entirely internal to the sphincter musculature, as was thought by Milligan and Morgan (1934), but between the internal and external sphincter or at a higher level between the circular and longitudinal muscle coats of the rectum, as pointed out by Eisenhammer (1958, 1961) (Fig. 126A). They are thus more correctly termed intermuscular or intersphincteric fistula. Rarely there is a fistulous opening at the upper end as well. Not infrequently a high intermuscular fistula occurs as an upward extension of an ordinary anal fistula (Fig. 126B).

Horizontal Disposition

Goodsall (1900) pointed out that if a transverse line were drawn across the mid-point of the anus, fistulae with their external openings anterior to this line usually run directly to the anal canal, whilst those with external openings behind the transverse line tend to take a curved course terminating in an opening in the midline of the posterior wall of the anal canal (Fig. 127). This generalization is known as Goodsall's rule. The curved track of a posterior fistula may be present on one side only, or may be bilateral, the two fistulae then converging on a single midline internal opening. These are known as 'single' and 'double' horseshoe fistulae respectively. As Parks et al. (1976) have emphasized, horseshoe fistulae may occur at different levels relative to the anus, anal canal and lower rectum.

Though the majority of fistulae probably do conform to Goodsall's rule, there are many exceptions to it, and every surgeon of experience will have encountered posterior fistulae that pursued a straight course to the anus, and anterior fistulae that were of horseshoe type. Posteriorly the exceptions are usually low anal fistulae which generally follow a direct course to the anus on whichever part of the anal circumference they may be situated. But posterior high anal or anorectal fistulae are more liable to follow the conventional horseshoe pattern. Though the main track of an ischiorectal fistula may be on one side there is always a tendency for an extension to take place through the retro-sphincteric space of Courtenay to the opposite side,

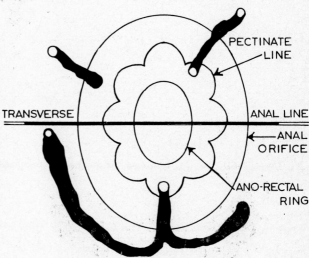

Fig. 127. Goodsall's rule that fistulae with their external opening in front of the transverse and line generally pursue a direct course to the anus, whilst those with external openings behind this line take a curved course to reach the posterior wall of the canal in the midline.

forming there a subsidiary horseshoe track. Whatever the situation of the internal or external opening with such posterior horseshoe fistulae the position of the actual horseshoe track is remarkably constant. *It hugs the puborectalis muscle as it forms a sling round the sides and back of the anorectal junction, lying external to the uppermost part of the external sphincter and below or external to the lowermost part of the levator ani muscle.* Its position on the vertical axis may therefore be defined as anorectal. Fortunately however any internal opening from it is usually situated quite definitely below the anorectal ring in the posterior wall of the anal canal, often at the pectinate line (Fig. 128). It is also important to note that

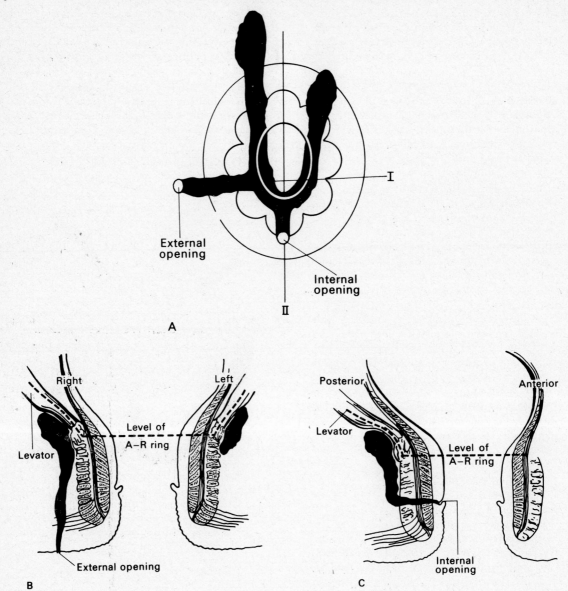

Fig. 128. The pattern usually assumed by a high posterior horseshoe ischiorectal fistula: (A) as seen in horizontal plane; (B) as displayed in coronal section, marked by line I in (A); and (C) as seen in sagittal section, indicated by line II in (A).

sometimes there may appear to be no internal opening at all, but the surgeon should be extremely reluctant to accept that this is so.

The forward extent of the two side limbs of a posterior horseshoe ischiorectal fistula is variable. Usually however the better developed of the two at least reaches beyond the transverse anal line. Milligan et al. (1948) have pointed out that the limbs of such a fistula may on occasion extend for-

ward above the urogenital diaphragm (triangular ligament) (Fig. 129).

CLINICAL FEATURES

The patient will usually give a history of having had an abscess which burst and has discharged inter-

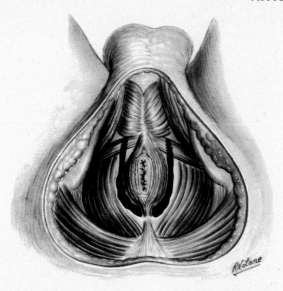

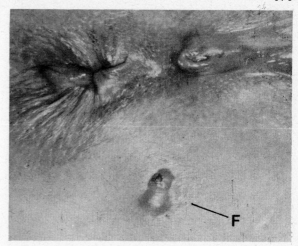

Fig. 130. View of the anal region showing single external opening of an anal fistula in the left anterior position, the opening being marked by a knob of granulation tissue (F).

Fig. 129. Pattern of the classical posterior horseshoe ichiorectal fistula with forward extension above the urogenital diaphragm.

mittently or continuously since, though occasionally in very long-standing cases the initial acute episode may be so remote that the patient has forgotten about it. In many cases there will also be a history of one or more operations for the original abscess or the subsequent fistula. At least half the patients seen by me with fistulae have already had one operation for this condition. Very occasionally the discharge will have arisen as a sequel to some other rectal or gynaecological operation or to a confinement at which the perineum was torn. Under these latter circumstances the fistula is situated anteriorly and often opens on to the posterior vaginal wall, with resulting leakage of flatus and faeces from the vagina if the opening is high enough to be above the sphincters. In any case of fistula, regardless of the cause, but especially if there has been previous surgical treatment for it, it is wise to ascertain by questioning whether the patient has normal anal continence or not.

An anal fistula is essentially a painless condition, though, if the discharge ceases temporarily and pus accumulates to form a recurrent abscess, pain is experienced till the abscess bursts, which gives immediate relief. Soreness and itching of the perianal skin, however, are common, due to pruritus resulting from the moist sodden condition of the skin.

With fistulae secondary to proctocolitis, Crohn's disease, actinomycosis or anorectal carcinoma there will often be additional bowel symptoms. These may be so slight that the patient has not really noticed them or at any rate does not mention them till questioned. Enquiry should therefore always be made as to bowel habits, passage of mucus and blood, abdominal pain and loss of weight. Similarly, whilst tuberculous fistulae may be associated with symptoms of pulmonary tuberculosis, they quite commonly occur in patients who appear to be in excellent general health, without chest symptoms of any kind, and who may or may not give a history of a previous pulmonary lesion.

Examination

INSPECTION

Inspection of the anal region will reveal any external opening or openings present. Whilst a single opening is the most common (Fig. 130), multiple sinuses are often encountered (Figs 131, 132), and sometimes these are so numerous as to give the 'water-can' appearance. Sometimes the opening may be relatively inconspicuous and only detected when pus is caused to escape by gentle palpation over some part of the surrounding skin. In many long-standing cases, however, the opening is situated on the summit of a little pink or red nodule of exuberant granulation tissue. Not infrequently the sinus is temporarily healed over, though its position is marked by a raised papilla such as has been mentioned or by a scar. The perianal skin may

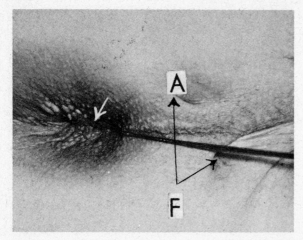

Fig. 131. View of the anal region showing double external fistulous openings anteriorly, the skin being indrawn at each opening (A and F). A probe has been laid on the surface to mark the course of one of the fistulous tracks to the anus, the latter being indicated by a white arrow.

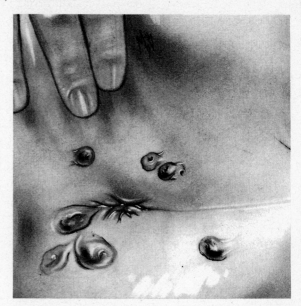

Fig. 132. View of the anal region showing seven external fistulous openings around the anus.

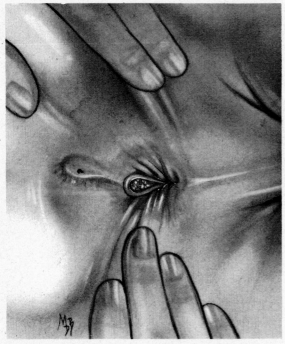

Fig. 133. View of the anal region showing a dorsal anal fissure with an associated posterior low anal fistula.

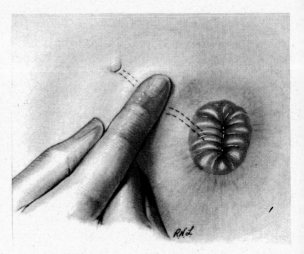

Fig. 134. Palpating the subcutaneous rod of induration produced by the fistulous track.

show the scars of previous operations undertaken for the fistula or some other condition; it may also be red, moist and thickened from secondary pruritus ani. When it is pruritic the thickened folds of skin tend to obscure small external fistulous openings situated close to the anal verge, so that they may easily be overlooked unless specially sought. A careful search should also be made for a dorsal anal fissure which is often the cause of posterior fistulae (Fig. 133). Finally the position of any fistulous openings and scars relative to the anus should be clearly recorded in diagrammatic form as in Figs 121–8 for this is more accurate and immediately intelligible than a written account.

leave a wide, shallow, saucerized, or guttered wound without overhanging edges.

THE MANAGEMENT OF THE SPHINCTER MUSCLES AND PRESERVATION OF CONTINENCE

It was Milligan's and Morgan's (1934) great contribution to the surgery of anal fistula that they focused the attention of surgeons on the precise anatomy of the anal region and on the patterns commonly assumed by fistulous tracks. We now know that except for the extreme lower end of the external sphincter the two sphincters lie parallel throughout their vertical extent and that exposure of fistulous tracks traversing them often necessitates severance of some of both sphincters. The significant thing in laying open fistulae by the classical method, as Milligan and Morgan (1934) have emphasized, is the height at which the track lies relative to the sphincters, and *particularly to the anorectal ring*. They claimed that, provided its integrity is preserved, the greater part of both sphincters may be divided without loss of continence, but that if the anorectal ring is inadvertently divided the effect is inevitably a total loss of anal control (and usually some degree of complete or partial rectal prolapse as well). As pointed out on pp. 35–41, this is to some extent an oversimplification of a complex subject, but is, in general, a sound principle. It is no exaggeration to say that the modern surgical treatment of laying open anal fistulae is dominated by this conception of continence depending ultimately on an intact anorectal ring and on the absolute necessity for preserving this structure.

The surgeon's first duty in planning treatment is therefore to define the relationship of the fistulous track to the anorectal ring, both preoperatively and again at the time of operation. In this connection it is important to stress that *light* general anaesthesia, which retains the tone of the anal musculature and facilitates accurate identification of the anorectal ring, is preferable to a full general anaesthetic using relaxants, or to low spinal anaesthesia, which used to be popular. If the fistula is of the subcutaneous, submucous or low anal variety its incision will clearly not endanger the anorectal ring in any way. Contrariwise if the fistula is of complete anorectal variety with an opening into the rectum above the anorectal ring its treatment by incision would inevitably divide the ring and render the patient incontinent; clearly this type of fistula is to be regarded as inoperable by the classical method. The really perplexing cases are those with a high anal or

anorectal fistula with an opening into the upper part of the anal canal; it may be extremely difficult to decide whether the internal opening is situated just below or above the anorectal ring. If the surgeon is quite satisfied that the former is the case then the fistula may be laid open with confidence that there will be no impairment of anal control. If he cannot make up his mind as to whether the opening is immediately above or below the ring his correct course is to refer the patient to someone of greater experience who may be able to reach a decision on this point.

An alternative method that is sometimes recommended in dealing with difficult high fistulae of the type just mentioned involves the use of a ligature of strong braided silk, No. 16, which is passed through the internal opening and round the sphincters—or their remaining upper portions if their lower parts have already been divided—and *tied tightly*. The object of this manoeuvre is to stimulate a fibrous reaction which is supposed to fix the sphincter muscles at this point so that when the ligature cuts out at the end of five or six days, or is eventually removed and the division of the sphincters com-

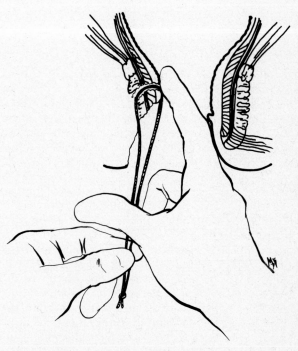

Fig. 138. The use of a loose-knotted loop of strong silk to mark the internal opening of a high anal or anorectal fistula whilst the anorectal ring is identified with the finger postoperatively.

pleted by scissors or scalpel, the cut ends are believed to be anchored by fibrous tissue and do not retract. Frankly I very much doubt the value of this method. I personally would not be prepared to divide the anorectal ring even by this technique; and I know from experience that division of the sphincters up to just below the ring can be accomplished, with preservation of a considerable measure of continence, by simple cutting in a one-stage operation.

There is, however, a variant of the two-stage operation which may sometimes be of value in doubtful high fistulae, not as a substitute for distinguishing between high anal and complete anorectal openings, but as an aid in making this distinction. At the initial operation a braided silk ligature is placed through the internal opening and knotted *as a loose loop* round the sphincters. This serves as a marker when the patient is re-examined postoperatively in a conscious condition. The ligature is rendered taut by gentle traction whilst the patient is asked to contract his sphincter and levator muscles. It is then usually possible with the finger in the rectum to decide whether the internal opening, marked by the silk, lies above or below the anorectal ring (Fig. 138).

DETAILED OPERATIVE TECHNIQUE:
SUBCUTANEOUS OR LOW-LEVEL ANAL
FISTULAE

First of all, the findings on preoperative clinical examination are confirmed by further probing, and, if the track was thought to be blind at its inner end, care is taken to establish whether this is in fact so or not. Sometimes a minute internal opening hitherto undetected may be demonstrated by a fine lacrimal probe passed from the external opening, or one may be found on inspecting and probing the wall of the anal canal with the aid of a bivalve speculum. Next, a probe-pointed fistula director is passed along the track into the lumen of the anal canal in a complete fistula (Fig. 139A), or so that its point projects against the skin or mucosa at the inner end in a blind fistula, possibly with the thickness of the internal sphincter intervening. In the latter case the end of the director can with a little force generally be made to emerge through the muscle and lining, thus converting the sinus into a fistula. The track is now laid open throughout its length by incision on to the director, the division of the overlying tissues being finally completed by sliding the scalpel with its blade uppermost along the groove on the upper aspect of the director (Fig.

139B). In the case of a low-level anal fistula, fibres of the lower part of the internal, and sometimes the external, sphincter will be severed in the process.

The skin edges are retracted with tissue forceps and, after careful haemostasis, the wound surface is closely inspected. With its characteristic velvety covering of granulation tissue the opened up track of the fistula is readily distinguished from the other tissues as a narrow strip running in a radial direction in the deepest part of the wound (Fig. 139C). Its recognition is useful in confirming that the director was correctly passed along the fistula and did not make a 'false' passage in the tissues. Using a sharp spoon the granulations are scraped off the exposed inner surface of the fistula, leaving the underlying pale tough fibrous base. Some of the granulation tissue and snippets of the fibrous wall are sent for histological examination for evidence of a tuberculous infection or Crohn's lesion, and also possibly for guinea-pig inoculation.

The fibrous layer is not excised but is left in the floor of the wound. Its surface should be closely examined throughout its length for any openings and these should be tested with a medium or fine lacrimal probe to determine whether they lead into subsidiary fistulous tracks. Similarly the soft fatty tissues on either side of the track are *palpated for nodules of induration* that might indicate the presence of divided fistulous offshoots, and any suspicious areas thus found are examined with a fine probe for an opening leading into a track. Finally, if no further fistulous openings are discovered, the sides of the wound are trimmed with scissors (Fig. 140A) removing skin and subcutaneous fat generously in order to leave a shallow concave raw area, more or less pear-shaped or conical with the apex usually entering the anal canal (Fig. 140B). If the original fistula was blind at its inner end and the apex of the wound does not actually reach into the canal it is an advantage to extend it to just within the anal orifice by removal of a small wedge of skin with scissors and possibly to snick the lowermost fibres of the anal sphincters, otherwise the fringe of skin between the anus and the wound is apt to become oedematous and painful during the postoperative period. I do not slavishly make a back cut of the type illustrated in Fig. 140, but prefer simply to excise a broad rim of skin and fat from the edges of the wound as required to give it a suitable shape; if the external opening of the fistula lies fairly far out it may not be necessary to enlarge the wound much or at all in a radial direction.

The wound is again surveyed for haemostasis and general configuration and again palpated to make

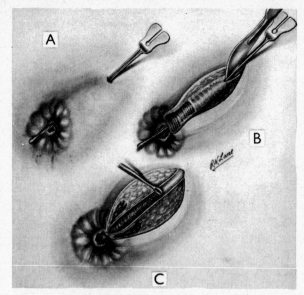

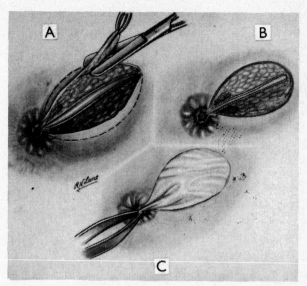

Fig. 139. Laying open *low anal* fistula: (A) Passage of probe-pointed director along the track from the external to the internal opening and emerging from the anus. (B) Incision on to the director has exposed the sphincter muscles—probably mainly or entirely the internal one—at the inner end; division of tissues is completed by sliding scalpel along the director with its blade uppermost. (C) The granulation tissue is being scraped off the opened-up track of the fistula with a sharp spoon.

Fig. 140. Laying open *low anal* fistula: (A) Trimming edges of wound with scissors. (B) The final, pear-shaped, guttered wound. (C) Packing the wound with flat gauze soaked in Milton or Eusol, the corner being tucked into the anal canal.

sure that no fresh areas of induration have been revealed by the process of trimming. Finally the dressing is applied; this consists of flat squares of gauze rinsed out of Milton or Eusol which are arranged to cover the wound surface, the corner of one square being tucked into the anal canal to provide a dressing for the apical part of the wound (Fig. 140C).

In the light of Parks' (1961) work showing that anal glandular epithelium sometimes forms part of the lining of the inner end of the fistulous track, it is open to question whether this end of the track should not be removed instead of merely laid open (Fig. 140). Theoretically, even if glandular epithelium does persist in the wall of the fistula, it ought to form part of the epithelial covering of the resulting fistula wound if the latter is to heal in an orderly fashion from its depths. But if this ideal is not achieved, the residual glandular epithelium might become buried and could lead to the formation of a further fistula. It might therefore be a wise precaution to excise the innermost 2–2·5 cm of the fistulous track as shown in Fig. 141, and perhaps to sacrifice a generous piece of the lower part of the internal sphincter, particularly in cases where the

fistula is blind at its internal end. However my experiences with simple laying open, without this addition, indicate that it is seldom followed by recurrence see (p. 187).

More complicated anal or subcutaneous fistulae with numerous subsidiary tracks and openings of course require additional incisions (Fig. 132A), and when these are amalgamated the effect may be to produce a much more extensive irregular wound (Fig. 132B). It is possible for a patient to have two entirely separate fistulae, but this is excessively rare, and it may be taken as a good working rule that all fistulous openings should be found to communicate with one another.

ISCHIORECTAL FISTULA (HIGH POSTERIOR HORSESHOE FISTULA)

This, by far the commonest type of anorectal fistula, is eminently amenable to well planned radical surgical treatment. There is nearly always an external opening and it is best to commence by using it to lay open the lateral limb of the horseshoe track on that side (Fig. 143). A director is passed into the opening and allowed to take its course. It may proceed towards the posterior wall of the anal canal and, if a definite internal opening has been identified there below the anorectal ring, it may be made to emerge through it into the canal; this part of the fistula is then laid open by incision. Otherwise, and

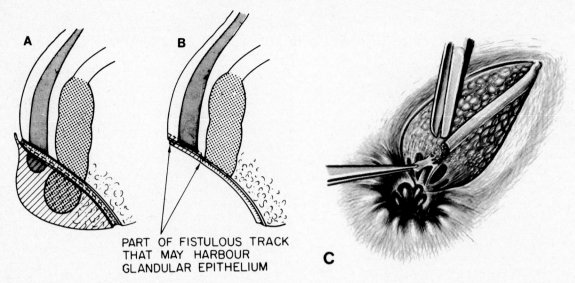

PART OF FISTULOUS TRACK
THAT MAY HARBOUR
GLANDULAR EPITHELIUM

Fig. 141. Modification of laying-open operation for fistula to excise anal glandular epithelium possibly present at the inner end of the track. The fistula has been laid open as in Fig. 140A and B. The innermost 2 cm of the opened-up track is now excised.

usually preferably, the point of the instrument is directed forwards and made to project against and penetrate through the skin at the side of the anus and slightly in front of it (Fig. 144A). An incision is then made on to the director releasing it and exposing part of the fistula. However, the latter lies deeply and is overhung by the fat of both walls of the wound and before proceeding farther it is wise to trim these walls generously of skin and fat. After haemostasis it is then possible for the assistant to separate the sides of the wound by fingers placed on two gauze swabs and bring the open track clearly into view. If oozing of blood proves a difficulty it

may be checked by pressing gauze soaked in a 1/1000 solution of adrenaline hydrochloride on to the wound surfaces for two or three minutes.

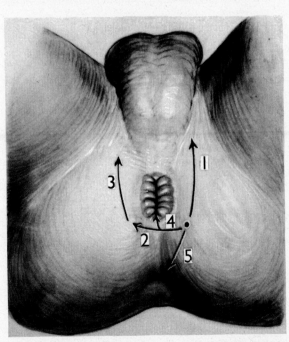

Fig. 143. The steps in the operation for a *posterior horseshoe ischiorectal* fistula: (1) Exposing lateral limb of track on one side; (2) Laying open posterior communication between the two limbs of the horseshoe; (3) Exposing the track on the opposite side; (4) Searching for any communication with the posterior wall of the anal canal; (5) (Only rarely required) incision towards side of coccyx and sacrum to assist in guttering of wound.

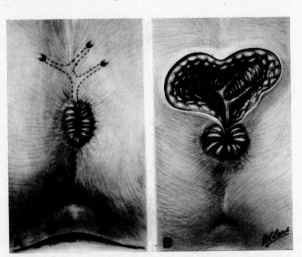

Fig. 142. (A) A more complicated *low anal* fistula with three external openings. (B) The wound resulting from laying it open.

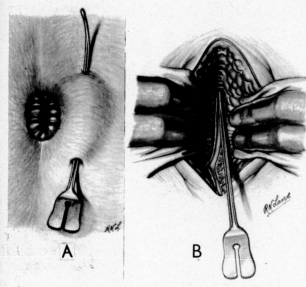

Fig. 144. Laying open *posterior horseshoe* fistula: (A) Probe-pointed director passed on left side. (B) Track on left side exposed by strong retraction of sides of wound, anterior extension being sought.

The granulations are removed with the sharp spoon, samples of tissue being sent for pathological examination. The fibrous base is now followed forwards, and probing at its anterior end (Fig. 144B) usually reveals prolongation of the track forwards for another centimetre or two at least, and occasionally even more, when its extremity may lie above the urogenital diaphragm. This anterior extension is incised and the wound in relation to it appropriately trimmed to avoid overhanging skin edges and fat.

Attention is next turned to the posterior extremity of the opened section of the fistula. It may be found by probing that the track extends transversely through the retrosphincteric space to the ischiorectal fossa of the opposite side. A director passed along it is forced through the skin of that side and the overlying tissues are incised (Fig. 145A). Thorough trimming of the walls of this newly formed part of the wound and control of bleeding with the aid of adrenaline packs allows proper exposure of the actual track. Two-thirds or three-quarters of the horseshoe track have now been opened. It remains to demonstrate and open any anterior extension on the second side, which is done in the same way as on the first side (Fig. 145B), and to search for an opening into the posterior wall of the anal canal. With the thorough exposure of the fistula now secured, it is possible to examine the posterior part of the main track and the anal canal

very carefully for an opening penetrating the anal sphincters. Fine lacrimal probes are especially useful but must be handled very gently if an artificial opening is not to be produced. It is possible to have a high posterior horseshoe fistula *without* a clearly demonstrable internal opening, but much the more usual arrangement is for an opening to be present in the posterior wall of the anal canal, often at the level of the pectinate line. It is most important not to miss such an opening if it exists, for to do so inevitably results in recurrence, however wide the unroofing of the actual horseshoe track may be. If an internal opening is found, the surgeon must satisfy himself that it lies below the anorectal ring. If he is happy on this point a director is passed (Fig. 145C) and the sphincter musculature superficial to it divided (Fig. 145D). If no internal opening can be discovered, it is probably wise—on the assumption that an anal glandular infection with resulting intersphincteric abscess formation was possibly the primary aetiological factor—to force a director through the posterior wall of the canal from the main wound into the lumen at the level of the pectinate line, and to divide the tissues below it.

It only remains now to carry out a general survey of the wound and to make sure, by further trimming if necessary, that the depths of the wide gutter that surrounds the posterior and lateral aspects of the anus can everywhere be easily exposed. Large gauze squares rinsed out in Milton are then applied so as to reach into the deepest parts of the wound; a corner of gauze is also tucked into the anus posteriorly. The dressing is completed with abundant dry gauze and wool and a firm T-bandage is applied.

PELVIRECTAL FISTULA

Blind Superiorly

On exposure at operation the track of this type of fistula is found to extend through a hole in the levator ani. The perforation in the muscle should be stretched by opening the blades of a pair of artery forceps in it or, if there is too much surrounding fibrosis, by incision with a scalpel. This is safely performed in a backward, lateral or forward direction, but not medially, the opening being enlarged as much as required to ensure free drainage of the supralevator portion of the track. The latter should be carefully explored and gently curetted, portions of tissue being sent for histological section and guinea-pig inoculation.

The external wound is now enlarged by wide trimming of the skin edges and fat, especially pos-

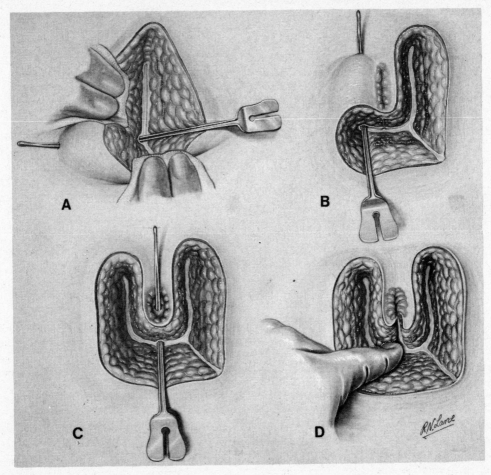

Fig. 145. Laying open *posterior horseshoe* fistula: (A) Probe inserted along posterior communication to opposite side. (B) Exposing track on right side. (C) Demonstration of communication with anal canal in mid-line posteriorly. (D) Resulting large horseshoe wound with division of part of sphincters in posterior wall of anal canal.

teriorly, to produce a deep gutter extending backwards towards the side of the coccyx. Provided there is no internal opening above the levator muscles and no unremoved chronic pelvic disease such as regional ileitis or a sigmoid diverticulitis, the prognosis with operation of this kind in these cases is good.

With Opening into Rectum above Levators
Apart from rectovaginal fistulae above the level of the anal sphincters, which may be regarded as essentially a form of anorectal fistula and the treatment of which is described on p. 191, these are fortunately very rare. Obviously it would be impossible to treat complete anorectal fistulae by incision and healing by granulation without producing incontinence, and they must be regarded as

inoperable or be treated by some other method (see. p. 190).

HIGH INTERMUSCULAR (SUBMUCOUS) FISTULA

The first essential in the treatment of a submucous fistula is for the surgeon to assure himself that it is in fact submucous or intermuscular and not extrarectal. Sometimes the induration that can be felt through the rectal wall of the blind upper end of an anorectal fistula (Fig. 146) closely mimics that of a high submucous or intermuscular track, and it is important not to confuse these two lesions, for treatment of an anorectal fistula by incision through the rectal wall would be disastrous.

If the fistula is submucous it should be treated by laying it open into the lumen of the rectum, and

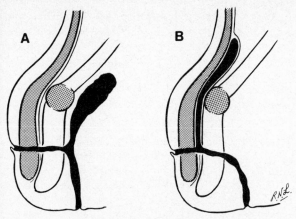

Fig. 146. Relative positions of the blind infralevator pouch of an ischiorectal fistula (A) and of a high intersphincteric fistula (B).

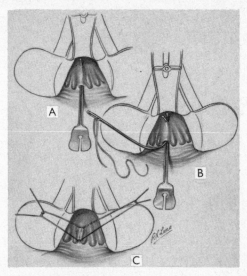

Fig. 147. Laying open *submucous or intermuscular* abscess and fistula: (A) Interior of anal canal and rectum exposed by bivalve speculum, and director passed through internal opening and along track to be forced through the intact mucosa at upper end of fistula. (B) Placing stout silk ligature by threading it on a malleable probe, which is passed along the director. (C) A second silk ligature has been similarly inserted and both are about to be tied tightly to produce slow necrosis of the tissue overlying the track.

anal canal and this obviously involves division of no muscle or, at most, of the upper part of the internal sphincter and the circular muscle coat of the rectum. A bivalve speculum is inserted and the opening of the fistula exposed at its usual site at or just above the pectinate line. A director is then passed into the opening and along the track to its blind upper end and forced through the intact mucosa at this point (Fig. 147A). If the bridge of tissue overlying the director is simply divided with scalpel or diathermy there is apt to be considerable bleeding from cut edges. To avoid this trouble it is perhaps better to accomplish the division gradually over a period five or six days by the necrosing effect of one or two tightly tied silk ligatures. They are most conveniently inserted threaded on a medium sized malleable silver probe (Fig. 147B, C). Submucous or intermuscular fistulae are perhaps more often found as an extension of some other variety of fistula than as an isolated lesion, and their treatment is therefore frequently only a part of the operation required.

In my experience, despite careful laying open of the tracks as described, submucous fistulae are liable to give trouble postoperatively from the development of residual pockets which may require further division of tissue. It is important therefore that progress after operation should be specially carefully reviewed by digital examination and if necessary by proctoscopy.

POSTOPERATIVE CARE OF THE WOUND

It is difficult to overestimate the importance of adequate attention to the wound during the postoperative period. Neglect of this aspect of treat-

ment may easily result in a recurrence of the fistula despite a well performed operation. The aim to be constantly kept in mind during this phase is *sound healing by granulation from the depths of the wound and the prevention of contact and premature healing between the opposing skin edges and granulating walls.* The regimen of baths, irrigations and dressings for achieving this end has been described in detail in Chapter 3 and it only remains to emphasize a few points of special relevance to fistula cases:

Removal of the Initial Dressing. In accordance with the routine for 'minor' rectal cases, the bowels are moved on the morning of the third postoperative day. The dressings inserted at the time of the operation may be left to separate at this event or at the subsequent irrigation with peroxide, but if the wound is of large size this may be a most uncomfortable proceeding, for the gauze has usually become firmly adherent to the raw surfaces and does not easily separate even with peroxide. It is preferable in these cases to remove the first dressing under a brief general anaesthetic given in the ward or dressing room, and then to insert a fresh one more loosely. This is best done the evening before the bowels are due to act. Thereafter irrigations and dressings are repeated morning and evening, and sedatives, such as 100 mg pethidine one hour before the dressing, may be required for the first few dressings. It is usually several days before baths can be undertaken in cases with really large fistula wounds.

Periodic Review of the Wound in the Theatre. Even when the dressings are being conducted by nurses specially experienced in the management of rectal cases, it is sometimes difficult during the first few days to ensure that the dressing has been inserted to the highest point of the wound. As a consequence the uppermost parts of the two sides of the wound may have fallen together and become adherent. Also the surgeon may not have been quite certain at the conclusion of the operation that he had in fact laid open every conceivable pocket of the track. It is therefore a good plan to review all but the most superficial fistula wounds under anaesthesia at the end of the first seven to ten postoperative days. If pus is found to be accumulating at any point this will suggest the possibility of an unopened pocket there, for which a determined search should be made. It will also be seen whether the wound is tending to fall together at any part and this can be corrected and the wound reshaped.

Subsequently the wound will be reviewed periodically, and not less frequently than once a week, by the surgeon in the ward at the time of a dressing. If at any stage, however, he should be dissatisfied with the course of healing, he should not hesitate to carry out a review in the theatre and do whatever seems indicated in the way of enlargement or reshaping.

Passage of a Finger or Anal Dilator. As they heal large fistula wounds lead to the production of a good deal of fibrous tissue, and narrowing of the anal opening may occur. It is essential to pass a finger occasionally to ensure that there is no stenosis; any incipient narrowing should be dealt with by regular daily passage of an anal dilator till healing is complete, and probably for some weeks thereafter, to guard against subsequent cicatricial contraction.

Maintenance of Continence. It may be a week or so before the patient learns to use his remaining musculature to maximum advantage, or perhaps before the muscles regain their normal tone and contractile power after the stretching and trauma of operation. There are thus apt to be occasional faecal leaks, especially when the motions are liquid as after purgation in the early postoperative period, and control of flatus may initially be imperfect. Thereafter, if the anorectal ring has been preserved, anal control becomes approximately normal; continued gross incontinence suggests an error of judgment in regard to the amount of muscle that was divided.

Time Required for Complete Healing. The process of healing after fistula operations is designedly slow and takes four or five weeks even for a relatively low fistula, and up to 12 or 16 weeks for a really high double horseshoe lesion. The patient need not be detained in hospital for all this time, for if satisfactory plans can be made for his dressings at home or in the out-patient department and he can attend the rectal clinic for weekly review of his wound, he may usually be discharged after the first two to three weeks. But, unless the surgeon is absolutely satisfied about the arrangements outside for attention to the wound, he should retain the patient in hospital till a stage is reached when sound healing can be confidently predicted. He should be quite adamant in his refusal to compromise on this issue, for to discharge the patient prematurely to unsatisfactory conditions may mean throwing away the chance of a successful result.

It is important that *before operation the patient should be made to understand the necessity for careful postoperative regimen.* It is *unwise to attempt an accurate preoperative forecast of the probable period of convalescence* after a fistula operation, for the fistula may be found on exploration to be much more extensive than was anticipated. Because of the prolonged period of hospitalization required for the cure of a high fistula by this method, some patients with this type of lesion may elect not to have an operation or to postpone it indefinitely. This is especially likely to happen if they have been operated on unsuccessfully before for the same condition and have already spent many weeks in hospital, all to no avail.

Secondary Skin Grafting. Thiersch grafts applied to the granulating surface as soon as it has reached the level of the surrounding skin, sometimes 'take', and even if only partially successful may expedite healing by three or four weeks in cases with very large wounds. Unfortunately the proportion of cases in which a reasonably satisfactory 'take' is obtained is in my experience scarcely great enough to warrant the discomforts associated with grafting in this situation.

RESULTS OF CLASSICAL LAYING-OPEN
OPERATIONS FOR FISTULA

Though it is clearly implied in the writings of many authors (Milligan et al. 1948 for example) that properly performed operations to lay open anal fistulae yield excellent results, there is remarkably little precise information as to the effectiveness of these methods in practice. One of the most revealing studies is that of Bennett (1962) who conducted a survey of 108 cases of pyogenic anal fistulae, treated in my department along classical lines during the preceding six years. The following information was disclosed:

Type of Fistula Treated. In 62% of the cases the fistula was of low anal type, in 25% high and, whilst other varieties were less common, horseshoe fistulae, usually of high anal or anorectal type, were present in 19%. A definite internal opening was found in 63% of the cases; no such opening was discovered in 28%, and in 9% the clinical notes contained no clear record on this point.

Duration of Convalescence. The length of time taken for completion of healing, which was fairly accurately reflected in the duration of the convalescence, naturally varied according to the size of the wound, which in turn could be gauged roughly from the type of fistula present. Thus the period during which patients were off work after operation ranged from five weeks on the average for low anal fistulae to 14 weeks for double horseshoe fistulae.

Imperfections of Healing and Recurrences. In eight patients troubles of this kind occurred. In six revision of the wound was necessary because of a tendency to pocketing of pus, observed either when the patient was still in hospital or soon after discharge; following this further operation, healing proceeded without incident and the patients subsequently remained well. In two other patients, however, the fistula recurred after healing had taken place and necessitated a second operation, and these are the only two cases that I would regard as genuine examples of recurrence in the 108 patients.

Functional Results. On questioning as to *changes in anal continence since operation*, 12% of the patients complained of occasional inadequate control of faeces, 16% of imperfect control of flatus, and 24% of frequent soiling of their underclothes. In all, 36% alleged that they suffered from one or more of these defects, which they stated had not been present before operation. With all defects, both the frequency and severity of poor control increased on passing from low anal fistulae to the high anal and horseshoe varieties. The incidence of patients with one or more defects after operation for horseshoe fistulae was approximately 55%. It must be emphasized that in the majority these defects were relatively mild, but in 10% of the patients they occurred daily and two persons constantly wore pads for protection. From this analysis it is clear that the classical methods of treating anal fistula are capable of affording a very good chance of cure with preservation of gross anal continence, but even when practised with the precautions prescribed by Milligan and Morgan (1934) they are likely to be followed by minor impairments of anal control in a proportion of the cases, particularly those with high horseshoe fistulae.

2. LAYING OPEN THE FISTULA, FOLLOWED BY IMMEDIATE SKIN GRAFTING

In this operation, which has been strongly championed by Hughes (1953) of Melbourne, the fistula is laid open *exactly as in the classical operation* and with the same precautions to saucerize the wound and avoid overhanging skin edges. After careful haemostasis Thiersch grafts taken from the medial aspect of the thigh are applied to the raw surface, being stitched in position and firmly affixed to the wound by a cotton wool pad. Full details of the operative technique, pre- and postoperative management, and results obtained by Hughes (1953), myself and Wilson (1969) are given on pp. 82 and 84.

When grafting is successful its advantages are obvious—it gives the patient a completely healed wound in 7 to 14 days and spares him the inconvenience of repeated dressings. As the fistula has been widely laid open before the grafts are applied, even if they do not take no harm results, for the wound is in a suitable condition for satisfactory healing by granulation to take place; survival of even a small part of the graft may expedite the latter process. The main drawback to immediate grafting is the time and trouble involved in applying and fixing the grafts, which in a moderately large fistula wound may amount to two or three hours. Another objection is the discomfort sometimes experienced in the donor site, particularly if the graft is taken from the posteromedial aspect of the thigh as recommended by Hughes (1953). This situation is attractively convenient when the patient is in the lithotomy position, but despite the trouble entailed by having to move the patient during the operation, I think it is better to take the skin from the front of the thigh or the anterior abdominal wall—sites not subjected to pressure when the patient is recumbent in bed. My own experience of the method, as explained on p. 84, has been confined to selected cases with large, relatively flat wounds following the laying open of superficial or low anal fistulae of an uncomplicated nature. For the majority of fistulae cases I still prefer to rely on healing by granulation, with periodic review of the wound as required during the healing process.

3. Laying Open of the Fistula, Excision of the Fistulous Track and Primary Suture

This operation has been recommended by Starr (1949) of Sydney, using sulphonamides or antibiotics for bowel antisepsis and systemically pre- and postoperatively (see also p. 81). The first operative step is to lay open the fistulous track by incision; skin and subcutaneous fat, however, should not be excised but preserved to facilitate the final closure of the wound. Obviously complicated high fistulae, where tissue may have to be fairly generously removed in order to assist exploration of the tracks, are technically quite unsuitable for primary suture, as are fistulae with numerous offshoots to the main track. The method is most readily applied to simple direct fistulae. To prepare the wound for suture it is necessary to *excise* the opened-up fistulous track as far as possible and *leave fresh wound surfaces free from granulations or fibrous tissue.* Suture implies the *complete reconstitution of the wound from the depths* using several layers of buried interrupted sutures of fine plain catgut as well as the surface sutures (see Fig. 61A–F, p. 81). The deepest layer consists of several mattress sutures in the divided parts of the sphincter muscles; subsequent layers appose the subcutaneous fat. The surface stitches comprise vertical mattress stitches of fine chromic catgut in the mucosa and skin of that part of the wound lying in the anal canal, and similar stitches of serum-proof silk in the skin of the perianal region. The wound is sealed by a plastic spray.

Postoperatively the bowels are confined for five or six days and then moved with one or two doses of cascara and liquid paraffin or an enema. The silk skin sutures are removed on the seventh day, the superficial catgut stitches eventually separate spontaneously.

Starr (1949, 1953, 1959) has recorded very gratifying results with primary suture, primary healing without complication being apparently obtained in practically all his cases so treated. My own experiences have been less happy. I have performed this operation on 20 cases, all with very straightforward, mostly low, anal or subcutaneous fistulae; 12 secured uneventful sound healing, but in the remaining eight sepsis occurred necessitating re-opening and re-fashioning of the wound, which was followed by satisfactory healing by granulation. It might be argued that these results are fairly good in that all the cases eventually had satisfactory results and over half of them achieved these with a convalescence of just over a week as contrasted with probably four or five weeks by classical methods. But several of the patients whose wounds became infected suffered a considerable amount of discomfort before their wounds were finally laid open again. There is also to be taken into account the disappointment to the patient of the temporary setback, for what the average patient with a fistula demands more than anything else is certainty of cure. So often he has already had one or more unsuccessful operations and cannot tolerate the possibility of yet another failure. I have no doubt at all that, despite its advantages when successful, primary suture is too uncertain in its results ever to be acceptable as a routine method for the treatment of anal fistula (but there are occasional circumstances when it has to be employed despite its unreliability as in the treatment of complete pelvirectal or rectovaginal fistulae—see pp. 189 and 191).

4. Conservative Operation Based on the Acceptance of Anal Glandular Infection as the Prime Cause of Fistula-in-Ano

As has been pointed out on pp. 154 and 163, a number of workers in the past have drawn attention to the possible role of the anal crypts and glands in initiating and perpetuating anorectal abscesses and fistulae; but Eisenhammer and Parks were the first to suggest amending the classical fistula operation to accord with this theory. Eisenhammer (1958, 1961) described the part played by an anal gland in producing an intersphincteric abscess, which he believed was responsible for feeding the fistula with further infection, and claimed that the laying open of this abscess into the anal canal by internal sphincterotomy was the essential step in surgical treatment. Admittedly, he also opened up the more peripheral part of the fistulous track, without apparently making any particular attempt to conserve sphincter

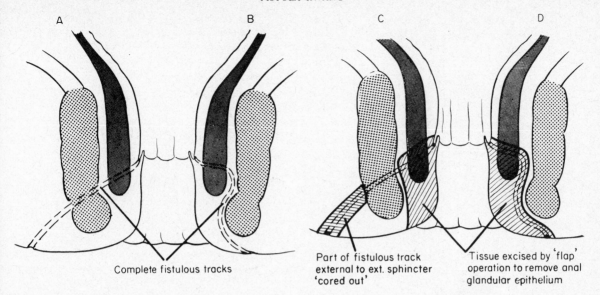

Complete fistulous tracks

Part of fistulous track external to ext. sphincter 'cored out'

Tissue excised by 'flap' operation to remove anal glandular epithelium

Fig. 148. (A, B) Relationship of complete low anal fistulae to the sphincter muscles; (C, D) Extent of tissue removed (shaded areas) in Parks' operation for these lesions.

muscle, but he subsequently sutured the latter wound, except for the inner end which was left to drain into the canal.

Parks (1961) was even more rational and conservative in his proposals. He suggested that it is insufficient merely to open the intersphincteric space by internal sphincterotomy. In addition the lining of the lower half of the anal canal, together with the related portion of the internal sphincter, is excised in order to expose the intersphincteric abscess and to remove the causally related anal gland (Fig. 148c). This step eliminates all the fistulous tracks internal to the external sphincter (Fig. 148c); and, if the track does not traverse the external sphincter (Fig. 148b)—as is frequently the case in low anal fistula—it may indeed remove the entire lesion (Fig. 148d). If, however, the fistula penetrates the external sphincter, this and the skin overlying the outer part of the track are not divided, but instead the peripheral portion of the fistula is 'cored-out' (or, alternatively, curetted) from its external opening as far as the external sphincter (Fig. 148c). The same principles are applied in the treatment of fistulae that are blind internally.

Results published by Parks (1961) in 38 cases suffering from various types of fistulae treated by this more conservative operation have been encouraging with satisfactory healing in all instances. My own experience with this method was confined to 34 patients with all types of fistula and led to the following conclusions:

For low anal fistulae it is difficult to see what advantages this method enjoys over simple laying-open. It is, in theory, a slightly more radical operation at the important inner end of the fistula, but we know from Bennett's (1962) survey that recurrence is extremely rare after the classical type of operation for these fistulae. So far as the functional results are concerned, the amount of sphincter musculature divided when the fistula is laid open is relatively small (Fig. 140), and disturbances of continence are uncommon and slight. The conservative operation certainly preserves the entire external sphincter, but it causes a good deal more damage to the internal sphincter (Fig. 149), which we now know often has an important role in the control of flatus and liquid faeces. I doubt if there will be much difference

in the effects of the two operations on function. Similarly the period required for healing and convalescence is much the same after both methods. In the treatment of low anal fistulae I cannot believe that there is anything to be gained, as a rule, by displacing the classical operation by this more difficult and tedious conservative operation—an opinion with which Parks (1962) himself agrees.

As for high anal or ischiorectal fistulae of posterior horseshoe variety, if it were applicable, the conservative technique would appear to be potentially most attractive. But in my experience the method proved impracticable in the few cases in which I tried it and I ended up by performing a classical horseshoe laying open operation but with an internal sphincter*ectomy* at the site of the internal opening on the posterior wall of the anal canal instead of a division of both sphincters up to that level. Clearly I could not recommend Park's method for these more complex fistulae.

Treatment of Certain Special Types of Fistula

COMPLETE PELVIRECTAL FISTULA

An anal fistula that has a track passing clearly above the anorectal ring to end in an internal opening in the lower rectum, is quite unsuitable for treatment by an orthodox laying-open operation, which would render the patient incontinent, and, in my experience, this would apply equally, whether the tissues were divided immediately or after a preliminary double ligation with strong silk ties. Four courses are open to the surgeon:

Expectant Treatment. If the fistula is left entirely alone, it may give the patient relatively little trouble apart from a slight continuous or intermittent discharge. Occasionally noisy escape of flatus may be an embarrassment, but the complication that most

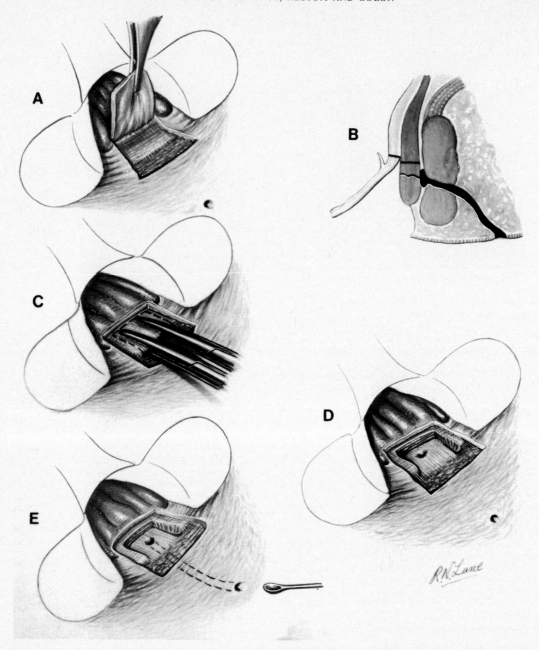

Fig. 149. Technique of conservative operation for *direct low anal fistula*. (A) Turning up flap of anal canal lining to just above pectinate line. (B) Amount of anal canal skin and mucosa and of internal sphincter excised, and the position of the fistula and anal gland. (C) Internal sphincter has been defined and a piece of lower half is being excised between forceps. (D) Intersphincteric space has been unroofed, exposing inner end of blind fistulous track. (E) Peripheral part of track about to be curetted through external opening.

often renders purely conservative management untenable is the development of recurrent abscesses. If these do not occur, the patient may continue indefinitely along expectant lines, keeping the part clean by regular baths morning and evening and possibly wearing a dry dressing or piece of cotton wool to protect his underclothes from soiling.

Establishment of a Temporary Colostomy. This may be regarded as an extension of expectant treatment. It might be hoped that the resulting defunctioning of the anorectum would at least lessen the risk of recurrent abscesses, but it would seem from the report of Williams (1968) that it may offer some prospect of healing the fistula, so that the colostomy may eventually be closed. I have not been able to confirm this experience as yet in my own practice, but the possible curative value of a simple colostomy is something to be borne in mind in the management of these worrying cases. As regards technique, my own preference would be for a divided left iliac colostomy—the distal end being closed and dropped back into the abdomen—rather than a loop colostomy, because it is easier to manage subsequently and gives more certain exclusion of the anorectum. It should be maintained for probably at least six to twelve months before contemplating its closure.

Repair of the Fistula. If expectant management proves irksome because of recurrent infection or chronic discharge, or if a proximal colostomy for a prolonged period fails to heal the fistula or is unacceptable to the patient, an attempt may be made to close the internal opening, but it is a difficult operation, which I have undertaken only thrice—two cases being successful, the third not. If not already present a preliminary defunctioning iliac colostomy should be established. The steps of the actual repair are similar to those adopted in laying open an ordinary high anal or ischiorectal fistula; that is to say, the tissues are opened widely on the affected aspect or aspects of the anal canal. The sphincter muscles may be divided below any subsidiary internal opening into the anal canal, but the musculature of the upper part of the canal is scrupulously preserved. The track leading to the high internal opening in the rectum proper is now followed up through the levator muscle, the latter being divided sufficiently to expose the hole in the rectal wall. The latter is then sutured, preferably with a non-absorbable material such as fine stainless steel or tantalum wire, or silk, linen or cotton, the sutures being inserted on the Lembert principle to secure good inversion of the edges of the opening. The sides of the whole wound are now trimmed—if this has not already been done to give good access for the suture of the rectum—to leave a wound cavity of roughly conical shape. Finally flat gauze dressings soaked in Milton are laid on the raw surfaces to the top of the wound and further gauze and wool are applied as required.

The postoperative treatment follows the lines adopted in the management of any open fistula wound, the aim being thus a combination of primary union of the actual opening in the rectum and healing by granulation for the rest of the wound cavity. The aperture in the rectal wall may re-open and the fistulous track reform, or fortunately the sutures may hold, at any rate long enough for the tissues to unite, so that, even if the wire or silk is subsequently extruded or plucked out during one of the dressings, the fistula does not recur and the wound heals soundly.

An alternative operative approach to a complete pelvirectal fistula would be through a Kraske type of incision (p. 503), with removal of the coccyx and last one or two pieces of the sacrum, the patient lying on the side opposite to that of the internal opening.

Excision of Rectum with Permanent Iliac Colostomy. If recurrent sepsis and discharge persist despite a defunctioning iliac colostomy and a direct attack on the fistula has failed or been decided against, the only alternative is rectal excision.

RECTOVAGINAL FISTULA

A rectovaginal fistula may result from extension of a carcinoma of the rectum, uterine cervix or vagina, or may be due to tissue necrosis produced by irradiation administered in the treatment of the latter two growths. Another important cause is obstetrical tears with infection following repair, or injury during gynaecological surgery. The condition may also occur as a complication of an anorectal abscess (or its treatment), ulcerative colitis or Crohn's disease.

Rectovaginal fistulae due to carcinoma clearly require very radical excision of the rectum and vagina (possibly with the uterus), if this is technically feasible (see p. 548). Failing that the patient will be made a good deal more comfortable by establishing a proximal iliac colostomy to stop the gross leakage of faeces and flatus through the vagina. Fistulae associated with ulerative colitis or Crohn's disease require treatment of the underlying bowel condition by abdominoperineal excision with or without colectomy (see p. 851). The management of rectovaginal communications due to irradiation proctitis and necrosis introduces special problems due to the reduced capacity of the surrounding, still viable tissues to tolerate operative trauma and yet survive, and is dealt with on p. 873. Post-traumatic (obstetrical or gynaecological) rectovaginal fistulas may be amenable to plastic repair and several approaches are possible depending on the exact circumstances.

A *high* fistula opening on to the upper part of the posterior vaginal wall is dealt with most conveniently, as a rule, through the abdomen, the two viscera being separated and the perforations in their related walls closed by an invaginating suture technique. It may be an advantage finally to attempt to rotate the rectum slightly to one or other side to bring intact rectal wall against the site of suture in the vagina, or alternatively to interpose a tail of greater omentum—specially mobilized, as described on p. 438, if necessary—between the two organs to separate them. Personally, I would always establish a temporary iliac colostomy at the conclusion of the operation as an additional precaution, but some would regard this as ultra-cautious. It must be mentioned, however, that Lawson (1972), who has had an unrivalled experience of treating rectovaginal fistulae arising as a result of difficult parturition, prefers the vaginal route even for some of the fistulae involving the upper half of the vagina. He frees the rectum from the vagina at the site of the fistula and opens into the pouch of Douglas. The upper edge of the rectal defect is drawn down for suture to the lower edge, and the lower vaginal flap is sutured over the rectal suture line, but some of the anterior rectal wall forms the new upper posterior vaginal wall.

A *low* fistula involving the lower part of the vagina necessitates an approach from below. If the opening into the bowel lies below the level of the anorectal ring (i.e. the fistula is really anovaginal rather than rectovaginal), the treatment is simple and consists of laying the track open in classical manner. If the opening is definitely above the anorectal ring this ready solution is not applicable and some form of reparative surgery has to be considered. The prospects of success must always be uncertain but they are probably enhanced by defunctioning the part with a preliminary iliac colostomy. Four main methods are available.

a. The fistula may be approached *transvaginally*, a close circumcision being made around the vaginal opening and deepened into the rectal wall. The cut edges of the vaginal and rectal walls are then defined and separated for 2 cm or more all round. Finally the opening in the rectum is sutured with one or two rows of fine catgut stitches inserted so as to invert the mucosa into the rectal lumen, and the vaginal wound is similarly closed with catgut turning the edges into the lumen of the vagina. This method is only technically feasible if the fistula lies 2 or 3 cm above the anorectal ring where the vaginal and and rectal mucosa are in fairly close apposition with little intervening tissue. Even then it may be difficult to strike a satisfactory plane of separation between the vagina and rectum. The great defect of the technique is that the suture lines in the two viscera are in apposition without any separating tissue. I have only performed this operation once; there was some subsequent breakdown, but eventually sound healing was secured.

b. Another method is the *transperineal*, in which through a slightly curved incision in the perineum the anal canal and rectum behind are separated from the vagina in front. The recto-vaginal communication is encountered and divided, and the posterior vaginal and anterior rectal walls are mobilized as widely as possible to facilitate suture of the apertures in these walls without tension. Fine catgut stitches are used for the latter purpose, the mucosa being well inverted first of all and then the muscle coat and fascia being drawn over it with a second row of sutures. If the rectum and vagina can be rotated slightly in opposite directions to prevent the respective sites of suture falling together again, this is doubtless an advantage. The transperineal technique is my favourite method. I have used it five times with a successful outcome in all cases.

c. Recently a *transanal* approach to low rectovaginal fistula has been advocated by Greenwald and Hoexter (1978), who describe 20 cases successfully treated in this way. The patient is placed in a prone jack-knife position, the buttocks being taped apart. Using a Ferguson–Hill retractor (see p. 90) or bivalve anal speculum (see p. 37), the anterior anorectal wall containing the fistula is exposed. A transverse elliptical circumcision is made in the rectal

mucosa around the opening and gradually deepened till it reaches the posterior vaginal wall, an ellipse of which is also excised. The vaginal mucosal defect is not sutured but instead left open to provide drainage. The rectovaginal septum is reconstituted by at least two layers of interrupted Dexon or chromic catgut sutures and then the opening in the rectal wall is closed by the same material.

d. Perhaps the most popular of the four operations is that of *laying open the fistula, excising the track and performing primary suture of the wound, including the sphincters.* The steps of this procedure are shown in Fig. 150. It is the technique employed by gynaecologists for rectovaginal fistulas, or more commonly for complete perineal tears, either just after parturition or months or years later (MacLeod and Howkins 1964). Though they have some failures, most of these wounds apparently heal by first intention, as they did even before the advent of sulphonamides or antibiotics and usually without the protection of a covering colostomy! The five patients dealt with by this type of operation by me were mostly recurrent cases, who had already had one or two unsuccessful attempts at repair, and they were all given preliminary iliac colostomies. Three healed without incident; in

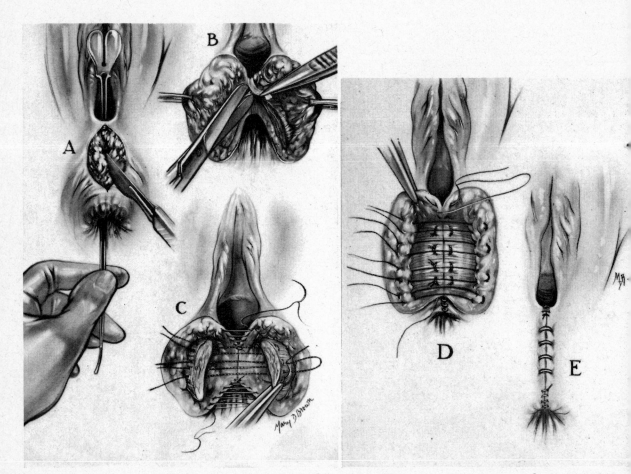

Fig. 150. Laying open suprasphincteric *rectovaginal* fistula, followed by primary suture. (A) Laying open fistula. (B) Excising fistulous track. (C) Suture of sphincter muscles. (D) Suture of fat and vaginal and anal skin. (E) Approximation of perineal skin with clips or sutures.

two infection and partial breakdown occurred, but a successful further repair was undertaken at a later date. Rectal function was satisfactory but not perfect in these cases.

RECTOURETHRAL FISTULA

A fistulous communication between the rectum and the male urethra may arise in several ways.

a. The condition may be *congenital*, in association with a high type of imperforate rectum, the end of the rectal stump opening into the prostatic urethra (see p. 264).

b. An important type of rectourethral fistula is that *resulting from trauma.* This is usually operative and most commonly occurs during prostatectomy. It was a notorious complication of perineal prostatectomy, but can occur after suprapubic and retropubic prostatectomy and other operations in this region. Thus Shackelford (1955), reviewing 57 cases of traumatic rectourethral fistula at the Johns Hopkins Hospital, Baltimore, found that 36 followed perineal prostatectomy (due to Hugh Young's teaching and example this operation was particularly popular in Baltimore), four suprapubic prostatectomy, two transurethral prostate resection, two rupture of the urethra during catheterization, one perineal cystolithotomy, one a Whitehead type of haemorrhoidectomy and two a fractured pelvis. Goodwin et al. (1958) report on a series of 20 prostatorectal fistulae following prostatectomy—15 after a perineal type of operation, three after a retropubic operation, and one each after suprapubic and transurethral prostatectomy.

c. Rectourethral fistula can also occasionally be *produced by infective processes.* For example it may be the result of a prostatic abscess bursting into the rectum, or of an extravasation of urine into the anal canal from behind a gonorrhoeal stricture of the urethral bulb. I have also seen a rectourethral stricture arising as a complication of Crohn's disease of the distal bowel.

d. Finally rectourethral fistula may be *secondary to malignant disease* of the prostate or of the lower rectum or anal canal. Actually, considering the great frequency of carcinoma in these organs, the remarkable thing is that a fistulous communication between them is so exceeding rare.

TREATMENT

For management of *congenital rectourethral* fistula in the neonatal period see p. 270. Rectourethral fistula *secondary to malignant disease* of the prostate or low rectum is generally incurable (except in the very rare case where a complete pelvic clearance proves feasible). As a rule the most that can be done is to establish a proximal iliac colostomy, which may help to reduce urinary infection. A *traumatic prostatorectal fistula* may close spontaneously with continuous catheter drainage for four to six weeks, as happened in nine of Goodwin et al.'s (1958) 22 cases. This is obviously more likely to happen with small fistulae. A proximal colostomy was not part of Goodwin et al.'s (1958) conservative management. If the fistula persists surgical repair will be required. Several methods are available for closing such fistulae; they may be grouped as follows:

Peranal Intrarectal Repair

Vose (1949) has treated these fistulae by the simple method of stretching the anal sphincters and using a bivalve speculum to expose the anterior rectal wall containing the fistulous opening (the patient being in a prone or lateral semi-prone position). An incision is made with a long-handled scalpel around the open-

ing and the cut mucosal edge is defined separately from the underlying muscle coat. A two-layer suture is then carried out with interrupted fine catgut, the deeper layer approximating the muscle and the more superficial one the mucosa. An indwelling urethal catheter is maintained in position for two weeks (longer would seem safer—J.C.G.).

Vose (1949) reported three cases treated by this method, all successfully though there was temporary leakage of urine *per anum* postoperatively in one of them. Goodwin et al. (1958) used the same principle in one case but without separately suturing muscle and mucosa, which was successful temporarily but had to be repeated before final closure was achieved.

Repair through a Perineal Approach

The simplest operation of this kind is that of Jewett (1955) in which a curved transverse incision is made in the perineum and deepened between the anal canal and urethral bulb. As this plane of dissection is followed upwards the fistula is exposed and divided, and the respective openings in the urethra and rectal wall are carefully sutured in layers with fine catgut and silk. The wound is then closed. Lowsley and Kirwin's (1944) method is similar, except that after the openings in the urethra and rectum have been closed an effort is made to prevent them falling together by rotating the site of the urethral repair 15° to the right and the site of the rectal repair 15° to the left and anchoring them in these positions by sutures.

A good recent report of the technique and results of the perineal method of repair of these fistulae is given by Goodwin et al. (1958). They do not consider that a covering proximal colostomy is necessary in the treatment of these cases, but a suprapubic cystostomy is part of their routine, being made either at the time of the repair or as a preliminary. Through a perineal incision the anal canal and rectum are separated from the urethral bulb and prostate, the fistula being exposed and boldly divided. The dissection is then continued upwards between the base of the bladder and the rectum till normal tissues are encountered, this wide mobilization being essential to facilitate the subsequent closure of the fistulous openings. The edges of these later openings in urethra and rectum are dissected to define an inner mucosal and an outer muscular and fascial layer, and the apertures are closed with two layers of fine catgut sutures. An indwelling urethral catheter may or may not be left in position in addition to the suprapubic cystostomy tube. After closure of the rectum, its anterior wall is drawn down towards the anus sufficiently to ensure that the former fistula sites in the two organs are no longer in apposition. The levator muscles are brought together with a few catgut sutures and the wound is closed with drainage.

Goodwin et al. (1958) used this technique in 12 cases of rectourethral fistulae with primary healing in all of them. In nine cases treated by a similar type of operation Wilhelm (1944) had two failures, but one of these was in a patient with advanced renal and vesical tuberculosis.

Young and Stone (1913) and Watson and Knapp (1943) describe further modifications of the perineal approach to rectourethral fistulae.

Repair through a Sacral Approach

Kilpatrick and Thompson (1962) have used a Kraske type of approach (see p. 503) for the repair of rectoprostatic fistulae following prostatectomy. They establish a preliminary iliac or transverse colostomy, if this has not already been done. The incision having been made and the coccyx and terminal one or two pieces of sacrum having been excised, the fascia of Waldeyer is incised exposing the rectum, which is mobilized from the sacral concavity and dissected off the back of the bladder and vesicles. During this anterior dissection it is a convenience to have a Young's prostatic retractor in position (introduced, opened and locked before the operation began) to assist in the identification of the prostate and bladder. The rectovesical peritoneal pouch may or may not be opened at this stage of the operation. The separation of the rectum from the urinary tract is continued downwards till the prostatorectal fistula is reached. The plane between the prostate and the rectum distal to the fistula is then opened up, and finally the communication is divided. The hole in the urethra is repaired with fine chromic catgut and the closure reinforced by suture of neighbouring tissues over the site. The edges of the opening in the rectum are trimmed to remove scar tissue and the aperture is closed with fine chromic catgut sutures, the mucosa being well inverted into the lumen. The rectum is then rotated slightly to have normal rectal wall, rather than the former fistula site, resting against the posterior urethra, and it is fixed in this position with a few stitches. The levator and subcutaneous fat are sutured with catgut and the skin wound closed, a drain being left down to the site of the repair. As a last step a suprapubic cystostomy is established, which is retained for two to four weeks as a rule if healing is uneventful.

Kilpatrick and Thompson (1962) have treated six patients along these lines with two temporary failures but eventual sound closure in all cases. Postoperative rectal function and urinary control were said to be excellent.

Repair through a Posterior Transsphincteric Approach

One of the best uses of the posterior transsphincteric approach to the lower rectum advocated by Mason (1970) is in the treatment of rectoprostatic fistulae (Kilpatrick and Mason 1969). The details of the approach are described on p. 355. The rectum having been opened and the fistulous opening on its anterior wall exposed, it is a simple matter to make a close circumcision round this opening and to deepen it down to the prostatic urethra. The prostatic capsule is then stitched with fine interrupted catgut or Dexon sutures, and the rectal wall similarly coapted to give good mucosal inversion into the lumen of the bowel. The posterior incision is then repaired. The operation is performed under cover of a preliminary iliac colostomy, and bladder drainage is secured by means of an indwelling urethral catheter—or, if preferred, by a suprapubic cystotomy—till the fistula has healed.

Mason (1970) reported four patients successfully treated by this method and his series of successful cases now stands at 9 (Mason 1979). But I know that in addition quite a number of unpublished cases have now been treated by this operation by numerous other surgeons throughout Britain with generally good results. For example, I myself have dealt with four patients in this way.

Repair as Part of an Abdominoanal Resection

Hampton and Bacon (1961) have used a pull-through technique for the closure of rectourethral fistulae, based on the latter's method of proctosigmoidectomy for rectal cancer (see p. 510). The advantage is that fresh healthy bowel is brought into apposition with the site of closure of the urethral opening, making re-establishment of the fistula more difficult. Before the proximal stump is drawn through the denuded anal canal, the opening on the back of the urethra is carefully sutured over an indwelling metal sound. The operation is done under a covering transverse colostomy and a suprapubic cystostomy. Hampton and Bacon (1961) reported the successful use of this operative plan in four cases of rectourethral fistula.

I have had two patients with postprostatectomy fistulae between rectum and urethra on whom I used a pull-through abdominoanal excision of the lower rectum with subsequent sound closure and satisfactory anal continence. The Turnbull-Cutait version of this operation was employed (see p. 514) and a covering transverse colostomy was established. In one case a suprapubic cystostomy was made, in the other reliance was placed on an indwelling urethral catheter for urinary drainage.

More recently a preferable alternative to the abdominoanal pull-through resection for repair of a prostatorectal fistula would be the abdominotransanal technique of resection (see p. 577 and also p. 874 for an account of the use of this operation in the treatment of post-irradiation rectovaginal fistulae—Parks et al. 1978).

Separation of Rectum from Prostate by Abdominal or Abdominoperineal Route and Interposition of a Tail of Greater Omentum

Turner-Warwick (1972, 1976) has recommended a purely abdominal operation, in which a plane of dissection is carried downwards between the seminal vesicles and prostate anteriorly and the rectum posteriorly, leading eventually to definition and division of the prostatorectal fistula. The resulting hole in the anterior rectal wall can usually be closed fairly easily by fine silk or catgut sutures, though sometimes it may be necessary to mobilize the rectum posteriorly and by division of the lateral ligaments in order to do so. Because of the rigidity of the tissues it is best as a rule not to attempt suture of the prostatic hole but simply to leave it open with the indwelling urethral Foley catheter in position and to tuck a long tail of greater omentum—prepared as described on p. 438—into the space between the prostate and rectum. To facilitate the insertion of the omental tail between the prostate and rectum O. V. Lloyd-Davies in one case (Miller 1977) made also a perineal incision and fixed the end of the omentum to the perineal fat, but more often this does not seem to be necessary. I personally elected to establish a loop iliac colostomy at the conclusion of the operation in the two cases that I treated successfully by this method, and it was not closed for six to eight weeks afterwards. The urethral catheter was retained for three weeks.

Conclusion

At the present time I consider that the two best methods available for dealing with these traumatic prostatorectal fistulae are the repair through a posterior transsphincteric approach, or the interposition of a pedicle graft of greater omentum through an abdominal (or abdominoperineal) approach.

TUBERCULOUS ANAL FISTULA

Many surgeons adopt a distinctly conservative approach to the treatment of tuberculous anal fistulae. For example Gabriel (1948), whilst admitting that relatively superficial tuberculous fistulae are amenable to operative treatment, counsels strongly against any attempt at radical operation in cases with higher tuberculous fistulae. Such lesions enjoy a sinister reputation and this may perhaps be partly due to the attempts often made by surgeons in the past to explain away their failures in the operative treatment of high complicated fistulae by suggesting that they were probably tuberculous. Frequently bacteriological confirmation of this allegation has been lacking, and it is strongly to be suspected that the majority of these failures have been due, not to tuberculosis having been the cause of the fistula, but to some part of the fistulous track having been overlooked at the operation.

I certainly cannot agree with this ultra-cautious attitude towards tuberculous fistulae, for my experience and that of Milligan et al. (1948) show that, provided an active pulmonary tuberculous lesion has been excluded or brought to a state of quiescence, these fistulae may be treated like any non-tuberculous fistula. This holds true even when the fistula is of a high complicated type. Moreover the operation can be conducted with exactly the same technique as for fistula operations in general, there being in particular no necessity to employ diathermy coagulation of the wound surfaces as recommended by some surgeons such as Gabriel (1948). These conclusions are based on the results obtained in treating some 27 cases with different varieties of tuberculous fistula. Satisfactory healing of the wounds was obtained in all, and though no complete follow-up survey has been possible it is known that nine patients treated more than five years ago have been perfectly well since—and incidentally in few of these cases was supplementary streptomycin and PAS or INH therapy used. Similarly it is known that one patient, after remaining well for 13 years following his operation, then developed a proven recurrent tuberculous fistula at the same site without an active pulmonary lesion. He is now well again 10 years after a further operation.

Clearly, however, the overall results in any large series of cases of tuberculous fistula will be considerably influenced by the success in controlling the chest condition. This is brought out in Granet's (1954) report on a series of 68 patients with tuberculous fistula-in-ano treated at the Sea View Sanatorium, New York City. Of these, 72% were cured, 12% died of their pulmonary lesion whilst their anal fistulae were still unhealed, 10% were discharged with arrest of their lung focus but with incompletely healed anal wounds, and 6% remained with a persistent sinus.

The first requirement in the treatment of tuberculous anal fistulae, then, is an accurate assessment by a chest physician of the activity of any pulmonary tuberculous focus present. If it is considered to be active, appropriate treatment with streptomycin and PAS or INH and rest should be instituted. Meanwhile no operation should be undertaken for the anal lesion, other than the opening by minimal incision of an abscess, if this has not already burst to produce an overt fistula. Only after the chest condition has become inactive, which will probably take two or three months, is the fistula subjected to formal surgical treatment for its cure. The course of this operation and post-operative management do not differ in any respect from that adopted for an ordinary fistula, except that it is now customary to continue streptomycin and PAS therapy for at least three months from the time of operation.

If at the time of initial examination the pulmonary lesion is quiescent or the chest is considered to be completely clear, surgical treatment can be undertaken for the anal condition right away, provided there is no other focus of tuberculosis, say in the hip or seminal vesicles, to account for the fistula.

ANAL FISTULA WITH CROHN'S DISEASE

The treatment required for these lesions depends on the site of the underlying enteritis in the intestinal tract. If it is located in the small bowel or proximal colon, with the distal large bowel normal, the surgical attack is two-fold; first the excision of the diseased intestinal segment, and secondly an appropriate 'unroofing' operation for the fistula. These measures are probably best carried out in that order if the underlying Crohn's

lesion has been detected before treatment has been commenced. Not infrequently, however, the fistula has already been treated surgically in the first instance and it is the failure of the wound to heal or the early recurrence of the condition that has led to the suspicion and eventual diagnosis of the regional ileitis (see also p. 834).

ANAL FISTULA WITH ULCERATIVE COLITIS

It is generally said that local surgical treatment of these fistulae, by ignoring the underlying bowel condition, is futile and even dangerous as it may be followed by an exacerbation of the colitis. This is not entirely true for I have had four patients with anal fistulae associated with mild distal proctocolitis in whom surgery resulted in complete, if tardy, healing despite the colitis. Some of these fistulae become quiescent as the colitis improves and occasionally the very superficial ones may heal and form skin-lined subcutaneous tracks. But very frequently fistulae arising in connection with colitis require radical surgical treatment with total proctolectomy and ileostomy.

ANAL FISTULA WITH CARCINOMA

Whether the carcinoma has been the primary condition or has arisen as a complication of the fistula, the prognosis is poor due to the, usually, wide spread of the lesion in the tissues of the buttock and to the inguinal lymph glands. Occasionally, however, excision is possible by means of an abdominoperineal excision of the rectum with wide ablation of the surrounding tissues on the affected side, and a subsequent block dissection of the glands of the groin. This may give a good palliative result for one or two years before recurrence takes place, and I have had one patient who survived for $5\frac{1}{2}$ years after such an operation. In inoperable cases super-voltage radiotherapy may be of some value, especially in cases of squamous epithelioma.

HIDRADENITIS SUPPURATIVA— INFECTION OF THE APOCRINE SWEAT GLANDS

Hidradenitis suppurativa is a chronic, indolent, inflammatory disease of certain areas of the skin and subcutaneous tissues, characterized by the formation of abscesses and sinuses, and due primarily to an infection of the apocrine group of sweat glands. As one of the sites where these glands occur is the perianal region, hidradenitis often presents to the rectal surgeon as a fistula-in-ano. The disease was first recognized clinically by Verneuil (1854), and its relation to the sweat glands was established by Pollitzer (1892) and Dubreuilh (1893). However, no clear account of the condition based on any substantial series of cases appeared in the English language till Brunsting's comprehensive report from the Mayo Clinic in 1939.

DISTINGUISHING CHARACTERISTICS OF THE APOCRINE AND ECCRINE SWEAT GLANDS

The following characteristics were described by Schiefferdecker (1921) and Woollard (1930):

The eccrine, or ordinary, sweat glands are simple tubular glands distributed over practically the whole skin of the body, being most abundant in the palms and soles. They are derived directly from the epidermis and become active within the first few months of life. They secrete sweat through their tortuous ducts which open on the epidermal surface independently of the hair follicles. The fluid they produce is clear and transparent, the chief constituents being water, salt, urea and fatty acids.

The *apocrine* glands are large compound tubular glands, 50 mm long, 2 mm wide and 3–5 mm deep, situated more deeply in the corium. They are restricted in their distribution to certain zones of the skin, normally only the axillary, mammary, inguinal, genital and perianal regions. They are developed from the hair follicles, but do not become active till puberty. They function by rupture of the cell membrane of the lining epithelial cells, cellular protoplasm being thus discharged into the ducts, which open either into the hair follicles or on the cutaneous surface immediately adjacent to the follicles. A close correlation therefore exists between the distribution of these glands and the hairs of the skin. The secretion of the apocrine glands is thicker in consistency than that of the eccrine glands; its precise composition is unknown, but it has a characteristic odour.

Clinical Features

Hidradenitis occurs after puberty, the majority of patients being in the second or third decades of life. As a rule it affects robust individuals who show no impairment of general health, but may have a rather oily skin and are predisposed to acne.

In the early stages the disease appears as a firm subcutaneous nodule. This may resolve slowly over a period of several weeks without producing any pus. More commonly adjacent nodules appear and coalesce to form a cord-like elevated band or plaque. The lesion then gradually extends to produce a considerable area of induration. Suppuration is usually slight; there may be one or more superficial pustules, but when opened only a few drops of thick creamy pus are evacuated. In other cases a slight amount of discharge persists and the affected region may show numerous sinus openings. In the latter stages ulceration may occur.

Pathological Changes

As described by Brunsting (1939) the earliest changes on histological section of the affected skin and subcutaneous tissues are

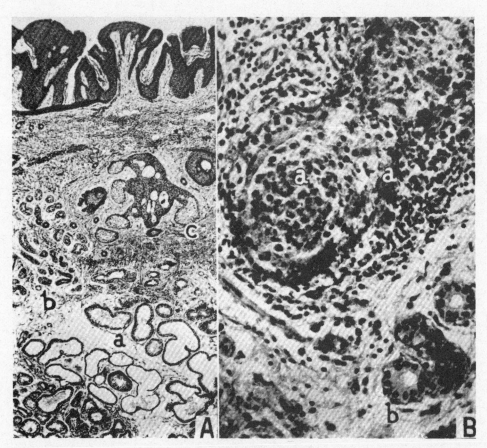

Fig. 151. (A) Normal relationship of glands in the skin of the axilla of a Negro; (*a*) apocrine gland; (*b*) eccrine gland; and (*c*) sebaceous gland; specimen stained with haematoxylin and eosin, ×34. (B) Early changes of hidradentis suppurativa, showing (*a*) acute inflammatory reaction within the lumen of the apocrine gland and in the peri-glandular connective tissue, and (*b*) absence of involvement of the neighbouring eccrine glands; specimen stained with haematoxylin and eosin, ×240. (*From Brunsting 1939*)

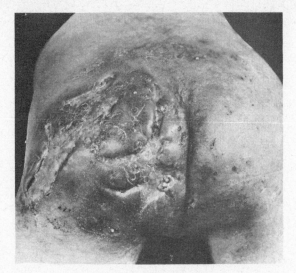

Fig. 152. Extensive hidradenitis suppurativa of the perianal region and left buttock. (*From Granet 1954*)

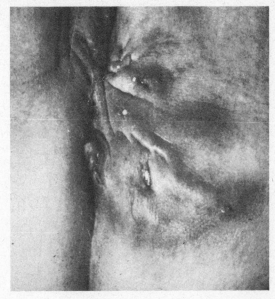

Fig. 153. Hidradenitis suppurativa of the anal region and left buttock (Mr V. P. McAllister's case).

seen to be a cellular reaction within the lumen of the apocrine glands, many such glands being distended with leucocytes, and cellular infiltration of the surrounding connective tissue (Fig. 151).

Distribution of the Lesions

Jackman and McQuarrie (1949) reviewed a series of 388 patients with suppurative hidradenitis, seen at the Mayo Clinic between 1940 and 1947 inclusive. Roughly half of the patients were men and half women. The axilla was the commonest site of involvement, being affected on one or both sides, alone or in combination with lesions in other sites, in 72% of the series. The mammary region was implicated in 8% of the cases, the groin in 24%, the back of the neck in 11%, and the perianal region in 32%, of which roughly one-third had anal lesions alone.

Diagnosis of Suppurative Hidradenitis of the Anal Region

Undoubtedly this disease has frequently been overlooked in the past, mainly because it has not been thought of. But once seen and correctly diagnosed, it leaves a vivid impression that cannot easily be forgotten or confused with any other condition. The characteristic features are the considerable extent of the lesion, the great thickening of the subcutaneous tissues, either diffusely or in a somewhat nodular fashion, the purplish discoloration of the overlying skin suggesting a subacute or chronic imflam-

matory condition, and the presence of numerous sinus openings which seldom discharge much pus (Figs 152, 153). If attempts are made to incise the affected part to lay open the sinuses, no real cavity or track is discovered and the subcutaneous tissues are seen to be thickened, oedematous, and fibrosed and to contain scattered, very small collections of purulent fluid. In many cases the existence of concomitant manifestations in the axillary or other regions will place the diagnosis beyond all doubt, but even without this aid the disease is easily recognized if it is simply borne in mind. Otherwise suppurative hidradenitis may be mistaken for furunculosis, an ordinary anal fistula, Crohn's disease of the perianal skin, or, if extending into the post-anal region, a pilonidal sinus.

Treatment of Anal Hidradenitis Suppurativa

Though Brunsting (1939) suggested that sulphonamides or X-ray therapy might be beneficial in assisting spontaneous resolution, there is no clear evidence of their value. Christensen (1950) found that penicillin was useful in controlling areas of more acute inflammation, but did not affect the ultimate need for surgical treatment. Operation requires *complete excision of the lesion* in single or multiple stages. The involved skin and subcutaneous tissues are excised down to the deep fascia. The resulting raw area may be very extensive; it is, however, a relatively flat superficial surface well suited to split-skin grafting, and this may often be practised with advantage.

REFERENCES

ALLINGHAM, W. and ALLINGHAM, H. W. (1901) *The Diagnosis and Treatment of Diseases of the Rectum.* London: Baillière.
BENNETT, R. C. (1962) A review of the results of orthodox treatment for anal fistulae. *Proc. R. Soc. Med.*, 55, 756.
BLOND, K. (1940) *Haemorrhoids and Their Treatment: The Varicose Syndrome of the Rectum*, trans. E. Stanley Lee. Bristol: John Wright.
BRUNSTING, H. A. (1939) Hidradenitis suppurativa; abscess of the apocrine sweat glands. *Archs Derm. Syph.*, 39, 108.

CHRISTENSEN, J. B. (1950) Hidradenitis suppurativa involving the peri-anal region. *Am. J. Surg.*, *79*, 61.

DUBREUILH, W. (1893) Des hidrosadénites suppuratives disséminées. *Archs Méd. exp. Anat. path.*, 5, 63.

DUKES, C. E. and GALVIN, C. (1956) Colloid carcinoma arising within fistulae in the anorectal region. *Ann. R. Coll. Surg. Engl.*, *18*, 246.

EISENHAMMER, S. (1958) A new approach to the anorectal fistulous abscess based on the high intermuscular lesion. *Surgery Gynec. Obstet.*, *106*, 595.

—— (1961) The anorectal and anovulval fistulous abscess. *Surgery Gynec. Obstet.*, *113*, 519.

GABRIEL, W. B. (1921) Results of experimental and histological investigations into seventy-five cases of rectal fistulae. *Proc. R. Soc. Med.*, *14*, 156.

—— (1948) *Principles and Practice of Rectal Surgery*, 4th ed. London: H. K. Lewis.

GOLIGHER, J. C. (1975) *Surgery of the Anus, Rectum and Colon*, 3rd ed., p. 209. London: Baillière Tindall.

—— ELLIS, M. and PISSIDES, A. (1967) A study of the rôle of intersphincteric abscess formation in the pathogenesis of anorectal abscess and fistula. *Br. J. Surg.*, *54*, 64.

GOODSALL, D. H. (1900) In *Diseases of the Anus and Rectum*, ed. D. H. Goodsall and W. E. Miles, part I. London: Longmans.

GOODWIN, W. E., TURNER, R. D. and WINTER, C. C. (1958) Rectourinary fistula: principles of management and a technique of surgical closure. *J. Urol.*, *80*, 246.

GORDON-WATSON, C. (1934) Progress in rectal surgery. *St Bart's Hosp. J.*, *41*, 104.

GRANET, E. (1954) *Manual of Proctology*. Chicago: Year-Book Publishers.

GREENWALD, J. C. and HOEXTER, B. (1978) Repair of rectovaginal fistulas. *Surgery Gynec. Obstet.*, *146*, 443.

HAMPTON, T. M. and BACON, H. E. (1961) Diagnosis and surgical management of rectourethral fistulas. *Dis. Colon Rect.*, *4*, 177.

HUGHES, E. S. R. (1953) Primary skin-grafting in proctological surgery. *Br. J. Surg.*, *41*, 639.

JACKMAN, R. J. and BUIE, L. A. (1946) Tuberculosis and anal fistula. *J. Am. med. Ass.*, *130*, 630.

—— and McQUARRIE, H. B. (1949) Hidradenitis suppurativa: its confusion with pilonidal disease and anal fistula. *Am. J. Surg.*, *77*, 349.

JEWETT, H. J. Quoted by Shackelford (1955).

KILPATRICK, F. R. and MASON, A. Y. (1969) Postoperative recto-prostatic fistula. *Br. J. Urol.*, *41*, 649.

—— and THOMPSON, H. R. (1962) Postoperative recto-prostatic fistula and closure by Kraske's approach. *Br. J. Urol.*, *64*, 470.

KLINE, R. J., SPENCER, R. J. and HARRISON, E. G., Jr. (1964) Carcinoma associated with fistula-in-ano. *Archs Surg.*, *Chicago*, *89*, 989.

LAWSON, J. (1972) Rectovaginal fistulae following difficult labour. *Proc. R. Soc. Med.*, *65*, 283.

LOCKHART-MUMMERY, J. P. (1934) *Diseases of the Rectum and Colon*, 2nd ed. London: Baillière.

LOWSLEY, O. S. and KIRWIN, T. J. (1944) *Clinical Urology*, vol. I, p. 695. Baltimore: Williams & Wilkins.

McANALLY, A. K. and DOCKERTY, M. B. (1949) Carcinoma developing in chronic draining cutaneous sinuses and fistulas. *Surgery Gynec. Obstet.*, *88*, 87.

McCUNE, W. S. and THISTLETHWAITE, J. R. (1959) Fistula cancer. *Am. Surg.*, *149*, 815.

MacLEOD, D. and HOWKINS, J. (1964) *Bonney's Gynaecological Surgery*, 7th ed. London: Baillière, Tindall & Cassell.

MASON, A. Y. (1970) Surgical access to the rectum—a trans-sphincteric exposure. *Proc. R. Soc. Med.*, Suppl. *63*, 91.

—— (1979) Personal communication.

MILES, W. E. (1939) *Rectal Surgery*. London: Cassell.

MILLER, W. (1977) A successful repair of a recto-urethral fistula: a case report. *Br. J. Surg.*, *64*, 869.

MILLIGAN, E. T. C. and MORGAN, C. N. (1934) Surgical anatomy of the anal canal with special reference to anorectal fistulae. *Lancet*, *2*, 1150, 1213.

—— —— LLOYD-DAVIES, O. V. and THOMPSON, H. R. (1948) In *British Surgical Practice*, ed. E. R. Carling and J. P. Ross, vol. 4, p. 102. London: Butterworth.

MILLIKEN, J. C. (1960) Squamous carcinoma arising in anal fistula. *Br. J. Surg.*, *48*, 224.

MORSON, B. C. and LOCKHART-MUMMERY, H. E. (1959) Anal lesions in Crohn's disease. *Lancet*, *2*, 1122.

NORBURY, L. E. C. and MORGAN, C. N. (1927) The value of lipiodol in determining the extent of fistulae-in-ano. *Proc. R. Soc. Med.*, *20*, 1274.

PARKS, A. G. (1961) Pathogenesis and treatment of fistula-in-ano. *Br. med. J.*, *1*, 463.

—— (1962) Personal communication.

—— ALLEN, C. LO., FRANK, J. D. and McPARTLIN, J. F. (1978) A method of treating post-irradiation rectovaginal fistulae. *Br. J. Surg.*, *65*, 417.

—— GORDON, P. H. and HARDCASTLE, J. D. (1976) A classification of fistula-in-ano. *Br. J. Surg.*, *63*, 1.

PENNINGTON, R. (1910) Quoted by Lockhart-Mummery (1934).

POLLITZER, S. (1892) Hidradenitis destruens suppurativa. *J. cutan. Dis.*, *10*, 9.

POTT, P. (1779) Quoted by Tuttle, J. P. (1903).

POWER D'ARCY (1910) *Treatise of Fistula-in-Ano, Haemorrhoids and Clysters*, by John Arderne. Oxford: Oxford University Press.

REDDING, M. D. (1956) Colloid carcinoma arising in chronic anal fistula. *Calif. Med.*, *85*, 250.

ROSSER, C. (1931) The aetiology of anal cancer. *Am. J. Surg.*, *11*, 328.

SCHIEFFERDECKER, P. (1921) Uber morphologische Sekretionserscheinungen in den ekkrinen Hautdrusen des Menschen. *Arch. Derm. Syph.*, *132*, 130.

SCHWARTZ, A. (1963) Anorectal fistula and cancer. *Dis. Colon Rect.*, *6*, 305.

SHACKELFORD, R. T. (1955) *Surgery of the Alimentary Tract*, pp. 1851–1862. Philadelphia: W. B. Saunders.

STARR, K. W. (1949) Chemotherapy in intestinal surgery. *Aust. N.Z. J. Surg.*, *19*, 72.

—— (1953) Primary closure in proctology. *Postgrad. Med.*, *14*, 365.

—— (1959) Personal communication.

STELZNER, F. (1976) *Die Anorectalen Fisteln*, 2nd ed. Berlin: Springer Verlag.

STOCKMAN, J. M. and YOUNG, V. T. (1953) Carcinoma associated with anorectal fistula. *Am. J. Surg.*, *86*, 560.

TURNER-WARWICK, R. (1972) The use of omental pedicle grafts in the repair of urinary tract fistulae. *Br. J. Urol., 44,* 644.

—— (1976) The use of the omental pedicle graft in urinary tract reconstruction. *J. Urol., 116,* 341.

VERNEUIL, A. (1854) Etudes sur les tumeurs de la peau; de quelques maladies des glandes sudoripares. *Archs gén. Méd., 94,* 447.

VOSE, S. N. (1949) Technique for repair of rectourethral fistula. *J. Urol., 61,* 790.

WATSON, E. M. and KNAPP, L. S. (1943) A simplified technique for the cure of urethro-rectal fistula. *J. Urol., 49,* 488.

WILHELM, S. F. (1944) Rectourinary fistula. *Surgery Gynec. Obstet., 79,* 427.

WILLIAMS, A. F. (1968) Pelvirectal fistula treated by temporary colostomy. *Br. J. Surg., 55,* 219.

WILSON, E. (1969) Skin grafts in surgery for anal fistula. *Dis. Colon Rect., 12,* 327.

WOOLLARD, H. H. (1930) The cutaneous glands of man. *J. Anat., 64,* 415.

YOUNG, H. H. and STONE, H. B. (1913) An operation for urethrorectal fistula: Report of three cases. *Trans. Am. Ass. genito-urin. Surg.,* 8, 270.

8

Pilonidal Sinus

In its more usual form this disease consists of a sinus or fistula situated a short distance behind the anus and generally containing hairs. It was first described by Anderson in 1847 in a paper entitled 'Hair extracted from an ulcer'. Warren in 1854 reported an 'Abscess containing hair on the nates', and Hodges in 1880 coined for it the expressive term pilonidal sinus (*pilus* = hair; *nidus* = nest). The condition seems to have increased greatly in frequency in recent years and appeared to be particularly common in Anglo-American Service personnel during the Second World War. The fact that many of the latter individuals had done a fair amount of travelling in Jeeps led some writers to refer to pilonidal sinus as 'Jeep disease'. Because of the uncertainty as to its aetiology and the considerable difficulties often encountered in its treatment, a formidable and controversial literature has arisen in connection with pilonidal sinus both in this country and in America.

INCIDENCE

The main facts in the natural history of *postanal* pilonidal sinus have been well brought out in a collective review by Kooistra (1942) of 350 cases of the condition. They can be summarized as follows:

Average age of onset of symptoms: 21½ years.

Average age at admission to hospital: 25 years.

Age distribution: Few cases were under 17 years; there was a great increase to a maximum at 19 years, continuing high to 25 years and steeply declining thereafter.

Sex incidence: 73·7% were males.

Effect of sex on age incidence: Women were affected at a slightly earlier age; 40% had symptoms before 20 years as compared with 19% of the men.

Race: The condition is rare in Negroes.

Bodily type: The majority of patients are dark hairy subjects, but pilonidal sinus occurs also in blonde, relatively hairless types.

Trauma: Riding in bumpy vehicles for long periods is apparently an exciting factor.

Associated congenital defects including spina bifida are rare; only 1·8% of Kooistra's (1942) series had such lesions.

OTHER SITES OF PILONIDAL SINUS FORMATION

Until recently pilonidal sinus was thought to be a lesion confined to the post-anal region. In 1946, however, Patey and Scarff reported a case of pilonidal sinus of the finger webb in a barber. Further examples of the condition in the hand have been described by Ewing (1947), Patey and Scarff (1948), King (1949), Currie et al. (1953) (who gave a good review of the literature and pathology of this variety of the condition), and by Oldfield (1956). Pilonidal sinus has also been observed in the axilla (Aird 1952), the perineum (Smith 1948), on a mid-thigh amputation stump (Shoesmith 1953; Gillis 1954), in the umbilicus (Patey and Williams 1956), and in the suprapubic region (MacLeod 1953; Patey and Curry 1962; Crosby 1962). It is not proposed to describe the pathological or clinical features of these forms of the condition further, but they will be briefly referred to later in discussing the aetiology of the disease.

CLINICAL FEATURES

A post-anal pilonidal sinus seldom presents itself till infection has supervened. A typical history is that a young adult develops an abscess at the base of the spine which bursts or is opened by his doctor. The discharge then ceases after a few days, though a nodule of induration may persist for a week or two. The patient remains well, possibly for several weeks or months, till another abscess occurs and the same course of events is repeated. He may have several recurring abscesses in this way before the condition is correctly diagnosed.

On examination the findings in the post-anal region are very characteristic. Situated *accurately in the midline* some 5 cm or so behind the anus, there is an opening or a series of openings, placed close together or spread out over a distance of perhaps 2–3 cm (A in Fig. 154). Sometimes they are so small

that they barely admit a fine lacrimal probe, but usually they are rather larger, more of matchstick size. The skin enters them so that they have a smooth edge, unlike that of an ordinary fistula. In addition hairs often project from the openings.

In some cases this is the only abnormality present, but in the majority there is another sinus opening 2–5 cm more superiorly, *almost always slightly to one or other side of the midline*, more commonly the left (c in Fig. 154). This does not differ in appearance from that of any other pyogenic fistula and frequently shows exuberant granulation tissue projecting from it. On palpation an elongated oval or irregular area of induration (B in Fig. 154) can usually be felt connecting orifices A and C, and pressure on it may cause pus or seropurulent fluid to escape from either opening. Occasionally the sinus opening (c in Fig. 154) has closed over and there may be a cystic swelling underlying it or occupying a position between it and the opening at A.

PATHOLOGICAL ANATOMY

This account of the pathological features is derived from the comprehensive accounts of Newell (1933), Patey and Scarff (1946), Kooistra (1942), Brearley (1955) and Spencer (1967), as well as my own observations, of the findings at operation and in excised specimens of the condition.

Main Features

The Primary Track. This commences in the skin-lined orifice or orifices at A, Fig. 155, and extends in the subcutaneous tissues in a headward direction for a distance of 2–5 cm, often expanding into a terminal small cavity. Most of the tracks apart from the actual opening appear to be lined with granulation tissue.

Hairs. Hairs are a striking feature of the condition and are nearly always found by the surgeon projecting from the sinus opening or lying in the primary track when it is laid open at or immediately after operation, but as he often removes them before the specimen goes to the pathology department hair is less frequently found by the pathologist. Thus Kooistra (1942) and Patey and Scarff (1946) discovered hairs in only 50% of the

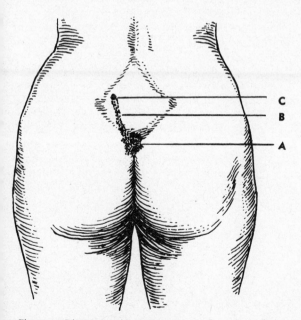

Fig. 154. Diagrammatic representation of a pilonidal sinus showing the essential features: (A) 'Developmental' holes. (B) Elongated area of induration representing the tracks and abscess cavity. (C) The fistula opening. (*From Newell 1933*)

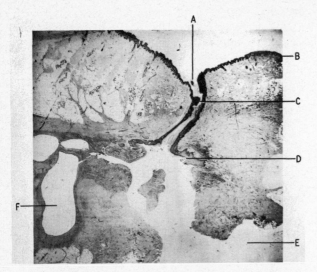

Fig. 155. A low-power microscopic section of a pilonidal sinus to show the connection of the primary sinus with the skin and deep tissues. (A) Tiny orifice situated in the median raphé. (B) Skin surface. (C) Primary sinus lined by squamous epithelium. (D) Termination of epithelium. (E) Main cavity and secondary sinuses lined with granulation tissue. (*From Newell 1933*)

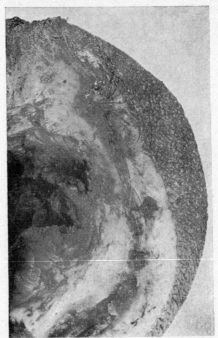

Fig. 156. Hairs converging on the sinus opening. (*From Brearley 1955*)

lesions examined by them. Nearly all the hairs lie loose, but a few are still attached to the wall of the track (Spencer 1967); some may grow into the sinus from the skin outside it (Fig. 156). If entirely free they are usually tapered at both ends like shed hairs, and according to Weale (1955) and Spencer (1967), generally lie with their bases directed towards the head.

Secondary Tracks. The secondary track, which connects the deep part of the primary track to the sinus opening lying to one or other side of the midline more posteriorly, has the appearance of any ordinary fistulous track when laid open. The skin does not enter it and often granulations project at the opening.

Further Microscopical Considerations

Lining. Though Gabriel (1948), Newell (1933) and Spencer (1967) have produced photomicrographs showing a well-defined squamous epithelial lining to a considerable part of the track in specimens of pilonidal sinus, it is a common experience that secondary tracks and the deeper expanded portions of the primary track are usually lined with granulation tissue. Indeed many writers find that an epithelial lining is a very inconstant feature even of the primary track; it was noted, for

example, in only eight of Patey and Scarff's (1946) 21 cases, and if present at all tends to be confined to its extreme lower end. Sheehan (1953) even goes so far as to say that he has never found the epithelial lining to extend more than 2 mm from the primary cutaneous opening in over 200 examples of pilonidal sinus examined by him.

Dermal Appendages. As already mentioned, hairs are frequently present in the lumen of the primary track. But the existence of hair follicles in the wall of that track, from which it might be postulated they have grown, or of sebaceous or sweat glands, has apparently never been conclusively demonstrated. Patey and Scarff (1946) and Sheehan (1953) could find neither hair follicles nor glands, but Spencer (1967), by careful serial sectioning, was able to display hair follicles in many of his specimens.

Malignant Change

Matt (1958) reported a case of malignant change in a pilonidal sinus—the tumour being of mixed basal and squamous celled type, and on searching the literature he was able to discover eight other instances of carcinomatous transformation. Another case of squamous celled carcinoma arising in a pilonidal sinus was reported by Goodall (1961).

AETIOLOGY

Five main theories have been advanced to explain the development of post-anal pilonidal sinuses:

1. THE PREEN GLAND THEORY

In 1931 Harvey B. Stone of Baltimore discovered in casual reading that in birds a preen gland is often present as a crypt near the anus, and he threw out the suggestion that possibly pilonidal sinus in man was some form of vestigial preen gland. But he produced no evidence or logical argument in favour of this highly imaginative theory, which need not be further considered.

2. THE MEDULLARY CANAL VESTIGE THEORY

The chief advocates of this hypothesis have been Mallory (1892), Rogers (1933), Gage (1935) and Kooistra (1942). They believe that caudal remnants of the medullary canal persist in the sacro-coccygeal region and develop into a pilonidal cyst, which in due course ruptures and becomes a sinus. It is known that epithelial-lined cystic vestiges of the medullary canal do occur beneath the skin of the sacral region during embryonic life, but, as Kooistra (1942) admits, the lining of these cysts is invarably cuboidal epithelium and not skin. The distinguished American embryologist, Streeter, is quoted by Stone (1924) as stating that the epithelium of the sacrococcygeal medullary remnant is already so far advanced that if it persisted into extrauterine life it could not be expected to give rise to skin. However, clinical cases are occasionally encountered in which a sinus is present with an opening situated in the skin of the sacrococcygeal region, and a track extends down between the sacrum and coccyx and along the sacral canal, to become continuous with the central canal of the spinal cord, and discharges cerebrospinal fluid from it (Kooistra 1942; Haworth and Zachary 1955). These sinuses are lined with skin but contain no hair. They usually open at a higher level than the ordinary post-anal pilonidal sinus, generally in the upper sacral region. Invariably they have been present since birth, and they are usually observed in young children. A varying degree of spina bifida is sometimes present. There is a great risk of meningitis in early life with these sinuses, and accordingly a high death rate. Though Haworth and Zachary (1955) consider that these lesions are juvenile versions of pilonidal sinuses, it is not clear that they are the same condition.

3. THE TRACTION DERMOID THEORY

This theory has been propounded by Newell (1933). He postulates that the tail bud is attached to the skin of the coccygeal region in the midline, and that during development, due to retrogression of the bud, the skin is drawn into the subcutaneous tissues in a cephalad direction to form a sinus which is present at birth and may become deeper due to further traction as the child grows. The condition remains symptomless till infection occurs, leading to abscess formation, the destruction of some of the epithelial lining, and the development of a secondary sinus track. If this theory were valid one would expect to find congenital dimples or sinuses not infrequently in the coccygeal region of infants and children. Hitherto it has been the general impression that such sinuses are excessively rare in childhood, but Haworth and Zachary (1955) in a survey of 500 children attending the Sheffield Children's Hospital, found that seven (1·4%) had a sinus overlying the coccyx, and 14 (2·8% had deep dimples in the same region. Six of the sinuses were excised and found to be lined with squamous epithelium and to be connected to the tip of the coccyx by a fibrous band.

4. THE INCLUSION DERMOID THEORY

Bland-Sutton (1922) asserted that pilonidal sinuses of the sacrococcygeal region were sequestration dermoids but produced no evidence in favour of this belief. Gabriel (1948) formerly shared this opinion, but has more recently accepted the view that pilonidal sinus is usually acquired (Gabriel 1963). In a recent comparison of barber's and post-anal pilonidal sinuses Weale (1964) has drawn attention to histological differences in the two lesions which led him to conclude that the former is an implantation dermoid, the latter a sequestration dermoid. If this theory were correct one would expect that a cyst, not a sinus, would be present from birth. In due course this might enlarge, become infected, suppurate and burst, discharging cheesy material, hairs and pus. It would be reasonable to expect that occasionally such a dermoid cyst would be encountered and removed before the occurrence of infection; also that after infection and discharge, the epithelial lining would be present in the deeper parts of the track rather than at the lower opening. As Fox (1935) points out, no one has in fact observed this sequence of events.

5. THE THEORY THAT PILONIDAL SINUS IS AN ACQUIRED CONDITION

This theory was originally propounded by Patey and Scarff in 1946. They were prompted to do so by the experience which they had in one case where, after they had removed a pilonidal sinus by an excision which they considered to be very generous and adequate, it recurred, presenting exactly the same features as those shown by the original condition. Further excision resulted in yet another typical recurrence. Even if they had inadvertently left some minute fragment of a hypothetical skin-lined tract after the first operation, it is hard to believe that they would have done so yet a second time. In recurrent lesions of this kind it is perhaps significant that the cutaneous lining in the track is not in the deeper part of the track where it might reasonably be expected to be found if it were an unremoved portion of the original track, but adjacent to the opening. An important point to Patey and Scarff (1946) is that hair follicles and glands have never been unequivocally demonstrated by them in the wall of a pilonidal sinus, so that if it were a congenital condition and the hairs had grown from the skin lining, it would be necessary to postulate that the follicles responsible had all been destroyed by the inflammatory reaction, which would indeed be remarkable. (But other observers such as Gabriel (1948) and Spencer (1967) do not agree on the absence of hair follicles.)

The alternative theory, which seemed more plausible to Patey and Scarff (1946), was that the hairs are derived from the surrounding skin and have somehow been introduced into the tissues causing the sinus. That this could occur was demonstrated by the discovery of pilonidal sinuses in other situations, such as the finger web, the axilla, and on an amputation stump, where no question of a congenital sinus arises. It could be objected that the hairs responsible for pilonidal sinuses of the interdigital webs of barbers' fingers are short and stiff and therefore more likely to penetrate the skin than the uncut naturally occurring hairs of the skin, so that the conditions here are different from those in the natal cleft. But on the other hand pilonidal sinuses in the axilla and umbilicus and on an amputation stump are presumably produced by the patient's own hairs.

How do these hairs make their way into the tissues? Brearley (1955) has suggested that the rolling movement which normally takes place between the contiguous surfaces of the buttocks at the natal cleft may result in hair still attached to the skin being twisted into a bundle which lies along the cleft and drills its way obliquely headwards through the skin (Fig. 156). Once the skin has been punctured, Brearley thinks that further penetration may be assisted by a suction mechanism, for, as he points out, separation of the buttocks in sitting or bending down renders taut the skin of the internal cleft and tends to lift off the underlying sacrococcygeal fascia with the creation of a negative pressure on the subcutaneous tissues. It is implied that eventually the hairs lose their attachment and become entirely free of the skin around the opening, thus allowing them to become completely or almost completely buried.

This theory of Brearley may explain some cases but is fairly clearly not the mechanism of entry of hair in the majority, for it would result in the hairs in the sinus always being placed with their root ends pointing caudally. According to Weale (1955) this is certainly not the usual finding, for generally the roots are directed headwards. This observation could be advanced as an argument for the congenital theory of origin of a pilonidal sinus, but Williams (1955) has offered an ingenious explanation as to how loose hairs from the surrounding skin could enter the tissues in this direction. He refers to the countryman's old trick of making a head of barley progress up someone's sleeve simply by introducing it base first, and points out that the scales of a hair are so arranged that their free ends point peripherally. As a result, if a hair is stroked from its root to the periphery there is little movement owing to the slight frictional resistance. If, however, it is stroked in the reverse direction there is considerable frictional resistance from the free ends of the scales and the hair is propelled in the direction of its root. These observations on the mechanics of the movement of hairs can be confirmed by placing a hair in the palm of the hand and rubbing to and fro along its axis with a finger of the other hand. It is interesting that in one case of pilonidal sinus of the umbilicus reported by Patey and Williams (1956)—where no doubt as to the acquired nature of the lesion arises—the hairs were placed with their root ends in the depths of the sinus.

The acquired theory fails to explain some aspects of the disease, for example: the occasional presence of hair follicles in the wall of the sinus; why the sinus itself usually points cranially; why it sometimes contains hairs that are much longer than any of those growing on the surrounding skin; and how a pilonidal sinus is produced, as it occasionally is, in almost hairless persons? But in general it seems to offer a more reasonable account of the aetiology of this condition than do any of the developmental theories. Having shared on three occasions Patey and Scarff's (1948) experience of recurrence of a pilonidal sinus in exactly similar form after a very thorough excision *by me personally in the first instance*, I am quite convinced that the acquired theory is the correct explanation of most recurrent lesions. There certainly seem to be plenty of loose hairs available in the perineal region between the buttocks, for, in patients who have developed a sinus in the perineal wound following abdominoperineal excision of the rectum, especially for colitis or

Crohn's disease, it is common in my experience to find quite a number of loose hairs in the track. I have no doubt that these hairs are often the factor responsible for preventing the healing of the sinus.

DIAGNOSIS

There is usually no difficulty about diagnosing a pilonidal sinus. As a rule the history of 'recurrent abscess at the base of the spine' is almost diagnostic in itself. The diagnosis is easily confirmed by observing the typical skin-lined sinus opening in the midline of the post-anal region, often with a secondary sinus opening higher up on one or other side. Difficulty in diagnosis may arise with very rare atypical cases, for example when the track runs caudally towards the anus and mimics an ordinary anal fistula, as it did in several patients seen by me and by Hughes (1961). The diagnostic feature in these cases was the finding of hairs in the sinus and the connection with a skin-lined opening in the midline of the post-anal region.

TREATMENT

The aetiology of the disease has been discussed at some length because it has an obvious bearing on treatment. *If the developmental conception of aetiology is accepted* and the existence of a skin-lined track with secondary infection is postulated, the essence of surgical treatment must be the complete excision of the track. *If the acquired theory is correct*, though it might still be argued that the best way to deal with the infected sinus is to excise it *in toto*, it has to be admitted that this step is no longer essential. Simple laying open of the fistula and removal of its contained hairs would seem to meet the theoretical requirements of surgery. But on this theory, whatever way the existing sinus has been treated surgically, the avoidance of recurrence depends on the prevention, if possible, of further drilling of the skin by hairs.

Complete Excision of the Sinus

Till 20 or 25 years ago this was the generally accepted mode of treatment and even now it is still the method favoured by very many surgeons. The actual excision is very simply performed; the difficulties arise in connection with the disposal of

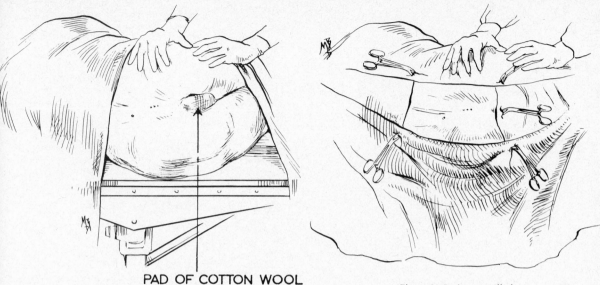

PAD OF COTTON WOOL

Fig. 157. Excision of pilonidal sinus: patient in left lateral position with the buttocks projecting beyond the edge of the table.

Fig. 158. Patient towelled.

the large resulting wound. Excision is best carried out when the lesion is in a quiescent phase. If there is an acutal abscess present with signs of acute inflammation in the surrounding tissues, the correct procedure in the first instance is to drain the abscess by a small incision. The actual excision can then be undertaken more satisfactorily two or three weeks later, when the inflammation has subsided.

Excision is most conveniently performed under a general anaesthetic. Some surgeons place the patient prone with the sacrococcygeal region elevated by pillows or angulation of the table. But I personally prefer the left lateral position with the buttocks projecting slightly beyond the edge of the table (Fig. 157). The skin is prepared by painting with iodine, chlorhexidine or some other skin antiseptic and a gauze swab or piece of wool soaked in alcoholic solution of chlorhexidine is placed over the anus to minimize the risk of contamination from this source during the operation. Towelling is then applied, care being taken to clip the mackintosh and towel covering the anal region and perineum to the skin immediately behind the anus as a further precaution against sepsis (Fig. 158). Lighting is best effected by a mobile light so placed that the light shines horizontally on the operation site. The assistant stands on the opposite side of the table and by firm traction with the fingers of both hands elevates the uppermost buttock, thus rendering the internal skin tense and more suitable for incision. As an immediate preliminary to operation some surgeons inject methylene blue or other dye into the sinus in order to stain all parts of the track, so that if it is inadvertently cut across at any point they will be made immediately aware of this fact. This technique may perhaps allow the excision to be carried out closer to the lesion and in a more selective manner than would otherwise be deemed advisable, but I personally have little experience of it and have preferred to keep well clear of the actual sinus and its ramifications when carrying out an excision.

The incision is an elliptical one so placed that it includes all sinus openings, and, if a secondary sinus lies unusually far laterally, the incision is extended to incorporate it either as a special offshoot or as an enlargement of the whole ellipse (Fig. 159). The incision is deepened at right angles to the skin through healthy fat to reach the fascia covering the coccyx and sacrum. Whilst traction is then applied to the isolated ellipse of skin and fat, it is separated from the fascia by scalpel or scissor dissection, commencing at the anal end and proceeding cranial-wards (Fig. 160). In the process numerous bleeding points are encountered close to the bone and are most easily dealt with by diathermy coagulation. True pilonidal sinuses invariably lie superficial to the coccyx and sacrum so that it is never necessary to remove any part of the bone in order to excise them.

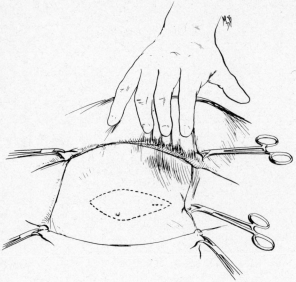

Fig. 159. Elliptical incision used for the operation.

The resulting wound is of considerable size and has steep shelving edges. It may be dealt with in several ways.

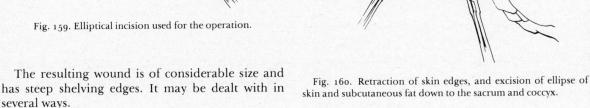

Fig. 160. Retraction of skin edges, and excision of ellipse of skin and subcutaneous fat down to the sacrum and coccyx.

1. PRIMARY SUTURE

This is perhaps the ideal to be aimed at, but there are often considerable difficulties in the way of accomplishing it. Whilst the skin edges can usually be brought together without too much tension, it is frequently difficult or impossible to secure firm apposition of the steep sides of the wound formed by the subcutaneous fat, particularly in the deeper parts adjacent to the coccyx and sacrum. If special care is not exercised, therefore, the result of primary suture may be to close the skin over a fairly large cavity which fills with blood or serum—the so-called 'tentage' effect. This state of affairs is incompatible with primary union and inevitably leads to sepsis or break-down of the wound. To avoid it, it is necessary to pass deep sutures through the whole thickness of the side walls of the wound on either side down to the bone. The actual suture technique used by me is as follows:

After careful haemostasis with diathermy and hot packs, a close series of deep sutures of strong braided silk (No. 16) or 5 kg braided nylon is inserted on large half circle or $\frac{5}{8}$ Hagedorn needles. These are passed at intervals of 2·5 cm from one another and 2 cm from the skin edge. Each stitch emerges in the wound at the junction of the fat with the fascia and peritoneum on the back of the coccyx and sacrum. It then takes a bite of this fascia roughly in the midline and is passed in the reverse direction from fat to skin through the opposite side wall (Fig. 161).

The ends of the deep sutures are clipped with forceps and left untied, whilst the actual skin edges and immediate subcutaneous fat are united by a close series of vertical mattress sutures of No. 4 serum proof silk, tied as they are inserted (Fig. 162). Finally when the skin wound has been completely closed a thick roll of gauze is applied and the deep sutures tied firmly over it, thus approximating the sides of the wound, not only to one another but to the back of the sacrum and coccyx (Fig. 163). Further gauze and wool are then placed over the anchored dressing and kept in position by several transverse strips of broad elastic strapping extending from one buttock to the other. Care is taken to see that the strips nearest to the anus make contact with the post-anal skin in the midline and so help to seal off the wound and dressing at this dangerous end. Finally a T-bandage is applied to reinforce the pressure of the strapping.

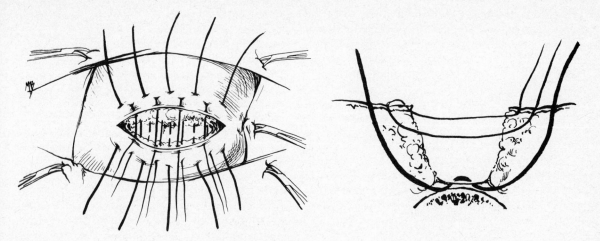

Fig. 161. Insertion of deep tension sutures of braided nylon down to the sacral fascia. (*Right*) Section showing arrangement of sutures.

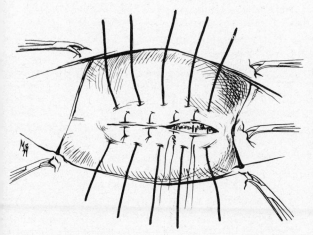

Fig. 162. Suture of skin edges with vertical mattress sutures of silk.

POSTOPERATIVE CARE

Strict bed rest is enjoined for nine to ten days after operation. The patient may be nursed partly on his back to exercise a gentle compression of the wound, but generally finds it more comfortable lying on one or other side. An effort is made to leave the bowels confined for six or seven days and during this time a low-residue diet is given. On the evening of the fifth or sixth day a retention enema of 225 ml of olive oil is given and the patient takes a dose of an aperient, such as three or four tablets of Senokot. The bowels move the following morning either spontaneously or with a soap and water enema.

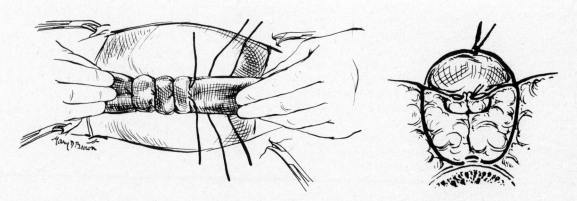

Fig. 163. Tying deep sutures over the anchor dressing. (*Right*) The effect of the suturing in obliterating the wound cavity.

The deep sutures are removed on the seventh day after operation for if left longer they generally cut into the tissues and may provoke some infection. The superficial sutures, however, are preferably retained till the tenth day. Sometimes pus may be seen escaping from one or more of the stitch holes before or after removal of the sutures. This may be relatively localized infection which may rapidly clear up on extraction of the stitch, assisted by suitable systemic antibiotic therapy. But it may indicate a more widespread condition necessitating re-opening of some or all of the wound and allowing it to heal by granulation. In certain cases a haematoma may form and similarly require that the sutures shall be cut and the wound laid open.

The advantages of primary suture, where it is successful, are immediately apparent. The entire period of hospitalization is reduced to 10–14 days at the most, and the patient is spared the necessity of frequent, sometimes painful, dressings during a long and tedious convalescence. But how often is suture successful? Different surgeons have given widely different answers to that question. Thus Ferguson and Mecray (1937), Bryne (1944), Bartlett (1945), and Holm and Hultén (1970) claimed some 90% of successes in their cases treated by primary suture. Gabriel (1948), on the other hand, had 12 failures in 25 consecutive patients so treated, the wounds becoming infected and having to be laid open subsequently to heal by second intention. My own experience with suture (36 cases with 17 failures) and that of most surgeons of my acquaintance corresponds closely with that of Gabriel. In fact these wounds have a notorious reputation for impaired healing after primary suture. As Gabriel (1948) rightly points out, the results of suture of these wounds depend to a considerable extent on the selection of cases for this method. Short thick-set males with tough inelastic tissues are generally unsuitable, as are very hairy individuals or those in whom the distribution of the sinus and secondary tracks has necessitated a particularly wide excision. The best results with suture are usually obtained in women with their more elastic tissues. Reserving primary closure for the specially favourable cases Gabriel (1963) has had a further series of 64 patients so treated with primary healing in 60. However, it is notable that in nearly two-thirds of his cases he prefers to leave the wounds open to heal by granulation.

It may be asked what harm results from attempting primary suture in all cases? If it fails the wound can simply be laid open with the loss of only a week or ten days and healing secured by second inten-

tion. That is certainly true of cases that are obvious failures. The trouble is that some cases are not so clearly unsuccessful in the first instance and there is a reluctance to dismiss them as complete failures. They show a little sepsis at two or three of the stitch punctures or at one point in the line of the incision, and this apparently subsides giving a false impression that sound healing has occurred. Within a few weeks, however, the patient returns with a further discharge and an obvious persistent sinus. Most writers fail to give any accurate figure of the *late* results in their cases, but Kooistra (1942), Block and Greene (1938) and Close (1955) state that some 20% of the cases recur subsequently, and this would accord roughly with my own observations. Though I have no careful follow-up report to offer, it is my impression that the late results are poorer when the wound has been successfully treated by primary suture than when it has been left open to granulate, and Rogers (1933) supports this contention. Gabriel's (1963) experience has been similar in that he had 4% of known recurrences in 89 cases treated by excision with primary suture, but only 2% in 147 cases treated by excision with subsequent granulation; these estimates were based on spontaneous re-attendances by patients and not on a special follow-up survey. However, Notaras (1970), in a 6–15-year follow-up of 43 patients treated by excision with primary suture, discovered five recurrences within the first year, and another four subsequently, which contrasted with no recurrences in the first postoperative year but four subsequently in 41 patients similarly followed up after excision and leaving the wound open to granulate. On the other hand, it must be noted that Holm and Hultén (1970), in their very careful and complete follow-up study of 48 patients with pilonidal sinuses treated by excision with primary suture, found recurrences in only 4%. They attribute their good results to the fact that the patients adopted a high standard of cleanliness in this region following operation.

2. CLOSURE BY PLASTIC PROCEDURES

The technical difficulties and uncertain results of simple suture of these wounds have induced several surgeons to devise plastic methods for achieving immediate closure. The simplest of these is that suggested by Lahey (1932) and Cattell (1934) of Boston, of relaxing tension on the sutures in the main elliptical wound by making a straight or angled relieving incision in the skin and fat of one buttock. The secondary wound is then closed by an advancement type of suture.

Another method is that of Davies and Starr (1945) of Sydney, and consists of rotating a flap of skin and subcutaneous tissue from the buttock into the defect, care being taken to make the width of the base of the flap at least half the length of its free edge. The secondary defect in the buttock can usually be closed by simple suture or a further small plastic procedure. Hirshowitz et al. (1970) have also used this technique with good results.

Pope and Hudson (1946) have described a more complicated method of closing pilonidal sinus wounds by mobilization of the gluteus maximus muscles to form sliding muscle grafts. In their experience primary union has followed this operation in 78 of 92 cases in which it was used.

Several other methods—for example Z-plasty (Monro and McDermott 1965; Middleton 1968)—have also been described, and the results claimed for them by their originators—as for the procedures outlined above—are generally excellent. The multiplicity of techniques, however, strongly suggests that these operations are neither simple to perform nor by any means invariably successful in their results. Furthermore they all suffer from the very serious disadvantage that, if breakdown should occur, secondary healing is then likely to take longer than if no attempt had been made to suture the wound at all. These considerations have dissuaded me from using any form of plastic closure after excision of a pilonidal sinus.

3. LEAVING THE WOUND OPEN TO GRANULATE

By this method, after haemostasis has been achieved, the wound is simply packed open with gauze soaked in 2·5% Milton, soft paraffin gauze or other dressing. The subsequent management is as for an ordinary fistula wound, with opening of the bowels on the third day, and thereafter the institution of baths morning and evening followed by wound irrigations and dressings. The usual pilonidal sinus wound treated by this open regimen takes up to eight or 10 weeks to heal completely, and hospitalization is usually necessary for the first four weeks of this time. The long period required for healing and the inconvenience of frequent dressings are the objections to this method. But it is far simpler and more reliable than any form of primary closure and, probably because of the broad hairless scar that it leaves in the post-anal region, is

TABLE 4. *Average Duration of Hospitalization, Wound Healing, and Unemployment after Three Methods of treating Pilonidal Sinuses*

Method	Period in hospital (days)	Time taken for wound to heal (days)	Period off work (weeks)
Excision with primary suture (43 patients)	16	12	6
Excision followed by granulation (41 patients)	26	70	8
Simple laying open (45 patients)	17	49	7

After Notaras (1970).

believed by some to be less liable to be followed by recurrence than is a successful primary suture, though this contention has been challenged by others (see p. 208). It is interesting that, in his comparative follow-up study of patients treated by excision with suture and by excision followed by granulation respectively, Notaras (1970) found that, though the average period in hospital was longer with the latter method, there was not much difference in the average period off work with the two methods—six and eight weeks respectively (Table 4).

THE USE OF A SILICONE FOAM SPONGE FOR PILONIDAL SINUS WOUNDS

Wood and Hughes (1975) have reported favourably on a method of using a sponge instead of ordinary gauze packing for the granulating wounds resulting from excision (or simple laying open) of pilonidal sinuses. The sponge is first introduced as a rule about four days after the operation, and most patients find it very comfortable and convenient. For details see p. 90.

4. THIERSCH GRAFTING OF THE OPEN WOUND

This may be performed as a primary procedure or carried out secondarily once granulations have filled the wound cavity. In primary grafting the sheets of skin are sutured in position as described for ordinary fistulae on p. 82, or inserted on a Stent mould which is likewise fixed by suture. I have not used primary grafting myself because I have been unhappy about the deep skin-covered depression which it would leave in the sacro-coccygeal region. To overcome this objection the application of the grafts may be postponed till the wound has filled with granulations, say after three or four weeks. Unfortunately grafts 'take' much less readily on granulation tissue than on fresh raw surfaces, and the percentage of completely successful results, or even partial 'takes', is very much lower than with primary grafting. A practical difficulty with grafting at this stage, moreover, is that by then the patient is mobile, is on a normal diet and has become accustomed to the routine of a daily motion and twice daily baths and dressings. He is therefore rather unwilling to accept strict bed-rest, a reduced diet and the discomforts of constipation for five or six days, in order that grafting may be carried out, and his displeasure is much augmented if, after all, the grafts fail to take.

Simple Incision of the Sinus

This operation, based on the theory of acquired aetiology, treats a pilonidal sinus like any other fistula in the anal region. It is performed with the patient in the left lateral position. A fistula director or probe is passed into the primary opening and made to emerge through any secondary fistulous opening, or is brought out through the skin at the posterior extremity of the track which, if it is blind, is opened to make a small snick in the skin. The skin between the two openings is then incised on to the director, and the track and cavity are laid widely open. Any hairs contained in the sinus are removed and the wall of the cavity scraped free of granulations with a Volkmann's sharp spoon. Occasionally other pockets and subsidiary tracks require to be explored further with the probe and laid open by additional incisions proceeding from the main wound. It may be advisable sometimes to trim the skin edges slightly to encourage the wound to remain widely open, but more usually no actual excision of skin is necessary. The cavity, which is relatively small and superficial as a rule, is packed with gauze soaked in Milton, and the after-care is as for any other fistula wound in the anal region. A silicone foam sponge may be used instead of gauze packing, as explained on pp. 90 and 209.

It should be emphasized that there is a considerable difference between the open wound resulting from simple incision of a pilonidal sinus and that left by complete excision of such a lesion. The former does not go nearly so deeply as a rule and there is almost always a substantial layer of fat between its floor and the coccyx and sacrum. It is also much narrower and on coronal section would be concave rather than rectangular in shape. The result is that it heals with much greater rapidity. Within 10–14 days of the operation it has filled with granulations almost to the surface, and after the first five to seven days the patient can be allowed home and the dressing of his wound entrusted to a district nurse or reliable relative. However, regular supervision by the surgeon on an out-patient basis is essential, with particular reference to bridging and the growth of hair in the post-anal skin; it is important to keep the area well shaved. Frankly I have been disappointed at how long it often takes these relatively small wounds to achieve complete healing with full epithelialization. Notaras (1970) too, though favouring this method, finds that it takes, on average, seven weeks for the wounds to heal and the patients are usually off work for this period of time (see Table 4). He also noted six recurrences in 45 patients, all after the post-operative year.

Marsupialization of Pilonidal Sinus

In some cases where a strong fibrous layer is present in the wall of the sinus, the operation of simple incision may be completed by the method of marsupialization introduced by Buie (1937). In this technique the edge of the skin wound is sutured all round to the margin of the opened up wall of the sinus with a series of interrupted fine chromic catgut or silk sutures (Fig. 164). This covers over the exposed subcutaneous fat and reduces the total raw area. Provided that separation does not occur subsequently, as sometimes happens, the healing time is reduced. I find that this method is practicable in about half the cases of pilonidal sinus under my care, but in the remainder the wall of the sinus is too insubstantial and friable to hold the sutures. Good accounts of the application and achievements of marsupialization are given by Marks (1947), Watters and Macdonald (1958), and Abramson (1960). As for latter results, Abramson (1960) reported recurrence in 6·9% of 159 patients followed up for one to eight years, and Goodall (1962) had a recurrence rate of 7·7% in 15 cases traced for (mostly) one to three years.

Primary Suture or Immediate Skin Grafting

These are alternative methods of dealing with the wound that results after simple incision and curettage, but I have little experience of either.

More Conservative Operative Measures

TREATMENT BY INJECTION OF PHENOL

Maurice and Greenwood (1964) have described a method of treating pilonidal sinuses by injecting

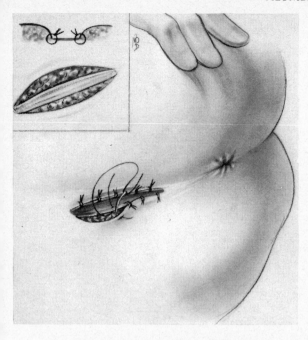

Fig. 164. Technique of marsupialization of a pilonidal sinus after simple incision. The edges of the skin wound are sutured all round to the margin of the opened up fibrous wall of the sinus, thus covering over the exposed subcutaneous fat. *Inset:* The state of affairs before the suturing is commenced, and a diagram to show the effect of the marsupialization in reducing the size of the raw area.

skin. The phenol is left in situ for about a minute; the needle is then withdrawn and the fluid together with the loose hair and debris is expelled by pressure over the track. This injection–expression sequence is repeated until the total period of contact of the tissues with phenol is approximately three minutes, after which the fluid is finally expressed. The orifice of the sinus is usually blanched by the phenol, but, if this has not occurred, the area of skin surrounding the opening is touched with phenol to destroy the epithelium. A light dressing of petroleum jelly gauze is then applied and covered with some dry gauze and wool. The patient requires to be in hospital for only 24–36 hours after this treatment and can resume work almost immediately. The area is frequently uncomfortable and discharges a little serous fluid for a few days or so before eventual healing occurs, which takes from three to over six weeks.

Maurice and Greenwood (1964) have treated 21 patients by this method, including a number who had had previous attacks of infection or previous operation. They have all been followed up for at least 18 months: 17 secured complete healing which has persisted; four developed abscesses or continued to discharge, so that operative treatment was required. Clearly further studies with longer follow-up periods will be necessary to evaluate this method properly, but these experiences are promising.

them with phenol to destroy the epithelium of the track and sterilize the cavity in the hope that after extrusion of the hairs the sinus would heal. A short general anaesthetic is required. They prefer to have the patient in the prone jack-knife position with the sacrum horizontal. The skin has previously been shaved, with particular reference to the natal cleft. It is now cleansed with spirit and the area is towelled off, a pad of cotton-wool being placed over the anus. An area of skin, approximately 15 cm in radius, around the sinus is generously smeared with petroleum jelly to protect it from inadvertent overflow of phenol.

The main sinus and its sidetracks are gently probed, particular care being taken that no new tissue planes are opened up, and a blunt-nosed coned needle (such as is employed for injecting into the ureteric catheter in retrograde pyelography) is inserted firmly into the orifice of the main track, its shape securing for it a very snug fit. Pure phenol is then injected slowly without pressure until the fluid is seen to issue from all the side openings. Excess is immediately wiped away from the surrounding

LIMITED EXCISION OF MIDLINE SINUS OPENINGS UNDER LOCAL ANAESTHESIA

Lord and Millar (1965) advocated treatment of pilonidal sinuses by a relatively limited operation which could be practised under local anaesthesia in the out-patient department. It consisted of excising the midline sinus openings to a depth of 0·5 cm only and then picking out hairs from the underlying cavity and from any lateral tracks by means of a tiny bottle brush with nylon bristles as used for cleaning electric razors. No attempt is made to pack the sinus cavity and reliance in after-care is placed on frequent baths and the application of a simple external dressing. It is also considered most important to keep the part shaved and to have the patient attend regularly at a special dressing clinic for periodic review.

In a five-year survey of 102 patients who have been treated by this method Edwards (1977) found recurrence in only 11% of those who had been diligent in their attendance at the dressing clinic, but in 43% of patients who failed to attend regularly.

The Prevention of Further Drilling of the Skin by Hairs

This would seem to be an essential additional requirement of treatment on the hypothesis of acquired aetiology. An obvious way of attempting to prevent further drilling would be to produce depilation of the post-anal skin *by postoperative irradiation*, as practised by Smith (1937), Turell (1940), Carvalho (1945) and Mathesheimer (1945). I am informed by radiotherapists and dermatologists, however, that such treatment, even if dangerously large doses are used, only produces a temporary arrest of the growth of hair lasting not more than six to 12 months. To be permanently successful therefore X-ray treatment would have to be repeated at intervals, but this would introduce a very serious risk of skin necrosis or even malignant change, and on this account no radiologist would ever countenance repetition of the irradiation. Because of these defects in the method I have not employed X-ray depilation in my cases.

The use of depilatory creams is another obvious method to be considered. Though various proprietary preparations for removal of superfluous hair are on the market, these are in fact notoriously unreliable in their results, as is shown by the fact that they have not succeeded in displacing the razor and other methods from feminine beauty culture. I have used some of these creams postoperatively on patients after pilonidal sinus operations with disappointing results as regards control of the growth of hair.

Electrolysis, as used for the removal of superfluous facial hairs, may also be employed, but has in fact seldom been applied in this situation.

Shaving if repeated frequently enough could presumably avoid the risk of further drilling by hairs. Its disadvantage is that the patient cannot shave himself and has to depend on some other member of his family to do it for him. Patients who can afford it may find it a convenience to have an electric razor specially for this purpose.

Simple scrubbing of the post-anal and internatal skin, if carried out daily and vigorously, ought also to be an effective method of preventing further drilling. It has the advantage that the patient can do it himself, and for that reason it is the method which I now recommend to my patients after surgical treatment of their pilonidal sinuses. Only if

he is exceptionally hairy is a patient also advised to shave the part occasionally, at any rate during the first few weeks after operation till the scar becomes tougher.

Author's Preference in Treatment

Due to the advocacy of Patey and his colleagues, which has been clearly summarized by him (Patey 1969), the method of simple laying open of pilonidal sinuses has become that most favoured in Britain at the present time. I personally have followed this trend, but I must admit that when I read of the excellent results obtained by Holm and Hultén (1970) and Lamke et al. (1974) with excision and primary suture, the vast majority of whose patients secured healing *per primam*, I cannot help feeling that this approximates more to the ideal. Unfortunately, in my hands primary closure is far less satisfactory and, under the circumstances, simple laying open is a very convenient and more reliable alternative. As in many other controversies regarding the choice of surgical treatment, I believe there is an urgent need for carefully controlled prospective comparative studies of the accomplishments of the different methods of treating pilonidal sinus, the patients being randomly allocated to the various techniques of treatment, all in the same centre or centres, and all assessed subsequently by the same group of observers, as we have done in comparative operations for duodenal ulcer (Goligher et al. 1968). I have no personal experience of the operative methods of Maurice and Greenwood (1964) or Lord and Millar (1965).

RARER FORMS OF SINUS WITH AN EPITHELIAL LINING IN THE ANAL REGION

Apart from the common post-anal pilonidal sinus just described several other varieties of sinus with an epithelial lining are occasionally encountered in the anal, perineal or sacrococcygeal regions.

ATYPICALLY PLACED PILONIDAL SINUS

Rarely sinuses with an epithelial-lined orifice and containing hairs occur in front of the anus, directed towards the perineum, or lateral to it and extending sometimes on to the buttock or the thigh (Smith 1948). Penetration of the skin by hair is presumably the initiating factor here and the treatment required is a thorough laying open of the sinus and any subsidiary tracks and, postoperatively, steps to control further drilling by hair.

CONGENITAL FISTULAE IN THE ANAL CANAL

Gabriel (1948) has described several cases of low anal fistulae with an internal opening in the skin-lined part of the anal canal, and with either a short straight track or a subcutaneous horseshoe track, which on laying open was found to be lined throughout with squamous epithelium. He has suggested that these fistulae were due to remnants of epithelial cells displaced during development from the junction of the ectodermal proctodeum and entodermal postallantoic gut into the anal and perianal tissues, but it is probable that these fistulae are simply atypically placed pilonidal sinus as described above.

EPITHELIALIZATION OF AN ORDINARY FISTULA-IN-ANO

It is well known that in very long-standing cases of anal fistula squamous epithelium may exceptionally rarely grow into the track from the skin so as to give it a partial covering. Usually this is a very incomplete process confined to the immediate vicinity of the external opening unless the fistula is a very short superficial one, when it may acquire a complete epithelial lining by this process. I have seen at least a dozen such epithelized subcutaneous fistulae, several of these being in patients who suffered originally from ulcerative colitis which completely subsided on a medical regimen.

DEVELOPMENTAL POST-ANAL SKIN DIMPLES IN CHILDREN

These have been well described by Haworth and Zachary (1955) and have already been referred to on p. 203. They are simply exaggerated dimples of the skin overlying the tip of the coccyx to which they are attached by a fibrous band. They are lined by normal skin and in childhood are free from hairs, but presumably will grow hairs later. If at all deep it might be a good plan to excise them as a prophylactic measure against septic complications, otherwise they would be better left undisturbed unless such complications occurred.

CONGENITAL FISTULAE ARISING FROM REMNANTS OF THE MEDULLARY CANAL

These have also been mentioned on p. 203. Here a communication exists through a spina bifida between the caudal end of the central canal of the spinal cord and the skin of the upper sacral region. The fistula is present at birth and discharges cerebrospinal fluid, so that infection and meningitis are practically inevitable if the fistula is not closed by operation. Haworth and Zachary (1955) report cases in which they dissected out the track to its communication with the dura and closed it, with a successful outcome.

INFECTED SACROCOCCYGEAL TERATOMATA AND DERMOID CYSTS

Sacrococcygeal teratomata or dermoid cysts, which are very liable to become secondarily infected, may cause post-anal abscesses and fistulae. These lesions are considered on p. 686.

REFERENCES

ABRAMSON, D. J. (1960) A simple marsupialization technic for treatment of pilonidal sinus: long-term follow up. *Ann. Surg., 151*, 261.
AIRD, I. (1952) Pilonidal sinus of the axilla. *Br. med. J., 1*, 902.
ANDERSON, A. W. (1847) Hair extracted from an ulcer. *Boston med. surg. J., 36*, 74.
BARTLETT, W., Jr. (1945) Pilonidal cyst and sinus; their management and operative treatment. *Surgery Gynec. Obstet., 80*, 69.
BLAND-SUTTON, SIR J. (1922) *Tumours Innocent and Malignant*, 7th ed. London: Cassell.
BLOCK, L. H. and GREENE, B. L. (1938) Pilonidal sinus; sclerosing method of treatment. *Archs Surg., Chicago, 37*, 112.
BREARLEY, R. (1955) Pilonidal sinus; a new theory of origin. *Br. J. Surg., 43*, 62.
BUIE, L. (1937) *Practical Proctology*. Philadelphia: Saunders.
BRYNE, R. V. (1944) Pilonidal cyst. *Nav. med. Bull., 42*, 386.
CARVALHO, N. (1945) *Revta Cirurg. S Paolo, 10*, 251.
CATTELL, R. B. (1934) Technic of operation for pilonidal sinus. *Surg. Clins N. Am., 14*, 1289.
CLOSE, A. S. (1955) Pilonidal cysts: an analysis of surgical failures. *Ann. Surg., 141*, 523.
CROSBY, D. L. (1962) Pilonidal sinus of suprapubic region. *Br. J. Surg., 49*, 457.
CURRIE, A. R., GIBSON, T. and GOODALL, A. L. (1953) Interdigital sinuses of barbers' hands. *Br. J. Surg., 41*, 278.
DAVIES, L. S. and STARR, K. W. (1945) Infected pilonidal sinus. *Surgery Gynec. Obstet., 81*, 309.
EDWARDS, M. H. (1977) Pilonidal sinus: a 5-year appraisal of the Millar-Lord operation. *Br. J. Surg., 64*, 867.
EWING, M. R. (1947) Hair-bearing sinus. *Lancet, 1*, 427.
FERGUSON, L. K. and MECRAY, P. M., Jr. (1937) Pilonidal cysts: excision and primary suture in ambulatory patients. *Am. J. Surg., 36*, 270.
FOX, S. L. (1935) The origin of pilonidal sinus, with an analysis of its comparative anatomy and histogenesis. *Surgery Gynec. Obstet., 60*, 137.
GABRIEL, W. B. (1948) *Principles and Practice of Rectal Surgery*, 4th ed. London: H. K. Lewis.
—— (1963) *Principles and Practice of Rectal Surgery*, 5th ed. London: H. K. Lewis.
GAGE, M. (1935) Pilonidal sinus: an explanation of its embryologic development. *Archs Surg., Chicago, 31*, 175.
GILLIS, L. (1954) Infected traumatic epidermoid cysts, the result of rubbing by an artificial limb. *Proc. R. Soc. Med., 47*, 9.
GOLIGHER, J. C., PULVERTAFT, C. N. and DE DOMBAL, F. T. (1968) Clinical comparison of vagotomy and pyloroplasty with other forms of elective surgery for duodenal ulcer. *Br. med. J., 2*, 787.
GOODALL, P. (1961) The aetiology and treatment of pilonidal sinus: a review of 163 patients. *Br. J. Surg., 49*, 212.
HAWORTH, J. C. and ZACHARY, R. B. (1955) Congenital dermal sinuses in children; their relation to pilonidal sinuses. *Lancet, 2*, 10.
HIRSHOWITZ, B., MAHLER, D. and KAUFMANN-FRIEDMANN, K. (1970) Treatment of pilonidal sinus. *Surgery Gynec. Obstet., 131*, 119.
HODGES, R. M. (1880) Pilonidal sinus. *Boston med. surg. J., 103*, 485.

HOLM, J. and HULTÉN, L. (1970) Simple primary closure for pilonidal sinus. *Acta chir. scand., 136*, 537.

HUGHES, E. S. R. (1961) Personal communication.

KING, E. S. J. (1949) Interdigital pilonidal sinus. *Aust. N. Z. J. Surg., 19*, 29.

KOOISTRA, H. P. (1942) Pilonidal sinuses: review of the literature and report of three hundred and fifty cases. *Am. J. Surg., 55*, 3.

LAHEY, F. H. (1932) A further suggestion for operative treatment of pilonidal sinuses. *Surgery Gynec. Obstet., 54*, 521.

LAMKE, L. O., LARSSON, J. and NYLÉN, B. (1974) Results of different types of operation for pilonidal sinus. *Acta chir. scand., 140*, 321.

LORD, P. H. and MILLAR, D. M. (1965) Pilonidal sinus: a simple treatment. *Br. J. Surg., 52*, 298.

MACLEOD, R. G. (1953) Pilonidal sinus of the suprapubic region. *Br. med. J., 1*, 710.

MALLORY, F. B. (1892) Sacrococcygeal dimples, sinuses and cysts. *Am. J. med. Sci., 103*, 263.

MARKS, M. M. (1947) Pilonidal sinus: treatment by eventration; report of 618 cases. *Sth. med. J., 40*, 844.

MATHESHEIMER, J. L. (1945) An ambulant method for the treatment of pilonidal disease: a preliminary report. *Am. J. Surg., 69*, 230.

MATT, J. G. (1958) Carcinomatous degeneration of pilonidal cysts. *Dis. Colon Rect., 1*, 353.

MAURICE, B. A. and GREENWOOD, R. K. (1964) A conservative treatment of pilonidal sinus. *Br. J. Surg., 51*, 510.

MIDDLETON, M. D. (1968) Treatment of pilonidal sinus by Z-plasty. *Br. J. Surg., 55*, 516

MONRO, R. S. and McDERMOTT, F. T. (1965) The elimination of causal factors in pilonidal sinus treated by Z-plasty. *Br. J. Surg., 52*, 177.

NEWELL, R. L. (1933) Coccygeal sinus. *Br. J. Surg., 21*, 219.

NOTARAS, M. J. (1970) A review of three popular methods of treatment of postnatal (pilonidal) sinus disease. *Br. J. Surg., 57*, 886.

OLDFIELD, M. C. (1956) A barber's interdigital pilonidal sinus. *Lancet, 2*, 1244.

PATEY, D. H. (1969) A reappraisal of the acquired theory of sacrococcygeal pilonidal sinus and an assessment of its influence on surgical practice. *Br. J. Surg., 56*, 463.

—— and CURRY, R. C. (1962) Pilonidal sinus presenting in the suprapubic region of a woman. *Lancet, 1*, 620.

—— and SCARFF, R. W. (1946) Pathology of postanal pilonidal sinus: its bearing on treatment. *Lancet, 2*, 484.

—— —— (1948) Pilonidal sinus in a barber's hand; with observations on post-anal pilonidal sinus. *Lancet, 2*, 13.

—— —— (1955) Pilonidal sinus. *Lancet, 1*, 772.

—— and WILLIAMS, E. S. (1956) Pilonidal sinus of the umbilicus. *Lancet, 2*, 281.

POPE, C. E. and HUDSON, H. W. (1946) Pilonidal sinus: a review of 130 consecutive cases in which patients were treated by closure; a new closed operative method and management. *Archs Surg., Chicago, 52*, 690.

ROGERS, H. (1933). Pilonidal sinus. *Surgery Gynec. Obstet., 57*, 803.

SHEEHAN, H. (1953) Quoted by Brearley, R. (1955).

SHOESMITH, J. H. (1953) Pilonidal sinus in an above-knee amputation stump. *Lancet, 2*, 378.

SMITH, R. M. (1937) Roentgen irradiation as an adjunct to surgical treatment of pilonidal cyst. *Am. J. Roentgen., 38*, 208.

SMITH, T. E. (1948) Anterior or perineal pilonidal cysts. *J. Am. med. Ass., 136*, 973.

SPENCER, J. A. (1967) Unpublished work.

STONE, H. B. (1924) Pilonidal sinus (coccygeal fistula). *Ann. Surg., 79*, 410.

—— (1931) The origin of pilonidal sinus. *Ann. Surg., 94*, 317.

TURELL, R. (1940) Radiation therapy for recurrent sacrococcygeal cysts and sinuses, *Surgery, St Louis, 8*, 469.

WARREN, J. M. (1854) Abscess, containing hair, on the nates. *Am. J. med. Sci., 28*, 113.

WATTERS, N. and MACDONALD, I. B. (1958) Marsupialization of pilonidal sinus and abscess: a report of 50 cases. *J. Can. med. Ass., 79*, 236.

WEALE, F. E. (1955) The hair of the pilonidal sinus. *Lancet, 1*, 230.

—— (1964) A comparison of barber's and postanal pilonidal sinuses. *Br. J. Surg., 51*, 513.

WILLIAMS, E. S. (1955) Quoted by Patey, D. H. and Scarff, R. W. (1955).

WOOD, R. A. B. and HUGHES, L. E. (1975) Silicone foam sponge for pilonidal sinus: a new technique for dressing open granulating wounds. *Br. med. J., 3*, 131.

9

Pruritus Ani

This condition of intense itching of the anal region is one of the commonest complaints encountered in the practice of rectal surgery, and, as regards understanding of its causation and treatment, unquestionably one of the least satisfactory. It is more frequent in men than women, and is rarely seen in childhood. It may be the patient's only complaint, or it may occur in conjunction with some other anorectal condition.

CLINICAL FEATURES

Pruritus may begin as a sensation of uneasiness or slight itching, often confined to one aspect of the anus. In time, however, the itching becomes more severe and usually spreads to the entire perianal skin, possibly extending on to the vulva or back of the scrotum as well, but it often continues to be experienced maximally at the anal verge and along the median raphe in front of and behind the anus. In many cases the itching is felt only or mainly at night and it would seem as if the warmth of the bed in some way acts as an exciting cause. A smaller proportion of patients suffer chiefly during the day, and various factors have been incriminated by different patients for precipitating their attacks of pruritus—mental strain, anxiety, overwork; certain items of food and drink such as strawberries, shellfish, coffee, several forms of alcohol; or a change of climate. Most patients agree that their pruritus is worse in summer weather than in winter, presumably due to the greater amount of sweating which increases anal moisture.

In the established case of severe pruritus the itching becomes well nigh intolerable. It has a tormenting, tantalizing, distracting character so that by comparison with it actual pain is almost a pleasure. The patient scratches himself incessantly during the more severe phases to try to stop the itching, but the relief obtained is only very temporary. After the condition has been present for some time he may be reduced to a state of complete nervous exhaustion due to the irritation and indignity of the complaint during the day and, even more so, to the constant interference with sleep at night. For many patients with severe pruritus ani life is rendered utterly miserable, and indeed some of them are brought to the brink of suicide.

EXAMINATION

Pruritus may present a variety of clinical appearances on inspection of the anal region. At one extreme there may be no evident changes at all in the anal and perianal skin, and yet the patient may suffer from quite severe itching. At the other extreme the skin around the anus may be raw, red and oozing and may make one feel uncomfortable even to look at it. More usually the significant abnormality is that the perianal skin is thickened and there is considerable exaggeration of the normal radiating creases and folds, which may be developed into anal skin tags. The actual skin surface is also altered and has a sodden dead-white appearance which is highly characteristic of pruritus ani. In addition there may be numerous excoriations of the epidermis due to scratching, and the skin often shows many radiating cracks and linear ulcers which tend to split even more when the buttocks are separated.

In all cases a complete rectal examination should be carried out; it will frequently reveal the existence of other anorectal abnormalities which may have a bearing on the pruritus or may be entirely co-incidental.

AETIOLOGY AND CLINICAL TYPES

Allingham and Allingham (1901), Tuttle (1903), Lockhart-Mummery (1934), Gabriel (1948) and most other authors recommend that pruritus ani should be regarded not as a disease but merely as a symptom, like headache or diarrhoea, and they claim that a cause, if carefully sought, will usually be found. I agree that pruritus is probably often secondary to some other condition, but in my experience in less than half the cases it is possible to find a primary cause to which the pruritus may conscientiously be attributed. There are thus many instances where the condition appears to be idiopathic. The aetiology may be conveniently considered under the headings of *secondary* and *idiopathic* pruritus respectively, though in practice this clear line of distinction is not always so easily drawn.

Secondary Pruritus

Condition to which pruritus ani is commonly secondary are the following:

LOCAL ANORECTAL LESIONS

Any disease of the anus, rectum, colon or even the upper intestinal tract that leads to excessive moisture in the anal region is liable to cause pruritus ani. Some of the more important lesions in this respect are anal fistula or fissure, anal papillomata or condylomata, all of which tend to produce a discharge resulting in a sodden perianal skin; prolapsing internal haemorrhoids, complete or partial prolapse of the rectum, and anal incontinence due to a badly executed fistula operation or to a Whitehead's haemorrhoidectomy, which all tend to cause a mucoid leak; diarrhoea and discharge of liquid faeces or mucus due to carcinoma or benign tumours of the rectum or colon, or to colitis or other causes, which may cause soreness and irritation of the perianal skin, as may leakage of liquid paraffin through the anus when taken in excessive dosage in the treatment of constipation. The role of anal skin tags and hyper-trophied anal papillae in the production of pruritus is much more debatable. In most instances skin tags are secondary to the pruritus and not its cause. Wallis (1911) believed that hypertrophied anal papillae played an important part in the aetiology of pruritus ani. A specially large papilla that projects at the anus might conceivably interfere with proper anal closure and thus predispose to leakage of mucus which could lead to pruritus. But with only moderately enlarged papillae it is hard to believe that there can be any causal relationship to prutitus.

LACK OF ANAL CLEANLINESS

In individuals of untidy personal habits faecal staining of the perianal skin or matting of the peri-anal hairs with inspissated faeces are often found and this lack of cleanliness sometimes seems to predispose to pruritus.

EXCESSIVE SWEATING

In men engaged in heavy manual labour excessive sweating, especially in hot weather, appears to be a factor causing pruritus ani by producing increased moisture of the anal skin. In this type of patient the condition is often aggravated by the wearing of thick woollen underpants of a rough kind.

PARASITIC INFECTIONS

Threadworms
Threadworms are a well recognized cause of pruritus ani and may occur not only in children but also in adults. The pruritus is produced by the wriggling movements of the worms in the lower part of the anal canal and at the anal orifice. The diagnosis of threadworms in such a case is usually made by noting the worms at the anus on simple inspection or in the anal canal or lower rectum on proctoscopy. The parasite is white in colour, about 6 mm long and of roughly the same thickness as a piece of cotton thread. Any doubt as to its animate nature when seen during examination is settled by noting its rapid movements. In cases where thread-worms are suspected but no evidence of them can be obtained on routine rectal examination a diagnostic enema of 115 ml of normal saline may be given at a time when the pruritus is severe, usually best in the evening. The enema is retained for five to

ten minutes if possible, and then passed into a clean chamber pot and inspected, preferably after being transferred to a black vulcanite photographic dish, which facilitates the detection of the white parasites. A negative result to be significant should be repeated two or three times.

Pediculosis Pubis

In some patients with pediculosis pubis the parasites may extend anal-wards and set up pruritus ani. The condition is readily recognized by noting the nits and the parasites themselves in the anal region, as well as in their usual site in the pubic hairs and skin.

Scabies

In cases of scabies the anal region may be affected causing pruritus ani which brings the patient to hospital. The diagnosis is established by noting the characteristic lesions elsewhere in the body, notably between the fingers and on the front of the wrists.

MYCOTIC DISEASE OF THE ANAL SKIN

Infection of the skin of the anal region with fungi (*Epidermophyton* or *Trichophyton*) or yeasts (*Candida albicans*) may produce pruritus ani. In its clinical appearances this pruritus may be indistinguishable from other types, but sometimes it differs in showing some definite cutaneous abnormality such as vesiculation or pustule formation, desquamation, moist or dry. A fungus infection is particularly to be suspected in cases where the skin lesion has *a well-defined border to its lateral extent*, and this suspicion is strengthened by finding evidence of a similar infestation of the skin between the toes, especially the fourth and fifth, with resulting desquamation and maceration, or by noting the presence of a tinea cruris or eliciting a history of this condition in the past. Obviously the toes and groins should always be carefully inspected in cases of pruritus in which a mycotic aetiology is suspected.

Proof of a mycotic aetiology may be sought by microscopical examination or culture of a scraping from the affected skin. The material is mixed with a little 10% potash on a slide, and gently warmed for a few minutes. A cover glass is then laid on and air bubbles eliminated by pressure. *Candida* appears as a series of refractile, double-countered, rounded bodies tending to grow in chains. *Epidermophyton*, on the other hand, grows as a delicate branching mycelium. There are also cultural differences.

My experience is that fungus infection in the anal region is rare, but that candidal infestation is more common. However, *Candida* is often a secondary invader on any moist excoriated skin so that it may well not be the primary cause in many of these pruritic cases.

It is also important to remember that it is predisposed to by topical steroid therapy applied to the perianal region (Winner and Hurley 1964).

BACTERIAL CAUSE

Erythrasma, which is due to *Corynebacterium minutissimum*, has been described as a cause of pruritus ani, particularly in chronic cases (Bowyer and McColl 1966). The diagnosis is made with the aid of an ultra-violet lamp which gives a very characteristic perianal fluorescence. The skin in other intertriginous areas (e.g. interdigital cleft, groin, umbilicus) may also be infected and should be tested by inspection under ultra-violet light.

GYNAECOLOGICAL CAUSES

In women pruritus vulvae may extend backwards to involve the anal skin and it is common to find a vaginal discharge or urinary incontinence as the responsible factor. Apart from these local causes pruritus of the anus or vulva is frequently encountered in women at the time of the menopause.

ANTIBIOTICS

It should be remembered that certain antibiotics, notably tetracyclines, taken by mouth are a potent cause of pruritus ani, partly by facilitating the development of a candidal infection in the perianal region.

Idiopathic Pruritus

In these cases, where no obvious cause is present, the aetiology of the pruritus is naturally obscure. Several more or less fanciful theories have been advanced to account for it but no really satisfying explanation has yet been provided. Certain American writers such as Tucker and Hellwig (1937), Bacon and Hardwick (1947) and Granet (1954) have claimed that the pruritus in these cases is due to irritation of the perianal skin by faecal contamination even when no gross soiling is evident. Numerous chemicals are present in the faeces which might conceivably irritate the skin. Among these are bacteria and their exotoxins, intestinal enzymes, and also the end-results of bacterial action on ingested proteins—the indoles and skatole. According to Granet (1954), in a number of patients with severe pruritus ani, solutions of indole, or skatole or faecal emulsions applied as patch tests in the axillary region (which closely approximates to the perianal region in its physical characteristics) produced a dermatitis. I suspect that the same experiment in non-pruritic patients might also cause an axillary dermatitis. To Bacon and Hardwick (1947) the irritating feature of the rectal contents in regard to the perianal skin is their strong alkalinity, which is apparently especially marked in cases of pruritus.

Frankfeldt (1948) has claimed that pruritus ani is often an allergic phenomenon due to sensitivity to items of diet or other allergies. It may occur in association with other allergic manifestations such as asthma or urticaria or may be the only manifestation of the condition. This may possibly explain an occasional case of pruritus ani, but in my experience is certainly not applicable to the majority of cases of idiopathic pruritus.

As with many other skin lesions for which no obvious organic cause can be discovered, the possibility of psychogenesis has to be considered. Many patients with severe idiopathic pruritus find that their attacks are more liable to occur at times of stress and tension. The anal skin is also one of the erotic areas of the body and it is claimed by Saul (1938), Drueck (1943), Rosenbaum (1945) and Granet (1954) that in some patients the sensation of itching with its resulting scratching arouses pleasurable sensations amounting even to sexual orgasm. They are thus reluctant to give up the symptom of intractable itching with its pleasure–pain component and retain it despite all local treatment.

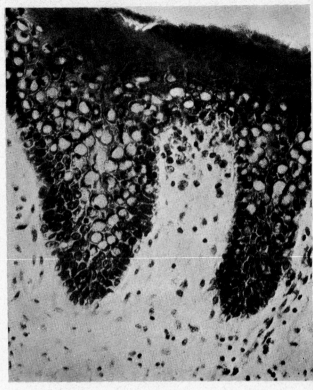

Fig. 165. Histological section of perianal skin in chronic pruritus ani, showing marked hydrops of the cells of the Malpighian layer. (*From Tucker and Hellwig 1937*)

mucosum and of the hair follicles, hyperkeratosis with plugging of the hair follicles and atrophy of the sebaceous glands (Fig. 165). In addition there is often oedema of the dermis itself and dilatation of the superficial blood vessels and lymphatics. The cutaneous nerves, however, invariably appear normal. Cocci are sometimes found beneath ulcerated areas but not underlying intact skin.

TREATMENT

As we are totally ignorant of the cause of pruritus ani in most cases it is not surprising that treatment should frequently be ineffective and disappointing. The result is that these patients often re-attend on many occasions showing little or no improvement. Indeed a rectal clinic is apt to be haunted by its pruritic patients in much the same way that an orthopaedic clinic is by its cases of low back pain! In the long run the surgeon's fund of sympathy is often drained dry and the patient is relegated to

PATHOLOGY

The histological appearances of the affected skin in cases of pruritus ani have been studied particularly by Montgomery (1931), Riddoch (1937) and Tucker and Hellwig (1937). It is clear from their accounts that the histological changes are in no way specific but resemble closely those observed in cases of chemical dermatitis. There is hydrops of the cells of the epidermis, irregular proliferation of the stratum

progressively lower strata of surgical care at subsequent visits.

Obviously if a clear cause can be found for the pruritus and effectively dealt with the outlook is much improved. But not infrequently if the pruritic condition has been present for a long time it may persist in modified form even after the initial cause has been eliminated. For that reason the prognosis should always be rather guarded. To avoid disappointment it is wise indeed to warn the patient that complete cure of pruritus ani is often beyond our powers and that the most that may be possible is some improvement in his condition. However he can fairly safely be promised that if he carries out the prescribed treatment conscientiously substantial amelioration often results.

The practical management of a case of pruritus can be considered along the following lines:

The Search for a Primary Cause and Its Elimination if Possible

The first step is a thorough examination for any of the numerous conditions that have been listed as possible causes of pruritus ani. In some cases where such a condition is present it may have an obvious and direct relationship to the skin lesion, as for example when a threadworm infestation or discharging fistula is discovered. In other cases the significance of an associated condition in regard to the aetiology of the pruritus may be more doubtful, as for instance when large internal haemorrhoids are found. Some of the conditions liable to be encountered, such as incontinence due to previous fistula operations, are unfortunately not amenable to effective treatment. But many others are, either by operation or other means. This may involve a variety of operations such as laying open of an anal fistula, haemorrhoidectomy or internal sphincterotomy for anal fissue. Pruritus in women, where a gynaecological cause such as vaginal discharge is discovered, demands expert gynaecological investigation and treatment. Parasitic or fungus infections will also require appropriate medical management as follows:

Threadworms
These may be effectively treated by piperazine citrate, conveniently given as a syrup, as, for example, in the proprietary preparation Antepar Elixir. It is administered thrice daily after food, the exact dosage depending on the age and weight of the patient as in the schedule shown in Table 5.

TABLE 5. *Dosages of Antepar Elixir (Piperazine) for Threadworms*

Age	Weight (kg)	Dosage to be continued for seven days
9–24 months	6–9.5	Half teaspoonful twice daily
2–4 years	9.5–12	Half teaspoonful three times daily
4–7 years	12–18	One teaspoonful twice daily
7–13 years	18–36	One teaspoonful three times daily
13 years and over and adults	Over 36	Two teaspoonfuls twice daily

Mycotic Infections
Fungal infections may be treated by various fungicidal preparations. A classical agent is Whitfield's salicylic acid ointment, of which several proprietary variants exist, some with a water-soluble basis such as chlorphenesin (Mycil). These are applied twice daily and their use is continued as long as required, usually several weeks, to eradicate the infection.

An essential item of treatment in cases of epidermophytosis is eradication of the interdigital infection of the feet. Unless this is done relapse is almost certain to occur. In this situation Whitfield's ointment is excellent.

Candidal infections can be cleared up by the regular application of nystatin ointment, but it is well to remember that the yeasts may only be secondary invaders and that strict hygienic measures may also be required to effect a substantial improvement in the pruritic condition (see below).

Pediculosis Pubis
An effective treatment of this condition consists of applying Esoderm lotion to the pubic and perineal regions for several days. Generally this avoids the necessity for shaving the affected parts and using a mercurial ointment.

Scabies
Scabies responds to 25% benzyl benzoate emulsion on two successive days, reinfestation being avoided by a complete change of underclothing and bedding which then require to be sterilized.

Erythrasma
This condition is usually effectively treated with oral erythromycin, 250 mg four times daily, for 10–14 days.

Attention to Anal Hygiene

This is a most important measure in all cases of pruritus ani and in itself is often capable of effecting considerable improvement even up to complete cure on occasions. *The anal region should be washed morning and evening and after defaecation* with luke-warm or cold water and ordinary white soap. Medicated soaps are to be avoided as sometimes proving irritating because of the contained anti-septic. After washing, the part should be gently dried with a soft towel, and a dusting powder of talc or zinc, starch and boric applied. *Greater ventilation of the body surface* is usually desirable and linen- or cotton-mesh underclothing with short pants is pre-ferable to woollen undergarments, especially those with long trousers. Similarly night wear should be light and airy. In hairy individuals *shaving of the peri-anal skin* is sometimes helpful in hot summer weather.

Dietetic Measures

Older textbooks attach great importance to the dietetic treatment of pruritus ani, but there are no clear indications in regard to diet except to avoid items which the patient suspects as aggravating causes of his condition. Generally speaking highly seasoned articles such as sauces, pickles and curries are better eschewed, and this often applies as well to shellfish, coffee and some forms of alcohol, notably champagne, sweet sherry and port.

Attention to Bowels

If the patient suffers from constipation and requires to take a regular aperient it is generally advised that he should avoid saline purgatives, phenolphthalein and aloes, for they seem to produce irritating stools. Similarly liquid paraffin is apt to leak through the anus and makes the perianal skin sodden. Small doses of senna preparations or milk of magnesia are usually satisfactory in pruritic cases.

Local Applications

In general lotions are preferable to ointments in the local medicinal treatment of pruritus ani. Cala-mine lotion may be used but even more effective are preparations containing phenol such as carbolic lotion (1 in 100) or Lotio Mag. Carbol. which is an old favourite and has the following composition:

Phenol	3·5 ml
Zinc oxide	7 ml
Pulv. calamin prep.	3·5 ml
Glycerini	7 ml
Spirit rect.	7 ml
Aq. rosae	14 ml
Milk of magnesia ad.	112 ml

These lotions are dabbed on the perianal region after washing night and morning or more fre-quently as required.

When the more florid phase of the pruritus has subsided on this regimen a talc or zinc, starch and boric dusting powder may be substituted for the lotion, at any rate during the day.

Alternatively, local corticosteroid preparations may be tried; though Brossy (1955) was not impressed with the value of 1% hydrocortisone cream, I have seen some dramatic results with it or with a 0·1% lotion or cream of the much more potent betamethasone. Actually *the efficacy of most local applications in pruritus seems to wane in time and one of the secrets of success in the management of this condition is to ring the changes on different medicaments.*

Sedatives

In many cases of pruritus, when the itching is particularly severe at night, it is necessary to pre-scribe sedatives to help to secure undisturbed sleep. Phenobarbitone 65–130 mg or butobarbitone 100–200 mg is useful, as is diphenhydramine hydro-chloride 100 mg at least one hour before retiring, its value as a soporific being enhanced by its anti-histamine, anti-oedema effect. Another useful anti-histamine drug is promethazine hydrochloride, which, if given in a 25–50 mg dose in the evening, has a short-acting sedative effect, which has worn off by the following morning, whilst the anti-pruritic effect continues for 24 hours.

Injection Treatment

Various solutions have been recommended for injection under the skin of the perianal region in cases of pruritus ani. The aim has been either to obliterate tissue spaces which are alleged to be present and to contain irritating fluid in this condition, or more commonly to produce cutaneous anaesthesia by temporary or permanent nerve block.

SCLEROTHERAPY

The practice of injecting a very dilute solution of hydrochloric acid into the perianal subcutaneous tissues has been advocated by Hanes (1922) in cases of pruritus ani, and Goldbacher (1930) has used a solution of phenol in oil for the same purpose; both these authors have claimed good results for this treatment. I personally am unconvinced of the rationale of sclerotherapy in pruritus and I have no first-hand experience of it in practice.

THE PRODUCTION OF PROLONGED CUTANEOUS ANAESTHESIA BY INJECTION OF ALCOHOL OR LONG-ACTING ANAESTHETICS

ALCOHOL INJECTIONS

The perianal injection of alcohol in cases of pruritus ani was first undertaken by Stone (1919, 1926) of Baltimore. His technique was to inject absolute alcohol through multiple punctures under general anaesthesia, a few millilitres or so being deposited in the subcutaneous tissues at each site. Further injections were given on subsequent occasions as required. Buie (1931) modified the technique by using 40% ethyl alcohol and injecting it in much larger quantities through a single puncture posterior to the anus, placing 15–20 ml on either side of the anus. Many other surgeons have further adapted Buie's method so that the injection is given by means of four punctures placed equidistantly about 10 cm part around the anus, the 40% solution being used, 7–10 ml being given at each injection (Fig. 166). This allows a more uniform distribution of the fluid under the perianal skin. As the alcohol is injected a slight puffiness develops in the appropriate quadrant of the perianal region but there should be no pallor of the skin. If the latter sign develops it indicates that the fluid is being placed too superficially and sloughing of the skin will probably result. As the alcohol is extremely irritating *a general anaesthetic is essential* for the injection. It is also important to maintain strict asepsis and the injection should be given in the operating theatre with *full aseptic ritual* and after preliminary shaving of the perianal skin.

Ferguson (1952) gives a useful report on the results of perianal injections of alcohol employing a technique similar to that outlined above. Of 28 cases treated 15 achieved substantial or complete relief of their pruritus. Abscess formation in the subcu-

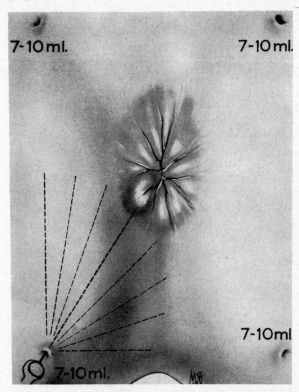

Fig. 166. Position of skin punctures relative to anus, and dosage of ethyl alcohol used, in the injection treatment of pruritus ani. A similar fan-shaped distribution of the fluid is sought in the other quadrants as well.

taneous tissues occurred in six cases, and some necrosis of the skin in five. These complications are a disadvantage of the treatment but they do not impair the final result, which is often particularly good in cases with such complications. My own experience confirms that this is a valuable method of treatment of severe pruritus provided that the patient is prepared to accept the risk of sloughing and sepsis.

INJECTION OF OIL-SOLUBLE ANAESTHETICS

In dealing with the treatment of anal fissure on p. 143 some comments have already been offered on the use of oil-soluble anaesthetics to secure prolonged anaesthesia. When these preparations were first introduced into rectal surgery an important indication for their use was held to be pruritus ani. A popular solution was Proctocaine which was injected either through a posterior puncture as in the treatment of anal fissure, using up to 10–15 ml on either side of the anus, or through four equidistant punctures as for the injection of alcohol,

5–7 ml being introduced at each site. As with alcohol injections the most scrupulous attention to asepsis is necessary. The injection could be given without a general anaesthetic if an intradermal weal was raised with 0·5% lignocaine or procaine as a preliminary to the main injection at each site.

I must say I was singularly unimpressed with the results of this treatment. In my experience the anaesthesia obtained by it was very incomplete and transitory as a rule, and within a few days or a week most of the sensation seemed to have returned together with the itching. As a consequence I soon discarded the use of oil-soluble anaesthetics, and most rectal surgeons of my acquaintanceship seem to have done likewise. I understand that the preparation of Proctocaine has now been discontinued by the manufacturers.

Tattooing of Perianal Skin with Mercuric Sulphide

This treatment has been advocated by Turell (1948) and he reports satisfactory results in many cases of pruritus ani. Other writers such as Bacon (1949) and Shapiro and Rothman (1945) found the method difficult to carry out and obtained no obvious improvement with it. It is difficult to discern any clear rational basis for the treatment and I have no personal knowledge of it.

Surgical Treatment

Apart from operations directed against other anorectal conditions to which the pruritus may be secondary, the surgical treatment resolves itself into operations to undercut and denervate the perianal and anal skin, or to excise it.

UNDERCUTTING OPERATIONS

BALL'S (1908) OPERATION

With the patient in the lithotomy position or on his side, semi-eliptical incisions are made in the skin on either side of the anus, some 5 cm lateral to the anal verge. The incisions leave a narrow strip of intact perianal skin in front and behind. The cuts are deepened through the subcutaneous fat and the flaps are dissected medially exposing the lower border of the external sphincter muscle. The dissection is continued into the anal canal separating the skin from the underlying internal sphincter up to the level of the anal valves, each side being done

in turn. When both flaps have been thoroughly mobilized in this way, the narrow bridges of intact skin in front and behind are undercut till the two lateral wounds communicate and the sphincter muscles have been exposed the whole way round. The skin on the outer side of the incisions is now dissected free for a distance of 6–12 mm and, after very careful attention to haemostasis in all parts of the wound, the skin flaps are stiched back in position with fine stitches of serum-proof silk. If there is any doubt about the completeness of the haemostasis—and perhaps indeed in any case—it is a good plan to place a fine rubber drain under each flap, projecting anteriorly and posteriorly. A firm dry dressing is applied. The drains are removed at the end of 48 hours, the sutures in eight to ten days. The bowels are confined for three or four days and then relieved by an enema. The operation should be preceded by a course of intestinal antiseptics and carried out under cover of suitable systemic antibiotic therapy.

Though Lockhart-Mummery (1934) reported favourably on the results of Ball's operation in a large series of cases of pruritus ani, most other surgeons, such as Gabriel (1948) and Bacon (1949), have been disappointed. Even when complete anaesthesia of the under-cut perianal skin is obtained, this is usually of short duration and in the course of time sensation and itching gradually return. Moreover, the convalescence in the past has often been marred by sepsis and separation of the wounds. My own experience of the operation is very limited, but it suggests that at the present time with very accurate haemostatis by means of diathermy and the use of antibiotics it is usually possible to secure uneventful primary healing. The result as regards control of the pruritus, however, is very variable and often bitterly disappointing.

MODIFICATIONS OF BALL'S OPERATION

Several surgeons have modified Ball's operation by using different skin incisions such as several small radiating incisions, or anterior and posterior circumferential incisions, to diminish the risk of sloughing. Bacon (1949) describes these modifications in some detail, but they suffer the disadvantage of making the undercutting and denervation of the skin more difficult and less efficient.

EXCISION OF ANAL AND PERIANAL SKIN

Years ago Wallis (1911), who held that hypertrophied anal papillae played an important part in the aetiology of pruritus ani, excised the papillae and the skin of the anal canal as far as the anal verge. This was done in circumferential fashion, the operation being completed by suture of the anal mucosa to the perianal skin with a continuous catgut stich. The operation never became popular and one imagines that it must frequently have been followed by separation of the suture line with resulting healing by granulation and stenosis.

More recently Hughes (1957) has advocated excision of the anal and perianal skin followed by immediate Thiersch grafting in the treatment of severe pruritus ani. The excision and grafting are best carried out in stages with intervals of several weeks or months between the stages, a segment of the anal circumference being dealt with at each operation. The actual technique of grafting is identical with that employed in connection with fistula wounds (see p. 187). Hughes claims encouraging results, but it will be interesting to see if the grafted skin ever becomes pruritic. I have no personal experience of the method to date.

Radiotherapy

Though radiotherapy applied to the anal region may give complete relief of pruritus ani for a time or even permanently, in the majority of cases it is ineffective or of only very transient value. In a few cases *serious X-ray burns have been produced in the perianal skin, which seems specially predisposed to this complication.* This danger is now well recognized and as a consequence most radiotherapists are extremely cautious in their treatment of this disease. *Under no circumstances should X-ray treatment of pruritus ever be repeated* if the patient has had previous radiotherapy to the anal region.

Summary

It may be helpful to summarize in a few words my present practice in regard to the treatment of idiopathic pruritus ani. Reliance is placed mainly on simple hygienic measures and the local use of various antipruritic lotions. Sedatives are also a valuable adjunct in severe cases. Only if these simple measures fail to produce substantial amelioration is anything more drastic contemplated, and usually this has consisted of alcohol injections, rarely Ball's operation. It is extremely difficult to become enthusiastic about the treatment of this disease.

REFERENCES

ALLINGHAM, W, and ALLINGHAM, H. W. (1901) *The Diagnosis and Treatment of the Rectum.* London: Baillière.

BACON, H. E. (1949) *Anus, Rectum and Sigmoid Colon,* 3rd ed., vol. 1. Philadelphia: Lippincott.

—— and HARDWICK, C. E. (1947) Pruritus ani. A biochemophysiologic entity. *J. med. Soc. N.J., 44,* 446.

BALL, SIR CHARLES. (1908) *The Rectum: Its Diseases and Developmental Defects.* London: Frowde; Hodder and Stoughton.

BOWYER, A. and McCOLL, I. (1966) The role of erythrasma in pruritus ani. *Lancet, 2,* 572.

BROSSY, J.-J. (1955) Pruritus ani. *Proc. R. Soc. Med., 48,* 499.

BUIE, L. A. (1931) Proctoscopic examination and the treatment of haemorrhoids and anal pruritus. *Mayo Clin. Monogr., 165.*

DRUECK, C. J. (1943) Essential pruritus perinei. *J. nerv. ment. Dis., 97,* 528.

FERGUSON, J. H. L. (1952) Alcohol injections in the treatment of pruritus ani. *Proc. R. Soc. Med., 45,* 391.

FRANKFELDT, F. M. (1948) Pyribenzamine: its role in the treatment of pruitus ani. *Am. J. Surg., 75,* 307.

GABRIEL, W. B. (1948) *Principles and Practice of Rectal Surgery,* 4th ed. London: H. K. Lewis.

GOLDBACHER, L. (1930) *Haemorrhoids, the Injection Treatment and Pruritus Ani.* Philadelphia: F. A. Davis.

GRANET, E. (1954) *Manual of Proctology.* Chicago: Yearbook Publishers.

HANES, G. S. (1922) Some observations, chiefly clinical, on infections of the rectum and adjacent structures, with special reference to pruritus. *Trans. Am. proct. Soc., 23,* 1.

HUGHES, E. S. R. (1957) *Surgery of the Anus, Anal Canal and Rectum.* Edinburgh: Livingstone.

LOCKHART-MUMMERY, J. P. (1934) *Diseases of the Rectum and Colon.* London: Baillière.

MONTGOMERY, H. (1931) Quoted by Buie, L. A. (1931).

RIDDOCH, J. W. (1937) Pruritus ani. *Lancet, 1,* 919.

ROSENBAUM, M. (1945) Psychosomatic factors in pruritus. *Psychosom. Med., 7,* 52.

SAUL, L. J. (1938) Incidental observations on pruritus ani. *Psychoanal. Q., 7,* 336.

SHAPIRO, A. L. and ROTHMAN, S. (1945) Pruritus ani; a clinical study. *Gastroenterology, 5,* 155.

STONE, H. B. (1919) A treatment for pruritus ani. *Bull. Johns Hopk. Hosp., 27,* 242.

—— (1926) Pruritus ani, treatment by alcohol injection. *Surgery Gynec. Obstet., 42,* 565.

TUCKER, C. C. and HELLWIG, C. A. (1937) Pruritus ani: histologic picture in forty three cases. *Archs Surg., Chicago, 34,* 929.

TURELL, R. (1948) Tattooing with mercury sulfide for intractable anal pruritus. *Surgery, St Louis, 23,* 63.

TUTTLE, J. P. (1903) *Diseases of the Anus, Rectum and Pelvic Colon.* New York and London: Appleton.

WALLIS, F. C. (1911) Pruritus ani. *Practioner, 87,* 417.

WINNER, H. J. and HURLEY, R. (1964) *Candida Albicans.* London: Churchill.

10

Prolapse of the Rectum

The term prolapse of the rectum implies a circumferential descent of the bowel through the anus. If this involves only mucous membrane, the condition is said to be one of *incomplete or mucosal prolapse*; if the entire thickness of the rectal wall is extruded the term *complete prolapse or procidentia* is used.

INCIDENCE

Age and Sex

It is traditional teaching that prolapse of the rectum is a disease of the extremes of life, the mucosal variety being commonest in young children, whilst complete prolapse is found chiefly in elderly patients. This generalization, however, is only partly correct, for rectal prolapse, complete or partial, also occurs at all ages of adult life.

In children, the incidence is highest in the first two years of life and thereafter declines, prolapse being very rare after the fifth or sixth year (Carrasco 1934). Boys are affected slightly more frequently than girls. The condition is usually of mucosal type, but sometimes complete prolapse occurs, as Hughes (1949) points out, and as I have found in my own experience (see Fig. 169).

In adults, rectal prolapse is more commonly of the complete type, though partial prolapse is also encountered. In the collective series of 231 cases of complete prolapse at St Mark's Hospital reported by Hughes (1949) 84% of the patients were women, and in a consecutive series of 100 cases of complete prolapse reported from my department (Küpfer and

Goligher 1970) 83 or approximately 85% were women. An interesting point brought out in these series was the difference in the age incidence of complete prolapse in the two sexes; in females the incidence was maximal in the fifth and subsequent decades, but in males it was evenly distributed throughout the age range (Küpfer and Goligher 1970) or maximal in the second and third decades (Hughes 1949). The very advanced age of many females with complete prolapse should be stressed; several of our patients were in their eighties and the oldest was 97 years of age.

Effect of Parturition

Carrasco (1934) and Gabriel (1948) both allege that complete prolapse is relatively commoner in women who have suffered the strain of parturition than in those who have not. I have been impressed rather by the fact that the condition occurs so frequently in single and childless women; thus no less than 39 of my 83 women patients with complete prolapse and 72 of Hughes' (1949) St Mark's Hospital series of 183 female cases were childless. When it is borne in mind what a small proportion of women of the fifth and subsequent decades in the general population are childless, these figures indicate that the incidence of complete prolapse in childless women is probably higher than in patients who have borne children.

COINCIDENT UTERINE AND RECTAL PROLAPSE

Though uterine and rectal prolapse may occur together, in my experience the combination has been relatively infrequent. Thus only 8 of my 83 female patients with complete rectal prolapse had uterine prolapse of sufficient severity to warrant operative treatment.

Mental State

It is commonly held that complete prolapse of the rectum is specially liable to occur in patients suffering from mental disease, and rectal prolapse is found surprisingly frequently amongst the inmates of asylums. As a matter of interest when a series of 100 cases of complete prolapse (Küpfer and Goligher 1970) was categorized according to their state of mental health—it being understood that this was a *surgeon's* and not a psychiatrist's assessment—the results were 64 cases apparently normal, 33 cases rather odd and 3 cases definitely psychotic.

AETIOLOGY

Partial Prolapse

In children predisposing factors that are generally held to be important in the development of prolapse are:

1. The absence of the sacral curve, so that in the sitting or standing position the rectum and anal canal form an almost straight tube.

2. Diminution in the amount of supporting fat in the ischiorectal fossae such as may occur in wasting disease or in conditions of malnutrition.

I think the second factor has been grossly overrated, for most of the children I have seen with rectal prolapse have been in a well-nourished and apparently healthy state. Exciting causes comprise those conditions leading to excessive straining at stool—diarrhoea, overpurgation, and constipation, particularly if combined with bad defaecatory habits, whereby the child is left sitting and straining ineffectively on the chamber pot for periods of 15–20 minutes each time. A chronic cough or severe attack of coughing as in whooping-cough is also said sometimes to be the exciting factor responsible for a rectal prolapse. In my experience it is usually difficult to attribute the prolapse to any particular cause and poor training in regard to defaecation is generally invoked as the explanation.

In adults prolapse of the mucosa on one or more aspects of the bowel circumference occurs with

third-degree internal haemorrhoids and if these are especially large and numerous the effect may be to produce a circular mucosal prolapse. In patients who have had a Whitehead's operation for haemorrhoids subsequent prolapse of the rectal mucosa is a common sequel. Mucosal prolapse is also found after fistula operations when the sphincters have been extensively divided, the unsupported mucosa on the opposite side of the anal canal tending to prolapse into the gap. If in a fistula operation or in a complete obstetrical tear of the perineum the anorectal ring has been severed, circular mucosal prolapse of the rectum normally results. In older patients an important cause of mucosal prolapse is atony and relaxation of the anal sphincters which, though occasionally due to organic disease of the nervous system such as tabes dorsalis, and tumours or injury of the cauda equina, more commonly arises idiopathically. The mechanism of this form of partial prolapse and incontinence has been studied by Parks et al. (1966).

Complete Prolapse

The factors that have been alleged to be important in the production of this form of prolapse are the following:

THE ABNORMALLY DEEP RECTOVAGINAL OR RECTOVESICAL POUCH OF PERITONEUM

This is a most striking and constant feature in all cases of complete rectal prolapse. The possible causal significance of the deep pouch was early emphasized by Jeannel (1896), Quénu and Duval (1910) and Moschcowitz (1912), who claimed that complete rectal prolapse was really a form of sliding hernia, the pouch of Douglas being the hernial sac, which presses the anterior rectal wall into the rectal lumen and then through the anal canal to the exterior (Fig. 167).

IDIOPATHIC INTUSSUSCEPTION OF THE UPPER RECTUM

The conception of complete prolapse as basically a sliding hernia has been challenged by Brodén and Snellman (1968), Devadhar (1965) and Theuerkauf et al. (1970). By a special cineradiographic technique with radio-opaque media in the rectum and

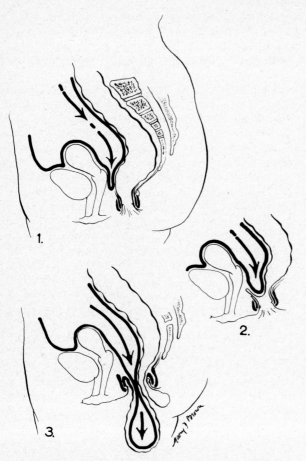

Fig. 167. Sagittal section of the pelvis to demonstrate the anatomy of complete rectal prolapse conceived as a sliding hernia of the pouch of Douglas. 1. Initial state with deep peritoneal pouch between rectum and vagina. 2. Pouch starting to invaginate anterior rectal wall into lumen of rectum. 3. The anterior rectal wall has been further invaginated so that it now protrudes through the anus as a complete rectal prolapse containing the pouch of Douglas. (*From Goligher 1958*)

distal colon, in the small bowel lying in the pouch of Douglas, in the vagina and in the bladder, Brodén and Snellman (1968) have analysed the visceral movements that take place when patients with complete rectal prolapse strain and produce their prolapse. They found that the initial step in the genesis of the prolapse is an intussusception of the rectum with its starting point usually about 6–8 cm from the anal verge and affecting the bowel not just anteriorly but *circumferentially*. The apex passes down into the lower rectum and through the anus to the exterior. When the prolapse is fully descended it may often be shown to contain pouch of Douglas with loops of small bowel protruding

through the anus, but in the early stages of the descent of the prolapse—and sometimes even after it has passed through the anal orifice—there may be no small bowel discernible in it. These cineradiographic studies, which Dr Björn Snellman very kindly demonstrated to me during a visit to Stockholm, seem to my mind to *dis*prove quite conclusively the idea that herniation of the pouch of Douglas into the rectal lumen, as shown in Fig. 167, is the primary process in the formation of a complete prolapse of the rectum. Instead the primary factor appears to be this intussusception of the rectum, though Brodén and Snellman (1968) offer no definite explanation for the initiation of the intussusception.

Devadhar (1965) bases his objection to the conception of complete rectal prolapse as a sliding hernia of the pouch of Douglas on the grounds that, contrary to what is usually said, the anterior wall of a complete prolapse is *not* longer than the posterior one, and the lumen of the bowel is situated *not* posteriorly but centrally (I would agree that this is often so when the prolapse first appears outside the anal orifice, but on maximal straining the anterior part usually becomes more prominent and the luman eccentric). Like Brodén and Snellman (1968), Devadhar believes that prolapse of the rectum is a symmetrical intussusception of the bowel.

LACK OF THE NORMAL FIXATION OF THE RECTUM TO ITS BED

Jeannel (1896), Pemberton and Stalker (1939), Muir (1955) and Ripstein (1965) have claimed that an abnormal mobility of the rectum in its bed is a factor in the causation of prolapse, but it seems not unlikely that such increased mobility is a consequence rather than a cause of the recurrent prolapse. Whether this is so or not, one principle employed in certain of the operations used for this condition is the promotion of adhesions between the rectum and its surroundings.

THE LAX AND ATONIC CONDITION OF THE MUSCULATURE OF THE PELVIC FLOOR AND ANAL CANAL

Most cases of complete prolapse show a remarkably weak and atonic condition of the anal sphincters and levator ani muscles. It has always been a matter for dispute whether this state of affairs is the cause or an effect of the prolapse, but it has usually been observed even in my early cases of prolapse in which there hardly seems to have been time for the prolapse to have produced such secondary changes in the musculature. On the other hand I have seen three patients with large complete prolapses in whom the anal sphincters and levator muscles were absolutely normal on clinical examination after the prolapse had been reduced. The role of laxity of the pelvic floor musculature and sphincters in the genesis of complete rectal prolapse is demonstrated *par excellence* in patients with cauda equina lesions with resulting paralysis of these muscles. In such cases complete rectal prolapse often develops, as pointed out by Butler (1954), Muir (1955) and Todd (1959). In the average case of rectal prolapse, however, no clinically obvious neurological abnormality is present to account for the relaxed state of the musculature of the anal canal and pelvic floor. But Porter (1962a) has demonstrated by means of electromyographic studies that these muscles behave somewhat differently in cases of complete

prolapse and in normal individuals. He finds that the reflex suppression of the resting activity of the external sphincter and levator muscles that occurs normally on distension of the rectum with a balloon (see p. 38)—and presumably also with faeces immediately before and during defaecation—is more profound and prolonged in cases of complete rectal prolapse. It may, thus, be that some subtle disorder of the sphincteric mechanism connected with defaecation is the primary aetiological factor, to which laxity of the muscles, the development of the deep pelvic peritoneal pouch, and the increased mobility of the rectum are all secondary, with the ultimate formation of a complete rectal prolapse.

On the other hand, the intussusception of the rectum, which Brodén and Snellman (1968) observed cineradiographically as the initial step in the development of a complete rectal prolapse, starts well above the pelvic floor, which would suggest that laxity of the pelvic musculature cannot be a primary factor in the causation of this condition. Further evidence against weakness of the pelvic floor being the initial cause of rectal prolapse is provided by cineradiographic studies during voluntary contraction of these muscles (Fry et al. 1966). In 12 of 15 patients with complete prolapse the pelvic floor moved normally.

CLINICAL FEATURES

Prolapse in Children

SYMPTOMS

The mother complains that when the child defaecates the bowel comes down and projects at the anus, sometimes reducing itself spontaneously at the end of the act, at other times requiring to be replaced digitally. Occasionally the prolapse is found to be irreducible by the parents and reduction has to be effected in hospital—usually an easy matter. Whilst the prolapse is down the child may experience some discomfort from anal distention and there may even be a slight discharge of mucus or blood. At other times the child is perfectly well and is normally continent.

ON EXAMINATION

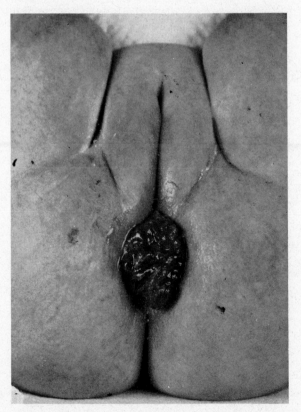

Fig. 168. Mucosal prolapse of the rectum in a child (Mr H. H. Nixon's case).

The prolapse may be down when the child presents, and it is seen to consist of a ring of mucosa projecting 2–4 cm beyond the skin of the perianal region (Fig. 168). If the index finger is inserted into the lumen and the protruding ring palpated between finger and thumb, there is no difficulty as a rule in deciding that it consists only of two layers of mucosa. If the prolapse has been unreduced for some hours there may be oedema adding to the thickness of the swelling. Generally very little pressure is necessary to reduce the prolapse, and when this has been accomplished examination of the anal canal by palpation reveals no abnormality of the sphincters.

More usually children with rectal prolapse are seen with the bowel already reduced, and with a history of one or several episodes of prolapse. Examination at this stage will be negative and it will often be difficult to decide whether the 'prolapse' of which the mother complains was a genuine one or merely the slight projection of the anorectal mucosa that occurs normally at defaecation. To settle the diagnosis *it is essential for the surgeon to see the rectum in its prolapsed condition*; this can easily be done by inserting a glycerine suppository and putting the child to stool. During the straining which this produces the prolapse is rapidly and fully reproduced and the diagnosis thereby established.

Rarely prolapse in children is of complete variety with a much larger projection of bowel, which may become irreducible or gangrenous as in Fig. 169.

DIFFERENTIAL DIAGNOSIS

Prolapse of the rectum in a child has to be distinguished from a *prolapsed rectal polyp* or the *apex of an intussusception* protruding through the anus. This is readily done by tracing the *outer* aspect of the swelling with the palpating finger up to the anal orifice. In rectal prolapse it is not possible to enter the canal at any point, but in an intussusception or prolapsed rectal polyp the tip of the finger can engage in the slit between the intussuscepted bowel or tumour and the wall of the canal.

Prolapse in Adults

SYMPTOMS

The symptoms produced by prolapse of the rectum in adults relate partly to the actual prolapse and partly to the disturbance of normal continence so often found in these cases. The prolapse at first occurs at defaecation only, but before long it happens after any slight exertion such as coughing or sneezing, and eventually may appear on standing or walking. When the bowel is prolapsed there may be a discharge of mucus from the exposed mucosa, leading to much soiling of the underclothes. Bleeding may also occur due to trauma or ul-

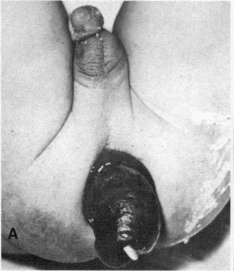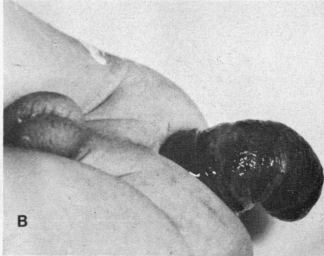

Fig. 169. Complete prolapse of the rectum in a child aged 1 year: (A) view from below; (B) side view. The prolapse was irreducible and the bowel almost gangrenous at the tip of the projection. Treated by rectosigmoidectomy.

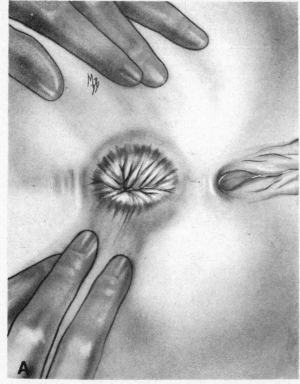

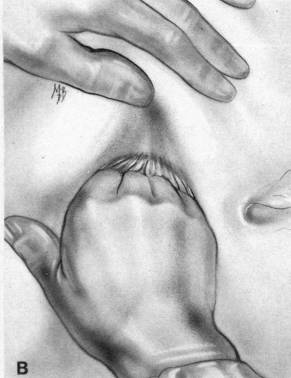

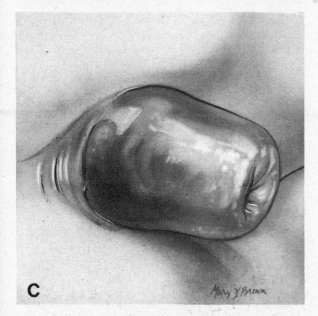

Fig. 170. Woman, aged 68, with a complete prolapse of the rectum: (A) Prolapse reduced, note patulous anus. (B) The great laxity of the anal sphincters is further demonstrated by the fact that four fingers can be inserted side by side without discomfort. (C) Rectum in prolapsed condition projecting 14 cm; note that the mucosa is fully stretched on this prolapse.

ceration of the surface of the prolapse. In addition there is usually some degree of incontinence of faeces and flatus. This occurs not only during the prolapse but at other times due to atony and relaxation of the sphincters, and possibly to some impairment of rectal sensation which is apparently a feature of many of these cases. Difficulty in regulating the bowel action is thus one of the most distressing symptoms. If the patient leaves the bowel to act spontaneously, the result is that she usually becomes constipated and in a rather peculiar way, that is to say she does not experience the normal call to stool, but by dint of much straining succeeds in passing several small motions a day, consisting mostly of faecal pellets. Sometimes these pellets are discharged also into her clothing when she walks around with the prolapse down. If on the other hand she attempts to secure a proper evacuation by taking a dose of aperient and produces diarrhoea, she is quite unable to control the liquid motions and is temporarily incapacitated. If an associated uterine prolapse is also present incontinence of urine may add to the patient's misery. Because of the discomfort from the prolapsing rectum and the uncertainty of their bowel function, these patients find it necessary to withdraw from most of their ordinary activities and lead secluded lives, devoted increasingly to the care of their lower intestinal tract. It is not surprising that they tend to become introspective and neurotic.

ON EXAMINATION

The prolapse is usually reduced when the surgeon commences his examination of the patient, but a valuable indication of the presence of a prolapsing rectum is generally afforded by noting the state of the anal sphincters. In many cases the anus is quite patulous, with lax mucosa showing at the anal orifice; in yet others, though the anal margins are in apposition, drawing the buttocks apart causes the anus to open widely (Fig. 170A). Only very few cases have an anal region that appears quite normal on inspection.

If the anus is now palpated, the surgeon is immediately struck by the deficient tone of the sphincter musculature and by the abnormally large size of the orifice. The atony affects most severely the internal anal sphincter, which often can scarcely be felt at all; but the external sphincter is also usually in a relaxed condition, though its lower edge can usually be distinguished by careful palpation at the anal margin. If the patient is asked to close the anus whilst the finger is held on the external sphincter, it is found that in most cases the contractile power of this muscle is grossly deficient or totally absent, the latter usually being in patients with patulous ani. The finger is then inserted farther into the anal canal and the state of the levator muscles determined by palpating the puborectalis sling. Again the tone of the muscle, as indicated by its prominence to the examining finger, is often subnormal, and its ability to contract voluntarily grossly impaired.

A further striking feature on palpation of the anus and rectum in these cases of prolapse is the relative lack of discomfort—so much so that two, three and even four fingers may sometimes be inserted side by side into the anus without causing any pain or sense of anal distention (Fig. 170B). Similarly there often seems to be some blunting of rectal sensation as determined by balloon distension of the lower rectum, much increased pressure being frequently necessary to evoke the normal sense of rectal distention.

The patient is now asked to bear down and the manner in which the bowel prolapses is observed. At first the mucosa appears hesitantly, as it were, at the anal orifice, but then as the expulsive effort is maintained, it emerges, often quite suddenly, to form a large red swelling. The mucosa on the swelling frequently appears thickened and is thrown into a series of concentric folds indicating its laxity and greater area relative to the underlying muscle coat (Fig. 171). But if the patient is asked to continue straining the prolapse undergoes further expansion and lengthening and these mucosal folds may become obliterated as in Fig. 170C. It often happens, too, with increased straining that the anterior part of the prolapse enlarges and lengthens more than does the posterior so that the lumen comes to occupy a somewhat posterior position. However severe the condition and however much

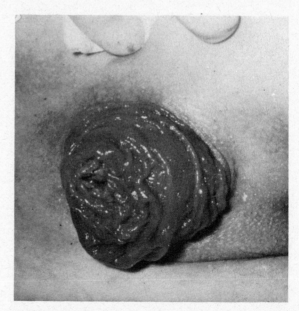

Fig. 171. Woman aged 50, with a complete rectal prolapse which projects about 7·5 cm. Note the circular folds in the mucosa.

the patient may strain it is unusual for the projection of bowel to exceed 10–12 cm from the anal skin. Often the mucosa covering the prolapse shows superficial ulceration due to repeat trauma against the clothing when the bowel is lying externally. Sometimes the scar of a previous unsuccessful rectosigmoidectomy is evident on the mucosa close to the pectinate line. Large dilated veins in the submucosa of the prolapse are usually evident whilst the patient is straining.

If the finger is now inserted into the lumen and the thickness of the prolapse palpated between finger and thumb, it will be immediately apparent that much more tissue is included than merely a double layer of mucosa. This is especially evident anteriorly, where the deep pouch of Douglas with its contained loops of small intestine adds greatly to the bulk of the prolapsing bowel. Actually, with large projections of over 5 cm in length it is fair to assume that the condition must be one of complete prolapse. But with swellings less than 4–5 cm long it may be difficult to decide whether one is dealing with a complete procidentia or simply a mucosal prolapse, and the findings on palpation are more important in making the differentiation.

DIAGNOSIS

In its grosser forms complete prolapse of the rectum is usually quite unmistakable for anything else, and even the less severe cases can as a rule be readily distinguished on careful examination from other conditions. Actually most adult patients referred to hospital with alleged rectal prolapse are found to be suffering not from prolapse, but from *large third-degree internal haemorrhoids*. The sphincter tone and contractility in these cases, however, are normal, or nearly so, and the findings on straining and on proctoscopy are quite different from those presented by a prolapse. Occasionally a *large polypoid tumour of the rectum or even the sigmoid colon* may prolapse and emerge at the anus giving the impression to the patient and doctor of a rectal prolapse. There may be other symptoms, such as bleeding and disturbance of bowel habits, to suggest the true nature of the condition, and rectal examination including sigmoidoscopy and possibly barium enema studies serves to confirm the diagnosis.

Perhaps the most difficult point that arises in connection with the diagnosis of rectal prolapse in adult cases is *the distinction between a purely mucosal prolapse and a small complete prolapse*. With the latter condition, if the patient fails to strain sufficiently during examination, the projection of bowel may not present the characteristic features of a complete prolapse. Though some degree of hypotonia of the sphincter apparatus is common in partial prolapse, a profound laxity of the sphincters should suggest that an early complete prolapse is present. If the patient can be encouraged to increase her expulsive efforts this impression can usually be confirmed at the initial examination or on a subsequent occasion. Having seen quite a number of patients who have been wrongly diagnosed as having mucosal prolapse in the first instance, I now regard this diagnosis with considerable suspicion. I would warn strongly against the danger of overlooking complete prolapse in its initial stages.

COMPLICATIONS

Irreducibility and Gangrene. Patients with complete prolapse are usually expert at reducing their prolapse, but occasionally urgent admission to hospital is required because the bowel has become oedematous and the patient cannot induce it to go back. By a firm manipulation in the out-patient department reduction can usually be achieved by the surgeon in such cases, but sometimes the condition is quite irreducible without an anaesthetic, and rarely even with an anaesthetic. In the latter circumstances there is generally doubt as to the viability of the bowel, or it may indeed be frankly gangrenous as in one case seen by me which had to be treated by an emergency rectosigmoidectomy (see Fig. 169). It is interesting to recall that the first case ever treated by this operation by Mikulicz (1889) also had an irreducible prolapse. Irreducibility with gangrene remains one of the few indications for rectosigmoidectomy at the present day.

Ulceration and Haemorrhage. Minor ulceration of the exposed mucosa of a complete prolapse is quite common and may be associated with some bleeding. Rarely the ulceration may be more extensive and severe haemorrhage may result if one of the large submucous veins is exposed and eroded.

Rupture of the Prolapse. This is an excessively rare complication which I myself have never seen and which has never been encountered by any of the numerous surgeons of my acquaintance interested in rectal surgery. Cases are, however, recorded by Quénu (1882), Ball (1908), Kelsey (1883) and McLanahan and Johnson (1945). The rupture apparently occurs usually during straining, as at defaecation or whilst lifting a heavy weight. The bowel gives way anteriorly with escape of loops of small gut through the rent. Most of the reported cases have terminated fatally. If this complication should occur it would obviously be an indication for urgent operation which could be conducted in several different ways, probably best through the abdomen.

TREATMENT
Prolapse in Children

It is important to appreciate, as Stephens (1958) has emphasized, that mucosal prolapse of the rectum in children is essentially a self-limiting disease, and moreover that it usually responds satisfactorily to simple non-operative treatment such as is detailed below. In certain cases, however, more active measures are required.

NON-OPERATIVE TREATMENT

Correction of Constipation and Institution of Proper Habits of Defaecation. If the child is constipated this should be corrected by the administration of small repeated doses of liquid paraffin, assisted if necessary by syrup of figs or cascara. A regular habit of defaecation is thus established, and the child is taught to defaecate promptly, no prolonged period of straining being allowed. In order to establish such a routine it is usually best to admit the child to hospital for a time so that proper discipline may be enforced in these matters. Occasionally a daily enema may be required at the commencement of this regimen to inaugurate a regular habit. In milder cases this treatment alone suffices.

Supporting the Anus Manually or by Strapping. In more severe cases the anus may also be supported during defaecation by the nurse or mother holding the buttocks together digitally or preferably by adhesive plaster. To be effective strapping must be adequate, painless and easily applied. A square of adhesive is applied almost to cover each buttock. The buttocks are then approximated. A piece of strapping 2·5 cm wide is placed across the natal cleft adhering only to the square of strapping on either side. This is left on even during defaecation, after which the strip is painlessly removed, the buttocks, covered with their squares of adhesive, cleansed, and a new transverse strip applied.

OPERATIVE TREATMENT

Submucous Injection of Phenol or Alcohol. Injection treatment may be employed in an endeavour to fix the lax mucosa to the underlying muscle coat. Usually a short general anaesthetic is required. I have invariably used a 5% solution of phenol in almond oil as the sclerosing fluid and have employed a technique very similar to that for injection of haemorrhoids (see p. 100). The fluid is injected into the submucosa at and just above the level of the anorectal ring, 1–2 ml being given at three or four places around the circumference of the bowel. A recent follow-up study of 28 children treated by me with phenol injections for rectal prolapse during the past 10 years was successful in tracing all but four of the patients. According to the parents the condition cleared up either immediately after the treatment or within a few weeks of it being given. The results thus appear very satisfactory, but they have been achieved at the price of a general anaesthetic. Sceptics might also say that the successes were due, not to the treatment, but to spontaneous cure—though I doubt this myself because of the rapidity of the change after the injections. Other surgeons such as Fraser (1930) and Stephens (1958) have favoured absolute alcohol as the sclerosing agent, 0·25 ml being injected into the submucosa on the anterior, posterior, and lateral walls of the anorectal junction, and have reported favourably on the results.

Insertion of a Subcutaneous Stitch of Catgut round the Anus. Stephens (1958) describes a method of treating partial rectal prolapse in children by inserting a stitch of stout chromicized catgut under the skin of the anus and tying it anteriorly so that the lumen of the anus is constricted to the size of the little finger. This procedure, which may be regarded as a sort of temporary Thiersch operation, is claimed by Stephens to be highly effective.

Perirectal Injections of Alcohol. Treatment of rectal prolapse in children by perirectal injections of absolute alcohol has been recommended by Findlay and Galbraith (1923). Two injections are given, one on either side on the posterolateral aspect of the anus 6 mm from the anal verge. The 7·5-cm needle used is directed upwards under the guidance of a finger in the rectum, towards the hollow of the sacrum; 1·5 ml of absolute alcohol are then injected slowly, the injection being continued as the needle is withdrawn. The same performance is repeated on the opposite side. The effect of these injections is to stimulate a periproctitis which may help to fix the rectum to the sacrum. Though good results have been claimed for this method by Findlay and Galbraith (1923), Brown and Drake (1924), and Potter and Wellman (1933), it is clearly not a rational treatment for purely mucosal prolapse. However, for the rare, more severe, cases of rectal prolapse in children in which it appears that the prolapse may be complete, perirectal injections are particularly suitable as an alternative to operative treatment.

Linear Cauterization of the Mucosa. The traditional operation of linear cauterization of the rectal mucosa, introduced by van Buren (1881), has been completely replaced in modern times by submucous injections of phenol, and I have never had occasion to use it.

Rectosigmoidectomy or Other Major Operation. In the treatment of complete rectal prolapse in children not responding to perirectal injections, operations such as those employed for complete prolapse in adults (see below) may have to be considered. I have twice had to carry out emergency rectosigmoidectomies for large irreducible complete prolapses of the rectum in young children.

Partial Prolapse in Adults

An important consideration in the treatment of partial prolapse in adults is whether the sphincter tone is normal or not. *In patients with normal or slightly relaxed sphincter tone* the partial prolapse may be treated in much the same manner as large third-degree internal haemorrhoids by means of a ligature operation. The circular prolapse of mucosa is caught by artery forceps placed in the right anterior, right posterior and left lateral positions respectively. By scissor cuts the prolapse is then divided into three main portions like primary piles with narrow skin–mucosa bridges intervening between them. Each of these parts is then ligated and excised as in haemorrhoidectomy. As the 'piles' are relatively broad-based it is a wise precaution to employ transfixion ligatures, and if necessary to use the Goodsall double transfixion technique (see Fig. 250). In the performance of 'haemorrhoidectomy' for mucosal prolapse it is often difficult to preserve satisfactory mucocutaneous bridges between the areas of mucosa being ligated. But the loss of one or two of the bridges may actually be beneficial in these cases, for it increases the raw area and thus predisposes to the development of some degree of anal stenosis, which may counteract the natural tendency to patulousness.

In older patients with partial prolapse associated with gross relaxation of the sphincters treatment is difficult and unsatisfactory. The main complaint in these cases is of incontinence due to the hypotonic sphincter apparatus rather than of prolapse, and removal of the prolapsing mucosa does little to improve the patients' incontinent condition. It is, moreover, liable to be followed by early recurrence of the prolapse leading to further disappointment. Efforts should obviously be directed to correcting the state of the sphincter muscles, but in fact there is very little can be done to improve their tone. Unlike Gabriel (1948) I have not been at all impressed by the results of voluntary sphincter exercises or of electrical stimulation, however assiduously carried out. Perhaps the best that can be done for these patients is to provide a substitute for the sphincter in the form of a circumanal ring of silver wire as recommended by Gabriel (1948). This Thiersch operation is not altogether an unmixed blessing, for unless the wire ring is made fairly tight it will not restrain the mucosal prolapse or offer much assistance in control of the incontinence. If sufficiently tight to assist in these ways it is liable to interfere with the passage of faeces and cause faecal impaction. But if the right degree of tightness is achieved and a good postoperative regimen established the patient with partial prolapse and poor sphincter tone may be benefited by a Thiersch operation, particularly if it is done with mono-filament nylon instead of wire (see p. 249).

Another treatment that may conceivably have something to offer in the future to these patients with mucosal prolapse is that of *continuous stimulation of sphincter tone by an electronic implant or anal plug*, which is under trial by Caldwell (1965), Hopkinson and Lightwood (1966) and Collins et al. (1968, 1969) (see below). Parks (1971) has introduced a *perineorrhaphy to tighten the puborectalis sling through a posterior intersphincteric approach*, which may be useful in some of these cases, if the patients are not too elderly (see p. 317).

Complete Prolapse in Adults

I. Methods Available

At the present time surgical treatment of complete rectal prolapse offers a good prospect of cure, but it has not always been so, and in the past the operative management of this condition has had the unenviable reputation of being all too frequently unsuccessful. Certainly it is by no means uncommon to find patients presenting with prolapse who have already undergone two or more previous operations for it. The unsatisfactory nature of the results is also reflected in the large number of operative procedures that have been proposed for this condition. A further cause of disappointment is the *poor functional state that often persists, sometimes in aggravated form*, after the prolapse itself has been successfully cured by operation.

It is difficult to provide a complete list of all the operations that have ever been devised for rectal prolapse, but the following account includes most of the more important ones. Some of these techniques, which have never enjoyed much vogue, are of little more than historical interest now and will not be discussed. Others, which are in current use or were at one stage popular methods of treatment, will be examined in more detail, an attempt being made to indicate their achievements and to describe their advantages and drawbacks.

PERINEAL OR SACRAL OPERATIONS

1. PLICATION OF THE ANAL SPHINCTERS AND LEVATOR ANI MUSCLES (Cunéo and Sénèque 1931)

2. RESTORATION OF ANAL SPHINCTER TONE BY ELECTRONIC IMPLANT

Caldwell (1965) employed an implanted electronic stimulator in relation to the anal sphincter to restore tone in cases of anal incontinence associated with partial or complete rectal prolapse. The implanted part of the apparatus consisted of a pair of electrodes sewn on to the external sphincter; insulated leads connected these to a radiofrequency transformer coil via a transistor rectifier. These latter components were contained within a Perspex box which could be sterilized. The box was secured subcutaneously at a convenient site—usually in the suprapubic region, stitched to the anterior rectus sheath—so that the external transmitter could be easily placed in apposition.

To avoid surgical implantation Hopkinson and Lightwood (1966) adopted the plan of connecting the external source of power directly by wires to an hour-glass-shaped plug* containing the electrodes, which is placed in the anal canal. Collins et al. (1968, 1969) have also used this method and found that the sphincter muscle responded for only a minute or so after the current was switched on, so that they preferred to arrange the electrical circuit to provide intermittent stimulation. There has also been some difference of opinion as to whether the plug should be worn for most of the day, or only for one or two hours daily. Duthie (1971) has given a useful summary of the results

* Made by Cardiac Recorders Ltd, 377 City Road, London EC1.

obtained in several centres using anal stimulation for various degrees of rectal prolapse with incontinence, including some patients with complete prolapse. Of 52 patients treated with intra-anal plugs, 21 were said to show some symptomatic improvement and one to be cured. My own experience of ten patients with mainly mucosal prolapse and lax sphincters, treated by intra-anal plugs for one to two hours daily, was that three or four were possibly slightly improved symptomatically, but this improvement could have have been largely a psychological effect. There was certainly no discernible objective change in the state of the sphincter muscles. All the patients tired of the treatment in time and asked to be allowed to discontinue using the plugs. Altogether, I am not at all impressed with the achievements of this form of treatment.

3. ENCIRCLEMENT OF THE ANAL ORIFICE WITH SILVER WIRE (Thiersch 1891), SILK (Henschen 1912), FASCIA (Henschen 1912; Schmerz 1918), TENDON OR MUSCLE (Schumacker 1934), POLYTHYLENE (Schwartz and Marin 1962), TEFLON (Haskell and Rovner 1963) OR NYLON (Plumley 1966)

The Thiersch Operation

This procedure had been largely discarded in the English-speaking world till 1951, when its use was reviewed by Gabriel, and since then it has become very popular in Britain and America. Thiersch (1891) had imagined that circumanal wiring would be beneficial in two ways: (a) by mechanically supporting and containing the prolapse, and (b) by provoking a reaction in the tissues of the anal region, leading to the development of a ring of fibrosis reinforcing the atonic sphincters. On this basis it seemed reasonable to hope that after a time, say in six or twelve months, it might be possible to remove the wire leaving the prolapse to be controlled solely by the fibrosed anal orifice. My experience of 24 cases treated by me by Thiersch wiring and some 25 others treated by my colleagues by this method, has shown that, on the contrary, the wire is relatively non-irritating and does not stimulate a significant tissue reaction around it. It is as easily and distinctly palpable after a year as it was at the time of its insertion, and, on its removal after such an interval, only a slight fibrous ring can ever be palpated. Its withdrawal is inevitably followed by recurrence of the prolapse. To be effective, therefore, it must be retained indefinitely. In many cases, particularly with smaller prolapses, this is quite possible without discomfort or other ill-effect. But in others, especially if the wire has been made rather too tight, there is interference with the passage of motions and a tendency to the occurrence of faecal accumulation, if great care is not taken in the postoperative regulation of bowel habits. Faecal impaction in the case with a Thiersch wire may be a singularly frustrating experience for the patient, and also very troublesome to the surgeon because of the impediment to disimpaction presented by the wire.

In patients with really large prolapses, however, it is unusual for the wire to remain indefinitely without complications. In most cases of this kind the wire eventually either breaks, with immediate return of the prolapse, or cuts through the tissues and becomes exposed in the perianal region. In the latter circumstances infection is inevitable, and in either event the wire must be removed. There is no reason why another ring should not be inserted at a later date and provide control of the prolapse for a further period. I have had three patients who have had the wire reintroduced in this way on two or three occasions and are reasonably comfortable.

One of the great virtues of the Thiersch operation is that it involves a minimal degree of surgical trauma and can if necessary be easily performed under local anaesthesia (for operative details see p. 249). It is thus specially suited for elderly patients in poor general condition, and no patient need be considered too frail to undergo this minor operation. Another attraction of the method is that if it does not produce a satisfactory result it can easily be undone by withdrawl of the wire. As against it is the fact that it does not, properly speaking, cure rectal prolapse but merely confines it within the anal canal. It is thus a palliative rather than a curative measure. For that reason I no longer use this method when the patient is fit to stand a more major operation which offers a chance of cure.

Recent Modifications of the Thiersch Operation

To overcome the risk of the wire breaking, which occurs not infrequently after the classical Thiersch operation, White (1961) has suggested the use of *a rigid stainless steel ring* (British Standard En 58 J) in place of wire. The ring consists of a hollow needle having a diameter of 2·5 mm, its length curving through five-eighths of a circle 2·5 cm in diameter. Into it slides a close-fitting stilette of the same curve but 2 cm longer. The stilette can be made to emerge from the sharp end of the needle and slide round until its point enters the tail end of the latter for 2 cm, thus forming a complete circle. The stilette moves with the needle with considerable friction so that there is no tendency for it to slip out of position once it has been set. The ring is introduced in the 'open' position (i.e. with the stilette mainly inside the hollow needle) through two small perianal incisions, and once in the tissues the stilette is manipulated, by means of special needle holders with circular notches cut into the jaws, into the 'closed' position. The manoeuvring is apparently somewhat clumsy and there is a real risk of perforating the lining of the anal canal with resulting infection as happened in one of White's (1961) seven cases. Also I would judge that the ring is a little too wide to provide proper control of a prolapse in the average patient. (The ring and forceps are made by Murphy Boyle of London.)

Plastic materials have been used instead of wire for the Thiersch operation: polyethylene (Schwartz and Marin 1962), nylon tapes (which are apt to give rise to sinus formation), and crimped Teflon tubes as used for arterial grafting (Haskell and Rovner 1963). The slight elasticity of the Teflon is said to give a particularly good functional result, but it also occasionally provokes sinus formation. Plumley (1966) has argued a good case for ordinary monofilament nylon as the structure material to employ for the Thiersch operation. No. 2 (22 SWG) is the size of the strand used and it is passed round the anus three times, being finally tied posteriorly with three reef knots. Baker (1970) reports that in 62 cases in which this technique with nylon was used, the suture broke (or the knot slipped) in three, cut out in eleven, had to be removed because of faecal impaction or infection in seven, and recurrent mucosal prolapse occurred in eleven. These results are certainly rather better than I have had using wire.

High or Supralevator Thiersch Operation

Notaras (1973) has devised a variant of the Thiersch operation, in which the surround of foreign material is placed, not in the subcutaneous tissue of the perianal region but at a higher level in the perirectal tissue immediately above the levator muscles. For the surround he uses a ribbon of Teflon (I personally have employed a strip of nylon mesh, rolled up like a cigarette).

The operation is performed with the patient in the lithotomy position under a general anaesthetic. After sterilization of the perianal, perineal and vaginal skin, suitable towelling and temporary closure of the anus by a subcutaneous pursestring suture of silk, two small transverse incisions, about 4–5 cm long, are made behind and in front of the anus. The posterior one is deepened through the fat and the superficial and deep anococcygeal raphes (see Fig. 3), to enter the supralevator region. The anterior wound is next deepened in the plane between the vagina and the anal canal, to reach the same level in front of the rectum as has been achieved behind, though it is important to emphasize that the anterior dissection is a good deal more difficult than the posterior one. The index finger can then be thrust forwards from the posterior wound, first on one side of the rectum and then on the other, immediately above the levators, to reach the upper end of the anterior wound in the space between the levators. Two large curved artery forceps or cholecystectomy forceps are now passed backwards on either side of the bowel from the anterior wound to emerge through the posterior one. They grasp the two ends of the nylon tube, which are pulled forwards as the forceps are withdrawn. The limbs of the nylon surround are then crossed anteriorly and pulled taut, so as to grip the bowel snugly, the perianal pursestring suture having meanwhile been removed and a size 18 Hegar dilator inserted into the anal canal and lower rectum to ensure the maintenance of an adequate lumen. The crossed limbs are sutured together—preferably with a 2–3-cm overlap—with at least five or six non-absorbable stitches, and the excess of plastic material is cut off. Finally the anterior and posterior wounds are closed with a few buried catgut sutures for the aponeurotic structures and fat, and silk stitches for the skin.

The averages of this technique over the classical Thiersch operation are that the surround seems less likely to cut out and appears to give more effective support to the bowel and control of the prolapse, especially when the latter is complete. On the debit side is the fact that, in order to introduce the plastic surround at this level, formal dissections are required, instead of two tiny stab wounds. These take at least 10–15 minutes and require a general anaesthetic. Of the four patients whom I have so far had the opportunity to treat by this method, one developed severe wound sepsis which, rather surprisingly, settled under systemic antibiotic therapy, without extrusion of the plastic material, and with a good eventual result. Another, who had an uneventful postoperative course in hospital developed recurrence of her complete prolapse some weeks after returning home. I suspect that this was due to giving way of the anterior fixing sutures, which in this instance were of silk, and since then have always used nylon for these stitches. The other two cases had uneventful convalescences and good results.

My feeling is that the high Thiersch operation may have a place in the therapy of complete prolapse as an alternative to the more certain method of abdominal repair or fixation in specially unfit subjects, for whom the latter would carry very grave risks.

4. NARROWING OF THE ANUS BY FIBROSIS PRODUCED BY A CIRCULAR INCISION IN THE PERINEAL REGION LEFT TO GRANULATE (Saraffof 1937, 1942)

This method, which makes use of a ring of cicatrical tissue instead of introducing foreign material, achieves an effect similar to that of the Thiersch operation. It was introduced by Saraffof (1937, 1942), and recent accounts of extended experiences with it have been given by Marchiori and Tomasini (1962) and Zängl (1965). The operation consists in making a circular incision around the anus (or a double concentric incision, with removal of a ring of skin about 1 cm wide) which is deepened into the perianal connective tissue just external to the sphincters to a depth of about 1 cm; the superficial ano-coccygeal raphe is divided posteriorly and some of the fibres of the external sphincter running forward to the perineal body are severed anteriorly. The resulting moat-like wound is then packed with gauze and assiduously repacked during postoperative management, to ensure that slow healing by granulation takes place. The consequence is that a firm ring of fibrous tissue forms which contracts the anal orifice. In some of the reported cases the opening would barely take the tip of the index finger, and massive complete prolapses were often well controlled by it (Marchiori and Tomasini 1962). Zängl claimed that in 23 cases treated by the Saraffof operation there were no operative deaths, and 21 patients had 'very gratifying' results, with only one recurrence.

5. SUTURE OF THE PUBORECTALES MUSCLES BY THE PERINEAL ROUTE (McCann 1928)

In this operation, which was introduced by McCann (1928), an incision was made into the perineum anterior to the anus, and, in the female, extending into the vagina as well. Through this approach the puborectales muscles were exposed and sutured together in front of the rectum. The external anal sphincter, which was also exposed in the wound, was also tightened anteriorly by sutures and the wound was then closed. *The pelvic peritoneum was not opened.* The whole operation very closely resembled the sort of perineorrhaphy employed by gynaecologists in the treatment of a rectocele. Twelve patients treated by McCann's operation at St Mark's Hospital were reviewed by Hughes (1949); the prolapse had recurred in all of them.

6. POSTERIOR FIXATION OF THE RECTUM FROM BELOW

Methods to accomplish this *by suture* of the posterior rectal wall to the sacrum and coccyx were described by Lange (1887), Verneuil (1891), Tuttle (1903), and Gant (1923). The better known procedure of this kind, however, is that of Sick (1909), popularized in Britain and America by J. P. Lockhart-Mummery (1910), in which the development of adhesions between the rectum and sacrum was stimulated *by temporary gauze packing* of the presacral space. The latter method was attractive because of its simplicity. With the patient lying on his side with his knees and hips flexed, a short transverse incision was made midway between the anus and the tip of the coccyx. This was deepened through the musculo-aponeurotic tissues to allow the finger access to the presacral space, which was thoroughly opened up. The resulting cavity was then packed with iodoform gauze for three weeks to promote the development of adhesions.

Lockhart-Mummery (1934) himself claimed excellent results from this operation, but Hughes (1949) managed to trace 29 of 32 patients treated by it at St Mark's Hospital and found that they had all had recurrence!

7. PARTIAL EXCISION OF THE RECTUM THROUGH THE ANUS

Two operations of this kind are available, *rectosigmoidectomy or amputation of the prolapse* (Mikulicz 1889; Miles 1933) and *mucosal sleeve resections* (Delorme 1900).

Rectosigmoidectomy (Amputation of the Prolapse)

Due to the firm advocacy of Miles (1933) and Gabriel (1948) this operation was, till a few years ago, the treatment most generally favoured in this country for complete rectal prolapse. The term 'amputation' applied to the method is unfortunate for it implies

merely an excision of the projecting portion of the bowel in the prolapsed condition. This gives an inaccurate conception of the procedure, which actually involves a much more extensive resection of bowel than would be effected by such a manoeuvre. Once the outer of the two tubes of rectal wall in the prolapse has been circularly divided it is possible to draw the inner tube of rectum down a considerable distance thus bringing the distal sigmoid down to the anal region, where it is divided and sutured to the anal remnant. The operation is thus aptly termed a recto-sigmoidectomy, the name given it by Miles in 1933. The specimen of excised bowel generally amounts to 15–25 cm at least, and there is certainly no slack rectum or distal colon at the conclusion of the operation to allow of further prolapse. (Full operative details p. 251).

Miles (1933) and Gabriel (1948) have claimed excellent results for this operation and in addition have emphasized its great safety—an important feature in any procedure for this non-lethal disease which so often affects elderly frail subjects. In 1949, however, Hughes surveyed the outcome in 150 consecutive cases of rectal prolapse treated by rectosigmoidectomy at St Mark's Hospital. He confirmed that this was indeed a very safe operation for there had been no operative deaths in this series. But that was the only good thing about the results. No less than 60% of the patients had suffered recurrences, and over half the cases—some with recurrence, some without—were also incontinent. It was thought by Hughes and myself (Goligher and Hughes 1951) that this incontinence was partly or mainly sensory in type, due to excision of the sensitive anorectal mucosa by the rectosigmoidectomy, but we recognized that another factor in its production was almost certainly the atrophied and atonic state of the anal sphincters and levator musculature. Possibly the risks of impairment of rectal sensation with resulting incontinence could be reduced by modifying the technique of operation to ensure retention of a cuff of at least 4 cm of anorectal mucosa in the anal remnant. It also seems probable that some of the imperfections of sensation in these cases represent an unavoidable continuation of a preoperative deficiency. But an operation that is followed by recurrence in over half the patients treated by it can scarcely be regarded as satisfactory.

A number of surgeons, such as Cohn (1942), Gabriel (1948), Morgan (1951) and, most consistently, Altemeier et al. (1952, 1964, 1971), have attempted to improve the results of recto-sigmoidectomy by inserting a few catgut or non-absorbable sutures in the puborectalis muscles during the course of the operation, if they can be easily identified, to bring them together in front of the rectum and thereby reinforce the pelvic floor. One might well doubt the durability and efficacy of such suturing in a potentially contaminated field. In fact, a collective report by Porter (1962b) on a further series of 109 cases of complete prolapse treated (at St Mark's hospital, London) by recto-sigmoidectomy between 1948 and 1960, in many of which such suturing of the levator muscles was practised, shows that the results are just as unsatisfactory as they were found to be by Hughes in 1949, with the recurrence rate still in the region of 60%.

Knowledge of the ultimately unfavourable outcome after rectosigmoidectomy has been followed by a considerable waning in the popularity of this operation in Great Britain in favour of abdominal repairs. But the method, with suture of the levator muscles for reinforcement, is apparently being used to an increasing extent in North America, where it is particularly associated with the name of Altemeier of Cincinnati. Though he writes with enthusiasm about this operation and has had excellent immediate results, with no operative mortality in 106 cases treated by it, I have been unable to discover in his writings (Altemeier et al. 1964, 1971) any clear account of the late results, based on a systematic follow-up of these patients. In a recent personal communication, however, Dr Altemeir tells me that he has had six recurrences in just over 200 cases.

Delorme's Operation

With the bowel fully prolapsed a circular incision is made through the mucosa 1–2 cm from the pectinate line. This cut is deepened down to the submucosa but no farther. The mucosa is then dissected off the underlying muscular coat as a sleeve, till the apex of the prolapse is reached where it is cut off. It will be readily appreciated that this manoeuvre may involve a fair amount of bleeding. The effect is to leave the outer aspect of the prolapse devoid of mucosal covering. Next the raw surface is closed by a series of sutures which pass through the cut edge of the mucosa at the base of the prolapse, then take several bites of the bared muscularis, and finally catch up the cut edge of the mucosa at the apex of the prolapse. When these are tied, they bunch up or reef the muscle coat and bring the edges of the mucosa together.

This procedure was at one stage employed not only in France but also in America, where it enjoyed the support of David (1947), Hayden (1947), Swinton and Palmer (1960) and Blair et al. (1963), and was at one stage widely used. But it leaves untouched the main anatomical defects and would seem in effect to be nothing more than a half-hearted amputation of the prolapse, which one would expect ought to carry most of the disadvantages of the latter operation, including a high recurrence rate in the long run. However, moderately encouraging early and medium-term results have been reported by Hayden (1947), Swinton and Palmer (1960) and Blair et al. (1963) on the basis of a small series of cases, and Nay and Blair (1972) have published the outcome of a 2–23-year follow-up on 30 patients treated by this method with only three recurrences.

8. APPROACH BY THE SACRAL ROUTE TO EXCISE SOME OF THE PELVIC PERITONEAL POUCH AND TO SUTURE THE PUBORECTALES, WITH OR WITHOUT RESECTION OF PART OF THE RECTUM

Jenkins and Thomas (1962) have strongly recommended the sacral or Kraske type of approach (see p. 503) in the treatment of complete rectal prolapse, as have Hagihara and Griffen (1975). With the patient in the prone or lateral, semi-prone position, one of the many incisions available for this approach is used, and the coccyx and lowermost two pieces of the sacrum are excised. The fascia of Waldeyer is then incised in the midline and the levatores ani are separated to expose the rectum. The dissection is carried round either side of the latter to reach the vagina or prostate and seminal vesicles anteriorly. These organs are separated from the front of the rectum, and as this process is continued downwards the superior surface and inner edges of the puborectales are defined with a view to subsequent suture. At a higher level the lateral fornix of the pouch of Douglas is encountered and opened. In their earlier cases Thomas and Jenkins (1965) resected the lower part of the sigmoid and the upper two-thirds of the rectum and restored continuity by end-to-end anastomosis, but more recently they have avoided excision of bowel. The next step is the suture of the puborectales opposite the space between the rectum and vagina. For this purpose No. 30 wire is used, from two to four sutures being inserted. Then the peritoneum of the pouch of Douglas is freed from the pelvic side walls and the vagina or bladder, the redundant portion of the sac is excised, and the peritoneal floor is reconstituted by suture at a higher level.

A few sutures may be placed between the posterior and lateral walls of the rectum and the fascia covering the sacrum and lateral pelvic walls to help to anchor the bowel in position. The levators are then closed in the midline posteriorly and over these the pelvic fascia and skin, the presacral space being drained with suction drainage for two or three days.

Davidian and Thomas (1972) report on the results obtained in 30 cases treated by this method. There were no operative deaths. In a few patients, on whom a partial resection of rectum and lower sigmoid was practised at the time of the repair, trouble-some wound infection or faecal fistulation occurred, necessitating the establishment of a temporary transverse colostomy. In the remaining patients, in whom no bowel was excised, the surgical complications were slight. There have been no recurrences of the prolapse to date, the period of follow-up ranging from one to eleven years. The functional results are claimed to be good, with satisfactory continence in 20 patients; however, some of the cases were mental defectives, which must have made assessment of rectal function difficult!

It will be seen that this operation accomplishes the same objectives as the better known abdominal (or abdomino-perineal) repair associated with the names of Roscoe Graham and Dunphy (see pp. 238 and 242), the only difference being in the method of approach. Probably, therefore, the results on a more extended trial will be similar to those of the later operation. The advantages which the sacral operation may possibly enjoy over the abdominal one are two-fold: that a wound in the sacral region may cause less disturbance of respiratory function than does an abdominal wound and may be associated with less morbidity and even a lower mortality rate than the latter; and also that the access is more direct from behind, possibly making the repair rather easier. But as against this is the fact that surgeons in general are very familiar with the abdominal approach from their experience in the treatment of malignant disease of the rectum, whereas very few are acquainted with the sacral approach.

ABDOMINAL (OR ABDOMINOPERINEAL) OPERATIONS

1. COLOPEXY

Jeannel (1896) endeavoured to hold the rectum up by fixing the taut pelvic colon to the peritoneum of the left iliac fossa. Ball (1908) and Hartmann (1931) adopted a similar technique. More usually, however, colopexy was employed in conjunction with other manoeuvres, as, for example, with suture of the pelvic peritoneal pouch (Quénu and Duval 1910; Bacon 1949) or with posterior fixation of the rectum (Pemberton and Stalker 1939) (see below).

2. OBLITERATION OR ELEVATION OF THE ABNORMALLY DEEP RECTOVAGINAL OR -VESICAL POUCH OF PERITONEUM

These operations are based on the conception that complete rectal prolapse is really a form of sliding hernia, the abnormally deep pouch of Douglas constituting the hernial sac, so that it became the main target for surgical attack.

The Moschcowitz Operation

This procedure was described first by the French surgeons, Quénu and Duval (1910), who usually combined it with a colopexy to fix the sigmoid colon to the left iliac fossa. But Moschcowitz (1912) of the Mount Sinai Hospital, New York, gave a very clear account of the rationale and technique, and the operation is now usually associated with his name in the British and American literature. He employed a series of purse-string sutures of silk running horizontally round the pouch of Douglas, placed in tiers at intervals of about 2·5 cm from the depths of the pelvis almost up to the pelvic brim. Great care was taken not to include the ureters in the bite of these stitches; to facilitate their identification and avoidance, it subsequently became the practice with some surgeons such as Rankin and Priestley (1933), to insert ureteric catheters immediately prior to the operation.

The long-term results of this type of operation are not very encouraging. Bacon (1949) treated 24 patients by a combined Moschcowitz operation and colopexy, with only three recurrences, but he failed to state how long the cases had been followed. Hughes (1949) managed to trace six of nine patients submitted to the Moschcowitz operation at St Mark's Hospital and found that one had died, four had recurred and one appeared well. Pemberton et al. (1953) reported on 55 cases treated by a modified Moschcowitz operation at the Mayo Clinic with one operative death; of 46 cases traced over two years, 29 or 63% had recurred.

The Mayo Operation

Mayo (1938) described a method in which the pelvic peritoneal pouch is elevated out of the pelvis and then supported in this position by strips of transplanted fascia stitched across the pelvic brim. No long-term results are available for this method, and from a later report from the Mayo Clinic by Beahrs et al. (1965) it does not seem that the operation has found favour even in the centre from which it originated.

3. PROCEDURES TO REPAIR THE PELVIC STRUCTURES AND FIX THE RECTUM

As most of these techniques involve two or more principles of treatment it is not easy to categorize them, and they will be referred to below mainly by eponymous designations.

The Roscoe Graham (or Dunphy) Operation

Roscoe Graham (1942) of Toronto recommended a purely abdominal approach to mobilize the rectum, expose and suture the levator muslces in front of the rectum, and remove the deep pouch of Douglas. In theory this would seem to be a much more satisfying operation than the Moschowitz procedure and it has been warmly favoured by Snellman (1954, 1961, 1965), Goligher (1958), Palmer (1961) and Küpfer and Goligher (1970). Goligher (1958) emphasized that an essential initial step in this operation is full mobilization of the rectum down to the anorectal ring and that if this is done suture of the levator muscles from above can be accomplished in a convincing manner (for operative details see p. 242).

But some surgeons, such as Dunphy (1948), now of San Francisco, Brintnall (1952), Newell (1954), Butler (1954) and Hughes et al. (1957), deterred by the anticipated technical difficulties of such a deep pelvic dissection, have employed a combined abdominoperineal technique for these repairs. Dunphy (1948) incorporated a rectosigmoidectomy in the perineal phase, but it seems preferable from the functional point of view to avoid removal of any part of the bowel and to rely on the repair above for cure of the prolapse. Though the perineal and abdominal dissections can be performed conclusively by the same surgeon, it is a convenience to have the legs supported on the Lloyd-Davies leg rests (see p. 526) so that the dissections from

above and below can be conducted simultaneously by two operators. For the perineal phase a transverse incision is made between the vaginal introitus and the anus and can if desired be prolonged up the posterior vaginal wall. The wound is deepened to expose the puborectalis parts of the levator muscles on either side. They are then approximated by three or four deep sutures of chromic catgut or other suture material. For this purpose Hughes and Gleadell (1962) of Melbourne use a specially long, almost straight, 15-cm needle which is passed upwards through the medial part of the levator muscle on one side to the abdominal operator, who then rethreads it and hands it back to the perineal operator. He uses it again to pass the other end of the catgut strand upwards through the opposite levator muscle. When all the sutures have been inserted they are tied from above. For the rest, the abdominal phase follows the lines of the Roscoe Graham operation.

The value of these operations for abdominal or abdomino-perineal repair has remained *sub judice* till recently, because insufficient cases so treated had been followed up for a long enough period of time. However, an impression is now beginning to emerge from reports in the literature on late reviews of 305 patients with complete prolapse submitted to these forms of repair *without bowel resection* (Table 6). The operative mortality was only 0·7% and the recurrence rate to date only 11·7%. It seems probable that the latter may increase in time but unlikely that it will ever reach the high figure found after rectosigmoidectomy. Information regarding the functional results in several of the reports is scanty, but I know from my own cases that rectal function is often far from perfect. I would say that about half the patients have apparently normal continence; in the remainder there is a varying degree of uncertainty of anal control, amounting to frank incontinence in approximately one-quarter. In most of the patients affected by incontinence, it seems to be due to a continuation of a pre-operative weakness of sphincter tone, which did not improve after operation, and to an inherent obtuseness of anorectal sensation dating from before operation. Occasionally there may possibly be some degree of sensory impairment attributable to the mobilization of the rectum during the repair (Goligher and Hughes 1951).

It is interesting to speculate as to how these repairs achieve a cure of rectal prolapse, and particularly as to the contribution made by the puborectalis suture. I have always felt (Goligher 1958) that the main mechanism of cure of the Roscoe Graham type of operation was probably the formation of firm adhesions around the rectum following the extensive rectal mobilization, which is an integral part of the technique of the repair. The value of the sutures in the levator muscles would appear to be very temporary. During the first few weeks after the operation the rectum can be felt on digital examination to be firmly gripped and even constricted by these stitches and the puborectalis sling, and I can believe that it would be difficult for the bowel to prolapse through this ring of narrowing (which is usually situated, incidentally, not at, but 1 or 2 cm above, the anorectal ring). On re-examination a year or so later the sutures can often be very distinctly felt anteriorly, but there is no suggestion of a constriction, which would prevent a recurrence of the prolapse. It would seem, therefore, that the most that can be expected from repair of the puborectalis is temporary support till such time as the rectum becomes fixed by adhesions.

The Pemberton–Stalker Suspension-Fixation Operation

In this operation, described by Pemberton and Stalker (1939) of the Mayo Clinic, the abdomen is opened and incisions are made

TABLE 6. *Collective Results from Literature of Abdominal and Abdominoperineal Repairs of Complete Rectal Prolapse Without Resection of the Bowel*

Author	Method used	No. of cases treated and followed up	Period of follow-up	Operative deaths	Recurrences
Palmer (1961)	Abdominal	23	3–22 years	0	0
Snellman (1965)	Abdominal	100	?	0	10
Butler (1962)	Abdominal	21	6 months to 8 years	0	4
Hughes and Gleadell (1962)	Abdomino-perineal mainly	84	3 months to 11 years	1	9
Porter (1962b)	Abdominal	14	1½–8 years	0	0
Küpfer and Goligher (1970)	Abdominal	63	12 months to 15 years	1*	5†
All authors combined		305		2 (0·7%)	28 (11·8%)

* From pulmonary embolism.

† One recurrence treated by low anterior resection, one by a second Roscoe Graham type of repair, one by Thiersch wiring and later abdominoperineal excision of the rectum and the remaining two by Ivalon sponge repairs.

in the peritoneum on either side of the lower sigmoid mesocolon and mesorectum. The hand is then passed down into the retro-rectal connective tissue space to lift the rectum upwards and forwards out of the sacral concavity. The sigmoid colon is then fixed in its elevated position by stitching it to the peritoneum of the anterior abdominal wall, pelvic brim, iliac fossa or uterus. Upward traction on the sigmoid and forward displacement of the rectum is thus maintained and the space which forms between the rectum and the sacrum is believed subsequently to fill with fibrous tissue fixing the bowel to the bone. The operation is thus a combined posterior fixation of the rectum and colopexy.

Pemberton et al. (1953) have reported on the late results of this operation in a series of 56 cases treated by it at the Mayo Clinic. There were no operative deaths, and in 44 of the cases traced over two years there were only five recurrences. The functional state of their patients was not discussed. However, a later report by Beahrs et al. (1965) on a longer follow-up of patients treated by the Pemberton operation gives a recurrence rate of 34·6% in 52 patients treated between 1951 and 1962, which is much less satisfactory. Rectal function was considered good in just over half the cases, and fair or poor each in approximately a quarter of the cases.

Moore (1969) of Exeter has described what might be regarded as a modification of the Pemberton–Stalker operation. The abdomen is opened by a long left oblique muscle-cutting incision. The rectum is freely mobilized and lifted strongly upwards and forwards, the left uterine tube and round ligament being divided to allow the straightened bowel to lie on the left side of the bladder. Sutures are then inserted between the lower rectum and the anterior pelvic wall, whilst the upper rectum and rectosigmoid are drawn out of the abdominal wound. Finally, the abdominal parietes are closed around the protruding bowel, the peritoneum, transversus abdominis and internal oblique being sutured behind the loop, the external oblique, fat and skin superficial to it. Moore (1969) has treated 12 patients by this method in a period of six years with no operative deaths but with two recurrences at three and four years respectively. Gordon and

Miller (1971) of Glasgow have also modified the technique of the Pemberton–Stalker operation, making the mobilization of the bowel much more extensive, and reported on 27 patients treated by this method over a 12-year period; there was only one recurrence.

Presacral Rectopexy by Simple Suture

This method, developed by Cutait (1959) of Sao Paolo, Brazil, also aims at posterior fixation of the rectum. The rectum is mobilized out of the sacral concavity as in the Pemberton–Stalker operation and pulled strongly upwards. No anterior dissection is performed and the lateral ligaments are not divided. Fixation of the bowel in its elevated position is then secured by passing four or five sutures of non-absorbable material or catgut between the rectal wall on one side and the fascia on the front of the sacrum. No attempt is made to obliterate or remove the pouch of Douglas or to fix the colon. No long-term follow-up seems to be available on the results of this operation.

In recent years I have adopted a modification of this operation in which the first instance the rectum is fully mobilized and freed down to the anorectal ring and then it is fixed by a series of silk sutures passed between the presacral fascia and the fascia, fat and muscle coat of the posterior rectal wall (Fig. 173). In 42 cases so treated there has been no significant morbidity or mortality and no recurrences to date, but the longest period of follow-up is only five years, so that the value of the method is still very much *sub judice*.

The Orr Operation

This procedure, which was introduced by Orr (1947) of Kansas City, aims at fixing the rectum by means of two strips of fascia lata, which are sutured above to the promontory of the sacrum and below to the sides and front of the rectum. The method does not seem to have secured much favour, but one surgeon, J. Loygue of Paris, has used a modification of it extensively and with very good results (Loygue et al. 1971). He emphasizes the importance of a full mobilization of the rectum as the first step in the operation. For the actual fixation he has abandoned the use of fascia lata in favour of two strips of nylon mesh. Each strip is sutured inferiorly to the side and front of the rectum, as far distally as possible, by eight to ten stitches over a length of 5–6 cm, and superiorly to the anterior longitudinal ligament on the front of the sacrum, as far from the midline as possible, by four to six sutures. The rectovesical or rectouterine pouch is obliterated by peritoneal sutures and the abdomen is closed with suction drainage to the presacral space. This procedure has been employed by Loygue et al. (1971) 146 times in 140 patients between 1953 and 1970 inclusive, with two operative deaths. On a careful follow-up, recurrence of the complete prolapse was found to have taken place in five patients (3·6%).

The Perirectal Implantation of Polyvinyl Alcohol Sponge

Impressed by the work of Schofield (1955) on the use of Ivalon (polyvinyl alcohol sponge) in the repair of abdominal herniae, Wells of Liverpool (1955) developed a technique employing this substance for the treatment of complete rectal prolapse. The principle is to mobilize the rectum fully through an abdominal approach and then to wrap a thin sheet of the plastic sponge round it to encourage subsequent fixation of the bowel to the surrounding parts (for operative details see p. 246). Some surgeons might feel reluctant to bury this amount of foreign material in the tissues because of the risk of intractable fistulation if sepsis should occur. It is also known that polyvinyl alcohol sponge is capable of stimulating the development of sarcoma in rats; but this species is very prone to produce malignant tumours when provoked by a variety of plastic substances, and it is unlikely that this risk applies to the human (Dukes and Mitchley 1962; Calnan 1963; Walter and Chiaramonte 1965). It should be appreciated by surgeons using this material that in the fullness of time it undergoes disintegration and slow absorption (Chen et al. 1969).

My own experience of the Ivalon sponge operation (Küpfer and Goligher 1970) comprises 35 patients treated by this method (combined in a few instances with a simultaneous abdominal repair of Roscoe Graham type), with one operative death due to coronary thrombosis. In four cases I am ashamed to record that pelvic sepsis occurred and did not clear up until the sponge was removed, but to date there have been no recurrences of the prolapse in these septic cases or in any others, the follow-up period being six months to four years. A survey of the results of the Ivalon sponge operation in a collective series of 101 cases treated by this operation at St Mark's Hospital, London, is given by Penfold and Hawley (1972). There were no operative deaths, but four patients developed postoperative sepsis, necessitating removal of the Ivalon in one. A follow-up of two to ten years was maintained on 95 cases; three have so far developed a recurrent complete prolapse and 31 a mucosal prolapse. Continence was improved in 20–30% of cases after operation. Stewart (1972) has reported on the results in a similar collective series of 40 patients treated by this operation at the Gordon Hospital, London, and folowed up for one to ten years (mean 5½ years). There were three complete recurrences and ten mucosal recurrences, whilst continence was enhanced in some two-thirds of the cases. Morgan et al. (1972) have recorded their personal experiences with the Ivalon sponge repair in 150 patients operated on between 1959 and 1972. There were four operative deaths and four cases were complicated by postoperative sepsis necessitating removal of the sponge. Follow-up information was available on only 93 cases; three had developed recurrent complete prolapses and eight mucosal prolapses. There was an improvement in anal control in roughly one-third of the patients after operation.

Ripstein's Operation

In 1952 Ripstein, now of Florida, described a technique for treating complete rectal prolapse. This involved full mobilization of the rectum, excision of the rectovaginal pouch of peritoneum and suture of the levator muscles in front of the rectum, exactly as in the Roscoe Graham repair (see pp. 242–5), but also included the placing of a sheet of fascia lata to reinforce the anterior repair of the levators, to support the pelvic peritoneum and to hold the rectum back against the sacrum. The fascial graft was V-shaped, the apex being sutured to the fascia at the base of the bladder in the male (or to the cervix uteri in the female) and the lateral edges to the levator muscles near their origin. The limbs of the transplant were brought round either side of the rectum, crossed behind it and sutured to the tissue overlying the sacrum. The edges of the defect in the graft were then sutured to the rectal wall, the effect being that the rectum was encircled by a new fascial pelvic floor which provided firm anterior support and also held the bowel back against the hollow of the sacrum. The pelvic peritoneum was then approximated over the graft.

In 45 patients treated by this operation by Ripstein and Lanter (1963) a supplementary high anterior resection of the redundant sigmoid and upper rectum was performed in nearly half, and in a few more recent cases a sheet of Teflon mesh was used instead of fascia. There was one operative death from pulmonary embolism, and one patient developed a recurrence of the prolapse three months after operation. All the other patients were said to be alive and well at the time of review or to have died without recurrence. No clear statement was made regarding the functional results, but it was admitted that in some patients the relaxed state of the anus had led to postoperative incontinence, which had been a problem, and a subsequent gracilis sling operation was undertaken in five older cases.

Despite these encouraging results, in 1965 Ripstein devised an alternative simpler operation, which is the one now usually associated with his name. The essential feature of this operation is the fixation of the rectum to the sacral hollow by means of a sling of Teflon mesh in much the same way as in the Ivalon sponge procedure. The rectum is first of all thoroughly mobilized by dividing the lateral peritoneal reflections and, after blunt dissection, lifting the bowel out of the sacral concavity. Whilst the rectum is held tautly upwards, a sling of Teflon mesh 5 cm wide is passed round it and the ends are sutured to the fascia and peritoneum on the front of the sacrum about 5 cm below the promontory. In addition a few stitches are passed between the edges of the sling and the anterior and lateral rectal walls. No attempt is made to repair the pelvic floor. The lateral peritoneal incisions are re-sutured and the abdomen is closed.

Ripstein (1965) had treated 30 patients by this method in the previous four years with no immediate mortality or recurrences, but no further details of the results were given. Even in his latest publication (Ripstein 1972), in which he reports that he has now treated 289 patients mainly by this method, he does not give any precise follow-up data.

Rectal Plication

As mentioned on p. 226 Devadhar (1965) of Bombay believes that rectal prolapse is simply an intussusception of the rectum. According to him the initial or 'crucial point' of the intussusception is constant and can be identified with confidence at operation as the junction between the thick-walled lower part of the rectum and the thinner upper part. There is also said to be a thickening of the peritoneum covering the rectal wall in this area. He has described an operative technique in which the rectum is exposed and mobilized from the abdominal aspect and the crucial point is located by palpation. A purse-string suture of heavy silk is now inserted in the anterior and lateral walls of the rectum surrounding the crucial point. The stitch does not enter the lumen of the bowel but only goes as deep as the submucosa. Whilst the anterior rectal wall at the centre of the area surrounded by the suture is invaginated upwards to the lumen of the rectum, the stitch is tied. Three or four Lembert sutures are now used to increase the invagination and produce a condition of reversed intussusception. Next, two longitudinal plicating sutures are inserted along the exposed lateral rectal walls from just above the level of the crucial point to as low as possible. When tied they reef the rectal wall making it shorter and more rigid. Finally some of the pelvic peritoneum is excised and the pouch is closed by suture.

Devadhar (1965) has treated 28 cases by this method with no recurrences, ten of the patients having been followed up for at least five years. He attributes his success to the suturing, but it would not be unreasonable to suggest that the main curative factor has been the mobilization of the bowel with subsequent formation of fixing adhesions.

4. PARTIAL OR COMPLETE EXCISION OF THE RECTUM

Low Anterior Resection

This procedure was introduced by Muir (1955) for the treatment of complete rectal prolapse. He was led to try this operation by finding, in common with other surgeons, that a subsequent abdominoperineal excision for recurrent rectal carcinoma after a previous anterior resection is technically extremely difficult because of the adherence of the rectum and colon to the sacrum, particularly at the site of the anastomosis. This applies even when the recurrence is not on the suture line, as is usual, but elsewhere in the rectal stump. As a result of this experience Muir deduced that a low anterior resection might be useful in the treatment of rectal prolapse, for in addition to removing any slack rectum and sigmoid colon, making the bowel taut as after a colopexy and excising or obliterating the pouch of Douglas, it would fix the rectum securely to the sacrum (for operative details see p. 563). By 1962 he had treated up to 50 cases of prolapse by this operation; he had one operative death but no other serious

complications and no recurrence of complete prolapse, though a few patients did develop mucosal prolapses subsequently.

Abdominoperineal Excision

Complete excision of the rectum may seem a very drastic treatment for rectal prolapse, and could only legitimately be considered as a last resort but occasionally when a patient has had repeated recurrences following previous operations and is grossly incontinent an abdominoperineal excision with permanent iliac colostomy may be very acceptable.

II. THE AUTHOR'S EXPERIENCE AND PRESENT PRACTICE IN THE TREATMENT OF COMPLETE RECTAL PROLAPSE

It may be helpful at this juncture to indicate more precisely my own personal experience in the treatment of complete prolapse and my present opinion as to the best choice of operation. Table 7 records the operations that I myself have used in the management of 194 cases of complete rectal prolapse which have come under my care during the past 30 years. It should be pointed out that, if the prolapse recurred, two or even three operations might be performed on the same patient.

In the earlier years rectosigmoidectomy was the operation chiefly employed because it was the generally accepted method. As the poor results of the operation emerged it was discarded in favour of the abdominal repair of Roscoe Graham, which has given very good results in my hands. But I recognize that it is a technically somewhat difficult operation, especially in the male patient, for the average surgeon who does not treat many cases of prolapse.

TABLE 7. *215 Operations Performed by Author in the Treatment of 194 Cases of Complete Rectal Prolapse from 1947 to 1977*

Type of operation	No. of times employed	No. of operative deaths	No. of recurrences
Rectosigmoidectomy	14	0	7
Thiersch operation	28	0	Suture had to be removed 15 times because of breaking, cutting out or sepsis
High Thiersch operation (Notaras)	4	0	1
Perineorraphy	3	0	2
Abdominoperineal repair	3	0	0
Abdominal repair operation	79	2	6
Ivalon sponge operation	23	1	0
Abdominal repair plus Ivalon sponge implant	12	0	0
Prescacral rectopexy by simple suture	42	0	0
Anterior resection	4	0	0
Abdominoperineal excision	3	0	0

For him I am sure that the Ivalon sponge or Teflon sling operation—or the Orr type operation, using plastic material instead of fascia—will be more suitable. In fact the Ivalon sponge operation is undoubtedly now the most popular method of treating complete prolapse in Britain, even with so-called experts. The published results suggest that these three forms of rectopexy will all prove about as satisfactory as the Roscoe Graham repair, but sepsis may prove something of a problem with the implant operations. Still more recently I have been using a presacral rectopexy by simple suture in the majority of my cases, but, as pointed out on p. 239, the really long-term results of this method remain to be answered.

Anterior resection is another useful operation, well within the range of all general surgeons, who are usually employing it regularly in the treatment of cancer of the upper rectum and rectosigmoid, but I feel sure that in any sizeable series of cases of rectal prolapse, it could not fail to be followed by more complications than are these other operations.

A further matter to be considered in connection with these various abdominal operations for complete rectal prolapse is whether a *supplementary sphincteroplasty* (as described on p. 317) is also indicated in an effort to mitigate persisting incontinence associated with the lax state of the anal sphincters so often present in these patients. Parks (1976) has argued strongly for this additional step in the one-third of the patients whose incontinence is not improved by rectopexy and has obtained encouraging results with it. I must say that I have been much less impressed with the achievements of a subsequent sphincteroplasty in my cases. Indeed, if there should be particularly gross incontinence in a case of complete prolapse and the incontinence is the patient's main complaint—especially if the prolapse has recurred after a previous abdominal repair or rectopexy—I am convinced that the most satisfactory procedure to adopt is an abdomino-perineal excision of the rectum with a permanent iliac colostomy, if the patient can be induced to accept it.

For especially frail, unfit subjects to whom any of these abdominal operations might prove altogether too dangerous—and I would relegate very few patients to this category—I would recommend the Thiersch operation, using nylon instead of wire (or even employing the Notaras high technique). I should also add that occasionally, in dealing with an irreducible complete rectal prolapse in an adult or child, rectosigmoidectomy is still required.

III. OPERATIVE DETAILS OF METHODS FAVOURED BY AUTHOR

THE ROSCOE GRAHAM OPERATION

The first method to be described will be the Roscoe Graham repair, not because it is the most popular, but because the initial dissection is common to other forms of abdominal repair for prolapse as practised by me (Goligher 1958). The approach to the lower abdomen is as for any rectal excision, namely through a long left paramedian incision extending from the pubis well into the epigastric region, the patient being in a moderately steep Trendelenburg tilt. The wound edges are retracted with a self-retaining retractor possessing a third blade to retain the packed-off small gut in the upper abdomen. The iliac colon is now held towards the right side by the assistant whilst the adhesions binding it and the iliac mesocolon to the posterior parietal peritoneum of the left iliac fossa are divided with scissors. This step restores the entire sigmoid loop to its embryonic median position with a free mesocolon.

Attention is next turned to the pelvis proper. It is a useful preliminary to hitch up the uterus and adnexa by two stay sutures passed under the uterine tubes and attached to the towelling in the pubis region or to the abdominal wall. The abnormally deep pouch of Douglas is now seen to fullest advantage (Fig. 172). The peritoneal cut for mobilization of the rectum begins on the right side over the main inferior mesenteric artery about the level of the bifurcation of the abdominal aorta (Fig. 172). It is particularly to be noted that as it is carried forwards it does not descend into the pouch of Douglas but describes a smooth curve along the brim of the pelvis eventually reaching the midline just behind the tip of the cervix uteri. The cut on the left side commences over the left common iliac artery and is carried forwards in a similar manner skirting the pouch of Douglas to join the right-sided incision at the cervix uteri (Fig. 172).

The outer edges of this circumferential incision are now elevated sufficiently to expose the ureter on either side. The upper end of the left ureter is then pushed firmly laterally to separate it from the inferior mesenteric vessels, as a safeguard against ureteric injury during the subsequent dissection. The inner edge of the peritoneal cut is now brushed inwards all round so that the pouch of Douglas is collapsed on to the rectum. As this flap of peritoneum is dissected up at the proximal end of the incision on the right side, the inferior mesenteric

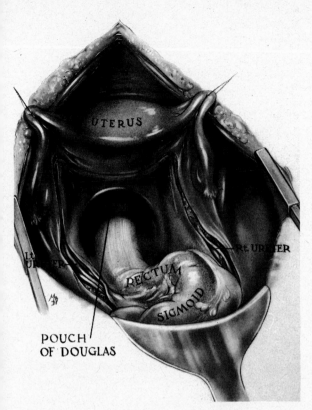

UTERUS

Lt URETER

Rt URETER

RECTUM

SIGMOID

POUCH
OF DOUGLAS

Fig. 172. View of the interior of the pelvis at laparotomy showing the deep pouch of Douglas and the peritoneal incision along the brim of the pelvis on either side. Note the exposure of the ureters in these sections. (*From Goligher 1958*)

to expose the posterior vaginal wall in front and the rectum behind. Further blunt dissection carries the separation down as far as the anorectal ring, bleeding from small vessels on the back of the vagina being checked by diathermy coagulation.

It only remains to divide the lateral ligaments to complete the freeing of the rectum. So far the front of the rectum and the connective tissues on either side of it, constituting the so-called lateral ligaments of the rectum, are still covered by the thin but very definite fascia of Denonvillier. A transverse cut is made in this fascia low down over the front of the rectum, and the lateral edge of the bowel clearly defined from the adjacent fat on either side by blunt dissection with the scissors. The hand is now re-introduced into the retrorectal space in front of the sacrum, and the index or middle finger worked forwards on the right side of the rectum to reach the point already established anteriorly, thus isolating the lateral ligament above the finger. This bulky band of tissue is then doubly clamped, divided and ligated close to the bowel. The lateral ligament on the opposite side is next isolated and severed in the same way.

The mobilization of the rectum has now been completed (Fig. 173). It will be seen that it differs from the dissection employed in an abdomino-perineal excision for carcinoma only in that particular care is taken to try to avoid damage to the autonomic nerves by dissecting out the presacral nerve and its branches above, and by keeping close to the rectum and as far away as possible from the parasympathetic nerves on the side wall of the pelvis when dividing the lateral ligaments.

The rectum is now drawn strongly upwards and slightly forwards and the point of junction of the bowel and the levator muscles examined posteriorly and laterally. Usually some further dissection of the connective tissue and fascia overlying this region is necessary with long curved scissors before the puborectalis sling can be clearly defined as it surrounds the bowel on these aspects (Fig. 174). The axis of traction of the rectum is then directed more backwards and the display of the muscles continued in front of the bowel on either side.

The scene is now set for the repair of the pelvic diaphragm. The sutures, which are of strong No. 15 silk or 5·5-kg braided nylon, may be introduced by a small stout half-circle needle on a long needle holder such as Mayo's, but are better placed by a small boomerang needle which can be much more easily manipulated in the depths of the pelvis. With the rectum pushed well backwards the initial stitch is inserted first in the left puborectalis muscle and

and superior rectal vessels are exposed. If the plane of dissection is now carried just deep to these vessels it will separate them from the presacral nerve. This plane of separation is followed downwards, the two terminal branches of the nerve being gently brushed off the rectum to which they cling very closely as they separate to run to either side of the pelvis. Long scissors can now be introduced between the rectum and sacrum to open up the soft presacral connective tissue sufficiently for the hand to be passed down behind the rectum as far as the tip of the coccyx. This completes the posterior mobilization.

Attention is next turned to the anterior dissection. The posterior edge of the initial cut in the peritoneum is seized by two long forceps on either side of the midline just behind the cervix uteri, and the corresponding anterior edge and cervix are drawn forwards by a wide deep retractor. A few scissor-cuts start the dissection which is then continued with gauze pushers on long forceps so as

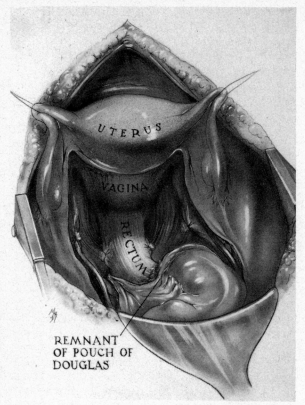

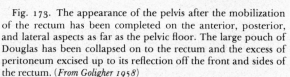

Fig. 173. The appearance of the pelvis after the mobilization of the rectum has been completed on the anterior, posterior, and lateral aspects as far as the pelvic floor. The large pouch of Douglas has been collapsed on to the rectum and the excess of peritoneum excised up to its reflection off the front and sides of the rectum. (*From Goligher 1958*)

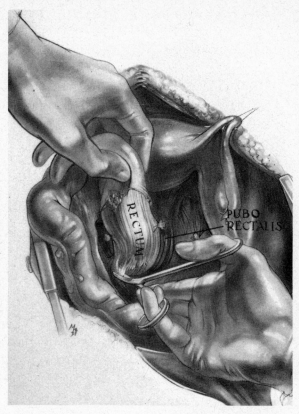

Fig. 174. Definition of the puborectalis sling. The rectum is drawn upwards and forwards, and strands of connective tissue proceeding from the rectal wall are divided with scissors to expose the puborectales clearly. (*From Goligher 1958*)

then in the right one, the point of penetration of the muscles being exactly lateral to the rectum (Figs 175 and 176). The result of siting the stitch so far back is that when it is drawn taut it sharply constricts the rectum and at first sight it would appear that it must be exerting injurious pressure on the bowel, but subsequent digital examination of the rectum per anum almost invariably reveals that there is still an ample lumen which admits three or four fingers easily. When this stitch is tied, the tails of the knot are kept long and clipped with forceps for traction, which brings the anterior portions of the puborectales muscles strongly into relief as two stout rods of muscle running forwards and laterally (Fig. 177). This step greatly facilitates the insertion of the remaining sutures. It is only at this stage that one realizes what substantial structures these muscles are despite their apparently atrophied condition on clinical examination. Usually three or four sutures

can be placed in the puborectales between the initial stitch and the vagina (Fig. 177 inset).

On a few occasions I have sutured the puborectales *behind* the rectum (Fig. 179) as originally suggested by Wookey of Toronto, according to Palmer (1961). It can be argued that this probably provides a more physiological arrangement in that it ought to accentuate the normal forward angulation of the anorectal junction. In one of the cases in which I employed this method I had had difficulty in completing the separation of the rectum from the prostate down to the top of the anal canal because of unusual bleeding. Under the circumstances it would have been difficult, if not impossible, to approximate or darn the puborectales in front of the rectum by suture, and this method of stitching them behind the rectum and pushing the rectum forwards against the prostate, from which it had not been separated, overcame this difficulty for me.

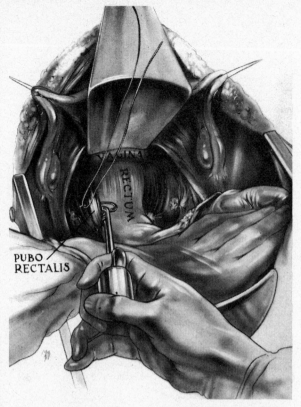

Fig. 175. Insertion of initial deep suture in puborectales. First stitch being placed in the left puborectalis with boomerang needle. (*From Goligher 1958*)

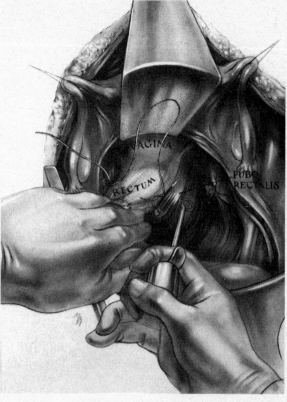

Fig. 176. Insertion of initial deep suture in puborectales. First stitch being carried through right puborectalis. (*From Goligher 1958*)

Reconstruction of the pelvic peritoneum is the next consideration. Some surgeons, such as Snellman (1961) and Hughes and Gleadell (1962), make an effort to reconstitute the rectovaginal septum at this stage, by suturing the front of the extraperitoneal rectum to the back of the vagina. I have never bothered to do so, but instead, at this stage I have simply sutured the cut edge of parietal peritoneum around the pelvic brim to the bowel, as in Fig. 180. The abdomen is usually closed without drainage of the pelvic cavity, but extraperitoneal suction drainage of the latter can be used for three to four days if desired.

Postoperative Management
Despite the fact that this operation involves an extensive pelvic dissection and much deep retraction, it seems to cause little shock and is well borne even by the elderly. In some cases 0·5 litre of blood has been transfused during or immediately after the operation but no more vigorous resuscitation has

ever been required. Parenteral fluids have generally been terminated in 36–48 hours, except when some degree of paralytic ileus develops necessitating continuation of the intravenous drip and gastric suction possibly for several days. Ambulation is usually commenced the day after operation. An indwelling urethral catheter is retained for four days, as after an excision of the rectum, and on its removal normal micturition is usually soon restored. The bowels are confined for three to four days and then opened with a purgative such as cascara or by an enema or glycerine suppository. This is followed by a period of irregularity often associated with some incontinence. The best management of this state of affairs has been found to be a daily enema to empty the distal colon completely. By the time the patient is ready to leave hospital at the end of two to two and a half weeks it has usually been possible to wean her off this routine on to natural evacuations with or without aperients, but in a few cases it is necessary to persist with the enema after discharge.

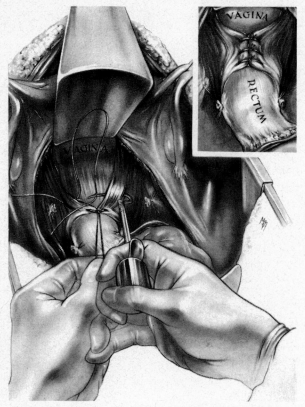

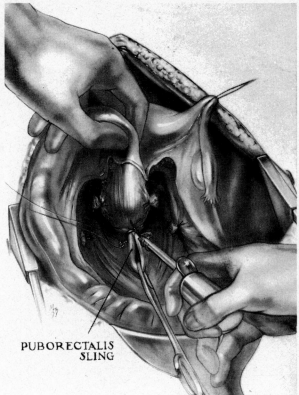

PUBORECTALIS
SLING

Fig. 177. Insertion of subsequent deep sutures in puborectales. Tails of the first stitch have been drawn taut, causing the puborectales to stand out as two prominent bars of muscle. This facilitates the insertion of the remaining sutures. *Inset:* the complete repair. (*From Goligher 1958*)

Fig. 178. Alternative technique of suture of puborectales *behind* the rectum. (*From Goligher 1958*)

THE IVALON SPONGE OPERATION

In performing this operation some surgeons are satisfied to free the rectum posteriorly as far as necessary to expose the upper half or two-thirds of the front of the sacrum, but leave the pelvic peritoneum and lateral ligaments mostly intact. However, I personally prefer to divide them as well and to mobilize the rectum more or less as in a Roscoe Graham type of repair (see above), except that it is not necessary to define the levator muscles as clearly as in this operation, which spares a good deal of operative effort.

When the rectum has been freed in this way, it is lifted upwards and forwards and held in this position by a deep pelvic retractor pressing strongly forwards (Fig. 181). The next step is to attach the sheet of Ivalon to the front of the sacrum. (Actually there is probably no special virtue in using Ivalon instead of other sheets of plastic material, such as

Teflon or Marlex mesh. It may in fact be more prone to be followed by infection than these other substances and in the presence of infection it disintegrates in a way that makes its subsequent removal very difficult.) A very thin rectangular sheet of this material is used, 160 × 110 × 3 mm. It is best cut from a block of Ivalon of these dimensions by a bacon-cutting machine, or if this is not available, by a large amputation knife. It is customary to snick a series of holes in the sheet with scissors as shown in Fig. 182, in the hope of facilitating its incorporation in the tissues. This piece of Ivalon is eventually going to be placed, with its long axis lying transversely, on the front of the sacrum, attached to the fascia in the presacral region by means of a vertical row of non-absorbable sutures, but, if these are inserted whilst the sponge rests against the sacrum, each insertion of the needle taking a simultaneous bite of the sponge and the fascia, there is a considerable risk that the middle sacral vessels may be punctured with resulting bleeding, which may be incompletely arrested by tying the suture and

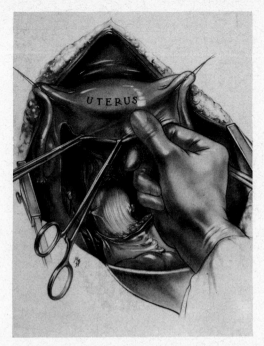

Fig. 179. Teasing out the fringe of pelvic peritoneum preparatory to suture. (*From Goligher 1958*)

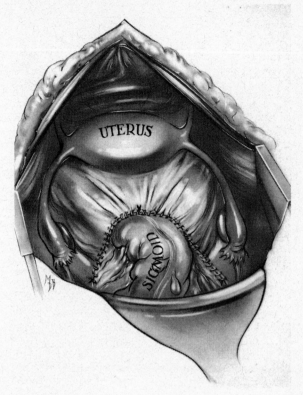

Fig. 180. Suture of pelvic peritoneum to sigmoid and mesosigmoid completed. (*From Goligher 1958*)

masked to some extent by the overlying sheet of Ivalon. For this reason I think it is better to insert these stitches in the presacral fascia before the Ivalon sponge is approximated to the sacrum, as advocated by Ellis (1966), so that any haemorrhage produced by spiking of presacral vessels can be immediately observed and checked by tying the causal stitch and by inserting further sutures, by diathermy coagulation or by applying oxycel, as required. My preferred routine for placing the stitches, for fixing the Ivalon to the sacrum and for attaching the rectum to it, comprises the following sequence of steps:

a. With the rectum retracted forwards, as already described, to give good access to the front of the sacrum, a row of five or six fine silk sutures is inserted in the presacral fascia, or preferably the anterior cortex of the sacral bone, at intervals of roughly 2 cm along the midline, starting as low down as is technically feasible and extending up to the sacral promontory just below the left common iliac vein. Each suture is 45 cm long and is threaded at either end on a small curved round-bodied needle. One of these needles is passed by means of a needle-holder through the presacral fascia close to the midline, the middle sacral vessels being carefully underrun or avoided. The thread is drawn

through until there are two tails of equal length, which are clipped with small artery forceps, the two needles being still attached (Fig. 181). This manoeuvre is repeated for each of the five or six sutures in turn. (Actually, if the stitch is to take a bite of the sacral bone, it is necessary to use a Mayo trocar-pointed needle. It will usually penetrate the bone of elderly females who constitute most of the sufferers from prolapse, but may fail in younger more robust males. I am indebted to my friend Mr Brian Morgan of Sydney for emphasizing the feasibility of this more secure form of sacral suturing to me.)

b. The sterilized sheet of Ivalon sponge, softened by being dipped in water for a minute or so, is held up in the pubic region above the lower end of the wound, whilst the two tails of each stitch are passed seriatim through it along its middle and re-clipped on the other side (Fig. 182). When the sponge has been traversed by all the sutures in this way the silk tails are held taut and the plastic sheet is slid down on them till it rests in contact with the front of the sacrum. Each stitch is then tied, fixing the

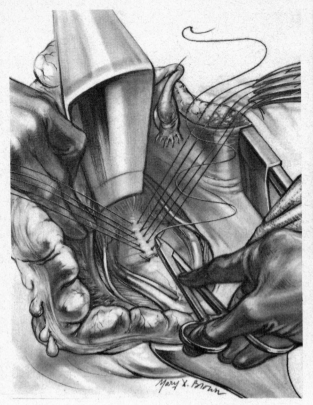

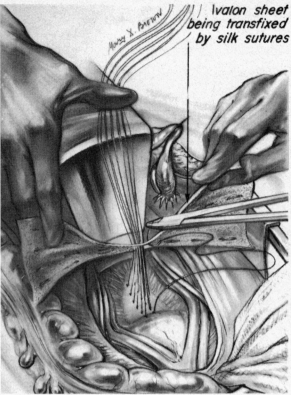

Fig. 181. Ivalon sponge fixation. Whilst the mobilized rectum is held forwards with a deep pelvic retractor, a series of fine silk sutures is inserted into the presacral fascia and clipped with forceps.

Fig. 182. Ivalon sponge fixation. The previously placed presacral silk sutures, which should be shown extending above the sacral promontory, are passed through the sheet of Ivalon sponge, which is then slid down on the silks to make contact with the front of the sacrum.

Ivalon to the presacral fascia, and the tails are cut short (Fig. 183).

c. The retractor is now removed and the rectum is allowed to fall back on the sponge, which is wrapped round the bowel. Usually it is necessary to trim off with scissors some of the anterior portion of the two 'arms' of Ivalon, so that the sheet just meets (or, as I now think is better, just fails to meet) in front of the rectum. Whilst the sigmoid and rectum are drawn tautly upwards out of the pelvis the anterior cut edges of the Ivalon are stitched partly to the rectal wall (but with only very superficial bites, so as to avoid entering the lumen) and partly to one another by five or six silk sutures (Fig. 184). The advantage of leaving a gap anteriorly is that it guards against the risk of subsequent stenosis. When that is done the anterior edges of the Ivalon are sutured only to the anterolateral wall of the rectum on either side.

d. Finally the pelvic peritoneum is reconstituted over the sponge surround and the rectum (Fig. 185),

and the abdomen is closed in the usual way. It is probably a good plan to lay a suction drain down to the extraperitoneal pelvic space for two or three days to remove any haemorrhagic exudate.

Postoperative Management

The after-care does not differ significantly from that given after an abdominal repair (see above), except that it is probably wise to administer a broad-spectrum antibiotic prophylactically to help to prevent the occurrence of infection in view of the presence of the buried plastic material.

PRESACRAL RECTOPEXY BY SIMPLE SUTURE

The initial stages of this procedure are identical with those of the Ivalon sponge operation up to the insertion of the silk sutures in the presacral fascia or anterior cortex of the sacral bone (see above and Fig. 181). Then, starting with the lowermost stitch and working upwards, each stitch in turn is taken

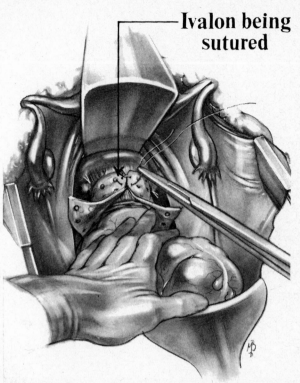

Ivalon being sutured

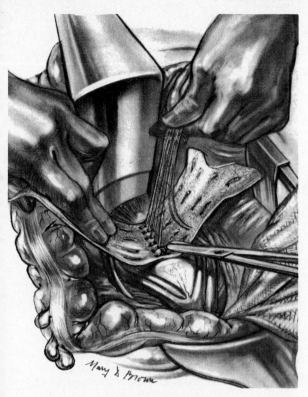

Fig. 183. Ivalon sponge fixation. Sutures being tied to fix the middle of the sheet of Ivalon to the sacrum.

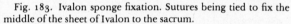

Fig. 184. Ivalon sponge fixation. The rectum is laid on the Ivalon sheet which, after trimming with scissors, is wrapped round the bowel as it is drawn strongly upwards, the edges being approximated anteriorly by silk sutures, or perhaps preferably a gap being left anteriorly and the anterior edges of the Ivalon being sutured to the anterolateral rectal wall on either side.

transversely by means of three or four bites with the needle through the fascia propria, fat and superficial part of the muscle coat of the posterior rectal wall (Fig. 186), the utmost care being exercised not to enter the lumen of the bowel. The lowest stitch is inserted into that part of the rectum that will stretch without undue tension (or laxity) to the front of the sacrum when the knot is tied. All the silk sutures are placed in the bowel before any is tied. When all have been tied and the tails are cut short, the pelvic peritoneum is re-sutured around the rectum, two suction drains usually being left down to the pelvic cavity.

There are no special points to be mentioned about the postoperative care.

ANTERIOR RESECTION

In the performance of anterior resection for prolapse essentially the same technique is used as when applying this operation to the treatment of carcinoma of the upper rectum (see p. 563). It is important, however, to carry out an extensive mobilization of the rectum down to the anorectal

ring with exposure of the junction of the rectum and the levator muscles laterally and posteriorly. Anteriorly the deep pouch of Douglas is dissected off the posterior vaginal wall and excised. The rectum is divided, leaving a 7-cm stump, and sufficient sigmoid colon is resected along with the upper rectum to remove any unnecessary 'slack'. When the anastomosis is completed the pelvic peritoneum is stripped off the back of the uterus and broad ligaments and sutured as high as possible on the front of the sacrum and colon so as to leave no pouch of Douglas.

The *postoperative care* is exactly the same as that after anterior resection for carcinoma (see p. 596).

THE THIERSCH OPERATION

With the patient in the lithotomy position and under light general anaesthesia, or if preferred, local infiltration of the perianal tissues, the anal region is cleansed and painted with a suitable anti-

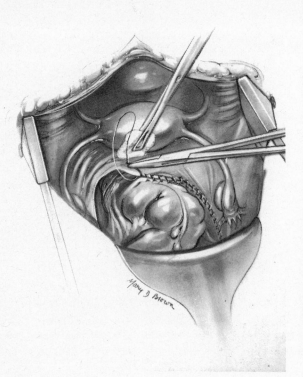

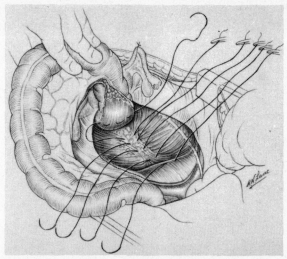

Fig. 186. Presacral rectopexy by simple suture. The rectum was fully mobilized down to the anorectal ring and displaced forwards whilst a series of fine linen thread sutures were inserted in the presacral fascia and left loose as in Fig. 181. The rectum is now allowed to fall backwards somewhat, whilst each of the linen sutures in turn, commencing with the lowermost, is placed in the fascia propria, perirectal fat and muscle coat of the posterior rectal wall. When all have been thus placed, they are tied and the tails are cut.

Fig. 185. Ivalon sponge fixation. The suturing of the Ivalon sheet has been completed and the pelvic peritoneum has now been largely reconstituted.

septic solution. Using a scalpel with a No. 10 Bard-Parker blade two small incisions, 6–12 mm long, are made in the midline 2·5 cm behind and in front of the anal verge. A fully curved handle needle of Doyen type is now passed from the posterior to the anterior wound on the left side of the anus (Fig. 187A). One end of a 30-cm strand of No. 20 SWG silver wire is threaded through the eye of the needle, looped back on itself, and withdrawn through the tissues. After unthreading the needle it is reinserted from the back to the front wound this time on the right side of the anus (Fig. 187B). The other end of the wire is threaded on to it and in similar manner drawn through to the posterior wound where the needle is again disconnected. The two ends of the wire are now lying on either side of the anus and projecting posteriorly, whilst the middle part of the wire forms a loop emerging from the anterior wound. By traction on the ends, the loop is gradually reduced to fit snugly round the anus; it is important to make sure that it does not become kinked in the process.

The wire is now ready to be tied posteriorly, but before doing so the assistant inserts his index finger or a No. 18 Hegar dilator into the anal canal and keeps it there whilst the two ends are twisted together. The ring should be made tight enough to grip the finger gently, but should allow the proximal interphalangeal joint to move comfortably through it (Fig. 187C). The twisted wire is cut to 1 cm and turned back with artery forceps so that its end is buried in the subcutaneous tissues and does not project towards the skin. The two wounds are closed with a couple of Michel clips each and sealed with a plastic dressing (Fig. 187D). The surgeon then confirms by palpation the tightness of the ring and the satisfactory position of the wire tail.

If monofilament nylon is being used instead of wire, a 60-cm strand of No. 2 gauge is employed. So far as the incisions and use of the handled Doyen needle are concerned, the technique is the same as when the operation is done with wire, except that the nylon is passed round the anus again and again till it is encircled by four thicknesses of suture material, each hemicircle having been pulled tight as it was inserted so that there was no slack. Finally the tails of nylon are tied tightly, with three reef knots, whilst a No. 18 Hegar dilator rests in the anal

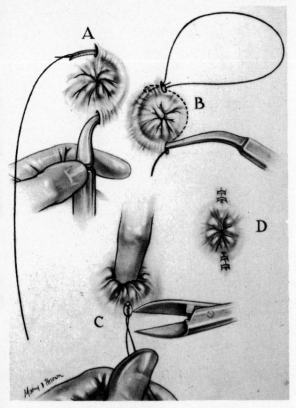

Fig. 187. (A–D). The Thiersch operation.

canal. The knots are pushed well into the tissues and the wounds closed with clips or sutures.

Postoperative Care

There is a distinct tendency to faecal impaction which should be countered by giving mild aperients such as paraffin or senna from the first post-operative day. A finger should also be passed frequently to ensure that accumulation is not occurring, and if necessary, glycerine or bisacodyl suppositories are ordered as well. The patient need only be in bed for a day or two but should not be discharged till a satisfactory bowel routine has been established. Skin clips can be removed on the sixth or seventh day.

RECTOSIGMOIDECTOMY

The patient should be placed in an exaggerated lithotomy position with the buttocks projecting well beyond the end of the table, and with a slight Trendelenburg tilt. A general anaesthetic with a relaxant is preferable to spinal anaesthesia which used to be popular for this operation but may lead to spasm of the bowel wall, including the longi-

tudinal muscle coat, and this interfere with adequate resection.

The Incision

The incision is a circular one placed circumferentially round the prolapse *not less than 3 cm distal to the mucocutaneous junction* (Fig. 188A). It traverses the mucosa and muscle coat of the outer layer of the prolapse and is usually attended by considerable haemorrhage till the bleeding points in the sub-mucosa have been secured. As the muscle coat tends to retract when it is divided and may be difficult to draw down for suture subsequently, it is a good plan to incise it 1 cm distal to the cut edge of the musosa. When these two coats have been completely divided all round, the distal cuff of bowel is brushed down with gauze, thereby opening up the incision, especially anteriorly.

Opening the Peritoneum

The peritoneum of the pouch of Douglas, covered with a layer of extraperitoneal fat, forms the floor of the wound anteriorly. It is incised transversely with the scalpel and then extended on either side round to the mesorectum or mesosigmoid, thus opening the pouch of Douglas widely (Fig. 188B).

Pulling Down the Sigmoid Colon

This is a most important step. The inner tube of bowel now exposed, which is usually upper rectum, is pulled down as strongly as possibly. This draws the sigmoid colon into the wound, and traction is continued till all slack colon has been delivered externally.

Closure of Pouch of Douglas by Suture

The open pouch of Douglas should now be closed by suturing the leaf of peritoneum in the anterior and lateral part of the anal cuff to the front and sides of the sigmoid *as high as is technically feasible*, so as to leave the rectouterine or rectovesical pouch as shallow as possible. This is accomplished by a continuous stitch of No. 1/0 chromic catgut mounted on a small half circle atraumatic needle held by a needle holder. As the fornices on either side of the colon, where the peritoneum in the cuff becomes continuous with the lateral leaves of the mesocolon, are the difficult parts, it is helpful to stitch them first by means of two separate stitches which meet in front (Fig. 188C, D).

Partial Division of the Colon

The anterior half or two-thirds of the bowel circumference is next divided obliquely with

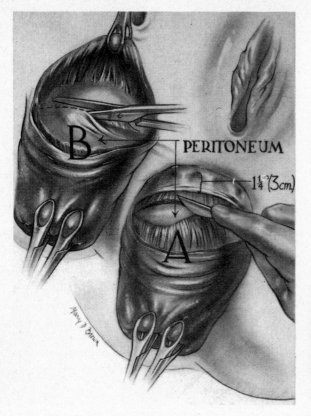
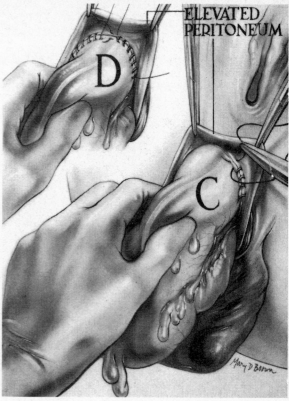

Fig. 188. Rectosigmoidectomy. (A) Circular incision being made on anterior aspect of prolapsed bowel 3 cm from the pectinate line. (B) The incision has been deepened down to the peritoneum of the protruded pouch of Douglas which is being opened with scissors. (C) The sigmoid colon has been drawn down forcibly through the peritoneal opening and stitched with continuous catgut to the everted upper flap of peritoneum. (D) The suture is commenced on either side posteriorly and finished in the midline in front.

scissors so as to leave a longer cuff of colon posteriorly than anteriorly, and not less than 2·5 cm of bowel should be retained distal to the peritoneal suture line (Fig. 189E).

Insertion of Stay Sutures and Performance of Anterior Part of Anastomosis

Three mattress sutures of No. 1 chromic catgut are placed between the mucosa and muscle of the anal cuff and the whole thickness of the colon wall on the anterior and both lateral aspects of the bowel. These are tied and their tails left long as stays whilst more accurate apposition of the cut edges of the anal canal and colon is secured by a series of fine interrupted catgut stitches (Fig. 189F).

Division of Posterior Part of Colon and Ligature and Division of Mesocolon

The remaining intact portion of the colon is now divided and the mesosigmoid or mesorectum exposed posteriorly with its contained vessels and divided between forceps (Fig. 189G, H). This step completes the separation of the segment of bowel to be resected. Ligatures of chromic catgut are now applied to the proximal cut edge of mesocolon which recedes, or is gently tucked back, into the pelvis out of sight.

Completion of the Anastomosis

An additional mattress stay suture is inserted to appose the cut edge of the colon and the muscle and mucosa of the anal cuff on the posterior aspect. By traction on this stitch and the two lateral stay sutures the contiguous cut edges are made prominent, and a close series of interrupted sutures of No. 1/0 chromic catgut is inserted, thus completing the anastomosis (Fig. 190I, J). The stays are now cut and the anastomosis recedes into the pelvis (Fig. 190K). A finger is passed to make sure that the suture line is sound everywhere. Finally a firm pad of gauze and wool and a T-bandage is applied.

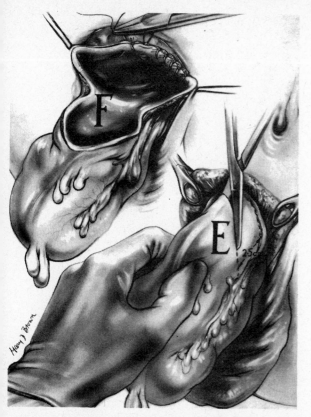

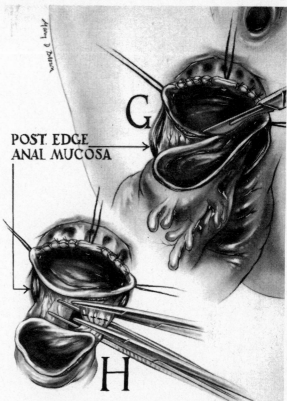

POST. EDGE
ANAL MUCOSA →

Fig. 189. Rectosigmoidectomy. (E) The colon is divided obliquely 2–2·5 cm distal to the peritoneal suture closing the pouch of Douglas. (F) When half to three-quarters of the circumference of the bowel has been opened, three mattress sutures of No. 1 chromic catgut are inserted as stays, anteriorly and on either side between the cut edges of the everted anal canal and the colon, whilst more accurate appostion is secured by a series of fine interrupted catgut sutures. (G) The posterior part of the colon is now divided. (H) Division of mesorectum or mesosigmoid between forceps.

Postoperative Care

If the patient has lost much blood during the operation a blood transfusion may be necessary in the theatre and postoperatively. Otherwise intravenous influsions are not usually required. A mild aperient should be given on the fourth day after operation and repeated as required to secure evacuation. Its action may be assisted by a bisacodyl suppository, but enemas should obviously be avoided. The integrity of the suture line should be determined by periodic rectal examination with the finger, commencing on the fifth or sixth day or sooner if a marked pyrexia suggests the presence of a leak and a resulting pelvic inflammation. If there is a gap in the suture line and a suppuration has occurred daily irrigations through a small proctoscope may be advised. Though a fair amount of dehiscence of the anastomosis is not uncommon, especially posteriorly, and may delay recovery, satisfactory healing eventually takes place in the majority without the need for a proximal colostomy. Sometimes, however, stenosis occurs if there has been much granulation. Some surgeons (Gabriel 1948) encourage sphincter exercises from an early stage in the covalescence but their value is highly doubtful.

SIGMOIDORECTAL INTUSSUSCEPTION

This condition, in which the distal sigmoid and upper rectum prolapse intermittently into the rectal ampulla (Fig. 191), is clearly described in many of the older textbooks, such as Allingham and Allingham (1901) and Tuttle (1903), and also more recently by Carrasco (1934) and Granet (1954). It is in effect an intussusception, but it differs from intussusceptions elsewhere in the intestinal tract in

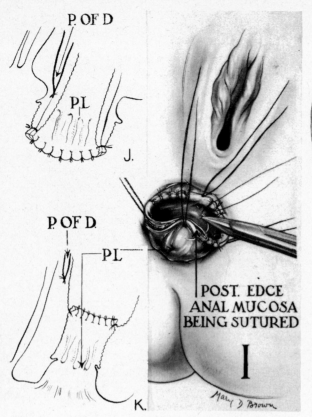

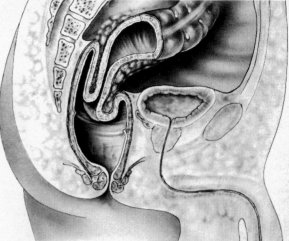

Fig. 191. Diagrammatic representation of the so-called, sigmoidorectal intussusception. (*From Granet 1954*)

Fig. 190. Rectosigmoidectomy. (I) A posterior stay stitch has been inserted between the cut edges of colon and anal canal and the circumferential suture is being completed. (J) Diagrammatic section of completed anastomosis; P of D = pouch of Douglas; PL = pectinate line. (K) Diagrammatic section of state of affairs after return of bowel to the pelvis.

that it rarely undergoes strangulation or causes complete obstruction, and that it reduces itself spontaneously. Even when developed to its maximum extent, the prolapse does not reach the anal canal, so that there is no external protrusion of bowel and the anus and sphincters remain normal.

AETIOLOGY AND INCIDENCE

In cases of carcinoma or benign tumour of the sigmoid, intussusception of this segment of colon into the rectum may occur with the neoplasm at the apex of the intussusception. The condition may thus be easily mistaken on digital examination for a carcinoma of the rectum, but on sigmoidoscopy it is usually found that the growth and the intussusception recede before the instrument as the rectum is inflated. This is a well-recognized, if rare, form of sigmoidorectal intussusception which most surgeons of experience have encountered.

The type of lesion to which the term sigmoidorectal prolapse is generally applied has no such definite cause and indeed is altogether a very dubious entity. It is regarded by Granet (1954) as an exaggeration of the slight projection of the terminal sigmoid into the upper rectum which occurs normally during defaecation. Conditions which are held to be responsible for the development of this more exaggerated intussusception are redundancy of the sigmoid loop, and an abnormally long mesosigmoid.

It is difficult to say how often this variety of sigmoidorectal intussusception occurs, for the symptoms associated with it are readily attributed to psychoneurosis or to a tumour, and the achievement of an objective diagnosis is far from easy. For this reason opinions vary widely as to the frequency of the disease, or indeed as to whether there is such a condition at all.

SYMPTOMS

The symptoms attributed to sigmoidorectal intussusception are varied and bizarre, but the most characteristic is said to be a sense of incomplete evacuation after defaecation. This feeling causes the patient to continue straining at stool, which possibly aggravates the tendency to prolapse. As a result of the frequent descent and recession of the sigmoid into the rectum, congestion and oedema of the mucosa may develop giving rise to a mucoid or blood-stained discharge. Another common symptom is said to be a heavy dragging sensation in the pelvis or lumbosacral region or a dull aching pain in the perineum or back of the thighs.

When the sigmoid is prolapsed into the rectum, the lumen of the intussuscepted bowel is considerably reduced, especially if there is superadded oedema, and this is held to be responsible for the obstinate constipation of which these patients usually complain. From years of experience they have found that to obtain an evacuation at all it is necessary to reduce the faeces to a fluid consistency by the regular use of aperients such as paraffin, cascara or saline purgatives.

Schapiro (1950) claims that sigmoidorectal intussusception is common in childhood and is indeed the most common form of rectal prolapse that occurs in children or infants. He emphasizes that it must always be borne in mind as a possible source of rectal bleeding in such young patients.

DIAGNOSIS

There is clearly nothing specific or particularly suggestive about the symptomatology of sigmoidorectal prolapse, and the symptoms could equally well be due to other organic lesions or to an anxiety neurosis. Unfortunately the findings on physical examination are also apt to be equivocal. An obvious source of fallacy is that if the patient is examined in the knee–shoulder position the intussusception reduces itself spontaneously and eludes detection. Granet (1954) claims that if the examination is conducted in the lateral or Sims position and the patient is asked to bear down, the apex of the prolapse can often be felt with the finger or seen with the sigmoidoscope. The difficulty is to decide whether the amount of sigmoidal projection is pathological or within the limits of normality. To be frank, I have never felt happy about a diagnosis of sigmoidorectal intussusception other than as a complication of carcinoma of the sigmoid. In my experience it has always been possible to explain the symptoms plausibly on the basis of some other diagnosis without having to postulate the existence of a recurrent sigmoidorectal prolapse.

TREATMENT

Most cases of alleged idiopathic sigmoidorectal intussusception have apparently been treated expectantly with aperients, antispasmodics and reassurance, which suggests that the diagnosis has usually been in doubt. There can obviously be no rational non-operative management for such a condition. If a case of sigmoidorectal prolapse were sufficiently definite to satisfy my diagnostic criteria,

I should advise operation either to resect the upper rectum and most of the sigmoid as in the treatment of rectosigmoid carcinoma by anterior resection, or to fix the sigmoid and upper rectum by some form of sigmoidopexy using Ivalon or a Teflon sling as in the treatment of complete rectal prolapse.

INTERNAL PROCIDENTIA

Ihre (1972) has applied the cineradiographic technique of investigation described by Brodén and Snellman (1968) (see p. 225) to many patients without obvious clinical prolapse of the rectum, but with rather vague symptoms, mainly a feeling of incomplete evacuation of the bowel, as are described with sigmoidorectal intussusception (see above). In a proportion of these cases he claims to have observed the occurrence of a rectal intussusception commencing about 6–8 cm from the perineum, as in the genesis of a complete rectal prolapse, and proceeding a varying distance down the rectum but not reaching the exterior. In a few cases it has also been possible to detect some degree of intussusception on digital examination of the bowel. To this condition Ihre (1972) has given the designation internal procidentia. As regards management of the complaint, if the symptoms have not been severe, he has adopted an expectant approach, and, incidentally, two of the patients so managed subsequently developed a complete rectal prolapse. For those with more severe symptoms he has employed a Ripstein type of rectopexy, apparently with very satisfactory results.

I have not knowingly encountered any example of this condition myself, but obviously, unless one employs a cineradiographic examination, internal procidentia is not really susceptible to diagnosis.

THE SYNDROME OF THE DESCENDING PERINEUM

Parks et al. (1966) describe a syndrome that may be related to rectal prolapse. In it there appears to be some loss of the normal tone of the pelvic floor musculature, which descends, distributing the normal mechanics of rectal function and elimination of stools. One of the features of the condition is excessive protrusion of the anterior rectal wall, which apparently impedes emptying of the rectum.

Patients with this abnormality complain of a sense of obstruction and of a dull, aching perineal pain. They experience tenseness and make frequent, unsuccessful efforts to empty the bowel. On digital examination of the rectum, muscle tone is found to be reduced, and with straining the puborectalis muscle descends, the upper anal canal becomes funnel-shaped, and the anterior rectal wall bulges downwards. Associated haemorrhoids are often present. Electromyography confirms that muscle tone is abnormal.

How genuine an entity is this alleged syndrome? Parks et al. (1966) encountered it in 12 of 100 consecutive proctological patients, but I must admit that I have not been able to recognize a syndrome of this kind in my practice. As for treatment, if the condition can be recognized, Parks et al. (1966) recommend avoidance of excessive straining at stool, sphincter exercises and the use of hydrophilic substances. Haemorrhoidectomy, with generous excision of the mucosa of the anterior rectal wall, may be useful in some patients.

REFERENCES

ALLINGHAM, W. and ALLINGHAM, H. W. (1901) *The Diagnosis and Treatment of Diseases of the Rectum*. London: Baillière.

ALTEMEIER, W. A., CULBERTSON, W. R. and ALEXANDER, J. W. (1964) One-stage perineal repair of rectal prolapse. *Archs Surg., Chicago, 89,* 6.

—— CULBERTSON, W. R., SCHOWENGERDT, C. and HUNT, J. (1971) Nineteen years' experience with the one-stage perineal repair of rectal prolapse. *Ann. Surg., 173,* 993.

—— GIUSEPPI, J. and HOXWORTH, P. (1952) Treatment of extensive prolapse of the rectum in aged or debilitated patients. *Archs Surg., Chicago, 65,* 72.

BACON, H. E. (1949) *The Anus, Rectum and Sigmoid Colon: Diagnosis and Treatment*, 3rd ed. Philadelphia: Lippincott.

BAKER, W. N. W. (1970) Results of using monofilament nylon in Thiersch's operation for rectal prolapse. *Br. J. Surg., 57,* 37.

BALL, C. B. (1908) *The Rectum: its Diseases and Developmental Defects*. London: Frowde; Hodder and Stoughton.

BEAHRS, O. H., VANDERTOLL, D. J. and BAKER, N. H. (1965) Complete rectal prolapse: an evaluation of surgical treatment. *Ann. Surg., 161,* 221.

BLAIR, C. R., NAY, H. R. and RUCKER, C. M. (1963) Surgical repair of rectal prolapse. *Surgery, St Louis, 53,* 625.

BRINTNALL, B. S. (1952) Surgical treatment of complete rectal prolapse. *Archs Surg., Chicago, 65,* 816.

BRODÉN, B. and SNELLMAN, B. (1968) Procidentia of the rectum studied with cineradiography: a contribution to the discussion of causative mechanism. *Dis. Colon Rect., 11,* 330.

BROWN, A. and DRAKE, T. G. H. (1924) Treatment of prolapse of rectum by alcohol injection. *Archs Pediat., 41,* 716.

BUTLER, E. C. B. (1954) Complete rectal prolapse following removal of tumours of the cauda equina; two cases. *Proc. R. Soc. Med., 47,* 521.

—— (1962) Intra-abdominal repair (of complete rectal prolapse). *Proc. R. Soc. Med., 55,* 1081.

CALDWELL, K. P. (1965) A new treatment of rectal prolapse. *Proc. R. Soc. Med., 58,* 792.

CALNAN, J. (1963) The use of inert plastic material in reconstructive surgery. I. A biological test for tissue acceptance. II. Tissue reactions to commonly used materials. *Br. J. plast. Surg., 16,* 1.

CARRASCO, A. B. (1943) *Contribution à l'Etude du Prolapsus du Rectum*. Paris: Masson.

CHEN, R. W., MUSSER, A. W. and POSTLETHWAITE, R. W. (1969) Alterations of and tissue reactions to polyvinyl alcohol sponge implants. *Surgery, St Louis, 66,* 899.

COHN, I. (1942) Prolapse of the rectum: a suggested operative procedure for use. *Am. J. Surg., 57,* 444.

COLLINS, C. D., BROWN, B. H. and DUTHIE, H. L. (1968) A basis for electrical stimulation for anal incontinence. *Scand. J. Gastroent., 3,* 395.

—— —— —— (1969) An assessment of intraluminal electrical stimulation for anal incontinence. *Br. J. Surg., 56,* 542.

CUNÉO, B. and SÉNÈQUE, J. (1931) Reconstitution de l'appareil sphinctérien dans le prolapsus du rectum. *J. Chir., Paris, 38,* 190.

CUTAIT, D. (1959) Sacro-promontory fixation of the rectum for complete rectal prolapse. *Proc. R. Soc. Med., 52* (Suppl.), 105.

DAVID, V. C. (1947) Surgery of the rectum and anus. In *Practice of Surgery*, ed. Dean Lewis, vol. 7. Hagerstown: Prior.

DAVIDIAN, U. A. and THOMAS, C. G. (1972) Trans-sacral repair of rectal prolapse. *Am. J. Surg., 123,* 231.

DELORME, R. (1900) Sur le traitement des prolapsus de la muqueuse rectale ou recto-colique. *Bull. Soc. Chirurgiens Paris, 26,* 459.

DEVADHAR, D. S. C. (1965) A new concept of mechanism and treatment of rectal procidentia. *Dis. Colon Rect., 8,* 75.

DUKES, C. E. and MITCHLEY, B. C. U. (1962) Polyvinyl sponge implants: experimental and clinical observations. *Br. J. plast. Surg., 15,* 225.

DUNPHY, J. E. (1948) A combined perineal and abdominal operation for the repair of rectal prolapse. *Surgery Gynec. Obstet., 86,* 493.

DUTHIE, H. L. (1971) Rectal prolapse. In *Modern Trends in Surgery*, ed. W. T. Irvine, vol. 3. London: Butterworth.

ELLIS, H. (1966) The polyvinyl sponge wrap operation for rectal prolapse. *Br. J. Surg., 53,* 675.

FINDLAY, L. and GALBRAITH, J. B. D. (1923) Injection of alcohol in the treatment of prolapse of the rectum in infancy and childhood. *Lancet, 1,* 76.

FRASER, I. (1930) Prolapse of the rectum in children. *Br. med. J., 1,* 1074.

FRY, I. K., GRIFFITHS, J. D. and SMART, P. J. G. (1966) Some observations on the movement of the pelvic floor and rectum with special reference to rectal prolapse. *Br. J. Surg., 53,* 784.

GABRIEL, W. B. (1948) *The Principles and Practices of Rectal Surgery*, 4th ed. London: H. K. Lewis.

GANT (1923) Quoted by Carrasco (1934).

GOLIGHER, J. C. (1958) The treatment of complete prolapse of the rectum by the Roscoe Graham operation. *Br. J. Surg., 45,* 343.

—— and HUGHES, E. S. R. (1951) Sensibility of the rectum and colon: its role in the mechanism of anal continence. *Lancet, 1,* 543.

GORDON, I. and MILLER, D. F. (1971) Surgical repair of rectal prolapse. *Scot. med. J., 16,* 393.

GRAHAM, R. R. (1942) The operative repair of massive rectal prolapse. *Ann. Surg., 115,* 1007.

GRANET, E. (1954) *Manual of Protology*. Chicago: Yearbook Publishers.

HAGIHARA, P. F. and GRIFFEN, W. O. (1975) Transsacral repair of rectal prolapse. *Archs Surg., Chicago, 110,* 343.

HARTMANN, H. (1931) *Chirurgie du Rectum*. Paris: Masson.

HASKELL, B. and ROVNER, N. (1963) A modified Thiersch operation for complete rectal prolapse using a Teflon prosthesis. *Dis. Colon Rect., 6,* 192.

HAYDEN, E. P. (1947) Prolapse of the rectum. *Surg. Clins N Am., 27,* 1062.

HENSCHEN, C. (1912) Über den Ersatz des Thierschschen Drahtringes bei der Operation des Mastdarmvorfalls durch geflochtene Seidenriemen, frei überpflanzte Gefäss-, Sehnen-, Periost- order Faszienstücke. *Münch. med. Wschr., 59,* 128.

HOPKINSON, B. R. and LIGHTWOOD, R. (1966) Electrical treatment of anal incontinence. *Lancet, 1,* 297.

HUGHES, E. S. R. (1949) In discussion on rectal prolapse. *Proc. R. Soc. Med., 42,* 1007.

—— and GLEADELL, L. W. (1962) Abdominoperineal repair of complete prolapse of the rectum. *Proc. R. Soc. Med., 55,* 1077.

—— —— and TURNER, J. (1957) Treatment of complete prolapse of the rectum. *Br. med. J., 2,* 179.

IHRE, T. (1972) Internal procidentia of the rectum: treatment and results. *Scand. J. Gastroent.*, 7, 643.

JEANNEL, D. (1896) Du prolapsus du rectum. *Clin. Fac. Méd. Toulouse*, *II*, 101; 121; 137.

JENKINS, S. G., Jr. and THOMAS, C. G., Jr. (1962) An operation for the repair of rectal prolapse. *Surgery Gynec. Obstet.*, *114*, 381.

KELSEY, C. B. (1883) *Diseases of the Rectum and Anus*, p. 182. London: Sampson Low.

KÜPFER, C. A. and GOLIGHER, J. C. (1970) One hundred consecutive cases of complete prolapse of the rectum treated by operation. *Br. J. Surg.*, 57, 34.

LANGE (1887) Quoted by Carrasco (1934).

LOCKHART-MUMMERY, J. P. (1910) A new operation for prolapse of the rectum. *Lancet*, *1*, 641.

—— (1934) *Diseases of the Rectum and Colon*, 2nd ed. London: Baillière.

LOYGUE, J., HUGUIER, M., MALAFOSSE, M. and BIOTOIS, H. (1971) Complete prolapse of rectum: a report on 140 cases treated by rectopexy. *Br. J. Surg.*, 58, 847.

McCANN, F. J. (1928) Note on an operation for the cure of prolapse of the rectum in the female. *Lancet*, *1*, 1072.

McLANAHAN, S. and JOHNSON, M. L. (1945) Spontaneous rupture of lower colon with evisceration of small intestine through anal orifice. A complication of advanced rectal prolapse. *Surgery, St Louis*, *18*, 478.

MARCHIORI, G. and TOMASINI, M. (1962) L'intervento di perineoplastica secondo Saraffof nella chirurgia del prolasso rectale. *Chir. ital.*, *14*, 637.

MAYO, C. W. (1938) Complete rectal prolapse; fascial repair. *West. J. Surg. Obstet. Gynec.*, *46*, 75.

MIKULICZ, J. (1889) Zur operativen Behandlung des Prolapsus Recti et Coli invaginati. *Arch. klin. Chir.*, *38*, 74.

MILES, W. E. (1933) Recto-sigmoidectomy as a method of treatment for procidentia recti. *Proc. R. Soc. Med.*, *26*, 1445.

MOORE, H. D. (1969) Complete prolapse of the rectum in the adult. *Ann. Surg.*, *169*, 368.

MORGAN, C. N. (1951) Personal communication.

—— PORTER, N. A. and KLUGMAN, D. J. (1972) Ivalon (polyvinyl alcohol) sponge in the repair of complete rectal prolapse. *Br. J. Surg.*, *59*, 841.

MOSCHCOWITZ, A. V. (1912) The pathogenesis, anatomy and cure of prolapse of the rectum. *Surgery Gynec. Obstet.*, *15*, 7.

MUIR, E. G. (1955) Prolapse of the rectum. Presidential address, Section of Proctology. *Proc. R. Soc. Med.*, *48*, 33.

—— (1962) The surgical treatment of rectal prolapse. *Proc. R. Soc. Med.*, *55*, 104.

NAY, H. R. and BLAIR, C. R. (1972) Perineal surgical repair of rectal prolapse. *Am. J. Surg.*, *123*, 577.

NEWELL, E. T. (1954) Combined abdomino-perineal herniorrhaphy for massive rectal prolapse. *Ann. Surg.*, *139*, 864.

NOTARAS, M. J. (1973) The use of mersilene mesh in rectal prolapse repair. *Proc. R. Soc. Med.*, *66*, 684.

ORR, T. G (1947) A suspension operation for prolapse of the rectum. *Ann. Surg.*, *126*, 833.

PALMER, J. A. (1961) The management of massive rectal prolapse. *Surgery Gynec. Obstet.*, *112*, 502.

PARKS, A. G. (1971) Anorectal disorders. *Med Ann.*, 15.

—— (1976) Anorectal incontinenece. *Proc. R. Soc. Med.*, *68*, 21.

—— PORTER, N. H. and HARDCASTLE, J. (1966) The syndrome of the descending perineum. *Proc. R. Soc. Med.*, *59*, 477.

PEMBERTON, J. DE J., KIERNAN, P. C. and PEMBERTON, A. H. (1953) Results of surgical treatment of complete rectal prolapse with particular reference to suspension operations. *New Engl. J. Med.*, *248*, 720.

—— and STALKER, L. K. (1939) Surgical treatment of complete rectal prolapse. *Ann. Surg.*, *109*, 799.

PENFOLD, J. C. B. and HAWLEY, P. R. (1972) Experiences of Ivalon-sponge implant for complete rectal prolapse at St. Mark's Hospital. *Br. J. Surg.*, *59*, 846.

PLUMLEY, P. (1966) A modification to Thiersch's operation for rectal prolapse. *Br. J. Surg.*, *53*, 624.

PORTER, N. H. (1962a) A physiological study of the pelvic floor in rectal prolapse. *Ann. R. Coll. Surg.*, *31*, 379.

—— (1962b) Collective results of operations for rectal prolapse [at St. Mark's Hospital 1948–1960]. *Proc. R. Soc. Med.*, *55*, 1087.

POTTER, E. B. and WELLMAN, J. M. (1933) Alcohol injection for prolapse of the rectum. *Am. J. Surg.*, *19*, 297.

QUÉNU, E. (1882) Quoted by Ball, (1908).

—— and DUVAL, P. (1910) Technique de la colopexie pour prolapsus du rectum. *Rev. Chir.*, *Paris*, *41*, 135.

RANKIN, F. W. and PRIESTLEY, J. T. (1933) Prolapse of the rectum. *Ann Surg.*, 9, 1030.

RIPSTEIN, C. B. (1952) Treatment of massive rectal prolapse. *Am. J. Surg.*, *83*, 68.

—— (1965) Surgical care of massive rectal prolapse. *Dis. Colon. Rect.*, *8*, 34.

—— (1972) Procidentia—definitive corrective surgery. *Dis. Colon Rect.*, *15*, 334.

—— and LANTER, B. (1963) Etiology and therapy of massive prolapse of the rectum. *Ann. Surg.*, *157*, 259.

SARAFFOF, D. (1937) Ein einfaches ungefährliches Verfahren zur operativen Behandlung des Mastdarmvorfalles. *Arch. klin. Chir.*, *190*, 219.

—— (1942) Über die Leistungsfähigkeit des Narbenringsverfahrens bei der Behandlung schwerster Mastdarmvorfälle sowie eines Vorfalles des Rectums und der Sigmaschlinge. *Dt. Z. Chir.*, *256*, 520.

SCHAPIRO, S. (1950) Occurrence of proctologic disorders in infancy and childhood. *Gastroenterology*, *15*, 653.

SCHMERZ, H. (1918) Die operative Behandlung des Mastdarmvorfalles mittels Fascienplastik. *Beitr. klin. Chir.*, *111*, 346.

SCHOFIELD, T. L. (1955) Polyvinyl alcohol sponge. An inert plastic for use as a prosthesis in the repair of large hernias. *Br. J. Surg.*, *42*, 618.

SCHUMACKER, Quoted by Carrasco (1934).

SCHWARTZ, A. and MARIN, R. (1962) Use of polyethylene in the Thiersch operation. *Dis. Colon Rect.*, 5, 302.

SICK, P. (1909) Heilung des Rektumprolapsus durch Tamponade. *Zentbl. Chir.*, *36*, 1225.

SNELLMAN, B. (1954) Twelve cases of prolapse of the rectum treated by the Roscoe Graham operation. *Acta chir. scand.*, *108*, 26.

—— (1961) Complete prolapse of the rectum. *Dis Colon Rect.*, *4*, 199.

—— (1965) Personal communication.

STEPHENS. F. D. (1958) Minor surgical conditions of the anus and perineum (in paediatrics). *Med. J. Aust.*, *1*, 244.

STEWART, R. (1972) Long-term results of Ivalon wrap operation for complete rectal prolapse. *Proc. R. Soc. Med.*, *65*, 777.

SWINTON, N. W. and PALMER, T. E. (1960) The management of rectal prolapse and procidentia. *Am. J. Surg., 99*, 144.

THEUERKAUF, F. J., Jr., BEAHRS, O. H. and HILL, J. R. (1970) Rectal prolapse: causation and surgical treatment. *Ann. Surg., 171*, 819.

THIERSCH, K. (1891) Quoted by Carrasco (1934).

THOMAS, C. G., Jr. and JENKINS, S. G., Jr. (1965) Results of the posterior approach in the repair of rectal prolapse. *Ann. Surg., 161*, 897.

TODD, I. P. (1959) Aetiological factors in the production of complete rectal prolapse. *Postgrad. med. J., 35*, 97.

TUTTLE, J. P. (1903) *A Treatise on the Diseases of the Anus, Rectum and Pelvic Colon.* New York and London: Appleton.

VAN BUREN, W. H. (1881) *Diseases of the Rectum*, p. 82. London: H. K. Lewis.

VERNEUIL, A. A. (1891) Quoted by Carrasco (1934).

WALTER, J. B. and CHIARAMONTE, L. G. (1965) The tissue responses of the rat to implanted Ivalon, Etheron and Polyfoam plastic sponges. *Br. J. Surg., 52*, 49.

WELLS, C. A. (1955) In Schofield, T. L. (1955) Polyvinyl-alcohol sponge. An inert plastic for use as a prosthesis in the repair of large hernias. *Br. J. Surg., 42*, 618.

WHITE, M. E. E. (1961) Operation for rectal prolapse using stainless steel ring. *Lancet, 1*, 858.

ZÄNGL, A. (1965) Utilization of the Saraffof operation for procidentia and prolapse. *Dis. Colon Rect., 8*, 39.

11

Congenital Deformities of the Anorectal Region

By H. H. Nixon

Congenital anorectal abnormalities are believed to occur about once in 5000 births. Some authorities consider this an underestimate. There is rarely any family history of similar defects.

TABLE 8. *The International Classification of Congenital Anorectal Anomalies*

	Male	Female
Low (translevator)	At normal anal site (a) Anal stenosis (b) Covered anus—complete	As for male
	At perineal site (a) Anocutaneous fistula (covered anus—incomplete) (b) Anterior perineal anus	As for male
	—	At vulvar site (a) Anovulvar fistula (b) Anovestibular fistula (c) Vestibular anus

Intermediate	Anal agenesis
	(a) Without fistula
	(b) With fistula—rectobulbar
		Anal agenesis
		(a) Without fistula
		(b) With fistula
		  (i) Rectovestibular
		  (ii) Rectovaginal—low

	Anorectal stenosis	As for male

High (supralevator)	Anorectal agenesis
	(a) Without fistula
	(b) With fistula
	  (i) Rectourethral
	  (ii) Rectovesical
		Anorectal agenesis
		(a) Without fistula
		(b) With fistula
		  (i) Rectovaginal—high
		  (ii) Rectocloacal
		  (iii) Rectovesical

	Rectal atresia	As for male
Miscellaneous	Imperforate anal membrane Cloacal extrophy Others	As for male

After Stephens and Smith (1971).

CLASSIFICATION

The differing nature of the anomalies has led to a confusion of classifications. An International classification was proposed at a meeting in Melbourne (Stephens and Smith 1971) (Table 9). It was slightly re-ordered before being used for the American Academy of Pediatrics National Survey of results of treatment (Santulli et al. 1970). Its 27 categories merely record the anatomical findings, avoiding as far as possible embryological implications, so that recording of results can be standardized between clinics.

The most important observation is that all were agreed on the fundamental practical importance of division into 'high' (supralevator) and 'low' (infra- or translevator) anomalies; with the inevitable smaller intermediate group. If the bowel passes through the levator before going wrong it will be

TABLE 9. *300 Consecutive Referrals of Anorectal Anomalies to One Unit, at the Hospital for Sick Children, Great Ormond Street, 1962–70*

Types of deformity	Male (%)	Female (%)	Total (%)
High	32·4	9·4	41·8
Intermediate	4·2	5·6	9·8
Low	20·9	26·5	47·4
Miscellaneous			1·0

seen later that the child should usually obtain normal continence after prompt and thorough treatment, but those with a high anomaly will rarely do so even though a socially satisfactory degree of control may usually be learned. Table 9 shows the proportions in a series of children referred to the author, and demonstrates the greater incidence of high anomalies in the male.

Embryological Considerations (Figs 192, 193)

The abnormalities can be differentiated further on embryological grounds following lines originally described by Sir Arthur Keith (1908) and applied to clinical surgery in 1953 by Stephens (see Stephens 1963) and Denis Browne (1955). Two concepts are important in this classification. *Failure of migration* of the anus from a more primitive site is one. The other is of *excessive fusion*—usually of the lateral genital folds, to cover the anus.

In this chapter a simpler classification based on embryological concepts will be used with references to the equivalents in the international classification.

Low Abnormalities

The main low abnormalities are the ectopic and covered ani.

ECTOPIC ANUS

The commonest varieties are the *vestibular* and *vulval ectopic anus* (Fig. 194) (or *fourchette anus*) of the female (anovestibular fistula and vestibular anus, International Classification). Both are externally very similar, but in the former the opening is immediately behind the vagina, and the bowel leads up parallel with it; in the latter the opening is just inside the vulva and the bowel extends back towards the normal anal site close under the skin. It has often been called an imperforate anus with low vaginal fistula but the opening is below the hymen. It is more helpful, however, to regard the opening as the anal orifice which has failed to migrate back to the usual position. The bowel passes through the pelvic floor which usually has a normal levator and puborectalis sling. A thickening of the muscle coat at its lower end represents the internal sphincter but the external sphincter—developed to a varying but usually reasonable extent—lies behind the orifice in its customary position.

If the failure of migration is less marked it will result in an anus placed farther forward than normal but on the skin surface of the perineum—*perineal ectopic anus* (anterior perineal anus, International Classification) (Fig. 196)—and may be seen in either sex.

Like all ectopic orifices these ani tend also to be stenotic which is of great importance in their management.

COVERED ANUS

The lateral genital folds should form the labia majora in the female or fuse to form the scrotum in the male. In this abnormality the folds appear to have fused over posteriorly to cover the anus. A track is usually left running forward to open some-

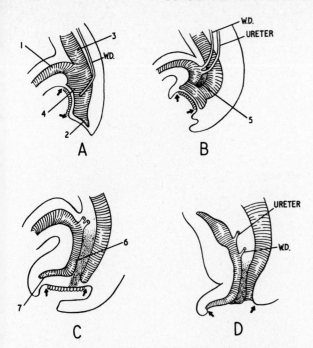

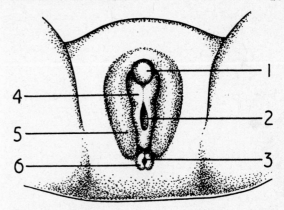

Fig. 193. Simplified diagram of parts involved in development of the perineum. (1) Genital tubercle → penis or clitoris. (2) Urogenital sinus → urethra, etc. (3) Anus. (4) Genital folds → penile urethra or labia minora. (5) Genital swellings (or lateral genital folds) → scrotum or labia majora. (6) Anal tubercles.

Fig. 192. Development of the rectum. (A) Allantois (1), tailgut (2) and hindgut (3) entering endodermal cloaca (4). Cloacal membrane extends between the two arrows. (B) 'Urorectal septum' (5) appears. According to Keith this occurs by migration of primitive anus down posterior wall of cloaca. According to many others it arises by craniocaudal fusion of lateral urorectal ridges arising from the walls of the cloaca. Tailgut is resorbed. (C) Migration of anus to perineum completed. (Alternatively stated as urorectal septum having reached perineum.) Urogenital sinus (6) separated from rectum and developing a phallic extension (7). (D) Cloacal membrane broken down. Ureter and Wolffian duct now opening separately into the urogenital sinus. (*After Keith 1908*)

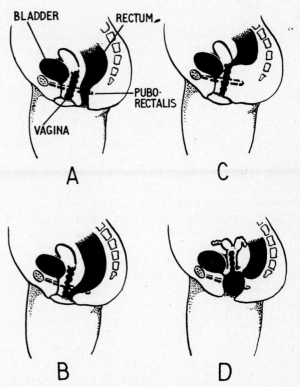

Fig. 194. Sectional diagram of (A) Normal female pelvis. (B) Vulval ectopic anus (Vestibular anus, International Classification). (C) Anorectal agenesis with rectovaginal fistula (High) (International Classification). (D) Cloaca (Anorectal agenesis with rectocloacal fistula, International Classification).

where along the perineal raphe. Usually it opens just behind the scrotum but it may extend as far forward as the tip of the penis (Fig. 197). The track may extend along the raphe for some distance bearing little pearl-like inclusions and often having such a thin cover that the dark green colour of the meconium shines through (anocutaneous fistula, International Classification).

In some cases the epithelial excrescence overlies the anus as a *median band* with a thin membrane on either side (covered anus, complete, International Classification). In these cases Bill and Johnson (1953) suggest that it is the anal tubercles which have fused abnormally. In others the cover narrows the anus to a *microscopic anus* at the normal site so that a careful search may be needed to see the telltale 'flyspeck' of meconium at the site of the anus (anal stenosis, International Classification).

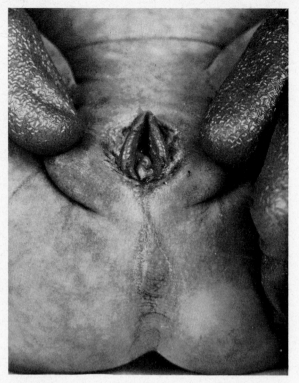

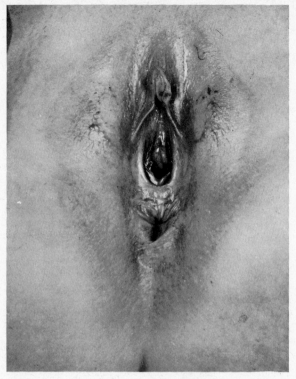

Fig. 195. A vulval ectopic anus (vestibular anus, International Classification). The edge of the anus just shows in the photograph at the back of the vulva.

Fig. 196. A perineal ectopic anus (anterior perineal anus, International Classification), farther forward in the perineum than normal and stenosed. Treated by dilatation only. Normal continence.

Fig. 198 shows a baby in whom the embryological derivation of the anal cover is particularly obvious.

In the female it will be appreciated that covering in this way could bring the anal outlet forward to the fourchette to produce a condition akin to the vulval ectopic anus already described. There is some reason to believe that 'vulval ectopia' may indeed be caused in either fashion, as will be mentioned later (anovulvar fistula, International Classification).

The sphincter equipment is usually normal in covered anus. It is thus particularly important to recognize this type and avoid unnecessarily elaborate and potentially destructive operations.

The 'anorectal membrane' of the older terminology usually relates to the type of covered anus in which a part of the cover becomes stretched, thin and bulging. Certainly such pictures as are available (e.g. Feggetter 1939) suggest that the membrane is really at the lower end of the anal canal and not at the anorectal junction—which would be 1 cm from the skin even in a newborn infant. True anorectal membrane is rare.

Intermediate Abnormalities

It is usual for an ectopic orifice to be stenotic. Certain forms of stenosis are met, however, in which the orifice is not displaced. The microscopic anus has already been described. Some other forms which are intermediate between the low and high groups will now be described.

ANORECTAL STENOSIS

A ring-like narrowing may also occur at the upper end of the anal canal—i.e. about 1 cm from the surface in a newborn increasing to about 2 cm in an older child. Its extent varies from a string-like stenosis in a normal canal to a diffuse fibrosis involving the internal sphincter. The external appearance is normal and hence the lesion may pass unnoticed for some time whilst the infant is having the soft stools of a milk-fed baby. It may not be until weaning is in progress that constipation becomes obvious and severe. By this time the

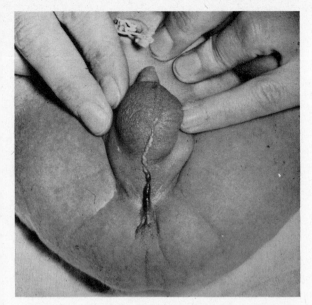

Fig. 197. A covered anus with track extending forward in the scrotal raphe (anocutaneous fistula, International Classification).

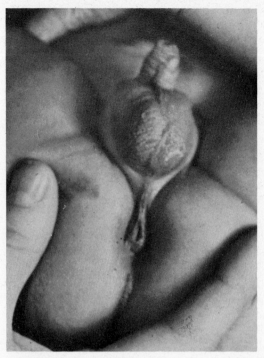

Fig. 198. A case of covered anus in which the embryological derivation of the abnormality is particularly clearly suggested.

rectum will already have suffered considerable secondary dilatation.

ANORECTAL MEMBRANE (IMPERFORATE ANAL MEMBRANE, INTERNATIONAL CLASSIFICATION)

This rare anomaly only occurred once in over 300 cases. The membrane crosses the anal canal at the upper end of the proctodeum and may rupture spontaneously, leaving the ring-like narrowing of the preceding type.

CONGENITAL FUNNEL ANUS

An apparently rare variant of anorectal junction stenosis has been observed on three occasions. I have not seen it described elsewhere. Normal skin extends up to the stenotic ring where it joins the rectal mucosa abruptly without the intervention of any transitional epithelium. The junction looks like a surgical rather than a natural one. Histological examination of the stenotic area reveals that the ring consists of fibrosed internal sphincter. The external sphincter feels deficient and the anus looks like a skin-lined funnel. The puborectalis feels normal. Intermediate forms exist between this type and the anorectal junction stenosis in an otherwise normally developed canal.

IMPERFORATE ANUS (ANAL AGENESIS WITHOUT FISTULA, INTERNATIONAL CLASSIFICATION)

This uncommon type only occurred once in our series of 300. The bowel extends to the pelvic floor and is cradled in the puborectalis sling. The skin covers the anus completely.

RECTOBULBAR FISTULA (ANAL AGENESIS WITH RECTOBULBAR FISTULA, INTERNATIONAL CLASSIFICATION

Sometimes associated with an atypical form of hypospadias, it may be caused by overfusion of the medial genital folds and related to a 'covering' anomaly (Nixon 1972b). Other fistulae entering the urethra low down may represent a low variant of the anorectal agenesis described later. It accounted for only 2·3% of our series.

RECTOVESTIBULAR FISTULA

Although the orifice is below the hymen only a narrow tube-like segment leads through the pelvic floor before entering the rectal ampulla. Distinguished from ectopic anus (anovestibular fistula,

International Classification) by inability to direct a probe posteriorly above the orifice on clinical examination.

High Abnormalities
(Anorectal Agenesis)

In this high group the rectum usually reaches to the upper surface of the pelvic floor but the anal canal which should traverse this is absent. The rectum usually opens into the prostatic urethra of the male (the classical atresia ani urethralis, Fig. 199; anorectal agenesis with rectourethral fistula, International Classification). This is an important group, representing 26% of our cases, and is a more primitive condition in which the cloaca has not divided into separate urinary and alimentary parts (owing to failure of migration of the primitive anus or to failure of development of the urorectal septum, depending on one's preferred interpretation of the differential growth pattern which should occur). In the female the interposition of the Müllerian system picks off the fistula to enter the posterior fornix of the vagina (anorectal agenesis with rectovaginal fistula, high, International Classification) (Fig. 194C, D).

The levator floor is usually well developed but the levator floor does not descend further than the bowel and hence the sling is higher than normal (Kiesewetter and Nixon 1967). The external sphincter muscle, perhaps only the subcutaneous portion of it, is usually present and may pucker the anal skin on stimulation. Alone it is insufficient to have any useful function, however, and may be displaced from the pelvic floor by a large fat pad lying across the midline. This fat seems to represent a coalescence of the ischiorectal fat pads. It is commoner for the usual anal site to be marked by a thickening of the raphe than by a dimple. The natal cleft is usually shallow because of the fat pad, and a bulging weak levator floor may accentuate this, when a neurological deficit accompanies sacral agenesis. Thin modified skin lies at the anterior end of the raphe at the normal anal site. It appears to represent anal lining skin. Stimulation causes reflex contraction of the external sphincter. Hence it seems to represent an everted proctodeum—admittedly of varying development—rather than an agenesis.

Variants of this anomaly occur. In the male the opening in the urinary tract is occasionally into the bladder (though most cases reported as such seem to be due to misinterpretation of neonatal anatomy) or less rarely into the membranous urethra. In the female it may open lower down the posterior vaginal wall. In either sex the bowel may end blindly and be attached to the above sites only by a fibrous cord (anorectal agenesis without fistula, International Classification). Rarely it may end higher in the pelvis suggesting absence of the greater part if not the whole of the rectum.

The pelvic splanchnic plexuses which normally lie to either side of the lower rectum fall together in the midline in these cases forming a cluster around the site of entry into the urethra (Scott 1959). It is not clear whether the rectum of these children commonly represents the whole organ or only the upper part but balloon and electromyographic studies have shown a normal sphincter response to rectal distension (Nixon and Callaghan 1964).

RECTAL ATRESIA

In this unfortunately uncommon type of high imperforation there is a normal anal canal and an atresia of the rectum just above it akin to atresias higher in the alimentary tract. The anal canal appears to correspond to the surgical canal, not only the proctodeum. There is no attachment to the urinary tract, and this seems to be a developmentally distinct kind of high anomaly.

PRIMITIVE CLOACA (RECTOCLOACAL FISTULA, INTERNATIONAL CLASSIFICATION)

In the female there may be a single external opening into a globular cavity. The cavity is entered by a short urethra anteriorly and by the rectum posteriorly. Between these there are usually two openings of the uteri, Müllerian systems having failed to fuse (Fig. 194D).

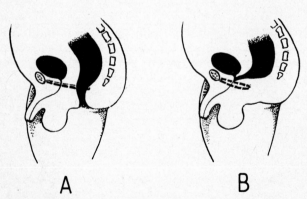

A   **B**

Fig. 199. Sectional diagrams. (A) Normal male pelvis. (B) Anorectal agenesis with rectourethral fistula.

VESICO-INTESTINAL FISSURE (CLOACAL EXTROPHY, INTERNATIONAL CLASSIFICATION)

In this rare and gross anomaly the symphysis pubis is separated and the genitalia bifid. The ectopic bladder is represented by two halves separated by a median intestinal field. Into this area bowel, usually ileum, opens proximally and a further opening leads to a shortened colon terminating above the pelvic floor. The amount of bowel 'lost' in this anomaly varies and there is often an associated exomphalos. Reconstruction will rarely be possible (Magnus 1969).

Associated Abnormalities

SACRAL AGENESIS

Partial failure of development of the sacrum is a common accompaniment of anorectal abnormality. The number of segments may be reduced or they may be deformed, or both. A short sacrum is likely also to be straight without the normal anterior concavity and with reduction of the usual lumbosacral angle.

The importance of this condition is that suppression of more than one segment is associated with a neurological deficit. Williams and Nixon (1957) found that every case studied with a sacrum of three or less segments had a neurological bladder neck disability. There were five such cases amongst 41 examined. Deformity of a segment seems to be as significant as its absence in this respect. Smith (1963), however, has found that the sacral nerves may occasionally develop in the absence of the corresponding vertebrae. A four-segment sacrum, however, was usually associated with an apparently normal innervation. A group was revealed which had only four segments in the sacrum but in which there was a compensating sixth lumbar vertebra. This condition of epistasis is a failure of specialization rather than suppression of a segment. It is not associated with neurological defect.

UROGENITAL DEFECTS

At least one-third of the high and a quarter of the low cases have some minor or major urogenital defect. Defects of the lower urinary tract such as urethral stricture or neurogenic bladder disorders occur. They may perhaps be considered as part of the defect rather than as associated phenomena.

Upper tract defects also occur. Hydronephrosis, megaureter, ectopic ureter, cystic kidney, horseshoe kidney, duplication, hypoplasia and aplasia of the kidney all occur. Fortunately unilateral conditions appear to be commoner than bilateral.

In the female, more commonly in the high deformities, some degree of division of the genital tract may occur. It may be only an incompletely septate vagina or an extensive division with two separate uteri. The vaginal orifice may be closed posteriorly so as to present such a small opening behind the clitoris as to appear to be a urethral orifice ('covered vagina'). A median cutback reveals the true state of affairs.

In the male, hypospadias may be associated with the anal abnormality but this is not a frequent association like that of bifid genital tract with rectal agenesis in the female.

Intravenous pyelography and voiding cystogram are always performed at an early stage in management.

OTHER ASSOCIATIONS

The association of oesophageal atresia with tracheo-oesophageal fistula with the congenital anorectal abnormalities is sufficiently frequent to justify the passage of a sterile catheter into the stomach routinely to exclude the proximal malformation.

Congenital cardiac defects also occur in a significant proportion (Stephens and Smith 1971). The VACTERL syndrome is a specific grouping of vertebral, anal, cardiac, tracheal, esophageal, renal and limb anomalies (Nora and Nora 1975).

To preserve a sense of proportion after discussing these possibilities it must be said that *most cases of 'imperforate anus' will not suffer from any abnormality other than the anal one*.

DIAGNOSIS

Inspection should reveal every case immediately after birth (except anorectal stenosis, imperforate anorectal membrane and the rare rectal atresia with an intact anal canal). Nevertheless they can be missed until obstruction with distension and biliary vomiting leads to further examination. This is particularly liable to happen when the abnormal orifice allows passage of enough meconium to produce a reasonable show on the napkin.

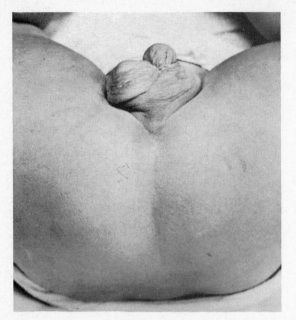

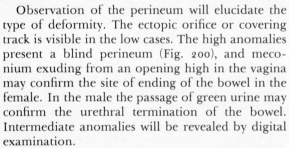

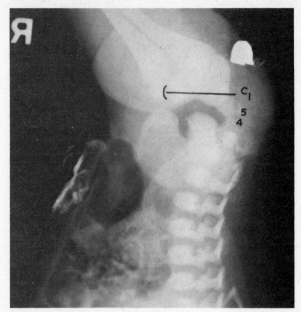

Fig. 200. The blind perineum with shallow natal cleft of a male cloaca: anorectal agenesis with rectourethral fistula.

Fig. 201. A lateral radiograph of pelvic area of the inverted baby. Stephen's pubococcygeal line is drawn in; bubble shows a high anomaly.

Observation of the perineum will elucidate the type of deformity. The ectopic orifice or covering track is visible in the low cases. The high anomalies present a blind perineum (Fig. 200), and meconium exuding from an opening high in the vagina may confirm the site of ending of the bowel in the female. In the male the passage of green urine may confirm the urethral termination of the bowel. Intermediate anomalies will be revealed by digital examination.

Radiographs of the inverted baby are widely used to confirm the level of obstruction. The lateral view of Stephens and Smith (1971) is preferable to Wangensteen and Rice's classical method because it relates the air shadow to skeletal markers which are more significant than the skin level. A line from the pubis to the expected site of the coccyx is just above the level of the puborectalis sling where the high anomalies end. The line passes through the comma-shaped ischial shadow just below the junction of the body and tail. The lowest visible point on the ischial shadow represents the level of the low anomalies (Kelly 1969). In the anteroposterior view the air shadow can also be related to the skeleton as the levator floor is at the level of the triradiate cartilage. However, there are many fallacies. If radiographs are taken too early, say in the first 12 hours of life, the gas may not have reached the end of the bowel. Later the shape of the shadow will usually make it clear that the end of the bowel has been reached. Even then, contraction of the levators may make the bowel end appear too high, whereas crying or paralysis of the pelvic floor may make it seem too low. Probably the most useful observation on the lateral radiograph is that of the development of the sacrum (Fig. 201). The lumbosacral angle is present from the third month of fetal life (Keith 1948) and is the most reliable marker for making a count of the sacral segments in the newborn. At least four should be present and free from deformity, otherwise bladder dysfunction and weakness of the pelvic floor are very likely.

MANAGEMENT

General Considerations

All anorectal anomalies except minor degrees of anterior perineal anus need immediate treatment. Those cases with a reasonably sized outlet may seem to offer scope for conservative management, but in practice there is nothing to be gained by such delay. Much may be lost when the rectum becomes overstretched by the extra effort needed to expel faeces through a small or inelastic orifice. The rectal inertia syndrome described on p. 295 may develop in a severe form which will need prolonged treatment. Indeed it is not uncommon to see a child with incontinence presumed to be due to sphincter deficiency which is in fact the result of the secondary rectal inertia.

The perineal anus may need only dilatation but most low anomalies require primary enlargement by a cutback. Furthermore delay may involve the baby unnecessarily in procedures at a psychologically vulnerable time after about the sixth month. The high anomalies need a colostomy to relieve the obstruction and given time for detailed analysis of the situation. Definitive surgery will usually be delayed between 6 and 12 months so that the pull-through procedure required can be performed with less trauma to the puborectalis sling.

In the high anomalies in the male with an orifice in the urinary tract an additional hazard present is urinary infection, particularly in those cases with concomitant abnormalities in this system. A colostomy should give adequate protection when the urinary tract is normal. A skin bridge colostomy with primary skin to mucosa suture (Nixon 1966) defunctions adequately. The distal loop should be emptied at operation and should be kept empty by weekly saline washouts until definitive surgery follows. Our past series did show a higher incidence of urinary problems with delayed surgery but I believe greater care of the distal loop in this manner would have avoided this.

The question of a permanent colostomy arises in more severe defects like anorectal agenesis in which a reliable bowel habit cannot be confidently anticipated. But even children who end up with a poor anus can often be taught a bowel regimen when they are, say, six or seven years old, like children with spina bifida paraplegia, although the absence of an internal sphincter with its constant tone makes soiling more of a problem for the anorectal anomalies. The writer feels that even this outcome is better than a permanent colostomy and justifies an attempt at repair in almost every case. The growing and developing child has totally different problems from the mature established adult in accepting a colostomy. The child may become seriously upset at puberty even if not before. I encountered one boy so well adjusted to a colostomy at 14 years of age that it seemed that further surgery would be unwise and he was advised against it. He returned a year later to ask for operation and is now pleased with the repair.

A middle course needs to be steered between persisting so long in attempts to achieve continence that the child loses heart and accepting a colostomy which may have been avoided had the child been given an opportunity of 'learned continence' when old enough to cooperate. There may be a place for longer term temporary colostomy to tide over a child incontinent after primary repair of a high anomaly until he is old enough to cooperate in a regimen after a secondary procedure.

Detailed Treatment of Individual Lesions

ECTOPIC AND COVERED ANUS

The basis of treatment is that the orifice which is present should be enlarged so that it can work where it lies. This usually means a simple 'cutback' or midline episiotomy. On occasion a course of dilatations alone is sufficient. Transplantation to the usual anal site is sometimes required later, but is never considered as a primary operation.

THE 'CUTBACK'

The usual vulval ectopic anus (Fig. 193) is treated by inserting one blade of a pair of scissors inside the orifice and passing it back as far as it will go under the skin without going deeper and then closing the blades to perform a midline episiotomy. The anus should then be dilated to take the fifth finger or Hegar 11 or 12. The raw surfaces are left to heal spontaneously. They do this with good supple epithelium. One or two sutures may be placed for haemostasis but the result is better than is obtained by precise suturing and avoids the risk of pocketing of infection. Daily dilatation is essential beginning 48 hours after operation. The mother is taught to pass the finger protected by a fingerstall, or Hegar's dilators up to size 12, but sometimes this needs to be supervised by the district nurse. At all events it is of supreme importance that dilatations continue daily for three months until the newly enlarged anus is settled and supple. The dilatations are then performed weekly for a month to be sure there is no tendency to re-stenosis.

Only in this way can constipation with consequent rectal inertia and overflow incontinence be avoided. Although this simple procedure does not bring the bowel properly through the subcutaneous external sphincter it allows of clinically normal continence. The result is what Denis Browne has called a shotgun perineum with both barrels alongside (Fig. 202). But it is usually functionally normal and the appearance improves as time passes and the posterior vaginal wall thickens up.

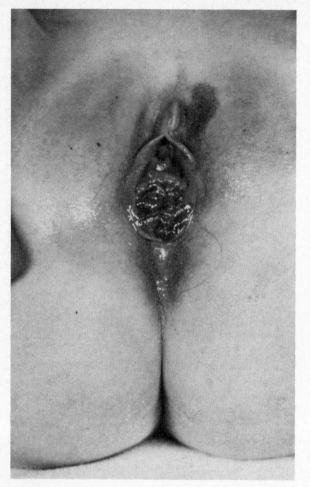

Fig. 202. The condition following a 'cutback' for vulval ectopic anus (vestibular anus, International Classification).

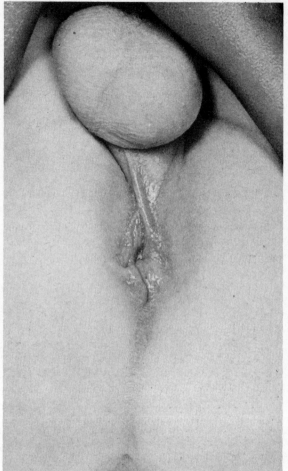

Fig. 203. Covered anus after 'uncovering' (same case as Fig. 197).

The covered anus is similarly treated by picking a track back from the orifice (Figs 197 and 203) until the anus is reached and then keeping it dilated. If there are epithelial excrescences left around the anus these are trimmed off.

DILATATIONS

Minor degrees of ectopia or covering may be adequately managed by dilatations alone. But these must be thorough and prolonged as above. The end result should be a bowel which does not have a sharp anterior curve at the lower end. If such a curve is left constipation results—apparently from a tendency to force a bolus down behind the opening on straining, producing a kind of ball-valve effect. If there is any doubt about the adequacy of the procedure it is better to cut back.

SECONDARY ANAL TRANSPLANTATION

In the majority of cases of ectopic anus the cutback procedure produces a definitively satisfactory anus. In a few, however, the anus remains tilted into the back of the vulva so that it is difficult to keep clean and to avoid soiling of the vagina. Urinary infections and even a tubovarian abscess have followed such a condition. In this minority a transplantation has been of great value. It has also seemed in some cases to have improved control. This is due more to the elimination of the forward curve at the end of the bowel and its replacement by the normal posterior angulation than to the course of the bowel now traversing the external sphincter material.

The transplantation is always done as a secondary procedure because the bowel in the neonatal period

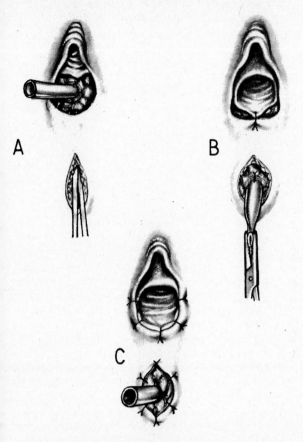

A

B

C

Fig. 204. Operation for transplantation of ectopic anus or fistula. (A) Ectopic anus circumcised and freed. Handling tube fastened in. Incision at usual anal site. Tunnel made forwards with forceps. (B) Bowel drawn through to anal site with the help of the rubber tube. (C) Suturing of bowel (in two layers) and of vulval gap (loosely) completed. (A cruciate incision at the anal site is now more customary.)

does not have a strong enough submucosa to resist the strains due to the contractions of the muscle coat. In spite of the most careful technique a proportion of anastomotic breakdowns occur as a result of transplantation performed at this period. Temporary colostomy does not avoid this hazard. The best time for transplantation is probably the fourth year. The child is less upset than it would be earlier during the toddler period and is more co-operative in after-care. There is still time for the child to get settled down to a routine before schooling starts in earnest. If circumstances dictate further delay from a psychological viewpoint this will in no way interfere with the performance of the operation.

The steps of the operation are as follows (Fig. 204):

1. The ectopic anus is circumcised.

2. A large-bore rubber tube is inserted through the anus and stitched into it. This device (suggested by Denis Browne) makes an excellent handle for manipulating the bowel, and by giving the bowel some content makes dissection around it easier. If the bowel is large enough it may be preferred to insert several stay sutures to spread the strain of handling and then performing the dissection with a finger in the rectum to make sure the recognition of the perirectal plane.

3. Dissection is continued upwards around the bowel for about 5 cm. Special care is needed in separating the anterior wall from the vagina. If the cut goes into the layers of the wall of the bowel then a fistula may result. Too extensive a dissection is also dangerous in that the residual blood supply may be inadequate and again lead to a fistula.

4. A cruciate skin incision 2–3 cm long is made over the usual site of the anus. By blunt dissection an opening is made through what exists of the external sphincter and is then carried forward in the subcutaneous tissues to the fourchette opening through which the bowel has been freed. The rubber tube is seized by the dissecting instrument and used to draw the bowel back and out through the new anal orifice. An anteriorly based 'trapdoor' incision in the skin may be preferred. It gives an oblique anastomosis less likely to stenose and extra tissue anteriorly where the bowel mobilizes less freely.

5. The bowel is now sutured to the new orifice. Several catgut sutures attach the bowel to the pelvic floor—taking bites of such pelvic fascia or muscle as can be exposed, and bites through muscle and submucosa of the bowel. The rubber tube is then removed. A layer of vertical Dexon mattress sutures joins the full thickness of the bowel to skin. The preliminary catguts take the strain off this layer and help to obtain primary healing.

6. The opening in the fourchette is loosely closed as a transverse line. Before this is done one or two loosely tied catgut sutures should be placed to draw the deep tissues together as a perineal body. If there is much of an oozing cavity around the mobilized bowel it is wise to put in a catheter and attach this to a suction drain for a few days. This will prevent an infected haematoma (yet another possible cause of fistula).

7. Postoperative care. If all seems well, *no rectal examinations or dilatations* are allowed for 14 days.

(Even if there seems to be some breakdown, because such examinations can only increase it.) On the fourteenth day, daily dilatations are begun and are continued for three months and then gradually discontinued; the formation of a 'string stenosis' at the mucocutaneous junction is thus avoided. From the third postoperative day to the fourteenth a few millilitres of oil are instilled daily through a small catheter to prevent any faecal masses forming.

In the uncommon cases of anal agenesis with low rectovaginal fistula, difficult to manage by cutback, this procedure is carried out at three to six months of age, following dilatations, and protective colostomy may then be wise.

Stephens prefers a sacral approach to these transplantations such as is described later as part of the operation for high lesions, and believes it allows better mobilization of the bowel and protection of the all-important puborectalis sling.

Rectovestibular Fistula

This is the only type with an opening below the hymen which cannot be primarily treated by cutback. Colostomy is required and followed later by perineal or sacroperineal transplant.

Anorectal Junction Stenosis

INTERNAL PROCTOTOMY AND DILATATIONS

The treatment is simple: division of the fibrous ring by internal proctotomies followed by persistent dilatations. The same applies to the funnel anus variant. Management, however, may be very tedious. This is because the external appearance of the baby is normal, and months or even years may pass before the lesion is discovered or its significance appreciated. A frequent sequence of events is, first, reassurance that constipation in a baby does not matter, then, as abdominal masses and distension appear, the use of paraffin and aperients, and when overflow occurs, courses of clear fluids and antibiotics for 'diarrhoea'; finally a rectal examination reveals the cause. The delay is apparently due to the belief, which I feel to be greatly exaggerated, in the psychological hazards of rectal examination. No psychological trauma follows digitation in the first few months of life. It certainly can later after about six months of age. If the lesion is discovered late, a gross rectal inertia will have developed requiring prolonged management

along the lines described in the next chapter. Dilatation of the funnel anus may leave an inelastic ring, so that soiling persists even after rectal inertia is cured. Isogel or similar bulk formers may help, and a gracilis transplant (see p. 275) has been useful.

Anorectal Membrane

Perforation may leave a fibrous ring stricture as in anorectal junction stenosis, so dilatations must be performed in the same way.

High Abnormalities

These are mainly rectal ageneses. The important feature is a bowel stopping above the pelvic floor, hence the basis of treatment is different from the methods previously described. There can be no question of 'making the orifice work where it lies' by enlarging or uncovering it. The bowel requires to be brought through the pelvic diaphragm at the correct point and an 'anus' constructed. Care is required to avoid damage to the musculature of the pelvic floor and sphincter. The classical advice to 'explore up the hollow of the sacrum' is disastrous in these high anomalies for it will inevitably divide the puborectalis sling which is the essential muscle in control. An abdomino-anal pull through operation after the lead of Rhoads et al. (1948) held the field for many years. We were only able to achieve 29% of good and 48% of satisfactory results. Stephens (1963) first used a posterior sacral approach to identify the puborectalis sling. Sometimes he now completes the operation from this posterior approach but at other times includes an abdominal phase adequately to mobilize the rectum. We and many others now use an elaborate abdominosacro-anal operation based on the technique described by Kiesewetter (1967). Although much room remains for improvement our results are better and are discussed later.

THE ABDOMINOSACRAL-ANAL OPERATION

Principles

1. Sacral approach to open the track in front of the puborectalis sling under direct vision.

2. Submucosal endorectal pull through (Rehbein 1959) to avoid dissection in the bladder neck region which is hazardous to the medially displaced pelvic splanchnic plexuses (Scott 1959). This also gives a

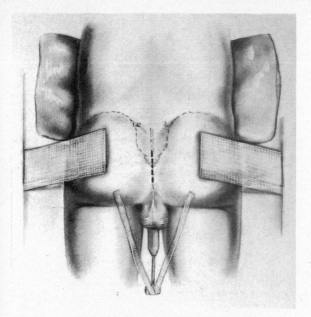

Fig. 205. Sacral phase. Prone 'jack-knife' position over sand-bag. Buttocks strapped apart. Sound strapped into urethra, so that it can be moved under the towels to aid identification of the site of the urethra.

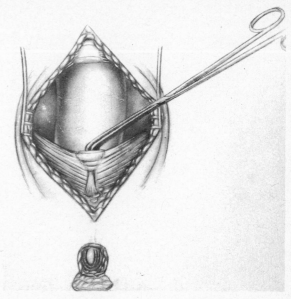

Fig. 206. Sacral phase. Coccyx cut off sacrum, and supra-levator space opened to dissect in front of levator sling. 'Trap-door' at anal site developed.

sound closure of the urethral fistula by drawing intact colon past it.

3. Inversion proctoplasty. Skin excision in front of and behind the newly constructed anus inverts the skin between them as a proctodeum lessening the tendency to mucosal prolapse and possibly helping with sensation (Nixon 1968).

Technique

An effective intravenous infusion is set up so that blood can be replaced as lost.

1. The child is placed prone with the pelvis elevated over a sandbag and with a sound in the urethra (Fig. 205).

A midline incision is begun over the lower part of the sacrum and carried to within 2–3 cm of the anal site. The coccyx is cut free from the lower end of the sacrum, thereby gaining entrance to the supralevator space (Fig. 206). The puborectalis sling is identified and is carefully eased off the urethra to develop a track down to the anal site. An anteriorly placed trapdoor of skin is reflected off the anal site and the instrument is passed through the anal orifice to allow a wide Penrose drain to be drawn through to the supra-levator space (Fig. 207) where it is left to be picked up in the next stage of the operation. The wound is repaired in layers.

(Kiesewetter does not cut the coccyx off the sacrum but incises through the diaphragmatic part of the supralevator to identify the puborectalis sling (Fig. 208). He also prefers a cruciate incision at the anal site.)

2. The patient is turned over and placed in the semilithotomy position on a small infant table made to strap on to the main table (see Fig. 215). The cross-bar between the leg pieces is not needed in this operation since there is no dirty field around the anus.

A transverse subumbilical skin incision is made and skin flaps retracted up and down with a Denis Browne retractor. It is deepened by a midline incision between the recti. Then a 'V' shaped peritoneal incision is made around the bladder which is largely an abdominal organ at this age. The bladder is drawn out of the wound with stay sutures attached to the retractor ring to improve visibility in the pelvis (Figs 209, 210).

The rectum is held up with stay sutures and divided across in its intraperitoneal part. The sigmoid is mobilized by division of the mesenteric vessels and laid aside under moist packs (Fig. 211).

The mucosal lining of the rectum is then peeled out by blunt dissection with broad tipped forceps and gauze pledgets. (The stay sutures will need to be removed in turn as they tether the submucosa if

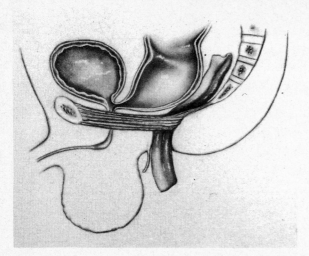

Fig. 207. Sacral phase. Wide Penrose drain drawn up from anal site into supralevator space.

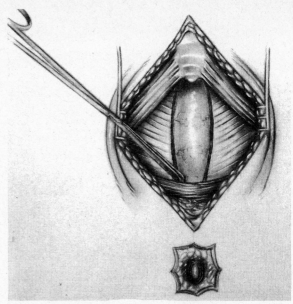

Fig. 208. Sacral phase. Kiesewetter's alternative approach through the median raphe of the diaphragmatic part of the levator to reach in front of the sling.

deep enough to hold satisfactorily.) Separation is surprisingly easy and the ooze of blood will always stop spontaneously. When the lining tube is freed as far as the fistula this is transfixed with a catgut suture and the lining cut away. (This closure is not important if the bladder is efficiently drained for ten days.)

An incision is then made in the bottom of the rectal muscle pouch and the Penrose drain is picked up and drawn into the abdomen (Fig. 212). Thus the drain demarcates the path from the anal site in front of the puborectalis sling and up through the rectal muscle tube. Lubricated Hegar's dilators are then passed through the drain in turn until it will accept a No. 12. This is wide enough to take the

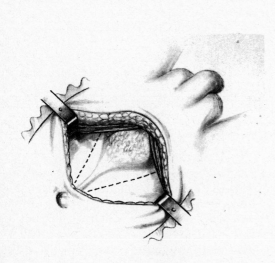

Fig. 209. Transverse skin incision. Recti separated. Peritoneal inverted V incision dotted in.

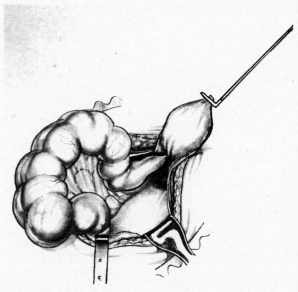

Fig. 210. Bladder drawn out and down to improve the exposure in the pelvis.

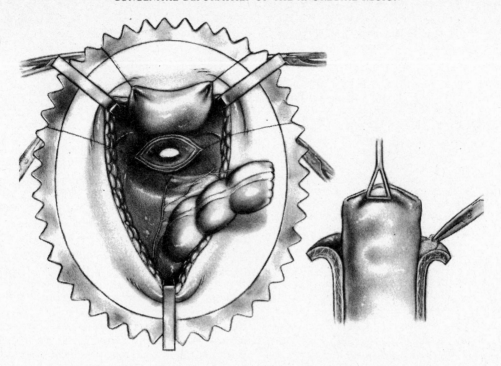

Fig. 211. Abdominal phase. Division of rectum above pelvic floor and coring our of lining in submucous plane.

intestine through and further stretching must be avoided to prevent trauma to the sling.

A tonsil forceps is a convenient instrument to pass next through the drain to catch the end of the mobilized sigmoid in the abdomen and draw it through to the anus.

3. *The anal phase.* The end of the sigmoid is then fixed with a few fine catgut sutures to the external sphincter muscle fibres (Fig. 213) and then trimmed so that the full thickness of the bowel wall can be sutured to the skin including the anterior trapdoor which avoids a ring scar. These sutures should be tied very slackly so that they do not cut out with

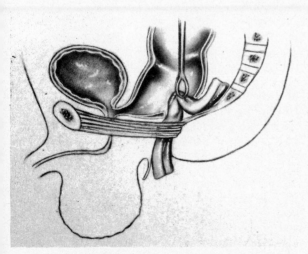

Fig. 212. Abdominal phase. Incision at bottom of rectal muscle tube to withdraw Penrose drain into rectal lumen as a guide for dilatation of the track through pelvic floor.

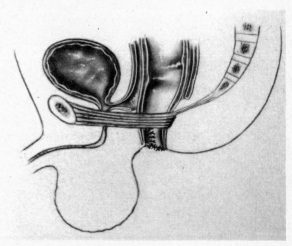

Fig. 213. Abdominal and anal phases. Mobilized sigmoid drawn through to anal site and sutured to anal tissues.

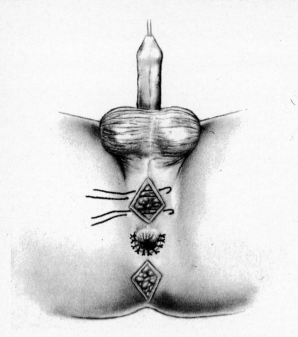

Fig. 214. Anal phase, completion. Kite-shaped incision in front of and behind the anus for inversion.

oedema. Swenson's suggestion that each stitch should be tied over the tip of a mosquito forceps is helpful.

Because I believe the proctodeum is everted rather than agenetic (admittedly in a variable degree of development) I prefer to invert the sensitive modified skin at the anal site in front of the usual epithelial excrescence. A kite-shaped skin incision is, therefore, carried out in front and behind the anus to advance and invert this skin into an anal canal (Fig. 214). These wounds are closed with deep tension sutures because swelling of the fat will otherwise disrupt the suture line.

Finally a plastic in-dwelling catheter is left through the urethra into the bladder for ten days.

Variations

In the *female* the procedure is simpler in that the vagina is interposed so as to protect the urinary system and there is rarely any urinary fistula. Unfortunately a congenital lesion of the bladder neck or urethra is not so uncommon. There may be a 'cover' of the vagina in addition to the rectal lesions so that a back cut of the small perineal opening is needed to expose a vagina with a urethral orifice inside it. The bowel needs to be brought through farther back. The fistula to the posterior fornix is easily approached from above without hazard to the bladder neck because of the interposed vagina. The dissection down to the pelvic floor is made immediately in front of the presacral fascia to avoid the pelvic splanchnic nerves. The rectum can be pulled through the pelvic floor immediately behind the vagina (checking with a finger or instrument in this structure) so that it must be in front of the sling.

In the rare *rectal atresia* the bowel stops above the pelvic floor but there is a normal anal canal. The dome of the anal canal reaches to the upper surface of the pelvic floor so that it can be opened from the abdomen over a Hegar's dilator inserted from below. The mobilized bowel can then be drawn through and sutured outside the anus to the skin. Catgut sutures are also placed above the pelvic floor from the abdominal side as a safeguard against retraction. For convenience these sutures should be placed before the bowel is drawn through the proctodeum and left untied until after this manoeuvre. The bowel will unite with the anal canal and dilatations are begun after 14 days to avoid contracture and continued for the usual three months before gradually reducing their frequency. One would expect to have to trim tags of excess bowel after healing, but in practice this excess material seems to shrink and retract and may need no treatment.

Postoperative Care

Gentle daily anal dilatations begin in 14 days after operation. When the anus will accept Hegar 11 or 12 the colostomy is closed. Daily dilatations continue for three months after operation and then weekly to check for recurrent stenosis for the next three months.

COMPLICATIONS

Excessive Protrusion of Mucosa from the Anus

In the abdominosacro-anal procedure the primary object is to make an adequate anus to avoid the ill effects of stenosis and consequent back pressure. In spite of anal inversion redundant mucosa may later develop and become exposed in the perineum. This can give rise to discomfort and straining. Secondary trimming of this material, drawing the perianal skin up toward the pelvic floor, is performed if necessary at or before four years of age. This seems to help in the attainment of control—probably mainly as a result of relief of discomfort and hence of habitual straining. It is also possible that the indrawn perianal skin helps by giving some measure of sensation. Minor degrees of mucosal excess and perianal irritation may be controlled by vigorous surface diathermy. The mucosa is replaced by stratified mucosa more akin to the natural transitional tissue.

Recurrent Urethral Fistula

A urethral fistula may recur after operation. In this case the track is usually from the congenital opening in the prostatic urethra down to the surgical junction between skin and mucosa at the anal verge. It can usually be excised from below. Diversion of urine (e.g. by posterior urethrotomy) for two weeks is essential. A colostomy may be considered wise in some cases but the essential in obtaining healing seems to be careful dissection so as to avoid devascularizing the mobilized bowel in the region of the fistula. The cuff of mobilized anterior rectal wall is drawn down over the track and re-sutured to the skin. The urethral end of the track retracts upwards after its division and is best left unsutured so that there is no buried suture material. As already mentioned urinary diversion is essential to this technique. A difficult fistula with pronounced local scarring may better be closed by Turner Warwick's technique of interposing mobilized greater omentum (see Fig. 318). But fistulas are exceptional after the endorectal pull-through now used.

Calculus Formation

In the classical abdomino-anal operation without endorectal pull through, the fistula may be divided at a distance from the urethra leaving a persistent pouch attached to the urethra. A urinary calculus may form in the pouch. This needs to be borne in mind should unexplained dysuria and straining occur. Removal by open operation should be accompanied by excision of the mucosal lining of the pouch and obliteration of the lumen. This will probably be easier to perform with safety than a radical excision of the pouch. Such a pouch may also become the seat of an abscess. These complications have not been seen since using the endorectal pull through.

Anal Stenosis

Necrosis, or breakdown of the suture line due to tension may cause anal stenosis. (It must be remembered that an inelastic anus with a mucocutaneous 'string' will act as a defaecation block even though a small finger may pass with ease.) The anus can be enlarged by the classical Z-plasties. The author has found the following procedure at least as satisfactory.

The posterior half of the mucocutaneous junction is excised. The posterior third of the rectal wall is mobilized for about 3 cm and a V of skin is excised behind the anus. Incisions upward at each side of the mobilized rectum allow a tag to be drawn out into the V. It is sutured to the skin after suitable trimming.

Elongated Inert Anal Canal

The presence in some cases of a considerable pad of fat in the perineum may have left the child with a long inert segment of bowel—as much as 7 cm—below the pelvic floor and surrounded by fat. Apart from the resistance to defaecation, trouble is caused because residual faeces in this tube is massaged out by activity after defaecation. Thus soiling occurs even when the child is reasonably successful in emptying the rectum proper. The anus can be made much easier to keep clean by excising the lower part of such a canal and drawing the perianal skin up towards the pelvic floor. Care should be taken not to dissect too high. Thus the bowel is left adherent in its course through the pelvic floor and any breakdown in the mucocutaneous suture is less serious. It may necessitate dilatations whilst secondary healing occurs but the pelvic floor will not be involved in the breakdown and the peculiarly resistant type of stricture which can occur at this higher level will be avoided.

Weak Pelvic Floor

This can be recognized by low pressures on anorectal manometry. The grip on the finger may feel deceptively good. *Levatorplasty* is the most useful secondary procedure.

A curved postanal incision with its apex above the sacrococcygeal junction allows reflection of a skin flap and by freeing the coccyx the levator floor can be assessed. If the bowel has been wrongly passed behind the puborectalis sling it can be rerouted in front. In my experience of secondary operations (usually following abdomino-anal procedures) it has been more common to find a deficient or scarred pelvic floor. Gross' levator plication (1970) has been combined with Kottmeier and Dziadev's (1967) levator liberation. The coccyx is allowed to drop forward or removed and the diaphragmatic part of the levator is freed laterally so that it comes forward as an additional sling. Silk sutures are then placed to plicate it in its anterior position. This operation also improves the anorectal angle (Nixon 1972a).

Should there be no adequate muscle for such improvement a *gracilis transplant* has been used. The original Pickrell procedure has not been very satisfactory in my hands and the addition of an implanted stimulator to maintain tone (Dickson and Nixon 1968) only helped about half the cases. Recent experience of the bilateral gracilis transplant (Hartl 1972) has been more effective, forming a more adequate muscular ring around the entire circumference of the anus. In some a permanent colostomy has still to be accepted.

Loose Stools

In some instances the bowel is overactive so that the stools are so loose that continence is more difficult to achieve. The use of loperamide (Imodium) to reduce the rate of transit and hence allow a more formed stool can be invaluable (0.1 mg/kg/day is the recommended starting dose though there has been a wide variation in the effective dose).

RESULTS

There is a vast difference between the results obtained in the low abnormalities and in the high ones. Covered anus and microscopic anus should give normal function and virtually normal appearance with thorough early treatment. Poor results are almost always the consequence of rectal inertia from delayed treatment or inadequate after-care.

The function of ectopic anus is equally good. The condition of the external sphincter makes one realize the crucial importance of the puborectalis muscle. Transplantation can certainly be undertaken as a secondary procedure without anxiety

about possible loss of control—and one has the impression that there may be a real improvement in some children who have previously had recurring bouts of loading and overflow. It may be that the change in direction removes a tendency for rectal contractions to waste their force in pushing faeces into a cul-de-sac behind the forward-turned anus. However, transplantation is not usually necessary and is more often indicated for hygienic reasons.

Anorectal junction stenosis gives good results if the muscles are well formed, but in the 'funnel anus' group a tendency to soiling may persist. One of our patients only achieved adequate control of soiling with a gracilis transplant and stimulator to substitute for the fibrous internal sphincter.

Naturally, an associated defect of the pelvic floor or its innervation such as is associated with agenesis of the sacrum will vitiate the result. But even these children can often be trained, like those with spina bifida, to a 'social control' by voluntary effort (perhaps with the help of enemas from time to time to ensure complete evacuation and avoid the development of retention and overflow). Dietary control, e.g. the avoidance of certain fruits, may also be needed in some. This is preferred to a colostomy. Surprisingly this may not be as easy to achieve as in the spina bifida patients—I believe because they do not have an internal sphincter to maintain persistent tone and prevent soiling. The distressing defect in these children is likely to be

TABLE 10. *Results of Surgical Treatment for Congenital Abnormalities of the Anus and Rectum**

		Results (%)†		
		Good	Satisfactory	Poor
Primary treatment	High abnormalities	36.5	58.5	5.0
	Low abnormalities	92	5.7	2.3
High abnormalities (primary and secondary referrals, i.e. not an unselected series)	Puborectalis seen (i.e. operation with sacral phase)	42	50	8
	Puborectalis not seen (i.e. abdomino-anal operation as used earlier)	14	18.7	67.3
Results related to period of follow-up‡	Under 6 years	37	33.3	29.7
	Over 6 years	43.1	49.5	7.4

* Patients referred to H.H.N., 1962–70; 171 for primary treatment and 129 for secondary treatment (total 300). Mortality 8.5%, of which 78% were cardiorespiratory and 22% due to sepsis.

† *Good* = no accidents. *Satisfactory* = occasional accidents or soiling. *Poor* = incontinence, impactions, etc. I am greatly indebted to Dr Gunther Willital of Erlangen for this analysis.

‡ Demonstrating improvement with age and development of a real interest in gaining control.

their urinary control which is not so easy to manage. This applies both in high and low anomalies.

Whilst virtually normal control is expected in the uncomplicated low cases it is exceptional in the high ones. In these latter socially acceptable control is often obtained by about school age, but it is an abnormal mechanism usually likely to break down to a varying degree under stress such as an unsuitable diet or infection. At times one gets the impression that the result in the high cases depends more on the mother's intelligence and capability than on the organic state of the bowel. Certainly an uncooperative and feckless mother can mar the progress of such a child and a period in a suitable hospital school may need consideration. Happily, at the other extreme, an observant and determined mother has often been able to help a child with what seems to be little better than a perineal colostomy to manage a normal school life.

An exception amongst the high anomalies is the rare type of rectal atresia with a normal anal canal traversing the pelvic floor. Here normal continence is to be expected.

Some of the surprising results may depend on variations on the sensory side of the defaecation reflex. Electromyographic records of striated sphincter responses to distension of a balloon in the rectum have shown that a response was present in all of ten high cases before operation; only one failed to show eventual inhibition. After abdomino-anal pull-through a sphincter response was present in only six, and none had eventual sphincter inhibition. Similar tests of 26 treated low anomalies showed coordinated responses in all, though a proportion of the cases treated late showed the changes of megarectum (Nixon and Callaghan 1964). The internal sphincter response was also demonstrated to be present in the cases of ectopic anus (Puri and Nixon 1976). Similar tests have not yet been completed on the high anomalies treated by abdomino-sacro-anal operation. Puri and Nixon (1977) have also carried out a longer-term follow up of high and low anomalies 13–20 years after treatment. An encouraging improvement in adult life was observed and a point of particular interest was a small group of neonatal primary abdomino-anal operations who had good control in adult life in spite of considerable trouble in childhood. They were operated on at a time when the importance of the puborectalis sling had been recognized so that the procedure was an advance on the original pull-through in which the external sphincter was considered of more importance. Perhaps in the long run Stephens' greatest contribution may prove to be the recognition of the importance of the puborectalis rather than the sacral approach to it.

The author believes that eventually a technique will be devised to bring the proctodeum up to the rectum without extensive mobilization. Uncomplicated cases have normal anal and rectal reflexes before operation so that continence akin to that of low cases might then be achieved, though an internal sphincter deficiency would remain.

REFERENCES

BILL, A. H., Jr. and JOHNSON, R. J. (1953). Congenital median band of the anus. *Surgery Gynec. Obstet.*, *97*, 307.

BROWNE, D. (1955) Congenital deformities of the anus and rectum. *Archs Dis. Childh.*, *30*, 42.

DICKSON, J. A. S. and NIXON, H. H. (1968) Control by electronic stimulator of incontinence after operation for anorectal agenesis. *J. pediat. Surg.*, *3*, 696.

FEGGETTER, S. (1939) Imperforate anus in identical twins *Newcastle med. J.*, *19*, 20.

GROSS, R. E. (1970) *An Atlas of Children's Surgery*, p. 44. Philadelphia: W. B. Saunders.

HARTL, H. (1972) A modified technique of gracilis plastic. *Pädiat. Pädol.*, Suppl. *2*, 99.

KEITH, A. (1908) Malformations of the hind end of the body. I. Specimens illustrating malformations of the rectum and anus. *Br. med. J.*, *2*, 1736.

—— (1948) *Human Embryology and Morphology*, 6th ed., p. 87. London: Edward Arnold.

KELLY, J. H. (1969) The radiographic anatomy of the normal and abnormal neonatal pelvis. *J. pediat. Surg.*, *4*, 423.

KIESEWETTER, W. B. (1967) Imperforate anus. II. The rationale and technic of the sacroabdomino-perineal operation. *J. pediat. Surg.*, *2*, 106.

—— and NIXON, H. H. (1967) Imporforate anus. I. Its surgical anatomy. *J. pediat. Surg.*, *2*, 60.

KOTTMEIER, P. K. and DZIADIEV, R. (1967) The complete release of the levator sling in fecal continence. *J. pediat. Surg.*, *2*, 111.

MAGNUS, R. V. (1969) Ectopia cloacae—a misnomer. *J. pediat. Surg.*, *4*, 511.

NIXON, H. H. (1966) Colostomy: a simple technique and observations on indications. *Z. Kinderchir.*, *3*, 98.

—— (1968) Principes d'une nouvelle opération pour l'agénésie rectale anus haut non perforé. *Revue Méd.*, *9*, 541.

—— (1972a) Possibilities in the treatment of anal incontinence. *Pädiat. Pädol.*, Suppl. *11*, 39.

—— (1972b) Anorectal anomalies: with an international proposed classification. *Postgrad. med. J.*, *48*, 465.

—— and CALLAGHAN, R. P. (1964) Anorectal anomalies—physiological considerations. *Archs Dis. Childh.*, *39*, 158.

NORA, A. H. and NORA, J. J. (1975). The VACTERL anomaly. *Archs envir. Hlth*, *30*, 17.

PURI, P. and NIXON, H. H. (1976) The internal sphincter in translevator (low) anomalies. *J. pediat. Surg.*, *11*, 553.

—— —— (1977) The results of treatment of anorectal anomalies: a thirteen to twenty year follow up. *J. pediat. Surg.*, *12*, 27.

REHBEIN, F. (1959) Operation der Anal- und Rectumatresie mit Recto-urethral-fistel. *Chiurg*, *30*, 417.

RHOADS, J. E., PIPES, R. L. and RANDALL, J. P. (1948) A simultaneous abdominal and perineal approach in operations for imperforate anus with atresia of the rectum and rectosigmoid. *Ann. Surg.*, *127*, 552.

SANTULLI, T. V., KIESEWETTER, W. B. and BILL, A. H., Jr (1970) Anorectal anomalies: a suggested International Classification. *J. pediat. Surg.*, *5*, 281.

SCOTT, J. E. S. (1959) The anatomy of the pelvic autonomic nervous system in cases of high imperforate anus. *Surgery, St Louis*, *45*, 1013.

SMITH, E. DURHAM (1963) In Stephens (1963).

STEPHENS, F. D. (1963) *Congenital Malformations of the Rectum, Anus and Genito-urinary Tracts*. Edinburgh: Livingstone.

—— and SMITH, E. DURHAM, (1971) *Anorectal Malformations in Children*, p. 133. Chicago: Year Book Publishers.

WILLIAMS, D. I. and NIXON, H. H. (1957) Agenesis of the sacrum. *Surgery Gynec. Obstet.*, *105*, 84.

12

Aganglionosis and Other Anomalies of the Colon and Rectum

By H. H. Nixon

MEGACOLON

The crucial advance in this field during the past 30 years has been the clear distinction of Hirschsprung's disease from other forms of megacolon and megarectum.

Hirschsprung's Disease

Hirschsprung in 1888 described his post-mortem findings in two infants; they had died of obstruction with grossly dilated colon and undilated rectum. He was describing a fatal condition. With the development of radiology it became possible to demonstrate 'megacolon' during life. This descriptive word was used as though it was a specific diagnosis to cover a variety of conditions, including the serious disease Hirschsprung originally described, as well as many cases with enlargement of the colon and severe constipation, but without any serious impairment of health. Dalla Valle described cases of 'true' Hirschsprung's disease in 1920 and 1924, noted their familial incidence, and observed that the undilated rectum contained no ganglion cells in its intramural plexuses. The papers seem to have excited little interest at the time and it fell to Swenson to devise an operation which gave these findings a clinical application. In 1948 he and Bill published the first results of his abdomino-anal 'pull-through' procedure to resect the undilated, but aganglionic, distal bowel; leaving the 'megacolon' to revert to normal after this functional obstruction had been removed. Further work

has confirmed the validity of the distinction of congenital aganglionic megacolon from the other forms of 'megacolon'. Since that minority of cases which have a lesion involving the entire colon do not have a megacolon, perhaps 'congenital intestinal anganglionosis' would be a more suitable name.

My views are based on 294 cases treated from 1949 to 1976. I am particularly indebted to the late Dr Bodian for sharing his great experience, and to our radiologists.

PATHOLOGY

All cases have shown absence of the ganglia of the intramural plexuses of the undilated distal bowel with hypertrophy of the dilated, but normally innervated, bowel proximal to it. Dr Bodian stressed the 'positive' histological criterion of the disease. The expected sites of the ganglia show instead abnormal collections of unmedullated nerve trunks (Fig. 21). Histochemical stains have added to our knowledge (Garrett et al. 1969; Gannon et al. 1969a, b). In the aganglionic zone the nerves which should terminate around the intramural ganglia spread instead through the muscle layers. Electron microscopy (Howard and Garrett 1970) shows terminals suggesting that these nerves are active. Although all cases are aganglionic the intensity of this abnormal intramuscular innervation varies greatly from case to case. The clinical severity coincided with this intensity in a series of 15 studied and explained why clinical severity does not

279

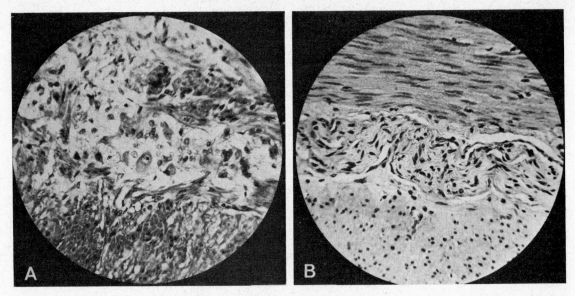

Fig. 215. (A) Normal Auerbach's plexus (×280). (B) Hirshsprung's disease. Aganglionic, showing abnormal nerve trunks (×300).

consistently correspond to the length of the segment. Aganglionosis in all cases causes obstruction by absence of coordinated peristalsis. The ganglia appear to act as a final common path for sympathetic and parasympathetic influences (Norberg 1964). In their absence the abnormal spread of cholinesterase positive fibres adds a varying degree of uncoordinated contraction. Also inability of the catecholamine positive fibres to reach ganglia removes an inhibiting influence.

Between the normal and aganglionic segments there is a transitional zone with scattered ganglia. Here the intramuscular nerves are even fewer than in normal bowel. Denervation hyposensitivity to acetylcholine could occur here as suggested by Ehrenpreis (1967) although it does not seem to apply in the aganglionic segment as he proposed.

Meier-Ruge (1974) has stressed the increased cholinesterase activity in the mucosa itself in aganglionosis—in the lamina propria and the

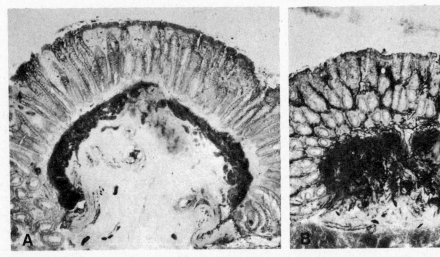

Fig. 216. Hanker's modification of Karnovsky and Roots' stain for acetylcholinesterase (Lake 1976). (A) Normal rectum. Suction biopsy obtained by Noblett apparatus. AChase nerves stain dense black. (B) Hirschsprung's disease. Greatly increased AChase-positive innervation in muscularis mucosae and in lamina propria of mucosal layer as well as in submucosa. (×50, *haematoxylin counterstain*)

TABLE 11. *Sex Incidence and Length of Segments*
(*Author's Series 1949–70*)

Segment	No. of cases*
Long	48
Usual	138
Short	48
Total	234

* 45 female and 189 male.

muscularis mucosae (Fig. 216A). It seems preferable to limit the term Hirschsprung's disease to congenital intestinal aganglionosis although other anomalies of the plexus are coming to light and are mentioned later in this chapter.

In about two-thirds of the cases the aganglionic segment includes the rectum and the lower part of the sigmoid colon. Some of the remainder have a shorter segment involving only a part of the rectum and others have a longer segment involving more of the colon or even extending into the small bowel. A rare variant has been seen in which the entire bowel from the duodenum down was aganglionic and also failed to show the excess of nerve fibrils of the usual lesion. In every case the lesion reached to the termination of the bowel. This is in keeping with Okamoto and Ueda's (1967) account of the craniocaudad migration of the ganglion cells from the neural crest ectoderm into the bowel wall. A segmental 'skip' lesion with normally innervated bowel below as well as above has been described in isolated case reports (Swenson et al. 1949; Tiffin et al. 1940; Perrot and Danon 1935) but not in Swenson's later series of 200.

CLINICAL PICTURE

The principal feature which distinguishes Hirschsprung's disease from other forms of megacolon and chronic constipation is that *symptoms date from early infancy* in almost every case, and usually from birth. Clinically there are three main types:

1. Neonatal low intestinal obstruction requiring colostomy for its relief.
2. Infant presentation when the neonatal obstruction is relieved by rectal examination or saline irrigations, but recurs, requiring surgical intervention.
3. Later presentation when the infant symptoms have been mild, or *very* rarely absent. Then the 'classical' picture is seen.

Basically the condition is a congenital functional intestinal obstruction—not just a form of constipation. About half of the children die in the first year of life and the great majority fail to reach adult life (Eek and Knutrud 1962).

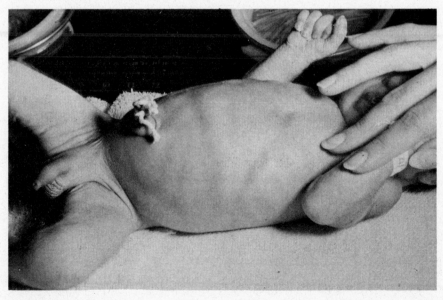

Fig. 217. A newborn with Hirschsprung's disease. Visible dilated transverse colon. The early stage at which aganglionosis should be diagnosed.

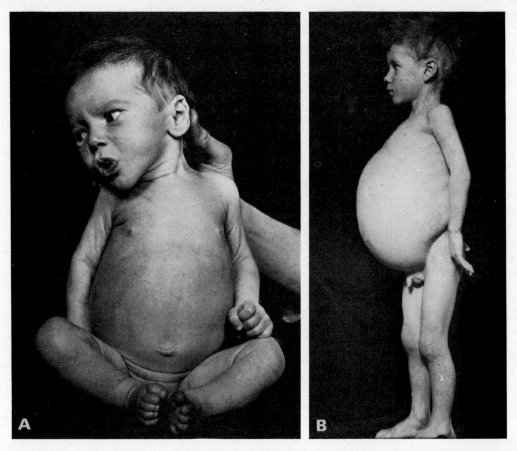

Fig. 218. (A) An infant with Hirschsprung's disease showing the gross abdominal distension; beginning of wasting (loose skin folds on arms and thighs); the flared ribs and downward displacement of the umbilicus resulting from the maximally upper abdominal gaseous distension. (B) An older child showing the chronic stage of Hirschsprung's disease with stunting, wasting (flat buttocks) and gross abdominal protrusion.

The first trouble will usually be failure of the newborn baby to pass meconium for the first two days or more. Abdominal distension will be noticed (Fig. 217) and difficulty in establishing feeding will be followed by bile-stained vomit. Visible peristalsis may be obvious. Gross abdominal distension at this age carries an additional hazard of causing respiratory distress by pressure on the diaphragm—for the newborn baby's respiration is almost entirely diaphragmatic. Cyanosis may be caused in this way.

Routine examination of such a baby will include a digital examination of the rectum using the fifth finger. This alone may be sufficient to cause the passage of a mucous plug followed by meconium and copious wind. Deflation may be dramatic and virtually diagnostic of the condition. If not, a rectal wash-out may be required, but treatment will be discussed later (p. 288). After spontaneous or

induced relief of the obstruction the baby may progress well for several months. But the majority will have frequent recurrent bouts and be constipated between them. It is important to realize that the infant's symptoms may be mild or, at the other extreme, so severe that medical management fails and colostomy is called for (Fig. 218A).

As infancy is passed the obstructive crises become less frequent. The child has stubborn constipation and fails to thrive. Few of these children maintain a decent standard of general health. The abdomen is grossly distended with wind, especially in its upper part. The big transverse colon may be easily felt and visible peristalsis and borborygmi are prominent. The umbilicus appears displaced downwards as a result and the ribs become flared with a wide subcostal angle. Poor basal aeration often leads to recurrent chest trouble. The buttocks and limbs are wasted so that the protuberant belly and flat buttocks may mimic the wasting of a coeliac syndrome (Fig. 218B).

The stools are often of a small, formed 'rabbit pellet' appearance and it is typical that overflow soiling does not occur. Rectal examination usually reveals an empty rectum but faeces can be felt higher up through the bowel wall. Of course by chance rectal examination may be carried out as a bolus is being forced through the segment, so that on about one-fifth of occasions digitation may reveal some faeces in the rectum.

Wyllie (1957) showed in his analysis of the Great Ormond Street Hospital series that the weights of these children were in general well below par; cf 109 cases satisfactorily measured the weight was under the third percentile in almost one-third. This interference with growth is important. Kempton's (1954) case also illustrates the general effect of the disease. This 20-year-old youth was still prepubertal when seen—after vigorous medical care he passed through a complete puberty. Hiatt (1951a) also quoted a girl suffering from the disease who weighed only 38 kg at 23 years of age and did not menstruate before operation.

ISCHAEMIC ENTEROCOLITIS

Crises which were called *putrefactive diarrhoea*, and now *enterocolitis*, may occur. The abdomen distends tensely within a few hours and the child vomits profusely. Offensive fluid motions which may contain blood are ejected. Dehydration is rapid, and requires intravenous therapy. Many patients used to die with mucosal necrosis. Despite the name 'putrefactive diarrhoea' there may be little stool passed. A flatus tube inserted high enough, however, will usually drain off copious frothing, offensive stool with dramatic improvement in the child's condition. The role of putrefaction is doubtful. The causes of these crises are not properly understood but sensitization to *E. coli* endotoxin has been considered (Fraser and Berry 1967). The primary lesion is an ischaemic necrosis of the mucosa of the bowel above the aganglionic segment. It may extend into the small intestine. Neglected it can lead to pneumatosis intestinalis, pericolic abscess, perforation or septicaemia. Histologically it is indistinguishable from the necrotizing enterocolitis of the premature and stressed newborns which is seen more often in recent years and in which asphyxia and hence mucosal ischaemia seem at least an important factor if not the entire cause (Bunton et al. 1977). This is the most serious complication and in the neonatal period is fre-quently fatal. Healing may be incomplete having a cuboidal epithelium deficient ion mucous glands and hence a persistently irritable colon (Berry 1969). Enterocolitis causes a paradoxical presentation of obstruction with diarrhoea and probably accounted for many diagnostic errors in the past. It occurs as frequently in short as in long segments.

ASSOCIATED DEFORMITIES

Associated deformities are not common. In particular we have found few genitourinary defects. Swenson described 'aparasympathetic bladder and mega-ureter' as a fairly common accompaniment. We carried out pyelography in 25 earlier cases and have inspected the lower ends of the ureters in all our cases at operation (over 300 now). No dilatation has yet been seen, nor has a follow-up over 20 years revealed any organic urinary trouble except one early case of operative damage to the pelvic splanchnics. Fortunately this was temporary in its effects. Also one megalocystis with pyelonephritis, and a unilateral renal agenesis. The only significant association is with Down's syndrome in 5%. (There has been an increased incidence of nocturnal enuresis. But as Wyllie (1957) pointed out it may not be unduly high for a series of children having the emotional upsets many must have experienced in early childhood.)

A family history of the disease may be found and the condition appears to be inherited by a recessive gene. In patients with the more common short aganglionic segment the condition is about five times more frequent in the male than in the female; 'long segment' cases show less sex differential and they recur more frequently in the family. The very rare complete intestinal aganglionosis also appears to occur very often within the family. These three types seem to breed true, and further cases in a family will fall into the same group (Bodian and Carter 1963; Passarge 1972). Earlier estimates of the frequency of Hirschsprung's disease, such as 1 in 20 000 births, were gross underestimates through failure to recognize the underlying lesion in severe cases dying in early infancy; 1 in 5000 is more likely.

DIAGNOSIS

Diagnosis depends first on the clinical picture described above. Barium enema usually confirms this and assesses the length of the aganglionic segment. Anorectal manometry may help in atypical cases and a rectal biopsy should clinch the matter. Aaronson and Nixon (1972) assessed the reliability of anorectal manometry, barium enema and formal biopsy in 100 consecutive cases. Each method as used at that time was about 85% reliable at first application, failures being mainly for technical reasons. In conjunction or on repetition they left no real doubt in the individual case.

BARIUM ENEMA EXAMINATION

This is made by a special technique worked out by B. C. W. Ward. The child is not prepared. Ir-

rigations should be avoided for a week before radiography or fallacies may be introduced. The tube is inserted just through the anus and the first flow of barium watched on the screen as it runs up through the rectum. As soon as it starts to spread out and outline the dilated bowel above the segment the flow is stopped. Pictures taken at this time and after evacuation will demonstrate the undilated segment and secondarily hypertrophied colon above (Fig. 219). The aganglionic segment is undilated but it may or may not be narrowed by

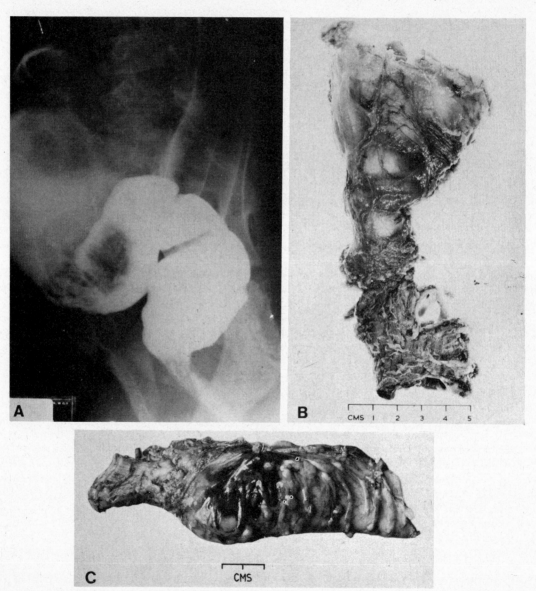

Fig. 219. (A) Barium enema in Hirschsprung's disease—a normal-sized rectum widening to join a grossly dilated colon. (B) The resected specimen from this case showing the cone of transition above the rectum (which is somewhat foreshortened by the pull-through procedure). (C) A shorter segment with the cone at the pelvic reflection.

spasm so that the phrase 'narrow segment' is misleading. To induce more barium may hide the aganglionic rectum behind a loaded sigmoid falling into the pelvis. Furthermore the barium may be difficult to get back from the colon and may encourage the formation of a faecolith. Filling of the hugely dilated colon has led to death from water intoxication—absorption can be so rapid from the large surface area.

If the child is prepared by irrigations the contrasting secondary dilation of the bowel above the segment will be reduced and hence the lesion may be missed—though a practised radiologist may recognize the pattern of loose mucosal folds of bowel which has recently been more dilated. Alternatively an irrigation may empty the bottom of a 'terminal reservoir' of faeces in a case of chronic constipation and produce a cone imitating the Hirschsprung picture.

It will be recognized that Ward's enema technique is a specialized one, used to confirm or deny the presence of the disease, and would be useless for the detection of other lesions—just as the routine enema techniques are almost useless in the detection of Hirschsprung's disease and may be dangerous. Some American clinics have developed their enema technique along rather different lines. They allow preparatory irrigations but accept that under these conditions it will often be necessary to

continue post-evacuation examinations up to 24 hours or more. Such delayed examination may reveal the aganglionic lesion by showing that the peristaltic waves die out at a constant point (the upper limit of affected bowel) or by showing a persistent hold-up of the residual barium bolus at the level of transition. This technique is particularly applicable to a child referred after emergency neonatal colostomy. For the defunctioning of the colon prevents the usual megacolon from developing and no 'cone' will be seen.

The hypertrophy and enlargement of the colon is a progressive condition occurring mainly after birth. It used to be thought that a barium enema would not reveal the lesion in the early weeks of life. With the present technique it has been found possible to demonstrate the proximal dilation contrasting with the undilated distal segment within a few days of birth (Fig. 220). However, it may not always be practicable to confirm the diagnosis by barium enema. When the clinical picture is severe, particularly in the newborn infant, it may be unjustified to attempt to leave the baby without irrigations and radiology may then be inconclusive (though the folded mucosal pattern may enable an alert radiologist to realize that the bowel above the segment, though not dilated, has recently been so). Or the baby may require an urgent colostomy, particularly in early infancy and if the segment is usually long. Following colostomy the distal bowel will collapse to a uniform calibre and again radiology may be inconclusive.

The barium enema may also reveal enterocolitis by the lack of normal haustrations and coarse or shaggy mucosa. The cone may be indistinct in the presence of enterocolitis, perhaps from inflammatory paresis of the muscle.

In some of the clinically milder cases radiology may also be inconclusive, especially if they have been cared for by an astute mother who has learned to recognize the early signs of acute exacerbations and has taken prompt action. If the segment is unusually short and the child older it may undergo considerable passive dilatation and render the radiological picture indeterminate.

ANORECTAL MANOMETRY

When the normal rectum is distended, the internal sphincter relaxes reflexly (see Fig. 216B). In aganglionosis this reflex is absent (Callaghan and Nixon 1964; Lawson and Nixon 1967; Schnaufer et al. 1967). This test is particularly useful in short segments where barium enemas may be difficult to

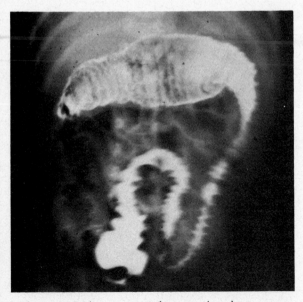

Fig. 220. Barium enema demonstrating long segment Hirschsprung's disease in the newborn with transition at the splenic flexure.

interpret, and may be the only convincing evidence in the *'forme anale'*, when the aganglionosis is minimal and approaches the normal variation in the level of the terminal ganglia. In the first week or so of life differentiation may be difficult from the functional obstruction seen in stressed newborn babies. The stress of anoxic delivery, particularly in the premature, causes temporary loss of reflex. This is usually associated with an abnormally low resting pressure. The normal response returns as the obstruction relents over the first two or three weeks but during recovery the picture of aganglionosis may be imitated both manometrically and clinically (Howard and Nixon 1968).

SUCTION BIOPSY

I have used the Noblett forceps but others may be equally suitable. Details of technique (Noblett 1969a) are important in obtaining sufficient submucosa. The knife must be sharp; suction must be maintained long enough to draw in the tissue and preliminary wash-outs should be avoided to prevent mucosal oedema. As one may be unfortunate enough to meet a lymphoid follicle which would spoil the picture, two specimens should be taken, and these should be 3 cm above the anal verge to avoid the normally aganglionic zone.

Meier-Ruge et al. (1972) claim clear differentiation by the increased cholinesterase staining of the mucosa itself with shallow specimens. We have found in 100 consecutive biopsies that this technique has been reliable using Hanker's modification of Karnovsky and Root's stain (Lake 1976). Although some cases of aganglionosis have few cholinesterase-positive nerves further up, we have not observed this at the lower end of the segment at the level used for diagnostic biopsy.

FORMAL RECTAL BIOPSY

Now rarely needed, it may be preferred occasionally if the suction biopsy is inconclusive or if the special stains or experience in interpretation are unavailable. The infant or child is placed in the left lateral position, and a Parks' retractor is used for exposure. It is our usual practice to take through the anus a strip of mucosa with its attached submucosa 3–5 mm wide (depending on the size of the patient); the strip is begun at the upper end of the anal canal (1 cm from the mucocutaneous junction in the infant) and extends upwards for at least 2 cm (Bodian's study showed that the ganglia normally cease 0·3–1·5 cm above the skin margin so that more than this height must be reached for the

findings to be significant). The wound is closed by catgut sutures for haemostasis. Histological search of the submucosa after simple H. and E. staining will show the absence of ganglia and the presence of the abnormal collections of nerve trunks. Many pathologists prefer to search between the muscle layers for Auerbach's plexus, and Swenson's (1955) biopsy technique removes the muscle coat only with this in view. But we have found the 'mucosal biopsy' completely reliable and, of course, its removal is a simpler matter. Full thickness biopsy may, however, be useful in the rare atypical case to exclude a plexus anomaly in ganglionic bowel as described later.

It is important to pin the specimen out flat as soon as it is taken or distortion may make the pathologist's task difficult. In carrying out transanal biopsy no difficulty is found in removing the submucosa with the mucosa, as the rectal wall splits naturally in this plane when bluntly dissected by scissor blades passed through the initial incision at the lower end of the proposed excision. It is important to remove the entire thickness of the submucosa, and this may be ensured by taking some fibres of the circular muscle coat. A submucosal injection of saline will demonstrate the plane if desired but usually the mucosa is in loose folds and lifts easily without this. The incision bleeds rather freely but haemostasis can be secured by continuous catgut suture closing the gap in the mucosa from the lower end upwards, using each stitch for traction to bring the next part of the incision into reach.

Disadvantages may be:

1. The incision may split at the subsequent pull-through operation. This has been a nuisance on occasion but has caused no untoward sequelae.

2. Frozen section technique cannot be used because the rigours of the preparation damage the more delicate tissue. This is of no importance in planned investigation of a case, but on the occasions when a biopsy may be urgently required during an exploratory operation (see p. 289) a muscle or full thickness specimen is needed. Such biopsies are usually taken from within the opened abdomen and are often obtained at specific levels to determine the extent of the segment rather than to reach a diagnosis.

3. General anaesthesia is necessary.

4. The newborn anus is too small for this technique. Unfortunately this is just the age at which a simple diagnostic test is needed to differentiate the functional obstruction of the 'stressed neonate' from aganglionosis.

BIOPSY IN THE NEWBORN

Formal biopsy may be undertaken by dilating the anus and drawing out a quadrant of the rectal wall by the serial insertion of stay sutures which include the entire thickness of the wall. When a strip 1 cm long starting 1 cm above the anal canal can be held outside the anus a section is removed between the two stay sutures. The wound is closed with catgut; the bowel is allowed to return within the anus and the stays are withdrawn.

This still requires general anaesthesia, undesirable in diagnosis from the stressed newborn with functional obstruction and fortunately the suction biopsy technique has rendered it rarely necessary.

DIFFERENTIAL DIAGNOSIS OF HIRSCHSPRUNG'S DISEASE

IN THE NEONATAL PERIOD

In early infancy the clinical picture is one of low intestinal obstruction and the differentiation must be from *other causes of obstruction*. The passage of a finger into the rectum may produce such a dramatic deflation that the diagnosis is virtually made. But such deflation has in the past been mistakenly attributed to the perforation of an intra-anal membrane or to the shifting of a meconium plug. The *meconium plug syndrome* does occur in the otherwise healthy newborn, but it is very rare and an infant with Hirschsprung's disease may rarely go several months before recurrence of symptoms. Suction biopsy is therefore indicated, since even these rare remitting cases are liable to the dangerous enterocolitis. An increasing number of *functional obstructions* are seen, presumably because better obstetrics and neonatal paediatrics allow more stressed babies to survive. Anoxic delivery, respiratory distress syndrome and exchange transfusion may each precede the syndrome. Half the patients are premature, though immaturity alone without stress does not usually seem to account for obstruction. Some settle on conservative management, but others seeming clinically similar at the onset proceed to frank necrotizing enterocolitis which still has a considerable mortality (Bunton et al. 1977). A few seem to be caused by immaturity of the intrinsic plexuses without stress (Bughaighis and Emery 1971). Low birth weight is rare in true aganglionosis.

The more difficult case is that with a long segment discovered at laparotomy for unrelieved intestinal obstruction. The cone may be in the ileum. *Meconium ileus*, caused by inspissation of the abnormal meconium in a baby with mucosis (cystic fibrosis), presents a similar picture in which a cone is found, most commonly in the lower ileum. In most cases palpation makes the diagnosis clear. The putty-like consistency of the meconium in mucosis is unmistakable. In advanced cases, however, considerable liquefaction of the meconium may occur by bacterial action and overdistension of the bowel causing intramural strangulation and the outpouring of sanguineous fluid. Then the diagnosis may be in doubt. The cone in meconium ileus tends to be more gradual over several centimetres and myohypertrophy of the ileal wall at this age is much grosser than in Hirschsprung's disease. Frozen section examination is not always practicable during an emergency operation. If Bishop and Koop's (1957) procedure (resection of the maximally dilated loop of ileum with end-to-side anastomosis and exteriorization of the open end of the distal bowel as an ileostomy) is performed, then suitable specimens for biopsy may be taken from the ileal wall at the site of section; these will be examined for ganglion cells and evidence of mucosis in the intestinal glands. Appendicectomy may also be done and the specimen sent for examination for ganglia; however, the appendix is a difficult organ to examine in this respect and a rectal biopsy is usually necessary. Noblett (1969b) has introduced the use of a gastrografin enema for diagnosis and treatment of clinically uncomplicated meconium ileus. By its surface tension and hygroscopic actions the enema loosens the meconium. Thus the differentiation may sometimes be made without recourse to laparotomy.

In the newborn period 30% of our patients with aganglionosis presented with diarrhoea. Infective gastroenteritis may produce abdominal distension if hypokalaemia develops, but the syndrome of diarrhoea with distension should always lead to consideration of underlying aganglionosis. The passage of a flatus tube and gentle saline irrigation gives prompt relief if carried out early enough, but the diagnosis is extremely important because delay may result in irreversible mucosal changes and death from septicaemia or other complications. Neonatal Hirschsprung's disease still carries a mortality from this complication of up to 20% in most centres.

Later in infancy more chronic enterocolitis has led to misdiagnosis and treatment as ulcerative colitis. Indeed there is an ulcerating colitis which can be demonstrated on the barium enema.

AFTER INFANCY

After infancy when *chronic constipation* looms larger in the picture the differential diagnosis is from other causes of such constipation. If the child is seen during one of the obstructive crises, or if they are well described by the parent, then the diagnosis will be in little doubt. In the usual case the puny body, grossly distended tympanitic rumbling abdomen, empty rectum, flared ribs, and constipation without overflow will also make the diagnosis quite clear and barium enema will confirm this. In milder cases doubt may remain between Hirschsprung's disease and rectal inertia (see p. 297). Then rectal biopsy will resolve it. Coeliac syndrome has already been mentioned as a possible misdiagnosis and aganglionosis needs to be remembered as an uncommon cause of malabsorption.

Treatment

Management consists in rendering the patient fit for resection of the aganglionic segment. Most of our patients are now diagnosed in the first few weeks of life, and the regimen will depend on the presence or absence of enterocolitis. Occasionally a laparotomy is performed for complete unrelieved low intestinal obstruction for which no organic cause is obvious. Then treatment may have to precede full diagnosis, though this situation should be rare with the radiological and other techniques now available for diagnosis. At laparotomy there is a gradual transition from dilated to collapsed bowel; the diagnosis rests between transient functional obstruction of the newborn, an incomplete mucosal septum, meconium ileus and Hirschsprung's disease. Meconium ileus is usually obvious from the inspissated chewing-gum-like meconium but with complicating volvulus the content may be liquefied. If doubt remains and frozen section is not available for biopsy then the Bishop and Koop (1957) Roux-en-Y anastomosis is useful. It is a definitive treatment for meconium ileus and gives a safety valve and time to investigate for aganglionosis.

THE INFANT WITH UNCOMPLICATED AGANGLIONOSIS

Daily saline irrigations will keep the baby with a normal or short segment well for definitive surgery at any time after, say, six weeks of age. *Any failure to maintain eager feeding and weight gain* or presence of established undernutrition is an indication for prompt colostomy.

No adjuvants should be used in the irrigations as irritation can precipitate peripheral circulatory failure and pulmonary oedema (Hiatt 1951*b*). (It should be mentioned that this kind of crisis may be precipitated in other conditions which cause faecal impaction as well as aganglionosis.) Nor should tap-water enemas be used as the retained fluid may be so rapidly absorbed as to cause water intoxication. Moving the child into the knee–chest position and advancing the catheter whilst the saline is running will help to negotiate corners. Force is never successful and I have seen perforation of the bowel three times. Irrigations must be continued daily or twice daily. One may use up to 10 litres syphoned in and out a few millilitres at a time in an older child, and a proportionate amount in babies. To use irrigations only when needed is unsatisfactory and fails to maintain progress. Irrigations will not succeed in keeping a long segment case deflated; colostomy is required. However, it is worth spending some time on nasogastric aspiration and irrigation to attempt to relieve the abdominal tension, making the operation easier and safer.

Some babies will already have had a colostomy performed elsewhere after exploration for unexplained unrelieved complete intestinal obstruction immediately after birth.

THE INFANT WITH ENTEROCOLITIS

This is an urgent condition. Antibiotics and blood or plasma infusions are used and an attempt made to deflate the abdomen by irrigation before colostomy. Wide-spectrum antibiotics should be given to minimize the risk of septicaemia and should include a drug active against anaerobes, e.g. kanamycin and metronidazole. The sudden response to colostomy in the acutely distended bowel may cause peripheral circulatory failure which typically develops about five hours after the operation (Fraser and Berry 1967). I believe without proof that this state is helped by hydrocortisone in large doses (100 mg six-hourly in the newborn) and that this should be given promptly before the rapid fluid infusions.

Rarely the bowel may perforate before birth leaving adhesions to the site of a secondary stenosis or atresia. Postnatal perforation is likely to be associated with enterocolitis and give the typical saddle-bag picture of free air under the diaphragm outlining the liver. The baby is very sick. Urgent exteriorization is needed and treatment for enterocolitis as described above.

Ehrenpreis (1970) points out that he has lost no cases from enterocolitis over a ten-year period and that conservative management without colostomy has sufficed. He attributes this to an efficient paediatric service and a more benign bacterial environment in Sweden. It remains a problem here and apparently in very many other countries throughout the world. However, my figures like those of Pellerin (1963) and Rehbein and Nicholai (1963) support an initial conservative approach before colostomy.

At least three months should be allowed for restitution of the mucosa before proceeding to definitive surgery.

THE OLDER CHILD

If the child is malnourished he is prepared by irrigations for colostomy. Three months or more are allowed for improvement in his general health. If the bowel is grossly enlarged, a similar period with a proximal colostomy is allowed for it to contract down and make anastomosis simpler. If there is enterocolitis, a similar regimen is advised as for the young infant, although the risk to life is less and our mortality from preoperative enterocolitis has been entirely in those presenting in the first month of life. If general health is good, one may prepare by irrigations for definitive surgery.

DETAILS REGARDING COLOSTOMY

Site. Colostomy immediately above the aganglionic segment is preferred in the neonatal period. Otherwise the unused bowel distal to a transverse colostomy has no stimulus to grow and lengthen its mesenteric vessels and the sigmoid vessels may remain too short to reach the bottom of the pelvis so that an extended colonic resection is needed. Ideally the site is confirmed by frozen section biopsy. Under emergency conditions this may not always be practicable, and then it seems safe to site the colostomy 5 cm above the upper end of the apparent cone if the cone is distal to the splenic flexure. In long segment cases in the newborn period the meconium may be packed into the bowel below the true site of transition to aganglionic bowel, so it is safer to perform an ileostomy if frozen sections are not available and the cone is proximal to the splenic flexure. Standard histology of a section from the colostomy or ileostomy site should then be able to confirm the presence of ganglia within 24 hours.

After the first few weeks of life when the sigmoid loop has already been stretched in a normal or short segment, a right transverse colostomy is preferred so that it can remain to protect the definitive operation.

Type. When the colostomy is performed just above the cone an end colostomy is fashioned and the proximal end is brought out as low in the abdomen as possible through a separate small incision. Primary skin to mucosa suture is used as for a formal ileostomy. This is easier than a loop colostomy to take down in an aseptic manner at the definitive operation. The distal end is brought out suprapubically at a site suitable for inclusion in the incision for the resection.

Proximal transverse colostomy is performed as a loop over a skin bridge with immediate opening and skin to mucosa suture.

A disposable plastic colostomy bag is applied to the stoma at the end of operation and the main wound sealed with collodion and a gauze strip.

Once a week the distal loop is washed out and a finger is passed into the anus to prevent disuse contracture.

PREOPERATIVE MEASURES

Mechanical cleansing by irrigations is considered most important. A recent controlled trial, however, has shown a significant benefit from metronidazole. In addition to irrigation we use a no-residue diet, with neomycin by mouth or into the distal loop of the colostomy if present, and metronidazole, usually by suppository, for two days before operation. The metronidazole is continued two days after operation. Systemic antibiotics are not used prophylactically but are reserved for use after operation only if complications arise. The haemoglobin is checked and should be over 10 g/100 ml. A reliable intravenous infusion is established to replace blood as it is lost.

CHOICE OF DEFINITIVE OPERATION

In my experience there are three satisfactory procedures—Swenson's (1964) abdomino-anal prolapse technique; Duhamel's (1963) retrorectal transanal pull through, and Soave's (1964) submucosal endorectal pull through. The following are my reasons for now preferring Duhamel's procedure in infants and young children and Swenson's operation for older children.

1. Swenson's operation is sound. The pelvic dissection is tedious but not difficult. Anastomotic breakdown can cause serious complications. Pelvic cellulitis may cause a frozen pelvis and damage the

pelvic nerves and hence bladder function. However, this should be avoidable if the operation is covered by colostomy. Residual symptoms including enterocolitis necessitate postoperative internal sphincterotomy in about 15% in spite of the lower anastomosis now used.

Pellerin's (1963) staged modification, akin to the Cutait operation (see p. 307) used in Chagas' disease, in my hands did not reduce the rate of complications in young children. Routine colostomy did avoid serious progress of any complications.

2. Duhamel operation: this is a simpler procedure and safer because of the minimal dissection below the pelvic floor. Postoperative residual symptoms of enterocolitis are rare. An anterior pouch may form if the spur is not completely divided. This may be avoided by Lester Martin's (Martin and Caudill 1967) modification or by use of the automatic stapler to divide the spur to the apex (Steichen et al. 1968). In older children one has the choice of a very long pouch necessitating application of the stapler from above as well as below, or of dissecting well below the peritoneal reflection to shorten the pouch. In these latter circumstances I prefer to complete the dissection and perform the Swenson operation.

The extra reservoir of the Duhamel resection makes it a clear choice in all with total colonic involvement. Postoperative stool frequency and soreness is much less than with a complete resection of the rectum. An ileostomy should be left for at least three months to colonize the small intestine before the pull through. Then postoperative fluid and electrolyte loss has not been a problem and I have not found it necessary to use the 'extended side to side ileocolostomy' also described by Lester Martin (1968).

3. Soave operation (1964): the procedure is simple and safe (Figs 221, 222). Postoperative dilatations are necessary for several weeks to prevent contracture of the non-suture anastomosis. This is both inconvenient and upsetting to a young child or infant. I therefore ceased to use the operation in spite of good end results. The Denda modification in which the colon is sutured to the upper end of the anal canal obviates this in my experience (Denda and Katzumata 1966; Boley et al. 1968). The submucosal stripping is usually simple but occasionally I have found the plane difficult to maintain, and this does not appear to have been related to prior enterocolitis.

4. Rehbein and Nicolai (1963) and others report good results of hemicolectomy with low anterior

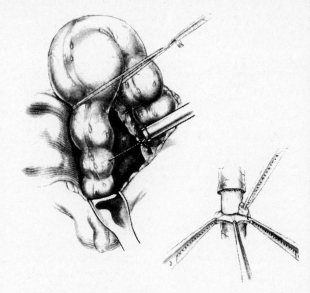

Fig. 221. Submucous (Soave) operation. Colon mobilized. Saline injected to assist blunt dissection, with occasional help of scissor points, in submucous plane (*inset*).

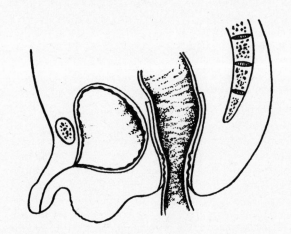

Fig. 222. Soave operation. Muscle coat of rectum stretched and colon drawn out through it and fixed by a few sutures at anus and around upper end of rectal muscle tube to avoid retraction.

resection and forcible divulsion of the sphincter. On theoretical grounds, since it would remove no aganglionic bowel in about a third of our cases which have a short segment, I have not used this procedure. I believe it is not uncommon to need to carry out repeated dilatations of the sphincter at intervals after the operation.

5. Anal myectomy: in a very few very short segments an anal myectomy without colostomy may

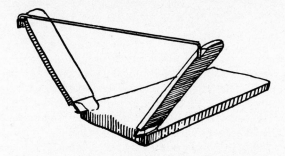

Fig. 223. The table used for rectosigmoidectomy (Swenson's operation) in the infant. Constructed in the hospital workshop.

strapped on to the main table. Slight Trendelenburg tilt is used with the buttocks kept well over the edge of the table. A pelvic wedge is not helpful in this operation because all the dissection is done from the abdomen and a downward tilt of the pelvis helps to give a straight view down the pelvis. The cheeks of the buttocks are drawn apart by broad adhesive strapping. A urethral catheter is inserted and left open to drain during the operation. The orifice of the colostomy if present is temporarily oversewn

A transverse lower abdominal skin incision may be used, retracting flaps up and down and entering

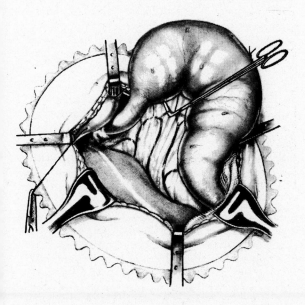

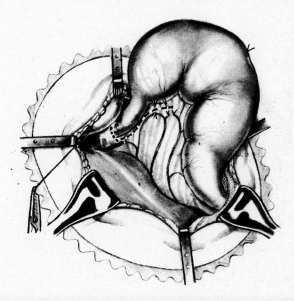

Fig. 225. Mobilization continued down to the peritoneal reflection where it continues around the bowel.

Fig. 224. The field is exposed and the 'cone' located. A suitable vessel has been chosen on which to mobilize the sigmoid colon and the arcade is being dissected with the divulsors prior to division. Note how the bladder is held forward by stay sutures steadied by haemostats clipped against the ring retractor. Case without preliminary colostomy.

avert the need for major surgery (Bentley 1966; Lynn and van Heerden 1975).

DETAILED OPERATIVE TECHNIQUE

Swenson Operation
The child is placed in the semilithotomy position with a towel between the legs to isolate the anal sphincter from the abdominal field. Lloyd-Davies type crutches are used in older children. For younger infants the simple table made by our hospital carpenter which is illustrated in Fig. 223 is

by a midline incision between the recti and carrying right down to the pubis. A Denis Browne self-retaining rectractor is invaluable especially in the small child where extra assistants cannot see, even if they are available. If there is a colostomy in the left iliac fossa a hockey-stick incision may be preferred to include it. In a longer segment case where one may need to operate in the upper abdomen a midline incision is easier to extend for additional exposure.

Abdominal Phase. The infant bladder reaches up into the abdomen so a V-shaped peritoneal incision is made around it after dividing the urachal ligament. The bladder is held up out of the wound by stay sutures clipped to the retractor.

If the diagnosis has not already been confirmed by suction biopsy, an extramucosal muscle biopsy is taken for frozen section before any irrecoverable steps are taken.

The colostomy is taken down and sigmoid vessels divided until it reaches the depths of the pelvis with sufficient slack to allow for peristaltic contraction without tension (Fig. 224).

Next the distal loop is mobilized and the peritoneal deflection incised around it. The ureters are identified. Dissection then proceeds to expose the muscle coat of the rectum above the pelvic floor (Fig. 225). From this point the rectum is freed by dividing the terminal branches of the vessels entering its muscular wall. Divulsers are useful for isolating these tissues. Larger vessels are divided between ligatures and smaller ones may be diathermied. The dissection continues to the levators (Fig. 226). I find it useful to palpate the coccyx which can be recognized by rocking it on the sacrum. The dissection should reach this level all round.

It should be stressed that the principle is the reverse of that in rectal resection for cancer. For cancer one wishes to remove all the pararectal tissues possible because of the danger of spread. In this benign lesion one must remain on the muscle coat throughout to avoid the pelvic splanchnic nerves and preserve bladder and nervi erigentes function.

The bowel is now clamped at the upper end of the rectum and at the chosen site for pull-through. The intervening segment is excised and the remaining end oversewn.

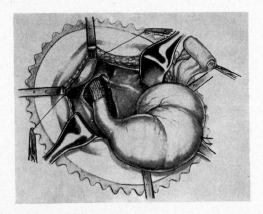

Fig. 226. Dissection has been continued down to the pelvic floor on the muscle coat of the rectum so that its fibres show clearly. Note the proximity of the ureters. Note also that a black silk marker stitch has been inserted in the bowel wall at a level where the blood supply remains good.

Anal Phase. The rectum is intussuscepted outside the anus. It should be so free that the entire anal canal can be everted by traction to eliminate the groove around the anus, but preferably not so slack as to lie out without traction. If it is not free enough it can be returned for further dissection. It is thoroughly disinfected.

Division of the rectum is carried out 1 cm above the anal canal in front and extends obliquely down to the anal canal posteriorly. (Swenson goes down to the dentate line posteriorly so as to include an upper partial sphincterectomy. I find it easier to remain above the anal canal and perform a sphincter division at the end of the anastomosis as described below). The anterior half of the division of the rectum is performed first. The proximal bowel is drawn down into the opening and held with interrupted 3/0 silk sutures which should include the submucosa of the colon and of the everted rectum in order to hold satisfactorily. Then the posterior half of the rectum is divided a little at a time to complete this outer layer of sutures. Then the anterior half of the colon circumference is opened and the mucosa and submucosa sutured with 3/0 catgut to that of the rectal stump. Next the posterior half is divided a little at a time as this layer is completed. A posterior paramedian suture is left long on each side to hold out the anastomosis. A midline incision is made down to the dentate line to divide the upper half of the internal sphincter, the edges are drawn aside and transverse closure obtained by suturing the colon into the gap.

Completion. The sigmoid mesentery is sutured to the posterior parietal peritoneum. The pelvic peritoneum is not closed. A drainage tube is inserted from a stab wound in the left iliac fossa down into the pelvis. A soft Jackson–Pratt suction drain appears very satisfactory and is used for two to three days. A proximal skin bridge loop colostomy is now made in all cases to protect for two or three weeks. The wound is closed in layers.

Modifications in Special Circumstances. A long segment may only require mobilization of the splenic flexure. A still longer segment may require left colectomy with mobilization of the right colon on the ileocolic vessels. The right colon can be brought down by rotation of the pedicle 180° to turn it down on the right side and this is preferable to attempting to draw it around in the coronal plane. If it is only possible to preserve the caecum and perhaps a few centimetres of ascending colon the bowel does not seem to take sutures well and it is preferable to

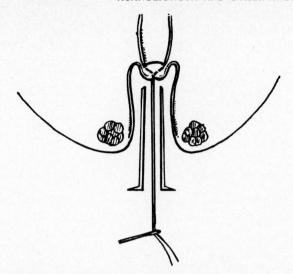

Fig. 227. Demonstrating the technique of pulling through the bowel by means of the loop of thick plaited silk and the sigmoidoscope to produce a complete prolapse through the anus. The 35-cm long needle has been pulled out through the lower end of the sigmoidoscope and the silk loop tightened around the bowel at the upper end of the instrument. By traction on the silk and sigmoidoscope together the bowel is guided down and through the anus.

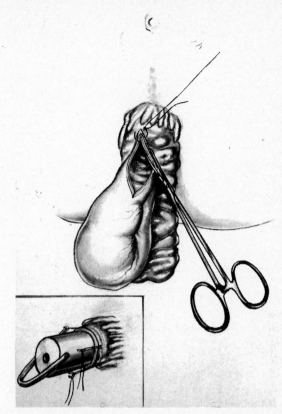

Fig. 228. The bowel has been brought out through the anus. Both layers have been opened in turn, the inner having been drawn down until the marker stitch appears. The layers are temporarily held together by the tissue forceps until the stay sutures are inserted. Four of these are placed around the bowel with the suture plug in place and the excess is cut away one quadrant at a time. The resection is made at the level of the upper end of the anal canal (1–3 cm depending on age). *Inset:* the stays attached to the plug ready for completion of the anastomosis.

remove all the large bowel and make an ileorecto-anal anastomosis by Duhamel's method.

If there is no preoperative colostomy or a transverse colostomy above a normal length segment, and the colon is not very grossly enlarged, Denis Browne's modification is preferred. The colon is mobilized and the rectum is freed without opening it. Biopsy confirms a safe level for division and the site is marked with a long black silk suture in the colon. The bowel is intussuscepted intact using the sigmoidoscope, long needle and thick silk loop technique illustrated in Fig. 227. The anterior half of the prolapsed rectum is divided outside the anus and the colon drawn down to expose the marker stitch. The colon is then opened anteriorly and fastened to the rectal stump with a long strong silk suture. Then one quadrant at a time the bowel is divided and three further stay sutures placed. These are tied to the suture plug shown in Fig. 228 so that the assistant can control the bowel with one hand whilst a complete ring of interrupted Denis Browne mattress sutures of silk are placed to complete the anastomosis in one layer (Fig. 229). Finally a proximal temporary colostomy is made and hence the entire procedure can be performed without opening bowel within the abdomen.

Aftercare. The catheter is removed 24 hours after operation. Rectal examination is avoided for seven days. If all is well a small contrast enema is given 10 days after operation and if no leak is revealed the colostomy is closed two weeks after the operation. If there is a leak, closure may be delayed for a month, the child returning home in the interval.

Duhamel Operation (Fig. 230)

The position, incision, exposure, selection of site for resection and mobilization of the colon proceed in the same way as for the Swenson operation.

Initial Abdominal Phase. The colon is divided at the chosen site and the ends oversewn. The rectum is drawn up into the abdomen with stay sutures.

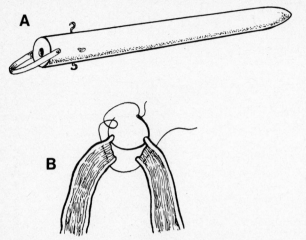

Fig. 229. (A) The 'suture plug' which facilitates handling of the bowel during the anastomosis. It is of plastic so that it is non-conductive and safe for diathermy, and hard so that a needle point will glance off it without getting caught during the suturing. (B) The type of mattress suture used for the single layer anastomosis. Both parts are placed from right to left and the thread is looped around the needle before drawing this through. Pulling the end bearing the needle apposes the mucosal edges and then pulling the other apposes the muscle layers.

The retrorectal space is opened by blunt dissection in the midline until a gauze pledget on a long curved artery forceps is able to evert the posterior half of the anal canal.

Anal Phase. The posterior half of the anal canal is everted by the application of Allis forceps at 3 and 9 o'clock and turning these back against the buttocks. A transverse incision is made across the anal canal just above the dentate line opening on to the pledget. The incision extends across the posterior half of the anal canal and leaves the lower part of the internal sphincter intact. The pleget is caught with a long curved artery forceps and traction on the abdominal forceps brings it up into the abdomen. The lower forceps is then used to catch the sutures closing the mobilized colon and draw this down behind the rectum and out at the anus. The posterior wall of the colon is then sutured to the lower edge of the anal canal incision with 3/0 silk sutures. The closed end of the colon is then cut off flush with these sutures. Further catguts may be placed to join the mucosa and submucosa to that of the anal canal. An Allis forceps is then applied to the adjacent posterior wall of the rectum and anterior wall of the colon. This forceps controls the edges whilst the ring of sutures is completed.

Second Abdominal Phase. The posterior wall of the rectum is then sutured to the anterior wall of the colon at the level of the peritoneal reflection. The rectum is cut across just proximal to these sutures and the residual colon discarded. The anterior wall of the colon is divided transversely at the same level to allow an end to side anastomosis of the rectum to the colon. Just before completing the anterior part of the anastomosis the anal operator passes a crushing clamp up with one blade in the rectum and one in the colon. When the upper ends of the

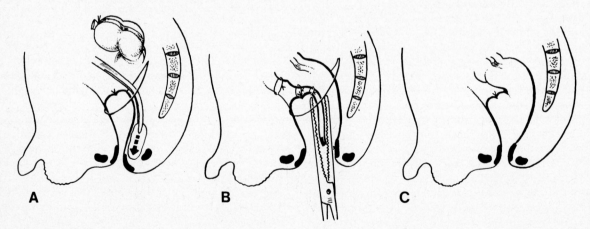

Fig. 230. Retrorectal transanal operation (Duhamel's operation). (A) Bowel divided and upper end of rectum closed. Path made behind rectum by blunt dissection. Gauze pack inserted on to which the transanal incision will be made. (B) Colon drawn down behind rectum and out through intra-anal incision. Colon sutured to anal canal, and spur crushed by insertion of a Kocher clamp. (C) Final result—a neorectum of which the anterior half is sensitive but aganglionic rectum, and the posterior half is ganglionic propulsive colon.

blades are seen to extend proximally beyond the end of the septum the clamp is closed and the anastomosis completed. (This is Lester Martin's (1967) modification and removes the risk of incomplete division of the septum and hence of later formation of an anterior pouch in which faecal impaction might occur.) I use a modified Lloyd-Davies colostomy spur crushing clamp. This avoids the inconvenience of a long handle projecting from the anus as occurs with the use of Kocher forceps

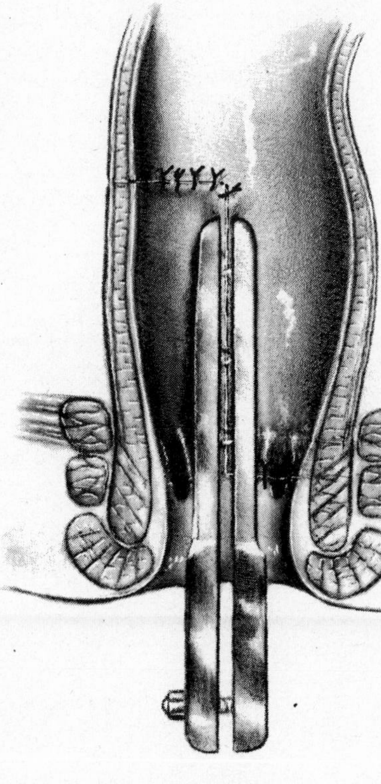

Fig. 231. Crushing clamp *in situ* and colorectal anastomosis completed in Lester Martin's modification of Duhamel's operation.

originally advised by Duhamel. The original technique also used two clamps placed as far apart as possible on the septum in the anal canal with their tips meeting at the top of the septum. This can cause ulceration of the anal canal especially in young infants. With the technique described of performing a complete sutured anastomosis at each end of the neorectum only one midline clamp is needed (Fig. 231).

Routine closure is made with a drain through a stab would in the left iliac fossa. A proximal colostomy is made if not already present.

Aftercare. The clamp is supported by strapping to the buttocks. It is tightened as far as possible 48 hours after operation. Some nurse the child in the gallows position until the clamp separates—usually on the fourth or fifth day—but with careful support of the clamp I have not found this necessary. The catheter is removed 24 hours after operation. The protective colostomy is closed two or three weeks later.

Variations in Technique. Duhamel's original technique of closing over the upper end of the rectum is simpler but care must be taken that the septum is crushed to the apex of the rectum, by reapplication of the clamp if necessary. The American Instrument Company's automatic stapler simplifies the operation further. The GIA model lays two rows of staples on each side and then cuts the septum between them. So the neorectum is formed at once and the unpleasant period with the clamp in the anus is avoided. The instrument only cuts a 5-cm length so that in an older child it will be necessary to insert it once from the anus and again from above. However, in my earlier experience with this instrument I have had some leaks which may have been attributable to forcing too long a segment of tissue into the instrument. In the presence of a covering colostomy these merely delayed its closure. In one case granulomas formed around the staples. There are two sizes of staples—paediatric and adult. In Hirschsprung's disease the bowel is so thick that the adult size is usually required.

In total colonic aganglionosis a preliminary ileostomy will have been performed. This should be given at least three months for colonization of the ileum before the Duhamel operation is performed. The mobilization of the blood supply is then easier and the likelihood of postoperative fluid and electrolyte problems is then greatly reduced. The increased reservoir function of the Duhamel neorectum is then adequate without the need for a specially long retained segment of rectum. Malabsorption has not been a problem when most of the ileum has been ganglionic as is almost always the case.

Postoperative Progress. Some soiling is not uncommon for a few weeks after operation but persistent staining has been rare and probably related to the irritable colon of chronic enterocolitis in neglected cases as much as to the sphincters. Recurrent obstructive symptoms have justified a further sphincterotomy in about one in seven Swenson procedures. Recently this has been performed by Notaras' subcutaneous technique (see p. 150). Sometimes vigorous dilatation is sufficient. Postoperative diarrhoea and distension suggesting enterocolitis is an important indication for dilatation or sphincterotomy. Fatal recrudescence of enterocolitis after operation has occurred—much less frequently after the Duhamel than the Swenson procedure.

Anal Myectomy

Some clinically mild cases with very short segments may not need major surgery. An anal myectomy—i.e. an extended internal sphincterotomy—may suffice. I have used Lynn and van Heerden's (1975) technique. A transverse anal incision is made and the internal sphincter exposed. A strip about 5 mm wide and 5–8 cm long is then excised submucosally.

A similar procedure may suffice following a badly performed Swenson procedure with the anastomosis too high.

RESULTS OF VARIOUS OPERATIVE METHODS

Table 12 shows my results to 1966. It will be seen that more than half the deaths were in those children who received no definitive treatment. This mortality is almost entirely due to the complications of enterocolitis. 109 of these cases presented in the neonatal period which may account for this high incidence. Table 13 shows the results of a further 80 cases up to 1970. The two postoperative deaths were both in cases who had Swenson procedures (one having a congenital heart defect and one Down's syndrome). In theory when signs of anastomotic failure arise prompt postoperative colostomy should suffice; but experience has led me now to advise routine protective colostomy. The end results of both the Swenson and Duhamel procedures have been good but secondary sphincterotomy has still been necessary after some of the Swenson pro-

TABLE 12. *Follow-up Survey to a Maximum of 17 Years (Author's Series 1949–66 Inclusive)*

Operation*	No. of cases	Cure	Control	Failure	Too early to assess	Death
Swenson						
1°	82	64	19	2	11	8
Ext.	18					
2°	4					
Duhamel						
1°	8	8	5	—	—	1
Ext.	4					
2°	2					
Soave						
1°	6	9	1	1	1	—
Ext.	4					
2°	2					
Pellerin						
1°	5	—	—	—	11	—
Ext.	5					
2°	1					
Sphincterotomy						
1°	1	1	—	—	—	—
2°	7					
No definite treatment	13	—	—	—	—	13
Total	155	82	25	3	23	9 + 13

* 1° = usual extent of operation, Ext. = extended resection for long segment, 2° = secondary operation after failed definitive operation (usually done elsewhere). The single 1° sphincterotomy case had a *very* short segment; in the seven 2° sphincterotomy cases the results are included with those of the definitive operation to which the sphincterotomy was secondary.

TABLE 13. *Results of Further 80 Cases (Author's Series 1967–70 Inclusive)*

	Duhamel		Swenson		Anal myectomy		Died before definitive treatment
	Primary	Secondary	Primary	Secondary	Primary	Secondary	
Good	18	1	25	0	5	2	—
Fair	5	1	9	3	1	0	—
Unsatisfactory	0	1	0	1	0	0	—
Died	0	0	2	0	0	0	6
Totals	23	3	36	4	6	2	6
Postoperative colitis	1	0	6	0	1	0	

'Secondary' cases were referred after unsatisfactory pull-through operations elsewhere.

cedures in spite of the low anastomosis. Anorectal manometry has shown that a long internal sphincter zone persists even when the anastomosis has reached down posteriorly to the dentate line. It appears that when the anal canal is everted for suturing, the muscle layer may slide on the mucosa so that it is divided higher than is intended.

Rectal Inertia (Secondary Megacolon)

There are many physical and psychological causes of chronic constipation. The lead to a common end result which has been called secondary megacolon. This is not a good name for there is no evidence that primary megacolon exists (Ehrenpreis 1946) and certainly the megacolon of true Hirschsprung's disease is secondary to the obstruction caused by the distal aganglionic segment of bowel. Terminal reservoir and tubular dilatation have been used to describe differing X-ray appearances but the significance of these variations in the type of dilatation is unknown. Dolichocolon is also no more than the name of an X-ray picture which could be altered by such measures as mixing the barium suspension with tannic acid (Figs 232, 233). Denis Browne has preferred the name colonic inertia which makes clear the essential difference between these children and those with aganglionic Hirschsprung's disease: their bowel is less active than normal contrasting with the gross functional obstruction of the aganglionic disorder. At the risk of further confusion of the nomenclature I would prefer to call the condition rectal inertia—for it seems that the failure to respond normally lies in the rectum and the colon usually makes a good effort to pack the faeces down into it. Physiological examination shows an increase in the faecal volume needed to stimulate a sensory or sphincter response. In severe

cases the reflex inhibition of the striated sphincter occurs before sensation arises—a reversal of the normal, clearly likely to encourage soiling (Callaghan and Nixon 1964). There is no reason to doubt that these changes are acquired, and treatment can induce reversion to normal.

However, recent work suggests that there is a condition of 'ultra-short' segment aganglionosis in

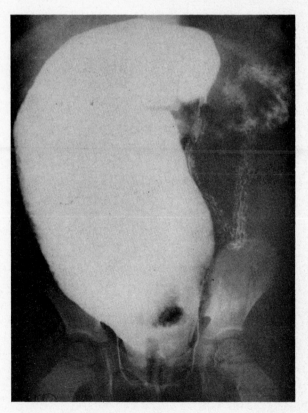

Fig. 232. Barium enema in rectal inertia showing the terminal reservoir with contracting colon above.

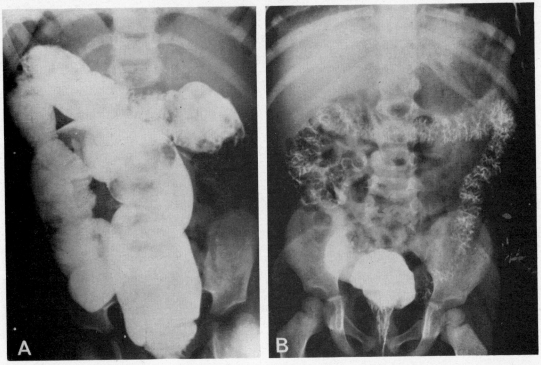

Fig. 233. (A) So-called dolichocolon. (B) The same colon a few minutes later after evacuation induced by tannic acid in the barium enema.

which the clinical picture may be more like rectal inertia—constipation without obvious abdominal distension or ill health, and even with overflow soiling. In some the terminal bowel is aganglionic though dilated and these are better called clinically mild Hirschprung's disease. In others ganglia extend down into the region of the normal variation in the level of the lowest ganglia but apparently their fibres do not reach and innervate the internal sphincter. These are perhaps better called anal achalasia (Hurst 1934). The former are recognizable on suction biopsy and the latter by anal manometry, the rectosphincteric reflex being absent as in Hirschprung's disease. The clinical importance is that anal myectomy (p. 296) or even anal dilatation may succeed as treatment.

CLINICAL FEATURES

The clinical picture of a patient with typical rectal inertia is of a rather tired-looking but not really ill child. The abdomen is quite flat and large masses of faeces are easily palpable—and perhaps visible. They often reach the costal margin and may be so hard that I have seen two cases referred as malignant tumours. Masses in the right iliac fossa are often described as 'faecal masses reaching back to the caecum' but in fact turn out to be masses in a very dilated and lengthened rectum and lower sigmoid which then lies over on the right side. I do not think I have seen faecal masses truly in the right colon as a result of chronic constipation. The rectum enlarges so greatly that it has on occasion been possible to deliver its upper end through an upper abdominal incision made for the preparation of a transverse colostomy. The spreading of the taenia to form a complete coat suggested that the organ was really all rectum and the sigmoid loop was still present above it. (Of course the opportunity to examine this type of case at operation is rare because it is usually managed medically and surgery is not indicated.)

Rectal examination will reveal perianal soiling in severe cases and the sphincter may have become lax. The finger immediately meets a large firm bolus in the grossly distended rectal ampulla.

The history will differ from Hirschprung's disease in that this acquired lesion will have developed some time after birth and the trouble is commonly dated from about the second year of life, except when it is the sequel to mismanagement of an anorectal anomaly (see p. 266) and in a few cases of precocious onset and doubtful aetiology (Nixon 1961; Coekin and Gairdner 1960). Overflow incontinence around the rectal mass is common in the later stages, making this an antisocial if not a dangerous disease, and may cause great upsets at school age. The early period of constipation may pass unnoticed in some families and the mother's first complaint is of diarrhoea. Many children are given chalk and opium and a series of antibiotics for recurrent diarrhoea before a rectal examination makes the true diagnosis obvious. The reluctance to perform a rectal examination in a young child is understandable but not justifiable. If properly done it is still unpleasant but need not be a distressing experience for any child except one of over-anxious and over-protective parents.

The primary cause of the rectal inertia may have gone by the time the child is seen. The syndrome persists and progresses by a vicious circle. Once the bowel becomes overstretched so that it does not evacuate completely, a residue builds up in the rectum which stretches it more and allows a large residue to collect. Overflow incontinence of fluid faeces then occurs around the impacted mass. Removal of the underlying physical or psychological cause alone at this stage will not result in cure because the secondary stretching makes the bowel physically unable to empty completely: the condition has become self-perpetuating.

UNDERLYING CAUSES

Rectal inertia without preceding organic cause is most often due to *training troubles*. To call them psychological causes is I think to overstate the case and raise unnecessary feelings of inadequacy in parents and doctors. It is easy to overstress the negative side of training a child—scolding for being 'dirty'—and forget the positive side of regular sitting out and brief approval for use of the pot. Coaxing with games and books whilst sitting on the pot is useless and gets the emotions involved in the potting habit in an undesirable fashion. Regular but brief potting without fuss should be persisted in even if the child seems uninterested in its use for some time. Fussing does not help. An early start to potting probably does not upset the baby providing the mother does not get upset when the early automatic defaecation reflex begins to be controlled by the baby, who is not able to maintain precocious

'regular' habits until he has learned real voluntary control. Some paediatricians and psychiatrists go so far as to say that 'constipation', i.e. missing days, is of no importance and should be neglected. This can be dangerous advice. When the baby is on a mixed diet it should produce enough residue for a daily stool. Upsets in its routine will certainly cause some missed days from time to time (and also the reverse). Such temporary upsets are rightly considered of no importance. But the regular missing of days is often due simply to a habit of putting off the act of defaecation when the call to stool is felt. This may lead to nothing more than an infrequent bowel habit, again of no importance. But in a minority it may lead to incomplete emptying of the bowel and then the vicious circle leading to rectal inertia may follow. A number of children have required many months of hospitalization in our wards for this reason and it seems as foolish to ignore training as to insist on perfect regularity.

In toddlers the habit of '*holding back*' is frequent. The original cause may have been fear of painful defaecation from say a fissure or a bout of acute constipation during a childhood fever, or from 'negativism'. Through holding back the motion becomes large and hard and it does hurt to pass it. Thus further holding back occurs and the trouble continues. It is goes on long enough the rectum may become stretched so that it cannot empty fully and the rectal inertia syndrome will follow.

Constipation from deeper *psychological maladjustments* does occur and in this minority expert advice may be required (Nurcombe 1972). Many psychiatrists now accept that even in these children the physical result of their upset also needs treatment and that correction of the emotional problem will not be successful unless the rectum is emptied and allowed to recover its normal physical state (Berg & Jones 1964).

The physical causes of the inertia syndrome include *anal fissure* as mentioned above. *Recumbency* especially in an illness causing anorexia and dehydration may start it. Several cases have followed orthopaedic care and the possibility of inertia needs regular consideration during the management of children undergoing prolonged immobilization in bed.

Congenital *anal stenosis* may cause the condition. It is important to realize that the stenosis may have been thoroughly corrected before the child is seen. The overflow incontinence may then be mis-diagnosed as due to sphincter inadequacy unless the importance of early correction with a careful follow-up is appreciated (see p. 270).

Neurological lesions such as spina bifida may cause the syndrome because the insensitive bowel fails to start a reflex. Recumbency and lack of training and management may be factors, and such children are often much dirtier than they need be because of mistaken kindness to a child who 'can't help himself'. Almost all these children can be trained to a clean habit, usually with the help of enemas once or twice a week, by the time they are about seven years old, if not before. Again the need is for measures which will prevent a residuum collecting thus adding overflow incontinence to the primary trouble.

An uncommon primary cause worth mention is *congenital mucocolpos* (imperforate hymen). The huge pelvic and abdominal mass formed in these babies can cause severe rectal inertia, apparently due to direct pressure interfering with defaecation in the early weeks of life (and perhaps in utero). In attending to the more dramatic side of this condition the incompleteness of evacuation may be overlooked at first.

Another mode of onset is that following an attack of a *dysenteric* infection in infancy. The bowel is apparently left atonic and constipation may occur and progress to the inertia syndrome; though in the great majority the bowel recovers its tone in time to evacuate fully before it has become enlarged by the residuum.

Retarded children appear to be particularly prone to rectal inertia. This seems to be due to failure to respond to the call to stool and inadequate socialization.

Congenital constipation is the name given by Coekin and Gairdner (1960) to a smaller group of children who have the typical clinical picture of rectal inertia but whose symptoms date from birth. Harris et al. (1954) have suggested that this may be the result of a congenitally tight fibrous ring at the lower end of the anal canal—something beyond the normal variation in this structure yet slight enough to be stretched to normal dimensions by repeated passage of stool or the examining finger. Some have abnormalities of the sphincter response on anorectal manometry and may have 'anal achalasia', but it is difficult to assess the significance of these findings and whether they are primary or secondary phenomena.

Plexus Anomalies Other than Aganglionosis
These are rare, tend to have a more insidious onset than Hirschsprung's disease and are not liable to enterocolitis.

Chagasic megacolon may develop in childhood (see p. 305). A unique form of constipation and megacolon has been described by Katz (1966) in Bantu children. There is a muscular atrophy of unexplained origin. The clinical similarity to Hirschsprung's disease can be close.

The rare *chronic adynamic ileus* which clinically mimics Hirschsprung's disease apart from absence of active peristalsis may be the same condition. Cytomegalovirus was isolated from a recent case and may be aetiologically significant. Yet another showed absence of acetylcholinesterase-positive nerves, and on electron microscopy vacuolated tracts and possible inclusion bodies. There was an absence of argyrophil neurones (Kapila et al. 1975; Puri et al. 1977). Tanner et al. (1976) have described a familial syndrome presenting with short small bowel malrotation and pyloric hypertrophy with delayed transit through the bowel in which failure of development of the argyrophil plexus was also found.

Colonic neuronal dysplasia is a rare cause of constipation with magacolon (Staple et al. 1964). Some have other stigmata of Von Recklinghausen's disease. Others may represent early manifestations of the syndrome of megacolon and 'apudomas' (Lichtenstein 1972). One of our children has already developed a medullary carcinoma of the thyroid at the age of four years, hence estimation of plasma calcitonin is advisable.

We have also observed 'colonic neuronal dysplasia' occurring above a typical Hirschsprung segment similar to those of Lassmann and Wurnig (1973).

Hypoganglionosis (Meier-Ruge 1974) is a condition rather like a long transition zone of Hirschsprung's disease without the aganglionic segment.

TREATMENT

The rectal inertia syndrome requires treatment of the enlarged bowel by similar methods whatever the primary cause may have been.

The basis of the treatment which has been found most effective is to empty the bowel completely and to keep it empty for at least two weeks to recover its tone. Then the second stage of training in regular habits of defaecation can begin. It is a long and tedious treatment for the child and the nurses. The temptation to abbreviate it is great but has only led to persistent or recurrent trouble and despondency of the child and his parents as well as the nursing and medical staff.

ATTENTION TO THE UNDERLYING CAUSE

The primary cause may be mal-training, psychological difficulties or a local physical cause such as anal stenosis or a painful anal fissure. In many cases this primary cause will have been resolved before the child comes to the surgeon for treatment of the secondary inertia syndrome. It is the radiographic discovery of a gross distension that often makes the doctor begin to think of surgical measures, and the possibility of true Hirschsprung's disease may need to be excluded as described above. If the rectal inertia syndrome is established, it cannot be stressed enough that surgery has little to offer.

MANUAL EVACUATION

A severe case will have large faecal masses in the bowel. These are best removed manually under an anaesthetic by a manoeuvre combining suprapubic pressure with a rotation of a finger in the rectum to break off pieces of faeces and assist them out of the anus. This unpopular treatment is kinder to the child than prolonged and probably only partly successful efforts to break up such masses by detergents or other medicaments. Manual evacuation without anaesthesia should never be undertaken in children.

RECTAL IRRIGATIONS

When the main masses are removed daily irrigations begin. Plain saline is used. Adjuvants become irritating in the prolonged courses these children are likely to need. The fluid is run in a little at a time from a funnel and drained back into a bucket before the next funnel full is poured in. This regimen reduces the risk of unpleasant or frankly dangerous reactions. As much as 7 litres for an infant or 11 for a child may be used, depending on the nurse's judgement of the child's tolerance. The irrigations continue daily whether or not spontaneous bowel actions occur. The object is to empty the bowel completely to give it the opportunity to recover tone. This may take as little as a week or perhaps as long as three weeks. It requires a patient and understanding attitude on the part of the nurses. Carried out by practised staff in this way it is surprisingly well tolerated—whereas the administration of an enema at home under makeshift conditions by a hurried district nurse can be a frightening experience indeed. (It is usually unfair to expect a district nurse to undertake the required course at home: she has neither the time nor the assistance needed to do it thoroughly.) The substitution of enemas is likely to be unsatisfactory as well as potentially dangerous. (It has been found that the term wash-out or irrigation may be wrongly used for the delivery of a single large volume of fluid by gravity instead of by syringe: the child being left to return the fluid by his own efforts.) However, hypertonic phosphate enemas can often be substituted in the later stages of treatment after hard masses have been removed; this is more convenient and in some cases allows the treatment to be continued at home.

APERIENTS

When the masses are removed the regular use of aperients is also begun to stimulate the bowel: Rae's mixture, Senokot or bisacodyl (Dulcolax) are often used. There is no specific virtue in any one aperient and one may suit a particular child better than others. The dosage has to be high in this condition, up to 8 ml of Rae's mixture or up to 10–20 ml syrup of Senokot or Dulcolax. I prefer a single daily dose increased as needed. Divided doses are less effective and more likely to cause colic.

After emptying the bowel the frequency of the irrigations or phosphate enemas is reduced. A minimum course would be daily for two weeks, alternate days for two weeks, then twice weekly for two weeks. In the more severe cases it is wise to continue a weekly phosphate enema for several weeks or months after clearance. The aperient also may need to be continued for many months in some cases. No evidence has been revealed that this leads to any undesirable habituation.

In some cases with a large but soft mass of faeces, it may be possible to avoid hospitalization by the use of Senokot or Dulcolax as a single daily dose increased to tolerance—which may mean four or more tablets—avoiding the need for wash-outs. Standard dosage is ineffective in this condition.

TRAINING

When the bowel is empty and has started to recover tone the most important part of the treatment begins. This is the training of the child to attempt defaecation at some suitable time (usually after a meal or a hot drink) twice a day. It is important that this effort should be made regularly and that the child should not be left to wait for a call to stool, for the overstretched rectum will comfortably accept large amounts of faeces without giving rise to any sensation of filling. So it is futile to expect the child to respond normally to a call to stool. For example balloon tests on one of our cases showed that 600 ml of water in a balloon in the rectum produced no sensation at all. Some time after successful treatment (which took over three months in his case) 60 ml in the rectum produced an urgent desire to defaecate. Radiology at that time confirmed the great reduction in calibre of the bowel allowing the sensory response to distension to be restored.

RESULTS

Results of this form of treatment have been good, but a three-year follow-up of a group showed that in severe cases a third will relapse and need a repetition of the treatment. Once a regular habit has been achieved, and the child has reached an age which allows intelligent cooperation, the results are lasting: 16 of the author's cases contacted eight years later had remained well.

There are disadvantages in this form of treatment. It is prolonged and tedious for the child. It would be better carried out at home from the purely psychological point of view. This is usually not practical, though an attempt may have to be made before the parents will appreciate the situation and accept the need for admission to hospital. We have observed no ill-effects from admission. Indeed the efficient treatment under less emotionally disturbed conditions seems to help many of them, and defaecation is seen to be an unimportant routine habit in the lives of the others in the ward and not a centre of emotional interest. Psychologists say that it is wrong to use local treatment which will centre the child's interest in the bowels, but the child's (and family's) interests are already centred on his bowels and the quickest way to get them elsewhere is to cure him. It goes without saying that such prolonged care should only be undertaken in a suitably staffed hospital with facilities for schooling and other activities. The worst place for these children is bed.

Some children relapse on returning home owing to parental attitudes—which were the primary cause of their trouble. It was noticed when follow-up appointments were being made for this study that many of the children failed to attend until social workers and health visitors had met the parents and explained the importance of after-care. Indeed parental ineffectuality is the main cause of difficulty in curing this condition. By contrast the children who had been treated for true Hirschsprung's disease came from great distances—for even those which we considered as imperfect cures were so grateful for relief from the constant ill health and recurrent crises of obstruction. The one begins as a purely physical condition whereas the other is often psychosomatic from the beginning and parental inadequacy is naturally commoner. With these difficulties in management it is understandable that resection of the dilated bowel has been proposed from time to time as a preferable alternative. If the operation is not followed by regular attention to re-training it merely provides a few weeks or months respite before the next piece of bowel dilates. Furthermore the most dilated part of the bowel is the rectum itself, so that to get rid of the 'reservoir' it is necessary to extend the operation beyond the abdomen into the pelvis and carry out a procedure very similar to that proposed for true Hirschsprung's disease. This gets rid of the reservoir but again will be followed by relapse unless training, and probably aperients, are given until the child has a well-established habit. I have carried out six such resections in very gross cases but would stress the dangers of the procedure. In a condition such as this it is clearly undesirable to remove the specific rectal sensation unless absolutely essential (e.g. Fig. 234).

Four of the resections have been fully successful and two have improved a lot. One of them, a girl who had had delayed treatment of a stenosed ectopic anus, was not resected low enough to remove the whole terminal reservoir. As a result of prolonged but ineffective treatment the child had become terrified of any local measures and wash-out treatment was out of the question. Fear of producing incontinence led me to perform an inadequate resection but even this has improved her and as she gets older it is becoming possible to obtain cooperation.

OTHER CONGENITAL ABNORMALITIES OF THE COLON

Duplications of the Colon

Duplication may occur at any level of the alimentary tract. Some thought it arose by persistence of pouches and extra lumina usually occurring transiently during the epithelial proliferation stage of early embryonic development (Lewis and Thyng 1970; Bremer 1944). It may also occur as part of the 'split notochord syndrome' (Bentley and Smith 1960). The duplication may be tubular and in-

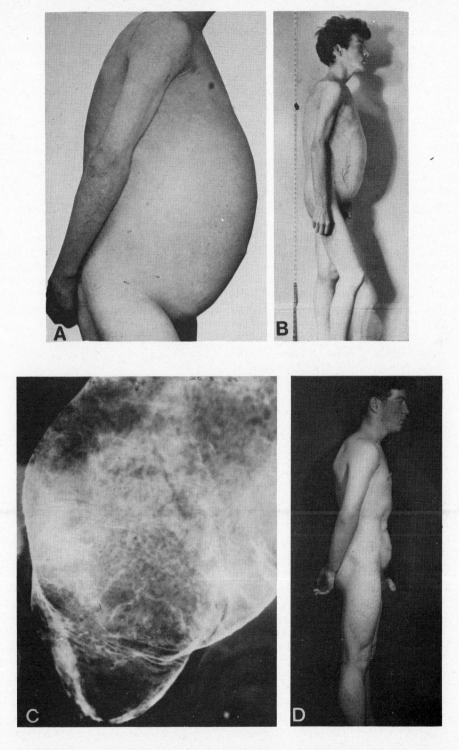

Fig. 234. An exceptional case of rectal inertia, showing gross wasting, abdominal distension, abdominal striae, ankle oedema and severe constipation. Biopsy confirmed that this was not Hirschsprung's disease. (A) On admission. (B) Condition after two weeks of medical care. (C) Barium enema. The apparent cone is merely the bowel filling the true pelvis and then expanding into the wider cavity of the false pelvis to diameter of 23 cm. (D) After treatment (see text); eight months later.

timately attached to the bowel so as to produce the 'double-barrelled colon' appearance. Or it may be more limited in its attachment producing the appearance of a cystic lesion on or in the bowel wall, or of a tubular diverticulum. The duplication may communicate with the bowel—usually at its proximal end—or be a closed sac. Its lining is usually that of the bowel to which it is apposed but may be from another part of the gastrointestinal tract, e.g. gastric mucosa.

Clinically these lesions may present in several different ways. A symptomless swelling may be noticed. The duplication may encroach on the lumen of the bowel causing obstruction. Volvulus of the duplication may cause recurrent obstruction and may terminate in an acute strangulation. Stagnation in the blind pouch may lead to inflammation and stercoral ulceration causing bleeding and anaemia. Distension of the pouch may cause reflex intestinal hurry and hence interfere with absorption. If it is lined with gastric mucosa peptic ulceration may occur causing pain, and the complications of haemorrhage or perforation may follow. An irregular mass of colonic tissue alongside a normal or ectopic anus may represent a terminal duplication. A rectal duplication may terminate in duplicated ani. Complete duplication of the colon and anus may be looked on as an abortive caudal twinning. The split notochord syndrome may also include coronally cleft vertebrae, mediastinal or intraspinal cysts or a dorsal sinus in addition to the duplication.

Treatment is governed by the fact that the blood supply to the two parts of the bowel is so intimately joined that separation at the common wall is impracticable. Resection of the bowel with its duplication is usual. If the lesion is very extensive an adequate stoma made at the distal end of the duplication, providing there is no ectopic mucosa, may be satisfactory. Such lesions may be treated by opening the duplication, peeling out the mucosa, and oversewing the muscular wall which is left *in situ*. Thus the resection can be limited to that part of the bowel which bears the stoma leading into the duplication.

Cystic duplications at the site of a sphincter (pyloric or ileocaecal valve) may also be better treated by coring out the mucosal lining to preserve sphincter function. The mucosa can be very adherent and tedious to dissect out in these non-communicating cysts, unlike the easily peeled lining of a communicating duplication.

Duplication of the rectum is a particular case where the laying open of the common wall forms one larger rectal structure which functions well. It avoids a difficult pelvic dissection and avoids sacrifice of a functionally specialized piece of the bowel in cases where the 'cyst' cannot be easily separated from the rectum.

'Anal Duplication Cysts'

Ectopic bowel may also occur externally with the mucosa on the exposed surface; usually adjacent to a normal or ectopic anus or on the labium majus. It is easily removed (Spitz and Rickham 1972).

Enterogenous Cysts

Enterogenous cysts arise in the mesentery and retroperitoneal regions. Their histology suggests an origin from the bowel but connection has generally been lost. They usually present as a symptomless swelling or as a cause of obstruction of the bowel stretched over them, or by volvulus. Treatment is by resection. The adjacent bowel may have to be sacrificed with the cyst.

Congenital Atresia and Stenosis

Atresia and stenosis are very rare in the colon, even as compared with their occurrence in the small bowel. If they occur, the lesions are similar to those of small bowel, i.e. an area of narrowing of normal-looking bowel wall; an area reduced to a cord-like remnant; a septum (complete or partial) across the lumen, or a complete gap between the blind ends of proximal and distal bowel, often with a V-shaped gap in the intervening mesentery. It must be remembered that there may be no external evidence of an intraluminal septum. A few centimetres of bowel proximal to the atresia are both enlarged and hypertrophied. Most appear to result from a late intrauterine accident to the bowel interfering with its blood supply and hence its development, as in the small intestine (Nixon 1956). However in an occasional case the accident may be perforation secondary to Hirschsprung's disease or meconium ileus. Treatment should therefore be primarily by colostomy. Secondary anastomosis will follow investigation to exclude aganglionosis or cystic fibrosis (rectal biopsy, sweat test, etc.).

There is a severe defect of the subumbilical ventral wall, commonly known as ectopia cloacae, in which a wide ectopia vesicae is associated with exposure of intestinal mucosa and an orifice between the two halves of the 'bladder'. It is usually found that the ileum terminates at this orifice and that beyond it there is only a few centimetres of gut ending blindly. The hindgut is commonly absent. Survival has been recorded after resection of the bladder halves, pelvic osteotomy, closure of the abdominal wall, ureterostomy and ileostomy. Variations in the extent of the bowel involvement are in keeping with Magnus' (1968) suggestion that the lesion results from snaring of prolapsed bowel. Vesicointestinal fissure is therefore a better name.

Microcolon

This should be considered a suspect diagnosis. It is true that the colon may be hypoplastic. Such a lesion is likely to be accompanied by great shortening of the bowel and other gross lesions which may be incompatible with life. But most of the cases which used to be considered as microcolon were merely unexpanded colons in unrecognized cases of meconium ileus, of long segment Hirschsprung's disease or of atresia proximal to the colon, as has already been mentioned. The bowel is only the diameter of a slate pencil in these cases but is capable of developing and functioning normally if the underlying lesion is treated.

ADDITIONAL NOTES ON MEGACOLON AND MEGARECTUM OCCURRING IN ADULT LIFE

By J. C. Goligher

Megacolon and Megarectum in Chagas' Disease

PATHOGENESIS AND COURSE OF CHAGAS' DISEASE

The disease described by Chagas (1916) is caused by *Trypanosoma cruzi*, which is transmitted to man by blood-sucking insects of the subfamily Triatominae. The trypanosomes multiply at the site of the initial infection and from there enter the blood stream. However, after a few days they disappear from the circulation and invade the smooth muscles of the body and the myocardium. In these tissues they proliferate in the form leishmania and form cyst-like cavities. When these pseudocysts rupture, most of the leishmania are destroyed by the natural defences of the body, but some of them reappear in the blood stream. This cycle is repeated many times during the first few weeks of the acute phase of the disease, during which the diagnosis can be confirmed by direct examination of blood smears or by means of xeno-diagnosis (that is, allowing a laboratory-bred insect to bite the patient, and examining its faeces 10 days later for the typanosome). The symptoms at this stage are those of an acute infection, with fever, generalized adenopathy, a slight enlargement of the liver and spleen, and often cardiomegaly with arrhythmia. About 10% of the patients die. Those who survive enter the chronic phase of the disease, which is mainly characterized by the occurrence of heart block and dysfunction and dilatation of many hollow viscera, particularly the oesophagus and large intestine. During this phase the diagnosis can be confirmed by the complement-fixation test of Machado-Guerreiro. Up to the present time no specific treatment has been discovered for acute or chronic Chagas' disease.

INCIDENCE

Chagas' disease occurs in many parts of Brazil, especially the central area of that country, and also in Argentina and Chile. It is believed to be the usual cause of the acquired form of megacolon and mega-oesophagus so often encountered in these regions. The great frequency of these latter manifestations in Brazil may be deduced from the statement of Ferreira-Santos (1961) of São Paolo that some 12% of his surgical beds are permanently occupied by patients with megacolon or mega-oesophagus, and, if a selective policy for admission to his hospital were not adopted, the proportion of sufferers from these conditions would be much greater. According to the same author about 50% of cases with mega-oesophagus suffer also from megacolon or megarectum, whilst nearly as many patients with megacolon or megarectum are found on radiological investigation to have mega-oesophagus. Indeed, if myographic recordings are employed an even higher incidence of associated peristaltic abnormalities is revealed in the oesophagus and large intestine respectively. Occasionally other hollow viscera, such as the stomach, duodenum, jejunum, gall bladder or ureters, may exhibit aperistalsis and eventually become dilated.

Megacolon and megarectum may occur at any age and in either sex. The oldest patient in Ferreira-Santos's (1961) series was 64 years, the youngest 10 months, and the average age 34·7 years. It follows that in Brazil megacolon in childhood may often be due to Chagas' disease rather than to Hirschsprung's disease or to ordinary rectal inertia.

PATHOLOGY

Though Cutait (1953) and Raia (1955) describe a distal aganglionic segment in all cases of Chagasic megacolon, as in Hirschsprung's disease, the researches of Köberle (1956a) show no completely aganglionic zone, but instead a relative reduction in the numbers of ganglion cells *throughout the whole large intestine* to about 4–6% of the normal. It is generally held that this relative aganglionosis is in some way caused by the *T. cruzi* infestation, though the exact mechanism has not been clearly defined. Köberle and Nador (1956) demonstrated that the muscular fibres of the hollow organs harbour the parasite in the leishmania phase. When the pseudocysts rupture they cause an inflammatory reaction in the tissues between the two muscle layers with partial or complete destruction of the ganglion cells resident there. Köberle (1956b) suggests that a neurotoxin, liberated after rupture of the pseudocysts and disintegration of the leishmania forms of *T. cruzi*, is the cause of the degenerative changes in the ganglion cells. Further evidence favouring the Chagasic aetiology of acquired megacolon in Brazil is provided by Nunan et al. (1952), who observed radiologically the development of motor incoordination and dilatation of the colon following the acute phase of Chagas' disease in a group of children who had previously been normal on fluoroscopy. In addition Okumura (1960) claims to have produced megacolon and mega-oesophagus in dogs and mice infected experimentally with *T. cruzi*.

Vieira et al. (1961) have found from pressure and motility studies of the colon in cases of chagasic megacolon that the first change is hyper-reaction to Mecholyl stimulation. It would seem that the initial dysfunction is hypertonicity and hypercontractility of the musculature of the intestinal wall, which occurs in an inco-ordinated way leading to impaired propulsive effort and considerable hypertrophy, especially of the circular fibres, and dilatation. Due to stagnation and desiccation of faeces the mucosa becomes inflamed and ulcerated and the bowel may even perforate. Occasionally acute volvulus of the tremendously dilated and elongated sigmoid loop occurs.

CLINICAL FEATURES

The salient symptom of aperistalsis of the colon and rectum is severe chronic constipation, and the patient may go for several days or many weeks without a motion. The tolerance which develops to this state of affairs is astonishing. Large hard faecal masses can be easily palpated as a rule on rectal and abdominal examination. Without aperients or enemas usually no bowel actions occur, and frequently manual disimpaction of the faeces under a general anaesthetic is required.

Barium studies after the colon has been cleared of its faecal accumulation show the gross dilatation of the bowel, confined usually to the sigmoid and rectum, occasionally extending farther proximally. Often an apparently contracted distal segment is seen corresponding to the terminal part of the rectum, but Ferreira-Santos (1961) emphasizes that this does not indicate the presence of a truly aganglionic functionally strictured portion of bowel, but is to be attributed to the fact that dilatation of the rectum here is hindered by the neighbouring structures, especially the pelvic musculature.

In about 10% of the patients, according to Ferreira-Santos (1961), the clinical picture is complicated by the occurrence of acute volvulus, which presents little difficulty in diagnosis.

It must be remembered that in patients with Chagasic megacolon dilatation of the oesophagus, and other parts of the alimentary tract—occasionally also the urinary tract—may occur with or without symptoms. Appropriate radiological investigation is thus indicated. The possibility of cardiac abnormalities must also be borne in mind and electrocardiographic studies made. Though the ECG often deviates from normal in these patients, Corrêa Netto et al. (1962) stress that instances of cardiac insufficiency are excessively rare, and these patients are practically invariably well able to withstand any major surgical interventions required in the treatment of their bowel conditions.

TREATMENT

Initial attempts to treat Chagasic megacolon and megarectum along surgical lines consisted of lumbar sympathectomy or pelvic splanchnicectomy. These were almost invariably unsuccessful as would be expected from our present knowledge of the pathogenesis of the condition, for they merely aggravated the pre-existing intramural denervation (Ferreira-Santos 1961). Another popular operation at one stage with Brazilian surgeons for this disease was external incision of the pelvirectal sphincter (Corrêa Netto 1934) combined with internal anal sphincterotomy, but recurrence was the rule (Raia and Campos 1948).

At the present time the popular surgical treatment is recto-sigmoidectomy (Cutait 1953; Raia 1955; Ferreira-Santos 1959),

to remove the dilated sigmoid and rectum, except for the terminal 4–5 cm or less of the latter organ. Sigmoidectomy alone, leaving all the rectum, has been found to be followed by dilatation of the left colon anastomosed to the rectal stump (Finochietto 1927; Riveros 1940).

It is important to carry the excision far enough proximally to remove all the dilated hypertrophied bowel, but even so the condition sometimes recurs (Ferreira-Santos 1961), for, as Köberle (1956a, b) has shown, the intramural neuronal changes are present in most cases through the length of the large intestine. So far, however, the results of rectosigmoidectomy have been generally good, though long-term follow-up studies will be awaited with interest.

As regards the choice of operative technique for achieving rectosigmoidectomy, there are considerable differences of opinion among Brazilian experts in this field. In treating young children Ferreira-Santos (1961) has employed the Swenson abdomino-anal technique as for Hirschsprung's disease (p. 291), but for all other cases he has preferred a purely abdominal technique, which is essentially that of a *low* anterior resection. Without personal experience of treating Chagasic megacolon, but from my knowledge of the management of rectal cancer, I am rather surprised that he has found it possible to achieve a low enough resection by this approach. A frequent complication has been dehiscence of the anastomosis, which occurred in 50% of the cases treated by one-stage resection. Since adopting a three-stage operation (preliminary transverse colostomy to allow of thorough emptying of the left colon of its retained faecal masses and sterilization; resection; and closure of the colostomy) the incidence of dehiscence has been reduced to about 12%. Ferreira-Santos (1961) has had no operative deaths in 58 cases treated by either one-stage or three-stage resection.

Corrêa Netto et al. (1962) have favoured an abdomino-anal type of operation for effecting rectosigmoidectomy, though their actual technique has undergone several changes to overcome difficulties and lessen the risk of complications. Originally they used a Bacon–Babock type of pull-through operation (see p. 510), but soon changed to a technique not unlike that of Swenson (p. 291) or Maunsell-Weir (p. 510). A very high incidence of dehiscence of the anastomosis after this operation when done as a one-stage procedure, led them to adopt a three-stage method with preliminary transverse colostomy. Despite the protection afforded by proximal colostomy, however, dehiscence remained a frequent complication, the operative mortality in 190 cases being approximately 7%. More recently they have employed a technique which re-establishes intestinal continuity without using a sutured colorectal anastomosis (Simonsen et al. 1960). In this operation the mobilization of the rectosigmoid from the abdominal aspect proceeds as usual. Then, working from below, the lining of the anal canal is incised all round *just above the pectinate line*, and the mucosa is freed by dissecting upwards in the submucous plane till a point is reached just above the anorectal ring. At this level the muscle coat of the rectal wall is divided, thus entering the field of the abdominal dissection and freeing the rectum from the retained anal sphincters, internal and external, and the levator muscles. The dilated bowel is then removed, and the colon stump is drawn down through the anal canal to project 6–8 cm beyond the anal verge. A few sutures are passed between the outer aspect of the colon and the pectinate line. The protruding colon is left in this position to act as a perineal colostomy for ten days or so. The second stage is then carried out, consisting of amputation of the colon stump beyond the pectinate line.

One of the advantages claimed for this last method is that it enables the surgeon to dispense with a transverse colostomy. The results are described as encouraging, but no detailed account of them is given. Though all the rectal mucosa down to the pectinate line is excised in this technique it is stated that the patients are able to appreciate some form of rectal sensation and to exercise satisfactory control of faeces.

Cutait and Figlioni (1961) have also favoured an abdomino-anal technique for rectosigmoidectomy, their operation being described in detail on p. 574.

Other Forms of Megacolon and Megarectum in the Adult

Megacolon encountered in adult patients in the temperate climates of Britain, western Europe and most parts of North America may be of several types:

HIRSCHSPRUNG'S DISEASE

It may seem remarkable that a disease process of this kind, originating in infancy or earlier, should persist undiagnosed or untreated into adult life. But I myself have met with two such cases, and Fairgrieve (1963) reports seven adult cases of Hirschsprung's disease from St Mark's Hospital and St Bartholomew's Hospital, London. One of my patients was a young woman, the other a lad of 18. All the patients in Fairgrieve's (1963) series were males in their late 'teens or early adult life. In all these cases there was a history of severe intractible constipation extending back to early childhood. In only three of these nine patients was the rectum empty and of normal calibre, suggesting that the condition might be one of Hirschsprung's disease with a distal aganglionic segment; in all the others the rectum was dilated and usually contained a large faeculoma. In five instances barium enema examination showed appearances diagnostic or suspicious of Hirschsprung's disease with a relatively contracted distal segment and a cone-effect. The most important investigation was rectal biopsy which was performed in seven of these nine patients and showed the histological features of Hirschsprung's disease in all cases (see p. 279).

MEGACOLON OR MEGARECTUM UNASSOCIATED WITH AGANGLIONOSIS (SIMPLE MEGACOLON OR MEGARECTUM, RECTAL OR COLONIC INERTIA)

This category, which may possibly embrace several different types of case, is much larger that the preceding one and for that reason more important, though unfortunately it is often dismissed very summarily in writings on the subject. Thus my own group of late adolescent or adult cases of megacolon or megarectum includes only two patients with Hirschsprung's disease but comprises ten without aganglionosis, whilst in Todd's (1961) collective series of 53 mainly adult patients with megacolon and megarectum, non-Hirschsprung cases heavily predominated.

Attempts have been made by Todd (1961) and Porter (1961) to subdivide these cases further according to the macroscopic appearances. Three subgroups may perhaps be recognized:

1. Megarectum without significant megacolon.
2. Megarectum with gross megasigmoid or more extensive megacolon.
3. Megasigmoid with a normal or only slightly dilated rectum.

The third group of megasigmoid associated with enlargement of the rectum is possibly a distinct entity and is sometimes complicated by the occurrence of attacks of abdominal pain and distension due to recurrent volvulus (see p. 929). But probably subgroups (1) and (2) are merely different stages of the same process, the aetiology of which is obscure. Possibly the condition is like rectal inertia in childhood (see p. 297), and due to habitual constipation, but it is perhaps remarkable (and disappointing) that prolonged conservative treatment with wash-outs is seldom followed by a return of the bowel to normal calibre. Indeed the dilatation and thickening of the wall of the rectum and lower sigmoid is sometimes so gross that it is hard to conceive of them ever returning to normal, and one cannot help wondering whether there is not some intrinsic physiological abnormality present which is responsible for this state of affairs. But we know from rectal biopsies there is no deficiency of intramural innervation. Studies by Todd (1961), Porter (1961) and Connell (1961) of the mechanism of defaecation and continence and of colon activity in these cases have failed to disclose any consistent abnormality. In some patients rectal sensation to balloon distension is greatly reduced or almost completely absent, but in other cases it is not very different from what it is in normal individuals. Also in some patients, but not in all, the normal inhibition of the external anal sphincter which occurs in response to prolonged distension of the rectum is absent or impaired. Pressure studies on the sigmoid colon show that its activity may be increased, diminished or normal.

Treatment (Goligher 1961)

The first question to be decided when the surgeon is faced with a case of megarectum or megacolon is whether the patient is suffering from Hirschsprung's disease or from one of the forms of megacolon unassociated with aganglionosis. In some instances the diagnosis may be clinically and radiologically evident, as, for example, when the barium enema plate shows an appearance typical of Hirschsprung's disease with a relatively contracted distal segment, or alternatively an enormous dilatation of the rectal ampulla extending down to the anorectal ring, suggesting that the condition is one of rectal inertia. However, the latter appearances may not be incompatible with Hirschsprung's disease when the aganglionic segment is exceptionally short, and for that reason it is *always wise to do a rectal biopsy* on these cases, as recommended by Swenson (1958). For details of this latter operation see p. 286. Anorectal manometry may also be helpful in eliciting evidence of aganglionosis (see p. 285). Once the diagnosis as to the type of megacolon present has thus been clarified, the plan of management can be decided upon.

FOR HIRSCHSPRUNG'S DISEASE

In this condition the rational surgical treatment is the removal of the distal aganglionic segment, but, as Todd (1961) has emphasized, there are considerable technical difficulties in the performance of an ordinary Swenson type of operation (p. 291) in the adult patient. These stem mainly from the grossly dilated, hypertrophied and loaded condition of the colon in long-standing Hirschsprung's disease, and the narrowness of the adult male pelvis, which greatly hamper the pelvic dissection and the subsequent suturing of the bowel. There would seem to be a strong argument for a two- or three-stage operation, the first step consisting of the establishment of a proximal defunctioning colostomy for three to six months to allow of thorough emptying of the left colon by washes-through and to permit the dilated colon to shrink to a more normal size. This colostomy may be made either in the right transverse colon—in which case it is closed as a third stage, after the resection has been successfully completed—or in the most distal part of the ganglionic colon, as determined by frozen-section biopsy at operation—in which case it is excised at the time of the resection.

The Turnbull–Cutait type of pull-through excision (see p. 574) was used in both of my adult cases, preceded by a preliminary transverse colostomy for several weeks, but the Parks abdomino-anal resection (see p. 577) would now seem to be a very suitable alternative.

It is only fair to add that in the series of seven adult cases with Hirschsprung's disease reported from St Mark's and St Bartholomew's Hospitals, London, by Fairgrieve (1963), a pull-through rectosigmoidectomy was employed on only one patient. All the others were treated by operations, such as colectomy and ileorectal anastomosis, descending and sigmoid colectomy with colorectal anastomosis, or anterior resection, each of which left a variable, but often substantial, amount of aganglionic distal large bowel. On theoretical grounds these are all quite inadequate operations, but all but one of these patients seemed on a follow-up of several years' duration to be doing well; the unsatisfactory case is one in which some degree of megaureter has developed following a colectomy and ileorectal anastomosis.

Another operation well worth considering, if the patient is prepared to accept the inconvenience of a permanent artificial anus, is a simple iliac colostomy. It has the advantage of avoiding the dangers of a difficult resection of the distal large bowel, not the least important of which in a young male patient is the risk of injury to the pelvic autonomic nerves with resulting impotence. Such a colostomy is best made by dividing the colon and placing the proximal end in the abdominal wall of the left iliac fossa, whilst the distal inactive end is brought out nearer the midline in the lower epigastric region.

FOR MEGARECTUM OR MEGACOLON
UNASSOCIATED WITH AGANGLIONOSIS

Surgical opinion in general is very much in favour of conservative management of the non-Hirschsprung type of megarectum and megacolon. Though operative treatment may occasionally be indicated, there is little consensus of opinion as to the precise indications for intervention or as to the form operation should take.

One type of case for which surgery should seriously be considered is that with a long dilated sigmoid but with a normal rectum, especially if there have been episodes of recurrent abdominal pain and distension to suggest recurring subacute volvulus of the loop (Hallenbeck and Waugh 1952; Todd 1961). For this condition an elective sigmoid colectomy with end-to-end anastomosis may be dramatically effective (see p. 460).

For the much more common cases with gross megarectum and a variable degree of megacolon conservative management should certainly be tried in the first instance. This consists of regular daily wash-outs and aperients (p. 301), and it is often a good plan to commence the treatment with a manual disimpaction of the faeces under a short general anaesthetic. Of aperients, Senokot is best (four or more tablets daily). Once the large bowel has been thoroughly emptied after 10–14 days in hospital, the patient may be discharged and the wash-outs continued at home. Later it may be possible to replace the wash-outs with bisacodyl suppositories or rely on Senokot alone. Regular follow-up examinations are needed to ensure that faecal impaction is not recurring. Often this treatment is successful in enabling the patients to avoid gross accumulation of faeces and incontinence, which were the symptoms that usually brought them to hospital in the first instance, though, as already mentioned it seldom results in much objective diminution in the rectal calibre. But it is a tedious regimen, and sometimes it fails to give even symptomatic relief, so that surgical measures may have to be considered.

In such cases it is tempting to resect the grossly dilated rectum and sigmoid by abdominal anal pull-through excision in the hope as it were of giving the patient a fresh start. I have only done this operation twice in patients with rectal inertia producing gross megarectum and megasigmoid and in neither case was the result encouraging. One unfortunately developed leakage, sepsis and a host of complications for which I had eventually to remove the rectal remnant and given him a permanent colostomy. The other had a smooth postoperative course, but he has had indifferent rectal function since and still has to have wash-outs. One would hesitate to draw conclusions from such a limited operative experience, but Nixon (1961) has also found that a continuation of the training regimen is usually necessary after Swenson type of resection in children with rectal inertia.

Todd (1961) reported a group of 14 patients with non-Hirschsprung forms of megarectum and megacolon treated by ileorectal, ileosigmoid or caecorectal anastomosis or by sigmoid and anterior rectal resection in the hope of producing a softer type of stool less likely to inspissate in the rectal stump. Unfortunately the results have not been impressive, for nine of the patients still have a loaded rectum and require regular enemas, and two have diarrhoea.

One operation can be relied upon to give a good result but at a price. That is a proximal iliac colostomy, as described in connection with Hirschsprung's disease on p. 307. I have now done this operation four times for severe rectal inertia. Preoperatively the idea of an artificial anus was naturally repugnant to these young people, but now they are all very satisfied with their colostomies, which seem to them like charms compared with the bother they used to have with their megarectum! I do not suggest that a colostomy should often be indicated in the management of rectal inertia, but when medical treatment has apparently failed to keep the patient reasonably comfortable, this simple and effective operation should be considered as an alternative to any form of resection, which is so frequently followed by serious complications or continued symptoms.

REFERENCES

AARONSON, I. and NIXON, H. H. (1972) A clinical evaluation of anorectal pressure studies in the diagnosis of Hirschsprung's disease. *Gut, 13*, 138.

BENTLEY, J. F. R. (1966) Posterior excisional anorectal myotomy in management of chronic faecal accumulation. *Archs Dis. Childh., 41*, 144.

—— and SMITH, J. R. (1960) Developmental posterior enteric remnants and spinal malformations. *Archs Dis. Childh., 35*, 76.

BERG, I. and JONES, K. V. (1964) Functional faecal incontinence in children. *Archs Dis. Childh., 39*, 465.

BERRY, C. L. (1969) Persistent changes in the large bowel following enterocolitis associated with Hirschsprung's disease. *J. Path., 97*, 731.

Bishop, H. C. and Koop, C. E. (1957) Management of meconium ileus: resection, Roux-en-Y anastomosis and ileostomy irrigation with pancreatic enzymes. *Ann. Surg., 145*, 410.

Bodian, M. and Carter, C. O. (1963) A family study of Hirschsprung's disease. *Ann. hum. Genet., 26*, 261.

Boley, S. J., Lafer, D. J. Kleinhaus, S., Cohn, B. D., Mestel, A. L. and Kottmeier, P. K. (1968) Endorectal pull through procedure for Hirschsprung's disease with and without primary anastomosis. *J. pediat. Surg., 3*, 258.

Bremer, J. L. (1944) Diverticula and duplications of the intestinal tract. *Archs Path., 38*, 132.

Browne, D. (1955) In *Abdominal Operations*, ed. R. Maingot, 3rd ed., p. 1269. London: Butterworth.

Bughaighis, A. C. and Emery, J. L. (1971) Functional obstruction of the intestine due to neurological immaturity. In *Progressive Pediatric Surgery*, Vol. 3. Baltimore: University Park Press.

Bunton, G. L., Durbin, G. M., McIntosh, N., Shaw, D. G., Taghizedeh, A., Reynolds, E. O. R., Rivers, R. P. A. and Urman, G. (1977) Necrotizing enterocolitis *Archs Dis. Childh., 52*, 772.

Callaghan, R. P. and Nixon, H. H. (1964) Megarectum: physiological considerations. *Archs Dis. Childh., 38*, 153.

Chagas, C. (1916) Trypanosomîase americana: forma acuda da moléstia. *Mems Inst. Oswaldo Cruz, 8*, 37.

Coekin, M. and Gairdner, D. (1960) Faecal incontinence in children: the physical factor. *Br. med. J., 2*, 1175.

Connell, A. M. (1961) In Discussion on megacolon and megarectum with the emphasis on conditions other than Hirschsprung's disease. *Proc. R. Soc. Med., 54*, 1040.

Corrêa Netto, A. (1934) Tratamento cirûrgico do megacolon pela ressecção dos chamados esfincteres funcionais do intestino grosso. *Revta Cirrurg. S Paulo, 1*, 249.

—— Haddad, J., de Azevedo, P. de A. V. and Raia, A. (1962) Etiology, pathogenesis and treatment of acquired megacolon. *Surgery Gynec. Obstet., 114*, 602.

Cutait, D. E. (1953) Tratamento do megasigma pela retossigmoidectomia. *Tese râ Fac. Med. Univ. S. Paulo Brasil, 1953.*

—— and Figlioni, F. J. (1961) A new method of colorectal anastomosis in abdominoperineal resection. *Dis. Colon Rect., 4*, 335.

Dalla Valle, A. (1920) Richerche istologische su di un caso du megacolon congenito. *pediatria, Napoli, 28*, 740.

—— (1924) Contributa alle conoscenza della forma famigliare del megacolon. *Pediatria, Napoli, 32*, 569.

Denda, T. and Katzumata, K. (1966) New techniques for Hirschsprung's disease. *J. Jap. Ass. pediat. Surg., 2*, 37.

Duhamel, B. (1963) Technique et indications de l'abaissement retrorectal et transanal en chirurgie colique. *Gaz. méd. Fr., 70*, 599.

Eek, S., nd Knutrud, O. (1962) Megacolon congenitum Hirschsprung. *J. Oslo Cy Hosps, 12*, 245.

Ehrenpreis, T. (1946) Megacolon in infancy. *Acta chir. scand., 94*, Suppl. 112.

—— (1967) Mortality in Hirschsprung's disease in infancy. *J. pediat. Surg., 2*, 569.

—— (1970) *Hirschsprung's Disease*, p. 94. Chicago: Year Book Medical Publishers.

Fairgrieve, J. (1963) Hirschsprung's disease in the adult. *Br. J. Surg., 50*, 506.

Ferreira-Santos, R. (1959) Symposium on mega-oesophagus and megacolon. *Inst. Med. Trop. S Paulo.*

—— (1961) Megacolon and megarectum in Chagas' disease. *Proc. R. Soc. Med., 54*, 1047.

Finochietto, R. (1927) Megasigmoideum: resultados alejados de la sigmoidectomia. *Revta Cirurg. B. Aires, 6*, 712.

Fraser, G. C. and Berry, C. (1967) Mortality in neonatal Hirschsprung's disease with particular reference to enterocolitis. *J. pediat. Surg., 2*, 205.

Gannon, B. J., Burnstock, G., Noblett, H. R. and Campbell, P. E. (1966a) Histochemical diagnosis of Hirschsprung's disease. *Lancet, 1*, 894.

—— Noblett, H. R. and Burnstock, G. (1969b) Adrenergic innervation of bowel in Hirschsprung's disease. *Br. med. J., 3*, 338.

Garrett, J. R., Howard, E. R. and Nixon, H. H. (1969) Autonomic nerves in rectum and colon in Hirschsprung's disease. *Archs Dis. Childh., 44*, 406.

Goligher, J. C. (1961) In Discussion on megacolon and megarectum with the emphasis on conditions other than Hirschsprung's disease. *Proc. R. Soc. Med., 54*, 1053.

Hallenbeck, G. A. and Waugh, J. M. (1952) The surgical treatment of megacolon. *Surg. Clins N. Am., 32*, 1203.

Harris, L. E., Corbin, P. F. and Hill, J. R. (1954) Ano-rectal rings in infancy, incidence and significance. *Paediatrics, Springfield, 13*, 59.

Hiatt, R. B. (1951a) The pathologic physiology of congenital megacolon. *Ann. Surg., 133*, 313.

—— (1951b) The surgical treatment of congenital megacolon. *Ann. Surg., 133*, 321.

Hirschsprung, H. (1888) Stuhlträgheit Neugeborener in Folge von Dilatation und Hypertrophie des Colons. *Jber. Kinderheilk., 27*, 1.

Howard, F. R. and Garrett, J. R. (1970) Electron microscopy of myenteric nerves in Hirschsprung's disease and in normal bowel. *Gut, 11*, 1007.

—— and Nixon. H. H. (1968) Internal anal sphincter. *Archs Dis. Childh., 43*, 569.

Hurst, A. F. (1934) Anal achalasia and megacolon. *Guy's Hosp. Rep., 84*, 317.

Kapila, L., Haberkorn, S. and Nixon, H. H. (1975) Chronic adynamic bowel stimulating Hirschsprung's disease. *J. pediat. Surg., 10*, 885.

Katz, A. (1966) Pseudo Hirschsprung's disease in Bantu children. *Archs Dis. Childh., 41*, 152.

Kempton, J. J. (1954) Hirschsprung's disease in a man aged 23. *Proc. R. Soc. Med., 47*, 545.

Köberle, F. (1956a) Pathologische Befunde an den muskulären Hohlorganen bei der experimentellen Chagaskrankheit. *Zentbl. allg. Path., 95*, 321.

—— (1956b) Über das Neurotoxin des Trypanosoma Cruzi. *Zentbl. allg. Path., 95*, 468.

—— and Nador, E. (1956) Mal de engasgo. *Z. Tropenmed. Parasit., 7*, 259.

Lake, B. D. (1976) A cholinesterase method for light and electron microscopy. *R. Microsc. Soc. Proc., 11*, 77.

Lassman, G. and Wurnig, P. (1973) Lokale Ganglionzellhyperplasie in der Submucosa an oralen Ende desaganglionare segmentesbei Morbus Hirschsprung. *Zschr. Kinderchir., 12*, 236.

Lawson, J. O. N. and Nixon, H. H. (1967) Anal canal pressures in the diagnosis of Hirschsprung's disease. *J. pediat. Surg., 2*, 544.

LEWIS, F. T. and THYNG, F. W. (1907) The regular occurrence of intestinal diverticula in embryos of the pig, rabbit and man. *Am. J. Anat.*, 7, 505.

LICHTENSTEIN, J. R. (1972) Syndrome. In *Birth Defects*, Part XIII, p. 166. Baltimore: Williams and Wilkins.

LYNN, H. B. and VAN HEERDEN, J. A. (1975) Rectal myectomy in Hirschsprung's disease. *Archs Surg., Chicago, 110*, 991.

MAGNUS, R. V. (1968) Ectopia cloacae—a misnomer. *J. pediat. Surg., 4*, 571.

MARTIN, L. W. (1968) Surgical management of Hirschsprung's disease involving the small intestine. *Archs Surg., Chicago*, 97, 183.

—— and CAUDILL, D. R. (1967) A method for the elimination of the blind rectal pouch in the Duhamel operation for Hirschsprung's disease. *Surgery, St Louis*, 62, 951.

MEIER-ROUGE, W. (1974) Hirschsprung's disease: its aetiology, pathogenesis and differential diagnosis. In *Current Topics in Pathology*, Vol. 59. Berlin: Springer.

—— LUTTERBECK, P. M., HERZOG, B., MORGER, R., MOSER, R. and SCHÄRLI, A. (1972). Acetylcholinesterase activity in suction biopsies of the rectum in the diagnosis of Hirschsprung's disease. *J. pediat. Surg.*, 7, 11.

NIXON, H. H. (1956) Intestinal obstruction in the neonatal period. *Gt Ormond St. J., No. 11*, 1.

—— (1961) In Discussion on megacolon and megarectum. *Proc. R. Soc. Med.*, 54, 1037.

NOBLETT, H. R. (1969a) A rectal suction biopsy tube for use in the diagnosis of Hirschsprung's disease. *J. pediat. Surg., 4*, 406.

—— (1969b) Treatment of uncomplicated meconium ileus by gastrografin enema. *J. pediat. Surg., 4*, 190.

NORBERG, K.-A. (1964) Adrenergic innervation of the intestinal wall studied by fluorescence microscopy. *Int. J. Neuropharmac., 3*, 379.

NUNAN, B., REZENDEN, Col. and CANELAS, A. (1952) Quoted by Ferreira-Santos (1961).

NURCOMBE, B. (1972) Psychogenic megacolon: the study of a psychosomatic relationship. *Med. J. Aust., 2*, 1178.

OKAMOTO, E. and UEDA, T. (1967) Embryogenesis of intramural ganglia of the gut and its relation to Hirschsprung's disease. *J. pediat. Surg., 2*, 437.

OKUMURA, M. (1960) Personal communication to Ferreira-Santos (1961).

PASSARGE, E. (1972) Genetic heterogenicity and recurrence risk of congenital intestinal aganglionosis. *Birth Defects Original Article Series*, 8, 63.

PELLERIN, D. (1963) *Nouvelle Pratique Chirurgical Illustrée*, fasc. XXI. Paris: Doin.

PERROT, A. and DANON, L. (1935) Obstruction intestinale de cause rare, chez un nourrison. *Annls Anat. Path., 12*, 157.

PORTER, N. H. (1961) In Discussion on megacolon and megarectum with the emphasis on conditions other than Hirschsprung's disease. *Proc. R. Soc. Med.*, 54, 1043.

PURI, P., LAUE, B. D. and NIXON, H. H. (1977) Adynamic bowel syndrome. *Gut, 18*, 754.

RAIA, A. (1955) Pathogenesis and treatment of acquired megacolon. *Surgery Gynec. Obstet., 101*, 69.

—— and CAMPOS, O. M. (1948) O tratamento do megacolon; estudo do follow-up de várias técnicas adotodas. *Revta Med. Cirurg. S. Paulo, 18*, 287.

REHBEIN, F., and NICOLAI, I. (1963) Operative treatment for Hirschsprung's disease. Results of 110 cases of intra-abdominal resection. *Dt. med. Wschr., 88*, 1595.

RIVEROS, M. (1940) Quoted by Ferreira-Santos (1961).

SCHNAUFER, L., TALBERT, J. L., HALLER, J. A., REID, N. C. R. W., TOBON, F. and SCHUSTER, M. M. (1967) Differential sphincteric studies in the diagnosis of anorectal disorders of childhood. *J. pediat. Surg., 2*, 538.

SIMONSEN, O., HABR, A. and GAZAL, P. (1960). Rectosigmoidectomia endoanal com ressecção de mucosa rectal. *Revta paul. med.*, 57, 116.

SOAVE, F. (1964) Hirschsprung's disease: a new surgical technique. *Archs Dis. Childh., 39*, 116.

SPITZ, L. and RICKHAM, P. O. (1972) Anal duplication cysts. *Z. Kinderchir., 11*, 433.

STAPLE, T. W., McALISTER, W. H. and ANDERSON, M. S. (1964) Plexiform neurofibromatosis of the colon simulating Hirschsprung's disease. *Am. J. Roentgen., 91*, 840.

STEICHEN, F. M., TALBERT, J. L. and RAVITCH, M. M. (1968) Primary side to side colorectal anastomosis in the Duhamel operation for Hirschsprung's disease. *Surgery, St Louis, 64*, 475.

SWENSON, O. (1954) Modern treatment of Hirschsprung's disease. *J. Am. med. Ass., 154*, 651.

—— (1955) Congenital defects in the pelvic parasympathetic system. *Archs Dis. Childh., 30*, 1.

—— (1958) In *Pediatric Surgery*. New York: Appleton-Century-Crofts.

—— (1964) Partial internal sphincterectomy in the treatment of Hirschsprung's disease. *Ann. Surg., 160*, 540.

—— and BILL, A. A. H., Jr. (1948) Resection of rectum and rectosigmoid with preservation of the sphincter for benign spastic lesions producing megacolon. *Surgery, St Louis, 24*, 212.

—— RHEINLANDER, H. F. and DIAMOND, I. (1949) Hirschsprung's disease: a new concept of etiology; operative results in 34 patients. *New Engl. J. Med., 241*, 551.

TANNER, M. S., SMITH, B. and LLOYD, J. K. (1976) Functional intestinal obstruction due to deficiency of argyrophil neurons in the myenteric plexus. Familial syndrome presenting with short small bowel, malrotationary pyloric hypertrophy. *Archs Dis. Childh.*, 51, 837.

TIFFIN, M. E., CHANDLER, L. R. and FABER, H. K. (1940) Localised absence of ganglion cells of the mesenteric plexus in congenital megacolon. *Am. J. Dis. Child., 59*, 1071.

TODD, I. P. (1961) In Discussion on megacolon and megarectum with the emphasis on conditions other than Hirschsprung's disease. *Proc. R. Soc. Med., 54*, 1035.

VIEIRA, C. B. et al. (1961) Personal communication to Ferreira-Santos (1961).

WYLLIE, G. G. (1957) Course and management of Hirschsprung's disease. *Lancet, 1*, 847.

13

Anal Incontinence

Patients about to undergo operation for minor rectal conditions such as haemorrhoids or fistula are apt to be worried particularly by two fears: that they may suffer intolerable postoperative pain or that they may be left incontinent. Certainly one of the foremost considerations in the mind of the surgeon in selecting and carrying out surgical procedures in the anal region is the preservation of normal continence, and defects of this function as a result of operative treatment are now relatively rare, which is fortunate because there is very little that can be done to remedy them. In practice anal incontinence is far more frequently found to be due to disease or non-surgical trauma. Most of the conditions that may give rise to incontinence are discussed in different chapters of this book, but it may be helpful to summarize the causes and comment further on a few of them.

CAUSES OF ANAL INCONTINENCE

Congenital Abnormalities of the Anus and Rectum

Various forms of anorectal deformity may be associated with some degree of incontinence before or after surgical treatment as mentioned in Chapter 11.

Trauma

ACCIDENTAL INJURIES

Severe lacerated wounds of the anal region due to impalement injuries with spikes, etc., or to military projectiles may result in complete division of the sphincter apparatus. Depending on circumstances it may be possible to carry out an immediate 'toilet' of the wound and repair of the damaged structures under systemic antibiotic therapy and possibly a covering iliac colostomy, or reconstruction may have to be delayed till a later date.

OBSTETRICAL TEARS

A complete tear of the perineum during childbirth will sever the sphincters. A primary suture of the tear including the sphincter muscles is often completely successful, but if infection and breakdown occur the patient will be rendered incontinent. This is unfortunately a fairly common state of affairs, for many middle-aged women who suffer from incontinence due to this cause are unable, because of the pressure of their domestic duties, to come into hospital for an elective perineorrhaphy. The disability, however, is often surprisingly slight. Late repairs of these tears are generally performed by gynaecologists without the protection of a proximal colostomy, but primary healing is secured in the majority. Though the functional results are usually claimed to be excellent, that was not my impression in a series of 50 patients in whom I investigated anal function after perineorrhaphy (Goligher 1956, unpublished). I found that between a quarter and a third of the cases had some imperfection of control for flatus or liquid faeces, even though the repair seemed sound on examination.

OPERATIVE TRAUMA

FISTULA OPERATIONS

As Blaisdell (1940) showed in his collective enquiry for the American Proctologic Society, operations for fistula-in-ano are those most commonly followed by postoperative incontinence. The avoidance of gross incontinence depends on preservation of the anorectal ring, and the ways in which this may be done have already been described in Chapter 7 (p. 179). But the later work of Bennett (1962) in my department has shown that lesser degrees of impaired anal control may occur after fistula operations, even when the anorectal ring has not been damaged (see p. 187).

OPERATIONS FOR ANAL FISSURE

As pointed out on p. 148, contrary to what was formerly believed, partial division of the internal sphincter by an open posterior internal sphincterotomy is followed in a proportion of the patients so treated by minor degrees of incontinence. Simple sphincter stretching for fissure is also occasionally, but much less frequently, complicated in this way, and the presently popular lateral subcutaneous internal sphincterotomy is perhaps even less likely to be followed by disturbances of this kind.

OPERATIONS FOR HAEMORRHOIDS

Formal Haemorrhoidectomy. Contrary to our earlier findings (Bennett et al. 1963), it seems that a modern ligature and excision operation for haemorrhoids, performed by a reasonably competent surgeon, is most unlikely to be followed by any impairment of continence, provided that the sphincters have not been deliberately stretched at the time of the haemorrhoidectomy (Goligher et al. 1969). The great offender in the past was Whitehead's operation, which is now seldom used. The impairment of continence often seen after that operation was due to two factors: to the loss of the anal and lower rectal mucosa which is considered by many to play an important role in the mechanism of continence, and to the fact that the remaining rectal mucosa was often stitched to the perianal skin—instead of to the anal canal skin at the level of the dentate line as recommended by the originator of the technique (Whitehead 1887)—and so pouted at the anal orifice causing a mucoid leak.

Manual Dilatation. Not perhaps surprisingly the very vigorous eight finger dilatation of the anal canal practised in the Lord procedure is followed in some cases by incontinence. But the precise frequency and inconvenience of this complication is a matter of some dispute (see p. 126).

SPHINCTER-SAVING RESECTIONS OF THE RECTUM

Though these operations preserve the sphincters, they are not all successful in retaining normal continence. Some of the failures have been due, at least in part, to damage to the sphincter apparatus itself, usually the internal sphincter, but most of them have hitherto been held to be caused by interference with the sensory side of the mechanism for anal control or by loss of the reservoir function of the rectal ampulla (Goligher 1951, 1958; Goligher and Hughes 1951; Goligher et al. 1965). However, more recent work by Winckler (1958), Walls (1959), Stephens and Smith (1971), Bennett et al. (1973), and Lane and Parks (1977), suggesting that 'rectal' sensation is mediated, at any rate in part, by nerve endings in the levator muscles and puborectales rather than in the mucosa or muscle coat of the rectal wall, calls for a re-appraisal of previous explanations of the impairment of function in some of these cases.

Anterior Resection. As generally performed this operation preserves not only the sphincters but also the lower third or more of the rectum, so that both the sensory and motor components for proper sphincter control are fully safeguarded. In practice *high* anterior resection, in which the pelvic peritoneum and lateral ligaments of the rectum are not divided, the rectum itself is not lifted out of its sacral bed and the anastomosis is to the upper rectum, is practically invariably followed by perfect continence for faeces and flatus. The only abnormality noticed after it is that at first motions are passed not once but three or four times a day, usually after each meal. This is due to loss of the normal sigmoid reservoir for faeces, and it gradually corrects itself as the remaining colon assumes this function. In *low* anterior resection, in which the rectum is fully mobilized down to the anorectal ring with complete severance of the lateral ligaments, the eventual suture line usually lies 6–8 cm from the anal verge, but may occasionally be as low as 4·5–5 cm, particularly if a stapling device was used. Fairly normal function seems to result from this operation as a rule, but there is often at first imperfect control for flatus and occasionally for liquid faeces in patients with particularly low anastomoses. These latter patients may well have to wear a protective pad over the anus at any rate for some weeks to avoid soiling their underclothes.

Abdomino-anal Resections. As the Bacon–Babcock type of pull-through abdomino-anal resection (see

p. 510) leaves a very small anal stump and denudes it of its lining—possibly damaging the internal sphincter in the process—and in some modifications of the operation actually divides both sphincters in the midline posteriorly and subsequently resutures them around the colon stump, it would perhaps be surprising on theoretical grounds if it gave perfect functional results. Bacon (1949) and Waugh et al. (1954) admit that continence is often grossly impaired after this procedure, but claim that in a proportion of their patients— perhaps about a third—normal control is retained. I must say that this was not my experience in the few cases that I treated by this operation—they were all quite incontinent and, if they had a bout of diarrhoea, were completely incapacitated by it.

Better types of abdomino-anal resection from the functional point of view have been held to be the Maunsell–Weir, Marden Black or Turnbull–Cutait operations (see pp. 510–13), all of which preserve the sphincters and the normal lining of the small anorectal remnant, though they may during the operation and subsequently subject this remnant to gross stretching or eversion. They are capable of giving full continence eventually, but a long period of rehabilitation may be necessary and many of these patients wear a pad for a long time. In our experience (Goligher et al. 1965) continence for flatus and liquid faeces was seldom normal unless an anorectal stump of at least 6 cm from the anal verge was retained, but some other surgeons, such as Bennett et al. (1972) have found that good control gradually develops after a considerable time in some patients with even smaller anorectal stumps.

The latest contender for surgical favour is the abdominotransanal resection (see p. 513) which usually removes the muscle coat of the rectal wall down to 4–4·5 cm and the mucosal lining to 2–2·5 cm, respectively, from the anal verge and finishes with a sleeve type of colo-anal anastomosis. Lane and Parks (1977) claim that in 7 of 12 patients so treated, continence was eventually perfect but often took several weeks to reach that state. My own experience of eleven cases on follow-up after abdominotransanal resection is that after six to nine months seven achieved full continence but of a rather precarious kind, whereby, if they suffered an attack of severe diarrhoea, their anal control broke down temporarily to some extent. Three of the remaining four are still partly incontinent for flatus and soft or liquid faeces and two of them wear anal pads constantly. One with severe anastomotic dehiscence has now a tight stenosis and retains a permanent colostomy (see p. 513).

Abdominosacral Resection. In this operation a colorectal anastomosis is achieved through a posterior or sacral approach usually at a level about 4·5–5 cm from the anal verge. It would appear from the reports of Localio (Localio 1975; Localio et al. 1978), who has had by far the greatest experience with this procedure in recent years, that the functional results eventually become entirely satisfactory in the great majority of cases, with full continence for flatus and faeces and no need to wear a pad, but he emphasizes that, as with most patients given very low colorectal anastomoses by other methods, there is usually a very tiresome immediate postoperative period of several weeks or months during which the patients experience great frequency of defaecation and sometimes a degree of incontinence. I can confirm these findings from observation on 18 of my own patients and a rather larger group of Dr Localio's patients whom he kindly allowed me to interrogate and examine in 1975 (see also p. 509).

Colectomy and Ileorectal Anastomosis. When this operation is performed for colitis or polyposis, even more of the rectum is preserved as a rule than in an anterior resection, so that the conditions for normal continence are in no way jeopardized. This is as well, because the more liquid motions resulting from the colectomy subject the mechanism of anal control to very exacting demands (see p. 367).

Colectomy, Mucosal Proctectomy and Ileo-anal Pullthrough Anastomosis. In this operation, designed by Ravitch (1948), the entire colon and upper half of the rectum are excised, the mucosa of the retained lower rectal segment dissected off the underlying muscle coat down to the pectinate line, and the terminal ileum drawn down through the denuded anorectal remnant for suture of its lower edge to the anal canal skin at the pectinate line. So far as anal continence is concerned the rationale of the procedure rests on the hypothesis that the nerve endings responsible for appreciating distension of the rectum are located not in the mucosa but in the muscle coat of the rectal wall and that the retention of the muscle coat should therefore ensure the conservation of rectal sensation. Even on the basis of the alternative more recent concept that the location of the relevant nerve endings is not in any part of the rectal wall but instead in the adjacent levator or puborectales muscles, there is equally good reason to postulate that the operation could be compatible with normal rectal sensation and continence. In actual practice, though Ravitch (1948) himself and Devine and Webb (1951) claimed good results with the operation my own limited experience with it nearly 30 years ago showed that the patients invariably suffered incessant diarrhoea and incontinence (Goligher 1951), but whether this was due to lack of rectal sensation or the loss of the normal rectal and sigmoid reservoir was not determined. It is also true that my patients were followed up for only a few weeks—and then converted to ileostomy. Recently a far more favourable assessment of the ileo-anal pull-through procedure has emanated from Martin et al. (1977) who reported that of 17 patients given ileo-anal anastomoses, 15 were completely continent, but it is to be noted that most of them had very considerable frequency of defaecation and some incontinence for several months following the operation (see Appendix C).

Colectomy, Mucosal Proctectomy, Creation of Ileal Reservoir and Ileo-anal Pull-through Anastomosis. This modification of the Ravitch (1948) operation, introduced by Parks and Nicholls (1978), is a very logical evolution to compensate for the lack of a rectal reservoir by providing an ileal pouch just above the ileo-anal anastomosis which might be expected to reduce some of the pressure on the mechanism of continence. In fact these patients usually have to intubate the ileal pouch per anum in order to evacuate the faeces and in between intubations are usually continent, though occasionally anal leakage has occurred especially at night (see Appendix C).

Rectosigmoidectomy for Prolapse. As pointed out on p. 236, this operation is followed by incontinence in fully 50% of the cases. Some of this may be due to the sacrifice at operation of a considerable part of the lower rectum, but much of it may be attributable to other factors—such as the unusual laxity of the anal sphincters, possibly combined with some blunting of normal anorectal sensation in cases of prolapse—and be a continuation of a preoperative defect of continence.

Rectosigmoidectomy for Aganglionic Megacolon. By contrast with the results of rectosigmoidectomy for prolapse is the excellent degree of continence often found after the similar operative manoeuvre performed in the Swenson operation (p. 296) for aganglionic megacolon—presumably due to the better state of the sphincter musculature and to the fact that these young patients have a better chance to adapt gradually to altered postoperative state than do elderly sufferers from prolapse. Also very relevant to the outcome of the Ravitch (1948) type

of operation for colitis are the generally good functional results afforded by the Soave (1964) form of rectosigmoidectomy for megacolon in which the mucosa of the distal anorectal remnant is 'cored out' and the colon drawn down through the denuded stump to the pectinate line (see pp. 291, 296).

OPERATIONS FOR CONGENITAL ANOMALIES OF THE ANORECTUM

The functional results after operations raise interesting points in regard to the mechanism of continence (see p. 276).

TRANSSPHINCTERIC EXPOSURE AND ABDOMINO-TRANSSPHINCTERIC RESECTION OF THE RECTUM

In both these procedures the external anal sphincter is divided and subsequently sutured; in the former the internal sphincter is also divided and sutured and in the latter most of the rectum is resected down almost to the top of this sphincter (Mason 1977). Yet the functional results are often eventually satisfactory, sometimes after a period of considerable frequency and some incontinence (see pp. 356, 509).

Disease of the Anorectum and Colon

CONDITIONS ASSOCIATED WITH ABNORMAL LAXITY, STRETCHING OR DESTRUCTION OF THE ANAL SPHINCTERS

Notorious in this respect is *complete or partial prolapse of the rectum*, and perhaps the most distressing feature of these conditions is the loss of normal anal control so frequently found with them. An obvious cause of the incontinence in these cases is the mechanical interference with closure of the anus by the protruding bowel. But probably equally important is the great laxity of the sphincters so often present, and possibly some hypoaesthesia of the lower rectum and anal canal, for after the prolapse has been cured by operation the incontinence not infrequently persists (see p. 229–38).

Large prolapsing third-degree internal haemorrhoids may also be associated with some measure of incontinence, mainly for flatus.

In cases of *ulcerative colitis* with associated abscesses in the anal region, the sphincter musculature may be so destroyed by the inflammatory process as to be rendered completely incompetent, and the same state of affairs may result from *amoebic and lymphogranulomatous* infections. A *carcinoma of the anal canal or lower rectum* extending down towards the anus may also cause incontinence partly from stretching and partly from infiltration and destruction of the sphincters.

IMPACTION OF FAECES

In children with so-called acquired or habitual forms of megacolon and megarectum, faecal impaction occurs with resulting overflow incontinence (see p. 298).

In adults impaction of faeces is met with chiefly in feeble, senile individuals who are disinterested in their personal habits, or in bedridden patients. It may also occasionally occur in younger patients as a complication of abdominal operations, and it sometimes complicates the convalescence after certain ophthalmic operations, such as removal of cataracts and fixation of detached retinae, when absolute immobility is considered essential, even to the extent of banning normal defaecatory efforts. Constipation is the first symptom but is followed by incontinence as aperients are taken to relieve the condition. This is accompanied by a feeling of incomplete evacuation. The diagnosis is readily established by digital examination, when the large hard mass is felt filling and distending the rectum, whilst liquid faeces trickle round it and through the anus causing the incontinence.

Aperients and enemas alone are quite ineffectual in the treatment of this condition. What is required in the first instance is a digital or instrumental evacuation of the rectum under general anaesthesia. This is a tedious and unpleasant operation, the classical instrument for which is the ordinary domestic dinner spoon! By means of it and the surgeon's finger the faecal mass is broken up and delivered through the anus. Thereafter a vigorous regimen of aperients and enemas should be instituted to establish regular habits and avoid a recurrence of the condition. Suppositories may also be useful to this end.

Neurological and Medical Conditions

Neurological conditions such as tabes dorsalis, spinal tumours (or injuries) or spina bifida may be associated with anal incontinence, as may also the later stages of wasting or malignant disease. But the commonest cause of anal incontinence is *old age and general debility*, and a major problem of geriatrics is incontinence.

TREATMENT

The treatment obviously depends on the cause of the condition and for the most part has already been described in the various chapters dealing with these causes. It only remains to say something about the surgical treatment of incontinence due to patulousness of the anus, whether arising idiopathically or as a result of injury or operation. A number of operations have been described for the treatment of this state of affairs and are considered below.

Suture of Sphincters

GYNAECOLOGICAL PERINEORRHAPHY

When the incontinence is due to an old third degree obstetrical laceration of the perineum, the treatment is by a formal perineorrhaphy, in which the cut surfaces of the sphincter muscles are approximated and the puborectales brought together by suture. For full details of the operative technique gynaecological texts should be consulted. Incidentally, though gynaecologists usually perform this operation without a covering colostomy, they manage to obtain healing per primam in the majority of their cases! The outcome of such repairs in terms of anal continence is not always perfect, but most patients have a reasonable measure of control and reckon that the result is fairly successful.

OTHER FORMS OF SUTURE

The other sort of case for which suture of the sphincters may be required is one in which these muscles have been completely or nearly completely divided in a fistula operation. Experience in the late repair of such cases has mostly been very disappointing, as was brought out by Blaisdell (1940). But a recent very valuable report by Parks and McPartlin (1971) paints a much more encouraging picture of the treatment of these patients. Of 16 cases treated by them all but two secured a very useful measure of anal control and were most grateful. The two failed cases had both been done without a covering colostomy, whereas all but one of the successful cases had been given a temporary colostomy. As a consequence Parks and McPartlin feel strongly that *an essential preliminary to the operation on the anal canal is the establishment of an iliac colostomy*, which is closed after the sphincter repair has soundly healed.

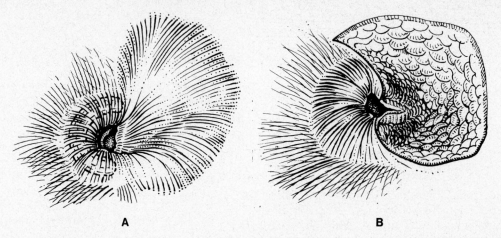

A   **B**

Fig. 235. (A) Following section of the sphincters the wound has healed with much scar tissue formation, the sphincters retracting to about half their normal circumference. (B) Excision of secondary epithelium and underlying scar tissue has been effected leaving large wound encompassing half the circumference of the anus and extending up into the anal canal itself. (*From Parks and McPartlin 1971*)

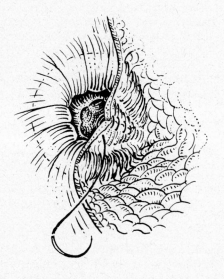

Fig. 236. Reconstruction of epithelial lining of anal canal. (*From Parks and McPartlin 1971*)

In the conduct of the repair itself, they emphasize the importance of *wide excision of the secondary epithelium and underlying scar tissue*. This creates a large wound (Fig. 235). The next step is to mobilize the normal mucosa of the anal canal and lower rectum by dissecting a 1-cm fringe of it free from the underlying muscle, so that it can eventually be sutured without tension. *The muscle ends are next sought.* Great judgement is required in defining them, for, if they are cleaned of all fibrous tissue, the sutures subsequently inserted in them will merely cut out. It is not necessary to identify the internal and external sphincter separately; all that is needed is to dissect the sphincter mass for a short distance on its outer side, to free it from fibrous tissue that may have formed in the ischiorectal fossa (Fig. 237A).

In *the repair* the mucosal tube is first reconstituted with a continuous stitch of 2/o chromic cat-gut (Fig. 236). The fibrosed cut ends of the sphincters are then brought together, preferably with a slight overlap, with horizontal mattress sutures of 40 SWG stainless steel wire rather loosely tied (Fig. 237B). No attempt is made to suture the perineal skin, and a large open wound is left to heal by granulation which it usually does satisfactorily, despite the fact that it has exposed muscles and wire sutures in its base. At first the circumference of the canal is reduced by about a half, but it gradually stretches in due course.

In the light of Parks and McPartlin's (1971) experience, it is clearly the surgeon's duty to offer to any patient, who has been rendered incontinent by operative or accidental division of the sphincters, the possibility of operative repair. No doubt some will be put off by the prospect of a colostomy—however temporary—but probably most of them will be anxious to avail themselves of this reasonable chance of having their continence restored.

Alternative Procedures

In view of the difficulty usually experienced in the past in securing a successful late suture of divided

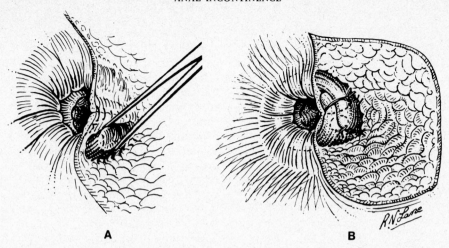

Fig. 237. Suture of sphincters. (A) Definition of muscle by dividing fibrous tissue connections with ischiorectal fat. (B) Suture of sphincters with fine stainless steel wire with slight overlap if possible. (*From Parks and McPartlin 1971*)

sphincters—and also to deal with the more numerous patients whose incontinence was due, not to any injury of the sphincter apparatus, but to an idiopathic laxity of the anal musculature and a resulting patulousness of the anal canal—various alternative forms of surgical treatment have been suggested:

POSTERIOR SPHINCTEROPLASTY AND SUTURE OF PUBORECTALES

A sphincter-pleating operation was practised by Lockhart-Mummery (1934) and Blaisdell (1940), in which a semicircular or curved incision was made behind or in front of the anus with its base on the anal verge, and a flap of skin and subcutaneous tissue was then dissected up towards the anal canal, exposing the posterior or anterior extremity of the sphincter ellipse. Three or four sutures, preferably of non-absorbable material, were then inserted to approximate the two limbs of the ellipse and narrow the anus till it fitted snugly round the index finger inserted into the anal orifice. Thereafter the skin was closed by suture.

A more satisfactory repair of this kind is that devised by Parks (1971), because it includes also suture of the limbs of the puborectalis sling behind the rectum, thus accentuating the forward angulation of the anorectal junction which is often somewhat flattened in such cases. The operation is conducted through a posterior curved incision (Fig. 238A). The plane between the internal and external sphincters is opened up (Fig. 238B), and the anal canal is lifted forward with its surround of internal sphincter away from the external sphincter behind and at the sides up to and beyond the level of the puborectales (Fig. 238C). The dissection is continued upwards till the layer of perirectal fat on the back of the rectum is clearly exposed. The limbs of the puborectalis sling are then opposed by a series of interrupted sutures of 40 SWG wire. Finally the external sphincter is similarly repaired and the flap of skin is sutured back with fine silk stitches. The skin wound is sealed with a plastic spray and systemic antibiotics are administered. The bowels are confined for three or four days.

It is important to emphasize that this type of repair can be performed in patients after they have had a rectopexy, say, by the Ivalon sponge method, if incontinence persists, but Parks (1971) does not recommend it for elderly patients, who unfortunately represent the majority with incontinence.

STIMULATION OF ANAL SPHINCTER TONE BY ELECTRONIC IMPLANT OR ANAL PLUG

The method of trying to restore sphincter tone by an electronic implant (Caldwell 1965) or an anal plug (Hopkinson and Lightwood 1966) was initially hailed with a good deal of enthusiasm, but I have been bitterly disappointed with its results in my patients, and a report by Duthie (1971) has been rather discouraging (see p. 234).

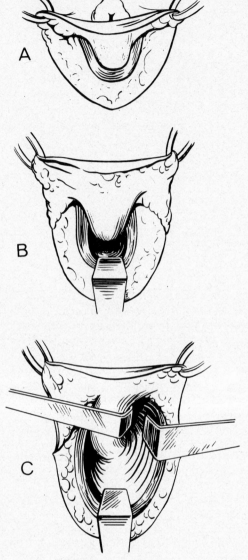

Fig. 238. Parks' posterior sphincteroplasty and suture of puborectales. (*From Parks 1971*)

OPERATIONS TO SUPPLEMENT THE SPHINCTER WITH MUSCLE GRAFTS OR FASCIAL SLINGS

Chetwood (1903) devised an operation in which the lower borders of both gluteus maximus muscles were exposed and freed as muscle strips except for their sacrococcygeal attachment. The two bands of muscle were then crossed just behind the anus and taken forward on either side of the anal canal to meet anteriorly where they were sutured together. Then Pickrell et al. (1952) and von Rappert (1952) developed operations on the same principle but using the gracilis muscle or adductor longus muscle, still attached by one end to the pubis, to encircle the anus and provide a substitute sphincter, and Mann (1970) has also had success with this technique. (See also p. 275 for discussion of use of gracilis sling operation in children after correction of imperforate anus.) State and Katz (1955) have described an alternative method using the superficial transverse perineal muscles, divided at their lateral ends and turned backwards to surround the anus.

Wreden (1929) and Stone (1929) have practised methods in which two slings of fascia lata or silk were passed between the lower borders of the gluteus maximus muscles in front of and behind the anus respectively. The tension in the slings was so adjusted that when the glutei were contracted the anus was firmly compressed between them.

I can claim no personal experience of these plastic operations, and have always been very sceptical—perhaps wrongly—of their value. I strongly suspect that any benefit derived from muscle grafting or fascial sling operations may have been due not to active compression of the anus, but rather to the formation of scar tissue, which subsequently contracted narrowing the orifice. It is a great deal simpler to secure such narrowing by the Thiersch method of perianal suturing with wire or nylon.

THIERSCH'S OPERATION

This operation was strongly recommended by Gabriel (1948) particularly for the elderly patient with incontinence associated with great laxity of the sphincters and some degree of mucosal prolapse. The technique is fully described in Chapter 10 (see p. 249). I have used it a few times and think that it is occasionally of benefit. Though it certainly does not restore normal continence, it seems to lessen the discharge of mucus and prolapse of the mucosa. (Distinctly better control has been claimed by Stanley et al. (1969) in experimental work in sheep with an operation involving implanting a surround of silicone rubber, covered with nylon velour, in the perianal tissues, and then placing an inflated balloon in the lower rectum, to act as a ball-valve. The method has not yet apparently been used in clinical practice.)

Colostomy with or without Rectal Excision

This is the final resort, when everything else has failed. But most patients with complete incontinence learn to regulate their bowel actions by attention to diet etc., in the same way as does a colostomy patient, and prefer not to have an abdominal anus. However, a few are so inconvenienced that they are prepared to accept a colostomy. This may take the form of either a loop colostomy or a divided colostomy in the upper sigmoid. The latter is preferable in that there is no possibility of subsequent trouble from recession of a spur or of stenosis, if the proximal active end is sutured to the skin. A moot question is whether the rectum should be left or removed. Removal of it undoubtedly adds to the risks of the operation, but if it is retained it often causes a good deal of trouble from leakage of mucus through the patulous anus, particularly if there is much prolapse of mucosa.

REFERENCES

BACON, H. E. (1949) *Anus, Rectum, and Sigmoid Colon*, 3rd ed. Philadelphia: Lippincott.

BENNETT, R. C. (1962) A review of the results of orthodox treatment for anal fistulae. *Proc. R. Soc. Med., 55*, 756.

—— BULS, J., KENNEDY, J. T. and HUGHES, E. S. R. (1973) The physiologic status of the anorectum after pull-through operations. *Surgery Gynec. Obstet., 136*, 907.

—— FRIEDMAN, M. H. and GOLIGHER, J. C. (1963) Late results of haemorrhoidectomy by ligature and excision. *Br. med. J., 2*, 216.

—— HUGHES, E. S. R. and CUTHBERTSON, A. M. (1972) Long-term review of function following pull-through operations of the rectum. *Br. J. Surg., 59*, 723.

BLAISDELL, P. C. (1940) Repair of the incontinent sphincter ani. *Surgery Gynec. Obstet., 70*, 692.

CALDWELL, K. P. (1965) A new treatment of rectal prolapse. *Proc. R. Soc. Med., 58*, 792.

CHETWOOD (1903) Quoted by Tuttle, J. P. (1903) In *Diseases of the Anus, Rectum and Pelvic Colon*, New York: Appleton.

DEVINE, J. and WEBB, R. (1951) Resection of the rectal mucosa, colectomy and anal ileostomy with normal continence. *Surgery Gynec. Obstet., 92*, 437.

DUTHIE, H. L. (1971) Rectal prolapse. In *Modern Trends in Surgery*, ed. W. T. Irvine, vol. 3. London: Butterworth.

GABRIEL, W. B. (1948) *Principles and Practice of Rectal Surgery*, 3rd ed. London: H. K. Lewis.

GOLIGHER, J. C. (1951) Functional results after sphincter-saving resections of the rectum. *Ann. R. Coll. Surg. Engl., 8*, 421.

—— (1958) Sphincter preservation in the radical treatment of rectal carcinoma. *Ann. R. Coll. Surg. Engl., 22*, 311.

—— DUTHIE, H. L., DE DOMBAL, F. T. and WATTS, J. M. (1965) Abdomino-anal pull-through excision for carcinoma of the middle third of the rectum: a comparison with low anterior resection. *Br. J. Surg., 52*, 323.

—— GRAHAM, N. G., CLARK, C. G., DE DOMBAL, F. T. and GILES, G. (1969) The value of stretching the anal sphincter in the relief of post-haemorrhoidectomy pain. *Br. J. Surg., 56*, 859.

—— and HUGHES, E. S. R. (1951) Sensibility of the rectum and colon: its role in the mechanism of anal continence. *Lancet, 1*, 543.

HOPKINSON, B. R. and LIGHTWOOD, R. (1966) Electrical treatment of anal incontinence. *Lancet, 1*, 297.

LANE, R. H. S. and PARKS, A. G. (1977) Function of the anal sphincters following colo-anal anstomosis. *Br. J. Surg., 64*, 596.

LOCALIO, S. A. (1975) Personal communication.

—— ENG, K., GOUGE, T. H. and RANSOME, J. H. C. (1978) Abdomino-sacral resection: 10 years experience. *Ann. Surg., 188*, 745.

LOCKHART-MUMMERY, J. P. (1934) *Diseases of the Rectum and Colon*, 2nd ed. London:Baillière.

MANN, A. (1970) Gracilis anoplasty: report of a successful case. *Aust. N.Z.J. Surg., 39*, 405.

MARTIN, L. W., LECOULTRE, C. and SCHUBERT, W. K. (1977) Colectomy, mucosal proctectomy and ileo-anal anastomoses for ulcerative colitis. *Ann. Surg., 186*, 477.

MASON, A. Y. (1977) Transsphincteric surgery for low rectal cancer. In: *Surgical Techniques Illustrated*, ed. R. Malt and F. Robinson, vol. 2, no. 2, p. 71. Boston: Little Brown.

PARKS, A. G. (1971) Anorectal disorders. *Med. Ann.*, 15.

—— and McPARTLIN, J. F. (1971) Late repair of injuries of the anal sphincter. *Proc. R. Soc. Med., 64*, 1187.

—— and NICHOLLS, R. J. (1978) Proctocolectomy without ileostomy for ulcerative colitis. *Br. med. J., 2.*, 85.

PICKRELL, K. L., BROADBENT, T. R., MASTERS, F. W. and METZGER, J. T. (1952) Construction of a rectal sphincter and restoration of anal continence by transplanting the gracilis muscle. *Ann. Surg., 135*, 853.

VON RAPPERT, E. (1952) Plastischer Ersatz des Musculus Sphincter Ani. *Zentbl. Chir., 77*, 579.

RAVITCH, M. (1948) Anal ileostomy with sphincter preservation in patients requiring total colectomy for benign conditions. *Surgery, St Louis, 24*, 170.

SOAVE, F. (1964) Hirschsprung's disease: a new surgical technique. *Archs Dis. Childh., 39*, 116.

STANLEY, T. H., KESSLER, T. R., WISEMAN, L. A. R. and BLUMLE, A. B. (1969) Artificial control of the anal colostomy in sheep. *J. surg. Res., 9*, 223.

STATE, D. and KATZ, A. (1955) The use of superficial transverse perineal muscles in the treatment of post-surgical anal incontinence. *Ann. Surg., 142*, 262.

STEPHENS, F. D. and SMITH, E. D. (1971) *Ano-rectal Malformations in Children*. Chicago: Year Book Medical Publishers.

STONE, H. B. (1929) Plastic operation for anal incompetence. *Archs Surg., Chicago, 18*, 845.

WALLS, E. W. (1959) Recent observations on the anatomy of the anal canal. *Proc. R. Soc. Med.*, Suppl. 52, 85.

WAUGH, J. M., MILLER, E. M. and KURZWEG, F. T. (1954) Abdominoperineal resection with sphincter preservation for carcinoma of the midrectum. *Archs Surg., Chicago, 68,* 469.

WHITEHEAD, W. (1887) Three hundred consecutive cases of haemorrhoids cured by excision. *Br. med. J., i,* 449.

WINCKLER, G. (1958) Remarques sur la morphologie et l'innervation du muscle releveur d l'anus. *Archs Anat. Histol. Embryol., Strasbourg, 41,* 77.

WREDEN, R. R. (1929) A method of reconstructing a voluntary sphincter ani. *Archs Surg., Chicago, 18,* 841.

14

Benign Polyps with Particular Reference to Adenoma and Papilloma of the Colon, Rectum and Anus

---

DEFINITION AND CLASSIFICATION

The term polyp is derived from the Greek words *poly* (= many) and *pous* (= foot), and means literally 'with many feet'. However it has come to be applied to a tumour or swelling arising from a mucosal surface by a *single* pedicle or stalk. Indeed even non-pedunculated or sessile swellings projecting from a mucosa are now accepted under the same title.

Strictly speaking the word gives no indication whatsoever of the intimate structure of the swelling, though it is often used by clinicians and even pathologists as a synonym for adenomatous polyp. So deeply ingrained is this habit of equating intestinal polyps with adenomas, that non-adenomatous or inflammatory polyps, such as occur in ulcerative colitis, are frequently referred to as 'pseudo-polyps'—a bastard expression if there ever was one! Adenoma is unquestionably a common variety of intestinal polyp—perhaps the commonest—but there are many other forms which should be borne in mind. It may be a good plan therefore to begin by classifying benign polypoid lesions of the colon and rectum. (It should also be emphasized that malignant tumours may likewise present in the form of polyps, see p. 379).

A comprehensive classification of benign polyps is provided below. In this chapter we shall consider only a few of the common lesions; the remainder are described in other parts of the book.

CLASSIFICATION OF BENIGN POLYPOID LESIONS OF COLON AND RECTUM

A. NEOPLASMS

Epithelial
Adenoma, including familial polyposis (pp. 325, 359)
Villous papilloma (p. 325)
Other
Leiomyoma (p. 679)
Lipoma (p. 678)
Neurofibroma (p. 681)
Haemangioma (p. 680)

B. HAMARTOMAS

Juvenile polyp (p. 322)
Polyps of Peutz–Jeghers syndrome (p. 323)

C. INFLAMMATORY

Ulcerative colitis (p. 717)
Segmental colitis (p. 699)
Crohn's disease (p. 829)
Dysenteries (p. 865)
Diverticulitis (p. 882)
Benign lymphoma (p. 678)

D. UNCLASSIFIED

'Hyperplastic' or 'metaplastic' mucosal polyps (p. 324)
Pneumatosis cystoides intestinalis (p. 930)
Hypertrophied anal papillae (p. 131)

JUVENILE POLYPS

The commonest type of polyp of the large bowel occurring in infants and children is the juvenile polyp. As Horrilleno et al. (1957), Knox et al. (1960), and Morson (1962a) have pointed out, it is a distinct pathological entity, easily distinguished histologically from other polypoid lesions of the colon.

Pathology

Juvenile polyps are invariably rounded or oval with a smooth surface which contrasts with the finely papillary or granular surface of an adenomatous polyp (Fig. 239). There is a slender stalk covered with normal colonic mucosa which is continuous with the adjacent lining of the colon; as it extends on to the body of the polyp the epithelium becomes replaced by granulation tissue. The polyp itself is composed of cellular vascular tissue, heavily infiltrated with acute and chronic inflammatory cells. In this tissue there are characteristic cystic spaces, vary-ing in size and lined by columnar mucus-secreting epithelial cells.

These polyps are regarded by pathologists not as tumours but as hamartomas—non-neoplastic errors of tissue development characterized by an abnormal mixture of tissue indigenous to the part (Willis 1958). A hamartoma is not necessarily congenital in the sense of existing prior to birth; on the contrary it may appear at any age, although it is commoner in younger patients.

Incidence

In a series of 43 patients with juvenile polyps reported by Knox et al. (1960) the ages ranged from 22 months to 20 years (mean $6\frac{1}{2}$ years), with some 80% of the patients aged less than 10 years; 27 were males and 16 females. Most of the polyps were situated in the rectum or rectosigmoid (Fig. 240) and were palpable on rectal examination in 44% and accessible to palpation or sigmoidoscopy in 71%. The lesion was single in 70% of the cases and multiple in 30%, the largest number of polyps pre-

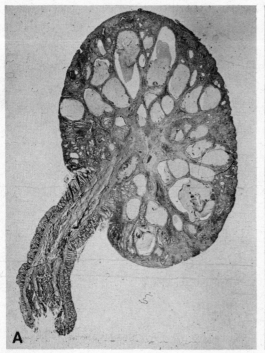
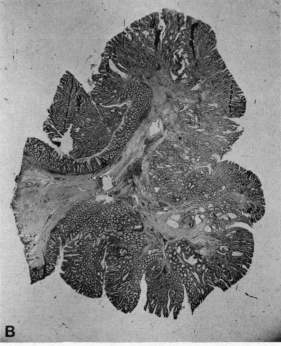

Fig. 239. Comparison of juvenile polyp and adenomatous polyp of colon. (A) Juvenile polyp. Note continuous smooth surface and presence of cystic spaces. (Haematoxylin and eosin. Original magnification ×8.) (B) Adenomatous polyp. The surface is finely papillary and the stroma is arborescent, delicate, and not abudant. (Haematoxylin and eosin. Original magnification ×10.) (*From Knox et al. 1960*)

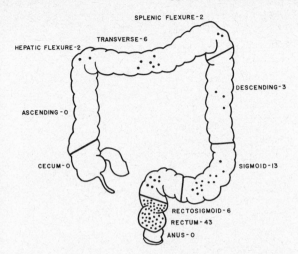

SPLENIC FLEXURE-2

TRANSVERSE-6

HEPATIC FLEXURE-2

DESCENDING-3

ASCENDING-0

CECUM-0

SIGMOID-13

RECTOSIGMOID-6
RECTUM-43
ANUS-0

Fig. 240. Distribution of 75 juvenile polyps in 43 children at St Luke's Hospital, New York City. (*From Knox et al. 1960*)

sent in an individual patient being nine. In no case were polyps located solely in the colon beyond the reach of the sigmoidoscope. Later reports by McColl et al. (1964), Veale et al. (1966) and Smilow et al. (1966) suggest that there is a familial tendency to develop juvenile polyposis.

Symptomatology

Juvenile polyps can cause three groups of symptoms: (*a*) those due to descent of the polyp itself (prolapse of the lesion through the anus, rectal mucosal prolapse, colonic intussusception); (*b*) those due to torsion of the pedicle (bleeding, auto-amputation with extrusion in the faeces); and (*c*) those attributable to inflammation or surface trauma (bleeding).

Prognosis and Treatment

Horrilleno et al. (1957), Cabrera and Lega (1960) and Knox et al. (1960) emphasize that follow-up studies on their own cases and a careful review of the literature *have failed to reveal any clear evidence that juvenile polyps are premalignant.* Lesions accessible to palpation or sigmoidoscopy should be removed either by breaking them off with the finger or by snaring, partly to prevent them prolapsing through the anus or causing other symptoms, and partly to provide a precise histological diagnosis. More proximally located polyps may safely be left if

biopsy of rectal or distal sigmoid lesions shows that they are juvenile polyps, but if they are unassociated with lesions within reach of sigmoidoscopic biopsy, colonoscopy and removal by polypectomy might be necessary to establish their exact nature.

Recurrence of juvenile polyps at a different site in the large intestine is by no means uncommon. Thus Horrilleno et al. (1957) have observed 10 such recurrences in their series of 53 cases followed up for 10 weeks to 10 years, and Knox et al. (1960) report three recurrences in 24 patients traced for periods up to 14 years. The recurrences were of the same histological structure as the original lesion and not malignant.

PEUTZ–JEGHERS SYNDROME

In this very rare disease, associated with the names of Peutz (1921) and Jeghers (1944), polyposis of the alimentary tract occurs in conjunction with pigmented spots in the skin and buccal mucosa. The condition shows a high familial incidence, but sporadic cases have been described (Neely and Gillespie 1967). The pigmentation has a fairly constant distribution and occurs as small irregular flecks of brown to bluish discoloration of the skin and mucous membrane of the lips, especially the lower lip, on the hard and soft palate and oral mucosa (but not on the tongue) and on the skin of the fingers and toes. The polyps are found more frequently in the small bowel, particularly the jejunum, and less often in the stomach and large intestine. Some patients have a solitary polyp or only a few polyps; more usually there are large numbers of polyps throughout the small gut, stomach and large bowel.

Macroscopically the polyps range from sessile nodules a few millimetres across to pedunculated tumours as much as 5 cm in diameter, and do not differ significantly in their gross appearances from adenomatous polyps of the large intestine. But microscopically they reveal, not the structure of adenomata, but that of malformation or hamartoma (Bartholomew et al. 1957; Rintala 1959; Morson 1962a). This applies equally to polyps in the colon and to those in the small intestine. The essential abnormality appears to be a malformation of the muscularis mucosae, which provides a tree-like structure bearing the epithelial elements. The latter, though abnormally disposed, show normally differentiated goblet cells with no evidence of hyperplasia (Fig. 241).

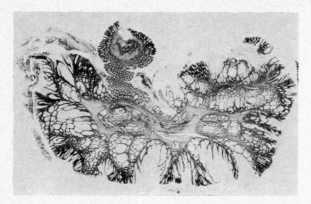

Fig. 241. A colonic polyp of Peutz–Jeghers syndrome showing the branching smooth muscle abnormality. (Dr B. C. Morson's case.) (Original magnification ×10)

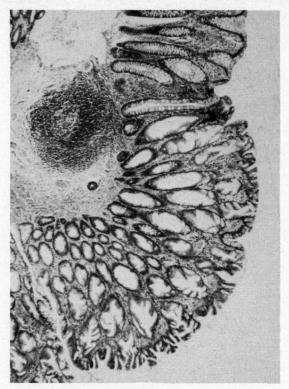

Fig. 242. Enlargement of metaplastic nodule showing cystic dilatation of the tubules, scalloping of the columnar epithelium, and the tiny papillary projections at the surface contrasted with the adjacent epithelium. (Dr B. C. Morson's case.) (Original magnification × 150)

It is of the utmost practical importance to distinguish between polyps of Peutz–Jeghers syndrome occurring in either small or large bowel, and those of familial polyposis of the colon and rectum. The latter are true adenomas and are well known to be associated with a strong tendency to development of malignant disease in the large intestine—though whether in the adenomas themselves or in the intervening mucosa is open to dispute (see p. 360). There has been much dispute as to whether the polyps of Peutz–Jeghers syndrome carry any malignant potential. Dormandy (1957), Bartholomew and Dahlin (1958), Rintala (1959) and Morson (1962a) considered that the evidence for malignant transformation in most of the reported instances of cancerous change was unconvincing. However, Bussey (1970) has collected from the literature and from his own experience 14 cases of genuine malignancy arising in association with this syndrome, the growth being situated in the stomach in five, in the pyloroduodenal junction in two, in the duodenum in five, in the jejunum in one and in the ileum in one. All the patients were below the age of 40 years. It seems, therefore, that Peutz–Jeghers syndrome is associated with an increased liability to cancer in the upper gastrointestinal tract at an early age.

The polyps are present during childhood and from this time onwards repeated complications due to their presence may occur. Intussusception and bleeding are the commonest of these occurrences, but rectal prolapse is also seen. The history of these patients often includes repeated episodes of acute upper abdominal pain which have remitted in two or three days, and it seems probable that these have been caused by intestinal invaginations which have undergone spontaneous reduction. More serious obstructive incidents may occur necessitating operative intervention. This should be confined to dealing with the actual obstruction, though this may necessitate a local resection. Because of the widespread nature of the disease radical surgical treatment to obviate further symptoms is out of the question and, even if the condition is to some extent precancerous, there is clearly no possibility of practising extensive excision of bowel as a prophylactic measure against the development of malignant disease.

METAPLASTIC OR HYPERPLASTIC MUCOSAL POLYPS

These terms are used to describe a type of polyp only recently recognized to be distinct from adenomatous and other forms of polyp (Morson 1962a; Arthur 1962). It is usually multiple and occurs as minute plaque-like excrescences, 1–2 mm in diameter as a rule, seldom more than 5 mm. These are seen most commonly in the rectal mucosa, less often in the mucosa of the colon. They are found at all ages and apparently are as likely to be present in individuals with an otherwise normal large bowel as in those harbouring a carcinoma of the rectum or colon.

Microscopically metaplastic polyps have a structure that can be clearly differentiated from that of adenomas according to Morson (1962a) (Fig. 242). There is lengthening of the mucosal tubules with a tendency to cystic dilatation. The lining epithelium loses its regular columnar and goblet-cell pattern and appears serrated, due to patchy flattening of its cells. The proportion of goblet cells is diminished and the lamina propria sometimes shows an increased number of plasma cells and lymphocytes. There may be fragmentation of the muscularis mucosae, some of the fibres extending into the lamina propria towards the mucosal surface.

Though minute polyps of 2 or 3 mm may occasionally be very small adenomas or lymphomas, it is possible that the great majority of polyps of this size fall into the category of metaplastic polyps. The term 'metaplastic' in this connection is used merely to indicate a difference in appearances from that of normal mucosa. So far as is known these polyps are unrelated to adenomas or to intestinal cancer, and we are quite ignorant of their pathogenesis. Presumably in the past, in the compilation of data on intestinal polyps, these tiny polyps have either been considered as very small adenomas or completely disregarded because of their minute size.

A very different account of the histopathological features of minute polyps of the large intestine is given by Pagtalunan et al. (1965), perhaps because their material was from biopsies and not autopsies. They studied 1000 polyps under 5 mm in diameter at the Mayo Clinic and do not seem to have encountered—or at least recognized—'metaplastic' lesions of the kind described by Morson (1962a) and Arthur (1962). Instead they found that 86·1% of the polyps were adenomas, and 13·9% a mixture of various pathological entities—hypertrophic tags of normal mucosa, inflammatory polyps, lymphoid nodules, hamartomas, leiomyomas, a carcinoid and a lipoma. The adenomatous polyps were further subdivided into different grades: 30·9% with minimal hyperplasia but no cellular atypism; 26% with mild hyperplasia and epithelial atypism; 23·4% with moderate hyperplasia and epithelial atypia; 5·2% with severe hyperplasia and epithelial atypia; and 0·6% with carcinoma-in-situ.

ADENOMA AND VILLOUS PAPILLOMA OF THE COLON AND RECTUM

Benign adenomas and papillomas of the rectum and colon may cause symptoms and necessitate treatment in their own right as it were, but undoubtedly the chief significance of these tumours lies in their association with the development of malignant disease. It seems probable that they play an important part in the pathogenesis of carcinoma of the large intestine, though this hitherto widely accepted belief has recently been the subject of bitter controversy.

Though it has been customary to describe adenomas and villous papillomas as if there were always clearly distinct from one another, it has long been known that occasionally a polyp may exhibit histological features of both lesions. A new classification of benign epithelial tumours of the intestine, incorporating such mixed tumours, has been proposed by Morson and Sobin (1976) for the World Health Organization. However, in this text, which is written primarily for surgeons rather than pathologists, the old terminology will continue to be used, because much of the information available in the literature on the clinical features, behaviour and treatment of these conditions has been documented in relation to these terms.

Pathology

GROSS FEATURES

These are often best appreciated when the tumour is examined clinically through the sigmoidoscope for the natural colouring is then preserved.

An *adenoma* may present several appearances. In its smallest form it is a tiny nodule in the mucous membrane about the size of a millet-seed or split pea, and of exactly the same colour as the surrounding mucosa. At its biggest an adenoma may reach the dimensions of a cherry, or very exceptionally that of a small plum, but most of them are in between these two extremes. Even the largest adenoma may be sessile, but with enlargement there is apparently an increasing tendency to acquire a pedicle. The latter may be 1–3 cm long or even

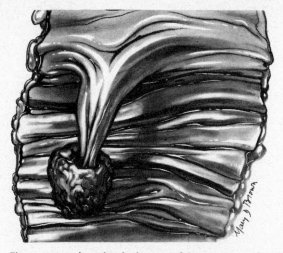

Fig. 243. A pedunculated adenoma of the rectosigmoid seen in the upper part of an anterior resection specimen, removed for a coincident rectal cancer not shown here.

longer; it is composed of normal mucosa, has a broad base and narrows distally so that at its junction with the adenoma proper it is somewhat constricted, often markedly, so as to give a mushroom-like appearance (Fig. 243, Plate IId and e). The adenoma itself is smooth or slightly lobulated; its colour in the smaller tumours is usually identical with that of the normal rectal or colonic mucosa, but in better developed adenomata is a darker red and may even have a purple tinge. On palpation simple adenomata feel soft.

A *villous papilloma* (styled *papillary adenoma* by many American authors) is a soft sessile tumour with a coarsely granular or shaggy surface and ill-defined edges (Figs 244, 245). Often it extends over a considerable area of the bowel mucosa and may be completely circumferential. Usually it is fairly closely applied to the intestinal wall, but sometimes it projects into the lumen as a big soft fleshly

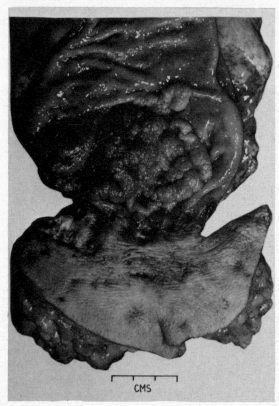

Fig. 244. Villous papilloma of the rectum removed by combined abdominoperineal excision. Histological section revealed a small focus of carcinoma.

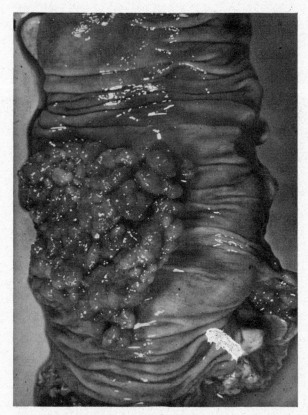

Fig. 245. Large villous papilloma of the upper rectum excised by anterior resection. Histological examination showed it to be wholly benign.

mass. Its colour is generally darker than that of the normal mucosa and it has often a somewhat bluish hue (Plate IIc).

HISTOLOGICAL APPEARANCES

The microscopic anatomy of an adenoma is quite different from that of a papilloma. An *adenoma* is composed essentially of masses of closely packed gland tubules of intestinal mucosa and nourished by a central connective tissue core drawn up from the submucosa. The epithelium covering the growth and lining the glands may be very similar to that of the normal rectum and colon or may show varying degrees of incomplete differentiation. The latter is revealed by the darker staining of the cell nuclei, by diminution or absence of mucus in the protoplasm, by the occurrence of mitotic figures, and by the arrangement of the cells not in a single layer lining the tubules but in several layers or in masses projecting into the lumen of the tubules and into the connective tissue core. In a more advanced stage of de-differentiation the tubular arrangement may be completely lost, the cells simply being grouped in piles without any attempt at gland formation. The process of de-differentiation in an adenoma is often confined to one or more foci whilst the rest of the tumour is composed of well-formed gland tubules of normal appearance (Fig. 246).

Potet and Soullard (1971), Eklund and Lindström (1974) and Kozuka (1975) have sought to classify adenomatous polyps into several categories according to the degree of differentiation and other histological features, culminating in so-called carcinoma-in-situ or even invasive carcinoma. Kozuka (1975) has paid attention particularly to the degree of epithelial pseudostratification and glandular branching in formulating five grades of premalignancy in adenomatous polyps. These three groups of workers have further examined the apparent influence of various other factors on the relative frequency of the different categories of polyp in large series of cases which they have studied. Eklund and Lindström (1974) found that the differentiation was on the average poorer the nearer the polyp lay in the large intestine to the anus or to an existing frank carcinoma; they also claimed that in general polyps tended to be less well differentiated in men than in women, but Potet and Soullard (1971) found the

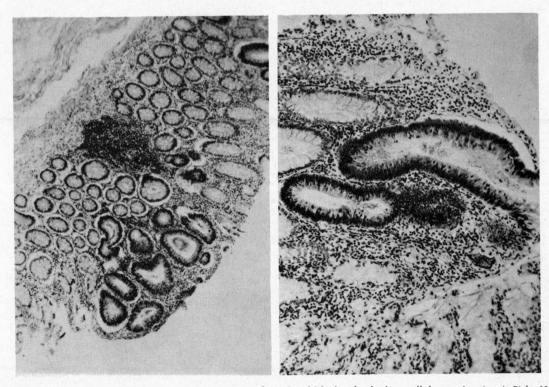

Fig. 246. *Left*, Adenoma of the colon containing tumour focus in which the glands show cellular atypism (×20). *Right*, Higher power view of the focus (×20). (*From Willis 1948*)

reverse to be the case. According to Kozuka et al. (1975) the average ages of patients increased with the advance of atypism in their polyps.

Microscopically a *villous papilloma*, as its name implies, consists of a central connective tissue core bearing numerous delicate frond-like branches or villi which are covered usually by a single layer of columnar epithelial cells. The latter may approximate in appearance to normal large intestinal epithelium and contain a variable amount of mucus, or they may be more active as indicated by their darker staining, by the occurrence of mitoses, and by stratification in their arrangement. As with adenomas de-differentiation is apt to affect a papilloma in a patchy or focal fashion.

Why two different forms of adenoma—villous and non-villous—should occur in the large intestine is not known. Dukes (1947) suggested that villous papillomas arise from the more superficial parts of the crypts of Lieberkühn of the normal colonic and rectal mucosa, whilst ordinary adenomas originate from cells at the bottom of the crypts. Other pathologists such as Helwig (1947) attribute the differing structure not to differences in the site of origin in the mucosa but to variations in growth potential.

Incidence

In Clinical Cases

Much useful information on many aspects of the incidence of these tumours, as seen in surgical practice, has been provided by Grinnell and Lane (1958). They surveyed the clinical records and pathological data on all adenomatous polyps and villous papillomas submitted to the laboratory of surgical pathology of the Presbyterian Hospital, New York, from 1928 to 1955 inclusive. Their study included adenomas and papillomas, the removal of which was the primary concern of the surgeon, and also such growths removed incidentally in a resection done for a separate coexisting carcinoma. Excluded from the the series were polyps removed from infants and young children, and diffuse familial polyposis. Altogether 1856 tumours were analysed in 1335 patients, and the following points emerged.

RELATIVE FREQUENCY OF ADENOMAS AND VILLOUS PAPILLOMAS

In most instances the gross and microscopic appearances enabled a clear distinction to be made between adenomatous polyps and villous papillomas, but very occasionally a tumour presented histological features of both lesions. In mixed cases of this kind the growth was apparently classified according to the predominant histological picture. Altogether 88·4% of the tumours were considered to be adenomas and 11·6% villous papillomas. It is interesting to note for comparison that an almost identical proportion—namely 12·2%—of all the benign intestinal polyps observed by Sunderland and Binkley (1948) were considered by them to be villous papillomas.

SIZE OF GROWTHS

The average size of adenomatous polyps was 1·2 cm in diameter, the minimum 2 mm and the maximum 7 cm. The corresponding figures for villous papillomas were: average 3·7 cm, minimum 5 mm maximum 9 cm, the tumours not infrequently being annular or very widespread on the bowel wall.

SESSILE OR PEDUNCULATED

68% of the adenomatous polyps were pedunculated, 32% sessile, the latter usually being lesions less than 1 cm in diameter. Pedunculated forms of villous papilloma also occurred but more than 90% of these growths were sessile.

MULTIPLICITY

Somewhat surprisingly only 26% of the cases of adenomatous polyp had multiple tumours. In the 311 cases with a separate coexisting carcinoma, 34% had multiple polyps, whilst in only 17% of the cases without associated carcinomas were the polyps multiple.

The villous papillomas were *almost invariably solitary*, and only 8 of the 216 patients with these lesions had multiple papillomas—five had two tumours and three had three, distributed equally in the rectum, sigmoid and caecum/ascending colon. It is interesting to note that some 30% of these 216 cases also had associated adenomatous polyps, and apparently about 10% had concomitant cancers of the colon or rectum.

SITE

The relative frequencies of the two forms of tumour in different segments of the large bowel is shown in Table 14 which also gives for comparison the site incidence of 2152 cases of carcinoma of the large intestine at the Presbyterian Hospital between 1916

TABLE 14. *Site of Adenomas, Villous Papillomas and Carcinomas of the Colon and Rectum at the Presbyterian Hospital, New York*

Site	Adenomatous polyps (%, n = 1640)	Villous papillomas (%, n = 216)	Carcinomas (%, n = 2152)
Caecum	1·0	4·2	5·1
Ascending colon	4·6	4·2	6·3
Hepatic flexure	0·8	1·4	2·0
Proximal transverse colon	3·1	1·4	3·9
Distal transverse colon	4·3	0·9	4·9
Splenic flexure	1·6	1·8	2·9
Descending colon	5·2	1·8	4·9
Sigmoid colon	51·0 } 79·4	30·5 } 84·1	26·7 } 70·0
Rectum	28·4	53·6	43·3

After Grinnell and Lane (1958).

and 1950. Though there are variations in the distribution of these three types of tumour in the large bowel it is notable that the great majority of all the lesions occurred in the rectum and sigmoid. Another point that emerges from this table is that, contrary to the clinical impression of very many surgeons, villous papillomas are not confined entirely to the rectum and sigmoid colon, but are found occasionally in other parts, especially the caecum and ascending colon.

AGE AND SEX OF PATIENTS

The ages of patients with adenomatous polyps, excluding those with separate coexisting cancers of the bowel, ranged from 13 to 87 years and averaged 61·9 years. The average age of patients with villous papillomas was 62·3 years, the range from 32 to 86 years.

Of the patients with adenomatous polyps 59% were males and 41% females; of those with villous papillomas 45% were males and 55% females.

FREQUENCY OF INVASIVE CANCER IN THE TUMOURS

Grinnell and Lane (1958) comment on the uncertainty as to the significance in adenomas and papillomas of what has been variously termed 'areas of atypism', 'focal carcinoma', 'carcinoma-in-situ' and 'intramucosal cancer' (Fig. 247A). They have therefore preferred to reserve the designation 'cancer' for cases in which there has been clear evidence of *invasion of the muscularis mucosae* (Fig. 247B).

Applying this criterion they found that the incidence of cancer in the whole group of 1856 lesions was 6·3%. In adenomatous polyps it

averaged 2·9%, whilst in villous papillomas it was 31·9%. There was a striking correlation between the size of adenomatous polyps and the frequency with which they contained areas of cancer—malignant changes were evident in 0·6% of those with a diameter less than 0·6 cm; in 4·7% of those with diameters between 1 and 1·9 cm; in 9·1% of those

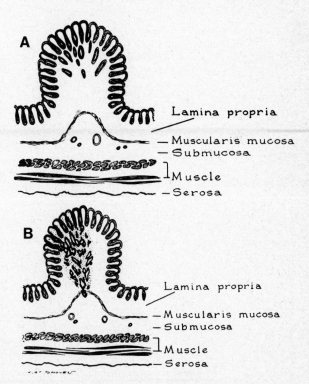

Fig. 247. Apparently benign adenomata containing foci of carcinoma. (A) Carcinoma-in-situ. (B) Invasive cancer. (*From Fisher and Turnbull 1952*)

with diameters between 2 and 2·4 cm; and in 13·8% of those 2·5 cm and more in diameter. By contrast, no very close association was evident between the size of villous papillomas and the likelihood of finding cancer in them.

Further evidence as to the truly malignant nature of areas of apparent carcinoma observed in these lesions would be provided by the discovery of metastases in the related lymph glands, but obviously these could only be sought in those cases in which the tumour was treated by segmental resection. 27 cases with carcinomatous areas in adenomatous polyps were subjected to resection; lymph node metastases were observed in only one of these patients (4%). (The tumour in this case was sessile, and the malignant portion had extended almost to the base of the broad pedicle but had not reached the adjacent muscle coat of the bowel wall.) By contrast, there were 15 instances of metastases to the regional nodes in 52 resections of villous papillomas, an incidence of 29%.

FREQUENCY OF SEPARATE COEXISTING CANCERS OF THE BOWEL

The exact case incidence of associated frank carcinoma of the rectum or colon is not given in Grinnell and Lane's (1958) study, but there were 311 carcinomas in the 1119 patients with adenomatous polyps (27·8%) and apparently about 15–20 such growths in the 216 cases with villous papillomas.

IN SYMPTOMLESS INDIVIDUALS SUBJECTED TO ROUTINE PROCTOSIGMOIDOSCOPY AND BARIUM ENEMA EXAMINATION

There have been a number of reports of the results of routine sigmoidoscopic examination for polyps in *symptomless individuals*. Some of the most comprehensive statistics of this kind have come from cancer detection clinics, where a part of the routine examination to which all the symptomless individuals attending are subjected is proctosigmoidoscopy, sometimes supplemented by barium studies. Working in such clinics Miller et al. (1950) found polyps in 6·4% of 7494 persons and Wilson et al. (1955) in 2·9% of 20 847 persons. A particularly detailed report is that of Enquist (1957) from the Detection Center of the University of Minnesota Hospitals. 7608 persons over the age of 45 were examined between 1945 and 1956, a majority of them re-attending again at one or more annual follow-up visits. At the original examination 876

(11·5%) of the patients were found to have one or more polyps in the rectum or colon. In another 586 patients (7·7%) rectal or colonic polyps were found at subsequent examinations, yielding a total of 1462 patients (19·2%) who had rectal or colonic polyps on at least one examination. In 1459 persons a total of 2363 polyps were discovered by proctosigmoidoscopy in the distal 25 cm of large bowel. Another 94 polyps were demonstrated by barium enema at a higher level in the colon in 68 of these patients. The site of maximum incidence was on the posterior wall 13–14 cm from the anus. Nearly half of the 2366 polyps seen on proctosigmoidoscopy were less than 3 mm in diameter (and this may be why the overall incidence of lesions was so much higher in Enquist's cases than in those reported from other detection centres). Only 454 of all the lesions were studied microscopically, usually those of 5 mm or more in diameter; most of them were found to be benign adenomas but 15 showed malignant foci, an incidence of 0·33% of malignancy in the material examined. The incidence of carcinoma was found to increase with the size of the polyp. With smaller polyps of less than 4 mm diameter spontaneous disappearance was common, the lesion being no longer detectable at a subsequent examination.

I never cease to be amazed at the frequency with which American surgeons discover polyps on sigmoidoscopy. My impression is that they are far less common in my patients, but I have no accurate figures to offer in support of this belief. As for the frequency of detection of polyps on barium enema study, it is interesting to note that Welin (1967) of Malmö, using his modification of the double-contrast method of examining the colon, found benign polyps in 2897 or 11·7% of 24 783 patients submitted to this examination—though it is not clear how many of these patients were symptomless.

THE INCIDENCE OF SUBSEQUENT POLYPS AND OF CARCINOMA IN PATIENTS WITH SYMPTOMLESS POLYPS

Rider et al. (1954, 1959) conducted an interesting survey of the incidence of polyps in the large intestine of 9669 patients who during a six-year period underwent proctosigmoidoscopy and radiological studies as part of a routine gastrointestinal examination at the University of Chicago Medical Clinic. 537 (5·5%) were found to harbour one or more adenomatous polyps, which were usually destroyed or removed by sigmoidoscopic diathermy or by laparotomy. A vigorous follow-up programme succeeded in getting 372 of the patients with polyps to attend for at least one re-examination four to nine years after their initial attendance; 153, or 41%, of these were found to have developed new polyps, which compares with an expectation for polyps in the general population of 5·5%. The predisposition to further polyps was more marked in patients who had originally had multiple polyps than in those with only one polyp, the rate of new formation in these two groups being 55·7% and 38·5% respectively.

The incidence of carcinoma of the large intestine in the 9132 patients *without* polyps was 2·1%. The original incidence of carcinomatous polyps in the 537 patients *with* polyps was 5·8%. In addition, 7·2% of the latter patients had an associated carcinoma of the rectum or colon, which means that 13% of the polyp-bearing patients had carcinoma either in a polyp or elsewhere in the large intestine. If the cases with what was regarded as carcinoma-in-situ were added to this figure, the percentage of patients with polyps who showed evidence of malignant disease was 32·2%.

Rider et al.'s (1954, 1959) study thus reaffirms that the presence of an adenomatous polyp in the colon or rectum is an indication of an abnormal large bowel mucosa prone to develop further polyps or carcinoma. Henry et al. (1975) also found an increased tendency to further polyp formation in patients who have had polyps, but claimed— surprisingly and not really convincingly— that the greater predisposition in such patients compared with the ordinary population holds only for four years after the initial polyps were removed.

In Routine Autopsies

Several pathologists have drawn attention to the fact that apparently benign polyps are frequently present at autopsy in the colon and rectum of individuals who during life had no symptoms referable to these lesions. However the estimates of the incidence of this occurrence have varied greatly from author to author, as shown in Table 15. There are perhaps several reasons for these variations. Some of the series of cases examined have included children or coloured patients, both of whom are generally held to develop polyps less often than does an adult white population. Another factor may have been a lack of uniformity as to the smallest size of lesion to be included as a polyp. Several of the authors such as Lawrence (1936) and Helwig (1947) do not quote a minimum size, but some were

between 3 and 6 cm in size. It seems likely from the work of Arthur (1962) that many of the minute polyps in these series may have been of the so-called 'metaplastic' variety (see p. 324).

The exact distribution of the polyps is not given in all these papers, but they appear to have been multiple in over half the cases and to have occurred in all parts of the large bowel, but especially in the sigmoid and rectum. The ages of the patients varied widely but they were mostly older subjects. As will be seen from Table 15 areas of apparent malignant change were observed in a variable proportion of the polyps, but it is not usually clear whether this referred to intramucosal or invasive cancer.

In Operative Specimens of Carcinoma of the Large Intestine

It is well known that in resection specimens of carcinoma of the rectum or colon there are often clusters of satellite polyps in the adjacent bowel (see Fig. 286, p. 382), the incidence being much higher than the 4–10% or so usually observed at routine autopsies in people without carcinomas of the large intestine (Table 15). Thus Stewart (1931) reported finding such polyps in 27% of 71 consecutive cases of carcinoma of the rectum or colon, Willis (1958) in 60% of 40 cases, and Bussey et al. (1967) in 28% of 3381 cases. My own experience is that approximately 30% of our operative specimens of large bowel cancer show satellite polyps. Once again, however, these variations in estimated incidence probably reflect differences in the minimum size of lesion recognized as a polyp for, in examining 34 resection specimens of rectal carcinoma, Arthur (1962) found that 32 contained nodules less than 2 mm in diameter—in 17 there were 15–25 such nodules, and in 15 up to 14. 71% of these lesions were 'metaplastic' polyps, 18% minute adenomas and 10·2% lymph follicles.

Relationship of Benign Adenomas and Villous Papillomas to Cancer

Adenomas

Till the late 1950s it was generally held that adenomas of the large bowel were premalignant lesions. There were several very suggestive pieces of evidence for this belief. (*a*) The distribution of adenomas and carcinomas in the large bowel is

TABLE 15. *Incidence of Polyps in Large Intestine at Autopsy according to Various Authors*

Author	No. of cases examined	Percentage with polyps	Comments
Dukes (1926)	127	9·4	Deaths due to causes other than cancer of bowel
Stewart (1931)	1815	4·19	
Susman (1932)	1100	6	
Lawrence (1936)	7000	2·37 / 0·42	Low incidence possibly because of large numbers of children. White and coloured patients included
Mayo and Schlicke (1942)	100	16	Death due to causes other than cancer of bowel
Atwater and Bargen (1945)	241	69	*Hand lens used to* examine bowel
Swinton and Haug (1947)	1843	7	Large number of cases of carcinoma of the gastrointestinal tract included
Helwig (1947)	1460	9·5	White and coloured patients included
Moore (1960)	119	27	

roughly similar, though with minor variations as pointed out by Berge et al. (1973) and Eklund and Lindström (1974), the maximal incidence being in the rectum and sigmoid colon (p. 376). (However, Spratt et al. (1958) dispute whether there is such a close correlation between the site incidence of these lesions.) (b) Adenomas are often found in association with carcinomas of the rectum and colon (p. 490). (c) Persons with polyps are apparently more likely to produce carcinomas of the large bowel than are other members of the population (p. 330), and patients with polyps in association with a carcinoma of the rectum or colon are twice as likely to develop a subsequent (metachronous) carcinoma after resection as are those who had no polyps at the time of their original operation (Bussey et al. 1967). (d) This tendency (c) is seen *par excellence* in familial polyposis where the risk of subsequent development of carcinoma, often multiple, is formidably high (p. 363). (e) Many pathologists have claimed to be able to demonstrate not infrequently the transition from a benign to a malignant neoplastic process on histological examination of polyps (see below; Dukes 1926; Westhues 1934; Willis 1948; Lockhart-Mummery and Dukes 1952; Fisher and Turnbull 1952; Welch et al. 1952; Dockerty 1958; Morson 1962b, c, 1970; Enterline et al. 1962; Potet

and Soullard 1971; Eklund and Lindström 1974). (f) Some observers have also stated that in a proportion of frank rectal and colonic carcinomas they have been able to recognize an origin from a pre-existing adenomatous polyp—for example in 14% of 827 cases studied by Swinton and Warren (1939).

There can be no gainsaying contentions b, c and d, that people with adenomas of the large bowel appear to be predisposed to the occurrence of intestinal malignant growths, but this could be so without the polyps themselves undergoing malignant change. The ideal way to determine whether the latter event took place would perhaps be to adopt a strictly expectant attitude towards clinically benign polyps and to see what happened to them under regularly repeated sigmoidoscopic reviews. Several isolated instances have been recorded in the literature where a carcinoma was found to arise at a site where a polyp had previously been noted (Jackman 1941; Mayo and Castro 1956; Scarborough 1960; de la Vussière et al. 1965; Smith et al. 1970). More systematic observations of this kind have been reported by Colvert and Brown (1948), who followed up two groups of cases with apparently benign rectal adenomatous polyps, one consisting of 117 patients who had their lesions dealt with in orthodox fashion, and another 43 who refused to have them removed. A careful follow-up during the succeeding five years failed to show that the cases with retained adenomas were any more likely to develop carcinomas than those without. But the number of cases in this enquiry was small so that its significance is doubtful. Further, in studies of this kind, unless a satisfactory biopsy is obtained at the start of conservative treatment of the polyp, the results could be vitiated by inclusion of cases with small polypoid cancers *de novo*.

However, the possibility of following the natural life history of adenomatous polyps has usually been denied by the current policy of removing or destroying them surgically as soon as they are detected. In exchange, as it were, this practice has provided pathologists with a wealth of histological material which, supplemented from other sources, has encouraged intensive histopathological study, resulting in the concept (referred to in *d* and *e* above) that foci of malignant degeneration not uncommonly arise in previously benign adenomatous polyps. This doctrine had acquired almost the character of a religious dogma when its validity was questioned on a number of grounds, not least the histological, by Spratt et al. (1958), who advanced the alternative opinion that adenomas in the colon are either simple from the beginning and remain so, or are carcinomas *ab initio*. Castleman and Krickstein (1962) have given their strong support to this belief and indicate that in their view three histological errors have been responsible for the frequent assumption that a large percentage of adenomatous polyps show malignant change:

The *first* consists of misdiagnosing as adenomas with areas of carcinoma cases of polypoid cancer with no evidence of origin from underlying benign polyps. In such cases it has often been assumed that the carcinoma had completely destroyed the benign elements. Castleman and Krickstein (1962) entirely reject this reasoning and consider it quite unjustifiable to assume that a grossly polypoid carcinoma has arisen from a polyp unless there is histological evidence of benign adenomatous tissue in the lesion. In this connection they emphasize that on careful histological examination of many hundreds of specimens of frank intestinal cancer they—and Spratt et al. (1958) and Enterline et al. (1962)—were unable to discover any unequivocal remnants of adenomatous tissue. Even in 20 carcinomas of the colon, all under 2 cm in diameter, Spratt and Ackerman (1962) could find no evidence of origin from benign adenomatous polyps in any of them.

The *second* error of histological diagnosis castigated by Castleman and Krickstein (1962) is failure to distinguish clearly between adenomas and villous papillomas. As will be mentioned presently (p. 334) the latter tumours, though initially benign, have a strong tendency to undergo malignant change.

The *third* error according to Castleman and Krickstein (1962) lies in misinterpreting the significance of apparent carcinomatous change in adenomatous polyps. They are not prepared to accord any malignant significance whatsoever to foci of 'atypism' of cellular structure and arrangement of areas of 'intramucosal cancer' without penetration of the lamina propria—an opinion that is shared by many other pathologists at the present day. Even in regard to such foci invading the connective-tissue core of the polyp they have some misgivings, for they point out that the presence of glands in the site does not always imply the existence of invasive cancer. As Fisher and Turnbull (1952) have previously emphasized, 'pseudo-invasion' of the core of a polyp can often be demonstrated in the most benign-looking adenoma by sectioning through a twisted stalk.

Castleman and Krickstein (1962) believe that, if a strict vigilance is exercised by the histopathologist against these sources of error, very few instances of genuine carcinomatous change will be encountered in adenomatous polyps. As an illustration of the truth of this remark, they describe the results of a review by them of the histological diagnosis in a much-quoted series of 60 adenomatous polyps with alleged carcinomatous change, originally reported by Welch et al. (1952). Castleman and Krickstein (1962) reclassified these lesions as follows:

Benign adenomatous polyp	33 cases
Benign adenomatous polyp with focus of carcinoma	1 case
Benign villous papilloma	4 cases
Benign villous papillomas with focus of carcinoma	5 cases
Polypoid carcinoma—no adenomatous polyp tissue present	14 cases

Perhaps the crux of the matter is whether, regardless of their classification as carcinoma by the pathologist, atypical foci in adenomatous polyps metastasize, as shown by deposits in the lymph nodes of resected specimens or by subsequent recurrence after simple local excision. Information on this score is somewhat contradictory but indicates that metastases do sometimes occur with invasive foci, but not with carcinoma-in-situ. Thus Enterline et al. (1962) examined 1700 adenomatous polyps of the colon and considered that 61 contained foci of invasive cancer, but in none of the

61 cases submitted to resection were lymph node metastases present, nor could any deaths be proved to have been caused by these lesions on a follow-up of five or more years. Grinnell and Lane (1958), as mentioned on p. 329, discovered lymph node metastases in one of their 27 cases of adenomatous polyp showing invasive cancer treated by resection. Fisher and Turnbull (1952) in a 3–13-year follow-up of 14 cases of adenomatous polyp—seven with 'intramucosal cancer' and seven with 'invasive cancer'—treated by local excision only, found no malignant recurrences in the former group, but three local recurrences of invasive cancer in the latter; however there were no deaths. Lockhart-Mummery and Dukes (1952) followed up 47 cases of adenomatous polyp with malignant change for from 2 to 18 years after treatment by local excision. The 17 who had focal cancer showed no recurrences, but 9 of the 30 with invasive cancer developed recurrence in the rectal wall, and in another three cases *metastases developed in the inguinal or mesorectal glands in the complete absence of any local recurrence* at the former site of the polyp in the bowel. Lockhart-Mummery and Dukes (1952) also mention that in 18 other cases with adenomatous polyps showing invasive cancer and treated by radical excision of the rectum, lymphatic metastases were found in several.

Histochemical Observations on the Polyp–Carcinoma Sequence

Though the biochemical aberrations that result in the transformation of a normal cell into a malignant one are not known, certain differences have been recognized. For example it has been noted that the content of deoxyribonucleic acid (DNA), which is the primary constituent of the chromosomes, is increased, and various enzymatic activities are often diminished in malignant cells as compared with the normal cells of origin. These observations suggested that a comparative study of certain histochemical features of epithelial cells of normal colon, of adenomatous polyps, of carcinomas-in-situ, and of frank carcinomas might show that the changes from normal cell to carcinoma cell pass through an intermediate phase in the cells of adenomatous polyps.

Cole and McKalen (1960) have estimated the DNA content of cells obtained from adenocarcinomas and adenomatous polyps of the large bowel as well as from the parent normal mucosa from which these lesions originated. They found the mean DNA value for cells of normal mucosa to be 2·83 ($\pm$ SE 0·14), of adenomatous polyps 3·23 ($\pm$ SE 0·19), and adenocarcinomas 4·32 ($\pm$ SE 0·33). The DNA figure for normal mucosa is a little higher than that recorded by Leuchtenberger et al. (1954) and Stich et al. (1960) for colonic mucosa from patients without adenomas and carcinomas.

Nachlas and Hannibal (1961) studied the activities of hydrolytic, proteolytic and respiratory enzymes in cells of normal colonic mucosa, of adenomatous polyps, of carcinomas-in-situ and of adenocarcinomas. In general, they found that they were diminished in polyps as compared with normal mucosa. In car-

cinomas some of them were equally diminished, but others were the same as, or greater than, in normal mucosa. Nachlas and Hannibal therefore conclude that their findings neither support nor reject the concept that adenomatous polyps are precancerous lesions.

CONCLUSION

It is very difficult for one who is not a professional pathologist to attempt to adjudicate on this perplexing problem. However it seems reasonable to me to conclude quite definitely from the foregoing conflicting evidence that invasive cancer can develop in benign adenomatous polyps and may sometimes cause lymph-node metastases. But this change of character is probably rarer than has usually been imagined in the past and may, in certain circumstances, be safely treated along relatively conservative lines. So-called 'focal' or 'intramucosal cancer' *per se* can be completely ignored. One of the most significant features of adenomatous polyps, in regard to the development of malignant disease, is that they indicate a diffusely abnormal state of the large bowel mucosa, which renders it more liable to produce further epithelial tumours of benign or malignant nature. Another is that they may be confused in diagnosis with villous papillomas and primary carcinomas.

VILLOUS PAPILLOMAS

There seems to be no disagreement whatsoever, even amongst those who doubt the malignant potential of adenomatous polyps, such as Wheat and Ackerman (1958) and Castleman and Krickstein (1962), that villous papillomas are precancerous lesions. This belief is based on the following considerations:

1. It is a well known clinical phenomenon for villous papillomas to undergo carcinomatous change after many years of apparently benign existence.

2. Histological examination of villous papillomas removed at operation often reveals the presence of malignant foci, though there is a considerable variation in the frequency with which they have been observed by different authors (Table 16). These varying estimates reflect in large measure differences in the pathological material examined—some series being made up entirely of macroscopically benign papillomas, others including growths with obvious malignant change—and differences in the criteria of assessment of malignancy—some pathologists interpreting areas of

TABLE 16. *Estimates by Various Authors of Frequency of Carcinoma arising in Villous Papilloma*

Authors	No. of cases of villous papilloma examined	Incidence of malignant change (%)
Ferguson (1957)	16	6·2
Hines et al. (1958)	71	8·5
Freund (1955)	20	10·0
Southwood (1962)	180	11·7*
Wheat and Ackermann (1958)	50	16·0*
Swinton et al. (1955)	35	31·4
Grinnell and Lane (1958)	216	31·8*
Enterline et al. (1962)	81	55·0*
Moran (1957)	32	56·2
Sunderland and Binkley (1948)	48	68·7
Fisher and Castro (1953)	4	75·0*

* Refers only to invasive cancer.

cellular atypism and carcinoma-in-situ as cancer, others reserving this term for cases showing clear evidence of invasive carcinoma. Furthermore, the likelihood of finding foci of malignancy increases with the number of sections cut, for these are often big tumours and a small area of carcinoma can easily be missed. For example, Fisher and Castro (1953) serially sectioned four villous papillomas and examined 150–200 sections from each tumour; they found invasive cancer in three of the cases.

That the foci of carcinoma revealed in villous papillomas—certainly in those showing invasive cancer—are biologically malignant is indicated by the not infrequent occurrence of metastases in the lymph nodes, and by the development of recurrence after radical excision of the tumour in a fair proportion of cases. Thus, in Southwood's (1962) 21 patients with histological evidence of invasive cancer in the primary growth, 12 were submitted to radical excision with removal of the related lymph glands; lymph node metastases were present in three of these cases. No follow-up report is available. Of Grinnell and Lane's (1958) 52 cases with villous papilloma containing foci of invasive cancer treated by resection, 15, or 29%, had node metastases. After excluding cases with a separate intestinal cancer there were 38 patients available for five-year follow-up; 9, or 23·7%, developed recurrent cancer. Enterline et al. (1962) had 45 patients with invasive cancer shown in their villous papillomas. 30 of these were treated by resection, and 13 were found to have deposits in lymph nodes; 11 cases died of recurrent cancer.

3. Pathological examination of large numbers of frank carcinomas of the rectum and colon discloses the presence in some of them of villous papillomatous tissue, suggesting that the cancer had originated in a pre-existing benign lesion of this kind. For example 98 of 969 malignant rectal growths removed by Gabriel (1952) were reported by the pathologist to have arisen in papillomas.

4. In cases of villous papilloma associated frank carcinoma elsewhere in the bowel is not an uncommon occurrence. Grinnell and Lane (1958) observed concomitant separate carcinomas in about 10% of their 216 cases of villous papilloma, Wheat and Ackerman (1958) in four (8%) of their 50 cases, Enterline et al. (1962) in 17 (21%) of their 81 cases, and Southwood (1962) in 12 (6·6%) of his 180 cases.

The evidence in favour of regarding villous papillomas as precancerous lesions is thus very strong. In addition, as with adenomatous polyps, it appears that the presence of villous papillomas also indicates a diffusely abnormal state of the large bowel mucosa, so that it is predisposed to produce other tumours as well.

Symptoms

ADENOMA

Adenomas of the large intestine may be *entirely asymptomatic* as shown by their not infrequent discovery during routine rectal examination in symptomless patients or in patients whose complaint is adequately explained by some other condition. But an adenoma can cause symptoms. *Bleeding* is the most common and may occasionally be severe; if the polyp is situated low in the rectum, it may *prolapse*, but this is most unusual. A *discharge of mucus* may rarely be noted but only with large or multiple polyps. *Diarrhoea* and sometimes *tenesmus* may occur due to the irritation of a large polyp in the lower rectum. Recurrent slight intussusception or spasm with a polyp of the colon may cause *colicky abdominal pain. Anaemia* may be produced in the long run by repeated slight haemorrhages.

VILLOUS PAPILLOMA

The most prominent symptom as a rule is a *discharge of mucus* which, with a large papilloma, may be profuse. The mucus is passed partly with the motions but often calls for separate evacuations causing a *spurious diarrhoea* and even *inconsistence. Bleeding* is usually a much later symptom and often indicates the development of malignant change. *Failure of general health and anaemia* may result, but the striking feature of most of the patients with villous papillomas is that despite the length of their complaint, they have remained well. Indeed a history of profuse mucoid discharge of long duration without impairment of general health is always strongly suggestive of a villous papilloma.

Severe Fluid and Electrolyte Depletion with Villous Papillomas. Certain patients may show serious metabolic disturbance as a consequence of the profuse mucous diarrhoea, with resulting dehydration, loss of electrolytes, circulatory collapse, prerenal azotaemia and metabolic acidosis. This syndrome, which was first reported by McKittrick and Wheelock (1954), is now well recognized and quite a number of cases have been recorded. Shnitka et al. (1961) were able to collect 16 examples from the literature and added two cases of their own. Since their paper another case has been published by Findlay and O'Connor (1961), and there must be many other unpublished encounters with this phenomenon, for I myself have had five patients under my care with severe fluid and electrolyte depletion associated with villous papillomas, none of which have been reported.

Nine of the 18 patients referred to in a paper by Shnitka et al. (1961) were dangerously ill or moribund when first brought to hospital, and eight of the remainder developed signs and symptoms of serious fluid and electrolyte loss during one or more stages of their illness. These patients displayed marked dehydration, lethargy, weakness, oliguria, acidotic breathing, mental confusion and hypotension. When a history of diarrhoea was not available, this clinical picture was apt to be attributed to diabetic coma, adrenaline insufficiency, or other cause of sudden collapse. The amount of mucous fluid estimated to have been lost per anum in the 18 cases varied from 375 to 3400 ml in 24 hours, figures of the order of 2000–3000 ml being very frequent. The concentration of sodium and chloride in this fluid was little different from that in the plasma, but the potassium concentration was 4 to 20 times the plasma value. Though hypokalaemia was frequent, sodium and chloride deficiences were also common, as was elevation of the blood urea nitrogen, acidosis and haemoconcentration. Of the 18 patients, 15 proceeded to some form of surgical excision of their tumour after fluid and electrolyte depletion had been corrected or lessened by suitable infusions; all recovered. In three cases, however, the diagnosis was missed or only supportive treatment given; all died.

Many explanations have been advanced to account for the profuse mucous diarrhoea in cases of villous papilloma. The careful studies of Duthie and Atwell (1963) of bidirectional rates of transport of fluid and electrolytes to and from the lumen of the bowel in such cases show that there is an increase in *ex*sorption of sodium and water, *in*sorption being relatively unaffected; the disposal of potassium was relatively unchanged (see p. 41). This reversal of the net movement of water and sodium refutes the theory that the diarrhoea might be due simply to an increased epithelial surface area and suggests that there is an intrinsic difference in the behaviour of the cells of the villous papilloma compared with the normal colonic mucosal cells.

Diagnosis

RECTAL EXAMINATION AND SIGMOIDOSCOPY

Fortunately the majority of villous papillomas and very many adenomas are within the reach of these two procedures so that direct confirmation of the diagnosis is frequently possible. It may be helpful to emphasize a few special points in regard to the detection of these tumours by digital and sigmoidoscopic examination:

1. A rounded polyp in the lower rectum may be an extremely elusive object to feel, for, if pedunculated, it slips about in an apparently unattached manner like a small faecal mass. With care however it is possible to demonstrate that, when its mobility is tested to its fullest extent, it is in fact restricted by a pedicle.

2. It is sometimes extremely difficult to distinguish between an adenoma and a villous papilloma, especially if the examination is beset by bleeding. However, the latter growth has a shaggy or very coarsely granular surface, is usually a much deeper red than the surrounding mucosa, and is generally extensive. Indeed any large soft tumour is more probably a papilloma than an adenoma.

3. An exact definition of the extent of a villous papilloma is often impossible because of the soft impalpable nature of its edges and its undulations and irregular surface. Usually it turns out to be more extensive than was thought on clinical examination.

4. Due to the tendency of benign tumours of the lower sigmoid or upper rectum to intussuscept into the rectal ampulla a polyp seen or felt in the latter may in fact arise at a very much higher level. Simi-

larly a long pedicle may occasionally allow an adenoma to descend a considerable distance from its origin and be within reach of the finger.

RADIOLOGICAL EXAMINATION

From what has already been said about the frequent coincidence of carcinoma (and additional benign tumours) in other parts of the bowel with either adenomatous polyps or villous papillomas, it will be evident that *a full investigation of the whole large bowel is essential* in every case of adenoma or papilloma. This implies barium enema studies to supplement digital examination and sigmoido-scopy (Fig. 248). Obviously radiological studies are also necessary in patients with suggestive symptoms in whom palpation and endoscopy have revealed no abnormality.

Though the reliability of a barium enema examination, even using a double-contrast technique, in the detection of colonic polyps has been criticized by Deddish and Hertz (1955) and Teicher and Abrahams (1956), there is little doubt that the accuracy of the X-ray diagnosis depends very much on the skill and enthusiasm which the radiologist brings to his barium enema work and particularly on his familiarity with the Welin technique (Welin 1967; Welin and Welin 1976; see also p. 69). If the latter conditions are satisfied (Simpkins and Young 1968), the radiologist can be astonishingly accurate in his detection and assessment of the character of polyps of the colon, as I well know from the magnificent radiological assistance which I have had from Dr Keith Simpkins and his colleagues in recent years.

FIBREOPTIC COLONOSCOPY

The introduction of fibreoptic colonoscopy in the last few years has provided a most important new diagnostic (and therapeutic) aid in the recognition and treatment of colonic polyps. *It should always follow and be regarded as complementary to the barium enema study.* Performed by an expert it can confirm, amplify or possibly correct information derived from radiological examination, but in less experienced hands it may prove inferior to radiology as lesions in the more proximal colon may not be reached or may be overlooked due to faulty technique. As explained on p. 70, colonoscopy allows piece biopsy or total excision biopsy of lesions depending on circumstances.

CRITERIA OF MALIGNANCY

The overriding consideration in the assessment of apparently benign epithelial tumours of the rectum and colon is whether they are in fact still simple or have undergone malignant change. The criteria on which this point is decided are as follows:

The Age of the Patient. A polyp in a young child is usually of so-called juvenile type (see p. 332) and can invariably be assumed to be benign, but at other ages it may be either simple or malignant.

The Local Characteristics of the Growth. The most important criterion in this regard is the presence or absence of *induration* in the polyp or its base. This is almost certain evidence of malignancy, whilst complete softness is in favour of a benign condition, though not entirely ruling out the possibility of a carcinoma. The *size* of the tumour is also important. Large polyps of, say, the size of a plum are more likely to exhibit carcinomatous change than are small adenomas. The *colour* of the growth is another helpful consideration. A pale colour like that of the surrounding mucosa usually indicates inactivity, whilst a dark red or purple colour suggests a vascular, active lesion which is more likely to undergo malignant degeneration. *Ulceration* of the tumour is also suggestive of carcinomatous change.

The Family History. In cases with multiple polyps careful enquiry should be made into the family history. If it appears that some relatives have died of bowel complaints the probability is that the condition being dealt with is a familial polyposis with the great likelihood of developing a carcinoma eventually.

The Histological Findings on Biopsy or Total Biopsy-Excision of the Tumour. It must be strongly stressed that *piece biopsy* is extremely unreliable as a means of determining whether an adenoma or papilloma is wholly benign or not. When carcinoma supervenes in these lesions it is usually confined to one part of the tumour in the first instance, and even though the surgeon may be guided to this area by suggestive induration it is not unlikely that his biopsy may miss the malignant focus. Consequently, though a positive biopsy for carcinoma is significant, a negative report is valueless. Undoubtedly in dealing with circumscribed adenomas, the simple nature of which is in question, the better plan is to practise a *total excision biopsy*, the entire tumour being removed by diathermy snare or other method

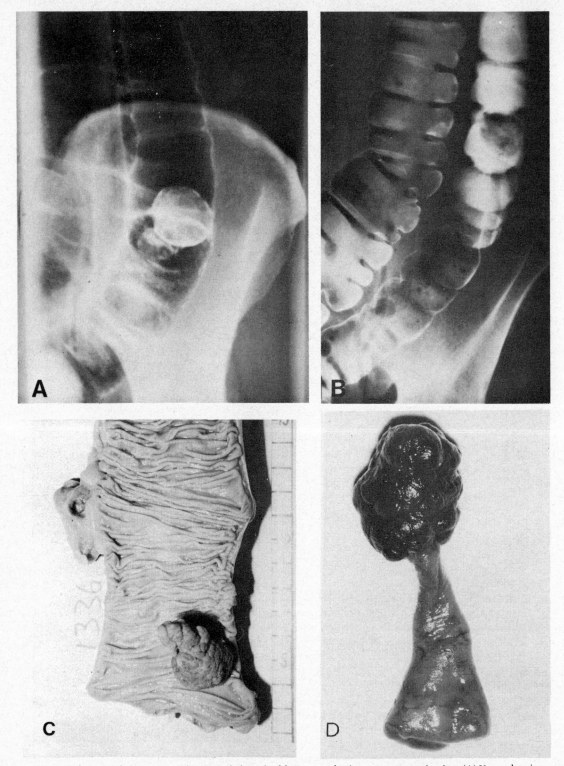

Fig. 248. Large benign adenomatous polyps revealed on double contrast barium enema examination. (A) X-ray showing a sessile polyp of the descending colon, and a resection of the part of the gut that was later removed. (B) X-ray showing a pedunculated polyp with a very long stalk. (C, D) The polyp which was later removed.

and submitted to complete histological examination. In carrying out this form of biopsy it is essential not to destroy the tumour tissue extensively by diathermy otherwise it may be rendered unsuitable for histological examination. With villous papillomas total removal of the growth in this way is only rarely feasible; more usually a decision as to the presence of carcinomatous change has to be made on clinical grounds for, if it is thought to be malignant, more radical treatment than simple local removal will be required.

Recurrence after Excision. The development of a persistent ulcer or nodule at the site of previous excision of a polyp should always raise the query as to whether the original lesion may not have been a carcinoma which has recurred. If the recurrence is indurated this is strong evidence in favour of a malignant condition. A biopsy of the nodule or ulcer should settle the diagnosis.

Treatment of Adenoma

The treatment of these tumours in the past has been dominated by the belief that they are in fact premalignant. For that reason it has usually been recommended that they should always be excised or destroyed. In view of the recent differences of opinion expressed by pathologists about the risk of carcinomatous change in adenomas, it may well be questioned whether this policy in treatment should still hold. However, if it is allowed that there is any malignant potential at all in these tumours—as I firmly believe there is—it would seem a wise preventive measure to remove them, if this can be accomplished with negligible risk. Another, perhaps even stronger, reason for advising excision of these lesions is that it may be difficult to be sure on clinical examination that the condition is in fact an adenoma and not some other form of polyp, such as a small villous papilloma—which carries undoubted considerable potentialities for malignant change—or a polypoid cancer *de novo*. On both these scores, therefore, I would continue to counsel excision as a general principle, but I think it is important to recognize that there may reasonably be some exceptions to this rule. These arise chiefly in connection with the size of the lesion and the magnitude of the hazards involved in removing it, relative to the possible diagnostic and therapeutic advantages of its excision.

As regards *size*, the information provided by Grinnell and Lane (1958) (see p. 329) shows that with lesions less than 1 cm in diameter, the risks of encountering malignant change in them are under 1%. Similarly it is most exceptional to meet with primary cancers of this minute size (Spratt and Ackerman 1962). It seems possible indeed that some of the tiny sessile 'split pea' or 'millet seed' polyps that one sees so frequently, with a colour indistinguishable from the surrounding mucosa, may be of the innocuous 'metaplastic' kind rather than true adenomas (see p. 324). My experience is that, whatever may be their exact histological structure, such small polyps usually remain unchanged in size or actually disappear over the years, and Enquist (1957) has found likewise. My practice, therefore, has been to leave these very minute lesions untouched even if within reach of the sigmoidoscope, and to keep them under observation, but they can often be removed *in toto* with one bite of the biopsy forceps.

As for the *risks of removal*, there were until recently largely proportional to the level of the polyp in the bowel. Thus a lesion in the lower rectum could easily be excised or destroyed by diathermy through the sigmoidoscope or otherwise removed per anum, with or without a short general anaesthetic, with infinitesimal risk and for that reason most surgeons have always taken the view that polyps located in this easy part of the rectum should be removed or destroyed as a routine. But endoscopic removal of a polyp in the peritoneal-covered upper rectum or lower sigmoid was associated with some hazards, whilst adenomas beyond safe reach of the sigmoidoscope required an abdominal approach for their excision, which could only be practised at the price of quite definite operative risks, especially in more obese relatively unfit subjects, as Kleinfeld and Gump (1960) and Castleman and Krickstein (1962) have emphasized. Some discretion, therefore, was indicated in pursuing smaller polyps in the colon proper. But the advent of the operating fibreoptic colonoscope, which in favourable circumstances permits snaring of suitable polypoid lesions from all parts of the colon, has altered these concepts and gone a long way towards bringing the management of colonic polyps into line with that of rectal polyps (Wolff and Shinya 1973a, b; Williams et al. 1973, 1974; Spencer et al. 1974; Shinya and Wolff 1975). Initially, the number of experienced colonoscopists available to undertake safe colonoscopic polypectomy was very small, but in the last few years the necessary expertise with the colonoscope has become much more generalized so that all patients in Britain at any rate can now be easily referred to appropriate centres for this treatment. As a general rule it may now be accepted that polyps of the colon, like those of the rectum should be subjected to endoscopic inspection before the final decision is reached regarding their treatment. In many cases immediate local removal of the lesion by endoscopic snaring will be possible, as when well pedunculated polyps are found. In other cases the evidence provided by colonoscopy, added to that derived from the radiological study and possibly from a biopsy, may indicate the need for laparotomy and colotomy or colonic resection, as when there are large sessile lesions in a peritoneal-covered part of bowel.

Occasional exceptions to this rule may arise, as when a very small symptomless colonic polyp of less than 1 cm in diameter has been revealed on radiological examination and its demonstration by colonoscopy might be expected to be more than usually hazardous because of the patient's poor general condition, or exceptionally difficult because the lesion is situated in the more proximal part of the bowel or there is a very redundant sigmoid loop intervening between the colonoscopist and it.

Under these circumstances it may be considered preferable to rely on repeat double-contrast barium enema studies at intervals of 6 to 12 months for a year or two to determine whether the polyps are undergoing enlargement. In this connection it should be stressed that a prolonged follow-up is required for all patients who have suffered from colorectal polyps, whether the original lesion was removed or not, in order to detect at an early stage the formation of further polyps or even a frank carcinoma, for it is clear that patients harbouring adenomatous polyps are predisposed to either of these developments (p. 330).

The following methods are available for the removal or destruction of adenomas of the rectum or colon: surgical excision *per vias naturales*; diathermy excision or coagulation through the sigmoidoscope; colonoscopic polypectomy; abdominal removal by colotomy and polypectomy, segmental resection, or subtotal colectomy. These will now be considered in turn.

LOCAL EXCISION PER ANUM

This is a method which is sometimes applicable to rather bigger polyps in the lower third of the rectum, occasionally in the middle third. When the anal sphincters are fully relaxed under general anaesthetic and a relaxant, a pedunculated adenoma in these situations can usually be hooked

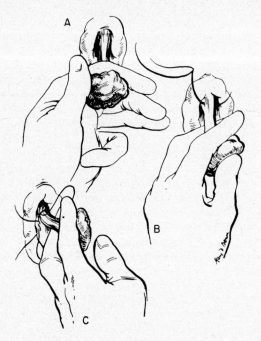

Fig. 249. Local excision *per anum* of a large pedunculated adenoma of the lower rectum: (A) Drawing the tumour down through the anus. (B) Transfixing the pedicle. (C) The ligature has been tied round part of the pedicle and the tails have been carried round the whole stalk for further tying.

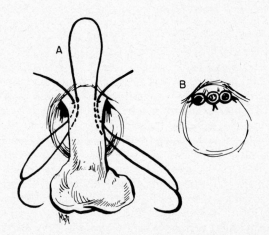

Fig. 250. The Goodsall stitch with double transfixion which is useful for broad pedicles: (A) Transfixion of pedicle with ligature on two needles. (B) After division of the ligature through the middle of the loop and immediately proximal to the needles, three separate strands are available for tying, the pedicle then being severed 1 cm distal to the ligatures.

down by the finger and delivered through the anus (Fig. 249A). Whilst the tumour is drawn strongly downwards, the pedicle is transfixed and tied with a No. 2 chromic catgut ligature as near as possible to its base (Fig. 249B and C), and then divided 1–1·5 cm distal to the ligature. If the pedicle is very broad it may be safer to use on it a Goodsall stitch which provides for double transfixion (Fig. 250A and B). A *sessile* tumour of the lower third can also be excised per anum using the technique shown in Fig. 255, but this manoeuvre is more appropriate to broader villous papillomas than to adenomas.

SIGMOIDOSCOPIC DIATHERMY, SNARING OR FULGURATION

This is the method used for the vast majority of rectal polyps. For its proper application certain items of equipment are essential:

Operating Sigmoidoscope. Though one or two small polyps can sometimes be satisfactorily dealt with by diathermy methods through an ordinary 2·5 cm bore sigmoidoscope (which has the advantage that the treatment can usually be carried out without a general anaesthetic), for most cases a specially wide operating sigmoidoscope is desirable. This gives more room for intraluminal instrumentation and affords a clear view to the operator whilst the snare etc. are in position. I prefer the Lloyd-Davies pattern of operating sigmoidoscope (Fig. 251A). It is 14 cm long and 3 cm wide, and has proximal lighting. In the latest model this is provided by a fibre-optic system from an outside source, instead of a small incandescent bulb on the head end of the instrument, which is a great advance for it gives a much stronger light. A suction tube is available for clipping to the sigmoidoscope after introduction, to evacuate smoke from the lumen during the course of diathermy treatment (Fig. 251B). This large sigmoidoscope can only be used on the anaesthetized patient. Welch Allyn make a specially wide bore sigmoidoscope with distal fibreoptic illumination very suitable for operative work (see p. 52).

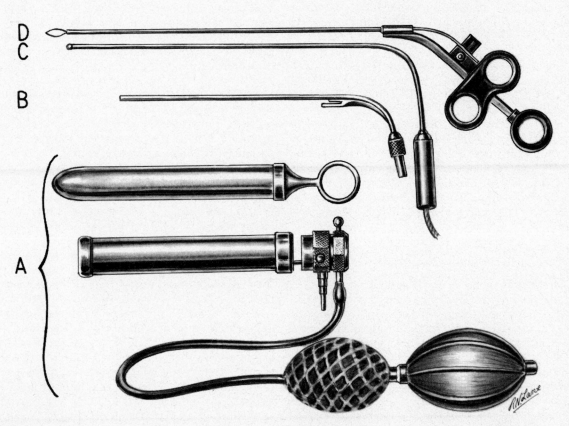

Fig. 251. Equipment for sigmoidoscopic diathermy. (A) Lloyd-Davies operating sigmoidoscope with proximal lighting. (B) Suction tube. (C) Button electrode with insulated shaft and handle. (D) Frankfeldt's diathermy snare with insulated shaft and handle.

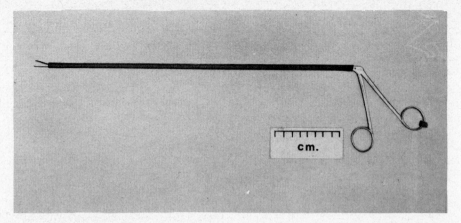

Fig. 252. Diathermy forceps improvised from ordinary sigmoidoscopic forceps by drawing a length of thin rubber tubing over the shaft as an insulator.

Diathermy Snare. Several patterns of wire snare with insulated shaft handle are available but I personally use that designed by Frankfeldt (Fig. 251D).

Diathermy Button Electrode. For sessile polyps that are unsuitable for snaring some form of button electrode with insulated shaft and handle is generally employed such as that shown in Fig. 251C.

Diathermy Forceps. The disadvantage of a button electrode is that it gives relatively superficial coagulation. A better instrument in some ways for piecemeal destruction of tumours is a diathermy forceps with insulated shaft such as Frankfeldt's. Actually quite an efficient forceps for this purpose can be improvised by drawing a thin rubber tube over the shaft of an ordinary long alligator forceps used for holding swabs during sigmoidoscopy (Fig. 252). The terminal blades are left uncovered whilst the shaft is satisfactorily insulated by the rubber covering.

TECHNIQUE OF SIGMOIDOSCOPIC DIATHERMY

With the patient anaesthetized and lying on his left side the sigmoidoscope is introduced, the light connected and the lesion brought into view. The window is next removed and the suction tube attached with its distal extremity projecting to the end of the sigmoidoscope. The appropriate applicator for the diathermy is then selected and connected to the diathermy machine which is set to give a slow coagulating effect.

For *pedunculated tumours* the snare is the ideal instrument to use. The wire loop is manipulated over the polyp and gradually tightened (Fig.

253A, B), the current being circulated during the terminal phases of the tightening. It will be found that it slowly cuts through the pedicle till the tumour is finally separated from the bowel wall, usually without haemorrhage. The resulting small coagulated area usually takes two or three weeks to heal. An alternative technique for a well-pedunculated tumour is to use diathermy forceps and to grasp the pedicle with the blades. When the current is put through the same effect is obtained as with a snare.

For a *sessile polyp or one with a very short squat pedicle*, snaring may still be possible but a rather different technique is needed. So that the wire may be kept on the pedicle or the surrounding mucosa as it is tightened, it is necessary that the polyp should be grasped by ordinary holding forceps and drawn strongly into the lumen through the loop (Fig. 253C, D). In this way a satisfactory diathermy snare-excision may often be accomplished with removal of an adequate stalk or disc of normal mucosa. However, this is a somewhat dangerous method for it may draw into the loop not only mucosa but also the muscle coat of the bowel wall. It may safely be used for tumours arising below the peritoneal reflection, but for sessile polyps of the peritoneal-covered upper rectum or sigmoid it requires to be employed with great caution and delicacy, and certainly only on small lesions (Fig. 253E). For most sessile lesions the preferable technique is to use a button electrode or diathermy forceps, the polyp being touched or grasped and the current then switched on for a few seconds (Fig. 253F). With a very small tumour one point of contact may suffice, but with larger lesions, the performance has to be repeated several times at different places on the

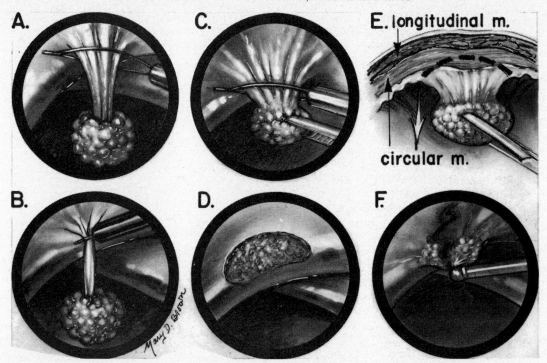

Fig. 253. Technique of sigmoidoscopic diathermy: (A and B) Snaring of pedunculated polyp. (C) Snaring of sessile polyp by drawing it into the lumen of the bowel by means of a holding forceps and snaring the short mucosal pedicle thus created. (D) Resulting raw area after snaring of sessile polyp may extend down to circular muscle coat (or even deeper) on occasions. (F) Alternative of diathermy coagulation *in situ* of sessile polyp.

tumour. It is not till the sigmoidoscopic review after two or three weeks that a clear idea will be obtained of the amount of destruction achieved. As this is often more extensive than was imagined at the time of application of the diathermy it is well to under-treat in the first instance.

COMPLICATIONS OF SIGMOIDOSCOPIC
DIATHERMY

Three dangerous complications may occur with diathermy treatment, all of them fortunately relatively rare—perforation of the bowel, intraluminal explosion and haemorrhage.

Perforation of the rectum or colon may result from deep snaring of sessile adenomas, especially if this method is used in the intraperitoneal part of the rectum or distal sigmoid where the wall is relatively thin and where the consequences of a breach are more likely to be serious than in the lower rectum. It may also be caused by ordinary contact diathermy if the amount of coagulation is allowed to become excessive and to extend too deeply. This latter form of injury is also more liable to occur in the upper rectum or lower sigmoid, but it is a more gradual process than perforation by snaring and by the time sloughing has taken place the diathermized part of the bowel may well be sealed off by the adherence of loops of small gut and greater omentum. A frank perforation produced by the snare and seen through the sigmoidoscope calls for immediate laparotomy and suture (or resection if the affected segment of bowel contains other polyps); a proximal colostomy should not usually be necessary. If the perforation is not suspected at the time of treatment the patient will rapidly or slowly develop the symptoms and signs of a pelvic or diffuse peritonitis and exploration will generally become necessary. With the more gradual type of perforation produced by diathermy coagulation the process may be very localized and may respond to a conservative regimen with antibiotics.

Intraluminal explosions due to the ignition of inflammable gases by the diathermy spark are described by Carter (1952) and Galley (1954). These gases may be the hydrogen methane or hydrogen sulphide which are usually found in the colon or rectum; alternatively they may consist of ethylene, acetylene or hydrogen produced by electro-coagulation of the tissues, or of anaesthetic gases such as cyclopropane derived by diffusion from the blood stream in the intestinal wall. In the prevention of such explosions it is obvious that the anaesthetist should not use inflammable anaesthetic gases; it is also important to evacuate the gases in the distal colon and rectum by the suction tube before diathermy treatment is commenced and to continue this process during the treatment. An even more certain method of prevention is to direct a flow of an inert non-inflammable gas such as nitrogen or carbon dioxide into the lumen throughout the course of the diathermy session, but as explosions have been so rare, few surgeons feel the necessity to use this last measure.

Secondary haemorrhage from the diathermized areas is the least uncommon of the three complications. It occurs about the seventh to tenth day during separation of necrotic tissue. It may follow defaecation or arise spontaneously, and the bleeding may amount to a mere streak or may be quite profuse. In the latter case the patient soon becomes exsanguinated and shocked. For slight haemorrhage all that is required is mild sedation, observation and subsequent iron therapy. For more severe bleeding the patient should be given morphine without delay and transfused. If the bleeding should continue, it will be wise to examine the rectum with the operating sigmoidoscope under a short general anaesthetic. After evacuation of fluid and clotted blood, this will show the site of the bleeding. It may then be possible to check the haemorrhage by a touch of diathermy or application of an absorbable haemostatic on sigmoidoscopic forceps.

OPERATIVE MORTALITY OF SIGMOIDOSCOPIC DIATHERMY

The safety of diathermy treatment of rectal polyps is shown by the absence of fatalities in 231 cases of polyps in the rectum treated in this way in the series reported by Grinnell and Lane (1958).

SIGMOIDOSCOPIC DIATHERMY REMOVAL OF POLYPS COMBINED WITH LAPAROTOMY

In order to extend the range of safe diathermy removal of polyps through the sigmoidoscope, Benjamin et al. (1967) proposed that the sigmoidoscopy should be combined with a laparotomy to guide the end of the instrument to the polyp and to supervise the safe removal of the latter by snaring. This operation was best performed with the patient in the modified lithotomy-Trendelenburg position (p. 85) used for synchronous com-bined excision of the rectum. A non-scrubbed-up surgeon manoeuvred the sigmoidoscope from below and another surgeon conducted the laparotomy and threaded the end of the instrument through the colon. Benjamin et al. (1967) claimed to have used this method of anotransabdominal polypectomy on 125 patients without significant complications, and in the process to have removed many polyps in the upper sigmoid and descending colon, even as far as the splenic flexure on occasions! This combination of sigmoidoscopy with laparotomy for the removal of colonic polyps has now been completely supplanted by colonoscopic polypectomy, which may also be combined with laparotomy if desired (see below).

COLONOSCOPIC POLYPECTOMY

The technique of colonoscopy in general has been described on p. 70, and here only special points relating to the performance of polypectomy with the aid of the colonoscope will be considered.

EQUIPMENT

Snares. Long wire snares with thin plastic sleeves for insulation (Fig. 57) are available from the firms of Olympus, ACM and Storz and I have found all of them satisfactory. The Storz snare is equipped with a channel for introducing carbon dioxide before circulating the current if desired.

Colonoscope. A colonoscope with two channels for instrumentation is advantageous, for it allows a snare to be passed down one channel and a holding or biopsy forceps down the other, but I have snared many polyps with a single-channel instrument.

TECHNIQUE

It is usually best to pass the colonoscope as far as considered desirable in the first instance and to deal with any polyps as the instrument is being withdrawn. This statement immediately begs the question as to whether a total colonoscopy should be attempted in all cases having this examination for radiologically detected polyps, as urged by Coller et al. (1975). I make a distinction between patients whose barium examination was done by my own hospital radiologists (or a few others), in the accuracy of whose large bowel work I have learnt to repose great confidence, and those whose X-ray examination was done elsewhere. In the former group I am prepared to restrict the colonoscopy to the left colon or sigmoid colon if the polyps shown radiologically are confined to these parts, but in the latter group I prefer as a rule to pursue the colonoscopy to the caecum in all cases.

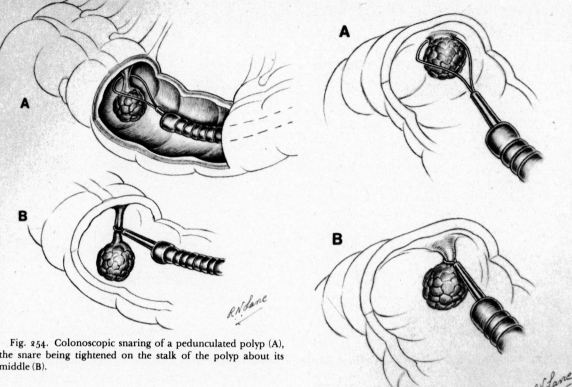

Fig. 254. Colonoscopic snaring of a pedunculated polyp (A), the snare being tightened on the stalk of the polyp about its middle (B).

Fig. 255. Snaring a sessile polyp, the snare being tightened on the base of the polyp (A), and traction being exerted on the polyp to draw it away from the colon wall creating a false pedicle (B) before the diathermy current is passed.

Actual Snaring

Before commencing withdrawal of the colonoscope, the snare is inserted into the intrument to the point where its distal end lies just inside the tip, ready for immediate projection when required. As the scope is slowly withdrawn, a close inspection is carried out for polyps or other lesions, the entire circumference of the bowel wall being brought into view as far as possible at every level, which may be quite difficult to do in some regions. When a polyp is encountered a decision has to be made as to whether it is likely to be benign or malignant and whether it is suitable for snaring or should simply be biopsied (and possibly diathermized). If snaring is decided upon, the insulating sheath of the snare is advanced so that it protrudes beyond the end of the scope and the snare is opened up so that wire loop can be slipped over the polyp (Fig. 254A). Sometimes in order to facilitate this step it is necessary to alter the position of the patient so that the lesion hangs from above. If it is a *well pedunculated lesion*, the loop is tightened about half way down the stalk (Fig. 254B). At the same time a coagulating current is circulated through the wire, preferably in a series of short bursts over a period of 8–10 seconds. In dealing with a *sessile polyp*, it is possible if the base is

not more than 1 cm across, to encircle it with the snare (Fig. 255A) and by traction on it to draw it somewhat into the lumen of the bowel, creating a pseudo-pedicle composed of lifted-up normal mucosa and submucosa (Fig. 255B). This false pedicle can then be cut across close to the actual lesion by a combination of further tightening of the snare and circulation of a coagulating current. It is in treating sessile polyps that the method of grasping the lesion with a biopsy forceps passed down one channel of the colonoscope and drawing it through the snare is often helpful. With a sessile lesion larger than 1·5 cm in diameter there is a risk with snaring that muscle coat and even serosa may be included in the bite with resulting immediate or delayed perforation of the bowel. For much bigger non-pedunculated polyps the safer course, therefore, is to snare the tumour piecemeal with a series of bites (Fig. 256A, B) and perhaps with some very cautious diathermy coagulation to the remaining

small basal segment. However, the safe and successful execution of this technique may test the skill and
resourcefulness of the colonoscopist to the utmost,
and if he is doubtful about his ability to deal with
the lesion endoscopically he should not hesitate to
advise laparotomy removal.

The largest polyp that can be easily snared
colonoscopically is about 4–5 cm, but whether it
will in fact be possible to remove it satisfactorily by
snaring will depend on whether it has a pedicle or
not and on other considerations. At the opposite
end of the scale it may sometimes be feasible to
snare sessile lesions of less than 0·5 cm in diameter,
but not infrequently this proves technically impossible. Under these circumstances the best plan is
either to take several biopsies and then coagulate
the lesion or leave it untreated. Williams et al.
(1974) have devised what they term a 'hot biopsy'
diathermy forceps which simultaneously biopsies
and destroys polyps up to 0·7 cm in diameter.

Recovery of a single snared polyp is normally
achieved by sucking the separated lesion up against
the end of the colonoscope and withdrawing it with
the instrument. When *several polyps* have been
snared at the same session—and there is no reason
why, say, four or five polyps should not be dealt
with at a single colonoscopy—only one or possibly
two can be retrieved in this way. In cases with
multiple polyps removed reliance has to be placed
on a subsequent saline or Veripaque enema with
careful examination of the returned fluid to recover
the lesions for histological examination. If the
polyps are very small, perhaps histological
confirmation of their benign nature may reasonably be omitted, but with larger lesions histology is
essential. If the passage of the colonoscope to the
site of the polyps has been particularly easy, it may
be preferable in dealing with two or three larger
polyps to snare and remove each one separately, the
colonoscope being re-inserted as required.

Unless there has been some special problem
about the polypectomy I allow my patients to
return home on the evening of the day of the
examination.

Per-laparotomy Colonoscopy in the Management of Polyps of the Colon

Espiner et al. (1973) suggest that peranal fibreoptic
colonoscopy may be of value during laparotomy for
neoplasm of the colon, by enabling a complete
inspection of the interior of the large bowel to be
carried out and additional polyps to be discovered
(and removed by snaring with the colonoscope or
by colotomy). Their advocacy of this method was at

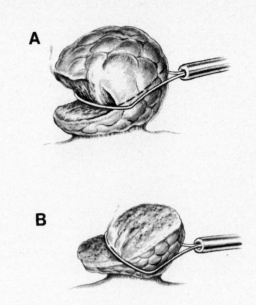

Fig. 256. Piece-meal snaring of a large sessile polyp unsuitable for complete snaring in one move.

a time when the technique of colonoscopy was not
as well developed as it now is and failure to reach
the proximal end of the large bowel during this
examination was more frequent. In the three cases
in which I used peroperative colonoscopy in the
way described by Espiner et al. (1973) I was dismayed by the amount of distension of the colon
that took place during colonoscopic inflation with
the abdomen opened and very apprehensive about
proceeding to resection of an associated carcinoma
with the bowel in this unfavourable condition. I
doubt if there is much place for Espiner et al.'s
(1973) manoeuvre at the present day.

COMPLICATIONS

The complications of colonoscopic polypectomy
are haemorrhage, colonic perforation (and,
theoretically, intracolonic explosion and perforation).

Haemorrhage

Bleeding is a well-recognized complication of polypectomy but usually ceases spontaneously and very
seldom assumes serious proportions. Greenen et al.

(1975) record five episodes of significant colonic bleeding in a collective series of 292 cases submitted to colonoscopic polypectomy; three patients were treated solely by blood transfusions with a satisfactory outcome and two required operative intervention to control the bleeding. Williams et al. (1974) admit to six instances of haemorrhage after 300 polypectomies; in all cases the bleeding stopped spontaneously with or without the need for blood transfusion. Wolff and Shinya (1973b) and Shinya and Wolff (1975) do not give a precise figure of incidence of haemorrhage in their unique experience of polypectomies but state that laparotomy was necessary to control bleeding in one case. As Shinya and Wolff (1975) and Williams et al. (1974) point out, if bleeding occurs, there is no colonoscopic manoeuvre that can be employed to stop it. Reliance has to be placed on spontaneous arrest, the patient meanwhile being transfused if required, or very rarely on surgical control at laparotomy.

Perforation

This complication occurred in two of the series of 292 cases of colonoscopic polypectomy collected by Greenen et al. (1975), one of which was fatal. Williams et al. (1974) had one delayed perforation in their series of 300 polypectomies; it was successfully treated by colonic resection. Wolff and Shinya (1973b) have apparently had only one perforation (which sealed itself) in their experience of 499 polypectomies. Clearly, if it is recognized that a perforation has occurred, the correct treatment is immediate laparotomy, but with delayed or sealed perforations a difficult problem of diagnosis may arise and there may be a place for conservative management.

Intracolonic Explosion

As mentioned on p. 343, there is a theoretical risk that during intrarectal or intracolonic diathermy procedures the combustible gases, hydrogen and methane, which are liberated by bacterial action on the faeces, might be ignited with a resulting explosion. This hazard provides the basis for the practice favoured by some people of routinely insufflating carbon dioxide into the colon immediately prior to colonoscopic polypectomy. But very many colonoscopists do not take this precaution and no intracolonic explosions have yet been recorded. Furthermore, as Ragins et al. (1974) and Bond and Levitt (1975) have demonstrated, the concentration of these gases in the colon at the time of colonoscopy is only a minute fraction of that needed for combustion. Presumably the vigorous preparation of the bowel before colonoscopy, by reducing the faecal content, keeps the gaseous concentration down and the alternating inflation and suction during the conduct of the examination largely replaces the natural intracolonic gas with air.

RESULTS

An exciting picture of what can be accomplished by first-class colonoscopy in the management of polyps of the colon has been provided by Wolff and Shinya (1973a). They removed 303 polyps from 218 patients, the greatest number of polyps from a patient at one session being five, which happened in three cases. The size of polyps removed ranged from 0·5 to 5 cm, the majority being 1–2 cm. They included both sessile and pedunculated lesions. The commonest sites of the polyps were the middle or proximal sigmoid and descending colon, but some were taken from virtually all parts of the large intestine. In only three cases was it found impossible to remove radiologically demonstrated polyps.

Williams et al. (1974) give a very similar account of their achievements with colonoscopic polypectomy, and very many other colonoscopists including ourselves have now (1978) had very substantial experience with this procedure.

THE PROBLEM OF THE APPARENTLY BENIGN
SNARED POLYP THAT IS FOUND ON
HISTOLOGICAL EXAMINATION TO BE
MALIGNANT

Surgeons are familiar with this problem arising in connection with rectal polyps snared through the sigmoidoscope and have been provided with good guidelines by Lockhart-Mummery and Dukes (1952), Carden and Morson (1964) and Morson et al. (1977) as to how to proceed under the circumstances (see also p. 358). Clearly a similar problem is going to arise with increasing frequency in connection with polyps snared at colonoscopy, and, as Williams et al. (1974) have stated, the same surgical pathological guidelines worked out for rectal polyps should apply (see p. 358), though obviously diathermy fulguration of the former site of the polyp at a subsequent endoscopy, which is safely feasible in the low rectum, is not practicable after colonoscopic polypectomy.

Wolff and Shinya (1975) give an interesting report on their experiences with this problem in colonoscopically snared polyps. Of 892 neoplastic polyps removed by them by this means 51 or 5% were subsequently found to harbour invasive carcinoma. Twenty-five of these patients with malignant polyps proceeded to laparotomy; 17 showed no residual cancer, whilst eight (five recognized incomplete endoscopic removal) had tumour in the bowel wall. In the remaining patients with malignant polyps the endoscopic polypectomy that had been performed was deemed to be adequate treatment and none have so far shown recurrent carcinoma on clinical and endoscopic follow-up, but admittedly the period of follow-up in many of the cases is relatively short. Gillespie et al.'s (1979) experience is very similar. Wolff and Shinya (1975) emphasize that nearly half of their malignant polyps were less than 2 cm in diameter and two-thirds were pedunculated.

EXCISION THROUGH THE ABDOMEN

As already explained, the indications for removal of polyps through the abdomen have recently undergone considerable shrinkage due to the capability of colonoscopic diathermy to deal with very many of the colonic polyps that previously required laparotomy for their treatment. But a need for abdominal removal still exists on rare occasions, as when the lesion proves inaccessible to the colonoscope or is large and sessile and unsuitable for colonoscopic snaring, or a considerable number of polyps are present. Several methods exist for excising colonic polyps at laparotomy, the choice in an individual case depending on the local circumstances and on the views of the surgeon concerned.

COLOTOMY AND POLYPECTOMY

This is the operation that has been most often employed. The colon is opened in the region of the polyp by a longitudinal incision 5–7 cm long in the line of one of the antimesenteric taeniae. If the adenoma is pedunculated its pedicle is transfixed and tied and the tumour excised. A sessile adenoma can be removed along with a circular cuff of mucosa, the mucosal gap being closed by suture, but, like many other surgeons, I have misgivings about the use of this method for sessile lesions. Finally the colotomy wound is sutured in two layers in either the longitudinal or the transverse axis of the bowel, additional security being provided by stitching adjacent appendices epiploicae over the suture line. It would be ideal to have a histological section of the lesion before the abdomen were closed, so that, if it were shown to be carcinomatous, an immediate radical resection could be performed. But frozen sections of intestinal polyps are technically difficult, and the surgeon has therefore usually to rely on the macroscopic features of the polyp—size, colour, consistency, and the possession of a pedicle—in making up his mind as to whether it is suitable for simple removal or not, confirmation of this decision being provided later by histological examination of an ordinary fixed section. If, however, this shows that carcinoma is present, he will bitterly reproach himself, particularly if the lesion was sessile, for not having performed a colonic resection in the first instance.

TRANSABDOMINAL COLOSCOPY (OR COLONOSCOPY) WITH THE RIGID SIGMOIDO-SCOPE AS AN AID IN THE DETECTION AND REMOVAL OF POLYPS OF THE COLON AT LAPAROTOMY

Because of their softness colonic polyps may be extremely difficult to detect with accuracy by palpation of the bowel at operation. They are very easily confused with small masses of faeces. Transillumination of the colon may be a help in searching for them, but even with this aid it is easy to miss polyps at laparotomy. To supplement simple palpation and transillumination Deddish (1953) and Bacon and Peale (1956) have developed the method of making two or more small longitudinal incisions in the line of a taenia—usually in the sigmoid and right transverse colon—and introducing a sterile sigmoidoscope in both directions at each colotomy wound to inspect the interior of the bowel for polyps or an early carcinoma. According to these authors colotomy and colonoscopy are easily performed and often very rewarding in their discovery of impalpable polyps, but my very limited experience of the method impressed me rather with the technical difficulty of obtaining a good view if there was any faecal loading, and with the tendency to gross contamination of the peritoneum. At the present time transabdominal colonoscopy has been largely replaced by transanal fibreoptic colonoscopy, which if desired can be performed at the time of laparotomy, though the resulting distension of the colon with air during the latter manoeuvre may prove something of an embarrassment if a colotomy or colectomy has to be employed (see p. 346).

Mortality, Morbidity and Late Results of Colotomy and Polypectomy with and without Coloscopy. A fair amount of information is available about the results of colotomy and polypectomy. In the 310 cases reported by Grinnell and Lane (1958) as being treated by this operation the immediate mortality was given as 0·6%. In another paper from the Presbyterian Hospital, New York City, dealing with 311 patients treated by colotomy and polypectomy, with or without coloscopy, between 1943 and 1959 Kleinfeld and Gump (1960) examined the hospital experience and morbidity with this operation in detail. The sigmoid was the site of the colotomy in 231 cases, the descending colon in 22, and one or other flexure in nine. In 60 patients more than one colotomy was performed. Sigmoidoscopy through one or more colotomies to find the polyp or exclude the presence of other polyps was carried out in 149 cases. The predominant pathological diagnosis was adenomatous polyp, noted in 256 cases; 33 cases were said to show foci of carcinoma in the polyp, 17 had villous papillomas, and in 11 no lesion was found. Prophylactic systematic antibiotic therapy was given in the great majority of the patients. A total of 81 postoperative complications developed in 61 patients, an overall complication rate of 20%. If complications relating directly to the performance of the colotomy only are considered, the rate in 14% was made up as follows: wound infections 6%, abscesses and fistulas 4%, bleeding 3% and ileus 3%. Twenty-three further operations were required in the management of these complications or their sequels. In six patients disrupted wounds had to be resutured; three diverting colostomies were performed for colotomy leakage or fistulas. In three cases chronic fistulas had to be excised, and in three other cases drainage of pelvic abscesses was required. Chronically infected sinuses from silk sutures were excised in three patients, and two cases with intestinal obstruction required division of adhesions. Only four deaths occurred; these were in poor-risk subjects and were not due to complications of the colotomy itself. Wound infection was three times commoner in cases in which coloscopy had been performed. On the other hand, Swinton and Weakley (1963) found no increased morbidity due to the use of coloscopy in conjunction with colotomy and polypectomy; their overall operative mortality in 245 cases was 0·4%. Bacon et al. (1963) give a similarly enthusiastic report.

Judd and Carlisle (1953) reported the early and late results in 246 consecutive cases of colonic polyps excised by colotomy at the Mayo Clinic and followed up for five years. In approximately 60% of the patients only one polyp was removed, in 15% three or more. The hospital mortality rate was only 0·8%. Recurrent polyps formed in 28% of the entire series, and in nearly 50% of those with four or more polyps. The recurrence took place usually at the original site or between it and the rectosigmoid junction. In addition in some 6% of the cases a definite carcinoma developed in the colon.

SEGMENTAL RESECTION

This operation has been advocated chiefly by Welch (1951) and Judd and Carlisle (1953) in an endeavour to improve on the late results of simple polypectomy (see above), particularly for *multiple* polyps. One can readily see its technical advantages in cases with several polyps, and how it might diminish the risk of further polyp formation or even the development of carcinoma by removing a generous segment, say 12–14 cm long, of large bowel mucosa predisposed to produce such lesions. It would also clearly be a vastly better primary operation in a case in which the polyp is subsequently shown to be cancerous. In the present safe state of colon surgery it would be not unreasonable to hope that it might be accomplished with little more hazard than a simple colotomy. Unfortunately this hope has not been realized in the published results of this operation to date. Thus in Grinnell and Lane's (1958) report there were 73 resections for polyps of the colon, with an operative mortality of 6·8%, which contrasts with 0·6% in the 310 patients treated by colotomy and polypectomy. In extenuation of these results it can be pointed out that, from the way in which patients were selected for the two operations in this series, more polyps with carcinoma were treated by resection than by polypectomy, which may have influenced the immediate mortality, and certainly makes it difficult to compare the late results. Also many of the cases were apparently treated over 20 years ago, and it might be expected that the risks of resection would have declined considerably in the interval.

In summary it would seem that for benign-looking polyps with a well defined soft pedicle, certainly when occurring singly, colotomy and polypectomy should be used, but for more dubious lesions, particularly if sessile, or for clusters of polyps a segmental resection is probably preferable. As will be appreciated, however, the lesions ideally suited for colotomy and polypectomy are also the one most suitable for colonoscopic polypectomy, which has now almost completely eliminated the use of the former method. As already mentioned (see p. 344) colonoscopic techniques can also deal effectively with many of the sessile polyps, even if multiple, provided that they do not have too wide a base, which thus limits the current indication for segmental colonic resection for polypoid disease.

TOTAL COLECTOMY WITH ILEORECTAL ANASTOMOSIS

The most drastic step of all to ensure that polyps are not overlooked at operation has been proposed by Lillehei and Wangensteen (1955) and consists of total colectomy followed by ileo-

rectal anastomosis. These authors used a similar operation in the treatment of many cases of carcinoma of the colon also, to avoid leaving associated polyps or a second carcinoma. They claim that it has been demonstrably successful in these aims, that the immediate mortality is low and that the postoperative functional condition is usually satisfactory (see p. 367). Total colectomy has also been used by Teicher and Abrahams (1956). A comparison of the findings on preoperative sigmoidoscopy and barium enema examination and on examination of the operative specimens in Teicher and Abraham's (1956) cases revealed many more polyps in the latter than had been suspected before operation, but these findings do not reflect the achievements of modern double contrast radiology of the colon and of colonoscopy. Total colectomy is regarded by most surgeons as altogether too radical a treatment for just a few polyps or indeed for carcinoma of the colon as a rule. I personally have reserved it for patients with frank and profuse polyposis—familial or nonfamilial—or with multiple polyps in two or three different segments of the colon but would probably now try colonoscopic polypectomy for the latter of these two indications unless the polyps were very numerous.

Treatment of Villous Papilloma

As already mentioned on p. 366, patients with villous papillomas may occasionally present in a profoundly disturbed metabolic state consequent upon fluid and electrolyte depletion. Clearly in such cases the prime indication in treatment is to correct this condition by suitable infusions, and only when this has been accomplished can the surgical management of the causal lesion be considered. It is well to bear in mind too that in the large majority of patients with villous papillomas who appear in excellent general condition, prolonged severe mucous diarrhoea may have led to a lesser degree of electrolyte imbalance and this should be corrected before operation. Estimation of the plasma electrolyte levels, therefore, should always be undertaken to investigate this point even in seemingly fit patients.

In treating these tumours it is important to bear in mind the considerable risk of malignant degeneration. This change cannot usually be detected by simple inspection of the lesion through a sigmoidoscope, nor, as it is a focal process initially, are ordinary *piece biopsies*, even if multiple, of much value. A *total excision biopsy*, on the other hand, is completely reliable and when feasible is a satisfactory mode of treatment in itself unless the subsequent histological examination of the removed specimen shows that the tumour has been incompletely removed or has undergone malignant change, when further measures will be required. But many villous papillomas are too large or otherwise unsuitable for this manoeuvre and in such cases valuable information regarding the probability of the lesion being still benign or partly malignant may be obtained by *simple palpation of the surface of the growth on digital examination of the rectum*, under a general anaesthetic with good relaxation, if necessary, to permit of the maximum reach of the finger. However, for this method of assessment to be reliable the *whole* tumour must be palpable. In formulating treatment on the basis of the palpatory findings it will thus be convenient to consider villous papillomas according to their availability for complete palpation.

VILLOUS TUMOURS LYING WHOLLY OR PARTLY BEYOND THE EXAMINING FINGER

Very rarely a villous tumour in this situation may be so small or so well pedunculated that it is amenable to safe total excision biopsy by sigmoidoscopic or colonoscopic snaring, and, if it is subsequently shown histologically to be benign and completely removed, that is all the treatment that is required. But much more usually villous papillomas at this level are too large and inaccessible for this simple solution. Under these circumstances, *as the lesion cannot be palpated completely if at all by the finger, it must be presumed from the therapeutic point of view to be malignant and treated as such by radical operation*. The form which this operation should take will depend on the exact situation of the growth and other factors as discussed on p. 520, but it should be emphasized that many villous papillomas of the upper and middle rectum are eminently suitable for anterior resection with anastomosis. In this connection it is worth remembering that, in dealing with papillomas extending down into the middle part of the rectum, if the lower part of the tumour is soft and apparently benign (as determined by digital examination before operation and again by palpation from the outside of the bowel at operation), the distal margin of clearance of normal rectal wall beyond the lesion need only be 1–1·5 cm, instead of the 4–5 cm generally considered desirable in carcinoma cases (see p. 520). If anterior resection is considered impracticable, several other possibilities are available: the Parks' type of peranal excision combined with anterior resection and colonic 'pull-through' (see p. 350), ordinary abdomino-anal pull through resection (see p. 574), abdominosacral resection (see p. 584) or abdominoperineal excision with iliac colostomy (see p. 525).

VILLOUS TUMOURS LYING ENTIRELY WITHIN REACH OF THE FINGER

If on careful palpation of the entire growth any area of induration is detected, the lesion must be presumed malignant and radical excision advised. The precise form which this operation might take will depend largely on the level of the tumour. A sphincter-saving method such as anterior resection or abdominoanal or abdominosacral resection, might be possible, but in many cases an abdominoperineal excision with permanent iliac colostomy will be required. *If, on the other hand, the tumour is felt everywhere to be soft, it may be presumed tentatively benign* and treated in many instances by measures that aim at purely local removal, though occasionally the size of the lesion or the technical difficulties necessitate more radical procedures. It must be stressed, however, that *after any form of local or conservative excision a meticulous histological examination of the operative specimen is required to confirm the innocent nature of the growth*. The following methods of treatment are available for apparently benign villous papillomas of the lower rectum.

LOCAL EXCISION PER ANUM

Under general anaesthesia some villous tumours of the lower rectum can be delivered through the anus on an artificial pedicle of normal mucosa and treated by transfixion ligation and excision (Figs 249, 250). This is a very acceptable operation but unfortunately is not practicable with really large papillomas.

DIATHERMY TREATMENT

Generally diathermy snaring is only practicable for relatively small stalked papillomas, which can usually be more easily treated by local excision. More often because of the extent and sessile nature of these tumours reliance has to be placed on contact diathermy with a button electrode or diathermy forceps. But, using this method, it is a tedious and difficult procedure to destroy an extensive growth, and usually several sessions are required with check sigmoidoscopies three weeks or so after each diathermization to see how much of the tumour remains to be treated.

PERANAL EXCISION ALONE OR COMBINED WITH ANTERIOR RESECTION OF RECTUM AND COLONIC 'PULL THROUGH'

As an alternative to diathermy treatment Parks (1968) has suggested using a peranal technique for

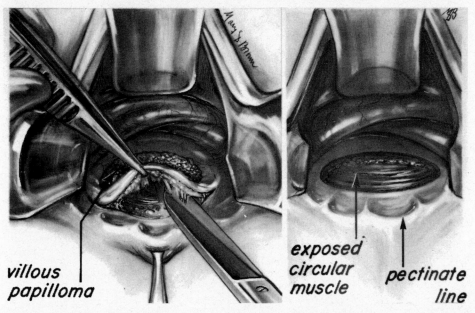

villous
papilloma

exposed
circular
muscle   pectinate
                        line

Fig. 257. (A) The tumour is elevated off the muscle coat. (B) The papilloma has been removed in one piece with a disc of mucosa, leaving exposed circular muscle.

excision of villous papillomas from the lower rectum. A bivalve anal speculum is inserted to open up the anal canal and explore the lower rectum and the tumour. Isotonic saline with or without adrenaline (1 part in 300 000) is injected into the readily distensible submucous layer of the rectal wall, lifting the tumour off the circular muscle coat. An incision is then made in the normal mucosa about 1 cm distal to the lower edge of the lesion, and, using scissors dissection, the tumour is elevated off the muscle coat (Fig. 257A). A small papilloma is removed in one piece with a disc of mucosa (Fig. 257B), but with large tumours, occupying, say, half the circumference of the rectum, it may be neces-

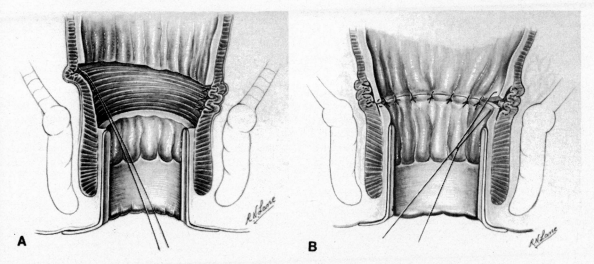

A   B

Fig. 258. Parks' method of dealing with circumferential raw area in rectal wall, following peranal excision of villous papilloma, by intramural suturing. (A) Through a trivalve anal speculum a close series of interrupted sutures of fine catgut or Dexon is placed in the muscle coat of the raw area. When tied they pucker it up. (B) It may even be possible to achieve mucosal apposition in some cases.

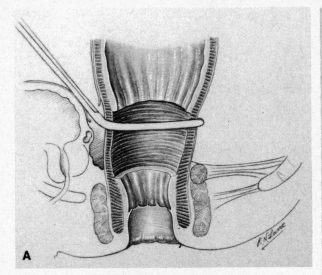

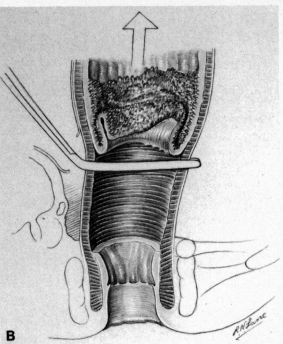

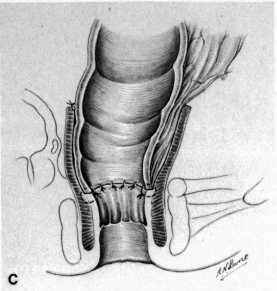

Fig. 259. Parks' abdominoperanal method of dealing with extensive circumferential villous papillomas of the rectum. Working from below through a bivalve anal speculum the papilloma is dissected off the underlying muscle coat either to the top of the lesion (A) or to at least 6 or 7 cm from the anal verge, the part separated being excised or pushed up into the upper rectum (B). Laparotomy is then performed and a low anterior resection carried out, the distal line of resection being taken to the top of the raw area thus created. The colon stump is passed through the denuded tube of rectum to be sutured below to the cut upper edge of anorectal mucosa (C).

sary to move the speculum round to expose a further portion of the lesion for excision as a separate piece. Even large bare areas of the rectal wall will heal with little trouble (as they do after diathermy destruction of big villous papillomas) and no suturing of the mucosa is necessary.

If the papilloma is very large and completely circumferential in its extent, the same tactic may be employed for its removal provided that the lesion is sufficiently accessible for an approach from below, but the consequence of so doing is that a complete segment of the lower rectum is denuded of its mucosal lining. To leave this raw area to heal spontaneously might well result in the formation of a

stricture, and to avoid this possibility it seems wise to attempt to reline the denuded segment. Parks and Stuart (1973) describe two techniques for so doing, the choice between them depending largely on the width of the gap between the cut edges of the mucosa.

Plication of the Raw Area by Intramural Sutures. Through a bivalve speculum a close series of interrupted sutures of 2/0 chromic catgut or polyglycolic acid (Dexon) is inserted into the exposed muscle coat of the rectal wall and tied in knots to plicate it and contract the raw area. These stitches are placed at intervals of 1–1.5 cm from above

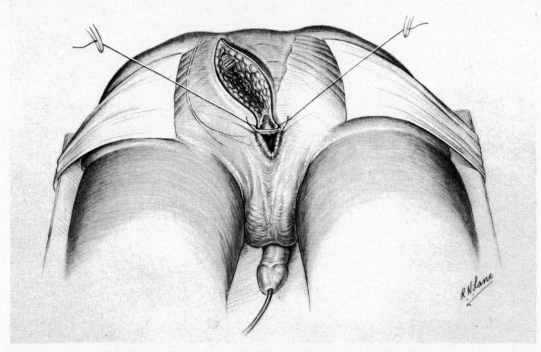

Fig. 260. The posterior transsphincteric (Mason) approach. The buttocks are retracted laterally with strapping. The incision runs from the posterior anal margin just to the left of the midline in a headward direction inclining slightly to the left to finish to the left of the coccyx over the lower margin of the gluteus maximus.

downwards and tied as they are inserted, the speculum being rotated round to expose the different sectors of the bowel in turn (Fig. 258A). Eventually, it may be possible to suture the upper and lower cut edges of mucosa, thus closing the denuded area completely, but, failing that, the mucosal edges should at least be considerably approximated, thus leaving a much narrower raw area. The final effect is to concertina the rectal wall somewhat as shown in Fig. 258B.

In my experience the peranal intrarectal suturing involved in this technique may be quite difficult to do, especially the higher up it takes place in the bowel. Accordingly, I think this method is only really suitable for relatively low lesions which are not too extensive in the long axis of the rectum.

Low Anterior Resection of the Rectum with Pull-through of the Colon Stump to Cover the Denuded Rectal Stump. If preoperative assessment of the lesion suggests that this more elaborate procedure, involving as it does a laparotomy, is likely to be required, the operation should be commenced with the patient in the modified lithotomy–Trendelenburg position (see p. 526). The circumferential villous papilloma has been removed, as already described, by submucosal dissection through the anal speculum from below—or at least dissected free from the underlying muscle coat to be level 6 or 7 cm from the anal verge. The abdomen is then opened, the rectum being fully mobilized and prepared for a low anterior resection, the distal line of the resection being carried across the bowel just below the top of the raw segment that was created in the lower rectum (Fig. 259A). Obviously if the growth had not been entirely separated at its upper end by the initial peranal dissection, the still-attached proximal part of the tumour, together with the freed lower portion delivered upwards with the lumen, is removed by the anterior resection (Fig. 259B). After thorough haemostasis in the anorectal stump, stay sutures are placed in the extreme lower end of the colon stump and passed through the anus for traction from below to draw the stump into the denuded muscle tube of rectum or anorectum down to the level of the lower cut edge of anorectal mucosa. The anal speculum is then reinserted into the anal canal and the lower end of the colon, and a circumferential row of 2/o polyglycolic acid sutures is inserted between the cut edges of the colon and

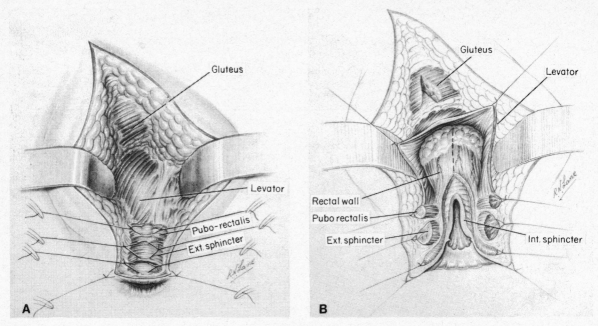

Fig. 261. The posterior transsphincteric approach. (A) The incision has been deepened to expose the external sphincter, levator and gluteus muscles. As the dissection proceeds the various structures exposed are marked by stay sutures on either side (as has been done in this illustration in regard to the external sphincter and puborectatis sling) before they are divided. (B) The external and internal sphincters and levator muscle have all been divided and the rectal wall is being cut in the midline.

the anorectal mucosa, a bite also being taken of the internal sphincter muscle with each suture. Working in the deep pelvis from inside the abdomen it is usually possible to pass a few stitches of 2/0 polyglycolic acid or 3/0 silk between the upper cut edge of the muscle tube of rectum and the serosal aspect of the colon stump as it passes through it. The final result of the pull-through is shown in Fig. 259c and further details about this type of coloanorectal anastomosis are given on pp. 581–4. To help safeguard the integrity of the anastomosis it is advisable to establish a covering right loop transverse colostomy at the end of the operation; it is retained for a few weeks. The new anorectum has two muscle coats and a colonic mucosal lining, and Parks (1968) claims that this technique of reconstruction yields satisfactory continence because, he believes, anorectal control depends on the sensory side, not on the rectal mucosa, but on nerve endings in the rectal muscle coat and perhaps also by the levator muscles (see also p. 34).

These are interesting and ingenious techniques, but depend for their efficient execution on a familiarity on the part of the surgeon with the method of intra-anal operation developed by Parks in connection with submucosal haemor-

rhoidectomy (p. 109). If the surgeon is not experienced in this approach to the anal canal and lower rectum, he will find it better to stick to other methods of dealing with villous papillomas. It is indeed difficult to see any great advantage in Parks' (1968) technique for small low papillomas, which can be easily dealt with by diathermy snaring or destruction or by delivery through the anus and ligature and excision. But for the expert colorectal surgeon dealing with extensive lesions which carpet virtually the whole circumference of the lower rectum, Parks' (1968) conservative type of peranal removal, combined with anterior resection and colonic 'pull through', is an attractive proposition, provided that one can feel confident that it has not undergone malignant change in its lower part, and this impression is confirmed by subsequent careful histological examination. As for the immediate results and subsequent continence I can only say that I have used this technique on five patients for large villous papillomas, with one temporary anastomotic leak, and all these patients had frequent urgent defaecation and some incontinence for flatus and faeces when the colostomy was at first closed, but after three or four months four of them developed pretty dependable continence.

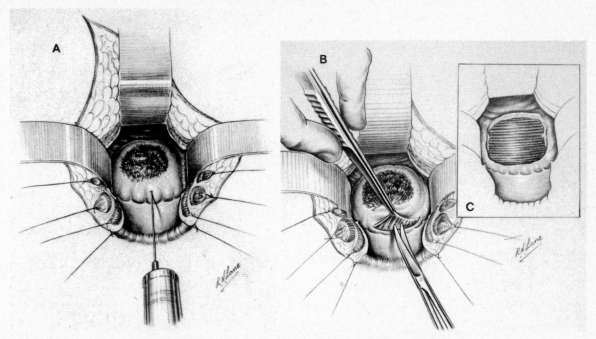

Fig. 262. The posterior transsphincteric approach. (A) Small sessile villous papilloma of the anterior rectal wall well exposed by this approach. Infiltration of the submucosa under the lesion with a weak adrenaline solution. (B) Dissecting the tumour off the underlying muscle coat with sharp pointed scissors. (C) The resulting raw area.

EXCISION BY POSTERIOR TRANSSPHINCTERIC
APPROACH

Another recent innovation designed to widen the scope of conservative surgery for these lesions has been the development by Mason (1970) of the posterior transsphincteric approach to the interior of the lower rectum—a method originally employed by Bevan (1917), but largely forgotten about till its recent revival. This technique, which involves complete division of the anal sphincters and puborectalis sling, may at first sight appear very destructive and likely to result in impairment of continence. But it is claimed that, if the sphincteric structures are accurately sutured, they heal well and normal anal control is retained.

For the performance of this operation the patient is placed prone on the operating table, which is slightly bent opposite the hips to produce a wide inverted V position (Figs 89, 260), the buttocks being strapped apart with adhesive plaster. The incision extends from the posterior margin of the anus just to the left of the midline obliquely upwards and to the left of the coccyx and lower sacrum (before making the incision it is an advantage to infiltrate the subcutaneous tissues with a dilute solution of adrenaline). The anatomical structures encoun-

tered as the incision is deepened into the anal canal and rectum are depicted in Fig. 261. The puborectalis–external sphincter complex presents as a large bundle of muscle, complete division of which is an essential step in obtaining adequate exposure. At a higher level, continuous with the puborectalis, is the levator ani sheet of muscle which has also to be divided to a variable extent. The fascia propria and muscle coats of the rectum are incised down to the submucous layer, the lower end of the circular muscle being noted to be thickened to form the internal sphincter. The main vessels in the submucosa should be controlled before the mucosa is divided. The exposure can be increased, if necessary, by dividing some of the lower fibres of the gluteus maximus muscle in the upper part of the wound, or further by excision of some or all of the coccyx. Meticulous haemostasis and the accurate marking of each layer, as it is divided, with stay sutures is essential, otherwise muscular structures retract and lose their characteristic appearances, making it difficult to identify them when the time comes for repair.

Using malleable copper retractors to hold the cut levator muscle and rectal wall aside the papilloma is brought clearly into view (Fig. 262A). If it is of relatively limited size, as in this illustration, it can be

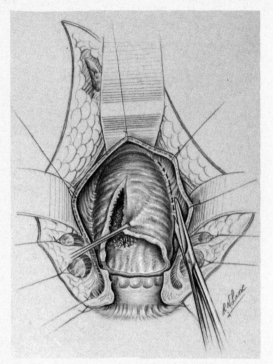

Fig. 263. The posterior transsphincteric approach. An extensive villous papilloma carpetting the lower rectum. After submucous infiltration with saline the mucosa has been divided below the tumour and the papilloma is being dissected off the entire circumference of the bowel leaving a large raw area surrounding the middle third or half of the rectum.

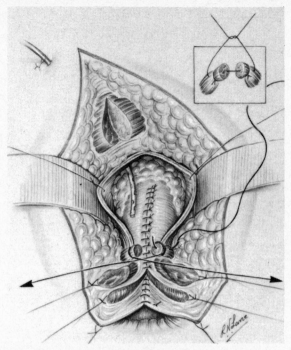

Fig. 264. The posterior transsphincteric approach: reconstitution of the rectal wall and the levator and sphincter musculature by suture. Note the sump suction drain to the perirectal space; I generally employ two.

conveniently removed employing a technique similar to that used by Parks in the peranal operation (p. 350), That is to say an infiltration with an adrenaline or saline solution is given into the submucosa underlying the tumour to 'float' it off the muscle coat. Then using slightly curved sharp-pointed Metzenbaum scissors the lesion can be dissected off in the submucous plane (Fig. 262B). If the resulting raw area is relatively small, it can sometimes be closed by suture, but often it has to be left open (Fig. 262C). With very extensive papillomas carpetting the lower rectum down to the pectinate line a much more time-consuming and tedious dissection is required to remove the lesion from the underlying muscle (Fig. 263) employing essentially the same principle as indicated in Fig. 262 but on a much grander scale. Because of the extent of the raw area produced by this operation, it is advisable to establish a temporary iliac colostomy at the conclusion of the operation—or as a preliminary procedure a week or so in advance if the size of the lesion suggests the necessity for it.

The wound is next closed in layers, using fine chromic catgut or polyglycolic acid (Dexon) throughout (Fig. 264). A continuous stitch is employed for the mucosa, interrupted sutures for the internal sphincter and muscle coat of the rectum together with the fascia propria. The levator ani, puborectalis sling and external sphincter are brought together by interrupted stitches of stronger catgut. The subcutaneous fat is approximated with fine catgut. The skin near the anus is closed with the same material, the rest of it with non-absorbable sutures. A suction drain is left down to the space in front of the coccyx for three or four days, and systemic antibiotic cover would seem a wise precaution during the immediate postoperative period. Mason (1970) had treated 10 cases of villous papilloma by this technique with no operative deaths, but with a certain amount of wound sepsis in several and a temporary faecal fistula in one. Eventually all healed satisfactorily and were said to have normal anal control. In my own experience of four cases submitted to this operation, three did well but one developed severe sepsis followed by incontinence and required a permanent colostomy.

This new technique is indeed a valuable addition to surgical resources in dealing with villous papillomas of the rectum (and also incidentally in the management of that therapeutically very difficult condition, prostatorectal fistula—see p. 194), but three points should be emphasized. Firstly, because this method is technically possible for lower rectal papillomas, it does not follow that they should all be treated by it. If such a lesion can be removed by diathermy snaring or fulgurized through a sigmoidoscope, or alternatively pulled down through the anus for ligation and excision, these older methods are, in my view, preferable, for they cause much less inconvenience to the patient and are likely to be followed by less postoperative morbidity. Secondly, if there are areas of induration in the papilloma on rectal palpation, indicating the development of malignant change, this method is no more suitable than any other technique of local excision in a fit subject, who ought to have an abdominoperineal (or other form of radical) excision of the rectum. Thirdly, it will be evident that for extensive villous papillomas of the extreme lower part of the rectum, which are deemed clinically to be benign (see p. 350). the methods of Mason and Parks are, as it were, in competition. One method divides and sutures the sphincters, the other forcibly stretches them during the insertion of the bivalve speculum. Which operation should be preferred will depend on the surgeon's personal inclination. Though I have used the Mason method, my own preference has generally lain with the Parks' technique.

ANTERIOR RESECTION, PULL-THROUGH
ABDOMINO-ANAL RESECTION,
ABDOMINOSACRAL RESECTION, SACRAL
RESECTION

As already indicated on p. 350, anterior resection has a most important role in the treatment of many villous papillomas of the upper or middle thirds of the rectum. Full technical details of this operation are given on p. 525, though a much lesser distal margin of clearance is acceptable when operating for a benign tumour. In other cases with still lower lesions, an abdomino-anal or abdomino-transanal resection (pp. 574, 577), abdominosacral resection (p. 584) or a purely sacral resection (p. 503) may be appropriate.

ABDOMINOPERINEAL EXCISION

For many really extensive villous tumours of the lower rectum a straightforward combined excision of the rectum will be found by some surgeons to be the simplest and most satisfactory treatment, and this will certainly apply if there is any doubt as to whether the lesion is still entirely benign.

RESULTS OF SURGICAL TREATMENT

As an indication of the relative use liable to be made in practice of the various methods of surgical treatment—and particularly of local removal or destruction versus bowel excision—it may be helpful to discuss my own experience in the management of 145 consecutive cases during a 30-year period up to 1977, which is partly described in Goligher and Graham (1967) and brought up to date in Table 17.

It will be seen that 70, or roughly half the cases, were treated by various forms of local removal. There were no operative deaths in this subgroup, but eight died later of intercurrent disease, nine required further local treatment for recurrence of the papilloma, and two developed a rectal carcinoma, requiring abdominoperineal excision.

Of the 74 patients who underwent a major bowel resection, it should be explained that 32 had malignant degeneration in their villous papillomas. It will be seen that the operation involved creation of a permanent colostomy in 17 cases. There was one operative death, and four patients died subsequently from intercurrent causes. Recurrent carcinoma developed in six cases, all of which ended fatally.

TABLE 17. *Primary Surgical Treatment of 145 Cases of Villous Papilloma*

Treatment	No. of cases
No treatment	1
(Discovery of villous papilloma after death from uraemia and electrolyte depletion)	
Local removal or destruction of papilloma	70
Snaring or fulguration by diathermy	39
Delivery through anus, ligation and excision	20
Peranal excision by Parks' technique	4
Transsphincteric excision by Mason's technique	4
Laparotomy, colotomy and polypectomy	3
Major Resection of Rectum or Colon	74
Left or transverse colectomy	2
Ordinary anterior resection	40
Anterior resection combined with Parks' pull-through manoeuvre	5
Turnbull–Cutait abdomino-anal resection	8
Abdominoperineal excision with ilial colostomy	19

Procedure to be Adopted in Cases with Apparently Benign Polyps Found after Local Excision to be Malignant

One of the most difficult problems that confronts a surgeon is when an apparently benign adenoma or villous papilloma has been removed by diathermy snare or other form of local excision and the pathologist reports that the lesion is in fact a carcinoma. If one could rely on the first evidence of 'recurrence' always being a local manifestation in the bowel wall, these cases might conceivably be treated expectantly in the first instance to see if the raw area remains unhealed (or closes temporarily, but subsequently breaks down to form an intractible ulcer), when it could be subjected to biopsy. Unfortunately the presence of lymphatic metastases is compatible with complete healing of the bowel wall after local removal, so that this simple solution would be unreliable, and it is essential to form some idea of the likelihood of such metastases occurring in any particular patient. Fortunately this subject has been carefully studied by a number of workers (Lockhart-Mummery and Dukes 1952; Fisher and Turnbull 1952; Grinnell and Lane 1958; Turnbull et al. 1961; Castleman and Krickstein 1962; Carden and Morson 1964; Morson et al. 1977) with the therapeutic problem specially in mind, and their researches make it clear that the surgeon can get good guidance from the pathological examination of the specimen.

1. Areas of cellular 'atypism' and of focal or intramucosal carcinoma can be completely disregarded, and no further operation is required.

2. If genuine invasive cancer is present the first point to be considered is its grade of malignancy. *High-grade carcinoma, however localized on section, carries a very poor prognosis, and probably the only prospect of cure lies with a radical excision which should be performed without further delay* (Lockhart-Mummery and Dukes 1953; Carden and Morson 1964; Bussey et al. 1977).

3. In dealing with the much commoner malignant polyps of average or low-grade malignancy, the decision whether to proceed to a radical operation depends chiefly on *whether the polyp has a pedicle or not and the extent to which the latter has been invaded by the growth*. The best insurance against local recurrence or lymphatic metastases after simple local removal would seem to be provided by the possession of a long stalk free from growth. If this state of affairs exists it can be assumed that the growth has been entirely removed and no further operation is required. On the other hand, if the stalk is exten-

sively invaded down virtually to the line of division, or the polyp is without a pedicle and the stroma is widely infiltrated, there is a distinct risk of local recurrence or of lymph node metastases being left unremoved if a formal radical excision is not performed. It is impossible to estimate the magnitude of this risk in any particular case, but Grinnell and Lane (1958) reckoned that, in general, the chances of lymphatic deposits being present in cases where the growth extends from the polyp down to the level of the adjacent bowel mucosa, were of the order of 14%.

4. Whilst the logical course is to recommend a radical excision to these latter patients, there may be good reasons in a few cases for refraining from taking this step. If the patient is generally unfit because of advanced age, obesity or bronchopulmonary or cardiovascular disease, such a radical operation might carry hazards greater than those of recurrence. Under these circumstances it may be preferable to accept the calculated risk of expectant management. An additional consideration, which is perhaps less valid in the eyes of the surgeon, but most compelling to the patient, is that with certain growths—namely those in the lower rectum— radical excision will mean sacrifice of the sphincter

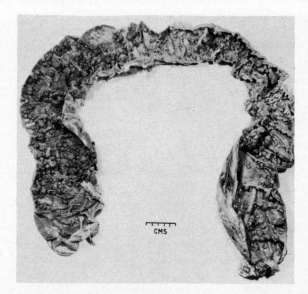

Fig. 265. The colon and rectum obtained by complete proctocolectomy in a girl of 19 with familial polyposis. A frank polypoid carcinoma was present in the sigmoid; one of the polyps in the rectum was found on biopsy to contain histological evidence of invasive carcinoma, and for that reason colectomy and ileorectal anastomosis was not performed. This patient died of recurrence 2½ years after operation.

apparatus and a permanent colostomy. In such cases the patient's reluctance to accept an artificial anus may be an additional serious obstacle in advising radical operation. As a consolation, it may be noted that it is with growths in this situation that further local operative treatment in the form of diathermy coagulation to the rectal wall can be practised, for what it is worth. Obviously this measure would not influence the course of lymphatic metastases already present, but it might lessen the risk of local recurrence in the bowel wall. After all it is a method of treatment that has been widely used in some centres for frank, early rectal carcinomas in unfit subjects, and has been shown sometimes to produce remarkably good results (p. 516).

FAMILIAL POLYPOSIS

Familial intestinal polyposis is a hereditary disease characterized by the development within the colon and rectum of large numbers of adenomatous tumours. The hereditary nature of the condition was first recognized by Cripps (1882), and it was J. P. Lockhart-Mummary (1925) who drew attention to the heavy predisposition to the development of carcinoma of the large intestine that exists in patients affected by familial polyposis. The subse-

quent monumental studies of Dukes (1952a, b, 1958) and others have served to emphasize the appalling magnitude of this risk. It is probably correct to say that polyposis is the most clearly defined pre-cancerous disease known in medicine.

Pathology

Intestinal polyposis consists in the formation of innumerable sessile and pedunculated adenomas throughout the large intestine. They may be uniformly distributed from caecum to anal canal, or may be more numerous in one part of the bowel than another; if anything the incidence is greater in the left colon and rectum than elsewhere. The polyps vary in size and shape (Figs 265–7). The smallest, when examined microscopically, appear as patches of epithelial hyperplasia. Larger lesions, worthy of being described as polyps, have the histological structure of adenomas. All the tumours are at first non-malignant and most of them remain so,

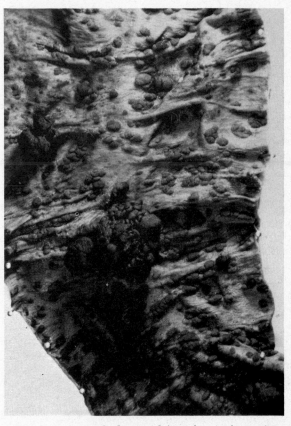

Fig. 267. 'Close up' of some of the polyps in the specimen shown in Fig. 266.

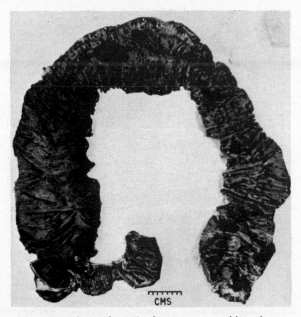

Fig. 266. Colon and proximal rectum removed by colectomy and ileorectal anastomosis in a boy of 17 with familial polyposis. None of the polyps examined showed signs of malignancy.

but after an interval of a few months or several years carcinoma develops in one or more sites, though whether they arise in pre-existing adenomas or in adjacent mucosa is uncertain. The onset of malignancy in an adenoma is said to be indicated by an increase in size of the polyp, by its acquiring a darker colour and a firmer consistency, and later by the occurrence of frank ulceration.

It has generally been held that the polyps in familial polyposis coli are restricted to the colon and rectum (Dukes 1952a; Morson 1969), but several cases of this condition have been reported more recently, in which polyps were also present in the small intestine, stomach or duodenum (Hoffmann and Goligher 1971; Utsunomiya et al. 1974). Clearly, unless the upper gastrointestinal tract is specially studied by radiological and endoscopic examination in patients with polyposis coli, these other lesions are unlikely to be discovered, and it seems likely that the failure to note the coexistence of gastric, duodenal and small intestinal polyposis in the past may often have been due to the fact that these special investigations were not undertaken.

Symptoms

Polyps are usually present for a number of years without causing any complaint. As a rule the disease does not manifest itself till later childhood or early adult life. The initial symptoms are extremely mild and consist of only slight looseness and frequency of the motions, which is readily ignored by the patient or dismissed as an individual peculiarity requiring no treatment. It is only when the diarrhoea increases in severity and is accompanied by a profuse discharge of mucus and some blood that it begins to interfere with the patient's daily life and can no longer be disregarded. Unfortunately by this time malignant change has often occurred; thus Waugh et al. (1964) have reported that of 86 patients coming to colectomy for polyposis at the Mayo Clinic 32.5% had developed invasive carcinoma of the colon.

In certain patients with polyposis there may be associated multiple sebaceous or dermoid cysts, bony exostoses or connective tissue tumours as pointed out by Gardner (1951), Gardner and Plenk (1952), Gardner and Richards (1953), Oldfield (1954), Weiner and Cooper (1955) and Dunning and Ibrahim (1965). This combination is now generally referred to as Gardner's syndrome, and it has been estimated by Waugh et al. (1964) that approximately 10% of sufferers from polyposis coli manifest this syndrome. Lockhart-Mummery (1967) put the incidence at 16.4% in 140 cases of polyposis at St Mark's Hospital. The osteomas have usually occurred in the cranial bones or mandible, but cortical thickening of a long bone has also been reported by Dunning and Ibrahim (1965), and was noted recently in a patient with Gardner's syndrome coming under my care. So far as can be gathered from the literature, though the dermoid cysts, subcutaneous fibrous tumours and osteomas are inherited as are the intestinal polyps, unlike the latter they do not appear prone to undergo malignant change. But malignant tumours of the central nervous system (Turcot et al. 1959) and primary sarcomas of bone (Hoffmann and Brooke 1970) have been described in association with polyposis coli. As the associated lesions in Gardner's syndrome may appear before the development of the polyposis, or at any rate before the occurrence of symptoms referable to them, they have a considerable diagnostic significance. When multiple soft or hard tissue tumours are encountered in clinical practice, the patient should always be examined—by sigmoidoscopy, etc.—to exclude polyposis of the rectum and colon (Laberge et al. 1957).

Utsunomiya and Nakamura (1975) have drawn attention to the quite frequent occurrence of localized radio-opacities on panoramic X-ray examination of the mandible (or rarely the maxilla) in patients with familial polyposis (Fig. 268). They found such opacities, of a size varying from 3 to 10 mm in diameter and either single or multiple, in no less than 93% of a series of patients with this disease; by contrast they were noted in only 16% of the members of polyposis families who were free of polyps and in only 6% of a normal control population. In the mandible the lesions were located mostly in the teeth-bearing part and never in the ramus, many being found near the dental apices but never fused with them. Utsunomiya and Nakamura (1975) consider that the finding of these localized radio-opacities on panoramic X-ray study is a useful aid in the detection of the polyposis carrier in the familial polyposis family, for they have often been able by this means to predict the presence of polyposis before rectal examination.

Another type of connective tissue lesion occasionally found with familial polyposis coli is desmoid tumour, of which we have given a full survey of the literature (McAdam and Goligher 1970). Most desmoids have arisen in the abdominal wall at the site of the laparotomy wound for the colectomy (Fig. 269), but some have arisen in other abdominal wounds (e.g. cholecystectomy), and a few have

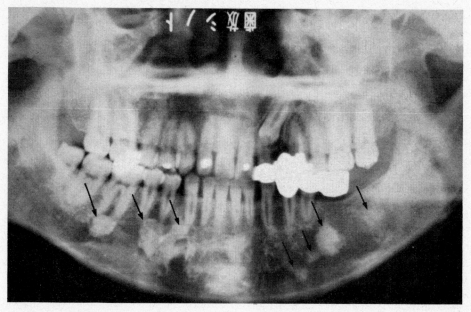

Fig. 268. Panoramic X-ray plate of the mandible of a patient suffering from familial polyposis, showing mutiple radio-opacities distributed in the body of the bone; an impacted canine tooth is also revealed. (*From Utsunomiya and Nakamura 1975*)

followed pregnancy or have occurred entirely spontaneously. In a certain number of cases fibrous lesions, of similar histological structure to that of classical desmoids, have developed inside the abdomen, either in the mesentery of the small bowel or in the retroperitoneal tissues. A few desmoids have also been described arising elsewhere than in the abdominal parietes or cavity. Weary et al. (1964) reckon that desmoids account for 45% of fibrous tissue neoplasms in Gardner's syndrome. Smith (1959) surveyed 150 cases of familial polyposis, who had undergone operation a long enough time previously for desmoids to form, and found that 3·5% developed these tumours, a much higher incidence of desmoids than is seen after other abdominal operations. In fact desmoids are so rare, except in patients who have polyposis coli, it is reasonable to suggest that the finding of a desmoid tumour (e.g. in an appendicectomy or cholecystectomy wound) in any patients, who is not already known to suffer from this disease, should lead to examination of the large bowel for evidence of this condition.

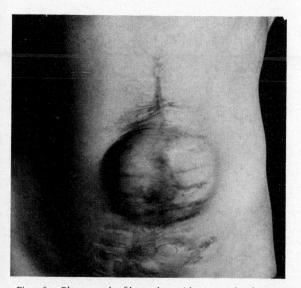

Fig. 269. Photograph of large desmoid tumour developing in the scar of the colectomy incision in patient operated on for multiple polyposis. The tumour was excised, but the patient subsequently developed an intra-abdominal desmoid, from which he eventually died 8 years later.

Diagnosis

The history of slight persistent or recurrent diarrhoea in a young subject without at first any impairment of general health is very suggestive of polyposis, especially if it emerges on questioning that a patient, or an aunt or uncle or other member of the family has succumbed to a bowel complaint. A mild, mainly distal, non-specific, proctocolitis, which is not uncommon in adolescents or young adults, can produce similar symptoms, but there is usually more bleeding in this condition. *The essential step in establishing the diagnosis is rectal examination and particularly sigmoidoscopy.* In polyposis the adenomas can be felt extending down into the lower rectum. Sigmoidoscopy shows the polyps, the intervening rectal and colonic mucosa being perfectly normal with a good vessel pattern and no contact bleeding. In proctocolitis, in which inflammatory polyps may occur due to hypertrophy of the remnants of mucosa surviving between the areas of ulceration, the polyps seldom affect the bowel farther distally than the rectosigmoid junction. Consequently if polyps can be felt on rectal examination they are almost certainly true adenomas of familial polyposis. On sigmoidoscopy in proctocolitis the rectal mucosa shows the absence of vascular pattern, the granularity and the tendency to bleed on contact which are characteristic of this condition, and it may be noted that there is pus or mucopus in the lumen as well as blood. At a higher level inflammatory polyps may possibly be observed.

A barium enema examination will usually confirm the diagnosis of polyposis though good radiological technique is required. In typical cases a striking picture is obtained particularly after evacuation of the barium and its replacement by air. The innumerable polyps are clearly outlined, and it is important to note that they occur in a colon of good calibre and normal haustration (Fig. 270). In ulcerative colitis, on the other hand, though non-adenomatous polyps may produce a rather similar appearance, the colon itself shows contraction, lack of haustration and other radiological signs of colitis, so that there is no difficulty as a rule in making a distinction (see Fig. 526). I would emphasize again that the diagnosis should already have been made on the basis of rectal and sigmoidoscopic examination before proceeding to barium enema, and that if polyps have not been demonstrated on endoscopy the condition is most unlikely to be one of familial polyposis, for in this disease the rectum is apparently virtually always affected to a greater or lesser degree—though Moertel et al. (1970) describe a number of cases of polyposis, mostly non-familial however, without rectal involvement. If what appear to be polyps are shown on radiological examination despite a negative sigmoidoscopy, it should be suspected that they are faecal masses and the barium enema should be repeated after further preparation.

Notwithstanding these disparaging remarks, radiological examination of the colon should always be undertaken in cases of polyposis because

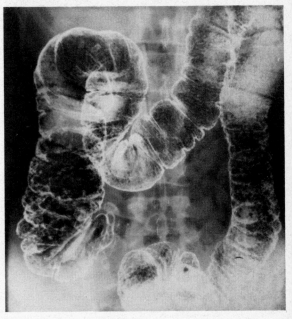

Fig. 270. X-ray plate after evacuation of barium enema and replacement with air in a case of familial polyposis. The numerous small polyps are clearly seen.

it may reveal the presence of one or more frank carcinomas in addition to the polyps, and this might affect the plan of treatment. Unfortunately a malignant growth among the welter of benign tumours is easily missed by the radiologist, for it may have the macroscopic structure of a large benign polyp in the first instance. Other indications that a carcinoma may have developed are provided by a recent increase in the severity of the diarrhoea, and the occurrence of more severe bleeding. Colonoscopy and biopsy of larger polyps may be informative.

Natural History

Our understanding of the natural history of familial polyposis has been greatly clarified by the comprehensive researches of Dukes (1952a, b, 1958) into the course of the disease in 57 polyposis families comprising some 700 members. For the more detailed genetical consideration of the subject reference should be made particularly to his paper in the *Annals of Eugenics* (1952a). It suffices for clinical purposes to summarize his main conclusions as follows:

1. Familial polyposis is a hereditary disease which is transmitted in accordance with Mendelian laws and follows the pattern of inheritance of a dominant gene.

2. It affects males and females equally and either may transmit the disease.

3. In most polyposis families *only half the children* are likely to inherit the abnormality, the remainder being normal.

4. As a rule *only those who have developed polyposis can transmit* it to the next generation.

5. There is a lack of accurate information as to *the time of first appearance of the polyps* in affected individuals, for sigmoidoscopy is not usually practised till symptoms occur to bring the patient to the surgeon, or till about puberty in asymptomatic relatives being investigated for evidence of the disease. The colon and rectum are apparently normal at birth, and it seems that the polyps usually develop during childhood, probably about the time of puberty.

6. The average *age at the onset of symptoms* of polyposis in Dukes' (1952b) series was 20 years. It was rare for symptoms to occur before the age of 10 and *exceptionally rare for them to develop for the first time after the age of 40.*

7. *Cancer* was diagnosed most frequently about 15 years after the commencement of symptoms of polyposis, that is to say on the average at about 35 years of age, though there were many patients in whom it became evident at an earlier age. There were a few in whom it did not appear at all, either because they died of intercurrent disease or, more rarely, because their disease seemed to run a specially benign course.

8. The average *age of death* of polyposis patients was 41·6 years. This is 26·3 years younger than the average age of death from rectal cancer in England and Wales in 1948, which was 67·7 years.

9. Occasionally only one member of a family is affected by polyposis. Dukes prefers to regard this condition as one of familial polyposis with an exceptionally low degree of 'penetrance' of the dominant gene, rather than as a separate form of non-familial polyposis.

Treatment

The management of familial polyposis resolves itself into two problems—the treatment of the individual patient, and the investigation and care of the family to which he belongs.

TREATMENT OF THE POLYPOSIS PATIENT

From the pathological point of view the ideal treatment for a patient with polyposis would be to remove the mucosa of the entire large intestine by performing a *total colectomy and excision of the rectum*, but this treatment would suffer the disadvantage of entailing the establishment of a permanent ileostomy. Now, an ileostomy may be fairly readily accepted by a patient with ulcerative colitis who has suffered severely from this disease, but it is a rather different proposition for a polyposis patient, who is often in excellent general health and has had only relatively slight bowel symptoms—or may indeed be entirely symptomless as when the condition has been discovered on routine examination of the members of a polyposis family.

It is for this reason that until recently, the great majority of surgeons have favoured the alternative less drastic procedure of *colectomy with preservation of the rectum and ileorectal or ileosigmoid anastomosis*. The polyps in the rectal stump are destroyed before or after the operation by diathermy applied through the sigmoidoscope. (Very occasionally such rectal polyps may undergo spontaneous disappearance after colectomy and ileorectal anastomosis, as pointed out by Hubbard (1957), Dukes (1958), Turnbull (1958), Dunphy (1959), Cole and Holden (1959), Localio (1962) and Waugh et al. (1964). It is perhaps wiser, therefore, to postpone diathermy treatment of these lesions till some months after the colectomy, in the hope that such regression may occur, but I must admit that this hope has seldom been realized in my patients, or, if the polyps did become smaller or disappear for a time, they ultimately recurred as a rule*). An essential item in the after-care of patients, following this plan of management with colectomy and ileorectal anastomosis for polyposis coli, has been regular repeat sigmoidoscopies every six months or so to detect any further polyps and destroy them by diathermy fulguration, on the hypothesis that any carcinoma arising in the rectum will probably originate in one of these polyps, so that, if they are promptly eliminated the subsequent development of rectal cancer can be prevented. However, it is by no means certain that rectal carcinoma in these cases

* De Cosse et al. (1975) have reported regression of adenomas in the rectal stumps of five of eight patients with familial polyposis following prolonged oral administration of slow-release capsules of ascorbic acid, but these results would need to be confirmed before accepting this regimen as an established method of treatment.

always commences in a polyp and may not spring de novo from an area of apparently normal mucosa. It must also be granted that, even if the polyp-to-cancer sequence does hold good, a polyp might develop and subsequently degenerate into a wide-spreading carcinoma all within the space of the few months that elapse between two consecutive sigmoidoscopic reviews.

When we turn from these theoretical misgivings regarding the adequacy of the protection against cancer afforded by colectomy and ileorectal anastomosis, followed by sigmoidoscopic supervision of the rectal stump with diathermy treatment of rectal polyps as required, to the results obtained by this regimen in actual practice, we encounter a conflict of evidence (Table 18). The findings at St Mark's Hospital, London, where colectomy and ileorectal anastomosis has long been the favourite procedure for familial polyposis, suggested that it is a fairly reliable operation, for, of 73 cases observed for up to 21 years (average 10·5 years) after this operation, only three (4%) developed rectal cancers (Bussey 1970), all of which were found on excision of the rectum to be Dukes' A lesions. By contrast, the results reported by some other authors, such as Everson and Allen (1954), Flotte et al. (1956) and Moertel et al. (1970), are a good deal less satisfactory, with incidences of subsequent rectal carcinoma ranging from 9 to 23%. Particularly significant, perhaps, is the experience of the Mayo Clinic, for in an earlier paper from there by Waugh et al. (1964) the frequency of rectal cancer in 46 patients followed-up was 4%, but in a recent more comprehensive study by Moertel et al. (1970), which comprises 143 patients, the incidence of rectal cancer was found to have arisen to 23%. (It is emphasized that these patients were submitted to regular sigmoidoscopic reviews and fulguration of rectal polyps as required, but a crucial point is how thoroughly this was done. Presumably not all the patients returned to Rochester every six months for

these examinations to be conducted by their original surgeon, which is the practice of St Mark's Hospital, London.) An important factor influencing the frequency of carcinoma seemed to be the length of the follow-up, for at 15 years the incidence was 25% and at 23 years over 50% (Fig. 271). Moertel et al. (1970) compared the incidence of rectal cancer during the 1785 years of follow-up in their series of cases with the age-specific rates of occurrence of this growth in the general population, as deduced from the records of the Connecticut and Alameda County tumour registries, and found that the ratio of observed rectal cancers in their study to those recorded in the registries was 94:1 and 100:1 respectively. Using the same comparative data they showed that the sex of the patient exercises a profound influence on the risk of cancer in their patients, for women appeared to be exposed to a five-fold increase in risk compared with men. The presence of carcinoma in the resected colon was also associated with a significantly increased risk of carcinoma occurring later in the retained rectum. The number of polyps in the rectum at the initial diagnosis of polyposis had a bearing, too, on the frequency of subsequent carcinoma, which was considerably reduced if there were less than 20 polyps in the rectum compared with over 100. One final point brought out by Moertel et al. (1970) is the extremely poor outlook for patients in whom rectal carcinoma develops. Only six of their 25 patients with rectal cancer who had proceeded to a five-year follow-up were still alive without evidence of malignant disease.

TABLE 18. *Incidence of Carcinoma of Rectum following Colectomy and Ileorectal Anastomosis for Polyposis of Large Intestine including Rectum*

Author	No. of patients treated	Patients who developed carcinoma of rectum	
Everson and Allen (1954)	122	11	(9%)
Flotte et al. (1956)	21	3	(14%)
Waugh et al. (1964)	46	2	(4%)
Bussey (1970)	73	3	(4%)
Moertel et al. (1970)	143	31	(23%)

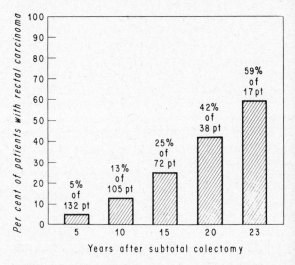

Fig. 271. Rising incidence of rectal carcinoma with increasing length of follow-up after colectomy and ileorectal anastomosis for polyposis coli. (*From Moertel et al. 1970*)

The practical implication of this study by Moertel et al. (1970) is that it casts grave doubt on the justifiability of recommending colectomy and ileorectal anastomosis with subsequent fulguration of rectal polyps for polyposis coli, and suggests that instead the standard operation should be a complete proctocolectomy with ileostomy, as for ulcerative colitis (see p. 734). It seems to me, however, that the very reassuring results reported from St Mark's Hospital for colectomy and ileorectal anastomosis are probably more relevant for those of us who practice in Britain, and so I still employ this operation as my standard treatment for familial polyposis. But surgeons practising in America may feel that the experiences of Moertel et al. (1970) are a more reliable index as to what is likely to happen to their patients and may therefore favour a complete proctocolectomy and ileostomy as the procedure of choice for most patients with familial polyposis. But even if this policy is adopted it must be acknowledged that, for the reasons mentioned on p. 363, a certain number of patients with asymptomatic or virtually symptomless polyposis will adamantly refuse an operation involving an ileostomy, and for them a colectomy and ileorectal anastomosis will still have to be employed. It must be accepted too that complete proctocolectomy carries some risk of damaging the pelvic autonomic nerves and thereby impairing sexual function in men—a danger that does not apply, at any rate to the same extent, to colectomy and ileal anastomosis to the upper rectum. It might be judicious, therefore, to consider using the latter operation in male adolescent patients and young men, at least as a temporary measure for eight to ten years until a family has been established, particularly when the number of polyps in the rectum is very small (less than 20) and where no carcinoma has already developed in the colon at the time of operation.

I suppose another operation that ought to be mentioned is a colectomy with mucosal proctectomy and ileo-anal pull-through anastomosis—the Ravitch operation—in view of some recent reports recording better functional results with it then had previously been obtained (see p. 738). But for a while it will certainly still be *sub judice*.

AGE AT WHICH PROCTOCOLECTOMY OR COLECTOMY SHOULD BE UNDERTAKEN

The average age of onset of symptoms of the disease is about 20 years, and the average age at which carcinoma is detected is 35. Cases are on record, however, in which malignant changes took place at the age of 20 or in the late teens. It would seem desirable therefore to carry out operation before this age, say about 14 or 15.

THE AMOUNT OF DISTAL LARGE BOWEL THAT SHOULD BE RETAINED IN A COLECTOMY AND ILEORECTAL ANASTOMOSIS

The less the amount of rectum retained, the less will be the area of potentially malignant large bowel mucosa to be supervised postoperatively. However, for a really good functional result it is necessary to retain not only the anal sphincters and some of the sensitive rectal mucosa to ensure normal continence, but also a good deal of the rectal segment to provide a faecal reservoir and avoid too frequent motions. At sigmoidoscopy a level of 12–14 cm from the anal verge, which means just below the rectosigmoid junction, is a satisfactory compromise and also makes for a technically easy anastomosis.

TECHNIQUE OF COLECTOMY AND ILEORECTAL ANASTOMOSIS

The technical details of colectomy are described on p. 748 in connection with ulcerative colitis, and only a few comments are required here. Through a long left paramedian incision the colon is completely

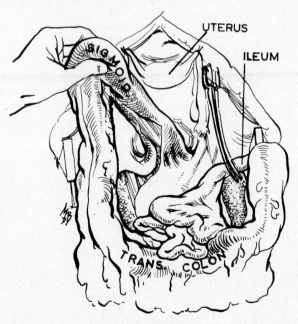

Fig. 272. Colectomy and ileorectal anastomosis: mobilization of colon completed. View obtained by surgeon on the left side of the patient and looking towards the pelvis.

mobilized from the ileocaecal junction to the lower sigmoid (Fig. 272). With the patient in a Trendelenburg tilt attention is then turned to preparing for the anastomosis. There terminal ileum is divided between two Parker-Kerr clamps applied slightly obliquely across the bowel 7–10 cm from the caecum. It will then usually be found that the distance from the mesentery to the resulting ileal stump is sufficient to allow the end of the ileum to stretch to the upper part of the rectum without tension. In a few cases it may be necessary to divide the mesentery slightly, possibly sacrificing one of the ileal arteries, in order to free the bowel sufficiently, or it may be found that a better place to divide the ileum in the first instance is 12–15 cm more proximally where the bowel is normally more dependent and the mesentery longer.

The freeing of the colon has proceeded to the lower sigmoid. The further mobilization down to the upper rectum may be carried out as in a high anterior resection for carcinoma of the lower sigmoid or rectosigmoid junction with division of the inferior mesenteric vessels above and, after mobilization of the bowel from the front of the sacrum, division of the superior haemorrhoidal vessels below on the back of the rectum (see p. 574). However, in the average polyposis case it is not necessary to sacrifice the main vessels in this way. Instead they may be preserved and the sigmoid branches divided between the inferior mesenteric and superior haemorrhoidal vessels behind and the sigmoid and rectosigmoid in front. This method is a little more tedious than the other technique but it is usually possible to free the bowel down to the upper rectum in this way without too much difficulty. The main superior haemorrhoidal supply to the rectal stump is thus preserved; an additional advantage is that the presacral nerve, which is specially important in younger male patients in regard to subsequent sexual function, is not exposed to injury.

The actual anastomosis has usually been conducted by me *end-to-end*, exactly as in an anterior resection except that it is an ileal stump instead of a sigmoid one that is being united to the rectum (see p. 574). The upper rectum is clamped with a Parker–Kerr forceps in the sagittal plane with the handles of the forceps lying anteriorly. The clamped ileal stump is then drawn to the left side of the rectum and a series of silk Lembert stitches inserted

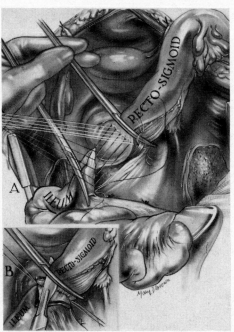

Fig. 273. End-to-end ileorectal anastomosis. (A) Insertion of row of Lembert sutures between ileal and rectal stumps. (B) Sutures tied approximating the ileum and rectum. Note that the lumen of the ileum is enlarged by cutting the bowel for 2–2·5 cm along its antimesenteric border.

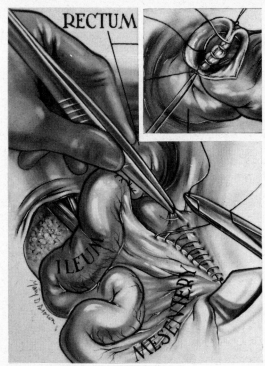

Fig. 274. First half of through-and-through suture inserted. *Inset:* Completed anastomosis, gap between the cut edge of ileal mesentery and posterior parietal peritoneum being closed by a running stitch.

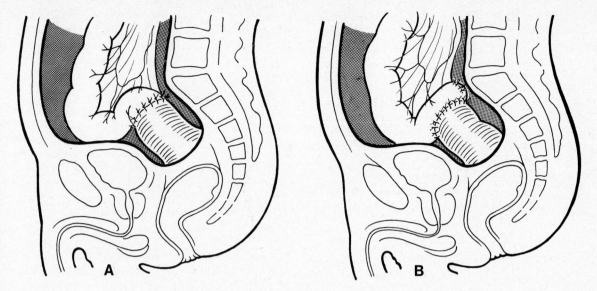

Fig. 275. Ileorectal anastomosis. (A) End-to-end. (B) Side-to-end.

and left untied till all have been placed (Fig. 273A). Next the ileal stump is slid down on these suture to make contact with the rectum and the silks are tied, the tails of the first and last being retained as stays. Thereafter the clamps are excised which, in the case of the rectal stump, means removal of the entire colectomy specimen (Fig. 273B). A continuous through-and-through catgut suture is then employed to unite the open ends of ileum and rectum, it usually being necessary beforehand to enlarge the ileal lumen by dividing the bowel for 2–2.5 cm along the antimesenteric border (Fig. 274, inset). The anastomosis is completed by the insertion of a row of silk Lembert sutures on the right side. A gap will now be found to exist between the cut edge of the ileal mesentery and the posterior parietal peritoneum, and this is closed by a running fine catgut stitch, the utmost care being taken to avoid pricking vessels in the mesentery (Fig. 274). A corrugated rubber drain or suction drain is left down to the site of the anastomosis and the abdominal wound is closed in layers. A diagrammatic representation of the complete end-to-end ileorectal anastomosis is shown in Fig. 275A.

But sometimes the lower ileum seems to lie more conveniently for a *side-to-end* anastomosis with the top of the rectal stump (Fig. 275). Under these circumstances I have not hesitated to employ this alternative technique. The open end of the ileum can be closed by several methods, but I have usually adopted the type of suturing shown in Figs 484 and 485 for closure of the open end of the rectum in doing a Hartmann's operation. Next the limits of the segment of the antimesenteric border of the ileal loop, 2–2.5 cm from the extreme end of the bowel, to be selected for the side-to-end ileorectal anastomosis, are marked with two Allis forceps. Whilst the ileal stump is held 12–15 cm from the clamped rectal stump, a row of 3/0 silk Lembert sutures is inserted between the ileum 0.5 cm behind the antimesenteric border and the left side of the rectal wall a similar distance below the sagitally placed clamp. These are left loose till all have been inserted and are then tied and cut except for the first and last, the tails of which are left long as stays. The ileum is then opened by a longitudinal diathermy incision along the selected portion of the antimesenteric border and the rectum is divided across with a scalpel immediately below the Parker–Kerr clamp, the blade actually cutting on the clamp itself. Thereafter the anastomosis is continued with a continuous suture of 3/0 chromic catgut or Dexon around the entire cut edges of bowel, and a row of interrupted 3/0 silk Lembert sutures on the right lateral side. Finally the mesenteric gap is closed and drainage established as with the end-to-end technique of anastomosis.

The *postoperative care* raises no special problems as a rule. The drain is retained for six or seven days in cases of leakage. The bowels may not act for 24 or 36 hours after the operation, then the motions are very liquid and frequent for a few days, but usually within a fortnight the frequency has reduced to six or seven motions in the day and one or two at night.

During the next two or three months further improvement takes place and the final functional state is three or four motions daily and one or none at night; continence is usually perfect throughout, though there may be a little uncertainty of control when the diarrhoea is at its height.

It is clear from the report of Moertel et al. (1970) on the immediate results of 203 colectomy and ileo-rectal anastomosis operations for polyposis that this procedure carries quite a few risks, for there was an operative mortality of 8% and a non-fatal complication rate of 13% in that series. Intestinal obstruction is a particularly common complication, as Lockhart-Mummery (1967) also emphasizes.

THE ALTERNATIVE OF SUBTOTAL COLECTOMY WITH CAECORECTAL ANASTOMOSIS

In doing a subtotal colectomy for polyposis it has been suggested by Lillehei and Wangensteen (1955) that the caecum should be retained in order to conserve the entire terminal ileum and the ileocaecal valve, and intestinal continuity should be restored by a caecorectal anastomosis. Rosi and Cahill (1962) describe the technical aspects of this operation in detail. The ascending colon is divided between clamps 3 cm above the ileocaecal junction and the caecal segment is then rotated through 180° in an anticlockwise direction as seen from the front, so that its clamped upper edge becomes inferior and the fundus uppermost, the ileum now entering the caecum from the right side. Thereafter it is a simple matter to construct an anastomosis between the cut under edge of the caecum and the top of the rectal stump, using whatever technique of suture the surgeon prefers. In 15 cases given caecorectal anastomoses by Rosi and Cahill (1962) the functional results were claimed to be excellent with most patients having only one or occasionally two formed stools per day.

I must confess that I have had little personal experience of caecorectal anastomosis and am indeed surprised that this technique of subtotal colectomy has found so little surgical favour to date, for there certainly is a good *a priori* argument on the grounds of function for its use. Incidentally, it should be a relatively simple matter to keep the retained caecum with its potentiality for producing further polyps under regular supervision by passing the sigmoidoscope through the anastomosis at the periodic sigmoidoscopic examinations which are a regular feature of the subsequent management of polyposis patients after operations retaining a rectal stump. Any polyps remaining in the caecum at the time of operation or subsequently developing there could presumably be easily dealt with by diathermy snaring or fulguration in the same way as are those occurring in the rectal stump.

TECHNIQUE OF SIGMOIDOSCOPIC FULGURATION OF RECTAL POLYPS

The equipment and general technique for rectal fulguration has been described on p. 341. In their application to cases of polyposis a few special points arise. Because of the extensive nature of the fulguration required and the resulting ulceration in cases of polyposis, it is very easy to produce strictures which may prejudice the usefulness of the rectal stump for an anastomosis. It is wise therefore to split the diathermy treatment into several sessions and to err in the direction of doing too little rather than too much on any one occasion. It is best to proceed from above downwards in the process of clearing the rectum, otherwise rigidity and narrowing of the fulgurized lower rectum at subsequent sessions may prevent the large sigmoidoscope from reaching the upper rectum to deal with remaining polyps. These sigmoidoscopic treatments are tedious and and may take up to 45–60 minutes on each occasion.

Postoperatively there may be some lower abdominal tenderness, a slight pyrexia, and aggravation of the diarrhoea with passage of a little muco-pus and blood for a few days due to the reactionary proctitis.

TREATMENT AND PROGNOSIS OF THE OTHER COMPONENTS OF GARDNER'S SYNDROME

Dermoid or Sebaceous Cysts. These are a considerable nuisance to the patient. For one thing, they constitute a major disfigurement on the exposed parts of the body. But even if a patient is prepared to overlook the blemish to his appearance—which is not easy to do, as the cysts may be very numerous on the face, scalp, neck and arms and legs—he has to endure the frequent, painful superadded attacks of sepsis that are apt to occur. Consequently operative excision of these lesions is often requested, not so much for cosmetic reasons, as for prophylaxis against further infection. Unfortunately, fresh cysts develop all the time. One of my patients regularly undergoes wholesale removal of 20 or 30 cysts under general anaesthesia every 12 months or so!

Osteomas. As these tumours occur usually on the mandible, they soon draw attention to themselves by their unsightliness, which may be a beneficial effect, in that it may lead to diagnosis of the previously unsuspected polyposis coli, as happened in one patient referred to me by a dental colleague! In this case the very hard exostoses were very conveniently removed, after suitable surgical exposure, by dental drills, with a very good cosmetic result.

Desmoids. The treatment of choice for *desmoids of the abdominal wall* is radical surgical excision, removing a margin of healthy tissue around the tumour. It is usually possible to close the resulting, often very large, defect in the parietes by suture, perhaps after fashioning flaps from the musculo-aponeurotic layers, but sometimes it proves necessary to implant a sheet of plastic or metallic mesh to bridge the gap (McAdam and Goligher 1970). Recurrences after surgical excision are generally regarded as evidence of incomplete surgery, but may represent fresh desmoid formation. When feasible, further excision for recurrence is worthwhile.

For *intra-abdominal desmoids* this principle of wide excision is very difficult to apply. Desmoids originating in the retroperitoneal tissues and extending diffusely in this region are quite unsuitable for surgical removal. A desmoid arising in the small bowel mesentery may occasionally be amenable to excision if it is quite small, so that its surgical removal, together with resection of the related portion of small bowel, is compatible with preservation of a major portion of the intestine. But more usually intramesenteric desmoids are very large by the time they come to operation and seem to involve most of the mesentery. To remove them would entail sacrifice of virtually all the small intestine and is quite out of the question as a rule.

The prognosis for the great majority of intra-abdominal desmoids that are unsuitable for surgical treatment is somewhat uncertain, for most authors who have reported these cases make no comment on this point. Admittedly a desmoid is basically a benign tumour, in that it does not invade adjacent tissues, such as intestine, but, from their great size, these intra-abdominal desmoids may impinge seriously on contiguous structures, such as ureters or bowel, and gravely impair their function. Certainly our impression (McAdam and Goligher 1970) is that the outlook for most patients with desmoids within the abdomen is very poor, and we have had four such cases who have died apparently from the effects of the desmoid—two from ureteric obstruction and urinary failure, one from peritonitis and one from intestinal obstruction. We have not found radiotherapy to be of any value in controlling the growth of these desmoids.

MANAGEMENT OF THE POLYPOSIS FAMILY

In addition to his ordinary clinical responsibilities to his patient the surgeon who treats a case of polyposis has important obligations to the other members of the family to which this patient belongs. It is his duty to search out the individuals in that family who might possibly be suffering from the same condition. The best way to do so is to see as many members as possible, and from the information supplied by them to construct a family pedigree as in Fig. 276. This may be a lengthy task, involving as it does a number of interviews and examinations at hospital as well as postal enquiries and domestic visits to outlying members. But the labour is worth while for it gives a picture of the present status of the family and the distribution of the disease amongst its members in one or two generations. From the family pedigree it will be evident which members might conceivably be affected by the disease and therefore require to be examined and kept under supervision. Particular importance attaches to the children of sufferers from polyposis. Though it would be interesting to sigmoidoscope them regularly from an early age to learn more of the beginnings of the disease, for psychological reasons this is not desirable, and instead the

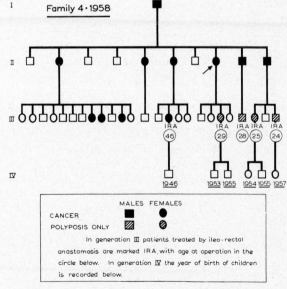

Fig. 276. Pedigree of polyposis family. (*From Dukes 1958*)

examination is usually postponed till the age of 13 or 14 unless symptoms occur earlier than this to suggest that polyps are already present.

Those who are found to harbour polyps at this initial survey are recommended to have treatment along the lines already mentioned. Those who are potential sufferers but do not as yet show evidence of the condition need regular supervision. It would seem, however, that, *if they have not developed polyps by the age of 40, they are unlikely to have inherited polyposis* (though Lockhart-Mummery (1967) has recorded a case in which polyposis and cancer began after this age).

Cronkhite–Canada Syndrome

Cronkhite and Canada (1955) have described an excessively rare syndrome, which is characterized by the development, usually in female patients after middle age, of an intractable diarrhoea, associated with generalized pigmentation, alopecia, onycho-trophia, hypoproteinaemia, oedema, cachexia, and low serum calcium and potassium. There is no family history of similar symptoms. The condition usually proves fatal within 18 months of onset, and at autopsy polyps (alleged by some to be adenomas, but this is doubted by others—see Lockhart-Mummery (1967)) are found scattered throughout the stomach, duodenum and large intestine, but not the small bowel. The detection of the polyps in the rectum and colon on sigmoidoscopy during life would necessitate differentiation from other forms of polyposis.

ANAL PAPILLOMA (ANAL WARTS, CONDYLOMATA ACUMINATA)

Papillomas arising from the skin of the anal canal and perianal region are not uncommon, especially in young men. Usually they are multiple and often completely surround the anus and extend into the lower part of the canal as seen in Fig. 277. The individual warts may be sessile or pedunculated and a mixture of the two is often present in any one patient. The moisture and warmth of the anal region results in the warts becoming sodden and whitened; usually an irritating discharge with a dis-agreeable odour results. The warts are often friable and when rubbed may bleed. Contrary to what is implied in some texts they are not due to a gonor-rhoeal infection. Their aetiology is uncertain, but probably like other cutaneous papillomas they are

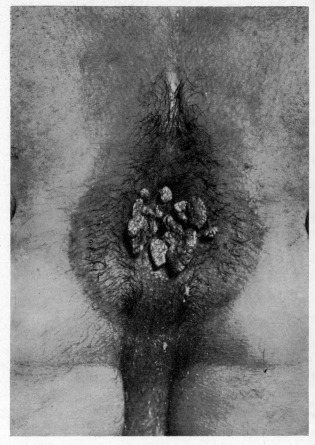

infective and due to an ultramicroscopic virus, which can be inoculated by intradermal injection of sterile filtrate material made from the warts. It is my impression that they occur with greater frequency in male homosexual patients, and Swerdlow and Salvati (1971) report that 46% of their male patients were homosexuals.

Diagnosis

In most cases the diagnosis is easy. But confusion may arise with the *condylomata lata* of secondary syphilis; they are fewer in number, smoother and flatter, and look more like areas of granulation tissue. Other clinical manifestations of syphilis may be present, and the diagnosis can be readily estab-lished by having a small quantity of the glairy dis-charge examined by dark ground illumination for the spirochaetes, which are usually present in large numbers. Another condition that may require to be differentiated is a *squamous-celled carcinoma* of the anus; it is more indurated, but a biopsy may be necessary to settle the diagnosis.

Treatment

As with penile and vulvar warts, *the local application of podophyllin* is sometimes an effective treatment. Kaplan (1942), who introduced this preparation, recommended that a 25% suspension of podophyllin in liquid paraffin should be used. Another vehicle for applying it is Tr. Benz. Co., a 12–15% suspension being employed as originally suggested by Marks (1947). The latter preparation has the advantage that it adheres better to the actual warts and is perhaps less likely to run on to the adjacent skin to which podophyllin is intensely irritating. The method of application is to paint the fluid accurately on the warts, avoiding the perianal skin as far as possible. To this latter end also the buttocks are kept separated so that the skin does not come into contact with the podophyllin on the warts. After 5–10 minutes the excess fluid is wiped off and a talc dusting powder applied to the surrounding skin. This is an out-patient treatment which is repeated at weekly intervals as required. In some cases the first application produces a dramatic response, the warts having almost completely disappeared by the next visit. One further treatment may then suffice to give the *coup de grâce* to the remnants. Other cases are more resistant and respond little if at all. Any warts remaining after four weeks should be treated by local excision. In some case podophyllin treatment has to be abandoned because the perianal skin becomes so sore.

Swerdlow and Salvati (1971) have proposed, as an alternative to podophyllin, *bichloracetic acid* (prepared by Kahlenberg Laboratories, Sarasota, Florida, U.S.A.). This caustic liquid is applied to the warts every seven to ten days, as required, for a few applications. I remain to be convinced that this treatment has any advantage over podophyllin.

Abcarian (1979), of the Colorectal Service of the University of Illinois Medical School, has used immune therapy. A vaccine, prepared by homogenizing, filtering and sterilizing an excised portion of wart, is injected weekly for six weeks. In 185 patients so treated the warts disappeared completely in 83%.

EXCISION OF ANAL WARTS

This little operation is most conveniently performed under a short general anaesthetic. A very useful initial step (Thomson 1979) is infiltration of the subcutaneous tissues of the affected anal and perianal regions with a generous amount of a weak adrenaline solution to stretch the skin and separate the warts, and also to help with haemostasis. Each wart is then lifted up with forceps and snipped off with fine scissors, conserving all normal skin between lesions. If necessary diathermy may be lightly applied to the raw areas for haemostasis but is better not used for the actual excision, because of the wider destruction of precious skin liable to be produced. *A special search should be made with a bivalve speculum for any warts lying in the anal canal.* Finally a Milton gauze dressing is applied. After-care follows conventional lines.

An alternative to excision is *cryodestruction* (O'Connor 1979), which can be effected without anaesthesia. But it may be followed by quite a lot of discomfort and discharge (see p. 126). I prefer surgical removal as more precise and certain.

REFERENCES

ABCARIAN, H. (1979) Personal communication.
ARTHUR, J. F. (1962) The significance of small mucosal polyps of the rectum. *Proc. R. Soc. Med.*, 55, 703.
ATWATER, J. S. and BARGEN, J. A. (1945) The pathogenesis of intestinal polyps. *Gastroenterology*, 4, 395.
BACON, H. E., HOLOMAN, M. B. and CHINPRAHAST, K. (1963) Pancolonoscopy: is it a valuable procedure? *Dis. Colon Rect.*, 6, 311.
—— and PEALE, H. R. (1956) Appraisal of adenomatous polyps of the colon, their histopathology and surgical treatment. *Ann. Surg.*, 144, 9.
BARTHOLOMEW, L. G. and DAHLIN, D. C. (1958) Intestinal polyposis and mucocutaneous pigmentation (Peutz–Jeghers syndrome). *Minnesota Med.*, 41, 848.
—— —— and WAUGH, J. M. (1957) Intestinal polyposis associated with mucocutaneous melanin pigmentation (Peutz–Jeghers syndrome). *Gastroenterology*, 34, 434.
BENJAMIN, H. B., KLAMECKI, B. J., HERZOG, J. V. and HARGARTEN, L. W. (1967) The anotransabdominal approach to polyps of the colon. *Surgery, St Louis*, 62, 411.
BERGE, T., EKLUND, G., MELLNER, C., PIHL, B. and WENCKERT, A. (1973) Carcinoma of the colon and rectum in a defined population. An epidemiological, clinical and postmortem investigation of colorectal carcinoma and co-existing benign polyps in Malmö, Sweden. *Acta chir. scand.*, Suppl. 4, 38.
BEVAN, A. D. (1917) Carcinoma of the rectum—treatment by local excision. *Surg. Clins N. Am.*, 1, 1233.
BOND, J. H., Jr. and LEVITT, M. D. (1974) Factors affecting the concentration of combustible gases in the colon during colonoscopy. *Gastroenterology*, 68, 1445.

Bussey, H. J. R. (1970) Gastro-intestinal polyposis. *Gut, 11,* 970.
—— Wallace, M. H. and Morson, B. C. (1967) Metachronous carcinoma of the large intestine and intestinal polyps. *Proc. R. Soc. Med., 60,* 208.
Cabrera, A. and Lega, J. (1960) Polyps of the colon and rectum in children. *Am. J. Surg., 100,* 551.
Carden, A. B. G. and Morson, B. C. (1964) Recurrence after local excision of malignant polyps of the rectum. *Proc. R. Soc. Med., 57,* 559.
Carter, H. G. (1952) Explosion in the colon during electro-dissection of polyps. *Am. J. Surg., 84,* 514.
Castleman, B. and Krickstein, H. I. (1962) Do adenomatous polyps of the colon become malignant? *New Engl. J. Med., 267,* 469.
Cole, J. W. and Holden, W. D. (1959) Postcolectomy regression of adenomatous polyps of the rectum. *Archs Surg., Chicago, 79,* 385.
—— and McKalen, A. (1960) Observations on cytochemical composition of adenomas and carcinomas of the colon. *Ann. Surg., 152,* 615.
Coller, J. A., Corman, M. L. and Veidenheimer, M. C. (1975) Colonic polypoid disease: need for total colonoscopy. *Am. J. Surg., 131,* 490.
Colvert, J. R. and Brown, C. H. (1948) Rectal polyps: diagnosis, 5 year follow-up, and relation to carcinoma of the rectum. *Am. J. med. Sci., 215,* 24.
Cripps, H. (1882) *Trans. path. Soc. Lond., 33,* 165.
Cronkhite, L. W. and Canada, W. J. (1955) Generalized gastro-intestinal polyposis; unusual syndrome of polyposis, pigmentation, alopecia and onychotrophia. *New Engl. J. Med., 252,* 1011.
de Cosse, J. J., Adams, M. B. and Kuzma, J. F. (1975) The effect of ascorbic acid on rectal polyps of patients with familial polyposis. *Surgery, St Louis, 78,* 608.
Deddish, M. R. (1953) Colotomy and coloscopy. *Cancer, 6,* 1021.
—— and Hertz, R. E. (1955) Colotomy and coloscopy in the management of mucosal polyps and cancer of the colon. *Am. J. Surg., 90,* 846.
Dockerty, M. B. (1958) Pathologic aspects in the control of spread of colonic carcinoma. *Proc. Staff Meet. Mayo Clin., 33,* 157.
Dormandy, T. L. (1957) Gastro-intestinal polyposis with muco-cutaneous pigmentation. *New Engl. J. Med., 256,* 1093, 1141, 1186.
Dukes, C. E. (1926) Simple tumours of the large intestine and their relation to cancer. *Br. J. Surg., 13,* 720.
—— (1947) Explanation of the difference between papilloma and adenoma of the rectum. *Proc. R. Soc. Med., 40,* 829.
—— (1952a) Familial intestinal polyposis. *Ann. Eugenics, 17,* 1.
—— (1952b) Familial intestinal polyposis. *Ann. R. Coll. Surg. Engl., 10,* 293.
—— (1958) Cancer control in familial polyposis of the colon. *Dis. Colon Rect., 1,* 413.
Dunning, E. J. and Ibrahim, K. S. (1965) Gardner's syndrome: report of a case. *Ann. Surg., 161,* 565.
Dunphy, J. E. (1959) The effect of colostomy and subtotal colectomy on cancer and polyposis of the colon. *Proc. R. Soc. Med.,* Suppl. 52, 53.
Duthie, H. L. and Atwell, J. D. (1963) The absorption of water, sodium and potassium in the large intestine, with particular reference to the effects of villous papillomas. *Gut, 4,* 373.
Eklund, G. and Lindström, C. (1974) Histopathological analysis of benign polyps in patients with carcinoma of the colon and rectum. *Gut, 15,* 654.
Enquist, I. F. (1957) The incidence and significance of polyps of the colon and rectum. *Surgery, St Louis, 42,* 681.
Enterline, H. T., Evan, G. W., Mercado-Lugo, R., Miller, L. and Fitts, W. T., Jr. (1962) Malignant potential of adenomas of colon and rectum. *J. Am. med. Ass., 179,* 322.
Espiner, H. J., Salmon, P. R., Teague, R. H. and Read, A. E. (1973) Operative colonoscopy. *Br. med. J., 1,* 453.
Everson, T. C. and Allen, M. J. (1954) Subtotal colectomy with ileosigmoidostomy and fulguration of polyps in retained colon. *Archs Surg., Chicago, 69,* 806.
Ferguson, J. A. (1957) Management of villous tumours of the rectum. *J. Ky med. Ass., 55,* 996.
Findlay, C. W. and O'Connor, T. F. (1961) Villous adenomas of the large intestine with fluid and electrolyte depletion. *J. Am. med. Ass., 176,* 404.
Fisher, E. R. and Castro, A. F. (1953) Diffuse papillomatous polyps (villous tumors) of the colon and rectum. *Am. J. Surg., 85,* 146.
—— and Turnbull, R. B., Jr. (1952) Malignant polyps of rectum and sigmoid; therapy based on pathological considerations. *Surgery Gynec. Obstet., 94,* 619.
Flotte, C. T., O'Dell, F. D., Jr. and Coller, F. A. (1956) Polyposis of colon. *Ann. Surg., 144,* 165.
Freund, N. L. (1955) Villous tumours of the rectum. *Am. J. Surg., 90,* 873.
Gabriel, W. B. (1952) The surgical management of large villous tumours of the rectum. *Proc. R. Soc. Med., 45,* 696.
Galley, H. G. (1954) Combustible gases generated in the alimentary tract and other hollow viscera and their relationship to explosions occurring during anaesthesia. *Br. J. Anaesth., 26,* 189.
Gardner, E. G. (1951) A genetic and clinical study of intestinal polyposis, a predisposing factor for carcinoma of the colon and rectum. *Am. J. hum. Genet., 3,* 167.
—— and Plenk, H. P. (1952) Hereditary pattern for multiple osteomas in a family group. *Am. J. hum. Genet., 4,* 31.
—— and Richards, R. C. (1953) Multiple cutaneous and subcutaneous lesions occurring simultaneously with hereditary polyposis and osteomatosis. *Am. J. hum. Genet., 5,* 139.
Gillespie, P. E., Chambers, T. J. and Chan, K. W. (1979) Colonic adenomas—a colonoscopy survey. *Gut, 20,* 240.
Goligher, J. C. and Graham, N. G. (1967) Traitement chirurgical des papillomes villeux. *Archs Mal. Appar. dig., 56,* 51.
Greenen, J. E., Schmitt, M. G., Jr., Wu, W. C. and Hogan, W. T. (1975) Major complications of colonoscopy: bleeding and perforation. *Am. J. dig. Dis., 20,* 231.
Grinnell, R. S. and Lane, N. (1958) Benign and malignant adenomatous polyps and papillary adenomas of the colon and rectum. *Int. Abstr. Surg., 106,* 519.
Helwig, E. B. (1947) Evolution of adenomas of large intestine and their relation to carcinoma. *Surgery Gynec. Obstet., 84,* 36.
Henry, L. G., Condon, R. E., Schulte, W. J., Aprahamian, C. and de Cosse, J. T. (1975) Risks of recurrence of colon polyps. *Ann. Surg., 182,* 511.

HINES, M. O., HANLEY, P. H., RAY, J. E. and BRALLIAR, M. (1958) Villous tumours of the colon and rectum. *Dis. Colon Rect., 1*, 128.

HOFFMANN, D. C. and GOLIGHER, J. C. (1971) Polyposis of the stomach and small intestine in association with familial polyposis coli. *Br. J. Surg., 58*, 126.

—— and BROOKE, B. N. (1970) Familial sarcoma of bone in a polyposis coli family. *Dis. Colon Rect., 3*, 119.

HORRILLENO, E. G., ECKERT, C. and ACKERMAN, L. V. (1957) Polyps of the rectum and colon in children. *Cancer, Philad., 10*, 1210.

HUBBARD, T. B. (1957) Familial polyposis of the colon; the fate of the retained rectum after colectomy in children. *Am. J. Surg., 23*, 577.

JACKMAN, R. J. (1941) The relationship of polyps of the colon to carcinoma. *Proc. Staff Meet. Mayo Clin., 16*, 11.

JEGHERS, H. (1944) Pigmentation of skin. *New Engl. J. Med., 231*, 88.

JUDD, E. S. and CARLISLE, J. C. (1953) Polyps of colon; late results of transcolonic removal. *Archs Surg., Chicago, 67*, 353.

KAPLAN, I. W. (1942) Condylomata acuminata. *New Orl. med. surg. J., 94*, 388.

KLEINFELD, G. and GUMP, F. E. (1960) Complications of colotomy and polypectomy. *Surgery Gynec. Obstet., 111*, 726.

KNOX, W. G., MILLER, R. E., BEGG, C. F. and ZINTEL, H. A. (1960) Juvenile polyps of the colon: a clinicopathologic analysis of 75 polyps in 43 patients. *Surgery, St Louis, 48*, 201.

KOZUKA, S. (1975) Premalignancy of the mucosal polyp in the large intestine: I. Histological gradation of the polyp on the basis of epithelial pseudostratification and glandular branching. *Dis. Colon Rect., 18*, 483.

—— NOGAKI, M., OZEKI, T. and MASUMORI, S. (1975) Premalignancy of the mucosal polyp in the large intestine: II. Estimation of the periods required for malignant transformation of mucosal polyps. *Dis. Colon Rect., 18*, 494.

LABERGE, M. Y., SAUER, W. G. and MAYO, C. W. (1957) Soft tissue tumours associated with familial polyposis. *Proc. Staff Meet. Mayo Clin., 32*, 749.

LAWRENCE, J. C. (1936) Gastrointestinal polyps: statistical study of malignancy incidence. *Am. J. Surg., 31*, 499.

LEUCHTENBERGER, C., LEUCHTENBERGER, R. and DAVIS, A. M. (1954) A microspectrophotometric study of desoxyribose nucleic acid (DNA) content in cells of normal and malignant human tissues. *Am. J. Path., 30*, 65.

LILLEHEI, R. C. and WANGENSTEEN, O. H. (1955) Bowel function after colectomy for cancer, polyps and diverticulitis. *J. Am. med. Ass., 159*, 163.

LOCALIO, S. A. (1962) Spontaneous disappearance of rectal polyps following subtotal colectomy and ileoproctostomy for polyposis of the colon. *Am. J. Surg., 103*, 81.

LOCKHART-MUMMERY, H. E. (1967) Intestinal polyposis: the present position. *Proc. R. Soc. Med., 60*, 381.

—— and DUKES, C. E. (1952) Surgical treatment of malignant rectal polyps, with notes on their pathology. *Lancet, 2*, 751.

LOCKHART-MUMMERY, J. P. (1925) Cancer and heredity. *Lancet, 1*, 427.

McADAM, W. A. F. and GOLIGHER, J. C. (1970) The occurrence of desmoids in patients with familial polyposis coli. *Br. J. Surg., 57*, 618.

McCOLL, I., BUSSEY, H. J. R., VEALE, A. M. O. and MORSON, B. C. (1964) Juvenile polyposis coli. *Proc. R. Soc. Med., 57*, 896.

McKITTRICK, L. S. and WHEELOCK, F. C. (1954) *Carcinoma of the Colon*, pp. 61–63. Springfield, Ill.: Charles C. Thomas.

MARKS, M. M. (1947) Condylomata accuminata: podophyllin in compound tincture of benzoin, an improvement in technic of treatment. *J. Mo. St. med. Ass., 44*, 749.

MASON, A. Y. (1970) Surgical access to the rectum—a trans-sphincteric exposure. *Proc. R. Soc. Med.,* Suppl. 65, 1.

MAYO, C. W. and CASTRO, C. A. DE (1956) Carcinoma of the sigmoid arising from a polyp first visualized 15 years previously; report of case. *Proc. Staff Meet. Mayo Clin., 31*, 597.

—— and SCHLICKE, C. P. (1942) Carcinoma of the colon and rectum; a study of metastases and recurrences. *Surgery Gynec. Obstet., 74*, 825.

MILLER, C. J., DAY, E. and L'ESPERANCE, E. S. (1950) Value of proctoscopy as routine examination in preventing deaths from cancer of large bowel. *New York J. Med., 50*, 2023.

MOERTEL, C. G., HILL, J. R. and ADSON, M. A. (1970) Surgical management of multiple polyposis. The problem of cancer in the retained bowel segment. *Archs Surg., Chicago, 100*, 521.

MOORE, J. M. (1960) The incidence and importance of polyps of the large intestine. *Scot. med. J., 5*, 83.

MORAN, T. F. (1957) Surgical treatment of villous tumours of the rectum. *J. int. Coll. Surg., 28*, 227.

MORSON, B. C. (1962a) Some peculiarities in the histology of intestinal polyps. *Dis. Colon Rect., 5*, 337.

—— (1962b) Precancerous lesions of the colon and rectum. *J. Am. med. Ass., 179*, 316.

—— (1962c) Precancerous lesions of the upper gastrointestinal tract. *J. Am. med. Ass., 179*, 311.

—— (1969) *Diseases of the Colon, Rectum and Anus*. London: Heinemann.

—— (1970) Some leads to the etiology of cancer of the large bowel. *Proc. R. Soc. Med., 64*, 959.

—— BUSSEY, H. J. R. and SAMOURIAN, S. (1977) A policy of local excision for early cancer of the colorectum. *Gut, 18*, 1045.

—— and SOBIN, L. H. (1976) *International Histological Classification of Tumours. No. 15. Histological Typing of Intestinal Tumours*. Geneva: WHO.

NACHLAS, M. M. and HANNIBAL, M. J. (1961) Histochemical observations on polyp-carcinoma sequence. *Surgery Gynec. Obstet., 112*, 534.

NEELY, M. G. and GILLESPIE, G. (1967) Peutz–Jeghers syndrome: sporadic and familial. *Br. J. Surg., 54*, 378.

O'CONNOR, J. J. (1979) Perianal and anal condylomata. *J. R. Soc. Med., 72*, 232.

OLDFIELD, M. C. (1954) Association of familial polyposis of colon with multiple sebaceous cysts. *Br. J. Surg., 41*, 534.

PAGTALUNAN, R. J. G., DOCKERTY, M. B., JACKMAN, R. J. and ANDERSON, M. J., Jr. (1965) The histopathology of diminutive polyps of the large intestine. *Surgery Gynec. Obstet., 120*, 1259.

PARKS, A. G. (1968) A technique for excising extensive villous papillomatous change in the lower rectum. *Proc. R. Soc. Med., 61*, 41.

—— and STUART, A. E. (1973) The management of villous tumours of the large bowel. *Br. J. Surg., 60*, 688.

PEUTZ, J. L. A. (1921) On a very remarkable case of familial polyposis of the mucous membrane of the intestinal tract and nasopharynx accompanied by peculiar pigmentation of the skin and mucous membrane. *Ned. Maandschr. Geneesk., 10*, 134.

POTET, F. and SOULLARD, J. (1971) Polyps of the rectum and colon. *Gut, 12*, 468.

RAGINS, J., SHINYA, H. and WOLFF, W. I. (1974) The explosive potential of colonic gas during colonoscopic electrosurgical poly-pectomy. *Surgery Gynec. Obstet.*, *138*, 554.

RIDER, J. A., KIRSNER, J. B., MOELLER, H. C. and PALMER, W. L. (1954) Polyps of the colon and rectum, their incidence and relation-ship to carcinoma. *Am. J. Med.*, *16*, 555.

—— —— —— —— (1959) Polyps of the colon and rectum. *J. Am. med. Ass.*, *170*, 633.

RINTALA, A. (1959) The histological appearance of gastrointestinal polyps in the Peutz-Jeghers' syndrome. *Acta chir. scand.*, *117*, 366.

ROSI, P. A. and CAHILL, W. J. (1962) Subtotal colectomy with caecorectal anastomosis for multiple adenomas of the colon. *Am. J. Surg.*, *103*, 75.

SCARBOROUGH, R. A. (1960) Relationship between polyps and carcinoma of the colon and rectum. *Dis. Colon Rect.*, *3*, 336.

SHINYA, H. and WOLFF, W. I. (1975) Colonoscopic polypectomy: technique and safety. *Hosp. Practice*, *10*, 71.

SHNITKA, T. K., FRIEDMAN, M. H. W., KIDD, E. G. and MACKENZIE, W. C. (1961) Villous tumors of the rectum and colon characterized by severe fluid and electrolyte loss. *Surgery Gynec. Obstet.*, *112*, 609.

SIMPKINS, K. C. and YOUNG, A. C. (1968) The radiology of colonic and rectal polyps. *Br. J. Surg.*, *55*, 731.

SMILOW, P. C., PRYOR, C. A., Jr. and SWINTON, N. W. (1966) Juvenile polyposis coli. *Dis. Colon Rect.*, *9*, 248.

SMITH, T. R., MAIER, D. M., METCALF, W. and KAPLOWITZ, I. S. (1970) Transformation of a pedunculated colonic polyp to adeno-carcinoma. *Dis. Colon Rect.*, *13*, 382.

SMITH, W. G. (1959) Desmoid tumours in familial polyposis. *Proc. Staff Meet. Mayo Clin.*, *34*, 31.

SOUTHWOOD, W. F. W. (1962) Villous tumours of the large intestine: their pathogenesis, symptomatology, diagnosis and management. *Ann. R. Coll. Surg. Engl.*, *30*, 23.

SPENCER, R. J., COATES, H. L. and ANDERSON, M. J., Jr. (1974) Colonoscopic polypectomy. *Mayo Clin. Proc.*, *49*, 40.

SPRATT, J. S., Jr. and ACKERMAN, L. V. (1962) Small primary adenocarcinomas of the colon and rectum. *J. Am. med. Ass.*, *179*, 337.

—— —— and MOYER, C. A. (1958) Relationship of polyps of the colon to the development of colonic cancer. *Ann. Surg.*, *148*, 682.

STEWART, M. J. (1931) Pre-cancerous lesions of the alimentary tract. *Lancet*, *2*, 565, 617, 669.

STICH, H. F., FLORIAN, S. F. and EMSON, H. E. (1960) DNA content of tumour cells. 1. Polyps and adenocarcinomas of the large intes-tine of man. *J. natn. Cancer Inst.*, *24*, 471.

SUNDERLAND, D. A. and BINKLEY, G. E. (1948) Papillary adenomas of the large intestine. *Cancer, Philad.*, *1*, 184.

SUSMAN, W. (1932) Polypi coli. *J. Path. Bact.*, *35*, 29.

SWERDLOW, D. B. and SALVATI, E. P. (1971) Condyloma acuminatum. *Dis. Colon Rect.*, *14*, 226.

SWINTON, N. W. and HAUG, A. D. (1947) The frequency of pre-cancerous lesions in the rectum and colon. *Lahey Clin. Bull.*, *5*, 84.

—— MEISSNER, W. A. and SOLAND, W. A. (1955) Papillary adenomas of the colon and rectum: a clinical and pathological study. *Archs intern. Med.*, *96*, 544.

—— and WARREN, S. (1939) Polyps of the colon and rectum and their relation to malignancy. *J. Am. med. Ass.*, *113*, 1927.

—— and WEAKLEY, F. L. (1963) Complications of colotomy and colonoscopy. *Dis. Colon Rect.*, *6*, 50.

TEICHER, L. and ABRAHAMS, J. I. (1956) The treatment of selected cases of multiple polyps, familial polyposis and diverticular disease of the colon by subtotal colectomy and ileoproctostomy. *Surgery Gynec. Obstet.*, *103*, 136.

THOMSON, J. P. S. (1979) Personal communication.

TURCOT, J., DESPRÉS, J.-P. and St PIERRE, F. (1959) Malignant tumours of the central nervous system associated with familial polyposis of the colon. Report of 2 cases. *Dis. Colon Rect.*, *2*, 465.

TURNBULL, R. B., Jr. (1958) Quoted by Dunphy (1959).

—— HAZARD, J. B. and O'HALLORAN, A. (1961) Occult invasive cancer on polypoid adenomas of the colon and rectum. *Dis. Colon Rect.*, *4*, 111.

UTSUNOMIYA, J. and NAKAMURA, T. (1975) The occult osteomatous changes in the mandible in patients with familial polyposis coli. *Br. J. Surg.*, *62*, 45.

—— MAKI, T., HAMAGUCHI, E. and AOKI, N. (1974) Gastric lesions of familial polyposis of the large intestine. *Cancer*, *74*, 745.

VEALE, A. M. O., McCOLL, I., BUSSEY, H. J. R. and MORSON, B. C. (1966) Juvenile polyposis coli. *J. med. Genet.*, *3*, 5.

DE LA VUSSIÈRE, G., JOURDE, L. and LOYGUE, J. (1965) Adénomes solitaires du colon gauch, dégénérés ou polypes malins? *Ann. Chir.*, *19*, 206.

WAUGH, J. M., HARP, R. A. and SPENCER, R. J. (1964) The surgical management of multiple polyposis. *Ann. Surg.*, *159*, 149.

WEARY, P. E., LINTHICUM, A. and CAWLEY, E. P. (1964) Gardner's syndrome. A family group study and review. *Archs Derm.*, *90*, 20.

WEINER, R. S. and COOPER, P. (1955) Multiple polyposis of the colon, osteomatosis and soft tissue tumours. *New Engl. J. Med.*, *253*, 795.

WELCH, C. E. (1951) The treatment of polyps of the colon. *Surgery Gynec. Obstet.*, *93*, 368.

—— McKITTRICK, J. B. and BEHRINGER, G. (1952) Polyps of the rectum and colon and their relation to cancer. *New Engl. J. Med.*, *247*, 959.

WELIN, S. (1967) Results of the Malmö technique of colon examination. *J. Am. med. Ass.*, *199*, 369.

—— and WELIN, G. (1976) *The Double Contrast Examination of the Colon: Experiences with the Welin Modification*. Stuttgart: Georg Thieme.

WESTHUES, H. (1934) *Die Pathologisch-anatomischen Grundlagen der Chirurgie des Rektumkarzinoms*. Leipzig: Georg Thieme.

WHEAT, M. W., Jr. and ACKERMAN, L. V. (1958) Villous adenomas of the large intestine. *Ann. Surg.*, *147*, 476.

WILLIAMS, C., MUTO, T. and RUTTER, K. R. P. (1973) Removal of polyps with fibreoptic colonoscope: a new approach to colonic poly-pectomy. *Br. med. J.*, *1*, 451.

—— HUNT, R. H., LOOSE, H., RIDDELL, R. H., SAKI, Y. and SWARBRICK, E. T. (1974) Colonoscopy in the management of colon polyps. *Br. J. Surg.*, *61*, 673.

WILLIS, R. A. (1948) *The Pathology of Tumours*, pp. 422, 425. London: Butterworth.

—— (1958) *Borderland of Embryology and Pathology*. London: Butterworth.

WILSON, G. S., DALE, E. H. and BRINES, O. A. (1955) Symposium on early diagnosis of tumors of rectum and colon; evaluation of polyps detected in 20847 routine sigmoidoscopic examinations. *Am. J. Surg.*, *9*, 834.

WOLFF, W. I. and SHINYA, H. (1973a) Polypectomy via the fibreoptic colonoscope. *New Engl. J. Med.*, *288*, 329.

—— —— (1973b) A new approach to colonic polyps. *Ann. Surg.*, *178*, 367.

—— —— (1975) Definitive treatment of malignant polyps of the colon. *Ann. Surg.*, *182*, 516.

15

Incidence and Pathology of Carcinoma of the Colon and Rectum

INCIDENCE

Some idea of the frequency of different forms of malignant disease may be obtained from the Registrar-General's Statistical Reviews which record the number of deaths from various causes occurring each year in England and Wales. Admittedly these figures give no indication of the number of individuals who develop carcinoma but are cured of it by treatment and die of other conditions. Considering the country as a whole, however, the proportion of such patients to those who are certified as dying of their growth is probably fairly small. An additional factor which probably minimizes the size of the former group is the tendency of practitioners in making out death certificates to incriminate a previously-treated carcinoma as the cause of death, when in fact the fatal outcome may have been due to intercurrent disease.

The Registrar-General records that during 1976 there were 17 268 deaths from carcinoma of the colon and rectum. By contrast carcinoma of the bronchus was responsible for 33 524 deaths during the same year, carcinoma of the stomach for 11 868 and carcinoma of the breast for 11 833. It will be seen, therefore, that carcinoma of the large intestine is one of the three or four really common cancers, being in fact only less frequent as a lethal condition than cancer of the bronchus and lung. Moreover, there has been very little change in the figures of deaths from carcinoma of the rectum and colon during the past 30-odd years—16 977 in 1945, 14 558 in 1957 and 15 758 in 1969.

The high incidence of colorectal cancer is at least as large a problem in the USA, for Silverberg (1970), on behalf of the American Cancer Society,

estimated a total of 79 000 new cases of carcinoma of the colon and rectum in that country during 1974, and approximately 45 000 deaths from that cause during the same period.

A more accurate assessment of trends in the incidence of cancer in various sites in the body, including the colon and rectum, has been worked out by Segi (1963) for several countries during the period 1950–9. His information was derived from mortality statistics relating to a selected population of standard composition according to age groups. He found that the total number of deaths from malignant disease at all sites in both sexes combined in England and Wales increased from 279·3 per 100 000 population in 1950–1 to 287·9 in 1958–9. But the age-adjusted mortality from carcinoma of the colon and rectum in both males and females diminished slightly during this time, as it did in many other countries (see Correa 1978).

Site Incidence

Of the 14 428 deaths in England and Wales in 1963 certified as due to cancer of the large intestine 8958 were attributed to carcinoma of the colon and 5470, or roughly 38%, to carcinoma of the rectum. Some hospital statistics show an even higher proportion of growths of the large intestine as occurring in the rectum. Thus in a series of 1644 cases of carcinoma of the large bowel admitted to the Leeds General Infirmary between the years 1938–43 and 1947–55 inclusive the lesion was found to be in the rectum in no less than 944 or 57·4% (Smiddy and Goligher 1957). The discrepancy between this figure and that of the Registrar-General's returns is doubtless explained partly by differences in interpretation of the position of growths lying in the vicinity of the rectosigmoid junction. It is often debatable whether such lesions should be categorized as carcinomas of the rectum or sigmoid colon. In the Leeds General Infirmary statistics growths in this controversial site have generally been classed as rectal lesions. It would probably be a fair conclusion to say that nearly half the carcinomas of the large intestine are situated in the rectum or rectosigmoid.

DISTRIBUTION OF CARCINOMAS IN THE COLON

The distribution of growths in the various segments of the colon has been the subject of many detailed clinical studies, several of the more comprehensive of which are summarized in Table 19. It will be seen that there is fairly general agreement that carcinoma of the sigmoid accounts for nearly half the growths of the colon proper, and carcinoma of the caecum and ascending colon for roughly a quarter. Thereafter the order of frequency for sites of carcinoma in the colon would appear to be transverse colon, splenic flexure, descending colon and hepatic flexure.

DISTRIBUTION OF CARCINOMAS IN THE RECTUM

There has been a great deal of controversy in the past as to the distribution of carcinomas in the *different segments of the rectum*. Several of the older writers such as Tuttle (1903), W. J. Mayo (1910), Rankin et al. (1932) and Gabriel (1948) claimed that

by far the commonest site is the rectosigmoid, but it is not always clear exactly what they meant by the rectosigmoid. Dukes (1940), in an analysis of 1000 operative specimens of adenocarcinomas of the rectum, worked out their frequency in different parts of the rectum most carefully. He found that the growth lay in the upper third in 30·8%, in the middle third in 32·6% and in the lower third and anal canal in 36·6%. However, these statistics can be criticized on the grounds that they refer to a selected group of cases, namely those suitable for excision of their growths. My own determination of the site of the lesion in a consecutive series of 1096 clinical cases of carcinoma recti at St Mark's Hospital avoided this source of error (Goligher 1941). The assessment was based partly on the site of the growth revealed in the operative specimens of operable cases, but mainly on the height of the lower margin of the growth above the anal verge as determined by sigmoidoscopy, lesions above 15 cm being considered to be not in the rectum but in the colon, those above 11 cm to be in the upper third of the rectum, those above 6 cm to be in the middle third of the rectum and those below that level to be in the lower third. According to these criteria 395 or 36% of the growths were regarded as being in the upper third, 314 or 28·7% in the middle third, and 387 or 35·3% in the lower third.

The relation of rectal growths to the reflection of peritoneum of the front of the rectum at the bottom of the rectovesical or rectouterine pouch is surgically important. It can only be determined in patients coming to operation. I examined the records of a series of 1500 cases treated by combined abdominoperineal excision at St Mark's Hospital between 1933 and 1947 (during which years this was almost the only operation used for

TABLE 19. *Distribution of Carcinomas in the Colon According to Various Authors*

Site of growth	No. of growths in each site				
	Körte (1900)	Judd (1924)	Fraser (1938)	Smiddy and Goligher (1957)	Collective series
Caecum	47 ⎫	159	171	101 ⎫	611 = 24·2%
Ascending colon	22 ⎭		63	48 ⎭	
Hepatic flexure	19	29	54	29	131
Transverse colon	44	75	126	77	322
Splenic flexure	31	24	90	50	195
Descending colon	10	46	27	45	128
Sigmoid colon	124	292	369	350	1135 = 45%
All sites	297	625	900	700	2522

rectal cancer at that hospital, anterior resection not having yet been adopted) and found that 713 or 47·5% of the growths lay above the peritoneal reflection and 787 or 52·5% partly or entirely below it.

As for the relative frequency with which carcinoma arises in the *different sectors of the rectal circumference*, in 1063 cases examined from this point of view the growth was found to be completely annular in 337 or 31·7% (Goligher 1941). In the remaining 726 cases with non-annular growths, though one, two or even three quadrants of the bowel circumference might be involved, it was assumed that the middle of the growth represented its starting point. It was found that 236 or 22·2% of the lesions were centred on the anterior wall, 265 or 24·9% on the posterior wall, but only 225 or 21·2% on the two lateral walls. This was a surprising finding, for one fully expected to discover that carcinoma originated with equal frequency in all four quadrants.

A POSSIBLE CHANGE IN THE RELATIVE INCIDENCE OF CARCINOMA IN COLON AND RECTUM

There is some evidence that the distribution of cancer within the large bowel is changing in the United States. Axtell and Chiazze (1966) first drew attention to this possibility when they reported that the ratio of colon carcinomas to rectal carcinomas in Connecticut had changed from 1:20 between 1935 and 1940 to 1:64 between 1960 and 1961 in males and 1:88 to 2:49 in females. Cutler (1969) reviewed much the same data and noted that the incidence of colon cancer had increased from 20 per 100 000 in 1940 to 30 per 100 000 in 1965, and accordingly the changing ratio as between colon and rectum was ascribed to this increased frequency of colon cancer.

Rhodes et al. (1977) analysed the distribution of colorectal carcinomas in the University of Kansas Medical Centre during the years 1946–75 and found that there was a statistically significant decrease in the percentage of distal (rectum, $P = 0·0192$) and an increasing percentage of proximal (caecum, $P = 0·0015$) large bowel lesions during this period of 30 years. Analysis of the numbers of deaths due to colorectal cancer in the State of Kansas from 1950 to 1975 showed a similar trend. Rhodes et al. (1977) conclude that the changing distribution is due to a swing of incidence away from the rectum to the more proximal bowel.

As indicated on p. 375, Registrar-General's records of death from cancer of the rectum and colon in Britain do not show any significant alteration in the relative incidence of carcinoma in these two subsections of the large bowel.

Sex Incidence

The Registrar-General's statistics show that of the 14 426 fatal cases of cancer of the large intestine in England and Wales in 1963, 6504 were men and 7924 women, and similar almost equal distribution between the two sexes is revealed in the returns for previous years. If, however, the deaths from carcinoma of the colon and rectum are considered separately a very considerable difference is disclosed. Of the 8958 deaths from carcinoma of the colon in 1963, 3567 occurred in males and 5391 in females, a ratio of roughly 7:11; whilst of the 5468 deaths from rectal carcinoma, 2935 were in males and only 2533 in females, a ratio of nearly 6:5. The records of the Connecticut Tumor Registry (Eisenberg et al. 1967), dealing with some 20 000 cases of cancer of the large bowel, give a male:female ratio of incidence of carcinoma coli of roughly 5:6 and of carcinoma recti of 6:5 approximately.

Clinical statistics also show differences in the behaviour of carcinoma of the colon and rectum in regard to sex incidence. In the series of 1644 cases of cancer of the large intestine reported by Smiddy and Goligher (1957) from the Leeds General Infirmary the incidence of carcinoma in the various segments of the colon was roughly equal in the two sexes, but carcinoma of the rectum occurred more frequently in males than females in the ratio of roughly 5:3 (see Table 20). Several other writers such as De Bovis (1900), Clogg (1908) and Fraser

TABLE 20. *Numbers of Growths in the Two Sexes at Different Parts of Bowel in Combined Series of 1644 Cases*

Site	No. of patients with growths in each site	
	Males	Females
Rectum	559	385
Sigmoid colon	176	174
Descending colon	18	27
Splenic flexure	25	25
Transverse colon	37	40
Hepatic flexure	20	9
Ascending colon	24	24
Caecum	48	53
All sites	907	737

After Smiddy and Goligher (1957).

(1938) also reported an almost equal incidence of carcinoma coli in males and females. Certain other clinical statistics show an even more marked preponderance of rectal carcinoma in men than women than was revealed in the Leeds General Infirmary series. Thus of the 1063 cases of cancer of the rectum analysed by me (Goligher 1941) 745 were males and 318 females, a ratio of 2 : 1.

Age Incidence

Cancer of the large intestine, like carcinoma elsewhere, is predominantly a disease of older patients though it may occur at almost any age. The general trend of incidence in relation to age is well shown in Table 21. It will be noted particularly that *more than half of these cases were over the age of 60*. The commonest decade for carcinoma of the rectum to occur was 60–9. Above that age the number of cases diminished, but it has to be borne in mind that there were fewer people alive in the general population in these higher decades, so that the tendency to develop rectal carcinoma may probably be considered to increase progressively with advancing age. It will be observed that there were many fewer cases below the age of 50, but that even below the age of 30 there were still 25 patients, who represented 2·1% of the entire series. Rankin and Comfort (1929) in a review of 1452 cases of rectal cancer found 3·85% to be under the age of 30, and in 4435 cases of carcinoma of the rectum at St Mark's Hospital 46, or approximately 1%, were under this age (Recio and Bussey 1965). Instances of carcinoma of the colon in children below the age of 20 years have been recorded by Fraser (1938), Saner (1946), Johnston (1947), Johnson et al. (1959), Salem and Postlethwait (1960) and Mayo and Pagtalunan (1963).

TABLE 21. *Incidence of Carcinoma of Rectum according to Age of Patients*

Age group	No. of cases	
20–9	25	
30–9	63	584 under 60
40–9	145	
50–9	351	
60–9	443	
70–9	139	587 over 60
80–9	5	

After Goligher (1941).

Dukes (1940) points out that carcinoma of the rectum tends to occur at an earlier age in women than in men. In the series of 1000 operable cases of rectal cancer studied by him, the mean age of the female patients was 55·1 as contrasted with 58·6 for the males; 11·2% of the women were under forty as compared with only 6% of the men; and the highest proportion of female patients occurred in the age group 40–59, whereas in men it was in the group 60–79. The fact that rectal cancer arises in general at a younger age in women than in men has an important bearing on the relative survival rate after its surgical treatment in the two sexes.

Familial Incidence

Many surgeons have noted the occurrence of colorectal carcinoma in two or more members of the same family. Lovett (1976) and Morson (1979) find that in such families the age of onset of the tumour is significantly earlier than in the general population and there is an increased incidence of multiple cancers. Though the patients do not have polyposis, the incidence of associated adenomas is somewhat increased compared with that in patients without a family history.

PATHOLOGY

Gross Appearances

In its initial stages cancer of the large intestine probably takes the form of a localized area of

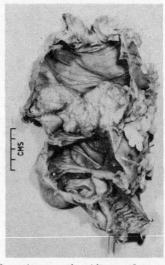

Fig. 278. A fungating or polypoid type of carcinoma of the caecum.

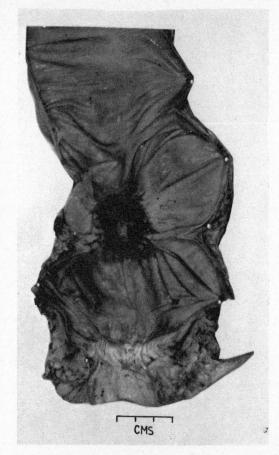

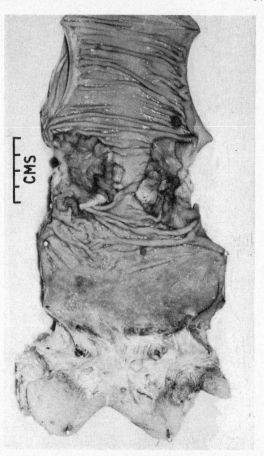

Fig. 279. A carcinoma of the rectum taking the form of a typical rounded malignant ulcer or plateau on the posterior wall.

Fig. 280. An ulcerating carcinoma of the rectum which is elongated in the transverse axis of the bowel. The growth lay on the anterior and lateral walls, and as the specimen was opened along the front, it has been bisected into two halves, the posterior poles of which are separated by a narrow strip of uninvolved rectum behind.

thickening of the normal mucosa or a hard nodule in a pre-existing adenoma or villous papilloma. As the growth enlarges it may assume a variety of appearances but tends to conform to one of five fairly distinctive macroscopic types—the polypoid, ulcerative, annular, diffusely infiltrating or colloid forms of carcinoma.

The Polypoid or Cauliflower Carcinoma produces a large fungating mass which projects into the lumen of the bowel, but is not usually associated with much infiltration of the intestinal wall (Fig. 278). The protruding surface of the lesion may be finely or coarsely nodular over most of its extent but, owing to rapid growth and resulting necrosis, there is usually ulceration at some point.

The Ulcerative Carcinoma presents as a typical malignant ulcer with raised irregular everted edges and a sloughing base. It may be roughly circular

and confined to one aspect of the colon or rectum (Fig. 279), but more often it is somewhat elongated in the transverse axis and may extend over two or more quadrants of the bowel circumference (Fig. 280). As this type of growth tends to infiltrate the bowel wall deeply there may be considerable deformity and often some narrowing.

The Annular or Stenosing Carcinoma. Clinical experience gained in following the course of untreated rectal cancer in certain patients who had declined to have an operation suggests that most annular carcinomas probably develop from an initially discrete malignant ulcer (see Miles 1926). This lesion gradually extends round the bowel wall and eventually its two advancing edges meet at the opposite pole so that it embraces the lumen and

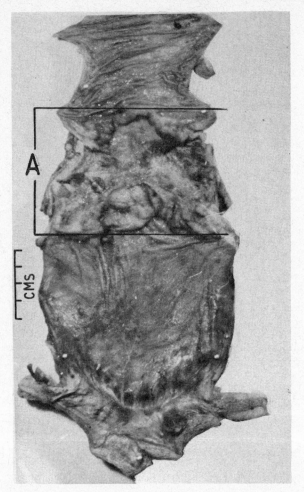

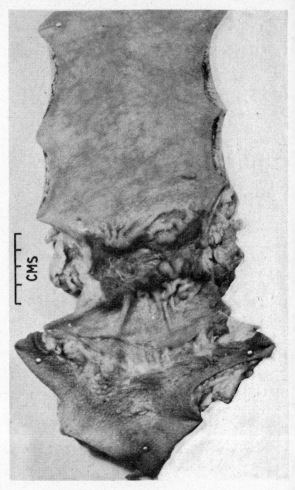

Fig. 281. An annular carcinoma of the rectum which, on opening up the specimen by division along its anterior wall, is seen to consist of a segment of ulceration roughly 6·5 cm long. A = the growth.

Fig. 282. An annular carcinoma of the rectum producing a short stricture 4 cm long.

forms a completely annular ulcerating growth. The extent in the long axis of the bowel is variable; in the rectum it often measures 5–8 cm (Fig. 281), but may be much less (Fig. 282), and in the colon it is usually relatively short (Fig. 283). As there is frequently a considerable amount of stenosis, the appearance of a completely annular carcinoma in the colon, as seen from the peritoneal aspect, is often highly characteristic; it looks as if the bowel had been deeply constricted by a string tied tightly round it (Fig. 284). This is the so-called *string-stricture carcinoma*, seen most typically in the sigmoid.

The Diffusely Infiltrating Carcinoma of the colon or rectum corresponds to the linitis plastica of the stomach (Fahl et al. 1960; Nelson 1965). It produces a diffuse thickening of the intestinal wall, usually extending for at least 5–8 cm and for the most part covered with intact mucosa. But there is usually ulceration at some point. This form of carcinoma is sometimes found as an extension of one of the other gross types of growth. It is also not infrequently the type of carcinoma that develops in ulcerative colitis.

The Colloid Carcinoma usually forms a bulky growth with a very suggestive gelatinous appearance. There may or may not be extensive ulceration and infiltration.

It is well known that the cauliflower type of growth tends to predominate in the right colon,

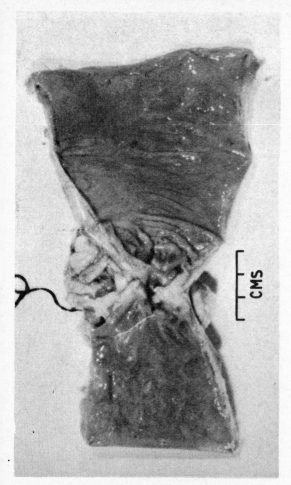

Fig. 283. A so-called 'string stricture' carcinoma of the sigmoid colon seen from the mucosal aspect on opening the bowel.

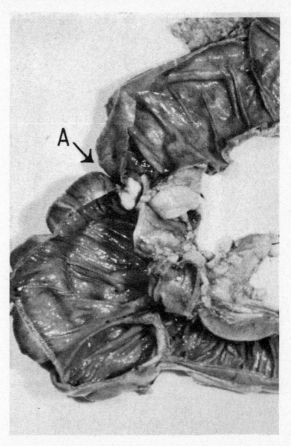

Fig. 284. A 'string stricure' carcinoma of the ascending colon. A = the growth.

whilst the more scirrhous, stenosing growths are commoner in the left colon, but this classical teaching should not be allowed to obscure the fact that any type of carcinoma may occur in any part of the colon. Rectal cancer usually assumes an ulcerating or annular form, but a polypoid type of growth, often with some ulceration, is not infrequent in the ampulla of the rectum (Fig. 285).

SECONDARY EFFECTS ON THE BOWEL

Obstruction. Depending on the type of growth and its situation in the large intestine there may be more or less interference with the passage of intestinal contents. Though bulky polypoid growths may seem to fill the lumen of the bowel almost completely they do not usually cause as much obstruction as annular constricting growths, especially as the intestinal contents are liquid in the right colon, where the former type of growth is most frequently found, whilst the faeces likely to encounter a 'string stricture' carcinoma of the left colon are semi-solid or formed. It is with this latter type of lesion that the effects of obstruction are usually most pronounced. At first the colon proximal to the growth becomes chronically dilated and loaded with liquid or solid faeces, and, due to exaggerated peristaltic efforts to overcome the impediment, its wall undergoes hypertrophy and thickening, so that it contrasts strikingly with the relatively collapsed thin-walled bowel distal to the growth. The proximal dilatation is usually limited to the large intestine, presumably owing to the action of the ileocaecal valve protecting the small gut from back-

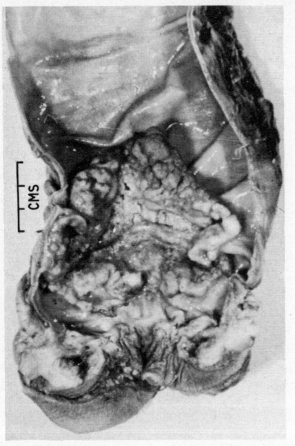

Fig. 285. A fungating carcinoma of the ampulla of the rectum.

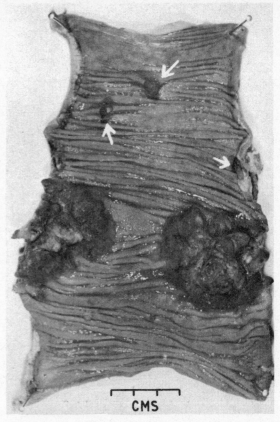

Fig. 286. A carcinoma of the rectum with associated adenomatous polyps (arrowed) in the adjacent bowel.

pressure. Even when acute obstruction has supervened owing to oedema of the growth, to the impaction of a faecal mass in it or to the bowel undergoing intussusception at this site, the small bowel usually remains undistended at first. But eventually this protective mechanism may break down, especially with growths of the right colon, and the ileum may also become dilated. The changes in the proximal colon in chronic obstruction are not confined to the muscle coat; in addition the mucosa may become ulcerated, showing numerous small 'stercoral' ulcers which give it a moth-eaten appearance.

Perforation. If acute obstruction supervenes the bowel sometimes gives way at the site of a stercoral ulcer, often in the caecum but sometimes elsewhere in the colon proximal to the growth. Contrary to popular belief, however, this is not the commonest form of perforation that occurs in connection with carcinoma of the colon and rectum. Far more frequent is perforation of the growth itself which takes place usually quite apart from acute obstruction (see Goligher and Smiddy 1957). This may develop suddenly with resulting diffuse peritonitis or more gradually with a localized peritonitis, the latter being especially common with growths in the ileocaecal region, the resulting mass or abscess often closely resembling the state of affairs found in appendicitis (Ewing 1951; Patterson 1956; Goligher and Smiddy 1957).

ASSOCIATED POLYPS

Adenomatous polyps are frequently found in the adjacent bowel in cases of carcinoma of the rectum or colon as pointed out on p. 331, and occurred in approximately 30% of my cases (Fig. 286).

Multiple Carcinomas

Occasionally carcinomas of the large intestine occur in multiple form, as many as two, three or more primary growths being present in the same patient. Thus in a series of 3220 specimens of cancer of the rectum and colon examined in the Pathology Department at St Mark's Hospital from 1928 to 1948 inclusive there were 98 examples of multiple tumours, an incidence of just over 3% (Goligher et al. 1951). In some cases the growths were placed close together in the same segment of bowel, in others they were widely separated, one growth being situated, for example, in the rectum and another at the splenic flexure or caecum. Sometimes the lesions present in these cases were of roughly the same extent and had apparently arisen more or less simultaneously as in Fig. 287A, but at other times one tumour was obviously much younger than the other as in Fig. 287B and had developed consecutively. It will be readily appreciated that in the latter cases the chronology of development and the location of the growths might have been such that the older carcinoma could have been detected and removed surgically before the other had appeared or was sufficiently large to be discovered by the surgeon at laparotomy. It would then show itself in the remaining portion of colon or rectum at a later date, as in the cases observed by Westhues (1934), Mayo and Schlicke (1942), Gilchrist and David (1947), Goligher et al. (1951), Devitt et al. (1969) and Bussey et al. (1967). It seems from the very careful analysis of the late results of radical operations for carcinoma of the rectum and colon by Bussey et al. (1967) that the incidence of further primary cancers in the large bowel is of the order of 1% on a 10-year follow-up and rises to over 3% when the follow-up is extended to 30 years.

Histological Features—Tumour Grading

Adenocarcinomas of the large intestine differ considerably in their histological appearances, some growths being relatively well differentiated, others more anaplastic. In general papilliferous growths tend to be better differentiated than those of a deeply ulcerating and infiltrating kind. A modification of the system of histological grading introduced by Broders (1925) has been extensively applied to the study of carcinomas of the large intestine by a number of pathologists, notably by Grinnell (1939) and Dukes (1940), and shown to bear a definite relationship to the extent of spread of the lesion and to the ultimate prognosis after surgical treatment. The actual grades recognized by different workers have varied somewhat. At one time Dukes (1940) distinguished five arbitrary grades as follows:

Grade I tumours closely resembled an adenoma in which there were signs of active epithelial proliferation, but were recognized as malignant because there was evidence of infiltration through the muscularis mucosae.

Grade II tumours were those in which the cancer cells were more crowded together but were still arranged in a fairly regular fashion one or two layers deep around glandular spaces. The nuclei stained deeply and irregular mitotic figures were fairly common.

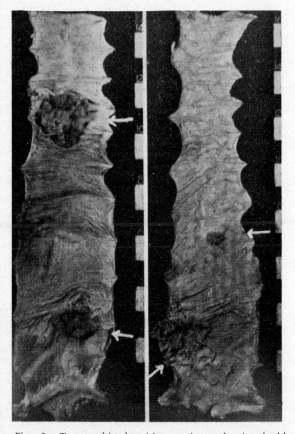

Fig. 287. Two combined excision specimens showing double carcinomas of the rectum. The growths are indicated by arrows. In specimen A both carcinomas are at approximately the same stage of development, but in specimen B one is obviously of much more recent origin than the other (*From Goligher et al. 1951*)

Grade III. The cells in this grade were less differentiated and were arranged in irregularly folded rings often two or three rows deep around glomerular spaces or in solid clumps. Mitotic figures were more numerous than in Grade II tumours.

Grade IV tumour cells were even more anaplastic and did not form glandular structures at all but pervaded the tissues singly or in small irregular groups or columns.

Colloid (or mucoid) tumours. These also varied considerably in their degree of differentiation, but satisfactory standards for grading them could not be devised and so they were all grouped together.

Applying this system of grading to 985 consecutive carcinomas of the rectum removed by radical operation Dukes (1940) grouped 6·7% of the tumours in Grade I, 56·7% in Grade II, 22·7% in Grade III, 1·4% in Grade IV, and 12·4% as colloid carcinomata. The distribution of the grades was roughly the same in the two sexes but tumours of high grade of malignancy (Grade IV and colloid growths) appeared to be slightly more common in young patients.

Applying the same system of grading to 331 carcinomas of the colon Dukes (1945) found that in general colon growths were rather better differentiated than carcinomas of the rectum. Thus Grade I tumours represented 16% of colon growths as compared with only 7% of rectal growths. Grinnell (1939) also concluded that carcinomas of the colon tended to be further differentiated than those of the rectum; in addition he thought that growths of the right colon were usually better differentiated than those of the left colon.

Dukes (1946) subsequently modified his system of grading so that it corresponded more to that of Grinnell (1939). It now comprises only four categories—low grade, average grade, and high grade of malignancy and colloid carcinomas. Low grade corresponds to his former Grade I, average grade to Grade II, and high grade to Grades III and IV (see Fig. 288).

Aetiological Factors

We are just as ignorant of the basic processes underlying the development of carcinoma in this site as elsewhere in the body, but among possible predisposing factors two appear to be incontrovertibly established and certain others may be mentioned:

INTESTINAL POLYPS

The role of adenomas and villous papillomas in the aetiology of carcinoma of the large intestine is discussed on p. 331.

INFLAMMATORY DISEASES

ULCERATIVE COLITIS

Recent work seems to have placed beyond dispute the fact that ulcerative colitis predisposes to the development of carcinoma of the colon or rectum (see p. 719), but whether Crohn's colitis induces any predisposition to malignant tumours is more debatable (see p. 831).

DIVERTICULOSIS OR DIVERTICULITIS

These conditions sometimes coexist with carcinoma coli (see Stewart 1931) but there is no clear evidence that the association is other than purely fortuitous. After all, diverticulosis of the distal colon is a very common condition in elderly subjects, and some degree of diverticulitis is by no means rare, so that its coincidence with carcinoma would be only natural in a fair proportion of cases.

OTHER INTESTINAL INFECTIONS

Amoebic and bacillary dysentery and tuberculosis do not predispose to cancer (Willis 1948). Though bilharzial infection of the bladder, which is prevalent in Egypt, is believed often to lead to vesical carcinoma, rectal bilharziasis, which is also common in that country, does not seem to predispose to rectal cancer (Dolbey and Moore 1924).

IRRADIATION

A few cases have been published by Slaughter and Southwick (1957), Smith (1962) and McMahon and Rowe (1971), in which, many years after irradiation treatment for carcinoma of the cervix uteri, there has developed a primary adenocarcinoma of the rectum—not to be confused with recurrence in the rectal wall of the original squamous celled carcinoma of the cervix. As the number of patients reported with such carcinomas is relatively small compared with the great many women who undergo radiotherapy for cancer of the uterine cervix, it is impossible to say whether the relationship is one of cause and effect or purely coincidental.

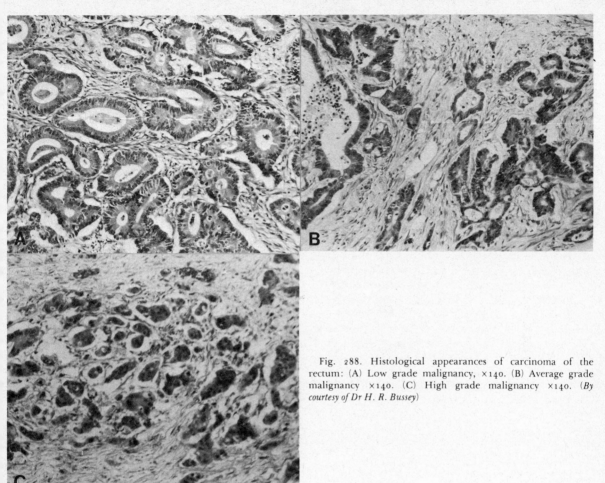

Fig. 288. Histological appearances of carcinoma of the rectum: (A) Low grade malignancy, ×140. (B) Average grade malignancy ×140. (C) High grade malignancy ×140. (*By courtesy of Dr H. R. Bussey*)

URETERIC IMPLANTATION INTO COLON

A number of reports have been published of tumours developing in the sigmoid colon many years after ureterosigmoidostomy, the lesions being found to arise in the bowel wall at the site of ureteric implantation. For example, Urdaneta et al. (1966) found that such tumours occurred in three of 23 patients surviving more than 10 years after ureterosigmoidostomy, and they were able to collect 11 more cases from the literature with the same complication of this operation. In this collective series of 14 cases the average length of follow-up was 13 years. The colonic tumour was

a carcinoma in 11 and an adenomatous polyp in three. In nine of the 14 cases the ureterosigmoidostomy was performed for a benign condition, such as extrophy of the bladder, which would make it unlikely that a carcinogen in the urine caused the original bladder cancer and later provoked the development of the colon tumour. More recently Kille and Glick (1967) have reported two further examples of such tumours occurring in the sigmoid after urinary diversion to this part of the colon (one of which was a benign adenoma), and I myself have encountered two such patients, the colonic growth in each being an adenoma. The precise significance of the ureterosigmoidostomy in the genesis of these growths is debatable (see discussion after paper by Urdaneta et al. 1966). Moreover the importance of any connection between this operation and sigmoid tumours has been greatly diminished in recent years by the trend of surgical fashion away from ureterosigmoidostomy as a means of urinary diversion to ureteric implantation into an ileal conduit.

The Possible Influence of Ingested Carcinogens and of Dietary Habits

From the work of Peacock and Kirby (1944) it seems possible that carcinogens may be produced in fats used repeatedly for frying. Other possible sources of ingested carcinogenic hydrocarbons are tobacco-tar, dust from tarred roads and domestic and occupational soots and smokes. Chemical carcinogens may also exist in the various drugs, colouring or flavouring materials, or preservatives that are consumed in our modern civilization. If any such carcinogens exist and are poorly absorbed they might play a part in the production of carcinoma of the large intestine. Naturally they would tend to exert their maximum effect so far as the intestine was concerned towards the distal end of the colon and in the rectum because of the slower passage and greater concentration of the faeces in these parts (Dukes 1945).

The possible role of regular ingestion of purgatives in the aetiology of intestinal cancer was investigated by Boyd and Doll (1954). They found that patients with carcinomas of the stomach or bowel had much more frequently been using liquid paraffin as a habitual aperient than had a control group of patients suffering from diseases other than gastrointestinal. But they pointed out that this substance is more commonly used by women than by men, yet the mortality from cancer of the bowel is less in the former than the latter. Further, there has been no striking increase in the mortality from gastrointestinal cancer since the medicinal use of liquid paraffin began during the period 1905–10. The case against paraffin seems to be unproven.

The possible relationship between dietary habits and bowel cancer has been specially stressed by Burkitt (1971), Hill et al. (1971) and Nigro and Campbell (1976). This hypothesis rests on the following facts:

1. Carcinoma (and adenoma) of the large intestine is extremely rare, almost non-existent in the indigenous black population of most parts of Africa (Hutt and Templeton 1971; Doll et al. 1966), but has an incidence in the white population in these countries roughly the same as that found in the peoples of Western European countries.

2. When the African native becomes westernized and abandons his customary diet and way of life, the frequency of cancer of the colorectum progressively increases (Burkitt 1971). Similarly in American Negroes there is a gradual rise in the incidence of bowel cancer accompanying their adoption of the feeding habits of the white population (Doll 1969).

3. There is a high roughage content in the maize meals eaten by native Africans living in their natural environment, which produces large soft frequent stools, compared with which the faeces of civilized white men seem small and constipated (Burkitt 1971; Burkitt et al. 1972).

4. Any potential carcinogen contained in the faeces will remain longer in contact with the colonic and rectal musoca in a constipated person (Oettlé 1967).

5. Bacteria can cause degradation of normal bile salts to form known carcinogens (Hill et al. 1971).

6. A greater proportion of bile salts can be recovered from the faeces of Bantu living on a high-residue diet in South Africa than from the faeces of Europeans taking a more refined diet (Antonis and Bersohn 1962), which suggests that part of the bile salts in the latter has somehow been disposed of, possibly by bacterial action.

7. Differences have been demonstrated between the bacterial flora of the faeces of Africans and of Europeans (Aries et al. 1969).

8. Though the lack of fibre in the diet of Western civilization has been particularly incriminated by Burkitt (1971) as the factor mainly responsible for the predisposition to carcinoma, it may be that another feature of aetiological importance in that diet is its relatively rich content of fat (Nigro and Campbell 1976; Correa 1978) and particularly cholesterol (Cruse et al. 1979). There may be a relationship between a high-protein content in the diet and the occurrence of colorectal cancer (Correa 1978).

Modes of Spread

Carcinomas of the colon or rectum may spread in five ways:

1. By direct continuity of tissue in and through the bowel wall.
2. Through the peritoneal cavity.
3. By way of the extramural lymphatics.

4. By means of the blood stream.
5. By implantation on to raw surfaces or suture lines in the bowel.

DIRECT SPREAD IN AND THROUGH THE BOWEL WALL

Spread in the plane of the bowel wall is an integral part of the process of enlargement of the growth. This marginal increase occurs in all directions, but seems usually to be more rapid in the transverse than the longitudinal axis of the bowel, and, as has already been explained, this is the mechanism whereby a small isolated growth eventually assumes a completely annular form. However, it may take very many months to reach this latter state. Miles (1926) reckoned that in the ampulla of the rectum the average carcinoma would require about six months to traverse each quadrant of the bowel circumference, so that when the lesion was found to be in a completely annular condition it might be assumed as a rule to have been present for at least two years.

Beyond the macroscopic margin of the primary growth there is a zone of microscopic spread in the lymphatic plexuses which are situated in the submucous, intermuscular, subserous or subfascial planes of the bowel wall. Many years ago Handley (1913) claimed that lymphatic permeation, particularly in the submucosa, could sometimes be very extensive, resulting in malignant cells being found a distance of several centimetres beyond the palpable edge of the tumour. But Cole (1913), Monsarrat and Williams (1913) and Leitch (1926) were unable to confirm this finding and concluded that such microscopic spread was usually a very limited process, seldom reaching more than a few millimetres beyond the growth. With the revival of sphincter-saving resections for carcinoma of the rectum this question has acquired a fresh relevance, for it is essential for the surgeon to know the minimum safe margin of apparently normal rectal wall that must be removed distal to the growth in such operations. Several very careful studies have been conducted to illuminate this point. Westhues (1934) found that microscopic spread never extended more than 15–20 mm distal to the lower edge of the growth, and Black and Waugh (1948) considered that it was even less extensive as a rule. Quer et al. (1953) agreed that in the vast majority of cases of rectal cancer distal microscopic spread in the wall of the rectum was very restricted and could be safely encompassed by resection of a margin of 25 mm of grossly normal wall beyond the growth,

but they emphasized that in very anaplastic growths intramural spread might sometimes be much wider, up to several centimetres. Grinnell (1954) also found that in some very advanced, essentially incurable, cases undergoing palliative excisions direct microscopic spread could be quite extensive. Even in the average more favourable cases he was able to observe carcinoma cells sometimes as far as 40 mm distal to the macroscopic edge of the lesion, and he advised that a margin of at least 50 mm of grossly normal bowel beyond the growth should always be insisted upon in a resection operation. Contrary to most other workers he considered that intramural spread took place by permeation of the lymphatic channels not of the submucosa but of the subserosa or perirectal fat, rarely by permeation of a vein or direct extension in the muscular coat.

As will be gathered from the above discussion there have been differences of opinion amongst the research workers concerned as to how great a margin of clearance of apparently normal rectal wall should be removed distal to the growth in a rectal resection specimen. There are certainly differences of opinion amongst surgeons, for whilst most aim at a margin of 4–5 cm, others, such as Localio and Eng (1975) feel that 3 cm should suffice. It could be argued that, if the peroperative biopsy shows a very well differentiated carcinoma, a small margin of say 3 cm, or even only 2 cm, would do, but I am not aware of any particular study of this point. Incidentally, it is not uncommon to find that the margin of clearance which the surgeon was confident was 5 cm wide at the resection, proves a good deal less when the specimen is examined immediately after removal. Accordingly if a somewhat narrower margin is accepted as adequate by the surgeon at his operation, the distal line of section might often subsequently be found uncomfortably close to the actual growth.

Spread radially through the bowel wall. Coincident with the circumferential expansion of growth a process of penetration of the bowel wall takes place, being usually most advanced at a point corresponding to the centre or oldest part of the tumour. As already mentioned, the amount of infiltration often varies inversely with the superficial bulk of the lesion. The submucosa and muscle coat are gradually invaded and eventually, unless the progress of the condition is interrupted by operative treatment, the growth reaches the perirectal or pericolonic fat or the peritoneum. According to Dukes (1940) this stage has already been reached by 85% of rectal carcinomas by the time they come to surgical excision. The proportion of carcinomas of

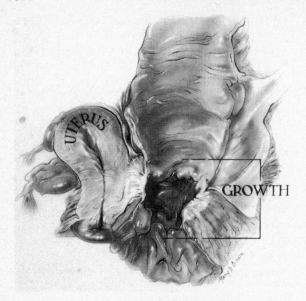

Fig. 289. Specimen obtained by combined hysterectomy and anterior resection of the rectum. Note ulcerating rectal carcinoma invading the uterus.

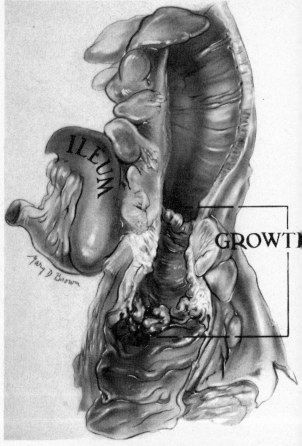

Fig. 290. Specimen of rectal carcinoma removed by anterior resection, an adherent loop of ileum being resected *en bloc* with the rectum.

the colon that have completely penetrated the bowel wall at the time of operation is probably a little less. The further progress of the process of direct spread depends on the precise situation of the growth. If it is *in the rectum and lying mainly posteriorly*, it extends through the perirectal fat, fascia propria and eventually reaches the fascia of Waldeyer. This certainly presents a considerable obstacle to further spread as Westhues (1934) emphasized, but in advanced cases it may also be penetrated and the sacral plexus, sacrum or coccyx are then liable to be invaded. If the growth is situated *in the extra-peritoneal part of the rectum on the anterior aspect*, it encounters relatively little perirectal fat, and the thin fascia of Denonvillier is apparently readily penetrated, with the resulting development of adhesions to the appropriate related viscera—the prostate, seminal vesicles or bladder in the male, the posterior vaginal wall or cervix uteri in the female. With a rectal growth *above the peritoneal reflection* direct spread anteriorly or laterally results in invasion of the peritoneal coat overlying the lesion. This may give rise to transperitoneal dissemination (see below), but what is perhaps more frequent is that other organs such as the uterus, uterine appendages, a loop of small gut, the sigmoid colon or the bladder become adherent to the peritoneal surface and are eventually invaded by the growth.

With *colon carcinomas* radial extension of the lesion if it is situated *on the retroperitoneal aspect* eventually results in infiltration of structures on the posterior abdominal wall such as the duodenum, ureter, perirenal fascia or fat, the iliacus or psoas muscle. If, however, it occurs anteriorly, or *possibly on either side*, it leads to invasion of the peritoneal covering often with secondary adherence to other abdominal organs such as the small or large gut, the stomach, pelvic organs, or abdominal parietes.

In fact, adhesion to other viscera or to the abdominal or pelvic wall is not at all uncommon with carcinoma of the rectum and colon and may present the surgeon with a formidable fixed mass implicating several viscera. Eradication of the growth will then necessitate excision in part or *in toto* of other adherent organs or removal of a portion of the abdominal parieties (Figs 289–91). However, it is important to stress that pathological

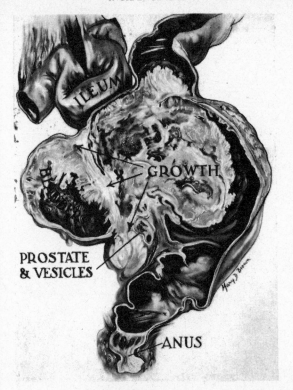

Fig. 291. Specimen of rectum, bladder, prostate, vesicles and ileum obtained by complete pelvic clearance. A rectal carcinoma was present which invaded the bladder in the trigonal region.

examination of the specimens obtained by such extended resection often shows that spread was much less extensive than was feared at operation; quite frequently lymphatic metastases are few or entirely absent and it is not uncommon to discover that the adhesions to adjoining structures are purely inflammatory and contain no actual growth (Goligher 1941; Dukes 1951; Goligher et al. 1951). In my cases of rectal and colon carcinomas requiring removal of other adherent organs I have found that only in one-third were the adhesions due to neoplastic involvement. The prognosis is thus often better than was imagined at the time of operation and this certainly provides an incentive to courageous surgery.

TRANSPERITONEAL SPREAD

Dissemination within the peritoneal cavity is one of the most serious forms of spread of carcinoma of the large intestine, for it quickly places the lesion beyond hope of surgical excision. In the earliest stages of peritoneal invasion transcoelomic spread may be confined to the immediate vicinity of the primary growth and may result in the development of discrete carcinomatous plaques in the adjacent peritoneum. It is possible indeed that some of these nodules may have arisen, not from transperitoneal spread, but from dissemination in the subperitoneal lymphatics, as claimed by Miles (1926). At a later stage the peritoneal deposits become more widespread till finally the parietal peritoneum, greater omentum and neighbouring viscera become studded with nodules of growth and there is abundant ascites. (See also Metastases by implantation of exfoliated cancer cells on to raw surfaces or the peritoneum, p. 399.)

SPREAD BY THE EXTRAMURAL LYMPHATIC SYSTEM

The importance of spread of carcinoma of the large intestine by means of the extramural lymphatic channels, with the production of metastases in the related lymph glands, needs no emphasis, for the direction and possible extent of such spread plays a decisive role in determining the scope of operation for radical excision. In this connection it should be pointed out that the glands draining lymph from the site of a carcinoma of the large intestine may be enlarged either from carcinomatous deposits or from septic absorption from the ulcerating surface of the growth. Usually septic glands are softer than malignant ones, but it is quite impossible at laparotomy to distinguish between them with accuracy (McVay 1922; Gabriel et al. 1935). Conversely, early glandular metastases may not be associated with any enlargement or induration of the glands at all, so that clearly the only safe course in essaying radical removal is always to excise the entire related lymphatic field along with the primary growth.

LYMPHATIC SPREAD FROM CARCINOMA OF THE COLON

Pathways

As already mentioned on p. 26 the usual drainage of lymph from the various segments of the colon was early studied by Poirier et al. (1903) and Jamieson and Dobson (1907). Clogg (1908) was one of the first to investigate systematically the actual distribution of lymphatic metastases from carcinomas in different segments of the colon, and his careful observations have been confirmed and

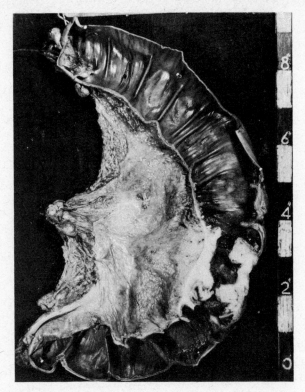
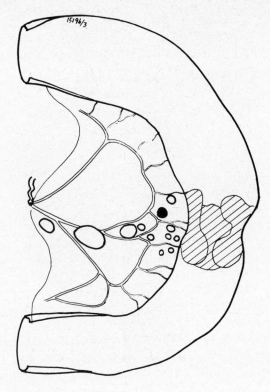

Fig. 292. A colectomy specimen and the related gland dissection chart showing a carcinoma of the descending colon with metastases confined to one paracolic lymph gland immediately adjacent to the primary growth. (Involved glands shaded black, uninvolved glands shown as clear circles; local spread indicated by hatching.) (*From Dukes 1951*)

amplified in more recent times by Hayes (1921), Rankin (1933), Rankin and Olson (1933), Raiford (1935), Coller et al. (1940), Dukes (1945, 1951) and Gilchrist and David (1947). These studies show that the first metastases usually occur in the paracolic glands nearest to the primary growth, frequently only one or two glands being affected (Fig. 292), though rarely the paracolic glands are missed and the first deposits occur in glands more proximally situated. As the condition progresses the glands on the lower main colic vessels to the affected part of the intestine are involved and the process extends gradually upwards through the chain of glands on the vessels (Fig. 293), eventually to reach the glands on the superior haemorrhoidal or inferior mesenteric arteries. It will be seen therefore that lymphatic spread follows closely the course of the blood vessels supplying the site of the carcinoma, and the appropriate fields of excision are readily worked out by reference to the arterial supply (pp. 20–21, Fig. 18). In the later stages of the disease, or in very active anaplastic growths, as is well known from experience at laparotomy and necropsy, glands may be widely involved along the abdominal aorta and elsewhere in the abdomen and other body cavities. Such findings indicate an incurable state of affairs (Grinnell 1966).

Frequency of Metastases

In a series of some 500 specimens of carcinoma of the colon removed by resection Dukes (1951) found lymphatic metastases in only 38%, and frequently these were confined to one or two glands in the immediate vicinity of the primary lesion. This was often so even when extensive direct spread had occurred to the abdominal parietes or adjacent viscera. There has been some difference of opinion as to the relative frequency of lymphatic metastases with growths of the right and left halves of the colon respectively. Gilchrist and David (1947) found metastases twice as commonly with growths of the right half as with those of the left half, but Rankin and Olson (1933), Coller et al. (1940) and Lloyd-Davies et al. (1953) reported no significant difference in the incidence with growths on the two sides of the colon.

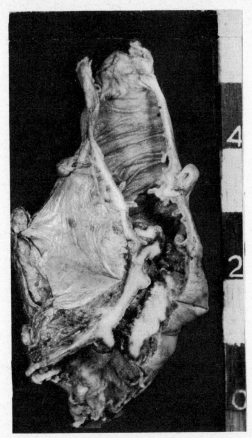 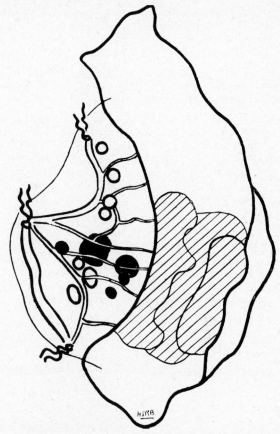

Fig. 293. A colectomy specimen and the related gland dissection chart showing a carcinoma of the sigmoid colon with extensive involvement of the paracolic glands and one gland along the sigmoid vessels. (Glands containing metastases shaded black, uninvolved glands shown as clear circles.) (*From Dukes 1951*)

LYMPHATIC SPREAD FROM CARCINOMA OF THE RECTUM

Pathways

Miles (1910, 1926) was the first to study this process in a really comprehensive manner. In his now classical researches he investigated the mode of spread of rectal cancer by the lymphatic system from several points of view: (a) by noting the position of metastases during the performance of operations for this disease; (b) by observing the sites of recurrence after operative treatment; (c) by studying the autopsy findings in patients dying of advanced and inoperable carcinomas of the rectum; and (d) by pathological examination of operative specimens of rectal cancer. From all these sources of information he concluded that lymphatic spread could take place in three directions, upwards, laterally and downwards, so that he recognized three zones of lymphatic extension (Fig. 23).

The Zone of Upward Spread. This comprised the lymphatics and glands lying alongside the superior haemorrhoidal and inferior mesenteric vessels as they lie in the mesorectum and base of the mesosigmoid, and ultimately connected with the glands situated on the front and sides of the abdominal aorta. Miles (1926) emphasized that this zone comprised also the whole of the sigmoid mesocolon, for the paracolic glands, lying in it close to the sigmoid colon, were in his experience very liable to be invaded.

The Zone of Lateral Spread. This consisted essentially of the lymphatics running in the lateral ligaments between the pelvic peritoneum and the levator muscles to end in the internal iliac glands on the pelvic side wall. Miles (1926) also depicted lymphatic glands interspersed in the course of these lymphatics between the rectum and the iliac glands, and reported that they and the levator muscles were not infrequently the seat of metastases.

The Zone of Downward Spread. This embraced the lymphatics traversing the sphincter muscles, the perianal skin, and the ischiorectal fat, and ultimately draining into the inguinal glands.

Miles (1910, 1926) emphasized the importance of the upward zone of spread but considered that the other zones were also frequently implicated. He believed that, regardless of the situation of the primary growth, spread could take place in all three directions, so that, for example, even with a carcinoma of the rectosigmoid junction evidence of lymphatic dissemination could be found in the lateral and downward zones as well as the upward zone of spread. It was on the strength of these observations that he advocated an extensive removal of the entire rectum and related structures by an abdominoperineal operation as the rational treatment for all cases of rectal cancer.

Miles' observations and teaching were accepted without serious question till Westhues (1930, 1934), Dukes (1930), Gabriel et al. (1935) and Wood and Wilkie (1933) published the results of their investigation of the modes of spread of rectal cancer, as revealed by a meticulous dissection of large numbers of operative specimens of the disease removed by sacral, perineal or abdominoperineal excision. These failed to confirm Miles' findings in several important respects. First of all, no evidence of lateral or downward spread could be demonstrated as a rule in their preparations. As for upward spread they agreed with Miles that this was a frequent mode of dissemination, but they found that it was usually confined very strictly to the chain of glands along the main superior haemorrhoidal and inferior mesenteric vessels. According to their observations the first glands to be implicated were the pararectal glands on the back of the rectum immediately adjacent to the growth (Fig. 294). From these the process of involvement extended steadily upwards in sequence along the chain of superior

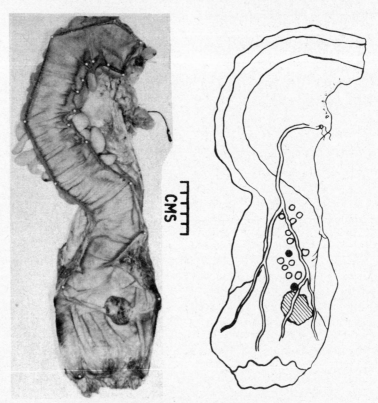

Fig. 294. A combined excision specimen with the related gland dissection chart, showing a rectal carcinoma with metastases in the adjacent pararectal glands on the back of the rectum. (Implicated glands shaded black, uninvolved glands shown as clear circles.)

haemorrhoidal and inferior mesenteric glands, eventually to the aortic glands (Fig. 295). Rarely *discontinuous* spread occurred, as stressed by Wood and Wilkie (1933), some glands high up on the superior haemorrhoidal or inferior mesenteric vessels being found to contain metastases whilst others closer to the growth were spared. Only very rarely, when all the glands along the superior vascular pedicle were choked with deposits, as in very advanced, probably quite incurable, cases, were the sigmoid paracolic glands affected, and only in such cases was any evidence of downward or retrograde spread likely to be found. The rarity of downward spread was further shown by continued research in Dukes' laboratory relating to no less than 1500 carefully dissected operative specimens removed by abdominoperineal excision (Goligher et al. 1951). Metastatic involvement of glands below the level of the primary growth was found in 98 or 6·5% of these cases. But in 68 of these the glands concerned lay within 6 mm of the lower margin of the growth (Fig. 296), and only 30 of the 98, or 2% of all the specimens, showed significant retrograde spread to 20 mm or more below the primary lesion (Fig. 297); practically all these cases had very extensive lymphatic spread in an upward direction as well. Glover and Waugh (1945) record an even lower incidence of retrograde lymphatic spread.

In regard to lateral spread it is, I think, important to appreciate that the average abdominoperineal excision specimen contains surprisingly little of the levator ani muscles and other tissues of the lateral zone of lymphatic extension. Contrary to the observations of Miles, the only constant glands in this zone are the internal iliac glands themselves, which are of course not normally removed in a combined excision, so that from the examination of the specimen it is not possible to adjudicate on the question of their involvement. My experience at operations for rectal cancer leaves me in no doubt

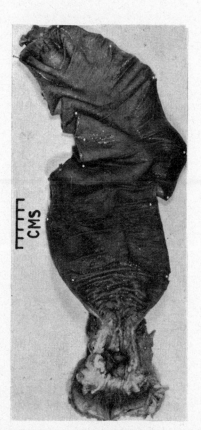
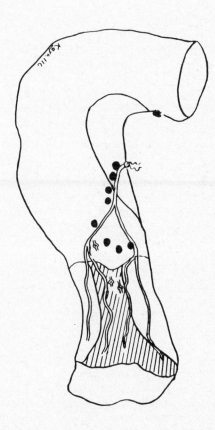

Fig. 295. A combined excision specimen with the related gland dissection chart, showing a rectal carcinoma with extensive involvement of the pararectal and superior haemorrhoidal lymph glands. (Glands containing metastases shaded black, uninvolved glands shown as clear circles.)

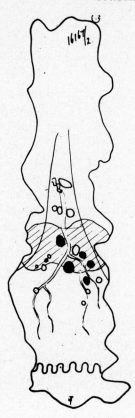

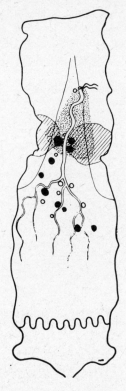

Fig. 296. The gland dissection chart of a combined excision specimen, showing a carcinoma of the rectum with metastases in the pararectal glands, one of the involved glands being situated just below the level of the inferior edge of the primary growth. (Involved glands shaded black.) (*By courtesy of Dr Cuthbert Dukes*)

Fig. 297. The gland dissection chart of a combined excision specimen, showing more extensive retrograde spread in the pararectal glands below the level of the lower margin of the growth. (Involved glands shaded black.) (*By courtesy of Dr Cuthbert Dukes*)

whatsoever that the internal iliac glands on one or both sides are fairly frequently the seat of metastases in cases with advanced growths of the extraperitoneal part of the rectum. When affected they can be quite clearly felt as hard enlarged fixed masses on the pelvic side wall, biopsy of which confirms the presence of carcinomatous deposits. Yet if a palliative abdominoperineal excision of the rectum is carried out in such a case, leaving the internal iliac glands, the pathological examination of the operative specimen usually shows no evidence of lateral spread. It should also be mentioned that Gilchrist (1940) and Gilchrist and David (1947), both from the dissection of operative specimens and from their finding of recurrences on follow-up of cases after operation, conclude that lateral spread is important with growths of the extraperitoneal part of the rectum, but probably not with intraperitoneal rectal growths.

But undoubtedly the most convincing evidence that lateral spread does occur has been provided by the attempts that have been made in recent years to extend the scope of ordinary combined abdominoperineal excision to include as a routine the removal of the internal iliac lymph glands. Sauer and Bacon (1952) performed 21 such operations for growths below the peritoneal reflection and found on pathological examination that metastases were present in the internal iliac glands in six. By contrast in none of 11 extended excisions for rectal carcinomas situated above the peritoneal reflection were deposits demonstrated in the glands removed from the pelvic sidewall.

It would seem therefore that lateral lymphatic spread can be disregarded with growths of the intraperitoneal rectum, the lymph drainage of which is apparently exclusively upwards, as claimed on anatomical grounds by Villemin et al. (1925), but it probably occurs more frequently with lesions of the extraperitoneal rectum than examination of operative specimens would imply. Indeed the absence of any sign of lateral spread as a rule in combined excision specimens of advanced ampullary growths is an indication of the inadequacy of this operation in dealing effectively with extension in this zone, rather than of the non-occurrence of such spread.

Frequency of Lymphatic Metastases

There is fairly general agreement among writers who have investigated this matter that, in about 50% of all cases of rectal cancer undergoing radical operation, lymphatic metastases have already occurred (*cf.* 38% of the colon, p. 390). Thus Dukes (1940) found metastases in the glands in 505 of 1000 consecutive operative specimens of carcinoma of the rectum. There was a significant difference in the incidence of metastases in the two sexes; they occurred in 57·7% of the female cases, but in only 46·6% of the males. In both sexes the percentage of cases with glandular metastases was much higher in young patients than in old, 71·8% of cases of both sexes between the ages of 20 and 39 years having metastases, as contrasted with only 46% of cases between 60 and 79. There was no correlation between the size or position of the primary growths and the presence of lymphatic metastases, but a close relationship existed between the incidence of glandular metastases and the histological grade of the tumour, metastases being much more frequent with growths of high grade malignancy. Cases with widespread lymphatic metastases *had almost invariably Grade III or IV growths or mucoid carcinomas.*

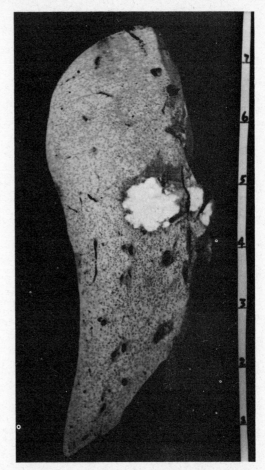

Fig. 298. Section of liver showing large central metastasis undetected at laparotomy—from a patient who died one week after a perineo-abdominal excision for carcinoma of the rectum. (*From Goligher 1941*)

SPREAD BY THE BLOOD STREAM

Blood-borne metastases are perhaps less common with carcinoma of the colon and rectum than with many other malignant growths, but they are by no means infrequent. They occur chiefly in the liver, more rarely in other organs and tissues:

LIVER METASTASES

The liver contains secondary deposits in about one-third to one-half of fatal cases. Thus in Brown and Warren's (1938) series of necropsies on 170 patients dying of carcinoma of the rectum 57 were found to have hepatic metastases. In Willis' (1948) series of 59 necropsies on fatal cases of rectal or colonic carcinoma 31 had liver deposits, 11 of them showing no other metastases. Naturally these post-mortem figures, relating as they do mainly to advanced inoperable cases, cannot be taken to indicate the frequency of hepatic metastases likely to be encountered in clinical practice. Clinically, however, it is only in patients submitted to laparotomy that accurate data exist as to the incidence of liver secondaries. My own analysis of a consecutive series of 893 cases of rectal cancer coming to laparotomy at St Mark's Hospital revealed that hepatic deposits were detected by the surgeon in 103 or 11·5% (Goligher 1941). Further, necropsy performed on 31 of the patients whose livers had been found to be smooth and free from palpable secondaries at operation, but who unfortunately succumbed in the immediate post-operative period due to various complications, revealed that in no less than five secondary growth was present in the depths of the liver (Fig. 298). This represents an incidence of concealed liver secondaries of roughly 1 in 6 in the cases coming to necropsy. If these findings apply to the other cases which were considered at laparotomy to be free from hepatic metastases (790), then as many as 127 of these may have had such metastases hidden in their livers. The total number of cases with secondary hepatic involvement would therefore be raised from 103 (11·5%) to 230 (25·8%). The significance of these buried metastases is that many patients are inevitably subjected to so-called radical excisions when actually the disease has extended beyond the scope of any such operations and has involved the liver. This fact no doubt accounts in large measure for the frequency with which 'recurrence' develops in the liver within two or three years of radical operation.

LUNG METASTASES

According to Willis (1948) the lungs contain secondary deposits in about one-fifth of fatal cases. Clinically such deposits are liable to be overlooked unless the chest is examined radiologically as a routine. Bacon and Jackson (1953) found pulmonary metastases in 5% of 600 clinical cases of carcinoma of the rectum or distal colon, but this is certainly more frequent than in my experience.

METASTASES IN OTHER TISSUES

In about 10% of fatal cases other organs—most often the adrenals, kidneys or bones—are involved (Willis 1948). In Bacon and Jackson's (1953) series of 600 clinical cases metastases were detected in the bones of 6% and in the brain of 1·3%.

EVIDENCE OF VENOUS SPREAD IN
OPERATIVE SPECIMENS

If the affected segment of bowel wall, removed either at necropsy or at operation, is carefully dissected and sectioned histologically, evidence of cancerous invasion of the veins can often be detected. Brown and Warren (1938) in their study of 170 necropsy cases of rectal carcinoma found venous invasion by growth in 41%. In operative specimens of clinical cases of rectal cancer Dukes found evidence of venous spread in approximately 17% (Dukes 1940; Dukes and Bussey 1941). According to him venous spread did not occur as a rule till the primary growth had penetrated through the bowel wall to reach the perirectal tissues, and it was the tributaries of the superior haemorrhoidal vein that were usually invaded. These then became palpable as solid cords of growth extending generally only a short distance, but sometimes a massive thrombosis was produced with solid fixed intravascular growth extending for several centimetres along the haemorrhoidal veins, as illustrated in Fig. 299. This latter, grosser, form is usually associated with secondary malignant tumours erupting on to the rectal mucosa above or below the primary growth, as shown in Fig. 300, due to a continuous cord of growth connecting the perirectal veins with the veins of the submucosa. Dukes (1940) found that venous spread was more common in cases showing lymphatic metastases; thus it was noted in 21·6% of the specimens with glandular deposits, but in only 13·7% of those without lymphatic involvement. He also found that there was a close correlation between the occurrence of venous spread and the activity of the growth as determined by histological grading. Thus venous invasion was detected in under 5% of the grade I growths, in 11·8% of the grade II growths, in 25% of the grade III growths, in 31% of the grade IV growths and in 19·5% of the colloid carcinomas.

A somewhat higher incidence of venous invasion in operative specimens of rectal or colonic carcinoma has been recorded by several other writers such as Grinnell (1942) 36%, Sunderland (1949) 27·6%, Barringer et al. (1954) 38%, and Moore and Sako (1959). This may be due partly to the fact that they, like Brown and Warren (1938), sought for evidence of vascular invasion partly by a histological technique whereas Dukes (1940) relied essentially on macroscopic examination. They agreed with him, however, that venous spread occurred much more often in cases with poorly differentiated growths.

Relationship between Venous Permeation and the Occurrence of Visceral Metastases

Brown and Warren (1938) found that all but one of their *necropsy cases* showing evidence of venous spread in the bowel specimen had visceral metastases, and in only one case with such metastases could invasion of vessels not be demonstrated. A similarly close relationship between the presence of venous spread in *operation specimens* and the occurrence of visceral metastases in clinical cases has *not* been observed. As Dukes (1940) pointed out, the non-discovery of intravascular growth does not exclude the possibility of venous spread, since malignant emboli may already have been carried away in the blood stream leaving no trace behind them. Certainly some patients whose specimens showed no evidence of venous invasion

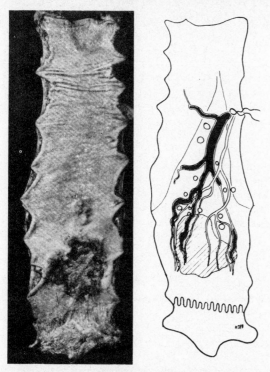

Fig. 299. An operative specimen of carcinoma of the rectum showing permeation of the superior haemorrhoidal vein with growth. (Invaded vein shaded black.) (*From Dukes 1940*)

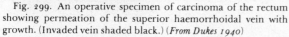

Fig. 300. A gross example of retrograde venous spread extending in the veins below the level of the primary growth and erupting on to the mucosal surface of the bowel as superficial nodules. (*From Dukes 1940*)

have subsequently died of hepatic metastases whilst others, whose specimens were found to have growth inside veins, have survived for five years and longer without signs of recurrence (Dukes and Bussey 1941; Sunderland 1949).

THE DEMONSTRATION OF CANCER CELLS IN THE CIRCULATING BLOOD IN CASES OF CARCINOMA OF THE RECTUM AND COLON

Work by Engell (1955) using a technique earlier employed by Pool and Dunlop (1934) has thrown fresh light on the mechanism of spread of carcinoma by the blood stream. He has succeeded in demonstrating tumour cells in samples of blood taken at operation from the veins draining the tumour site in 59% of 107 patients with cancer of the rectum or colon. Contrary to the opinion previously expressed by Cole et al. (1954) and Fisher and Turnbull (1955), that disturbance of the tumour by handling at operation is probably an important factor in releasing malignant cells into the portal circulation, he found no increase in the number of positive samples immediately after operative manipulation of the growth. Nor was

there any clear correlation between the proportion of positive results and the extent of spread of the growth. But a relationship seemed to exist between the histological grade of malignancy of the lesion and the chances of finding tumour cells in the venous blood draining from it. Thus cells were found in 35% of the cases with grade II carcinomas, in 78% of those with grade III growths, and in all those with grade IV lesions. This would make it appear likely that tumour cells are escaping practically constantly into the blood stream from poorly differentiated growths, and not infrequently even from better-differentiated lesions, perhaps as a result of peristaltic activity. Accepting that that is so, particular interest therefore attached to the follow-up study conducted by Engell (1955) on the patients who formed the basis of his investigation. He found that amongst those who had been demonstrated to have cancer cells in the venous blood from the tumour site there were as many surviving in good health at between six months and four years as had developed metastases, and this was confirmed by a subsequent 5–9-year follow-up study (Engell 1959).

Engell (1955) also attempted to demonstrate tumour cells in the peripheral blood, as obtained from the median cubital vein or the brachial artery, in 93 cases with carcinomas in various situations, not only in the large intestine but also the stomach, lung etc. In 14 of those patients suffering from advanced inoperable growths with widespread manifest metastases cancer cells were found in the peripheral blood in seven. In 79 patients with operable growths cancer cells were demonstrated in the systemic blood in 19, most of whom had poorly differentiated growths. It is not clear what the subsequent fate of these 10 patients was on follow-up, but it seems probable that tumour cells can negotiate the capillary beds of the liver and lungs without producing metastases in either of these situations.

Subsequently tumour cells have also been demonstrated by other workers in the peripheral blood and in the blood draining from the rectum and colon in cases of rectal and colonic cancer (Moore et al. 1957; Moore and Sako 1959; Long et al. 1960; Roberts et al. 1961; Sellwood et al. 1965; Forrest 1965). Moore and Sako (1959) found cancer cells in *surgical* blood specimens in 60 such patients but, contrary to the observation of Engell (1955), they were more frequent in more advanced lesions, being noted in six (37%) of 16 inoperable growths but in only seven (16%) of 44 resectable cancers. There was no difference in the proportion of positive samples before and after operative manipulation of the primary growth. Moore and Sako (1959) were much less successful in recovering malignant cells from the peripheral blood; none of 40 resectable cases and only one of 17 non-resectable cases of rectal or colonic carcinoma had demonstrable tumour cells in the peripheral blood (six curable cases and one incurable case had atypical, doubtful cells). They gave no long-term follow-up data. Long et al. (1960), working in Warren Cole's laboratories, concentrated mainly on examination of the peripheral blood. They found cancer cells in 25% of 59 patients classified as curable, and in 39% of 119 incurable patients, the growths included in these series not all being confined to the intestinal tract. In five of their patients, specially studied during operation, there was a striking increase in the frequency of malignant cells recovered from the peripheral blood during operative manipulation of the tumour. A two- to five-year follow-up study of Warren Cole's cases by Roberts et al. (1961) did not reveal any difference in the survival rates of those with or without demonstrable circulating cancer cells. Sellwood et al. (1965) examined the peripheral blood of 192 patients with malignant growths in

various organs, including the rectum and colon. They found that samples were positive for cancer cells in 7% *before* operation, in 6% *during* operation, and in 9% *after* operation. In only one patient—with an enormous carcinoma of the bladder—was there a clear indication that the number of circulating cells was increased by operative manipulation. Forrest (1965), using Seal's (1959) millipore filtration technique, found abnormal cells in the peripheral blood of 36% of patients with advanced, mainly gastrointestinal and breast, tumours. The regional blood in six cases with large bowel cancer showed malignant cells in five.

In interpreting the results of these researches, it is important to remember certain points:

1. They are all cytological studies of stained cells usually after incubation, repeated centrifugation and suspension for long periods, which may produce considerable cellular distortion and degenerative changes, leading possibly to misinterpretations. Unless the strictest cytological criteria are observed confusion with megakaryocytes and a variety of other non-malignant cells may occur (Rebuck 1947).

2. There is no conclusive evidence that these free 'malignant' cells are in fact alive. If they could be grown in tissue culture or as autoimplants in patients with advanced inoperable growths their viability would be established, but efforts to do so have been unsuccessful (Moore 1960).

3. No workers apart from Warren Cole's group have confirmed the contention that operative manipulation of the primary growth increases the risk of 'showering' malignant cells into the circulation, and they have done so only in a very small group of patients, mostly with non-alimentary tumours. In this connection it should be realized that, if numerous tumour cells can be isolated from a 5 ml sample of venous blood taken from near the tumour site, there must be millions of cancer cells released into the blood stream daily, particularly in association with bodily movement and peristalsis. An extra quota of cells dislodged into the draining veins by handling of the growth at operation would seem to be of relatively little importance. However, on the basis of experimental work, showing an increase in the number of hepatic metastases produced by injecting malignant cells into the portal circulation when the animal is under stress, Cole postulated that cancer cells escaping into the circulation at the time of operation have a much better chance of surviving and establishing themselves as secondary deposits in the liver than at other times (Buinauskas et al. 1958). It was to protect

the patient over this vulnerable period that *adjuvant chemotherapy* was introduced, cytotoxic agents being administered intraportally and intraperitoneally at the time of operation and intravenously during the first two postoperative days (McDonald et al. 1957; Mrazek et al. 1959).

4. The important fact remains that the discovery of malignant cells in the blood stream does not influence the ultimate prognosis, and it must be presumed that almost all these cells eventually perish without establishing themselves as metastases.

METASTASIS BY IMPLANTATION OF EXFOLIATED CANCER CELLS ON TO RAW SURFACES OR THE PERITONEUM

Most pathologists, such as Borrmann (1910) and Willis (1948), reject the possibility of metastases occurring by implantation from tumours of the alimentary tract, and consider that supposed instances of metastasis by implantation are susceptible of other and preferable explanations—either as examples of multiple primary growths or metastasis by other well-known routes. However, certain experiences which some of my colleagues and I have had strongly suggest that implantation metastases do occasionally arise from engrafting of exfoliated malignant cells in the lumen below or above carcinomas of the rectum or colon on to the raw surfaces of an operation wound or to raw areas in the lining of the bowel lower down (Morgan 1950; Lloyd-Davies 1950; Goligher et al. 1951). In several patients who underwent resections of carcinomas of the rectum, completed by anastomosis or by Hartmann's technique leaving a blind rectal stump, recurrences were found to develop subsequently on the suture line of the anastomosis or of the top of the rectal stump—areas where a raw area existed at the time of the operation, so that malignant cells might well have had the opportunity to become implanted. In some instances it was frankly debatable on the pathological material available whether this was the mechanism or whether the recurrence was due simply to inadequate excision, and Morson et al. (1963) have expressed their belief that most of these further manifestations of growth were in fact ordinary recurrences. But in a few of the cases the initial carcinoma for which the resection had been performed was a relatively early lesions, confined to the bowel wall itself (A case), and the amount of bowel and other tissues resected distal to the growth

appeared to have been perfectly adequate for thorough excision as judged by examination of the operative specimens. In one case, in addition, a discrete nodule of growth was found to have developed in the abdominal wound, which could hardly have arisen in any other way than by implantation at the time of operation. Five other examples of deposits in the parietal wound have since come to my attention.

I also have records of a case with rectal bleeding wrongly diagnosed as due to haemorrhoids which were treated by haemorrhoidectomy. The bleeding continued and three months later the patient presented at another hospital, where a carcinoma of the upper rectum was discovered on sigmoidoscopy. An implant of growth was also found in one of the haemorrhoidectomy wounds. Killingback et al. (1965) report five similar cases of anal deposits from carcinoma of the rectum or colon—one each at the site of a recent haemorrhoidectomy wound, an anal fistula and an anal fissure, and two arising apparently spontaneously in the anal or perianal region. They consider that three and possibly four of these cases were examples of implantation.

Certain other surgeons in recent times, such as Cole (1952), Lofgren et al. (1957), Le Quesne and Thomson (1958) and Keynes (1961), have also seen recurrences after resection for carcinoma of the rectum, which they also consider can be most logically explained as implantation metastases. Actually, as Keynes (1961) points out, the idea that loose, viable cancer cells might implant in freshly cut tissues apparently originated with Sir Charles Ryall, who in two papers (Ryall 1907, 1908) recorded seven examples of what he took to be implantation metastases from carcinoma of the large intestine (as well as others after operations for breast cancer). This was before the general use of rubber gloves, and he claimed on cytological examination to have recognized cancer cells lodged under his finger nails and on his scalpel. Cole et al. (1954) have shown that loose malignant cells can be demonstrated in the faeces below a carcinoma of the rectum or colon, especially after handling of the growth at operation. If tapes are tied tightly round the bowel, above and below the growth, before the latter is manipulated in any way, the number of carcinoma cells found in the lumen outside the confines of the tapes is greatly reduced.

It has certainly been demonstrated that there are exfoliated malignant cells in the lumen of the bowel and it would be reasonable to suppose that they might implant themselves on raw areas and suture lines. But a recent study by Rosenberg et al. (1978)

casts considerable doubt on this hypothesis by demonstrating that these shed cells are invariably non-viable, not only when recovered from washings of the tumour surface in excised operative specimens, but also when obtained from irrigation of the bowel in practising colonic exfoliative cytology for the diagnosis of colonic cancer. As against this evidence may be set the fact that Vink (1954) has succeeded in producing experimentally implantation metastases in the intestine of rabbits. He exposed a loop of bowel at laparotomy, and injected into it a suspension of malignant cells derived from a Brown-Pearce rabbit testicular tumour. Immediately afterwards the bowel was divided across at this same level and an end-to-end anastomosis performed, thus affording the tumour cells a chance to become engrafted on the suture line. This was done in 23 rabbits. In a second series of 27 rabbits the same experiment was carried out after a preliminary course of intestinal antisepsis with oral sulphasuccidine and streptomycin. The animals were killed after six to eight weeks and autopsies performed. In the first series metastases were present in 14 of the 23 rabbits—11 in the peritoneum and three in the anastomosis. In the second series metastases were found in 15 of the 27 rabbits—in three in the peritoneum and in 12 on the suture line. Vink concludes from this work that the practice of intestinal antisepsis now routinely employed in the preparation of patients with carcinoma of the large intestine for operation may favour the development of secondary deposits in the bowel suture lines after resection. Cohn et al. (1963) repeated this type of experiment with similar results. It is only fair to point out that the frequency of implantation tumours observed by Vink (1954) and Cohn et al. (1963) under experimental conditions is vastly greater than any reported clinical incidence of this form of metastasis; one may well question how far it is reasonable to go in applying results obtained with Brown-Pearce tumour in rabbits to the problems of bowel cancer surgery in the human.

Pomeranz and Garlock (1955) demonstrated cancer cells in smears, made at laparotomy, of the serosa in two of 20 cases of carcinoma of the colon, in which the tumour had invaded the full thickness of the intestinal wall. They commented on the grave danger of dissemination and implantation within the peritoneal cavity of malignant cells exfoliated from the serosal surface. Boreham (1958) was unsuccessful in isolating malignant cells from serosal smears of bowel cancers at operation, but he reported four or five cases of recurrence of rectal or colonic cancer in the main parietal wound or in the vicinity of the colostomy, which he believed could most plausibly be explained as due to implantation of carcinoma cells exfoliated from the peritoneal aspect of the growth during operation. Quan (1959) assayed the *cul-de-sac* fluid from patients with cancer of the colon or rectum by preparing smears directly from swabs. Among 133 specimens considered technically suitable for study, 33 (15%) were positive, 40 suspicious and 60 negative. It is interesting to note that 15 of the negative smears were from patients with visible intraperitoneal deposits and eight of the positive smears from patients without evidence of abdominal metastases.

The most detailed investigation of the phenomenon of exfoliation of cancer cells into the peritoneal cavity, however, is that of Moore et al. (1961), who studied 727 surgical patients with malignant disease of the stomach, colon, rectum, ovary, uterus and cervix, and, as a control, 166 surgical patients with benign lesions. Routine washings were obtained of the peritoneal cavity both before and after operative manipulation, 20 ml of saline being sprayed against the viscera and peritoneal surfaces adjacent to the tumour, and subsequently recovered from the gutters or *cul-de-sac*, using a long curved aspirating syringe with a rubber bulb. The fluid was then centrifuged and multiple smears were made of the deposit, using both Wright–Giemsa and Papanicolaou preparations. The slides were examined by a number of experienced cytologists. In the 166 non-malignant cases a false positive diagnosis was made on 9 occasions. In patients with carcinomas the prospect of finding tumour cells in the peritoneal washings varied with the extent of the lesion, for in 166 cases with 'curable' cancers of the rectum or colon smears were positive in 17·5% and there was an equivocal result in 5·4%, whilst in 95 cases with incurable rectal or colonic cancers, smears were positive in 40%, with an atypical result in another 6·3%. Positive smears were more likely to be obtained from cases with growths which had erupted on the serosal aspect with or without the production of serosal or other secondary deposits, than from patients with an intact peritoneal covering and no obvious dissemination; but positive results were sometimes found with the latter type of case. A comparison of the results of smears made before and after operative manipulation provided no support for the thesis that spread into the peritoneal cavity from serous surface of a growth is increased by handling of the tumour. Attempts to grow cancer cells isolated from peritoneal washings in tissue culture were mostly unsuccessful, which contrasts with the ready growth on culture of tumour cells from established ascitic fluid; the success with the latter is probably due to the large cancer cell population in ascitic fluid and to the previous adaptation of these cells to growth in a liquid medium. Moore et al. (1961) were able to attach a precise prognostic significance to the finding of isolated cancer cells in the peritoneal cavity. Of 42 patients with positive washings who had also serosal involvement, ascites or other distant abdominal metastases, 60% are already dead in a follow-up extending to three years and mostly of shorter duration. By contrast, of 42 patients with positive washings but no gross evidence of distant spread, only 14% have so far succumbed in a similar period of follow-up.

The whole concept of metastasis by implantation is still highly debatable but has aroused much surgical interest, and has led to the adoption of various precautions at operation to guard against its occurrence (see p. 444).

STAGING OF CARCINOMAS ACCORDING TO THE EXTENT OF SPREAD

It is convenient for assessing the results of surgical treatment to classify carcinomas of the rectum and colon according to the extent of spread. The classification originally proposed by Dukes (1930, 1940) for rectal carcinomas, based on the extent of direct spread and on the occurrence of lymphatic metastases, is very satisfactory and is widely used. In it growths are divided into three main categories—A, B and C. 'A' cases are those in which the growth is confined to the rectal wall, there being no extension into the extrarectal tissues and no metastases in the lymph-glands. In 'B' cases the growth has spread by direct continuity into the extrarectal tissues, but the lymph-glands are free from metastases. 'C' cases are those in which lymphatic metastases are found (Fig. 301). It may be added that with very few exceptions lymphatic metastases occur only after the growth has extended to the perirectal tissues, so that a 'C' case is in fact a B case with lymphatic metastases. In 1935 Dukes (see Gabriel et al. 1935) suggested that the C cases should be further subdivided according to the extent of glandular spread. If only a few glands are involved near the primary growth leaving some glands in the chain free from metastases below the main ligature on the superior haemorrhoidal or inferior mesenteric vessels, this is known as a 'C1'

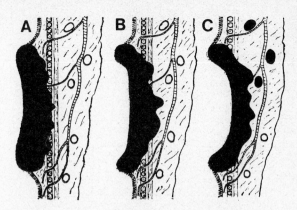

Fig. 301. The Dukes classification of carcinomas of the rectum (or colon): (A) Growth limited to wall of rectum. (B) Extension of growth to extrarectal tissues but no metastases in regional lymph glands. (C) Metastases in regional lymph glands. (*From Dukes 1936*)

case. If on the other hand there is a continuous string of glands containing metastases right up to the ligature, the case is considered to be 'C2' (Fig 302).

In Dukes' (1940) extensive experience over many years, of the cases of rectal cancer accepted by surgeons as operable about 15% are in category A as regards extent of spread, 35% in category B, and 50% in category C. About two-thirds of the C cases

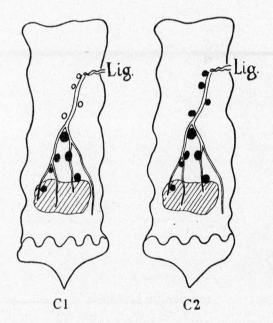

Fig. 302. Typical gland dissection charts in C 1 and C 2 cases of rectal carcinoma. (*After Dukes*)

TABLE 22. *Relation of Extent of Spread to Histological Grade (985 Cases)*

Grade	A cases (n = 144)	B cases (n = 342)	C cases (n = 499)
I	28 (19·4%)	20 (5·8%)	16 (3·3%)
II	97 (67·4%)	233 (68·1%)	232 (46·4%)
III	8 (5·5%)	57 (16·7%)	159 (31·8%)
IV	—	1 (0·3%)	13 (2·7%)
Mucoid	11 (7·7%)	31 (9·1%)	79 (15·8%)

correspond to the definition of C_1, one-third to that of C_2.

As might be expected, there is a close connection between the histological grade of malignancy of a carcinoma and the extent of spread. Grading may be regarded as an approximate gauge of the pace of growth of a tumour, and the A, B, C classification as a measure of the distance reached. The two methods are naturally interrelated as is shown by the analysis of 985 rectal carcinomas in Table 22 (Dukes 1940). The A cases (limited to the rectal wall) contained the largest percentage of grade I growths (slow-growing tumours), whereas the C cases (with metastases) contained the highest percentage of the more malignant grades.

Naturally also the extent of spread of the growth and its histological grading exert a profound influence on the prospects of cure by operative excision, and there is an intimate relationship between the A, B and C classification (and the histological grade) and the ultimate outcome of the case, as will be made clear on p. 641, Fig. 509.

This method of staging according to the extent of spread of the growth has been worked out most accurately and on a prodigious scale by Dukes (1940, 1944) in regard to rectal carcinoma. It has also been applied to carcinomas of the colon (Dukes 1945, 1951) and similar correlations have been found with the histological grade and the prognosis after surgical treatment, but not so much detailed information is available. In general colon carcinomas tend to be less advanced than do rectal carcinomas, as shown by a smaller proportion of C cases (see also Table 31). The ratio of A, B and C cases is roughly the same in all parts of the colon.

MODIFICATIONS OF THE DUKES' SYSTEM OF GRADING AND AN ALTERNATIVE TNM SYSTEM

The commonest modification in Britain is simply the addition of a D category to indicate patients who were noted at operation to have distant metastases or very extensive local or nodal spread

making their lesion quite incurable whatever the ABC categorization recorded by the pathologist on his dissection of the operative specimen. In America at least two groups of workers (Kirklin et al. 1949; Astler and Coller 1954) have introduced systems of grading which in their format bear a strong superficial resemblance to the Dukes' system, but on a more careful study are seen to differ from it in several very important respects. Thus, in the Kirklin et al. (1949) system, category A refers to growths that have not yet penetrated through the muscularis mucosae—in other words, carcinomas-in-situ, which were not regarded by Dukes (1930, 1940) as true invasive cancers at all and were not budgeted for in his system of grading. Kirklin et al. (1949) recognize two B categories, B_1 and B_2, for growths that have penetrated superficially and deeply respectively into the muscle coat of the rectal wall but *have not reached* the perirectal tissues. Clearly, therefore, their categories B_1 and B_2 correspond to Dukes' category A. There is no category in the Kirklin et al. (1949) system corresponding to Dukes' category B for growths that have spread to the perirectal tissues, but have not produced lymph node metastases.

Unfortunately, several American textbooks of surgery (Birnbaum and Schrock 1975; Egdahl et al. 1972; Storer and Lockwood 1969) have given prominence to these 'modified Dukes' systems' of classification without indicating how widely they differ in several respects from Dukes' (1930, 1940) original definition of his categories. Such differences could be a serious source of error in considering the effects of different forms of treatment. For example, patients with B growths according to Kirklin et al.'s (1949) classification ought to do much better in general after surgical treatment than those with growths classified on the proper Dukes' (1930) system as B lesions, for in fact they are Dukes' A tumours, removal of which offers an almost normal expectation of life. As has recently been argued by me (Goligher 1976), if an ABC style of categorization is to be used, there is a lot to be said for sticking to the original Dukes' categories, the significance of which in relation to ultimate prognosis has been so well established by the extensive follow-up studies at St Mark's Hospital (see above, and pp. 641, 642). But another possibility would be to abandon the ABC grading entirely and make a fresh start with a more comprehensive TNM classification, as used for other carcinomas, in which a great deal more information is recorded about the primary tumour (T), the regional lymph nodes (N) and distant

TABLE 23. *TNM Classification and Staging of Carcinoma of the Colon*

T: Primary tumours

T0	No tumour clinically demonstrable
T1	Clinically benign lesion, or confined to mucosa or submucosa
T2	Involvement of muscular wall or serosa, no extension beyond
T3	Involvement of all layers of colon with extension to immediately adjacent structures and /or organs and no fistula present
T4	Fistula present with any of the above degrees of tumour penetration
T5	T3 or T4 with direct extension to other organs or structures
TX	Depth of penetration not specified

N: Regional lymph node involvement

N0	Nodes not believed involved
N1	Nodes believed involved (distal to origins of the ileocolic, right colic, middle colic and inferior mesenteric arteries)
NX	Nodes not assessed or involvement not recorded

M: Distant metastases

M0	No known distant metastases
M1	Distant metastases present
MX	Not assessed

Non-invasive carcinoma (in situ)

Stage 0	Carcinoma in situ as demonstrated by histological examination of tissue (biopsy or other)

Invasive carcinoma

Stage I T0, 1/N0/M0 T0, 1/NX/M0	Tumour confined to mucosa or submucosa, with no demonstrable metastasis to regional lymph nodes and no evidence of distant metastasis
Stage II T2-5/N0/M0 T2-5/NX/M0	Tumour penetrating the muscularis of beyond, with no demonstrable metastasis to regional lymph nodes and no evidence of distant metastases
Stage III Any T/N1/M0	Any penetration of bowel or rectal wall by tumour, with metastasis to regional lymph nodes, but no evidence of distant metastases
Stage IV Any T/Any N/M1	Any penetration of bowel or rectal wall by tumour, with or without evidence of metastasis to regional lymph node, but with evidence of distant metastasis

After Beart et al. (1978).

metastases (M). The American Joint Committee for Cancer Staging and End-Results-Reporting has recently recommended a new TNM classification for colorectal carcinomas (Table 23) which covers all possible permutations of spread of large bowel tumours and, if accepted, would hopefully end confusion and yet allow comparison with earlier studies (Beart et al. 1978).

REFERENCES

ARIES, V., CROWTHER, J. S., DRASAR, B. S., HILL, M. J. and WILLIAMS, R. E. O. (1969) Bacteria and the aetiology of cancer of the large bowel. *Gut, 10*, 334.

ANTONIS, A. and BERSOHN, I. (1962) The influence of diet on facial lipids in South African white and Bantu prisoners. *J. clin. Nutr., 11*, 142.

ASTLER, V. B. and COLLER, F. A. (1954) The prognostic significance of direct extension of carcinoma of the colon and rectum. *Ann. Surg., 139*, 846.

AXTELL, L. M. and CHIAZZE, L., Jr. (1966) Changing relative frequency of cancers of the colon and rectum in the United States. *Cancer, 19*, 750.

BACON, H. E. and JACKSON, C. C. (1953) Visceral metastases from carcinoma of the distal colon and rectum. *Surgery, St Louis, 33*, 495.

BARRINGER, P. L., DOCKERTY, M. B., WAUGH, J. M. and BARGEN, J. A. (1954) Carcinoma of the large intestine: a new approach to the study of venous spread. *Surgery Gynec. Obstet., 98*, 62.

BEART, R. W., Jr., VAN HEERDEN, J. A. and BEAHRS, O. H. (1978) Evolution in the pathologic staging of carcinoma of the colon. *Surgery Gynec. Obstet., 146*, 257.

BIRNBAUM, W. and SHROCK, T. R. (1975) Large intestine. In *Current Surgical Diagnosis and Treatment*, ed. J. E. Dunphy and L. W. Way, 2nd ed, p. 619. Los Altos, California: Lange Medical Publications.

BLACK, W. A. and WAUGH, J. M. (1948) The intramural extension of carcinoma of the descending colon, sigmoid and rectosigmoid. *Surgery Gynec. Obstet.*, *87*, 457.

BOREHAM, P. (1958) Implantation metastases from cancer of the large bowel. *Br. J. Surg.*, *46*, 103.

BORRMANN, R. (1910) Die Beurteilung multipler Karzinoma im Digestionstraktus; mit besonderer Berücksichtigung des Einbruchs karzinomatöser Metastasen unter Vortäuschung primärer Tumoren. *Beitr. path. Anat.*, *48*, 576.

BOYD, J. T. and DOLL, R. (1954) Gastro-intestinal cancer and the use of liquid paraffin. *Br. J. Cancer*, *8*, 231.

BRODERS, A. C. (1925) The grading of carcinoma. *Minn. Med.*, *8*, 726.

BROWN, C. E. and WARREN, S. (1938) Visceral metastasis from rectal carcinoma. *Surgery Gynec. Obstet.*, *66*, 611.

BUINAUSKAS, P., McDONALD, G. A. and COLE, W. H. (1958) Role of operative stress on the resistance of the experimental animal to inoculated cancer cells. *Ann. Surg.*, *148*, 642.

BURKITT, D. P. (1971) Possible relationships between bowel cancer and dietary habits. *Proc. R. Soc. Med.*, *64*, 964.

—— WALKER, A. R. P. and PAINTER, N. S. (1972) Effect of dietary fibre on stools and transit-times, and its rôle in the causation of disease. *Lancet*, *2*, 1408.

BUSSEY, H. J. R., WALLACE, M. H. and MORSON, B. C. (1967) Metachronous carcinoma of the large intestine and intestinal polyps. *Proc. R. Soc. Med.*, *60*, 208.

CLOGG, H. S. (1908) Cancer of the colon: a study of 72 cases. *Lancet*, *2*, 1007.

COHN, I., Jr., FLOYD, E. and ATIK, M. (1963) Control of tumor implantation during operations on the colon. *Ann. Surg.*, *157*, 825.

COLE, P. P. (1913) The intramural spread of rectal carcinoma. *Br. med. J.*, *1*, 431.

COLE, W. H. (1952) Recurrence in carcinoma of the colon and proximal rectum following resection for carcinoma. *Archs Surg., Chicago*, *65*, 264.

—— PACKARD, D. and SOUTHWICK, H. W. (1954) Carcinoma of the colon with special reference to prevention of recurrence. *J. Am. med. Ass.*, *155*, 1549.

COLLER, F. A., KAY, E. B. and MACINTYRE, R. S. (1940) Regional lymphatic metastasis of carcinoma of the rectum. *Surgery, St Louis*, *8*, 294.

CORREA, P. (1978) Epidemiology of polyps and cancer. In *The Pathogenesis of Colorectal Cancer*, ed. B. C. Morson. Philadelphia: W. B. Saunders.

CRUSE, P., LEWIN, M. and CLARK, C. G. (1979) Dietary cholesterol is co-carcinogenic for human colon cancer. *Lancet*, *2*, 752.

CUTLER, S. J. (1969) Trends in cancer of the digestive tract. *Surgery, St Louis*, *65*, 740.

DE BOVIS, R. (1900) Le cancer du gros intestin, rectum excepté. *Rev. Chir., Paris*, *21*, 673; *22*, 773.

DEVITT, J. E., RORTH-MOYO, L. A. and BROWN, F. N. (1969) The significance of multiple adenocardinomas of the colon and rectum. *Ann. Surg.*, *169*, 364.

DOLBEY, R. V. and MOORE, A. W. (1924) The incidence of cancer in Egypt: an analysis of 671 cases. *Lancet*, *1*, 587.

DOLL, R. (1969) The geographical distribution of cancer. *Br. J. Cancer*, *23*, 1.

—— PAYNE, P. and WATERHOUSE, J. (1966) *Cancer in Five Continents*. Berlin: Springer.

DUKES, C. E. (1930) The spread of cancer of the rectum (Subsection in paper by Gordon-Watson, C., and Dukes, C. E.). *Br. J. Surg.*, *17*, 643.

—— (1936) Histological grading of rectal cancer. *Proc. R. Soc. Med.*, *30*, 371.

—— (1940) Cancer of the rectum: an analysis of 1000 cases. *J. Path. Bact.*, *50*, 527.

—— (1944) The surgical pathology of rectal carcinoma. *Proc. R. Soc. Med.*, *37*, 131.

—— (1945) Discussion on the pathology and treatment of carcinoma of the colon. *Proc. R. Soc. Med. 38*, 381.

—— (1946) Personal communication.

—— (1951) The surgical pathology of tumours of the colon. *Med. Press*, *226*, 512.

—— and BUSSEY, H. J. R. (1941) Venous spread in rectal cancer. *Proc. R. Soc. Med.*, *34*, 571.

—— —— (1958) The spread of rectal cancer and its effect on prognosis. *Br. J. Cancer*, *12*, 309.

EGDAHL, R. H., MANNICK, J. A. and WILLIAMS, L. F., Jr. (1972) *Core Textbook of Surgery*, p. 113. New York: Grune and Stratton.

EISENBERG, H., SULLIVAN, P. D. and FOOTE, F. M. (1967) Trends in survival of digestive system cancer patients in Connecticut, 1935 to 1962. *Gastroenterology, 53*, 528.

ENGELL, H. C. (1955) Cancer cells in the circulating blood: a clinical study on the occurrence of cancer cells in the peripheral blood and in venous blood draining the tumour area at operation. *Acta chir. scand.*, Suppl. 201.

—— (1959) Cancer cells in the blood. A five to nine year follow-up study. *Ann. Surg.*, *149*, 457.

EWING, M. R. (1951) Inflammatory complications of cancer of the caecum and ascending colon. *Postgrad. med. J.*, *27*, 515.

FAHL, J. C., DOCKERTY, M. B. and JUDD, E. S. (1960) Scirrhous carcinoma of the colon and rectum. *Surgery Gynec. Obstet.*, *111*, 759.

FISHER, E. R. and TURNBULL, R. B., Jr. (1955) The cytologic demonstration and significance of tumour cells in the mesenteric venous blood in patients with colorectal carcinoma. *Surgery Gynec. Obstet.*, *100*, 102.

FORREST, A. P. M. (1965) Personal communication.

FRASER, SIR JOHN (1938) Malignant disease of the large intestine. *Br. J. Surg.*, *25*, 647.

GABRIEL, W. B. (1948) *The Principles and Practice of Rectal Surgery*, 4th ed, p. 309. London: H. K. Lewis.

—— (1952) The surgical management of large villous tumours in the rectum. *Proc. R. Soc. Med.*, *45*, 696.

—— DUKES, C. and BUSSEY, H. J. R. (1935) Lymphatic spread in cancer of the rectum. *Br. J. Surg.*, *23*, 395.

GILCHRIST, R. K. (1940) Fundamental factors governing lateral spread of rectal carcinoma. *Ann. Surg.*, *111*, 630.

—— and DAVID, V. C. (1947) A consideration of pathological factors influencing five-year survival in radical resection of the large bowel and rectum for carcinoma. *Ann. Surg.*, *126*, 421.

GLOVER, R. P. and WAUGH, J. M. (1945) Retrograde lymphatic spread of carcinoma of the 'rectosigmoid region'; its influence on surgical procedures. *Surgery Gynec. Obstet.*, *80*, 434.

GOLIGHER, J. C. (1941) The operability of carcinoma of the rectum. *Br. med. J.*, *2*, 393.

—— (1976) The Dukes' A, B and C categorization of the extent of spread of carcinomas of the rectum. *Surg. Gynec. Obstet.*, *143*, 793.

—— DUKES, C. E. and BUSSEY, H. J. R. (1951) Local recurrences after sphincter-saving excisions for carcinoma of the rectum and rectosigmoid. *Br. J. Surg.*, *39*, 199.

—— and SMIDDY, F. G. (1957) The treatment of acute obstruction or perforation with carcinoma of the colon and rectum. *Br. J. Surg.*, *45*, 270.

GRINNELL, R. S. (1939) The grading and prognosis of carcinoma of the colon and rectum. *Ann. Surg.*, *109*, 500.

—— (1942) The lymphatic and venous spread of carcinoma of the rectum. *Ann. Surg.*, *116*, 200.

—— (1954) Distal intramural spread of carcinoma of the rectum and rectosigmoid. *Surgery Gynec. Obstet.*, *99*, 421.

—— (1966) Lymphatic block in carcinoma of colon and rectum. *Ann. Surg.*, *163*, 272.

HANDLEY, W. S. (1913) The dissemination of rectal cancer. *Br. med. J.*, *1*, 584.

HAYES, J. M. (1921) The involvement of the lymph-glands in carcinoma of the large intestine. *Minn. Med.*, *4*, 653.

HILL, M. J., CROWTHER, J. C., DRASAR, B. S., HAWKSWORTH, G., ARIES, V. and WILLIAMS, R. E. O. (1971) Bacteria and aetiology of cancer of large bowel. *Lancet*, *1*, 95.

HUTT, M. S. R. and TEMPLETON, A. C. (1971) The geographical pathology of bowel cancer and some related diseases. *Proc. R. Soc. Med.*, *64*, 962.

JAMIESON, J. K. and DOBSON, J. F. (1907) Lectures on the lymphatic system of the caecum and appendix. *Lancet*, *1*, 1137.

JOHNSON, J. W., JUDD, E. S. and DAHLIN, D. C. (1959) Malignant neoplasms of the colon and rectum in young persons. *Archs Surg., Chicago*, *79*, 365.

JOHNSTON, J. H., Jr. (1947) Carcinoma of the colon in childhood and adolescence. *Am. J. Surg.*, *73*, 703.

JUDD, E. S. (1924) A consideration of lesions of the colon treated surgically. *Sth. med. J., Nashville*, *17*, 75.

KEYNES, W. M. (1961) Implantation from the bowel lumen in cancer of the large intestine. *Ann. Surg.*, *153*, 357.

KILLE, J. N. and GLICK, S. (1967) Neoplasia complicating uretero-sigmoidostomy. *Br. med. J.*, *3*, 783.

KILLINGBACK, M., WILSON, E. and HUGHES, E. S. R. (1965) Anal metastases from carcinoma of the rectum and colon. *Aust. N.Z. J. Surg.*, *34*, 178.

KIRKLIN, J. W., DOCKERTY, M. B. and WAUGH, J. M. (1949) The role of peritoneal reflection in the prognosis of carcinoma of the rectum and sigmoid colon. *Surgery Gynec. Obstet.*, *88*, 326.

KÖRTE, W. (1900) Erfahrungen über die operative Behandlung der malignen Dickdarm-Geschwulste. *Arch. klin. Chir.*, *61*, 403.

LE QUESNE, L. P. and THOMSON, A. D. (1958) Implantation recurrence of carcinoma of rectum and colon. *New Engl. J. Med.*, *258*, 578.

LEITCH, A. Quoted by Miles, W. E. (1926).

LLOYD-DAVIES, O. V. (1950) Discussion on conservative resection in carcinoma of the rectum. *Proc. R. Soc. Med.*, *43*, 706.

—— MORGAN, C. N. and GOLIGHER, J. C. (1953) The treatment of carcinoma of the colon. In *British Surgical Practice*, Progress Volume 1953, Edited by Sir Ernest Rock Carling and Sir James Paterson Ross. London: Butterworth.

LOCALIO, S. A. and ENG, K. (1975) Malignant tumours of the rectum. In *Current Problems in Surgery*, ed. M. M. Ravitch. Chicago: Year Book Publishers.

LOFGREN, E. P., WAUGH, J. M. and DOCKERTY, M. B. (1957) Local recurrence of carcinoma after anterior resection of the rectum and Sigmoid relationship with the length of normal mucosa excised distal to the lesion. *Archs Surg., Chicago*, *74*, 825.

LONG, L., JONASSON, O., ROBERTS, S., McGRATH, R., McGREW, E. and COLE, W. H. (1960) Cancer cells in blood. Results of a simplified isolation technique. *Archs Surg., Chicago*, *80*, 910.

LOVETT, E. (1976) Familial cancer of the gastrointestinal tract. *Br. J. Surg.*, *63*, 19.

McDONALD, G. O., LIVINGSTON, C., BOYLES, C. F. and COLE, W. H. (1957) The prophylactic treatment of malignant disease with nitrogen mustard and triethylenethiophosphoramide (ThioTEPA). *Ann. Surg.*, *145*, 624.

MacMAHON, C. E. and ROWE, J. W. (1971) Rectal reaction following radiation therapy of cervical carcinoma: particular reference to subsequent occurrence of rectal carcinoma. *Ann. Surg.*, *173*, 264.

McVAY, J. R. (1922) Involvement of the lymph-nodes in carcinoma of the rectum. *Ann. Surg.*, *76*, 580.

MAYO, C. W. and PAGTALUNAN, R. J. G. (1963) Malignancy of colon and rectum in patients under 30 years of age. *Surgery, St Louis*, *53*, 711.

—— and SCHLICKE, C. P. (1942) Carcinoma of the colon and rectum: a study of metastasis and recurrences. *Surgery Gynec. Obstet.*, *74*, 83.

MAYO, W. J. (1910) Removal of the rectum for cancer: statistical report on 120 cases. *Ann. Surg.*, *51*, 854.

MILES, W. E. (1910) The radical abdomino-perineal operation for cancer of the rectum and of the pelvic colon. *Br. med. J.*, *2*, 941.

—— (1926) *Cancer of the Rectum*. London: Harrison.

MONSARRAT, K. W. and WILLIAMS, I. J. (1913) Intramural extension in rectal cancer. *Br. J. Surg.*, *1*, 173.

MOORE, G. E. (1960) The circulating cancer cell. *Lancet*, *2*, 814.

—— and SAKO, K. (1959) The spread of carcinoma of the colon and rectum: a study of invasion of blood vessels, lymph nodes and the peritoneum by tumor cells. *Dis. Colon Rect.*, *2*, 92.

—— —— KONDO, T., BARDILLO, J. and BURKE, E. (1961) Assessment of the exfoliation of tumor cells into the body cavities. *Surgery Gynec. Obstet*, *112*, 469.

—— SANDBERG, A. and SCHUBARG, J. R. (1957) Clinical and experimental observations on the occurrence and fate of tumor cells in the blood stream. *Ann. Surg.*, *76*, 755.

MORGAN, C. N. (1950) Discussion on conservative resection in carcinoma of the rectum. *Proc. R. Soc. Med.*, *43*, 701.

MORSON, B. C. (1979) Prevention of colorectal cancer. *J. R. Soc. Med.*, *72*, 83.

—— VAUGHAN, E. G. and BUSSEY, H. J. R. (1963) Pelvic recurrence after excision of rectum for carcinoma. *Br. med. J.*, *2*, 13.

MRAZEK, R., ECONOMOU, S., McDONALD, G. O., SLAUGHTER, D. P. and COLE, W. H. (1959) Prophylactic and adjuvant use of nitrogen mustard in the surgical treatment of cancer. *Ann. Surg.*, *150*, 745.

NELSON, P. G. (1965) Primary linitis plastica carcinoma of the colon. *Aust. N.Z. J. Surg.*, *34*, 288.

NIGRO, N. D. and CAMPBELL, R. L. (1976) Bile acids and intestinal cancer. In *The Bile Acids*, ed. P. P. Nair and D. Kritcharsky. New York: Plenum.

OETTLÉ, A. G. (1967) Primary neoplasms of the alimentary canal in whites and Bantu of the Transvaal, 1949–53. A histopathological series. *Natn. Cancer Inst. Monogr., 25*, 97.

PATTERSON, H. A. (1956) The management of cecal carcinoma discovered unexpectedly at operation for acute appendicitis. *Ann. Surg., 143*, 670.

PEACOCK, P. R. and KIRBY, A. H. M. (1944) Attempts to induce stomach tumours; action of carcinogenic hydrocarbons on stock mice. *Cancer Res., 4*, 88.

POIRIER, P., CUNÉO, B. and DELAMERE, G. (1903) *The Lymphatics*, p. 351. London: Constable.

POMERANZ, A. A. and GARLOCK, J. H. (1955) Postoperative recurrence of cancer of colon due to desquamated malignant cells. *J. Am. med. Ass., 158*, 1434.

POOL, E. H. and DUNLOP, G. R. (1934) Cancer cells in the bloodstream. *Am. J. Cancer, 21*, 99.

QUAN, S. H. Q. (1959) Cul-de-sac smears for cancer cells. *Surgery, St Louis, 45*, 258.

QUER, A. E., DAHLIN, D. C. and MAYO, C. W. (1953) Retrograde intramural spread of carcinoma of the rectum and rectosigmoid. *Surgery Gynec. Obstet., 96*, 24.

RAIFORD, T. S. (1935) Carcinoma of the large bowel. Part II: the rectum. *Ann. Surg., 101*, 1042.

RANKIN, F. W. (1933) Curability of cancer of the colon, recto-sigmoid and rectum. *J. Am. med. Ass., 101*, 491.

—— BARGEN, J. A. and BUIE, L. A. (1932) *The Colon, Rectum and Anus*, p. 514. Philadelphia: W. B. Saunders.

—— and COMFORT, M. W. (1929) Carcinoma of rectum in young persons. *J. Tennessee St. med. Ass., 22*, 37.

—— and OLSON, P. F. (1933) The hopeful prognosis in cases of carcinoma of the colon. *Surgery Gynec. Obstet., 56*, 366.

REBUCK, J. W. (1947) The structure of the giant cells in the blood-forming organs. *J. Lab. clin. Med., 32*, 660.

RECIO, P. and BUSSEY, H. J. R. (1965) The pathology and prognosis of carcinoma of the rectum in the young. *Proc. R. Soc. Med., 58*, 789.

REGISTRAR-GENERAL. *Statistical Reviews for England and Wales for 1935–63, Parts I and II*. London: HMSO.

RHODES, J. B., HOLMES, F. F. and CLARK, G. M. (1977) Changing distribution of primary cancers in the large bowel. *J. Am. med. Ass., 238*, 1641.

ROBERTS, S., JOHASSON, O., LONG, L., McGRATH, R., McGREW, E. A. and COLE, W. H. (1961) Clinical significance of cancer cells in the circulating blood: two- to five-year survival. *Ann. Surg., 154*, 362.

ROSENBERG, I. L., RUSSELL, C. W. and GILLES, G. R. (1978) Cell visibility studies on the exfoliated colonic cancer cell. *Br. J. Surg., 65*, 188.

RYALL, C. (1907) Cancer infection and cancer recurrence: a danger to avoid in cancer operations. *Lancet, 2*, 1311.

—— (1908) The technique of cancer operations with reference to the danger of cancer infection. *Br. med. J., 2*, 1005.

SALEM, M. and POSTLETHWAIT, R. W. (1960) Malignancy of colon and rectum in patients under 20 years of age. *Ann. Surg., 151*, 335.

SANER, F. D. (1946) A case of *carcinoma coli* in a child. *Br. J. Surg., 33*, 398.

SAUER, I. and BACON, H. E. (1952) A new approach for excision of carcinoma of the lower portion of the rectum and anal canal. *Surgery Gynec. Obstet., 95*, 229.

SEAL, S. H. (1959) Silicone flotation: a simple quantitative method for the isolation of free-floating cancer cells from the blood. *Cancer, 12*, 590.

SEGI, M. (1963) *Trends in Cancer Mortality for Selected Sites in 24 Countries—Graphic Edition*. Sendai, Japan: Department of Public Health, Tohoku University.

SELLWOOD, R. A., KAPER, S. W. A., BURN, J. I. and WALLACE, E. N. (1965) Circulating cancer cells: the influence of surgical operation (abstract). *Br. J. Surg., 52*, 69.

SILVERBERG, E. (1970) *Cancer of the Colon and Rectum: Statistical Data*. New York: American Cancer Society.

SLAUGHTER, D. P. and SOUTHWICK, H. W. (1957) Mucosal carcinoma as a result of irradiation. *Archs Surg., Chicago, 74*, 420.

SMIDDY, F. G. and GOLIGHER, J. C. (1957) Results of surgery in treatment of cancer of the large intestine. *Br. med. J., 1*, 793.

SMITH, J. C. (1962) Carcinoma of the rectum following irradiation of cancer of the cervix. *Proc. R. Soc. Med., 55*, 701.

STEWART, M. J. (1931) Precancerous lesions of the alimentary tract. *Lancet, 2*, 565, 617, 669.

STORER, E. H. and LOCKWOOD, R. A. (1969) Colon, rectum and anus. In *Principles of Surgery*, ed. S. I. Schwartz, D. M. Hume, R. C. Lille Rei, G. T. Shires, F. C. Spencer and E. H. Storer, p. 980. New York: McGraw-Hill.

SUNDERLAND, D. A. (1949) The significance of vein invasion by cancer of the rectum and sigmoid: a microscopic study of 210 cases. *Cancer, 2*, 429.

TUTTLE, J. P. (1903) *A Treatise on Diseases of the Anus, Rectum and Pelvic Colon*, p. 762. London and New York: Appleton.

URDANETA, L. F., DUFFELL, D., CREEVY, C. D. and AUST, J. B. (1966) Late development of primary carcinoma of the colon following ureterosigmoidostomy: report of three cases and literature review. *Ann. Surg., 164*, 503.

VILLEMIN, F., HUARD, P. and MONTAGNÉ, M. (1925) Recherches anatomiques sur les lymphatiques du rectum et de l'anus; leurs applications dans le traitement chirurgical du cancer. *Rev. Chir., Paris, 63*, 39.

VINK, M. (1954) Local recurrence of cancer in the large bowel: role of implantation metastases and bowel disinfection. *Br. J. Surg., 41*, 431.

WESTHUES, H. (1930) Über die Entstehung und Vermeidung des lokalen Rektumkarzinom-Rezidivs. *Arch. klin. Chir., 161*, 582.

—— (1934) *Die Pathologisch-anatomischen Grundlagen der Chirurgie des Rektumkarzinoms*. Leipzig: Thieme.

WILLIS, R. A. (1948) *The Pathology of Tumours*, pp. 422, 425. London: Butterworth.

WOOD, W. Q. and WILKIE, D. P. D. (1933) Carcinoma of the rectum. An anatomico-pathological study. *Edinb. med. J., 40*, 321.

16

Clinical Features and Diagnosis of Carcinoma of the Colon and Rectum

Broadly speaking there are three main ways in which patients with carcinoma of the large intestine may present to the clinician: (a) as non-urgent cases with insidiously developing chronic symptoms chiefly affecting bowel function or general health; (b) as emergencies with acute intestinal obstruction; or (c) as emergencies with perforation of the colon and peritonitis. The proportion of patients in these three categories seen by any individual surgeon will depend on the type of practice in which he is engaged. If he is working at a private clinic or specialized hospital he will encounter relatively few cases with acute obstruction or perforation. On the other hand if he is attached to a large city general hospital with a busy receiving room service but relatively little consulting work, he may see a disproportionately large percentage of cases complicated in this way. I think the experience of the General Infirmary at Leeds may be instructive in this respect, for it was formerly the main hospital of the region which it serves and responsible for the care of the majority of both acute and chronic cases in that region. In a series of 1644 patients with carcinoma of the colon or rectum dealt with at the General Infirmary over a period of 15 years, it was found that 1239 or 75·2% had been non-urgent cases referred to the out-patient clinics or consulting rooms, 290 or 18% were admitted as emergencies with acute obstruction, and 115 or 6·8% were admitted with perforation and peritonitis (Goligher and Smiddy 1957).

CARCINOMA OF THE COLON OR RECTUM WITHOUT ACUTE OBSTRUCTION OR PERFORATION

Symptoms

The commoner symptoms that may be produced by a carcinoma of the rectum or colon comprise the following: alteration of bowel habit in the form of constipation, diarrhoea, or a combination of the two; the passage of blood or slime; abdominal pain; dyspepsia; flatulent distension; audible borborygmi; a palpable abdominal mass; and impairment of general health as shown by loss of weight and strength, and anaemia. In any particular case the symptoms may vary from none to most of those mentioned, the reasons for the variations not always being clear. However, there is a fairly definite correlation between the symptomatology and the site and type of growth, carcinomas in certain situations being as a rule more prone to produce symptoms than those in others.

CARCINOMAS OF THE RIGHT COLON

With growths of the caecum, ascending colon and hepatic flexure, *bowel symptoms are usually completely absent*, and, if present, more usually take the form of mild *diarrhoea* than of constipation. In many instances the only manifestation may be a vague *deterioration of general health with loss of weight and anaemia*. Naturally such symptoms are very susceptible to misinterpretation; for example, the anaemia, which may be quite severe without obvious loss of blood in the stools, may at first be thought to be an idiopathic condition of Addisonian or pernicious type. In other cases, probably the majority, some constant not very severe *abdominal pain* is experienced in the right iliac or subcostal region or in the epigastrium, often associated with some local tenderness. In many of these cases there is also a complaint of abdominal fullness and eructation after meals, so that a misdiagnosis of dyspepsia due to cholecystitis, chronic appendicitis or peptic ulcer may be made. *An abdominal mass* is not infrequently palpated, usually in the right iliac region, and in a few cases it is the detection of such a mass by an otherwise symptomless patient that leads him to take medical advice. The passage of blood or slime, recognizable to the naked eye, is excessively rare with carcinomas of the right colon (though *occult* blood may be demonstrated by suitable tests in the majority of instances, see p. 76).

CARCINOMAS OF THE TRANSVERSE OR LEFT COLON

With these growths disturbances of bowel habit are more often found, this being particularly so the farther distally the lesion lies in the colon (Muir 1956). *Increasing constipation* is the more usual complaint, so that the patient finds that he has to start taking aperients or to increase the amount normally taken. Progressively larger doses are required, and eventually even these cease to be effective and merely produce griping abdominal pains. Occasionally *diarrhoea* is more prominent or there may be an alternation of diarrhoea and constipation every few days. *Blood* and *mucus* may sometimes be recognized by the patient in the motion, and are more often observed the closer the lesion approximates to the rectum. Exaggerated peristalsis may cause loud and embarrassing *borborygmi*. Some patients complain of flatulent distension or actual pain and as this often appears worst after meals a dyspepsia may be mimicked, but passage of flatus per rectum tends to relieve the pain and sense of fullness. At first the patient may feel quite well in himself, but in the long run his general health becomes impaired and loss of weight occurs. Rarely an abdominal mass may be felt by the

patient himself, and very exceptionally, as with carcinoma of the caecum, this may be the only symptom.

CARCINOMAS OF THE DISTAL SIGMOID OR RECTUM

It is undoubtedly growths of the distal sigmoid and rectum that produce the most characteristic train of symptoms as a rule, which is perhaps fortunate in view of the high incidence of cancer in these parts of the bowel. It should be emphasized, however, that these lesions also may very exceptionally be entirely symptomless, as in the rare case where a carcinoma of the rectum or rectosigmoid is discovered on routine examination of a patient attending for some other obvious lesion, such as an anal fissure or an anal haematoma.

Perhaps the most frequent symptom of a carcinoma of the rectum or distal sigmoid is bleeding per rectum. This may be slight and may accompany the motion, or the patient may have to go to stool to pass blood alone on occasions. On careful interrogation, however, it will nearly always be found that there is also some disturbance of bowel habit. This may take the form of *increasing constipation* but more usual is *diarrhoea*. This tends to occur chiefly in the morning; almost as soon as the patient stands out of bed he experiences an urgent call to stool, but on acceding to it he passes only a little slime mixed with blood and a small amout of faecal matter and accompanied by a great deal of flatus. He is left with a feeling of incomplete evacuation as he resumes his interrupted toilet. Then perhaps a quarter of an hour later he has another urgent call with equally unsatisfactory results. This performance may be repeated four or five times during the first few hours of the day, often with some tenesmus and straining, till finally a rather more satisfactory faecal motion may be obtained. This diarrhoea has been aptly termed a '*morning diarrhoea*', because of its time relationship, but in some cases it continues throughout the day as well, especially after meals and even at night, so that the patient may have 10–12 or more motions in the 24 hours and his sleep may be disturbed by it. It is well also to stress that it is a '*spurious diarrhoea*', for the patient is passing mainly mucous and blood, and so far as faeces are concerned is actually constipated, so that he has to take aperients.

A slight amount of colicky abdominal pain and flatulent distension may occasionally occur with a constricting growth, but *pain in the rectum is not as a*

PLATE II

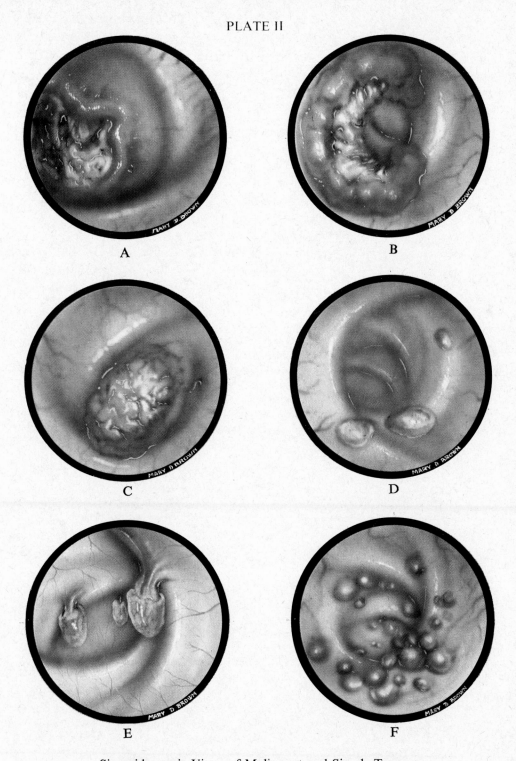

Sigmoidoscopic Views of Malignant and Simple Tumours

A, B, Ulcerating carcinoma of the rectum   D, E, Sessile and pedunculated adenomas
C,   Villous papilloma   F,   Multiple adenomas in familial polyposis.

rule a feature of rectal carcinoma till a late stage of the disease has been reached. The patient may then suffer sacral or sciatic pain due to implication of the sacral plexus. A growth of the lower end of the rectum, even at an early stage, may also cause severe pain if it extends down the anal canal to invade the skin-lined part of it or the perianal region. This pain is felt chiefly at defaecation, in much the same way as the pain of an ordinary anal fissure. In such cases the patient may detect an actual swelling or induration at the anal orifice due to a projecting tongue of growth.

As with other forms of carcinoma of the large intestine, the general health may be relatively unaffected at first and the patient may feel quite fit and strong, but in the course of time he loses strength and weight, often dropping 10–12 kg or more in a period of, say, 18 months.

Other symptoms that may occur are dependent on the involvement of neighbouring organs by the growth. For example, if the bladder or prostate are invaded symptoms of cystitis or urethritis may be experienced, and if an actual rectovesical fistula becomes established the patient may find that he passes flatus per urethram. In the female the posterior vaginal wall is occasionally infiltrated and a rectovaginal fistula may result with discharge of faeces and flatus per vaginam.

Diagnosis

From the foregoing remarks it will be seen that the history in a case of carcinoma of the colon or rectum may sometimes prove unhelpful in reaching a diagnosis, or actually misleading, in so far as it may point rather to a lesion of the stomach, duodenum, biliary tract or appendix, or to some more general ailment. A carcinoma of the colon should certainly be borne in mind as a possible cause of atypical dyspepsia or other vague abdominal symptoms in a patient over middle age. Similarly growths of the right colon should always be remembered as a possible cause of otherwise unexplained ill-health and anaemia. Carcinoma of the stomach is well known to produce a clinical picture very like that of pernicious anaemia; but it is not perhaps sufficiently recognized that a 'silent' carcinoma of the caecum may present in a similarly deceptive manner.

Fortunately, in the great majority of cases of cancer of the rectum or colon a well-taken history reveals some symptoms indicative of an intestinal lesion, and in very many instances a pretty firm tentative diagnosis can be reached on the patient's symptoms alone. It cannot be too strongly stressed that *any alteration of bowel habit which persists for more than two or three weeks in a patient over 40 years of age* should be regarded as highly suspicious of an intestinal growth and in urgent need of full investigation. Suspicion of an organic lesion will be heightened to the level of certainty if there is in addition a history of *passing slime and blood* with, or apart from, the motions, and, though it remains to be decided by further examination whether this is a carcinoma or, say, a colitis, in older patients the odds are naturally heavily loaded in favour of a new growth.

The passage of blood, which is such a frequent symptom of carcinomas of the rectum or distal colon, is usually attributed by the patient—and sometimes, it is to be regretted, by his doctor as well—to piles. Actually by far the commonest cause of rectal bleeding is haemorrhoids; if it occurs in association with constipation the likelihood of it being haemorrhoidal in origin is perhaps increased, for most patients with piles find that their bleeding is aggravated when they are constipated. But any rectal bleeding—with or without constipation—may well be due to a carcinoma of the rectum or colon or to several other organic lesions, and the only correct course is for it to be properly investigated as a prelude to effective treatment.

Routine Investigation

GENERAL AND ABDOMINAL EXAMINATION

A general examination may reveal facts of value in regard to diagnosis and to the assessment of the patient's fitness for operative treatment. The general physique and state of nutrition will be observed and any evidence of loss of weight noted. The state of the mucous membranes will give some indication as to the presence of anaemia.

If the abdomen is distended out of proportion to the patient's build and obesity, this may be due to chronic intestinal obstruction, or to the presence of free fluid secondary to peritoneal metastases. Percussion will usually distinguish fairly reliably between them by demonstrating dullness in the flanks in the cases with free fluid, and a general tympanites, maximal perhaps in the flanks, in chronic obstruction of the colon. With chronic obstruction also the caecum may form a more localized swelling in the right iliac region, and visible peristalsis may be observed if carefully and patiently sought. On palpation an abdominal mass may be felt in the line of the colon. This is more likely to be found on the right side than on the left, owing to the more bulky character of right-sided growths in general. Any mass felt in the left abdomen, especially in the region of the iliac colon, will more probably be due to hard faeces impacted in the bowel above an impalpable 'string-stricture' carcinoma of the sigmoid colon. However, a loaded iliac colon is such a common state of affairs in perfectly normal people, who are merely somewhat constipated, that no great significance can be attached to this finding. A carcinomatous mass is usually hard and irregular, whilst inspissated faeces, though possibly also coarsely nodular, are not so firm in consistency and can often be indented slightly by the finger. Thorough palpation of the splenic and hepatic flexures requires a very deliberate and forceful bimanual palpation of the loins whilst the patient inspires and expires deeply; neglect of this precaution may result in a potentially palpable growth being missed.

The liver should be examined and any obvious enlargement, firmness or nodularity noted. It is not usually possible to be confident clinically about the presence of secondary deposits, unless the liver is not merely enlarged, but actually studded with palpable nodules. In cases with a history of anal pain or swelling it is as well to palpate the inguinal lymph glands for enlargement or induration. Lastly it is a useful routine also to feel quickly the axillae and supraclavicular regions to determine the state of the lymph nodes in these situations; exceptionally metastases occur in these glands in connection with advanced intestinal cancer.

In all but an occasional case the general and abdominal examination will fail to reveal any significant abnormality, and the establishment of the diagnosis will then depend essentially on the correct use of three further investigations—digital palpation of the rectum, sigmoidoscopy, and radiological examination after a barium enema. It is important to insist, firstly, that *these three diagnostic methods are complementary*, and, secondly, that they *should preferably be carried out in this order*. Though possibly as many as 75% of all rectal carcinomas, or 35% of carcinomas of the entire large intestine, lie within reach of the examining finger, a negative digital examination alone is clearly of only limited value in excluding a growth of the large bowel. Even when it is followed by a sigmoidoscopy to the full length of 25 cm this still leaves a considerable part of the sigmoid colon and all the rest of the large intestine unexamined, and a barium enema is obviously essential to complete the investigation. The reason why it is desirable to perform these investigations in the order mentioned is that if the digital examination is followed by a barium enema without sigmoidoscopy it is all too easy for this latter then to be omitted entirely, leaving the upper rectum possibly inadequately examined, so that a rectosigmoid growth might be overlooked.

DIGITAL PALPATION

As described on p. 378, a rectal carcinoma may assume several forms and the findings on digital palpation will vary accordingly; but two features characterize all rectal carcinomas—*induration* and a *raised edge*. The following are some of the more detailed findings commonly encountered:

1. An early growth may be felt as an indurated disc-like lesion raised like a small plateau with a flat surface and a definite edge.

2. Another type of lesion is a nodular friable protuberant growth, which is usually softer, but generally has some areas of induration and ulceration, if it is a frank carcinoma.

3. A very common finding is of a typical malignant ulcer with raised nodular everted edges and a very deep excavated crater.

4. Almost equally common is an annular carcinoma, the lower edge of which is felt by the examining finger as a complete ring of growth. If the growth lies low enough down and is not too tightly constricting, the tip of the finger can be inserted into its lumen, feeling its concave ulcerated walls, and even, in favourable circumstances, reaching the upper edge of the lesion or the rectal mucosa above it. If, however, the growth is situated at a higher level the fingertip may barely engage in it as it projects downwards rather like the cervix uteri, and may not be able to trace the normal rectal mucosa up to its junction with the growth on all aspects of the bowel circumference. If the lower edge extends downwards a little more in front than behind, the impression may easily be obtained not of an annular carcinoma, but of an anterior wall ulcer, the lumen of the lesion simulating an ulcer crater, and the fornix of the normal rectal cavity palpable posteriorly suggesting that the rectal lumen extends upwards past the growth (Fig. 303). I have many times had cases of rectal carcinoma referred to me with such a faulty assessment of the anatomy of the lesion present.

5. Sometimes a malignant ulcer, which is just

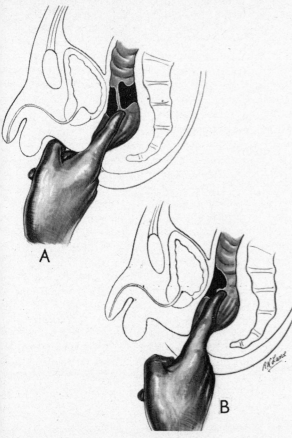

A

B

Fig. 303. Diagram illustrating how an annular carcinoma of the rectum, just within reach of the finger, may be wrongly assessed as an ulcerating growth confined to the anterior wall. The reason for this mistake is that the 'posterior fornix' of the rectum with the annular lesion (A) is not thoroughly palpated and traced up to the growth, and is thought to represent the lumen, as in an anterior wall carcinoma (B).

beyond the reach of the finger along the lumen of the rectum, may none the less be *palpable through the intact anterior rectal wall,* as the upper part of the rectum or lower portion of the sigmoid in which it is situated hangs down into the rectouterine or rectovesical pouch.

If a rectal carcinoma is present it is important before withdrawal of the finger to establish its precise situation and extent, its mobility, and the extent of spread, so far as can be determined by palpation:

a. Situation of the Growth. The circumferential extent of the lesion on the walls of the rectum should be noted and also the position of its lower edge relative to the anorectal ring, the cervix uteri, the upper border of the prostate, or the tip of the coccyx. If the growth lies low enough down, and a finger can be passed over or through it to reach the upper edge, its position is also recorded. (In female patients it is usually desirable also to palpate the growth if possible from the vaginal aspect. This reveals whether the vaginal mucosa over it is smooth and mobile or attached and possibly ulcerated. It may also be possible on vaginal examination to feel the upper limit of an annular lesion which would not transmit the finger on rectal examination.)

b. Mobility. It is valuable, as regards the prospects of surgical treatment, to record the mobility of fixity of the lesion. Very early lesions may be surprisingly mobile on the actual muscle coat of the rectal wall. More deeply ulcerated growths are generally fixed to some extent by penetration or fibrous adhesions to the extrarectal structures—the prostate, vesicles, bladder, posterior vaginal wall or uterus anteriorly, or to the sacrum or coccyx posteriorly. Still more advanced growths, particularly those of an annular type, are usually firmly fixed on several aspects and may give an impression of rock-like immobility. As a matter of fact, however, even these firmly fixed carcinomas can often be successfully excised (see p. 524), so that the surgeon should be very reluctant to declare a growth inoperable because of local fixation without proceeding to laparotomy (see Goligher 1941).

c. Extent of Spread. This is gauged partly by the size and characteristics of the primary growth and partly by its mobility or fixation. Other evidences of wide spread may, however, be detected in some cases. Induration may be felt below or above the main growth, due either to *submucous spread,* usually from extensive permeation of the superior haemorrhoidal veins, or to *extrarectal spread* from extensive direct spread in the perirectal tissues. Very rarely, hard enlarged pararectal glands on the back of the rectum can be felt against the sacrum, and sometimes extensive induration can be appreciated in one or other lateral ligament indicating spread of the growth in that direction. With any of these developments the prognosis as regards cure must be regarded as very poor or actually hopeless.

Finally, as the finger is withdrawn at the conclusion of the digital examination, it is noted whether blood is present on the examining finger. Such blood, usually rather dark and venous in character and having a peculiarly sickly and offensive smell, provides confirmation of the existence of a carcinoma, or, when no lesion was actually palpated, strengthens the probability that one lies beyond the reach of the finger.

PROCTOSCOPY AND SIGMOIDOSCOPY

If a rectal carcinoma has already been detected by palpation, proctoscopy may usually be omitted, but where no lesion has been felt it is as well to pass the proctoscope to determine whether any internal haemorrhoids are present, for these may provide an alternative explanation for the patient's bleeding. Occasionally also with a palpable growth of the lower part of the posterior rectal wall, proctoscopy may give a better view of the lesion for purpose of biopsy than does sigmoidoscopy.

It is, however, on the sigmoidoscope that the surgeon relies chiefly for endoscopic information. It is an indispensable diagnostic aid in cases where no lesion has been felt on digital examination, and not without value also in cases where the growth has already been diagnosed by palpation. In such cases it provides useful confirmation of the type, situation and extent of the lesion, especially when the latter was only just within reach of the finger and its thorough exploration by palpation was difficult.

The appearance of a rectal carcinoma on sigmoidoscopy is as a rule quite distinctive. The first thing that usually catches the examiner's eye is the raised everted lower edge of the lesion, which invariably appears a different shade of red from that of the surrounding pale pink mucosa—sometimes it is a brighter red, at others a darker, more purple, hue. If the instrument is advanced a little further, the grey sloughing base of the growth may be seen in those cases with an ulcerating or annular carcinoma, or the nodular protuberant surface may be observed in those with a more papilliferous type of lesion. Two characteristic views of rectal carcinomata are depicted in Plate IIA, B. A note should be made of the gross features of the growth, its circumferential extent on the walls of the rectum, and the sigmoidoscopic height of its lower margin. With non-constricting growths it may be possible to follow the lesion to its upper edge and note its exact position also, but with annular lesions this is usually impossible. If the sigmoidoscope can be passed above the growth it should be introduced as far as possible and the mucosa examined for polyps or a second carcinoma. Finally it should be mentioned that useful information can be obtained by the sigmoidoscope *about the mobility* of growths beyond

the reach of the finger. If the distal end of the instrument is engaged against the growth and gentle pressure exerted in the long axis of its shaft, some idea of the fixity of the lesion can be secured. The slightly yielding sensation of an early mobile growth is quite different from the rigid feel of a fixed carcinoma.

These various sigmoidoscopic manoeuvres are often much beset in a patient with a rectal carcinoma by the discharge of blood, slime and liquid faeces descending from above and obscuring the view. The bleeding is usually much increased as soon as the growth is touched by the end of the sigmoidoscope, but, by judicious swabbing or the use of a suction tube, and perseverance, it is generally possible to obtain a sufficiently good view of the lower margin of the lesion to make a sigmoidoscopic diagnosis and to secure a biopsy. It is wise to make the biopsy the last step in the examination, for the difficulties from bleeding are naturally aggravated by it.

In cases where no carcinoma is revealed by sigmoidoscopy, information suggestive of the presence of a growth beyond the reach of the instrument may be provided in the form of obvious blood or mucus in the rectal lumen, apparently coming from a higher level. It is important, of course, to observe the state of the rectal and colonic mucosa,

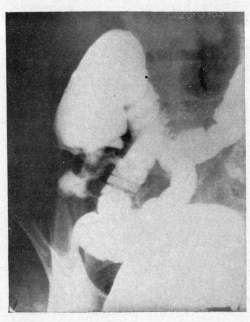

Fig. 304. Radiograph after a barium enema showing typical filling defect in the caecum due to fungating carcinoma.

to make sure that the blood and slime are not derived from the inflamed, granular, bleeding mucosa of a proctitis or proctocolitis. In cases in which the sigmoidoscopy does not show any immediate evidence of growth it is important to press the examination to the fullest possible extent and to make a determined effort to negotiate the rectosigmoid flexure, or if this proves impossible to remember the limitation of the sigmoidoscopy in interpreting the barium enema report. If the latter examination does not give good views of the rectosigmoid region *a repeat sigmoidoscopy under general anaesthesia* may be desirable.

BARIUM ENEMA EXAMINATION

From what has already been said it will be clear that *radiology has little place in the diagnosis of carcinoma of the rectum*, and usually of carcinoma of the distal sigmoid, for the recognition of growths in these situations should normally rest with digital and endoscopic examination. With the majority of colonic carcinomas, however, the diagnosis depends in large measure on radiology, and the method of choice as explained on p. 69 is the barium enema. The cardinal radiographic sign of a colonic carcinoma is a filling defect in the barium shadow, but other features that may be present are disturbances of the mucosal pattern, rigidity of the colon wall, colonic obstruction, or fixation of the gut.

The filling defect may take several forms depending on the size and gross characteristics of the growth. A bulky tumour that projects into the lumen of, say, the caecum or ascending colon produces a *filling defect usually with an irregular edge* as in Figs 304 and 305. In the majority of cases, however, the filling defect is represented by a very striking narrowing of the bowel—the so-called *napkin-ring* appearance (Fig. 306). In this the normal lumen is abruptly interrupted by a narrowed portion of 2·7–7·5 cm in length. The line of barium in the stenosed part is often slightly eccentric due to the greater bulk of the tumour in that part of the bowel wall in which it originated. Two features that distinguish such a narrowing from any form of colon spasm are its sharply defined, rather jagged or irregular outline,

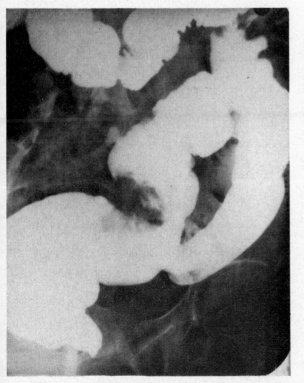

Fig. 305. Large polypoid growth of the rectosigmoid shown on barium enema examination.

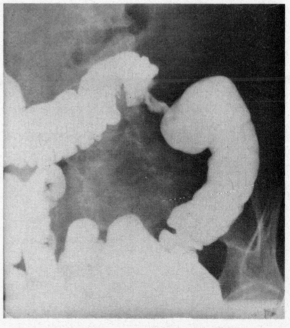

Fig. 306. Characteristic 'napkin-ring' appearance of an annular carcinoma of the colon on barium enema examination, well shown in this case with a growth in the left end of the transverse colon.

and its constancy. When an annular scirrhous growth is of classical *string-stricture* type, the narrowed segment may be very short indeed, sometimes even less than 2 cm in length. Even in this defect the involvement of the adjacent wall may be shown by a slight constant irregularity of the contours of the bowel as they dip into the constriction.

With stenosing carcinomas it will usually be found on screening that during the introduction of the barium enema there is a temporary hold-up of the opaque medium at the site of the lesion, which first draws the radiologist's attention to the growth. After a few moments the barium may then pass through the obstruction with a varying degree of difficulty, depending on the degree of narrowing present, and the lesion may then be more accurately defined. Its mobility or fixation may also be determined by palpatation under the screen. Sometimes the clear definition of the growth may be impaired by the fact that other coils of bowel filled with barium tend to overlap and obscure the segment containing the lesion. This is particularly liable to happen in the sigmoid and a growth just above the rectosigmoid junction may be completely hidden in a posteroanterior view, and may only be clearly demonstrated by the right or left oblique view. Another situation where difficulties from overlapping are liable to occur is in the region of the splenic flexure due to the fact that the rather redundant left end of the transverse colon lies exactly in front of and parallel to the uppermost few centimetres of the descending colon. Again the difficulty can be resolved usually be obtaining an oblique view.

So much for the grosser lesions, which are all fairly easily demonstrated by *a simple barium enema technique* (see p. 69). It is a good deal more difficult with small localized growths that do not cause stenosis and are confined to one small area of the bowel circumference (Fig. 307). These may easily be missed by this technique unless they happen to be caught in profile view. It is in the diagnosis of this type of growth and of the large polyp, that may or may not be malignant, that the *double contrast, air inflation, technique* mentioned on p. 69 is so valuable, for it gives a picture of the mucosal relief and may outline small lesions in full face view. Ideally also this method should be used even in cases in which a gross carcinoma has already been demonstrated to be present in the colon or rectum by the ordinary type of barium enema study or by clinical or sigmoidoscopic examination, in order to exclude the presence of associated polyps or

another primary carcinoma, but there are often technical difficulties in the presence of an annular growth in getting the bowel adequately prepared for a good double contrast examination.

PROCEDURE TO BE ADOPTED IN CASES WITH A NEGATIVE BARIUM ENEMA EXAMINATION

The standard of accuracy achieved by modern radiological methods in the diagnosis of carcinoma of the colon is very high, and it is only occasionally that the radiologist errs, either by diagnosing a growth that does not exist or by failing to detect a small early lesion. With a first-class radiological department the range of error in either direction should be small, but the radiologist is not infallible, and this is exemplified by a report by Lauer et al. (1965) from the Mayo Clinic on the accuracy of radiological examination in the diagnosis of carcinoma of the colon. They record 0.8% of false

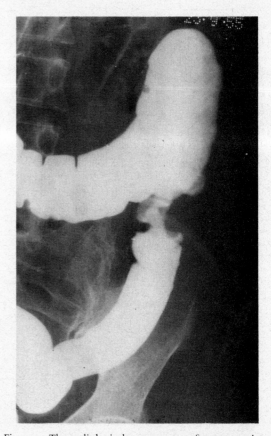

Fig. 307. The radiological appearances of a more polypoid type of carcinoma of the descending colon seen in profile.

positive and 6·9% of false negative diagnoses (mostly in connection with carcinomas of the caecum or sigmoid) in a large series of cases. It is well to bear constantly in mind therefore that the radiologist is sometimes wrong, and particularly to remember this when he returns a negative report. It is important for the surgeon to consider carefully what should be his plan of procedure in the face of such a negative radiological verdict:

1. He should make quite sure that the areas examined by sigmoidoscopy and the barium enema meet and overlap so that no segment of large intestine has been left unexamined in the region of the rectosigmoid junction. The further steps *depend almost entirely on the degree of clinical suspicion of a carcinoma.*

2. *If no strong suspicion exists* and if, for example, the barium enema had been performed almost as a gesture because of constipation that was merely a slight aggravation of a chronic condition, and there were no other very suggestive symptoms, the negative radiological report can be accepted as final. If there has also been rectal bleeding, *but no mucus,* and an adequate explanation for this latter complaint has been found in the form of internal haemorrhoids, these should be injected. The effect of the injections is of considerable diagnostic significance, for, whatever the degree of haemorrhoids present, bleeding will certainly be stopped for some weeks or months by injection treatment if in fact it was coming from the piles. Failure to arrest the haemorrhage in this way will raise afresh the suspicion of another cause for the patient's symptoms and demand a careful review of the case.

3. *If the symptoms are more suggestive* with, say, more severe constipation or diarrhoea or both, with some blood in the stools and perhaps a doubtful history of passing mucus, matters should not be allowed to rest with a single negative barium enema. Further investigation is certainly required. First of all a more proximal cause for the symptoms, in the form of a regional ileitis, should be excluded by a barium progress meal, supplemented if necessary by a fat balance. Secondly, if there were the slightest doubt about the manner in which the rectal examination and sigmoidoscopy had been performed, particularly if they had been entrusted to a less experienced assistant, it should be repeated by the surgeon himself. Thirdly, it may be wise to have the barium enema repeated after an interval of two or three weeks. If no abnormality is

discovered by these examinations and clinical suspicion remains strong, the question of *exploratory laparotomy* arises. Admittedly, before resorting to exploration, some surgeons would in the past have had the stools tested on two or three occasions for occult blood, as described on p. 76, or have had colon washings examined for exfoliated malignant cells (see p. 76). Unfortunately, neither of these investigations—especially the former—is entirely reliable, as Cameron et al. (1961), Knoernschild et al. (1961), Oakland (1961) and Raskin et al. (1962) have shown, and false positive or false negative results may be obtained in a small proportion of patients with either method, the false negatives being the serious ones. A much more important diagnostic step that is now available and should certainly always be taken before proceeding to exploratory laparotomy is *fibreoptic colonoscopy* (see p. 70). If a satisfactory examination of the entire colon round to the caecum can be achieved with it, this should provide a firm diagnosis regarding the presence or absence of any organic large bowel lesion. However, if for technical reasons this examination is incomplete and leaves more or less of the proximal colon uninspected, the surgeon will again be thrown back on his clinical suspicion in deciding whether to advise exploration or not.

EARLIER DIAGNOSIS

It would seem obvious that the earlier a carcinoma of the rectum or colon is detected and treatment initiated the better, but in practice this is rarely achieved (Holliday and Hardcastle 1979). More often an interval of 6 or 12 months or longer elapses between the onset of symptoms and the arrival of the patient at hospital. This delay is due usually to the patient's reluctance to seek advice, but also sometimes to a belated appreciation by the family doctor of the sinister significance of his symptoms.

CANCER EDUCATION OF THE LAY PUBLIC

In an endeavour to induce patients to report at an earlier stage symptoms suspicious of cancer—not only of the rectum but of other organs—many authorities have advocated so-called cancer education of the lay public. This is already in force in parts of the United States, and the idea has apparently received the blessing of our own Department of Health. I very much doubt its wisdom and value, which remain to be proven. As I see it, the effect if any may be to convert a small proportion of the population into cancerophobes, and to leave the majority quite untouched. Even if one did succeed in convincing most people by such propaganda, I am not convinced that it would influence their behaviour very much when they were unfortunate enough to develop cancer, for in my experience doctor patients—who are presumably better educated in regard to cancer than even well-informed lay people—do not behave very differently from ordinary patients when they fall victims to malignant disease. Though there are exceptions, in general they find much the same excuses as lay people for not coming to have their symptoms promptly investigated, and there is much the same delay in initiating effective treatment.

EARLIER REFERENCE OF PATIENTS WITH SUSPICIOUS SYMPTOMS TO HOSPITAL BY THEIR GENERAL PRACTITIONERS

It must be quite impossible for a medical student to proceed to qualification without having instilled into him on many occasions the paramount importance of regarding symptoms such as persistent constipation, or diarrhoea, and the passage of blood or slime in patients of middle age or over as due to carcinoma till proved to the contrary. Yet on entering practice he seems to forget this advice all too quickly, if one can judge from the numbers of patients with cancer of the rectum or colon who are labelled as 'piles' or 'colitis' by their doctors and treated as such for 6 or 12 months or longer before being referred to hospital. Some of these patients may have a rectal examination by their practitioner without any lesion having been discovered, which serves to emphasize that a *negative digital palpation alone means exactly nothing*, for the growth may well be beyond the reach of such an examination, particularly if it has not been expertly performed. For that reason I regard as unrealistic the criticisms often levelled at general practitioners for not having 'passed a finger' on their patients with rectal symptoms, for whatever he finds he ought still to refer his patient to hospital—either for treatment of the carcinoma he has detected by palpation or for further investigation by sigmoidoscopy and barium enema, as required. My fear—which is borne out by events—is that the doctor may sometimes forget the strictly limited diagnostic significance of simple examination with the finger, divorced from the other complementary investigations, and may allow himself to be dissuaded by it from referring the patient promptly to hospital for these additional examinations. For this reason it may happen that a keen practitioner, who always examines his patients most carefully but overrates the value of his own rectal examination in this way, sometimes gives them poorer service than does his less conscientious colleague whose immediate reaction to a case with a rectal complaint is to dismiss it forthwith, unexamined, to the nearest rectal clinic. I must say I think the latter is the correct disposal, for, whatever symptoms the patient may have and whatever their cause—be it carcinoma, colitis, diverticulitis, or simple piles—hospital facilities are needed for their proper elucidation and treatment.

THE POSSIBLE ACHIEVEMENTS OF EARLIER SYMPTOMATIC DIAGNOSIS

On the question of earlier diagnosis, which seems such a desirable aim, I feel it my duty to say that I regard some of the hopes that have been expressed of improvement in the results of treatment of cancer, if earlier diagnosis could be achieved, as altogether too sanguine. Nearly all surgeons can recall cases of carcinoma, operated on within a few weeks of the onset of symptoms, where wide dissemination has already taken place, and it seems probable that some active growths are incurable almost from their onset. In more slowly growing lesions it is possible that earlier diagnosis might improve the prospects of cure somewhat, but these are often already quite good even after considerable delay in this type of case. I strongly suspect that in general, the most important factor determining the outcome of treatment of a carcinoma is the histological type and activity of the growth rather than the time at which it is detected. This contention is supported in regard to carcinoma of the rectum by a correlation of the histological grading of the growth and the extent of spread at the time of operation (see p. 641). This shows that most of the C cases had relatively poorly differentiated growths, whereas the A cases included a very high proportion of the well-differentiated lesions. Moreover, the patients with the most advanced lesions and the poorest prognosis often have the shortest history (Slaney 1971). I agree, however, that in any particular case the sooner the carcinoma can be removed the better, and a delay of a few weeks might make the difference between the occurrence of hepatic metastases and a growth that can still be completely eradicated by surgery.

PRE-SYMPTOMATIC DIAGNOSIS

The ideal would be to achieve diagnosis at the very earliest stages, even before the onset of symptoms.

During the past two decades attempts have been made to accomplish this in America by means of periodic routine examination of apparently healthy people of cancer age. For this purpose cancer detection clinics have been established in a number of centres, such as the Memorial Hospital, New York (O'Donnell et al. 1962), and the University of Minnesota, Minneapolis (Gilbertsen and Wangensteen 1963). Symptomless individuals over the age of, say, 45 or 50 are encouraged to attend these clinics every six months for a complete physical examination, including: routine blood and urine examination; radiograph of chest; gastric analysis; proctosigmoidoscopy to 25 cm; testing of the stools for occult blood after a three-day meat-free diet; pelvic examination for women; and Papanicolaou examinations of cervical and vaginal smears as well as any sputum resulting from a productive cough. Depending on the results of these examinations, further radiological studies may be ordered to investigate the stomach (in patients with achlorhydria or hypochlorhydria, with occult blood in the stools, with anaemia, or with vague gastric symptoms); the colon (in patients with abnormal findings on sigmoidoscopy, with occult blood in the stools or unexplained anaemia; with a family history of bowel cancer, with marked weight loss, or vague symptoms referable to the bowel); the kidney (with haematuria or palpable mass in the renal region). One form of cancer where pre-symptomatic diagnosis is most promising has apparently been carcinoma of the large intestine, because of its relative accessibility, and of the possibility of detecting pre-malignant polyps which can be destroyed by sigmoidoscopic diathermy, preventing their development into frank carcinoma (Enquist and State 1952; Enquist 1957). Thus, in a group of 10 771 patients seen at the Cancer Detection Center of the University of Minnesota between 1948 and 1963, on whom a total of 44 324 examinations were performed, 375 cancers were discovered (Gilbertsen and Wangensteen 1963), a detection rate of 1 in 29 patients or 1 in 110 examinations. Of these, 31 were in colon, 29 in rectum, 22 in stomach, 25 in breast, and 45 in prostate, to mention only a few. The outcome of radical treatment for some of these growths, for example gastric cancer, does not seem to have been significantly better than that obtaining in ordinary clinical practice; but for others, notably the tumours of breast and large intestine, it is apparently much better than average. Thus, for the 18 cases of colon cancer seen and treated up to 1957, there was a 50% five-year survival rate, compared with the national figure of 30% for the USA.

For the 20 patients with rectal cancer detected before 1957, the five-year survival rate was 75%, the usual overall five-year survival rate for patients diagnosed to have this tumour in ordinary practice bing 25%. Of special note are the survival data for the six cases with rectal cancer found on follow-up examinations; each of the six patients has survived five years. However, one of the difficulties encountered in cancer detection surveys of this kind is that patients sometimes refuse to have radical operative treatment for the tumours thus revealed (St John et al. 1944; Roach et al. 1952; Wigh and Swenson 1953). It may also be that patients are occasionally induced to undergo unnecessary operations on a wrong diagnosis. It is difficult to say whether the yield in terms of cancer prevented or detected at an early more curable stage justifies the organization needed to undertake the very large numbers of routine examinations, but these Centers represent a very logical and commendable effort, and, so far as cancer of the large intestine (or breast) is concerned, do seem on the information available to be warranted. No clinics of this kind exist in Great Britain but in any well-run rectal clinic sigmoidoscopy is performed on all patients regardless of their symptoms, and any adenomatous polyps discovered are treated by diathermy. So far in Britain, therefore, we rely essentially on the clinical acumen of our general practitioners to set the diagnostic ball rolling.

Mass Screening for Colorectal Cancer using Guaiac-impregnated Slides

Recently a simpler method of screening asymptomatic people for colorectal cancer has been proposed by Greegor (1967, 1971) and employed in several centres (Glober and Peskoe 1974; Hastings 1974; Hardcastle 1978). It involves routine testing of stools for occult blood, using guaiac-impregnated slides (Hemoccult*). Subjects taking part in the survey are sent guaiac-impregnated slides by post and instructed to take two portions from each of three consecutive stools and smear each portion on a separate guaiac-impregnated slide, taking care not to spread the faeces too thickly on the slide (slides stained with mud are sent as examples of how thick the faecal smear should be). The subjects are told not to do the test if there is

* Made by Smith Kline Diagnostics, Sunnyvale, California.

obvious blood on the stool or in the toilet bowl and to report these findings to their doctor or the diagnostic centre. A stamped addressed envelope is enclosed for returning the slides. On receipt of them at the centre, two drops of developer (stabilized hydrogen peroxide and denatured alcohol) supplied by the manufacturer are placed on each slide and the results read within 20 seconds. The intensity of the colour, if present, is graded 1+, 2+, or 3+.

Negative results are reported by letter to the subject and his doctor. Subjects having positive results are sent six more slides together with instructions regarding a meat-free high-bulk diet for 24 hours prior to and during the collection of two portions from each of three more stools. These are returned in due course to the centre and tested as described. Subjects with negative results were discharged from suspicion and they and their doctor were notified accordingly. As regards subjects with positive results, they and their doctors were informed and they were advised to undergo thorough clinical examination and investigation by sigmoidoscopy and barium enema study.

In a report of a survey by Glober and Peskoe (1974), of 1539 subjects sent Hemoccult slides, 400 (25.7%) had at least one slide positive. Three-hundred and forty-four of these 400 proceeded to a further test whilst on a meat-free diet, 53 being found positive. Thirty-two of the 53 were fully investigated and four were found to have carcinoma coli, a yield of colon cancers of 0.2% of the original 1539 subjects. The great attraction of this method of screening is that it is easily done on an out-patient basis by paramedical staff in the first instance. Only when suspicion has been narrowed down to quite a small group of individuals are medical staff involved.

CARCINOEMBRYONIC ANTIGEN ASSAY AS A
SCREENING TEST FOR CANCER OF THE LARGE
BOWEL

In 1965, Gold and Freedman of Montreal discovered a specific antigen in adenocarcinomas of the entodermally-derived epithelium of the gastrointestinal tract. They were also able to demonstrate the same antigen in embryonic and fetal digestive tissues up to the end of the first six months of pregnancy. This new antigen was aptly designated by them the 'carcinoembryonic antigen' (CEA). Circulating antibodies to it were found in the sera of a high proportion of women throughout pregnancy, in postpartum women, and in 70% of patients who had non-metastasizing cancers of the ailmentary tract (Gold 1967; Gold and Freeman 1965a, b).

Thomson et al. (1969) developed a radio-immunoassay capable of detecting minute quantities of CEA in the serum, and with it demonstrated the presence of the antigen in 10 of 11 preoperative cases of cancer of the colon or rectum (the single negative case was shown at operation to have a volvulus of the sigmoid, not a carcinoma!), and in all of 24 postoperative cases of colorectal cancer with residual or recurrent growth. None of 26 postoperative cases without residual cancer was positive. Thomson et al. (1969) suggested that the finding of circulating CEA in the serum might be of diagnostic or prognostic significance.

Moore et al. (1971) further investigated this suggestion in a survey of 279 persons. CEA was found in the sera of 32 of 35 patients with carcinoma of the large intestine, of all of 13 patients with carcinoma of the pancreas, of six of 14 patients with other gastrointestinal cancers, of six of 8 patients with bronchogenic carcinomas, of 24 of 46 patients with severe alcoholic liver disease, and of seven of 13 patients with uraemia. By contrast, 79 assays on 40 young normal control subjects all gave negative results. Despite these occasional false positive and false negative findings, Moore et al. (1971) felt that the CEA assay test was of sufficient reliability to be of some value in the diagnosis of cancer of the large bowel and of some other parts of the gastrointestinal system including the pancreas, though its results needed to be interpreted with caution, especially in elderly patients. They were not so sure of its usefulness in monitoring tumour behaviour after operation.

Further experience in several laboratories in North America and Britain has cast further doubt on the value of CEA assay in the diagnosis of colorectal cancer (Laurence et al. 1972). Not only large bowel cancers but a wide variety of other malignant tumours of differing histogenesis can give positive responses, and also some non-neoplastic conditions such as ulcerative colitis and hepatic or renal failure. In addition, it is only the large advanced colorectal carcinomas—already easily diagnosed on clinical grounds as a rule—that produce fairly consistently high levels of CEA. As for the role of the test in monitoring patients for recurrent or metastatic disease, its value in detecting hepatic metastases seems to be established (Livingstone et al. 1974; Mackay et al. 1974), but a combination of CEA assays and liver function tests may be a more sensitive guide (Cooper et al. 1975).

CARCINOMA OF THE COLON OR RECTUM WITH ACUTE OBSTRUCTION

As already pointed out on p. 381 some degree of partial obstruction, causing severe constipation and other symptoms, is a frequent effect of carcinoma of the large intestine, especially when situated in the left colon. In about a fifth of the patients, however, complete obstruction occurs, either as an aggravation of this chronic state of affairs—the so-called 'acute on chronic' obstruction—or as an entirely fresh development. As with chronic obstruction, acute obstruction is far more commonly encountered with carcinomas of the left colon than with those of the right colon. As indicated on p. 380 there are good pathological reasons why the scirrhous type of growth found chiefly on the left side of the large intestine should be particularly liable to undergo complete blockage, and it would be reasonable to expect a greater tendency to acute obstruction with such lesions. Actually, however, there is quite a considerable risk of acute obstruction occurring with growths of the right colon as well, the main reason why this is not so apparent clinically being that there are many fewer carcinomas in that part of the large intestine to become obstructed. This fact was clearly brought out in our analysis of 1644 consecutive cases of carcinoma of the colon and rectum treated at the General Infirmary at Leeds (Goligher

and Smiddy 1957). Of the 290 cases complicated by acute obstruction in that series, only 70 had their growths in the right or transverse colon, as contrasted with 180 with growths in the left colon and sigmoid (Table 24). But when these figures were related to the total number of growths in each of these segments it was found that the incidence of acute obstruction with carcinoma of the right and transverse colon was 27·4%, and with carcinoma of the left colon 40·4%. It is also interesting to note that, though the rectum was the commonest site for malignant disease, the incidence of acute obstruction there was lower than elsewhere in the large intestine—only 4·2%.

Symptoms

Complete obstruction from carcinoma of the large gut is *often entirely insidious in its onset*, particularly if it is of the 'acute on chronic' variety, and the patient has been having increasing difficulty with his bowels for some weeks or months beforehand. With the development of acute obstruction he simply finds that he goes for two or three days or longer without a motion, despite the use of aperients. He has probably had similar episodes in the past which have responded eventually to purgation, so that he is not at first unduly worried and merely takes a larger dose of medicine. But this only causes further 'wind pain' and colic, without producing any motion. Moreover he finds that he is not able to get rid of flatus per rectum and his abdomen is becoming progressively more distended. But despite this he may be able to continue taking fluid and some food without nausea or, at any rate, actual vomiting. This state of affairs may continue with slowly increasing abdominal discomfort and distension over a period of six or seven days or longer before he finally comes to hospital, and even then, depending on the site of the growth and other factors, he may have only just started to vomit.

In certain cases, however, the acute obstruction is more sudden in its manifestation, particularly when the growth lies in the right colon. These patients have had little in the way of bowel symptoms before the development of acute obstruction. They are then suddenly seized with severe abdominal pain of colicky type, which persists and is liable to be followed by nausea and vomiting, which also continues. Fortunately these more acute and disturbing symptoms usually lead to the patient's early transfer to hospital.

TABLE 24. *Proportion of Patients with Carcinoma in Different Sites in Large Intestine presenting with Acute Obstruction*

Site	No. of growths	No. complicated by acute obstruction	Incidence of obstruction (%)
Caecum Ascending colon Hepatic flexure	178	50	28·1
Transverse colon	77	20	26·0
Splenic flexure Descending colon Sigmoid	445	180	40·4
Rectum	944	40	4·2
Total	1644	290	17·6

After Goligher and Smiddy (1957).

Examination

The general condition of patients with acute obstruction due to carcinoma of the colon or rectum is often excellent, because vomiting with its resulting dehydration and electrolyte depletion is usually a late phenomenon.

In all but the earliest cases there is obvious abdominal fullness, which may be very gross indeed. With obstructed growths of the sigmoid or descending colon the distension—which is usually confined to the large bowel and, due to the competence of the ileocaecal valve, does not involve the small gut—is particularly marked in the periphery of the abdomen, especially in the flanks. The absence of central distension may give a 'plateau-like' appearance to the abdomen. Visible peristalsis may be evident, especially in patients with 'acute on chronic' obstruction, the waves of peristalsis occurring every few minutes synchronously with spasms of pain and often loud borborygmi, clearly audible without a stethoscope. Palpation of the abdomen confirms that it is tense but not tender. The distended segments of intestine may be felt to harden with peristalsis. Only rarely can an actual tumour mass be palpated in these distended abdomens, or an enlarged liver clearly felt.

In all cases *the hernial orifices should be examined* to exclude a strangulated external hernia as the cause of the obstruction.

Rectal Examination.

On digital palpation, the most characteristic sign is 'ballooning' of the rectum, which is frequently elicited when the acutely obstructed growth lies in the sigmoid or upper rectum, but is seldom found with more proximally situated lesions. Exceptionally a rectal carcinoma causing acute obstruction is directly palpable; much more commonly the growth is beyond the reach of the finger. Sometimes, however, a carcinoma of the sigmoid responsible for acute obstruction may be felt through the anterior rectal wall as it hangs down in the rectovesical or rectovaginal pouch. A mass felt in either of these pouches may alternatively be a secondary deposit of growth in the pelvic peritoneum from a carcinoma at a higher level. Another finding that should be looked for is the presence of blood or mucus on the examining finger on withdrawal. Sigmoidoscopy should not be omitted, for it will sometimes clinch the diagnosis by revealing the lower edge of a constricting annular growth of the rectosigmoid or distal colon.

Diagnosis

It is not usually difficult to decide that the patient is suffering from an acute or subacute intestinal obstruction; the distended abdomen, free from tenderness, the colicky pain, and non-passage of faeces and flatus, and possibly vomiting all points to obstruction. Nor is there much difficulty as a rule in reaching the conclusion that the obstruction is probably due to a carcinoma of the large intestine, for this is one of the commonest causes of acute obstruction. Indeed, after exclusion of a strangulated external hernia, cancer of the colon or rectum remains as the most likely cause of an acute intestinal obstruction in a patient over middle age.

In many cases there will be a very suggestive history of irregularity of bowel habits, the passage of blood or slime, and a failure of general health, for some time before the occurrence of the more acute symptoms, to strengthen the tentative diagnosis of obstruction due to intestinal cancer. In a few cases there may be direct evidence in the form of a palpable mass in the abdomen or pelvis, or at least strong presumptive evidence such as ballooning of the rectum on digital examination and blood and slime on the examining finger, to confirm the existence of a growth and indicate with some accuracy its probable site. In the absence of such evidence, however, it may be assumed that the growth is situated in the sigmoid, which is by far the commonest site for an acutely obstructed carcinoma.

FURTHER DIAGNOSTIC MEASURES

PLAIN X-RAY EXAMINATION OF THE ABDOMEN

This is of the greatest possible value in diagnosing the presence of an obstruction and determining the exact site of the neoplasm. In acute obstructions due to carcinoma of the colon the normal colonic gas shadow proximal to the growth becomes greatly widened. In addition, in plates taken in the erect or sitting position, there are usually fluid levels in relation to the colonic gas—an occurrence that is met with so rarely in the normal colon that it may be regarded as pathognomonic of obstruction. A careful study of the distal extent of the colonic gas shadow will localize the lesion with fair accuracy. Sometimes, however, with obstructing growths in the sigmoid colon, the distension of the descending colon is not well shown and an erroneous diagnosis of carcinoma of the splenic flexure may be made.

In volvulus of the sigmoid, which is a possible source of confusion in diagnosis—but which may already have been suggested on clinical examination by the enormous distension of the abdomen—plain X-ray examination usually demonstrates clearly the grossly dilated sigmoid loop extending almost to the diaphragm, with in addition dilatation of the obstructed more proximal colon (p. 927).

The amount of distension of the small gut in cases of obstructed colonic carcinoma is very variable, but in many cases with growths in the left colon the ileocaecal valve may remain competent till a late stage and there may be no gas shadows or fluid levels in the small intestine. With carcinomas of the transverse and right colon, radiological signs of small bowel obstruction, though often absent in the initial phases, become increasingly evident later, and with obstructed growths in the caecal region the only gas shadows and fluid levels seen may be in the ileum and jejunum.

EMERGENCY BARIUM ENEMA EXAMINATION

If desired, and if appropriate radiological skill is available in the emergency, plain X-ray examination of the abdomen may be supplemented by a barium or gastrografin enema examination. In cases of real doubt this may be necessary, but usually sufficient information is obtained from the clinical and plain X-ray examination to enable the surgeon to make a decision regarding the plan of treatment to be adopted.

CARCINOMA OF THE COLON OR RECTUM WITH PERFORATION

According to the statistics of the General Infirmary at Leeds some 7% of all cases of carcinoma of the large intestine present with perforation of the bowel and consequent peritonitis (Goligher and Smiddy 1957). Many surgeons seem to believe that this complication of cancer of the colon or rectum occurs most frequently as an addition to an already existing acute or subacute obstruction, in association with a growth of the left colon, and that the perforation takes place through a stercoral ulcer, usually in the caecum, less commonly closer to the growth, with resulting faecal peritonitis. But in the series of 115 cases of carcinoma of the large intestine presenting with perforation at the Leeds General Infirmary between 1937 and 1949, only 20 were of this type. A far more common occurrence, which was found in 95 of the Leeds cases, was for the perforation to take place *apart from obvious obstruction*, at or very close to the growth itself, and to give rise either to a generalized peritonitis (57 cases) or to a localized peritonitis or abscess (38 cases). As Table 25 shows, these three types of perforation and peritonitis may be found with carcinomas at any site in the colon, but perforation of stercoral ulcers is commonest with growths of the left colon, and perforation of growths themselves with the production of a localized peritonitis seems specially liable to occur with lesions of the right colon, particularly in the caecal region, as Ewing (1951) and Patterson (1956) have also emphasized.

TABLE 25. *Proportion of Patients with Carcinomas in Different Sites in the Large Intestine presenting with Perforation and Peritonitis*

Site of growth	No. of cases in each site	Obstructed cases with perforation of stercoral ulcer	Unobstructed cases		All cases with perforations and peritonitis
			With perforation of growth and general peritonitis	With perforation of growth and local peritonitis	
Caecum Ascending colon Hepatic flexure	178	1	6	15	22 (12·9%)
Transverse colon	77	1	1	3	5 (6·5%)
Splenic flexure Descending colon Sigmoid colon	445	9	32	14	55 (12·3%)
Rectum	944	9	18	6	33 (3·5%)
All sites	1644	20	57	38	115

After Goligher and Smiddy (1957).

Clinical Features and Diagnosis

Obstructed Cases with Perforation of a Stercoral Ulcer and Faecal Peritonitis

These patients are usually in a desperately ill condition on admission to hospital and are obviously suffering from a general peritonitis with abdominal distension, diffuse tenderness, vomiting, gross dehydration and electrolyte depletion. The underlying carcinoma coli and acute obstruction may or may not be suspected from the history or physical examination. In the majority of cases with this form of perforation the condition rapidly deteriorates and ends fatally, without any opportunity being vouchsafed to the surgeon to carry out the exploratory laparotomy which the abdominal signs certainly demand.

Unobstructed Cases with Perforation at the Growth and Resulting *General* Peritonitis

Many of these patients are also gravely ill when they reach hospital and show the signs of general peritonitis, but, owing to the absence of a previous acute obstruction, the contamination of the peritoneum is a good deal less virulent, and the condition usually responds more satisfactorily to measures designed to correct dehydration and electrolyte loss. The majority of the cases can thus be made fit for exploration. It may or may not be possible to deduce from the history and findings on clinical examination that a growth has been present for some time before the development of this acute complication.

Unobstructed Cases with Perforation at the Growth and Resulting *Local* Peritonitis

These cases often occasion much confusion in diagnosis. If the carcinoma and perforation occur in the sigmoid colon they may easily mimic a diverticulitis with localized peritonitis and abscess formation, unless a previous history of bowel irregularity with the passage of blood and slime and loss of weight points strongly to growth. Cases are on record where the only presenting symptom or clinical sign of a carcinoma of the left colon which had perforated was the development of subcutaneous emphysema (Shambaugh and Burgert 1962), of a subcutaneous abscess of the abdominal wall (Shucksmith 1963) or thigh (Mair et al. 1977), or a left perinephric abscess (Feldman et al. 1968). With caecal carcinomas, which are notoriously prone to septic complications of this kind, obviously the condition may simulate an appendicitis with abscess formation or with a mass of adhesions. Indeed in some cases there may actually be an obstructive appendicitis due to blockage of the base of the appendix by a caecal growth as pointed out by Ewing (1951), Patterson (1956), Hossain (1962) and Miln and McLaughlin (1969). The clinical appearances may so closely resemble those of appendicitis that the surgeon may have little doubt that he is dealing with the latter disease. This conviction may be corrected at laparotomy when a carcinoma of the caecum is recognized as the cause of the mass and of any related inflammatory changes, but in some instances, as Patterson (1956) has emphasized, the clinical misconception may even survive operation, when this has taken the form of simple drainage of an abscess, any induration noted in the caecal wall being dismissed as due to inflammatory oedema. A faecal fistula is then likely to develop, but this often closes and the patient may then be discharged. Several months later he returns on account of an abscess or a discharging sinus in the right iliac region and is likely to have carcinoma growing along the old drainage track. Since the original operation was done as an emergency, many of these patients turn up at another hospital subsequently. The similarity with Crohn's disease will also be evident.

REFERENCES

Cameron, A. B., Knoernschild, H. E. and Zollinger, R. M. (1961) Detection of cancer and adenomas of the colon. *Am. J. Surg., 101,* 23.

Cooper, E. H., Turner, R. and Steele, L. (1975) The contribution of serum enzymes and carcinoembryonic antigen to the early diagnosis of metastatic colerectal cancer. *Br. J. Cancer, 31,* 111.

Enquist, I. F. (1957) The incidence and significance of polyps of the colon and rectum. *Surgery, St Louis, 42,* 681.

—— and State, D. (1952) Rectal and colonic polyps. *Surgery, St Louis, 32,* 696.

Ewing, M. R. (1951) Inflammatory complications of cancer of the caecum and ascending colon. *Postgrad. med. J., 27,* 515.

Feldman, M. A., Cotton, R. E. and Gray, M. W. (1968) Carcinoma of the colon presenting as left perinephric abscess. *Br. J. Surg., 55,* 21.

Gilbertsen, V. A. and Wangensteen, O. H. (1963) The results of efforts for asymptomatic diagnosis of malignant disease. *Surgery Gynec. Obstet., 116,* 413.

GLOBER, G. A. and PESKOE, S. M. (1974) Outpatient screening for gastrointestinal lesions using guaiac-impregnated slides. *Dig. Dis.,* *19*, 399.

GOLD, P. (1967) Circulating antibodies against carcinoembryonic antigens of the human digestive system. *Cancer, 20,* 1663.

—— and FREEDMAN, S. O. (1965*a*) Demonstration of tumor-specific antigens in human colonic carcinomata by immunological tolerance and absorption techniques. *J. exp. Med., 121*, 439.

—— —— (1965*b*) Specific carcinoembryonic antigens of the human digestive system. *J. exp. Med., 122*, 467.

GOLIGHER, J. C. (1941) The operability of carcinoma of the rectum. *Br. med. J., 2*, 393.

—— and SMIDDY, F. G. (1957) The treatment of acute obstruction or perforation with carcinoma of the colon and rectum. *Br. J. Surg., 45*, 270.

GREEGOR, D. H. (1967) Diagnosis of large-bowel cancer in the asymptomatic patient. *J. Am. med. Ass., 201*, 943.

—— (1971) Occult blood testing for detection of asymptomatic colon cancer. *Cancer, 28*, 131.

HARDCASTLE, J. D. (1978) Personal communication.

HASTINGS, J. B. (1974) Mass screening colorectal cancer. *Am. J. Surg., 127*, 228.

HOLLIDAY, H. W. and HARDCASTLE, J. D. (1979) Delay in diagnosis and treatment of sympathetic colorectal cancer. *Lancet, 1*, 309.

HOSSAIN, M. A. (1962) Unrecognized carcinoma of caecum presenting as acute appendicitis or appendix abscess. *Br. med. J., 2*, 709.

KNOERNSCHILD, H. E., CAMERON, A. B. and ZOLLINGER, R. M. (1961) Millipore filtration of colonic washings in malignant lesions of the large bowel. *Am. J. Surg., 101*, 20.

LAUER, J. D., CARLSON, H. C. and WOLLAEGER, E. E. (1965) Accuracy of roentgenologic examination in detecting carcinoma of the colon. *Dis. Colon Rect., 8*, 190.

LAURENCE, D. T. R., STEVENS, U. and BETTELHEIM, R. (1972) Role of plasma carcinoembryonic antigen. *Br. med. J., 3*, 605.

LIVINGSTONE, A. S., HAMPSON, L. G., SHUSTER, J., GOLD, P. and HINCHEY, E. J. (1974) Carcinoembryonic antigen in the diagnosis and management of colorectal carcinoma. *Archs Surg., Chicago, 109*, 259.

MACKAY, A. M., PATEL, S. and CARTER, S. (1974) Role of serial plasma CEA assays in the detection of recurrent and metastatic colorectal carcinomas. *Br. med. J., 4*, 382.

MAIR, W. S. J., McADAM, W. A. F., LEE, P. W. R., JEPSON, K. and GOLIGHER, J. C. (1977) Carcinoma of the large bowel presenting as a subcutaneous abscess of the thigh: a report of 4 cases. *Br. J. Surg., 64*, 205.

MILN, D. C. and McLAUGHLIN, I. S. (1969) Carcinoma of proximal large bowel associated with acute appendicitis. *Br. J. Surg., 56*, 143.

MOORE, T. L., KUPCHIK, H. Z., MARCON, N. and ZAMCHECK, N. (1971) Carcinoembryonic antigen assay in cancer of the colon and pancreas and other digestive tract orders. *Am. J. dig. Dis., 16*, 1.

MUIR, E. G. (1956) The diagnosis of carcinoma of the colon and rectum: a review of 714 cases. *Br. J. Surg., 44*, 1.

OAKLAND, D. J. (1961) Diagnosis of carcinoma of the large bowel by exfoliative cytology. *Br. J. Surg., 48*, 353.

O'DONNELL, W. E., DAY, E. and VENET, L. (1962) *Early Detection and Diagnosis of Cancer.* St Louis: C. V. Mosby.

PATTERSON, H. A. (1956) The management of cecal cancer discovered unexpectedly at operation for acute appendicitis. *Ann. Surg., 143*, 670.

RASKIN, H. F., KIRSNER, J. B., PALMER, W. L. and PLETICKA, S. (1962) The clinical value of negative gastrointestinal exfoliative cytologic examination in cancer suspects. *Gastroenterology, 42*, 266.

ROACH, J. F., SLOAN, R. D. and MORGAN, R. H. (1952) The detection of gastric carcinoma by photo-fluorographic methods. Part III: findings. *Am. J. Roentgen., 67*, 68.

ST JOHN, F. B., SWENSON, P. C. and HARVEY, H. D. (1944) An experiment in the early diagnosis of gastric carcinoma. *Ann. Surg., 119*, 225.

SHAMBAUGH, P. and BURGERT, P. H. (1962) Subcutaneous emphysema in cancer of the colon. *Archs Surg., Chicago, 85*, 344.

SHUCKSMITH, H. S. (1963) Subcutaneous abscess as the first evidence of carcinoma of the colon. *Br. J. Surg., 50*, 514.

SLANEY, G. (1971) Results of treatment of carcinoma of the colon and rectum. In *Modern Trends in Surgery, 3*, ed. W. T. Irvine. London: Butterworth.

THOMSON, D. M. P., KRUPEY, J., FREEDMAN, S. O. and GOLD, P. (1969) The radioimmunoassay of circulating carcinoembryonic antigen of the human digestive system. *Proc. natn. Acad. Sci. U.S.A., 64*, 161.

WIGH, R. and SWENSON, P. C. (1953) Photofluorography for the detection of unsuspected gastric neoplasms. *Am. J. Roentgen., 69*, 242.

17

Treatment of Carcinoma
of the Colon

THE EVOLUTION OF RADICAL
SURGICAL TREATMENT

Rankin (Rankin et al. 1932; Rankin 1945) has traced for us the early steps in the development of surgery for cancer of the colon. Though the first successful resection of a colonic growth was performed by Reybard of Lyons, in 1823, it was not till after the discovery of general anaesthesia and the introduction of antisepsis and asepsis that the operative treatment of cancer of the colon really began. The pioneers in abdominal surgery, such as Billroth, Czerny and von Mikulicz, naturally turned their attentions also to this part of the intestinal tract and, as familiarity with the technique of intestinal suture grew, an increasing number of colonic resections was attempted. By the close of the nineteenth century sufficient experience had accumulated to show that resection and anastomosis in the large gut, and especially in the left half of the colon, was much more hazardous than the same procedure elsewhere in the gastrointestinal tract, and carried a considerable risk of leakage and infection. The subsequent history of the surgery of carcinoma of the colon is mainly a record of the efforts that have been made to overcome these hazards as follows.

Extraperitoneal Resection (Bloch–
Mikulicz–Paul)

Bloch of Copenhagen reported in 1894 that he had resected a carcinoma of the sigmoid by an extraperitoneal technique. At the first stage he merely exteriorized the sigmoid loop containing the growth without removing any bowel, and inserted a tube to drain the proximal limb. A few days later, when the colon had become firmly fixed in the abdominal wall, the protruding loop was excised, and at a still later stage the resulting double-barrelled colostomy was closed by means of an enterotome. In another case he mobilized a carcinoma of a fixed part of the colon, and treated it in a similar manner. In neither of these cases did he attempt any extensive removal of the regional lymph-glands.

Paul of Liverpool (1895, 1912) and von Mikulicz of Breslau (1903) devised similar methods apparently quite independently

of Bloch or of one another. Von Mikulicz's technique was practically identical with that of Bloch, the carcinomatous segment, usually sigmoid, being exteriorized and intubated at the first stage and subsequently excised; whilst in the operation developed by Paul the exteriorized loop was excised at the time of the operation and specially large right-angled glass tubes were tied into each of the two limbs of bowel projecting at the wound. The final stage to close the double-barrelled colostomy was the same in the two operations, and consisted of destroying the spur formed by the contiguous walls of the two limbs of bowel, by means of an enterotome, after the method of Dupuytren. The remaining fistula sometimes closed spontaneously, but more often required a small plastic operation for its closure. Von Mikulicz was able to point to a reduction in his operative mortality from 42·9% for resection with primary anastomosis to 12·5% for the method of resection with exteriorization, and undoubtedly it was his advocacy that popularized this method on the Continent and in America; Paul's influence in this country was no less powerful.

As originally practised, the Mikulicz–Paul operation did not provide a wide removal of regional lymphatics, though, as lymphatic spread with carcinoma of the colon is often very localized, this restricted removal frequently gave adequate clearance and yielded good ultimate results. But with more extensive spread recurrence was liable to occur, and often took place in the wound, as emphasized by Rankin (1926) and Sistrunk (1928), due either to glandular metastases in the mesocolic edges stretching up to the abdominal wall or to implantation of cancer cells from the primary growth in the incision, when the original technique of Mikulicz was employed. But, as Rankin (1926), Devine (1931), Lahey (1932), Lloyd-Davies (1945) and many others showed, there was no reason why the scope of the operation should not be broadened to include practically as much tissue as would be excised in a resection with anastomosis. They also stressed that the method was often applicable, after suitable mobilization, to growths of the fixed parts of the bowel as well, such as the splenic flexure or descending colon. Devine (1931) and Lahey (1932) even employed extraperitoneal resection in the right colon, but they were almost alone in this respect, for most surgeons found that this technique applied here gave rise to troublesome digestion of the abdominal skin from the escaping ileal contents, and preferred a sutured anastomosis in the right colon, which appeared to be much safer than in the distal colon.

As regards the possible risk of implantation of malignant cells in the wound, it was obviously better to use Paul's technique with immediate excision of the growth, than that of Bloch and von Mikulicz with temporary retention of the growth in an exteriorized form; and Rankin (1926), who became one of the chief supporters of staged resection in America, introduced a modification of the former method, known as *obstructive resection*. In this version, instead of intubating the bowel at the conclusion of the operation, crushing clamps were left on the two limbs of colon for 48 hours or longer, the temporary obstruction being well tolerated as a rule in the left colon. The operative mortality in 387 colonic resections, mostly of staged type, recorded by Rankin from the Mayo Clinic was only 8%.

Intraperitoneal Resection with 'Aseptic' Anastomosis

Another development, designed to minimize the risks of infection after sutured anastomosis in the colon, was the introduction of various methods of 'aseptic' anastomosis, by which it was hoped to carry out the resection and suture in an entirely sterile manner without opening the bowel lumen till the union was completed. Much ingenuity was shown in devising these techniques, some of the better known methods being those of Halsted (1898), O'Hara (1900), Parker and Kerr (1908), Schoemaker (1921), Fraser and Dott (1924), Pringle (1924), Rankin (1928) and Wangensteen (1940). A good review of the subject is given by Monro (1950), from whom the illustrations in Fig. 308 depicting the technique of O'Hara (1900), which used to be popular, are taken.

It is manifestly impossible to make any method of anastomosis in the colon thoroughly aseptic (unless complete sterilization of the gut contents has been achieved in advance), for some of the burying Lembert sutures must inevitably penetrate more deeply than intended and enter the lumen of the bowel, so that faecal contamination is conveyed by them to the surface. But an 'aseptic' technique might well reduce the amount of soiling at the time of operation. However, the main argument against this method (Moynihan 1926) was that it was held to be founded on an erroneous conception of the factor chiefly responsible for postoperative sepsis in such cases, which is not contamination during the operation itself, but subsequent leakage (but see p. 437).

Intraperitoneal Resection in the Left Colon after Defunctioning by a Preliminary Transverse Colostomy (Devine)

It was common practice with surgeons, such as Cheever (1931), Whipple (1931), Wilkie (1934) and Rowlands and Turner (1937), who still favoured intraperitoneal resection, to establish a temporary caecostomy (or alternatively to pass a stout rectal catheter upwards per anum through the anastomosis at the time of operation and retain it for four or five days), in order to relieve tension in the colon and reduce the strain on the suture line. Such an opening usually closed spontaneously on withdrawal of the caecostomy tube after 14 days or so. But, dissatisfied with the accomplishment of caecostomy employed in this way, Devine in 1931 went a step farther and suggested that intraperitoneal resection for growths in the left colon should always be preceded by a preliminary transverse colostomy, done two or three weeks before the main operation. This opening, unlike a caecostomy, provided a complete diversion of faeces to

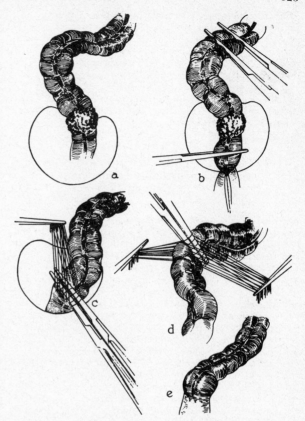

Fig. 308. O'Hara's method of 'aseptic' intestinal anastomosis. (*From Monro 1950*)

the surface, and also allowed irrigation to be carried out from the colostomy to the anus and *vice versa* to empty the left colon completely. In this way it was possible for the surgeon to perform his resection on a collapsed, 'defunctioned and debacterialized' distal colon, so that, even if partial dehiscence of the suture line should occur, the consequences would probably not be serious. Devine (1931, 1935, 1938) stressed particularly the advantage of a defunctioning colostomy before resection with a sutured anastomosis for lesions of the distal sigmoid, which in any case were too low for extraperitoneal resection, and its great value also as a preparation for conservative resection of carcinomas of the upper rectum. He recommended that the colostomy should be sited as far as possible to the right in the transverse colon, close to the hepatic flexure, so that it was out of the way of the incision that would be required in the left abdomen for the subsequent resection, and did not impede the mobilization of the greater part of the transverse colon, if this should be found necessary as part of that operation. Devine also emphasized that the loop of bowel used for the colostomy should be completely divided at its summit so as to give two separate openings, which could be implanted independently into the abdominal wall with a skin bridge intervening between them, to ensure that no faeces could pass over the colostomy spur into the distal colon. Actually, though Devine's teachings were widely accepted in the 1930s and early 1940s, most surgeons who adopted his methods found a simple loop transverse colostomy perfectly adequate to secure defunctioning of the left colon, without having to resort to Devine's rather complicated colostomy technique (an impression that has been completely confirmed by a recent radiological study by Rombeau et al. (1978)). It was the feeling at the time that the surgery of the distal colon was greatly facilitated and made much safer by the application of the principle of 'defunctioning', but it is not easy to produce statistical evidence on this point. In none of his writings, not even in his book on *Surgery of the Colon and Rectum* (Devine and Devine 1948), did Devine publish any comprehensive statement of his results.

Intraperitoneal Resection after Intestinal Antisepsis with Sulphonamides and Antibiotics

Nowhere in surgery did the introduction of sulphonamide drugs and antibiotics exert a greater influence than in the colon and rectum, because of the prospects which these antibacterial substances seemed to offer, not only for systemic therapy but also for sterilizing the gut. By means of them the surgeon appeared to have within his reach the possibility of intestinal antisepsis as a prelude to operations on the large bowel, and this profoundly affected surgical practice in the treatment of carcinoma of the colon. At first, whilst their efficacy as intestinal antiseptics was on trial, non-absorbable sulphonamides, such as sulphaguanidine, succinylsulphathiazole and phthalylsulphathiazole, were often used as a supplement to a defunctioning transverse colostomy, for instillation as an emulsion or suppository into the distal colon to complete its sterilization. Later, as confidence was gained in them, and as antibiotics such as streptomycin, the tetracyclines and neomycin became available for intestinal use, reliance was placed on them entirely and a preliminary colostomy was eventually omitted.

During the decade following World War II therefore a complete change of surgical fashion took place in the operative treatment of carcinoma of the colon in favour of simple straightforward resection with immediate intraperitoneal anastomosis. Though the intestinal and systemic use of sulphonamides and antibiotics undoubtedly played a major part in securing this state of affairs, other factors probably contributed—namely the improvement in transfusion methods, the greater understanding of the problems of fluid and electrolyte balance, and the considerable advances in general anaesthesia which gave the surgeon well-nigh ideal operating conditions, allowing a much more careful and meticulous operative technique.

As a result of all these factors, resections with immediate anastomosis became remarkably safe. Thus, Lloyd-Davies et al. (1953) reported that resection with immediate anastomosis and without any form of proximal decompression had been performed in 109 cases of carcinoma of the distal colon during the preceding five years at St Mark's Hospital, London, with only three postoperative deaths, none of which was due to sepsis. It may be added that the resectability rate during this period at St Mark's Hospital was between 90 and 95%.

It was clear from such reports and many unpublished experiences that staged resections of the Paul–Mikulicz type or the Devine procedure could no longer claim the merit of greater safety. They were certainly much more tedious and uncomfortable for the patient than a straightforward intraperitoneal resection. In addition, if the Paul type of operation was to be thoroughly radical, it required a more extensive mobilization of the colon than a resection with direct anastomosis, since the ends of bowel had to be exteriorized without tension. This extra mobilization might sometimes be difficult to obtain—as in obese

subjects with a short fat-laden mesentery, or when the growth lay in the lower sigmoid and there was insufficient bowel on the distal side. Under these circumstances, if the surgeon persisted in his plan to perform an extraperitoneal resection, he might compromise his chances of eradicating the disease. Altogether, then, every argument seemed to favour resection with immediate intraperitoneal anastomosis as the procedure of election for all non-obstructed carcinomas of the colon, wherever situated, and this has been my almost invariable practice for the past 25 years.

Ironically enough, once resection with immediate anastomosis had been firmly established—largely with the aid of non-absorbable sulphonamides and oral antibiotics—as the operation of choice for cancer of the colon, many surgeons began to have second thoughts about the value of intestinal antiseptics, particularly the more potent antibiotics. The trouble with them lay in the apparent tendency for their use to be followed postoperatively by the development of severe enterocolitis due to the emergence in the intestinal flora of dominant strains of antibiotic-resistant staphylococci. Specially incriminated in this respect have been the tetracyclines and neomycin, but other antibiotics commonly used for this purpose shared in the obloquy. As a consequence there was in many centres a trend away from antibiotics towards preparation with non-absorbable sulphonamides alone, combined with particular attention to cleansing of the colon with aperients and irrigations (Gabriel 1963; Hummel et al. 1964; McKittrick 1965; Morgan 1967). Some surgeons, indeed, have relied entirely on mechanical preparation (Tyson and Spaulding 1959; Wangensteen and Gilbertsen 1963; Grant and Barbara 1964; Black 1968) and it did not seem that the safety of their suture lines suffered as a result; but it is very difficult to secure reliable comparative data on this point. However, recently there has been a swing of the pendulum back towards the use of oral antibiotics, including those active against anaerobes (see p. 449).

SCOPE OF EXCISION REQUIRED FOR RADICAL REMOVAL OF CARCINOMAS IN VARIOUS SEGMENTS OF THE COLON

The extent of resection required for growths in different situations in the colon is determined, as explained on p. 389 by the necessity for wide removal of the extramural lymphatics which accompany the main colic vessels supplying the segment concerned. With regard to *growths of the right colon*—that is the caecum, ascending colon, hepatic flexure and right half of the transverse colon, all supplied by the superior mesenteric artery—resection involves ligation of the appropriate colic branches as close as possible to their origin from this parent vessel. Conventional resection along these lines is illustrated in Fig. 309B, C. However, the ileocolic, right colic and middle colic arteries all arise very close together so that there is at least a theoretical risk that glands related to the stems of all three vessels may be implicated by a carcinoma anywhere in the right colon. For that reason I prefer to practise the more extensive right hemicolectomy portrayed in Fig. 309D for all operable growths of the right colon, except when the patient's general condition is such as to compel restriction of the resection to the minimum that offers a reasonable chance of cure.

With growths of the left colon—that is, the left end of the transverse colon, the splenic flexure, and the descending and sigmoid colon, all deriving their blood supply from the inferior mesenteric artery— resection may follow the general plan used for right colon growths, with ligation of the colic vessels feeding the site of the lesion as close as possible to their origin from the mesenteric stem. Resections of this kind are shown in Fig. 309E, F. However, in dealing with growths of the left half of the colon it is possible to be even more radical and to sacrifice the main inferior mesenteric vessels as well, up to the point where the artery springs from the point of the abdominal aorta under cover of the third part of the duodenum. This step obviously improves the lymphatic clearance and seems a reasonable extension of the operation. It means, however, cutting off the main blood supply to the rectum through the superior haemorrhoidal artery, so that it and any part of the distal colon retained *below* the growth have to be nourished entirely by the middle (and inferior) haemorrhoidal vessels. As mentioned on p. 24 my experience shows that this latter supply is certainly sufficient to maintain in a viable condition the upper rectum and rectosigmoid for a distance of about 10–12 cm above the peritoneal reflection off the front of the rectum after inferior mesenteric ligation, but it would probably be unwise to rely on it to supply any greater extent of bowel. Clearly, therefore, when the more radical step of removing the inferior mesenteric artery is taken, the resection must be prolonged distally to ensure that the distal stump of bowel is not too long to have an adequate blood supply, and usually takes the form shown in Fig. 309G. This means that the final anastomosis has to be conducted in the pelvis, so that the dissection involved extends from the extreme upper abdomen to the pelvic cavity. In other words, this more radical form of left hemicolectomy imposes a greater strain on the patient than does the older style of limited resection with preservation of the inferior mesenteric vessels. In certain unfit cases this immediate disadvantage may more than outweigh any possible later gains from the wide scope of the excision. For that reason, though, my preference for all carcinomas of the left colon, wherever situated, is for this extended type of left hemicolectomy, I still employ more limited resections on poor-risk patients, particularly if they suffer from obesity.

Removal of Adherent Related Viscera and Abdominal Parietes

It will be appreciated that, in addition to the formal resection of bowel, mesocolon and lymphatic tissues already indicated, it will sometimes be necessary, in dealing radically with carcinomas of the colon, to excise part or all of a related viscus, such as the stomach, a loop of small gut, the uterus or appendages, or a portion of the abdominal parietes to which the growth has become adherent. As pointed out by Cooke (1956), Jensen et al. (1970a) and Ellis (1971), not infrequently the adhesions are inflammatory and not due to malignant infiltration, so that the prognosis is often much better than might have been imagined at the time of operation. In fact many cases are now on record in which lasting cure has been afforded by such multivisceral resections (Gilchrist and David 1947; van Prohaska et al. 1953; Brunschwig 1961; El-Domeiri and Whiteley 1970). The surgeon should, therefore, not readily allow himself to be deterred from carrying out a resection for carcinoma of the colon by finding that the growth is fixed to surrounding structures. By bold surgery it is usually possible to effect an excision with or without partial removal of adjoining tissues, often with reasonable prospects of cure.

The Problem of Distant Metastases

HEPATIC METASTASES

The presence of deposits in the liver affects the prospects of ultimate cure, but is not normally a contraindication to excision of the primary growth. In most cases with hepatic metastases it is still advisable to remove the primary lesion for palliative purposes, and many such patients have lived in comfort and reasonably good health for as long as 18 months or two years after palliative excision, and an occasional patient may even survive for three or four years or longer (Cady et al. 1970; Ellis 1971). In my opinion excision of the primary lesion would only be *in*advisable if it appears that the liver has been two-thirds or more replaced by growth, so that but a few weeks of life remain to the patient.

If hepatic metastases are very small it is sometimes difficult to decide on palpation alone whether one is dealing with deposits of growth or tiny cysts. The exact diagnosis of these nodules may not be of great practical significance, if one accepts the policy of almost invariable palliative excision of the primary in the presence of hepatic metastases, but it is usually desirable to know their nature for certain in order to keep clinical records accurate and to allow more precise prognosis. It is a considerable help in making a decision if a view can be obtained of the metastases, should they be situated on the anterior surface of the liver, by elevating the upper edge of the wound with a long pelvic retractor (see Fig. 383). A secondary deposit generally has a characteristic pearly white appearance, whilst a cyst is bluish in colour. If, after the nodule has been brought into view, doubt

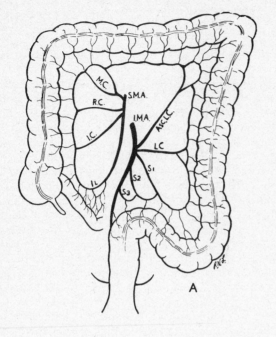

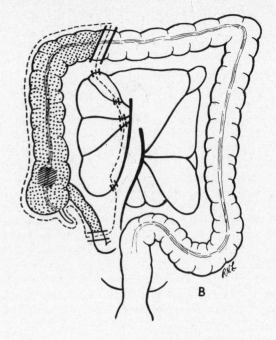

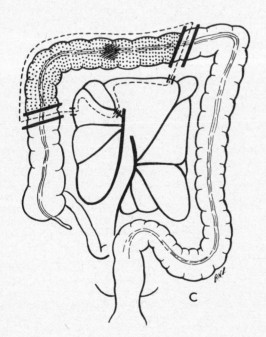

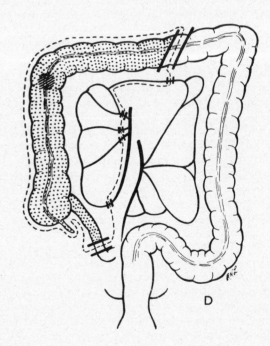

persists as to its exact nature, a biopsy specimen may be obtained by long sigmoidoscopic biopsy forceps passed up through the abdomen, or by means of a needle inserted through the abdominal wall overlying the debatable lesion, whilst the left hand simultaneously feels the nodule and guides the needle to it.

In certain cases with a solitary palpable hepatic metastasis (or close cluster of metastases) the possibility should be borne in mind of its removal, either by a wedge excision if it is situated near the free edge of the liver, or by a formal left or right hepatic lobectomy if less advantageously sited. Needless to say, local

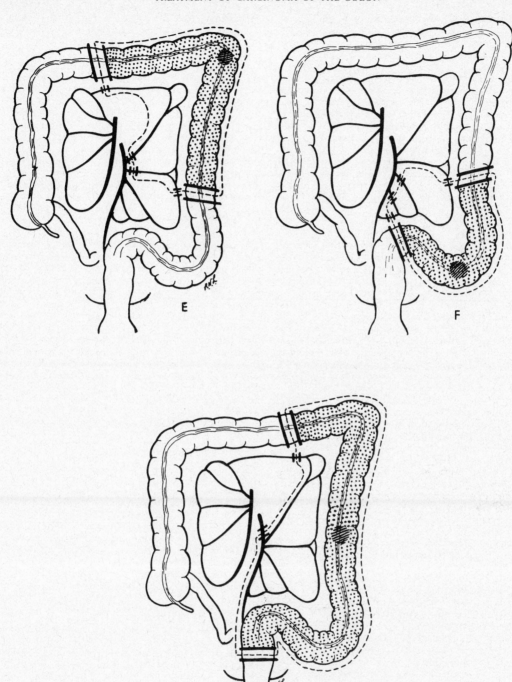

Fig. 309. The extent of resection of bowel and related vessels considered necessary in the radical removal of carcinomas in various sites in the colon.

excision or partial hepatectomy are speculative undertakings, in that it is impossible to exclude the presence of other impalpable metastases in the rest of the liver; however, if any surgical attack on the liver is postponed till a second intervention, a radioactive liver scan (Davies et al. 1974) in the interval between the two operations, possibly supplemented by hepatic arteriography or computerized axial tomography, may reveal other secondary deposits. Positive findings by these two investigations are valuable, but negative ones are not significant, for very small metastases would almost certainly be missed by scanning or arteriography. Lortat-Jacob and Robert (1952), Pack and Baker (1953), Raven (1957), Lloyd-Davies and Angell (1957), Quattlebaum (1962) and Wilson and Wolf (1966) have shown that *excision of the right lobe* of the liver is an eminently praticable surgical procedure, compatible with excellent health afterwards, but the fact remains that it can never be devoid of considerable immediate risks. *Removal of the left lobe* of the liver is even more of a gamble as regards the risk of other undetected metastases being present in the remaining very much larger right lobe, but technically it is a much simpler procedure. Raven (1957) and Wilson and Wolf (1966) give useful accounts of the technique. Both Lloyd-Davies (1947) and Morgan (1957a) record cases in which a supplementary left hepatectomy seems to have been entirely successful. I myself have performed only three right hepatectomies for metastatic cancer, but have removed the left lobe of the liver in connection with large bowel cancer on five occasions; the longest period of survival was 4½ years. Brunschwig (1961) reports seven left and seven right hepatic lobectomies for liver deposits in association with carcinomas of the rectum or colon, with three operative deaths, the longest period of survival being 27 months. Peden and Blalock (1963) recorded a five-year survival following right hepatectomy for a metastasis from bowel cancer. However, as Gaston (1966), Bengmark (1968) and Wilson and Adson (1976) point out, limited wedge excisions or segmental resections for metastases have more often been successful than has formal right or left hepatic lobectomy.

Actually a very interesting and encouraging report is provided by Wilson and Adson (1976) of the Mayo Clinic on 60 patients with colorectal cancer and associated hepatic metastases, who, during the years 1949–72 inclusive, underwent excision of the metastases in addition to removal of the bowel lesion itself. In 40 of the cases the liver deposits were solitary, in 20 multiple. They varied in size from 1 to 15 cm in diameter, but in three-quarters were 5 cm or less. In 39 patients the metastases were amenable to removal by wedge excision, in 10 cases segmental resection was necessary, and in 11 the lesions were so large as to require standard hepatic lobectomy. Approximately 80% of the causal colorectal cancers were well differentiated, and just over 50% had associated lymph node metastases.

Only one patient died in the immediate postoperative period, the cause of death being gastric stress ulceration. Follow-up data are available on all the survivors for periods of 2 to 23 years. No patients who had multiple hepatic metastases survived for five years, but 15 of the 36 with a single metastasis and eligible for five-year follow-up lived for five years or more, and eight patients were alive without evidence of recurrence 10 or more years after operation.

For comparison the authors have put together retrospectively a 'control' group of patients with colorectal cancer and associated metastases, who, during the same period, due to differences in the attitude of the various members of the surgical staff to the management of metastases, merely had colorectal resection without excision of the hepatic lesions. In making up this so-called control series, cases with very gross, obviously quite irremovable liver metastases were excluded, and only those with metastases roughly comparable to those in the operated series were chosen. Obviously such a concocted group is open to criticism as a control series, but, for what it is worth, it is to be noted that none of the 'control' cases survived five years.

A similarly encouraging report comes from the Memorial Hospital, New York (Wanebo et al. 1978) describing a 28% five-year survival rate in 27 patients with colorectal cancer and solitary hepatic metastases, treated by resection of bowel and removal of the liver secondary by local excision (13), wedge resection (10) or hepatic lobectomy (four, one right, three left).

My present feeling regarding the possible removal of apparently isolated small hepatic metastases would be to attempt this manoeuvre by a very limited wedge resection at the time of the colon resection, if the deposit is at or near the liver edge, if the findings at laparotomy suggest that the growth is otherwise a favourable one, if the patient's general condition is good, and if the exposure at laparotomy gives good access to the liver or can easily be made to do so. If, on the other hand, the metastasis is less conveniently placed on the liver or in relation to the abdominal incision (as when the primary bowel lesion is in the lower sigmoid or rectum), no attempt should be made to deal with it at the initial operation. Instead, following recovery from the colonic resection, further information should be sought by liver scanning and hepatic arteriography. Attention should also be given to the histological grading and extent of spread of the carcinoma, as revealed by dissection of the operative specimen. Unless the growth is a well differentiated one, which is no further advanced than Dukes' category B, or possibly early C, any form of hepatectomy is unlikely to be rewarding. Finally, it is important to take into account the patient's psyche and his probable reaction to the information that he has growth in the liver and requires a further major operation to attempt to deal with it. The proportion of cases in which it will be deemed advisable to proceed to a further operation to deal with the metastatic condition of the liver will probably be small, but perhaps not as small as previously imagined.

PERITONEAL INVOLVEMENT

Though obviously it affects the prognosis adversely, the invasion of the peritoneum overlying the growth, if unassociated with more widespread peritoneal involvement, is compatible with excision with some prospect of cure. A few discrete plaques in the parietal peritoneum adjacent to the growth, though probably placing the condition beyond the hope of lasting cure, can often be included within the scope of an excision, and such a removal should usually be undertaken as a palliative measure. But the presence of widespread peritoneal deposits invariably means that the period of survival will be short, and it, therefore, contra-indicates any attempt at palliative excision.

EXTENSIVE LYMPH NODE METASTASES

It is often extremely difficult for the surgeon at laparotomy to be confident whether the related lymph nodes contain metastases or not, for nodes may be quite enlarged from an inflammatory reaction without necessarily containing any growth. But on other occasions, when the nodes are not only enlarged but stony hard in consistency, it is possible to be quite sure that they are the seat of carcinomatous deposits. Even when the nodal involvement obviously extends well beyond the reach of a potentially curative resection for the growth, this should not as a rule preclude the performance of a palliative excision of the bowel lesion, leaving many of the implicated nodes behind.

PULMONARY METASTASES

As pointed out on p. 396, deposits in the lungs are relatively rare in connection with carcinoma of the large bowel. Obviously they place the case beyond hope of cure, but depending on circumstances they may be compatible with a palliative removal of the primary colonic condition. For example, if the bowel symptoms are very troublesome and the pulmonary involvement is apparently restricted to a single nodule in one lung, the patient might live for 9 or 12 months before the intrathoracic lesion proved fatal. There are cases on record where a pulmonary lobectomy has been performed as an additional palliative step in such circumstances (Clagett et al. 1964).

Treatment of Synchronous Adenomatous Polyps and Carcinomas and Prevention of Development of Metachronous Tumours

As explained on p. 331, there is strong evidence for the belief that in patients with carcinoma of the colon and rectum the mucosa of the large bowel is in a diffusely abnormal state predisposing it to epithelial hyperplasia, as shown by the occurrence of satellite adenomatous polyps in some 30% of cases, and of one or more synchronous frank carcinomas in another 3%. A second primary carcinoma should be readily detected if a systematic careful palpation of the entire large intestine is carried out as part of the initial abdominal exploration in all such patients, as it ought to be. The coexistence of adenomatous polyps, however, is less easily established, for on palpation of the colon at laparotomy such polyps, being soft, are easily confused with particles of faeces. As Deddish and Hertz (1955) have emphasized, these lesions have often been missed also in the preoperative barium enema examination. Consequently they and Bacon and Peale (1956) have strongly advocated that *peroperative colonoscopy* should be performed as a routine at operation on cases of carcinoma of the colon, a sterile sigmoidoscope being passed into either open end of bowel after resection of the obvious carcinoma and before completing the anastomosis (p. 348). They have found this an easy manoeuvre, which has often been rewarded by the discovery of impalpable radiologically-undetected polyps, which can then be removed by snaring or through a separate colotomy over the polyp. I must record that in my experience peroperative colonoscopy has proved a difficult and unreliable method owing to faeces obscuring the view, particularly in patients whose colon has not been entirely empty because of the impediment imposed by the carcinoma. It seems clear also, from the report of Kleinfeld and Gump (1960), that it can add considerably to the morbidity of a colon resection. My own practice, therefore, in searching for polyps is to rely essentially on the preoperative radiological examination—which with modern double-contrast technique has in my experience been much more dependable than formerly—supplemented by *preoperative fibreoptic colonoscopy* and by palpation of the colon at operation.

It can be argued that the polyp population of the colon is not static, so that, even if one succeeds in removing all polyps present at the time of operation, others may develop later and may be transformed into malignant growths, or a carcinoma may arise *de novo* in any part of the large bowel mucosa in such cases without having to pass through the intermediate stage of polyp formation. This reasoning induced Lillehei and Wangensteen (1955), Teicher and Abrahams (1956) and Rosenthal and Baronofsky (1960) to advocate routine *subtotal colectomy and ileorectal anastomosis* in the treatment of colonic carcinoma, leaving only a short segment of large bowel readily accessible to periodic sigmoidoscopic review. They have claimed that the prophylactic value of the procedure in avoiding further colonic carcinomas at a later date more than compensates for the slightly increased severity and risks of this operation, compared with a conventional resection. This raises the question of the magnitude of the risk of metachronous carcinomas arising subsequently in patients after conventional resections for large bowel carcinoma. Bussey et al. (1967) have provided a very clear answer in their report on the follow-up of 3381 patients who survived conventional resections for carcinomas of the colon and rectum at St Mark's Hospital, London, between 1928 and 1957. They found that the overall incidence of metachronous carcinomas was 1·5% approximately. In those patients who had been followed for at least 20 years since operation the incidence rose to some 3%, and in those who had been followed for this length of time and had had associated adenomatous polyps in their original operative specimen it reached the level of 5%. But the majority of patients having a colon resection for carcinoma are already advanced in age so that they are liable to succumb from intercurrent conditions within 10 years of their operation. According to Bussey et al. (1967) the incidence of metachronous carcinomas arising in that period was only 0·7%. It has to be remembered, moreover, that the incidence of metachronous growths is not the same as the mortality from them, for most of these second carcinomas will presumably be submitted to excision with at least an even chance of cure. Altogether, then, the findings of Bussey et al. (1967) would certainly not justify wholesale subtotal colectomy in the management of carcinoma of the large intestine, but they do stress the need to keep these patients under supervision and possibly to arrange for occasional air-contrast barium enema studies or colonoscopy.

My own practice in the treatment of carcinoma of the large bowel is to use conventional patterns of resection in virtually all cases and to reserve subtotal colectomy for exceptional circumstances, for example when there are two or more carcinomas in widely separated parts of the colon and rectum, or when there are associated polyps not merely in the immediate vicinity of the carcinoma but some distance away, particularly in another segment of the intestine. Possibly, it should also be considered in young patients with a strong family history of large bowel cancer, and it may occasionally be the most satisfactory way of managing cases of colonic cancer complicated by acute obstruction (see p. 478).

GENERAL TECHNIQUE OF COLONIC RESECTION WITH ANASTOMOSIS

Mobilization and Division of Colon and Colic Vessels

An essential preliminary to the wide resections of colon and potentially invaded lymphatic tissue that have been recommended is thorough mobilization of the bowel. This is readily accomplished as a rule because, apart from pathological adhesions due to the growth, both the ascending and descending colon are but loosely attached to the posterior abdominal wall by the process designated by Toldt as 'physiological fusion'. Once the peritoneum on

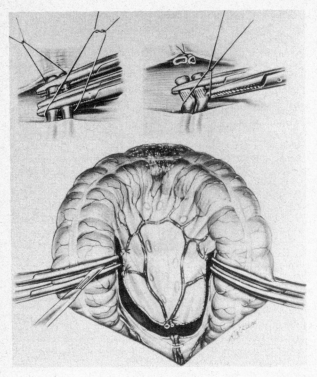

Fig. 310. Standard resection with anastomosis for carcinoma of the colon: the loop has been mobilized, the main colic vessels supplying it divided and the bowel above and below doubly clamped and about to be divided. *Inset:* The three-clamp method of dividing the vessels.

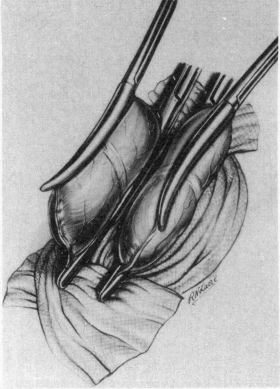

Fig. 311. After removal of the carcinomatous segment the two colon stumps, each controlled by a terminal crushing clamp and a spring clamp, are brought together in preparation for anastomosis.

their outer sides has been divided they may be stripped up almost to the midline of the abdomen, reproducing the fetal condition; they then remain attached only by the medial leaf of peritoneum which carries the vessels supplying the bowel. After being freely lifted up in this manner it is an easy matter (assisted by transillumination if necessary because of obesity) to see and secure these vessels, or, after a little additional dissection in the case of the left colon, to define and tie the main inferior mesenteric stem itself. The leaf of 'mesentery' may now be completely severed from the posterior parietal peritoneum right up to the colon at the proximal and distal side selected for its division. The bowel is then divided between two crushing clamps at either extremity of the portion to be resected, and the cancerous segment with its related lymphatics is entirely freed, leaving the two cut ends of remaining bowel each controlled by a clamp (Figs 310, 311).

The Anastomosis

GENERAL CONSIDERATIONS

PRINCIPLES OF INTESTINAL SUTURE

The traditional teaching in regard to intestinal suturing, dating from the pioneer work of Travers (1812), Lembert (1826), and Dieffenbach (1826; see Leonardo 1943), was that serosal apposition was essential for secure union and that mucosal eversion at the suture line was very liable to result in leakage. Usually this objective was achieved by two layers of suture. The first was an *inner through-and-through stitch*, usually of continuous catgut or polyglycolic acid or interrupted silk, to secure rough apposition of the cut edges of the bowel and good haemostasis. The second was an *outer seromuscular or Lembert stitch*, often interrupted and of non-absorbable material such as silk, to produce inversion and bring the peritoneal coats together (Fig. 317A). Halsted (1887) stressed that the stitch should penetrate deeply enough to secure a good bite of the submucosa, which is the toughest layer of the intestinal wall. Admittedly Halsted (1887) counselled against too much inversion, as did Gambee (1951), who sought to avoid it

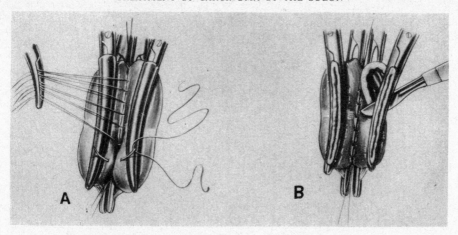

Fig. 312. (A) Insertion of posterior row of Lembert sutures of interrupted fine serum-proof silk. (B) Excising controlling crushing clamp together with the fringe of crushed bowel wall.

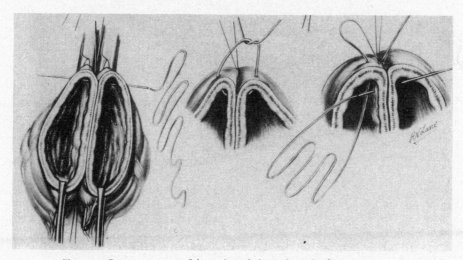

Fig. 313. Commencement of through-and-through stitch of continuous catgut.

largely or entirely by employing a special type of single-layer suture designed to secure accurate end-to-end apposition of the cut edges of bowel (Fig. 317B, C). But both these authors accepted the need to prevent pouting of the mucosa to the exterior through the suture line.

It came as something of a shock, therefore, to learn from experimental work by Getzen et al. (1966) that inversion, so far from being an advantage in an anastomosis, apparently resulted in a weaker union than did an everting technique. In an extensive series of anastomoses in the small and large intestines of dogs, they found that a technique of suture consisting of a single row of interrupted silk stitches, so introduced as deliberately to produce eversion at the site of anastomosis (Fig. 317D), was superior on several scores to the conventional two-layer inverting technique (Fig. 317A). It was easier and quicker to perform, it maintained a wide lumen at the site of suture, it was followed by more secure healing as determined by histological

examination and by studies of tensile strength at various stages after operation, and the resulting mortality was certainly no higher than with the inverting technique.

This work by Getzen et al. (1966) excited a flurry of activity in other surgical laboratories designed to test their surprising claims (Ravitch 1966; Healey et al. 1967; Hamilton 1967; Loeb 1967; Ravitch et al. 1967a, b; Buyers and Meier 1968). The majority of these further experimental studies up to early 1968 seemed to support the conclusions of Getzen et al. (1966), so that in March of that year we instituted a controlled clinical trial of everting versus inverting suture in large bowel surgery (Goligher et al. 1970). This trial had to be terminated prematurely 17 months later because by then there had emerged a significant difference in the results of the two methods, unfavourable to the everting technique. A higher proportion of patients had developed wound infection or peritonitis after it, and faecal fistulation was much more frequent. These experiences left us in

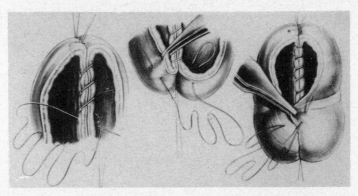

Fig. 314. Further steps in the insertion of the through-and-through suture. Note that the stitch returns along the anterior wall as a Connell stitch.

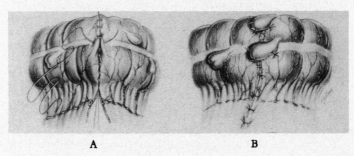

A   B

Fig. 315. (A) Insertion of anterior row of Lembert sutures of silk. (B) Suture of appendices epiploicae over the anastomosis for additional security.

no doubt that an everting technique of suture of the large intestine was too unreliable and dangerous to be recommended in clinical practice. Whilst this clinical study was in progress, incidentally, several other experimental studies were reported (Canalis and Ravitch 1968; Mellish et al. 1968; Singleton et al. 1968; Hargreaves and Keddie 1968; Gill et al. 1969; McAdam et al. 1969; Orr 1969; Rusca et al. 1969; Trueblood et al. 1969), most of which came out strongly in support of the conventional inverting technique and against the everting method.

The principle of avoiding mucosal eversion seems thus to have been firmly re-established, but whether it is necessary to use the conventional two-layer inverting technique of suture is more debatable. It could be argued that a single layer of interrupted sutures, say, of Gambee type (Fig. 317B, C) producing end-on apposition of the cut edges of bowel (with at most minimal inversion but avoiding protrusion of the mucosa) might be as safe or safer, in so far as it might interfere less with the blood supply to the ends of the bowel, a particularly important consideration in colon surgery. However, in some controlled experimental studies in dogs and rabbits respectively McAdam et al. (1970) and Irvin and Edwards (1973) were unable to demonstrate any significant difference in the incidence of anastomotic dehiscence depending on whether a single layer or a two-layer inverting technique of suture was used for colonic resections. Gambee et al. (1966) reported a 10-year experience with single layer silk inverting suture technique in 163 cases of colonic resection (36 right hemicolectomies, 31 transverse colectomies and 96 left hemicolectomies or sigmoidectomies). They had five fatal and six non-fatal anastomotic leaks, a total incidence of suture line dehiscence of 6–7%. As there were no cases of low anterior resec-

tion in their series, I think it could reasonably be suggested that these results are probably not much different from those obtained by most surgeons using a conventional technique of suture. Fortunately more precise information is now available from a controlled clinical trial in my Department (Irvin et al. 1973a) of a one-layer inverting technique of suture with silk contrasted with a conventional two-layer suture technique for intraperitoneal colonic anastomoses. No significant difference was shown in the incidence of anastomotic dehiscence as between these two techniques.

For completeness, it should be mentioned that a recent controlled trial by Everett (1975) of one-layer inverting suture (of interrupted 4/o Supramid with the knots on the mucosa) against two-layer inverting suture (inner continuous fine catgut, outer in interrupted 4/o Supramid) for anterior rectal resection showed an interesting difference depending on whether the resection was high or low (see p. 514 for definition). With high anterior resection with a rectal stump with a peritoneal coat there was no significant difference in the incidence of anastomotic dehiscence as between one- and two-layer techniques of suture, postoperative small opaque enema studies (see p. 604) being used to determine the integrity of the suture lines. But with low anterior resection, using the same criteria, there was a significantly lower incidence of anastomotic dehiscence after the one-layer technique. Matheson and Irvine (1975) also had a remarkably low incidence of dehiscence with a one-layer technique with interrupted sutures of braided nylon inserted from outside the bowel, not including the mucosa, and with the knots tied on the serosal surface, but not in a controlled trial. In sharp contrast are the findings of our recently completed controlled trial (Goligher et al.

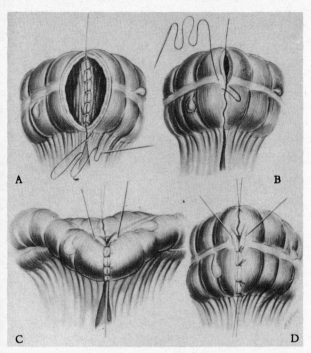

A   B

C   D

Fig. 316. Alternative *preferred* technique of suture, suitable when the colon stumps can be freely rotated, as is usually possible. The through-and-through suture is inserted first (A and B); this suture line is then buried by Lembert stitches, first posteriorly (C) and then anteriorly (D), and these sutures are inserted very deeply, usually through all coats and often embracing the catgut suture.

1977) of one- versus two-layer inverting technique for high and low anterior resection (by the methods shown on pp. 566–7, 568–70). We had a slightly greater incidence of dehiscence with the one layer technique for both high and low resections, the difference in high resections just being significant, that in low resections not being so, mainly because of the smaller number of cases.

CHOICE OF SUTURE MATERIALS

As regards the influence of different suture materials on the incidence of anastomotic dehiscence, there is remarkably little controlled clinical information on this question, though there have been variations in the suture material used in controlled trials in which other factors, such as the number of layers of suture, are being assessed. But Clark et al. (1978) have shown in a controlled clinical comparison that polyglycolic acid is superior to catgut for the inner layer of a conventional two-layer colonic or colorectal anastomosis, a conclusion that is supported by Deveney and Way's (1976) recent animal study. There have been strong claims by Kratzer and Onsanit (1974) and Trimpi et al. (1976) for the superiority of a single layer of interrupted 5/0 stainless steel wire for colonic or colorectal anastomoses, and Trimpi et al. (1976) have adduced evidence to support this belief from animal experimental work, but their clinical use of wire has not been within the framework of a controlled trial. This material is also favoured by some leading thoracic surgeons for oesophageal suture, which presents problems similar to those of rectal suture (Belsey 1971; Collis 1971; Goligher 1976). But many surgeons are daunted by the technical difficulties of using wire for anastomoses; these are somewhat lessened by choosing braided (Trimpi et al. 1976) rather than monofilament wire (Kratzer and Osanit 1974) for the purpose.

STAPLING DEVICES

Consideration of wire sutures leads naturally to an examination of automatic stapling devices for the construction of anastomoses. The instruments available in America and western Europe have been mostly those produced by the United States Surgical Corporation of New York and they in turn are based essentially on the brood of stapling machines elaborated in Russia during the 1950s (Ravitch 1974; Ravitch and Steichen 1972; Ravitch and Rivarola 1966; Ravitch et al. 1974; Steichen 1968, 1971). There are two main patterns of USSC instruments—the TA or monkey-wrench type of clamp, which is intended primarily for closure of duodenal, gastric or intestinal stumps, and the GIA type, which is designed to produce a side-to-side anastomosis. There are two phases in the operation of either pattern of device. The first is the closing of the jaws of the clamp sufficiently to secure the close apposition—but without crushing—of the walls of the viscus or viscera to be joined. The second phase is the driving through the tissues held in the clamp of the fine stainless steel staples. The latter initially have a ⊔

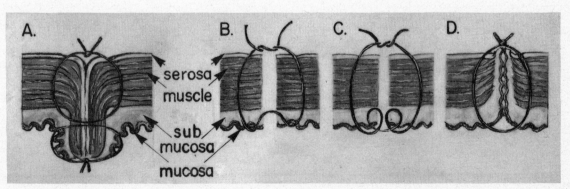

A.   serosa   muscle   B.   C.   D.

sub
mucosa

mucosa

Fig. 317. Some methods of intestinal suture. (A) Conventional two-layer inverting. (B) Gambee (1951) single layer designed to produce end-on apposition of the cut edges of bowel without mucosa pouting. (C) Modification of Gambee stitch, devised by De Almelda (1971), which is technically easier to insert. (D) Single layer everting suture.

shape; when they are inserted they are automatically closed into the shape of a capital B lying on its side—so ◯. The tissues held by the closed staples are not intended to be grasped so tightly as to occlude the small vessels in their substance passing through the openings in the B. The TA stapler inserts a double row of staples in the terminal fringe of bowel which it is closing, and the GIA instrument places a double row on either side of the lateral anastomosis which it creates.

It will be obvious that the TA stapler produces a mucosa-to-mucosa apposition of bowel walls. It has been claimed by Getzen et al. (1966) and by Ravitch et al. (1967a, b) that healing with an everting apposition of the intestinal edges is just as secure as that with the classical inversion and serosal apposition produced by Lembert sutures. However, many surgeons would doubt the validity of this claim, and certainly in our controlled clinical trial (Goligher et al. 1970) an everting technique of suture for colonic anastomosis gave a significantly higher incidence of leakage than did a conventional inverting technique, and a review of the published experimental work on the subject indicated that the weight of evidence was against the everting technique. As for the GIA stapler, admittedly it gives a serosa-to-serosa apposition of the viscera being laterally anastomosed, but the two holes through which the jaws of the device are introduced into the lumina have to be closed, and, if this is done by stapling, it involves using the TA stapler with resulting mucosal apposition.

End-to-end anastomosis of the intestine, and in particular of the colon, can be achieved by a combination of these two instruments, using one of several techniques worked out by Steichen (1968) and Ravitch et al. (1974). The effect of these methods is to convert what is essentially a side-to-side anastomosis into a functional end-to-end anastomosis. Alternatively an end-to-end anastomosis may be accomplished by the TA stapler alone if the lumen at the site of junction of the two intestinal stumps is triangulated by three stay sutures. The contiguous cut edges of the bowel stumps corresponding to one side of the triangle are clamped and stapled *from within* the lumen, producing serosal apposition and inversion of the mucosa, but the clamping of the other two sides of the triangle has to be done by the clamp applied *from without* with eversion of the cut edges and mucosal apposition. There will thus remain in some surgeons' minds strong theoretical objections to this technique. But it must be admitted that many surgeons use these stapling devices with apparently very satisfactory results in their practice.

More recently another type of stapling device has become available—the Russian SPTU instrument* for circular suture in the gastrointestinal tract. It employs the same general principles already outlined in association with the TA and GIA instruments—namely the apposition of, but not crushing by, the clamp of the tissues to be united and the insertion of ⊔ - shaped metal staples (actually of tantalum), which are converted to capital Bs on closure. It differs in two important respects. Firstly, it provides for a *completely circumferential row of staples*, and, secondly, it secures *apposition of the ends of the bowel in inversion*. It can be used in several parts of the alimentary tract, but it is specially well suited for constructing colorectal anastomoses, for in making anastomoses in this situation the device can be introduced to the anastomotic site through the anus from below and is thus particularly convenient for low rectal anastomoses (Fain et al. 1975; Goligher et al. 1978). But it can be employed for anastomoses anywhere in the colon—or elsewhere in the alimentary tract—by making a side cut in the wall of one of the

* Marketed in Great Britain by Geistlich Sons Ltd Pharmaceuticals, Chester. A very similar instrument is now made by the U.S. Surgical Corporation of New York and sold in Britain as the E.E.A. automatic stapler.

stumps of bowel participating in the anastomosis and passing the barrel of the instrument through it to the anastomotic site, the side hole being separately sutured by hand after the anastomosis has been completed and the instrument withdrawn. Our experience (Goligher et al. 1978) certainly suggests that the suture gun is capable of providing anastomoses at least as secure as those constructed by hand suture. It seems, too, that it may enable rectal anastomoses to be made at a lower level than would be possible by conventional low anterior resection using hand placed sutures. Accordingly, it is in my view a valuable addition to our repertoire for the treatment of rectal cancer. The instrument and the technique for using it are described on p. 570.

THE ROLE OF THE PERITONEAL CAVITY IN MAINTAINING THE INTEGRITY OF INTESTINAL ANASTOMOSES

Another fact that has emerged from recent experimental work on intestinal suture is the important part apparently played by the intrinsic peritoneal defences in maintaining the integrity of an anastomosis. Certainly a number of observers have found that experimental anastomoses in dogs and rabbits, if excluded partly or completely from the peritoneal cavity by wrapping them with oxidized cellulose or gelatin (Laufman and Method 1948), polyurethane foam (Trowbridge and Howes 1967), Silastic gauze (Canalis and Ravitch 1968), polyethylene (Rusca et al. 1969), or latex (Hawley et al. 1970), exhibited a greatly increased tendency to break down. Canalis and Ravitch (1968) and Rusca et al. (1969) found, moreover, that anastomoses made by an everting technique were much more susceptible to the deleterious effects of this manoeuvre than were those made by the conventional inverting method.

The way in which the peritoneum assists in the healing of anastomoses is not quite clear. The conventional teaching is that the greater omentum plays a useful part in protecting intestinal anastomoses. Experiments by Carter et al. (1972) in rabbits have cast doubt on the value of omental wrapping, but similar experimental work in dogs by McLachlin and Denton (1973) has reinforced traditional belief in the role of the omentum. The explanation suggested by Rusca et al. (1969) is that the peritoneal defences are normally capable of dealing effectively with organisms spilled during the anastomosis, but, when the defences are hindered by the plastic or other covering material, the resulting infection in the vicinity of the anastomosis may be sufficient to bring about a separation of the suture line. Hawley et al. (1970) found that the bursting pressure seven days after operation of intraperitoneal anastomoses in the rabbit colon, which had had an abscess in relation to them, was significantly less than that of similar anastomoses in the uninfected rabbits. They believe that the presence of infection in relation to a colonic suture line results in increased collagenase activity in the colon wall with consequent weakening of the important submucous layer, which depends for its strength on its collagen content.

Against this hypothesis, however, must be set the experimental work of Ryan (1969, 1970), who prepared an experimental model in dogs by bringing out a loop of descending colon in continuity into the subcutaneous tissues. The animal was then left for at least two months, at the end of which time the loop of colon was exposed in its subcutaneous pouch and either divided and sutured end-to-end or incised longitudinally and sutured. At this second operation concomitant 'pouch abscess' formation adjacent to the colonic suture line was encouraged by not preparing the bowel preoperatively, by the use of a non-aseptic technique with gross faecal soiling, and in some cases by deliberate contamination of the pouch at operation with a suspension of exogenous coliform organisms. In 16 or 18 dogs with contaminated pouches, abscesses formed in relation to the anastomoses or colotomy wounds, but in no instance did the suture line give way. Ryan (1970) also adduces evidence from the clinical field in the form of his own successful experience, and that of Madden and Tan (1961), Large (1964), Smiley (1966), Herrington and Graves (1968) and Roxburgh et al. (1968), with emergency resections for acute diverticulitis in the presence of diffuse peritonitis, to show that colonic anastomoses can heal well in the presence of florid peritoneal sepsis. But Botsford and Zollinger (1969) have reported a high incidence of leakage of anastomoses after primary resections for acute diverticulitis.

Altogether, it seems difficult to decide whether the suture line gives way usually as a sequel to pericolonic infection resulting from contamination at the time of operation, or whether the primary factor is anastomotic dehiscence, occurring some time after the operation (from necrosis of tissue or cutting out of sutures from excessive mechanical stress), and this in turn leads to most of the pericolonic sepsis and peritonitis, as believed by Halsted (1887), Moynihan (1926) and perhaps the majority of surgeons. Possibly both mechanisms operate, in some cases one of them being mainly responsible, in other cases the other.

TO DRAIN OR NOT TO DRAIN?

Another matter that has come under review recently has been the value of drainage in relation to colonic anastomoses. Probably most surgeons consider that drainage of the operative site is desirable after a colonic resection, not only when there has been significant faecal contamination at the time of operation, but even when soiling has been quite minimal. In the latter circumstances, whilst the drain may conceivably serve a useful purpose in avoiding any accumulation of potentially infected fluid in the neighbourhood of the anastomosis, which might predispose the latter to disintegration, its main objective is probably prophylactic—to encourage the escape of colonic contents to the surface instead of throughout the peritoneal cavity, if the suture line should give way. But to have this effect, it would seem necessary to retain the drain for at least five or six days, and many surgeons remove it after 48 hours. It must be admitted, also, that when anastomotic dehiscence has occurred, the escape of intestinal contents has not always followed the drain, but has sometimes taken place through the main wound. Drainage, then, seems not always to achieve its intended aim, and it could be argued further that the continued presence of the end of the drain in the neighbourhood of the anastomosis for several days might be detrimental by provoking an inflammatory reaction, which could predispose to dehiscence of the suture line and leakage from the bowel. In this connection an interesting experimental study of the possible ill-effects of surgical drains on anastomoses after colonic resection has been reported by Manz et al. (1970). They found that, in 15 dogs with undrained anastomoses, the bowel suture line healed *per primam* with only filmy adhesions and no stricture formation in all; but, of 20 dogs having Penrose drains left down to the site of the resection, nine developed anastomotic dehiscence and peritonitis and the rest had extensive adhesions and varying degrees of stricture formation. However, Manz et al. (1970) admit that, when drains of Teflon tape were used instead of Penrose drains in a further seven dogs, the gross and microscopical appearances of the anastomoses were similar to those of the control animals.

Personally I would doubt the alleged ill effects of retaining a drain for a considerable time in relation to an intestinal suture line in clinical practice, because, when Polya subtotal gastrectomy used to be the standard elective surgical treatment for duodenal ulcer some 15 years ago, I performed several hundreds of these operations and always used to leave a corrugated rubber drain down to the closed duodenal stump for seven days. Yet the incidence of dehiscence of this stump in my experience was quite negligible. I should also maintain that at one stage I started a controlled trial, in which patients undergoing colonic resection with end-to-end anastomosis for a variety of conditions were randomly allocated to two groups—one, in which a Zimmer suction drain was laid down to the anastomotic site for at least four to five days and sometimes seven or eight days, and the other, in which no external abdominal drainage was provided. However, after only 38 patients had been included without any striking difference emerging in the incidence of anastomotic dehiscence or intra-abdominal sepsis, the trial was abandoned because we were anxious to institute trials of other factors that seemed more likely to influence the healing of an anastomosis.

THE NUTRITIONAL STATE OF THE PATIENT

Some degree of malnutrition is recognized to be a fairly frequent accompaniment of colorectal cancer and it would be reasonable to suppose that this state of affairs might have a deterious effect on the healing of colonic anastomoses. Certainly it can be shown experimentally in rats that really gross malnutrition is associated with an abnormally low collagen content (Irvin and Hunt 1974) and tensile strength (Daly et al. 1970, 1972; Mukerjee et al. 1969) in healing colonic wounds. There is also a strong clinical impression that malnourished patients have an increased incidence of anastomotic dehiscence after colon resections (Irvin and Goligher 1973). Various uncontrolled clinical observations (Hadfield 1965; Vogel et al. 1972; Voitk et al. 1973) have suggested that improvement of the nutritional state of malnourished patients by intravenous feeding or elemental diet may have a favourable effect on intestinal healing, but unfortunately good objective evidence on this point is lacking.

THE POSSIBLE DELETERIOUS EFFECT OF
NEOSTIGMINE ON RECENTLY CONSTRUCTED
INTESTINAL ANASTOMOSES

It is common practice for anaesthetists to give an injection of neostigmine to reverse curarization and to combine with it an injection of atropine to block the muscarinic action of the neostigmine on smooth muscle, which otherwise would stimulate the bowel to increased activity. It has been suggested by Bell and Lewis (1968) that simultaneous administration of atropine does not completely eliminate the muscarinic effect of neostigmine, so that in patients whose operation has involved the creation of an intestinal anastomosis, the contraction produced in the bowel might be sufficient to cause disruption of the suture line. As evidence for this hypothesis Bell and Lewis (1968) reported a 36% anastomotic dehiscence rate in patients undergoing colectomy and ileorectal anastomosis. Hannington-Kiff (1969) claimed that, if the atropine were given *before* the neostigmine, a more efficient neutralization of the muscarinic action of the latter might be achieved.

The precise effect of neostigmine with atropine on intestinal activity was carefully studied by Wilkins et al. (1970), who recorded intraluminal pressures within the ileum, colon and rectum on conscious and anaesthetized patients. They found that in *unanaesthetized* patients atropine and neostigmine, in doses normally used by anaesthetists to reverse muscle relaxation, produced a pronounced increase in bowel activity, and this response occurred whether the atropine was given before or simultaneously with the neostigmine. The response still occurred in 38% of patients *anaesthetized without halothane* and might possibly expose

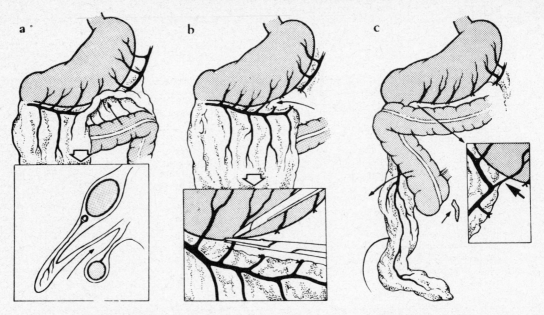

Fig. 318. (a) Greater omentum has been turned up to allow of its separation from the left end of the transverse colon and meso-colon. (b) The omentum is being detached from the greater curvature of the stomach. After the left gastroepiploic vessels have been ligated and divided well to the left, the line of omental division is carried to the right between the gastroepiploic arcade and the stomach, vessels passing between the two being meticulously clipped, divided and tied. (c) The freed greater omentum, hanging as a pedicle nourished by the right gastroepiploic artery, can now be extended down to the pelvis along the right paracolic gutter or taken to any other part of the abdominal cavity where its presence is required as a viable cover for an anastomosis.

a recently created anastomosis to undue strain. The ileum appeared particularly prone to neostigmine stimulation, so that anastomoses involving this part of the bowel would seem especially at risk. In patients *anaesthetized with halothane* the intestinal response to neostigmine was completely absent.

USE OF AN OMENTAL WRAP TO PROTECT COLORECTAL ANASTOMOSES

A debatable issue in abdominal surgery is the value of wrapping round intestinal anastomoses a piece of greater omentum, either in the form of a free graft without blood supply or as a pedicle graft with an intact arterial supply. Carter et al. (1972) were unimpressed by the effect of reinforcing intestinal anastomoses with omentum in the rabbit; a free graft seemed to increase the chances of anastomotic leakage, and a pedicled omental graft did not improve the survival rate of the animals. In further experimental work on dogs, McLachlin and Denton (1973) confirmed the uselessness of a free omental graft, but found that a pedicle graft of omentum wrapped round a devascularized anastomosis of small bowel considerably lessened the incidence of leakage. Subsequently, McLachlin et al. (1976) were able to demonstrate in the dog that wrapping a pedicle graft of omentum round a devascularized anastomosis after anterior resection in the dog was similarly beneficial. Of course the conditions produced by McLachlin in his experiments are distinctly artificial in that the blood supply to the bowel taking part in the anastomosis has been deliberately impaired, whilst in clinical practice every effort is made to ensure that the supply to the end of bowel being joined in the anastomosis is adequate. But it would be reasonable to suppose that, if an omental pedicle graft can help in one

situation it might be helpful in avoiding or restraining leakage in the other situation.

Despite the conflict in the experimental evidence, a number of surgeons have strongly advocated the use of a pedicle graft of omentum to wrap round suture lines in clinical practice, and particularly those resulting from anterior resection of the rectum, oesophagectomy and certain urological conditions (Turner-Warwick et al. 1967; Turner-Warwick 1976; Silen 1975; Localio 1975; Localio and Eng 1975; Goldsmith 1977). In certain patients with an abundant greater omentum it is a relatively simple matter to wrap a portion of this structure round even somewhat inaccessible anastomoses, such as those resulting from anterior resection: but in other cases, if omentum is to be used for this purpose, it is necessary to detach it from the transverse colon and most of the greater curve of the stomach to make a long omental tail deriving its blood supply from the right gastro-epiploic artery (Fig. 318). The omentum can as a rule most conveniently be passed down to the pelvis in the right paracolic gutter. There does not appear to be any really objective clinical information that establishes beyond doubt the protective value of omental wrapping, but, for an outlay of 10–12 minutes of operative time to prepare the graft, it is perhaps worth adopting this relatively simple and innocuous practice.

TECHNICAL DETAILS OF ANASTOMOSIS

The method of closing both cut ends of bowel after a resection and performing a *side-to-side anastomosis*, which is favoured by many surgeons for both

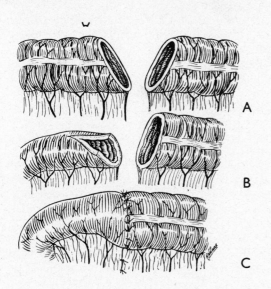

Fig. 319. (A) Oblique section of the colon ends ensures a good blood supply to all parts of the cut edge. (B and C) Enlargement of the lumen of the small bowel by division along the antimesenteric border for 2–2·5 cm to adapt it to the wider lumen of the colon.

small and large gut, has the theoretical advantage that it uses only completely peritonealized surfaces of bowel for the actual union. But it suffers certain drawbacks. It is more extravagant in bowel—a consideration of little significance in the small gut but often of some importance after colon resections where only a limited amount of bowel is available—and the blind ends are subsequently liable to undergo dilatation, which may give rise to discomfort and on occasion perforation. *End-to-end anastomosis* is simpler to perform and more physiological, and the excellent results obtained by it in clinical practice seem to show that the traditional dangers of the 'mesenteric angle' (Soresi 1919) and of unperitonealized bowel surfaces have been overrated. Disparity in the size of the lumens of the two pieces of bowel being anastomosed need not occasion any difficulty in the performannce of an end-to-end anastomosis; it can be easily corrected by a more oblique section of the bowel with the smaller lumen, or by enlarging the opening by a longitudinal cut for 1–2 cm along the antimesenteric border (Fig. 319). The same devices enable one to avoid narrowing at the site of anastomosis.

My own personal preference is strongly for end-to-end anastomosis, which I generally use even for ileotransverse colostomy after right hemi-colectomy, instead of end-to-end or side-to-end approximation as favoured by many surgeons in this situation. Aseptic methods of intestinal suture, which were popular in the period between the two world wars, have been largely abandoned in recent years in favour of 'open' techniques for anastomosis and, like the majority of surgeons at the present time, I employ the latter exclusively in colonic resections.

The blood supply to the large intestine requires special attention in the performance of resections. A good supply is provided by the main colic vessels, but advantage may sometimes be taken of the fact that the colon can often be nourished for considerable distances by the marginal artery alone. But in every case the surgeon must be completely satisfied that the blood supply at the site of proposed anastomosis is adequate. Though the colour of the bowel and the presence of arterial pulsation indicate a satisfactory blood supply, the only sure guide is the occurrence of arterial bleeding from the cut edge of the intestinal wall at the point of division, or from a small mural vessel specially divided to determine the state of the arterial supply before sectioning the colon. When the bowel is divided it is advisable to make the cut run obliquely so that a good arterial supply is obtained to all parts of the cut edge (Fig. 319A); this also has the advantage of obviating any narrowing of the lumen by the subsequent suturing. The terminal fringe of colon wall, which has been devitalized by the crushing clamp applied during the resection, should be excised.

Interrupted stitches probably interfere less with the blood supply to the ends of the bowel than does a continuous suture, and are therefore preferable, at any rate for the outer seromuscular row. In tying them it is important to avoid excessive force which increases the amount of strangulation and necrosis of tissue.

Finally it is essential at all costs to avoid tension on the site of anastomosis, and if necessary one or both limbs of colon must be further mobilized to relieve any tautness.

The standard method used by me for end-to-end anastomosis after resection is a two-layer inverting technique (Figs 312–6). As regards suture materials, for the *inner through-and-through* stitch continuous No. 3/0 chromic catgut mounted on a fine atraumatic needle has usually been employed, but more recently I have switched to 3/0 polyglycolic acid, the suture being lightly smeared with bone-wax to make its passage through the tissues smoother. In its posterior half it is inserted as a simple over-and-over stitch, but in the anterior half it changes to a 'loop on the mucosa' or Connell (1893) stitch to secure good inversion of the mucosal edges. For the *outer so-called seromuscular* stitches I have invariably used non-absorbable material such as No. 3/0 or 4/0 serum-proof silk, fine linen or cotton on atraumatic needles. These are inserted preferably after the inner catgut suture has been placed by rotating the anastomosis to give access to the posterior aspect (Fig. 316). The stitches penetrate the bowel wall deeply, not just the serosa and muscle layer, but all coats and include the catgut suture as well. As shown by sigmoidoscopy after low colonic or rectal anastomoses, the silk sutures are usually extruded into the lumen, and may give rise to granulomas which may mimic adenomas or nodules of recurrent growth.

THE PROBLEM OF FAECAL LOADING

Ideally patients coming to elective operation for carcinoma of the large bowel should, after suitable mechanical preparation, have a virtually empty colon, containing only a minimal quantity of faecal material. Unfortunately this ideal is not always achieved, for, despite a vigorous course of catharsis, enemas and washouts for five days, nearly half of my patients, particularly those with annular constricting growths, are found at laparotomy to have a fair degree of loading with soft or solid faeces proximal to the lesion. With carcinoma in the right colon and transverse colon this finding is not of much significance, since a right hemicolectomy or extended right hemicolectomy removes all the loaded colon and finishes with an anastomosis between the small bowel and the empty colon beyond the growth. But with tumours of the left colon and sigmoid colon a real problem arises, the solution to which depends partly on the severity of the loading and partly on the surgeon's personal preference.

1. Preliminary Transverse Colostomy. If there is very gross loading, the safest course is to establish a right transverse colostomy (or caecostomy, if the surgeon favours this operation) and leave the resection of the tumour for a subsequent operation two or three weeks later. In the interval the left colon is emptied by frequent washes through from colostomy to anus and *vice versa*.

2. Paul–Mikulicz or Hartmann's Operation (see pp. 465–7). Another perfectly valid solution is to perform an extraperitoneal type of resection, avoiding an anastomosis and leaving the patient with a temporary double- or single-barrelled colostomy respectively, the continuity of the intestinal tract being restored at a subsequent operation. But, as explained on p. 424, many surgeons feel—I think wrongly—that these methods may restrict the radical scope of the excision and are to be avoided, if possible.

3. Draining the Colon during the Resection and before the Anastomosis. Muir (1968) has advocated a method of washing out the obstructed colon at operation, to permit an immediate anastomosis on an empty bowel. All the usual steps of an elective resection are first taken (except for division of the bowel above the growth) and must include mobilization of the splenic flexure and the left half of the transverse colon. The colon (or rectum) is divided between clamps below the growth, and the stump of bowel containing the tumour and controlled by the proximal clamp is placed in a sterile polythene bag, which is tied with tapes above the lesion. A special wide short glass tube (made by Down Bros., London) with a side arm is securely tied into the bowel 5–9 cm above the top of the bag (Fig. 320). A long length of Paul's rubber tubing is attached to the broad end of the tube, and a rubber tube of the size used in blood-giving sets is fitted on to the side opening. Irrigation of the colon is now carried out, using 500–1000 ml of the detergent solution dioctyl sodium sulphosuccinate—or other soapy solutions as preferred—which is introduced through the fine tube and side opening, whilst the Paul's tubing is compressed. Five to ten minutes are allowed for the solution to mix with the faeces, and a certain amount of manipulation of the colon is carried out during this time to help to break up the faecal masses. Then the fluid contents are allowed to escape through the Paul's tube into a suitable receptacle, the colon being 'milked' with the fingers to assist in the emptying process. If necessary the irrigation may be repeated. Finally, the colon stump is clamped and divided at the appropriate site proximally, and the anastomosis is performed.

Though I have occasionally used this method, more often I have adopted the plan outlined in (4) or resorted to (1).

4. Emptying as Much of the Faeces as Possible into the Segment of Bowel to be Resected, Immediate Resection, and usually Right Transverse Colostomy. By a 'milking' manoeuvre with the fingers it is sometimes possible to move some of the faeces from the left transverse and upper descending colon into the distal colon to

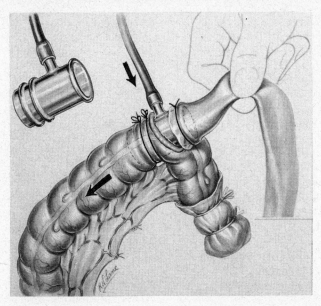

Fig. 320. A 26 or 32 mm glass tube with side arm for irrigation is tied securely into the proximal end of the opened bowel. The solution is dioctyl sodium sulphosuccinate, 0·2%, sterilized by autoclaving in a standard transfusion bottle. (*After Muir 1968*)

be resected. This method never accomplishes anything like a complete emptying of the colon at the site of anastomosis, but it may reduce the faecal content to an acceptable level. If a right transverse colostomy is then established, though a fair amount of faecal matter remains between it and the anastomosis, further addition of flatus and faeces is prevented, which probably has some protective effect on the suture line. Clearly, if there is really gross faecal loading, this method would be inadequate, and should give way to (1), (3) or (5).

5. *Subtotal or Total Colectomy with Ileosigmoid or Ileorectal Anastomosis*. Another rather drastic solution is to remove the entire loaded colon and anastomose the normal ileum to the undistended colon or rectum beyond the growth (see also p. 477).

MANAGEMENT OF FAECAL CONTAMINATION

Some degree of contamination with the intestinal contents is almost unavoidable with any open colonic anastomosis—and perhaps even with so-called 'aseptic' or closed anastomoses—but, as commonly used, the term 'faecal contamination' implies major soiling with obvious faecal material. This may occur during the conduct of the anastomosis if the bowel is heavily loaded, or may result from accidental rupture of the colon at the site of the growth or elsewhere. Though the patient may

have been treated preoperatively with bowel antiseptics (see p. 477) and the faeces may be relatively sterile, such severe faecal soiling is liable to result in subsequent infection in the peritoneal cavity or parietal wound (Rosenberg et al. 1971). How can contamination be best dealt with in order to lessen the risk of sepsis?

Irrigation and Local Antiseptic Applications to the Peritoneal Cavity
Apart from mechanical cleansing of the operative field with dry or moist swabs or irrigation with saline, it is natural to consider the use of various antiseptic agents. In the early days of sulphonamides and antibiotics it was a common practice with many surgeons to place in the abdomen at the site of the anastomosis a quantity of sulphanilamide or penicillin–sulphanilamide powder as a bowel antiseptic. As antibacterial agents with a broader spectrum of activity became available it was logical that they should be tried for this purpose. Polybactrin spray (Calmic), which consists of bacitracin, polymyxin and neomycin, was a popular topical antiseptic (Gibson 1958) and has been used intra-abdominally though no accurate assessment of its value in this connection has been made. Neomycin in a 0·5 or 1% solution has also been recommended as an irrigant by Poth (1954) and Hoffmann (1959), 50–100 ml of the fluid being used and eventually sucked or swabbed out of the peritoneal cavity before the abdomen is finally closed.

Singleton et al. (1959) found that neomycin was more effective than other irrigants, such as normal saline, 3% iodine or 20% sulfamylon, in preventing wound infection from colon organisms. However, there appears to be a risk of absorption of the neomycin, with subsequent toxic effects on the kidney, or respiratory arrest (Pittinger and Long 1959). Poth (1963) emphasizes that neomycin has a neuromuscular blocking effect, but that this can be reliably neutralized by an injection of neostigmine, if the anaesthetist is warned that a neomycin irrigation is about to be given. (The use of neostigmine in the presence of a recent anastomosis is not without danger, unless covered by an appropriate dose of atropine; see p. 437).

Cohn (1960) studied the relative toxicity of three antibiotics following intraperitoneal injection in anaesthetized and unanaesthetized animals. He found that tetracycline caused too much peritoneal reaction. Neomycin was better tolerated, but the mortality associated with larger doses was excessive. Kanamycin was safe even in very big doses in anaesthetized animals, and Cohn (1960) has used it intraperitoneally also in patients with satisfactory results. But Poth (1963) points out that this antibiotic, used in this way, also possesses a hypotensive and neuromuscular blocking action, which is not neutralized, but rather potentiated, by neostigmine. More recently cephalothin, 4 g to 1 litre of saline, has been employed as a continuous peritoneal irrigant for several days using 4 litres or so of the solution (Peloso et al. 1973), but in an experimental study in animals Sharbaugh and Rambo (1974) were unable to demonstrate that this intraperitoneal use had any significant advantage over intravenous cephalothin. Most recently of all povidone-iodine has been recommended as a peritoneal irrigant (Gilmore and Sanderson 1975), but I am not aware of any good evidence as yet to establish its value for this purpose in clinical practice.

In Britain at the present time a very popular peritoneal irrigant for cases with faecal contamination or severe peritonitis is noxythiolin (Noxyflex). This is not an antibiotic but a chemotherapeutic substance, which possesses remarkable antibacterial and antimycotic properties. Practically all Gram-positive and Gram-negative bacteria are affected by it. Noxythiolin is virtually non-toxic. It comes in powder form and should be dissolved in distilled water immediately before use. For peritoneal irrigation between 2·5 and 5 g are employed in 100–200 ml of fluid. The lotion is poured into the abdomen just before closing the wound, and left there for five to ten minutes, being finally removed by suction immediately prior to completion of the peritoneal suture. Alternatively, if a suction drain is inserted, the fluid may be left to find its way out through it. Though several surgeons of my acquaintance have, like myself, had some dramatic recoveries in cases of faecal peritonitis treated with noxythiolin, and Browne and Stoller (1970) have reported encouraging results with this agent in similar cases, unfortunately no controlled clinical observations are available. A possible beneficial effect of noxythiolin is that it may be cytotoxic to cancer cells (Jamieson 1972).

Frankly, on the evidence available I am not convinced that antibiotics or antiseptics introduced into the peritoneal cavity as an irrigant have any real merit over a vigorous lavage with 3 or 4 litres of normal saline alone at the conclusion of the operation, combined of course with systemic antibiotic therapy of suitable dosage according to the amount of contamination (see below).

Topical Application of Antibiotics or Antiseptics to the Parietal Wound

Not only the peritoneum but also (and perhaps even more so) the wound in the abdominal parietes is exposed to the risk of infection from faecal contamination. As for the prevention of this complication, the various antiseptic solutions such as noxythiolin or kanamycin, used for irrigating the peritoneal cavity, may also wash over the abdominal wound to some extent, though according to Bird et al. (1971) and Stoker and Ellis (1972) noxythiolin is relatively ineffective in combating parietal wound sepsis. In addition, as soon as the parietal peritoneum has been sutured, the exposed tissues in the wound may be sprinkled with 1 g of sterile powdered ampicillin, as recommended by Nash and Hugh (1967), Mountain and Seal (1970) and Andersen et al. (1972). They have shown by controlled trials that topical application of ampicillin in patients undergoing colon surgery or appendicectomy is effective in avoiding wound sepsis in the great majority of cases. Stoker and Ellis (1972) have demonstrated by a similar trial that ampicillin in the parietal wound is more effective than is penicillin and sulphadiazine. Evans et al. (1974) have shown by a controlled trial that instillation of 1 g of cephaloridine in 2 ml of water into the parietal wounds at the conclusion of colon resections significantly reduced the incidence of postoperative wound sepsis. A slight disadvantage was that, if infection occurred, more resistant organisms were encountered in the cephaloridine treated wounds than in the control wounds. More recently povidone-iodine sprayed into the potentially contaminated parietal wound has been shown to be quite effective in controlling subsequent sepsis (Gilmore and Sanderson 1975) but in a controlled trial Pollock et al. (1978) demonstrated that 1 g of cephaloridine intraincisionally is superior to irrigation of the wound with saline or spraying it with providone-iodine.

Drainage

Whatever divergence of views there might be about the advisability of instituting drainage in cases of colonic resection where there has been negligible soiling at the time of resection (see p. 437), surgical opinion would be unanimous in regarding drainage of the peritoneal cavity—and possibly the parietal wound—as essential when there has been a significant degree of faecal contamination during the operation. This may take the form of an *open* drain of corrugated rubber, a simple rubber or plastic tube, a Penrose drain, or a sump suction drain, or of a *closed* suction drain of Zimmer or Redivac type, my present preference being for sump drains. One or more drains may be used and are better brought out through separate stab wounds rather than through the main laparotomy wound. If desired, a further drain may be laid along the rectus muscle inside the rectus sheath in this latter wound and brought out at its lower end.

Systemic Antibiotics

Surgical opinion is divided on the usefulness of administering systemic antibiotics to 'cover' clean operations like a hernia repair, or even relatively clean ones such as a colon resection and anastomosis with minimal soiling after suitable mechanical and antibacterial preparation. But there would be general agreement on the desirability of systemic antibiotic therapy following a resection of large bowel in which much faecal contamination took place, even if the patient had had a full course of bowel preparation using bowel antiseptics and the faeces were in fact non-odorous and on bacteriological examination were found to be relatively sterile. In such circumstances the ideal antibiotic to use systemically is one with a broad spectrum of activity likely to be effective against the common intestinal organisms—for example, ampicillin, cephaloridine, cephalothin or gentamicin and lincomycin. Depending on the amount of soiling, it may be thought wise to commence the administration with a loading dose (e.g. 2–4 g cephalothin), given intravenously during the opera-

tion, and to continue thereafter with normal dosage intravenously or intramuscularly. It is also a good plan to take a swab of the faeces at the time of operation for urgent bacteriological examination to show which are the organisms and to indicate their sensitivity to various antibiotics as a guide to further therapy.

Polk and Lopez-Mayor (1969) have shown a spectacular reduction—and Evans and Pollock (1973) a less striking one—in the wound infection rate in colorectal cases with the routine intramuscular injection of three 1 g doses of cephaloridine, the first given immediately preoperatively or during induction of the anaesthetic, the second five hours and the third 12 hours later. Stokes et al. (1974) were able to demonstrate a similar advantage for a prophylactic regimen involving intramuscular injection of two doses of lincomycin 600 mg plus gentamicin or tobramicin 80 mg, one given with the anaesthetic premedication and the other eight hours later.

Precautions Against Tumour Dissemination and Implantation During Resections of the Colon for Cancer

As has been pointed out on p. 397 it is believed by some surgeons that malignant cells may be displaced into the venous blood draining the part by manipulation of the primary growth during operation, and may give rise to hepatic and other blood-borne metastases. There would also seem to be a risk that exfoliated carcinoma cells in the lumen of the colon adjacent to the tumour may become implanted in the suture line in the bowel, or engrafted in the peritoneal cavity or wound following spillage at operation (p. 399). In addition, seeding of tumour cells into the peritoneum or wound surfaces may take place at an earlier stage from the serosal aspect of the lesion, due to handling, particularly when the growth has erupted through the peritoneal coat. A great deal of attention was devoted to these possible hazards and to means of lessening them, notably by Warren Cole of Chicago, Moore of Buffalo and Cohn of New Orleans.

AGAINST VENOUS DISSEMINATION

PRELIMINARY LIGATION OF THE COLIC VESSELS

Because they were able to find carcinomatous cells in saline washings of the vessels of operative specimens of colorectal carcinomas, Cole et al. (1954) and Fisher and Turnbull (1955) deduced that the risk of malignant embolism might be accentuated by handling the growth during operation and might be obviated by preliminary venous ligation—as indeed, had been suggested by Miles in 1926 in the treatment of rectal cancer. Long et al. (1960) provided support for this idea by claiming to be able to show an increased outpouring of malignant cells into the portal venous system co-incident with handling of the tumours at operation. But in their careful studies Engell (1955) and Moore and Sako (1959) were unable to confirm this observation, and emphasized that there is a continual release of cancer cells from the growth into the veins draining the site throughout the life of the lesion. Altogether, their work seemed to invalidate the rationale of preliminary ligation.

But Turnbull et al. (1967) have reported on the late results obtained by him, employing this *no-touch, early ligation* technique, for radical resection of carcinomas of the colon in 664 cases at the Cleveland Clinic from 1953 to 1964, comparing them with the long-term results secured in 232 patients with colonic carcinoma submitted to radical operation by five other staff members at that Clinic during the same period using *conventional* technique. No cases or carcinoma of the rectum were included in either series. Excluding purely palliative resections, the crude five-year survival rate was 68·85% after the no-touch, early ligation technique, but only 52·13% after conventional technique. A comparison of the survival rate after the two operative methods when applied to patients with A and B growths showed no significant difference, but a comparison in regard to cases with C growths revealed a striking disparity—the crude five-year survival for C cases after the no-touch technique (57·84%) being roughly twice that for C cases after conventional technique (28·06%).

Coming from one of the outstanding centres for colonic surgery in America, these findings must command the closest attention. It is important to remember, however, that this study bears no relationship to a controlled trial, for patients were not allocated randomly to the two series of cases and different surgeons treated the two groups. It is certainly very difficult to understand why the technique of preliminary ligation of the vascular pedicles should make such a marked difference to the survival rate in C cases but none at all to that in A and B cases. The great pity is that, instead of treating 623 consecutive patients by the no-touch, early ligation technique and having to rely for comparison on cases treated by other methods by his colleagues at the Cleveland Clinic, Turnbull did not institute a properly controlled trial, in which he operated on some of his own cases by one method and on others by the other method. The results he would be able to produce now on such a basis would have been far more convincing.

It may also be appropriate to mention in this connection some experiences at St Mark's Hospital, London, on the effect of tying the superior haemorrhoidal/inferior mesenteric vessels before or after mobilization of the rectum in carrying out combined abdominoperineal rectal excision for carcinoma. At that hospital for many years two techniques were in vogue for performing combined excision of the rectum—the perineo-abdominal method in which the rectum and its contained growth are completely mobilized from below and the superior haemorrhoidal vessels are only tied through the abdomen after this has been done (see p. 504); and the synchronous combined excision, in which one of the first steps is ligation of the inferior mesenteric vessels by the abdominal operation before the growth is handled (see p. 504). A long-term follow-up study of many hundreds of cases treated by each method shows no significant difference in the survival rates for the two techniqes (Bussey et al. 1960). Admittedly patients were not randomly allocated to each method and the choice of operation depended on the personal preference of the surgeons concerned, but the comparison was at least as valid as that made by Turnbull et al. (1967).

For these reasons I have not adopted Cole's method of preliminary ligation of the colonic vessels as a routine in the resection of colonic cancers for, whilst sometimes easy to apply, on other occasions it can involve considerable technical difficulties.

AGAINST IMPLANTATION ON THE SUTURE LINE, PERITONEUM, OR WOUND

MECHANICAL MEASURES

Cole et al. (1954) recommended that, *before the tumour is subjected to any operative handling or mobilization*, strong tape ligatures should be applied to the colon several centimetres above and below the lesion respectively, but within the area of intended resection, to restrict the dissemination of exfoliated carcinoma cells in the bowel lumen (Fig. 321). They have shown that faecal smears taken proximal and distal to the ligatures are invariably negative, whilst those obtained from within the isolated segment are usually positive, for malignant cells. Once the bowel has been tied off in this way, however much exfoliation may occur into the lumen during the subsequent manipulation and dissection to free the tumour, the surgeon can feel confident that this will be prevented by the ligatures from extending to the sites of division of the bowel. But even so, the growth itself should be handled as little as possible, because of the risk of seeding malignant cells into the peritoneal cavity and wound. It would also be logical to tie a pack firmly round the bowel at the site of the lesion or to apply to it from an early stage of the operation a thin sheet of malleable metal in a gauze swab (as recommended by Boreham 1958) to minimize this danger from an early stage of the operation.

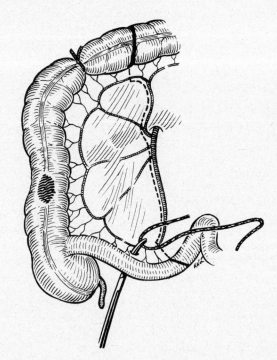

Fig. 321. The method of preliminary ligation of bowel above and below the growth, before commencing its resection. A ligature of strong braided silk has already been tied round the colon a few centimetres distal to the lesion in the ascending colon, and the proximal tie is just being inserted round the terminal ileum. The scope of the subsequent colectomy is indicated by the heavy, black, continuous and interrupted line.

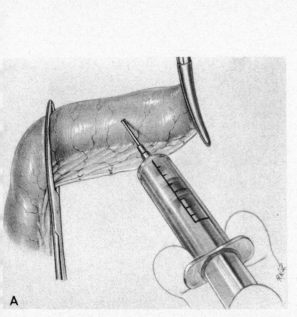
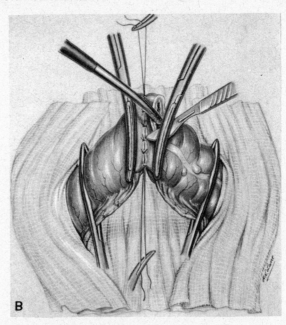

Fig. 322. One method of treating the ends of bowel with cytotoxic agents, preparatory to anastomosis. (A) A spring clamp is applied across the bowel and mesentery 10 cm or so from its extremity, held in a Parker–Kerr crushing clamp, and 20 ml of nitrogen mustard, 2 mg/100 ml saline, are injected into the isolated segment. The same procedure is then carried out on the other stump of bowel to take part in the anastomosis. (B) The two ends of bowel, still containing the nitrogen mustard, are brought together and the posterior row of Lembert sutures is placed and tied. The crushing clamps are then cut off and the escaping fluid which is released in the process is immediately taken up by a sucker.

CHEMICAL IRRIGATION

Though the method of ligation of the bowel before handling the growth might be successful in keeping malignant cells, displaced into the lumen during the operation, away from the parts of the colon to be used for the actual anastomosis, it would seem likely that in some cases exfoliated cells might already be present in the faeces beyond the sites of application of the ligatures, especially on the distal side. As an additional precaution, therefore, to destroy such cells the two colon stumps may be irrigated with a cytotoxic solution just before they are anastomosed. Convenient techniques for so doing are illustrated in Figs 322 and 323. Agents that have been used for the purpose include: mercury perchloride 1 in 500, as first recommended by Lloyd-Davies (1944) but found in animal experiments by McDonald et al. (1960) to be relatively valueless; sodium hypochlorite 0·5% and nitrogen mustard 1–2 mg/100 ml both of which McDonald et al. (1960) found to be effective; and 1% solution of cetrimide, which Gibson and Stephens (1966) demonstrated to be very useful and not at all detrimental to wound healing. Whichever method is used, some spilling of the cytotoxic agent into the peritoneal cavity during the anastomosis is inevitable, so that it is important to examine its effect on malignant cells spilled or exfoliated into this cavity. Atik et al. (1960) and McKibbin and Gazet (1964) showed that sodium hypochlorite, so far from discouraging malignant cells from implanting in the peritoneum, *actually enhanced their growth in this situation.* Nitrogen mustard was found by McCredie and de Peyster (1959) to inhibit the establishment of malignant cells in the peritoneum, but Cohn et al. (1963) demonstrated that it was relatively ineffective in suppressing the growth of such cells, not only in the peritoneal cavity, but also in the vicinity of the anastomosis in the bowel. Indeed, the latter workers were sceptical of the value of irrigations of the type advocated by McDonald and Williamson (1960). Instead Cohn et al. (1963) favoured the use of iodized catgut for the construction of the anastomosis for they found, like Gubareff and Suntzeff (1962), and Herter and Sbulz (1966) that this material acted as a deterrent to the growth of tumour cells implanted at suture lines. On the other hand Douglas and Le Veen (1971) were unable to confirm this beneficial effect of iodized catgut, and instead recommended the application of 10% formalin to the cut edges of bowel, which they had found effective in discouraging the growth of malignant cells in the suture lines of experimental animals.

What lessons has this experimental work for the clinical surgeon treating cancer of the colon? First of all the findings are to a considerable extent contradictory, and, secondly, it must be remembered that results obtained in connection with explanted tumours in rabbits may not apply to human carcinoma of the large bowel. But altogether, it is not unreasonable to feel very sceptical about the value of these measures that have been proposed to lessen the risk of implantation at operation—and indeed apprehensive as to the use of some of them. My own feeling is to continue with mechanical control by early proximal and distal ligation of the bowel (Fig. 321), for at worst it is a harmless practice. As for irrigations, for several years I have used a solution of nitrogen mustard 1 or 2 mg/100 ml for irrigating the bowel, the peritoneal and pelvic cavities, and the wound, without encountering any ill-effects. I would be inclined to continue to use it for these purposes, but I must agree that it might be preferable to employ saline, or no irrigation at all. Possibly, there may be a good case for using iodized catgut instead of ordinary chromicized catgut for the inner layer of the anastomosis, for it is difficult to see how any detriment could result, but iodized catgut is not easy to come by nowadays.

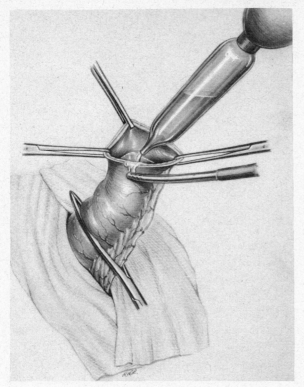

Fig. 323. Alternative method of applying a cytotoxic agent to an end of bowel before anastomosis. After applying a spring clamp across the bowel and mesentery, the Parker–Kerr forceps is removed and the cut edge of the intestine is held apart with Allis's forceps. The lumen is then mechanically cleansed of faeces by pledgets of gauze soaked in cetrimide 1%, and finally the nitrogen mustard solution is instilled by a glass Asepto syringe with rubber bulb.

ADJUVANT CHEMOTHERAPY

Believing that malignant cells are particularly liable to be released into the venous circulation by handling of growths during operation, Warren Cole (Cruz et al. 1956; Mrazek et al. 1959) suggested the practice of injecting nitrogen mustard immediately after curative resection of carcinoma into a tributary of the portal vein and into a peripheral vein, in the hope of minimizing the incidence of distant metastases. However, comprehensive multi-centre controlled trials of this form of adjuvant therapy using triethylene thiophosphoramide as the cytotoxic agent revealed no advantage for the treatment (Dwight et al. 1969; Holden and Dixon 1962). A further trial with 5-fluorouracil (5-FU) as the adjuvant drug showed a slight trend in favour of treated patients but no really significant difference in results (Higgins et al. 1971).

Rousselot et al. (1972) adopted a somewhat different technique for adjuvant therapy, the *drug (5-FU) being injected intraluminally* at operation into the cancer-bearing segment of bowel sequestered between tapes immediately before resection, and also given intravenously on the first and second postoperative days. No significant increase was observed in morbidity or mortality due to this practice, and there seemed to be a trend towards increased survival at five and eight years in treated patients with C growths, but not in those with A and B lesions. However, a long-term report by Lawrence et al. (1978) on a similar controlled trial of intraluminal injection of 5-FU, supplemented by five postoperative oral courses of 5-FU, is that there was no significant advantage in the treatment.

Yet another form of adjuvant chemotherapy directed at lymph node metastases rather than potential blood-borne metastases is that of Rob et al. (1963) who attempted to improve the prospect of radical operation for cancer of the colon by injecting into the lymph vessels draining the site of the tumour either 5-FU or radioactive gold, with the object of destroying small clumps of cancer cells in the nodes and lymphatics outside the zone removed by the surgeon. Adams et al. (1970) have conducted a trial of this form of adjuvant therapy in a group of hospitals in Rochester, N.Y. The operative mortality was approximately 4% in treated and untreated cases. As regards five-year survival rate, this was 51·2% in 136 control cases, 57·6% in 107 cases receiving 5-fluorouracil and 61% in 58 cases treated with radioactive gold. Thus the patients who had gold, but not those who had 5-fluorouracil, achieved a statistically significant advantage over the control patients.

Administration of a Prophylactic Course of Ordinary Chemotherapy

However, the only form of adjuvant chemotherapy now at all commonly practised is the administration simply of a course of chemotherapy for some weeks or months after resection of the growth in patients thought at operation to have been left with some residual tumour or known to have advanced Dukes' C lesions. The popular drugs are 5-FU, methyl CCNU and possibly vincristine. A number of trials of this regimen are in progress in several centres, but results so far available are rather disappointing (Higgins et al. 1976; Grage et al. 1976). Bearing in mind the not infrequent disturbing side effects of chemotherapy (see p. 473), I would certainly not consider recommending it as a routine to my patients after removal of C lesions until more positive advantages have been demonstrated in current trials. The indication would be different in a patient with known residual disease—say hepatic metastases, though, if these are extensive, not much benefit is likely to accrue from the chemotherapeutic agents at present available.

A further development in regard to adjuvant chemotherapy is the combination of *immunotherapy*, using the BCG vaccine, and chemotherapy, using 5-FU (Mavligit et al. 1976). Though some apparent improvement occurred in the five-year survival rate in the cases treated, it must be emphasized that these results would need to be extended and confirmed before definite conclusions could be drawn.

DETAILED MANAGEMENT OF CARCINOMA OF THE COLON WITHOUT ACUTE OBSTRUCTION OR PERFORATION

Assessment of Suitability of Patient to Proceed to Laparotomy

As already pointed out on p. 427, in the treatment of carcinoma of the large bowel the surgeon starts off with a strong bias in favour of excision of the lesion, if at all possible, even if only for palliative purposes. When, as occasionally happens, removal of the primary growth presents insuperable difficulties, it may still be feasible to carry out a short-circuiting operation to relieve or anticipate partial obstruction. There is thus a very compelling desire to proceed to abdominal exploration in dealing with patients suffering from colonic cancer, and in the vast majority of cases this is in fact the course followed and the state of the growth is assessed at laparotomy.

Rarely—certainly in my practice—the tumour has advanced to such an extent by the time the patient reaches hospital, it is only too evident on clinical examination that the period of life remaining to him is probably too limited to justify even the simplest palliative operation. This state of affairs arises most notably when there is widespread peritoneal dissemination with ascites. A more difficult decision is called for when there is clinically obvious involvement of the liver, with hard nodular enlargement of this organ. In some such cases the surgeon will find difficulty in making up his mind whether to turn the patient down for operation or to proceed to laparotomy in the hope that there may be sufficient uninvolved hepatic parenchyma to justify a palliative excision of the primary growth in the bowel. In these cases he will naturally also be influenced by the patient's general condition. As for pulmonary deposits, if these are numerous they will be a strong deterrent to operation, but, if only one or two metastases are evident in the lungs and the patient's bowel symptoms are really troublesome, particularly if they indicate an increasing degree of intestinal obstruction, laparotomy will be warranted.

The majority of patients with carcinoma of the large bowel are elderly, many of them are decidedly frail, and a fair proportion suffer in addition from cardiovascular or respiratory disease—all conditions which conspire to augment the hazards of a major laparotomy. But bearing in mind the lethal nature of the intestinal lesion, considerable hazards are acceptable in order to offer a chance of cure or significant palliation, and in fact it is only very rarely that a patient cannot be accepted as a reasonable operative risk.

A debatable issue is to what extent patients should be investigated preoperatively by more sophisticated means for the presence of clinically imperceptible hepatic metastases, for, unless the involvement is massive, which is unlikely under the circumstances, laparotomy and palliative excision would be required in any event. Claims that the presence of hepatic metastases is strongly suggested by alterations in the serum levels of certain liver enzymes such as gamma glutamyl transpeptidase alkaline phosphate (Baden et al. 1971) and 5'-nucleotide phosphodiesterase (Pollock et al. 1979), or of various plasma proteins (Milano et al. 1978), have not all been substantiated (Irvin et al. 1973b). Furthermore, the surgeon needs to know also the distribution of any metastases in the liver, information which can only come from some form of scanning. In the past ordinary scinti-scanning and arteriography have not been always very reliable and it remains to be seen whether CAT-scanning or ultrasonography—which have the additional advantage of being non-invasive—will prove more helpful in the future.

Preoperative Care

BOWEL PREPARATION

MECHANICAL CLEANSING

Unquestionably there are great advantages in operating on an empty colon, and preoperative mechanical bowel preparation is designed to secure that end as far as possible, by cleansing the colon of faeces retained above the growth by means of

TABLE 26. *Mechanical and Dietary Preparation for Elective Colon Resection*

Days before	Diet	Aperients	Enemas, wash-outs, suppositories
5	Ordinary	Magnesium sulphate 5 g thrice daily	Soap-and-water enema or two bisacodyl suppositories in evening
4	Ordinary	Magnesium sulphate 5 g thrice daily	Soap-and-water enema or two bisacodyl suppositories in evening
3	Ordinary	Magnesium sulphate 5 g thrice daily	Soap-and-water enema or two bisacodyl suppositories in evening
2	Light	Castor oil 45–60 ml at 6.0 a.m.	Soap-and-water enema or two bisacodyl suppositories in evening
1	Mainly fluid	Nil	Veripaque enema (1 phial containing 3 g in 1·5 litres of water) in morning and again in the evening
0 (day of operation)	Nil	Nil	Nil

are used for access to the right or left colon it is a great advantage to have the *patient tilted 25–30° to the opposite side*, which is also the side on which the surgeon should stand for the operation. This tilt causes the loops of small gut to gravitate away from the uppermost half of the addomen on which one is operating, either into the dependent part of the peritoneal cavity or into a suitable receptacle of moist packs and towels fashioned for them outside the abdomen (Fig. 327A, B); Lahey (1953) actually designed a special rubber bag for this purpose, and I have used a plastic one (made by Aldington Laboratories of Ashford, Kent) with a purse-string tape in its neck for gently tightening to retain the bowel in the bag. This manoeuvre enormously facilitates the exposure and mobilization of the colic flexures, particularly the splenic flexure. Only very rarely have I found it necessary to enlarge a paramedian incision by means of a transverse extension across the rectus muscle in order to secure adequate access for a left hemicolectomy. It will be appreciated that the final anastomosis after an extended left hemicolectomy with sacrifice of the inferior mesenteric vessels will take place in the pelvis, so that for this stage of the operation a moderate Trendelenburg tilt will be required.

ANAESTHESIA

This follows the lines of anaesthesia for abdominal surgery in general, and usually consists of a general anaesthetic aided by relaxants. By this means very satisfactory conditions are provided for the surgeon with complete relaxation of the abdominal muscles. Spinal anaesthesia, which used to be popular for colon surgery before relaxants were introduced partly because it gave a relatively bloodless field by lowering blood pressure, is now quite obsolete as it was undoubtedly somewhat more hazardous and less predictable in its results. However, epidural anaesthesia, which avoids the special risks of spinal anaesthesia but causes a fair degree of hypotension, is preferred by some surgeons. It has the additional advantage that, if administered by a plastic catheter, the latter may be left in situ during the first postoperative day or two and further anaesthetic solution may be injected as required to relieve pain (Thorne et al. 1954; Simpson et al. 1962).

EXPLORATION OF ABDOMEN

The first step on opening the abdomen is a careful exploration to determine the presence and extent of the lesion. It is a wise precaution to make the examination of the suspected site of the primary growth the last item in the systematic palpation of the abdominal cavity, for once the primary lesion has been felt there is a natural tendency for the surgeon to forget to explore elsewhere as thoroughly as he should, and, for example, palpation of the liver may inadvertently be omitted. Deferring the examination of the growth itself till the end of the exploration may also possibly diminish the risk of disseminating carcinoma cells in the peritoneal cavity. The liver is first palpated, then a hand is passed down into the pelvis to feel for deposits in the pelvic peritoneum. The greater omentum is next inspected and palpated for the presence of tiny 'seedling' deposits. As some 3% of all cases of carcinoma coli have two or more primary growths it is important that the whole colon and intraperitoneal rectum should be thoroughly palpated in

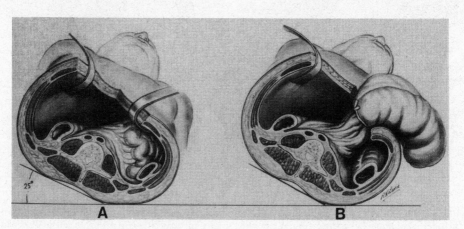

Fig. 327. A 20–25° lateral tilt of the operating table is valuable in displacing the small gut into the opposite half of the abdomen (A), or into a plastic bag outside the abdominal cavity (B).

search of additional carcinomas or associated adenomatous polyps. Finally the primary lesion is examined. The points to be noted in connection with it are: its size and fixity; whether it has involved the peritoneum over it or produced plaques in the adjoining peritoneum; if adherent, to which organs or structures it has become attached; and whether the related lymphatic glands are enlarged or indurated. The degree of obstruction and faecal loading present should also be noted as it may influence the choice of operation.

ASSESSMENT OF RESECTABILITY AND MANAGEMENT OF UNRESECTABLE CASES

As already mentioned it should be rare at the present day for a growth of the colon to be found unresectable because of local fixation and implication of adjacent viscera. A determined surgeon will nearly always be able to carry out a resection of the primary lesion, and, even if it appears doubtful whether a satisfactory clearance of the related lymphatics has been achieved, such a removal of the ulcerating growth in the bowel is generally well worth while on the grounds of palliation. The relief of bowel symptoms and the temporary improvement in general health is usually most gratifying. Even if hepatic deposits are present it is often preferable to perform a deliberate palliative resection if it appears that the patient may have six or nine months of life before him (and, very rarely, it may even be possible to contemplate a subsequent right or left partial hepatectomy—see p. 427). My own resectability rate for carcinoma coli is approximately 95%, and this includes 15–20% of palliative excisions in the presence of liver metastases.

If, however, *the growth is quite irremovable or extensive peritoneal deposits outside the scope of any excision contraindicate even a palliative resection*, a decision will have to be made as to the advisability of any alternative operative procedure for palliation. If there is a considerable degree of chronic obstruction present and it seems likely that acute obstruction is imminent, steps should be taken to relieve it. When feasible the operation of choice is a short-circuiting lateral anastomosis between the bowel proximal and distal to the lesion, as for example between the ileum and the transverse colon with a growth of the right colon, or between the transverse and descending or sigmoid colon with a growth of the splenic flexure; but a proximal colostomy close to the growth may be unavoidable with lesions in the lower sigmoid. More usually in cases with inoperable colonic growths a relieving opera-

tion for obstruction is not required, and is better avoided if it involves the creation of a colostomy. Finally *in an inoperable case a biopsy should be obtained if at all possible*, for histological confirmation of the diagnosis, even when the nature of the lesion appears to be beyond doubt.

RADICAL RESECTIONS

Before commencing the resection of a carcinoma of the colon, ligatures of strong braided silk may be tied round the un-mobilized bowel 10 cm or so above and below the growth, as recommended by Cole (Fig. 321), to confine malignant cells, that may be exfoliated into the lumen of the gut during the subsequent manipulation of the primary tumour.

RIGHT HEMICOLECTOMY

The parietal peritoneum of the right paracolic gutter is divided from below the caecum to just above the hepatic flexure (Fig. 328). As it contains numerous fine vessels, especially on the upper and outer aspect of the flexure, which tend to bleed when cut, I prefer to conduct the peritoneal division in piecemeal fashion between artery forceps, which are then replaced by ligatures. Division by diathermy may be used instead, but is less reliable. The process of division of the peritoneum is continued in similar manner horizontally above the proximal 7–10 cm of transverse colon, where it rests directly against the posterior abdominal parietes. The next step is to open the lesser sac by holding up the stomach and more mobile central part of the transverse colon and dividing the greater omentum between forceps as far as required (Fig. 329). This completes the separation of the peripheral peritoneal attachments of the whole right colon, so that the bowel with its medial leaf of peritoneum and colic vessels can be elevated from the posterior abdominal wall and mobilized towards the midline (Fig. 330). The ureter, spermatic vessels and retroperitoneal portion of the duodenum tend to adhere to the peritoneum and should invariably be carefully sought and, if necessary, gently swept back out of harm's way. By holding up the mobilized colon and viewing the artificially created mesocolon against the light, the ileocaecal, right colic and middle colic vessels are clearly displayed for division close to their origins from the main superior mesenteric trunk. Of the several techniques available for securing and dividing such vessels, the one I favour is the 'three-clamp method', in which three

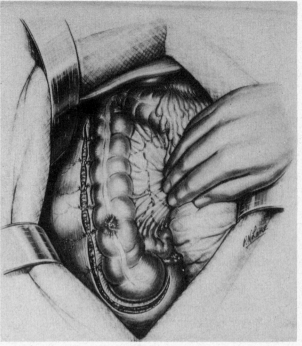

Fig. 328. Right hemicolectomy: division of posterior parietal peritoneum below and lateral to the caecum and ascending colon.

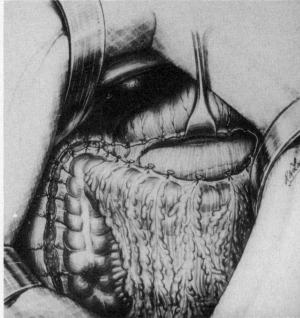

Fig. 329. Extension of the peritoneal cut round the hepatic flexure and through the greater omentum, opening the lesser sac.

strong artery forceps are applied close together and the vessel is divided between them leaving the more important end controlled by two of the clamps (Fig. 310, *inset*). Ligation of the stump is then accomplished by linen thread (No. 60) or catgut (No. 1 or 2 chromic), the forceps nearer the ligature being gradually removed as the latter is tightened so that the tie settles in the groove of crushed tissue made by the forceps. Finally, the second forceps is released just before the knot is tied. The effect is that a good wad of tissue is retained distal to the ligature so that it is not likely to slip, and I have found this a very quick and reliable method of dealing with important vascular pedicles in many fields of abdominal and general surgery.

The remaining portions of the medial leaf of peritoneum and the transverse mesocolon between the sites of division of the colic vessels are now divided. The peritoneal cut is then continued below into the mesentery of the ileum 15 cm or so from the ileocaecal junction. As it nears the small bowel this incision exposes the communicating vessel between the terminal ileal branches of the superior mesenteric artery and the ileocolic artery; this is ligated and divided and the ileum severed between

crushing clamps (Fig. 331). Attention is now turned to the upper part of the wound, and the cut in the transverse mesocolon is continued up towards the colon at a convenient point; in the process it exposes the marginal vessels between the two branches of the middle colic artery or between the middle and ascending left colic arteries 1 cm or so from the bowel wall, and these have to be secured and divided (Fig. 331). It only remains to continue the division of the greater omentum to the same level in the transverse colon, and the bowel can then be divided between clamps.

Probably the most popular method of restoring continuity between the ileum and transverse colon after right hemicolectomy is by end-to-side anastomosis which commends itself particularly in this situation because of the disparity in size of the small and large gut. However, for many years I have employed end-to-end anastomosis here as elsewhere in the colon and have never had any difficulty in adapting the small to the large intestine by cutting it along its antimesenteric border to enlarge the lumen as required (Fig. 332). Whichever technique is used, the gap between the cut edge of the ileal mesentery and the transverse mesocolon is finally closed by continuous or interrupted fine catgut sutures (Fig. 333). I usually make no effort to reperitonealize the raw area on the right side of the posterior abdominal wall.

A valuable modification of the ordinary technique of ileotransverse colostomy after right hemi-

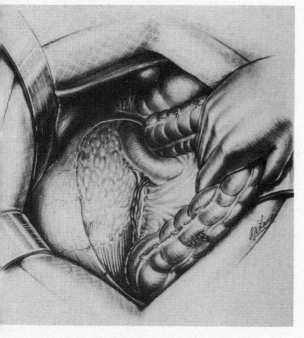

Fig. 330. Right colon has been swept medially exposing the extraperitoneal fat, quadratus lumborum, ureter, spermatic vessels and second and third parts of duodenum.

colectomy has been introduced by Muir (1947) for use in cases where the resection has been undertaken in the presence of acute or subacute obstruction (Fig. 334). Continuity is re-established by side-to-side or end-to-side (ileum to colon) anastomosis; a rubber catheter with multiple holes is then passed through the stoma well into the lower ileum and brought out through one edge of the invaginated end of the colon, which is again invaginated around the emerging tube. The end of the catheter is now drawn through a small incision in the abdominal wall immediately overlying the anastomosis, preferably with a tail of omentum intervening, and the colon is sutured to the parietes at this point to fix it in place. A skin suture secures the catheter.

The advantage of this method is that is provides decompression of the ileum above the anastomosis by gentle suction applied to the catheter, and this protects the suture lines from dangerous tension and minimizes the risk of paralytic ileus. When the catheter is finally withdrawn after 7–14 days the resulting fistula rapidly closes.

RESECTION OF TRANSVERSE COLON

First, the greater omentum is divided above or below the gastroepiploic arterial arcade along the greater curvature of the stomach for a distance corresponding to the proposed extent of the resection (Fig. 335). The omentum is then divided on

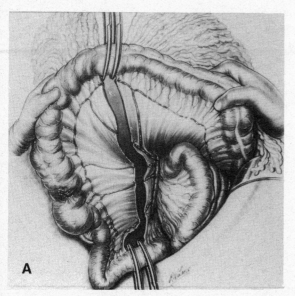

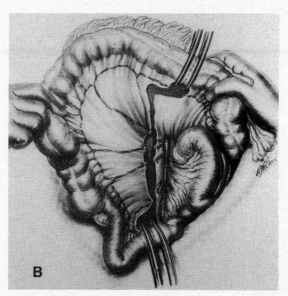

Fig. 331. Division of colic vessels and medial leaf of peritoneum, mesentery and mesocolon up to the bowel at the proximal and distal limits of the resection; (A) with preservation of the left branch of the middle colic vessels; (B) with sacrifice of the entire middle colic artery and more extensive removal of the transverse colon.

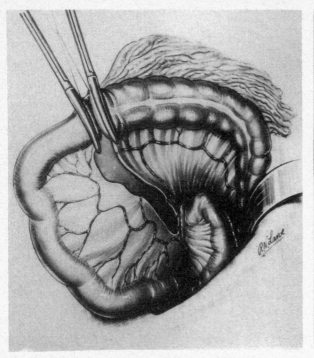

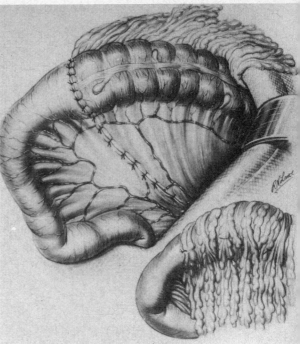

Fig. 332. End-to-end ileotransverse colostomy being continued.

Fig. 333. Completion of anastomosis between ileum and transverse colon, the mesenteric gap being closed by suture. *Inset:* Suture of greater omentum over the anastomosis.

either side to reach the colon at the sites corresponding to the proximal and distal extremities of the resection. Holding the bowel up to render the transverse mesocolon taut, the stem of the middle colic artery is now secured and severed close to its origin from the superior mesenteric trunk, and the mesocolon is divided in a V-shaped manner from this point towards the transverse colon at the places previously chosen as the limits of the segment to be resected (Fig. 336). The marginal vessels are crossed by these cuts close to the bowel and have to be secured. Finally, the colon is divided between crushing clamps above and below and continuity is restored by end-to-end anastomosis

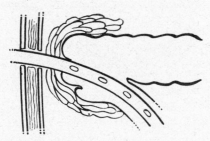

Fig. 334. Muir's method of ileotransverse colostomy and decompression of terminal ileum. (*From Lloyd-Davies et al. 1953*)

between the hepatic and splenic ends of the transverse colon; to avoid tension at the suture line, it will often be necessary to mobilize the colic flexures (Fig. 337). As previously explained, I frequently combine this operation with a right hemicolectomy when operating for carcinoma of the hepatic flexure or right end of the transverse colon.

RADICAL LEFT HEMICOLECTOMY WITH
SACRIFICE OF THE INFERIOR MESENTERIC
VESSELS

The mobilization of the left colon proceeds as in a right hemicolectomy, but the splenic flexure, lying at a higher level than the hepatic flexure, is more difficult to free. The approach to the flexure itself is best postponed till the descending and sigmoid colon and the transverse colon respectively have been freed of their peripheral peritoneal attachments. In the case of the sigmoid colon this involves first of all the separation of the lateral aspect of the iliac colon and mesocolon from the parietal peritoneum of the left iliac fossa, to which they have normally become adherent during development making the iliac colon a 'fixed' part of the large intestine. Once these developmental adhesions have been severed, preferably by scissor dissection (Fig.

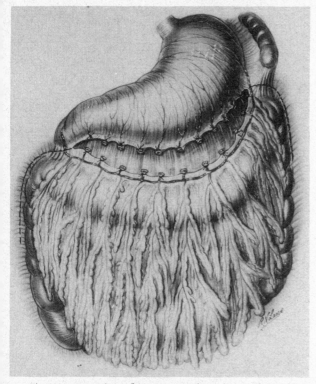

Fig. 335. Resection of transverse colon: division of greater omentum along the greater curvature of the stomach, above the gastroepiploic arcade.

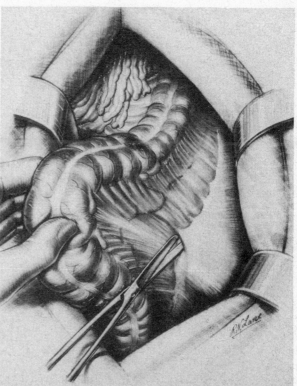

Fig. 336. The transverse colon has been turned up and the middle colic vessels and transverse mesocolon are being divided.

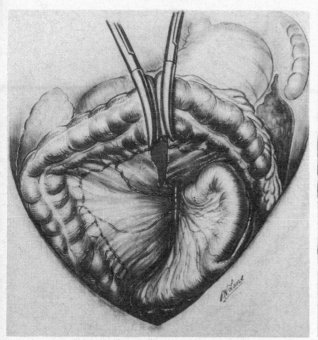

Fig. 337. After removal of the cancerous segment of colon the ends of bowel are brought together for anastomosis.

Fig. 338. Radical left hemicolectomy: separation of developmental adhesions on the outer side of the iliac colon.

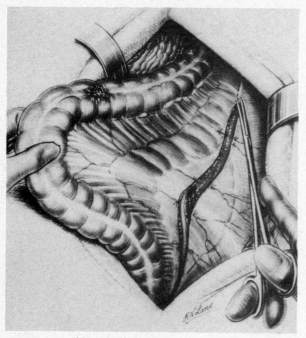

Fig. 339. The sigmoid mesocolon has been completely freed of adhesions and an incision is being made in its outer leaf and upwards along the 'white' line.

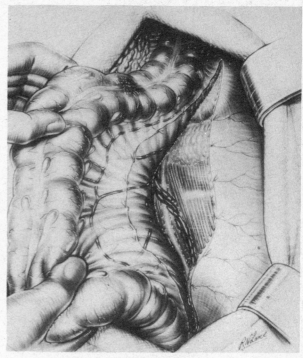

Fig. 340. The descending and sigmoid colon is swept medially exposing the quadratus, psoas, ureter and spermatic vessels.

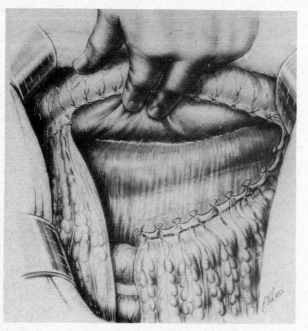

Fig. 341. Division of the greater omentum transversely between the stomach and the gastroepiploic arcade, and then vertically to the transverse colon at the proposed proximal limit of the resection.

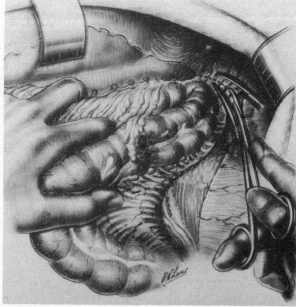

Fig. 342. Whilst the transverse and descending colon is drawn downwards and to the right and the lateral margin of the wound is retracted strongly laterally, the peritoneum and subjacent vessels above and lateral to the splenic flexure are clamped and divided.

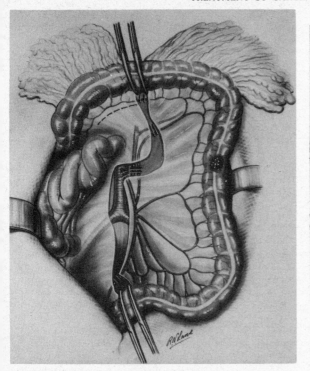

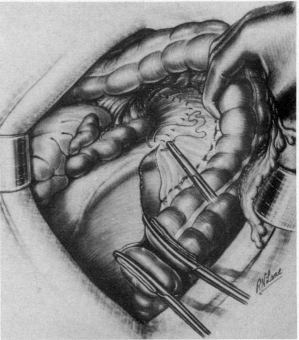

Fig. 343. The posterior parietal peritoneum overlying the abdominal aorta is incised, and the inferior mesenteric artery and vein divided at the level of the origin of the artery. The peritoneal incision is then carried upwards, exposing and dividing the ascending left colic and marginal vessels on its way to reach the mid-transverse colon, which is then clamped and divided.

Fig. 344. The left colon has been removed and the transverse colon stump is being drawn down into apposition with the sigmoid stump, whilst the edge of the transverse mesocolon is stitched to the right cut edge of peritoneum overlying the aorta.

338), the whole sigmoid colon has its natural mesocolon 'restored' to it. A cut is now made in the base of the left leaf of the sigmoid mesocolon and this is extended upwards in the peritoneum of the left paracolic gutter close to the descending colon to a point 7–10 cm below the splenic flexure (Fig. 339). This allows the colon and its medial leaf of peritoneum to be swept medially off the posterior abdominal wall, the same care being exercised as during mobilization of the ascending colon in right hemicolectomy to displace the ureter and the spermatic or ovarian vessels posteriorly to avoid damage (Fig. 340). As for the transverse colon, the greater omentum attached to it is divided close to the greater cure of the stomach as far to the right as necessary, and then the line of resection is carried down to the colon at the proposed proximal limit of the resection (Fig. 341). The two mobilized limbs of large bowel—the transverse and the descending colon—are then held in the left hand whilst an assistant exposes the flexure with a deep retractor.

The remaining intact peritoneum of the extreme upper end of the left paracolic gutter and the underlying connective tissue, containing a number of small vessels, are divided *seriatim* between forceps; the line of section is then continued round the top of the splenic flexure into the small undivided portion of the greater omentum lying below the interval between the spleen and the stomach (Fig. 342). During this manoeuvre care must be taken not to tear the spleen by rough traction on the peritoneum adherent to it.

The splenic flexure can now be displaced downwards and medially and the entire left colon lifted away from the posterior abdominal wall, to which, however, it remains attached by the left end of the transverse mesocolon, the medial leaf of peritoneum of the descending colon and the sigmoid mesocolon. In this partly real, partly artificial mesentery the main colic vessels can as a rule be clearly seen—the ascending left colic running obliquely upwards to the splenic flexure, the main left colic stretching directly to the lower descending colon, and the sigmoids proceeding downwards with varying degrees of obliquity to the sigmoid loop. Lying along the base of the mesentery is the main inferior mesenteric vein just to the left of the abdominal aorta.

The next step is to incise the posterior parietal peritoneum over the abdominal aorta from the lower edge of the third part of the duodenum down to a point a little below the level of the aortic bifurcation. Opening up this wound exposes the inferior mesenteric artery and vein and allows the former to be tied flush with the front of the aorta; the vein is taken by a separate ligature at about the same level or rather higher (Fig. 343). The uppermost 6–8 cm of these mesenteric vessels with their related lymph glands can now be displaced forwards off the aorta, and the latter may be further cleared by dissection of para-aortic glands if so desired, though I am sceptical as to the likelihood of such additional glandular ablation often making much difference to the prognosis. The upper end of the peritoneal cut is next continued upwards round the left side of the duodenojejunal junction to enter the transverse mesocolon, in which it is prolonged upwards parallel with, but 2·5 cm or so away from, the middle colic vessels, and then to the left along the marginal artery as long or as short a distance as required by the needs of the resection. For a growth of the splenic flexure itself the mesocolic incision is usually terminated about the middle of the transverse colon. At this point the cut is taken across the marginal vessel, which is secured, to the mesenteric edge of the colon, which is then divided between crushing clamps. The entire left colon can now be displaced forwards and downwards out of the wound, so that it lies on the towelling in front of the thighs, its sigmoid end being connected through the lower part of the incision with the rectum. The clamped stump of proximal transverse colon is then drawn towards the pelvis, its remaining greater omental attachment to the stomach being divided if necessary to allow this to be done. The cut edge of the mesocolon beyond the marginal vessel is conveniently sutured at this stage by a running fine catgut stitch to the right edge of the posterior parietal peritoneal wound in front of the aorta, to close the gap behind the bowel in its new situation (Fig. 344). The extension of the peritoneal cut downwards almost as far as the promontory of the sacrum and then forwards in either leaf of the upper mesorectum to reach the rectosigmoid junction, with subsequent ligature and severance of the superior haemorrhoidal vessels on the back of the rectum and clamping and division of the bowel, is better deferred till a later stage of the operation, when the patient has been placed in a slight head-down tilt

and the surgeon has taken his stance on the left side looking into the pelvis (see Fig. 438).

So far the patient has been in a horizontal position and tilted 25° or so to the right with the surgeon standing on that side. For the remainder of the operation the side tilt is undone, a moderate Trendelenburg position is produced, and the surgeon takes his stand on the left side. After the small gut has been packed off into the upper abdomen or turned out of the wound, the lower end of the incision in the posterior parietal peritoneum overlying the aorta is extended downwards on to the right leaf of the sigmoid mesocolon, exposing the inferior mesenteric vessels almost as far as the promontory of the sacrum, at which level they are ligated and divided. From this point the right and left leaves of the sigmoid mesocolon are divided in a line running directly forwards to the back of the rectosigmoid and on to the bowel for a short distance on either side (see Figs 456, 457). The gut can now be clamped and divided between crushing forceps, and the transverse colon stump and rectal stump united by end-to-end anastomosis (see Figs 458, 459), the anastomosis thus following the lines adopted in connection with high anterior rectal resection. There is usually no difficulty in securing a tension-free apposition of the two stumps, but, if necessary, the rectal stump can be further mobilized by manual separation from the front of the sacrum without interfering with its blood supply through the lateral ligaments; this manoeuvre usually enables the upper end of the stump to be drawn upwards for another 5–8 cm at least.

MORE RESTRICTED RESECTION OF THE LEFT
COLON WITH PRESERVATION OF THE
INFERIOR MESENTERIC VESSELS

This follows the lines of the more radical left hemicolectomy just described up to the point where the left colon has been separated from all its peripheral peritoneal attachments and lifted forwards and medially out of the flank. The vessels to the loop are displayed, with the aid of transillumination if necessary, and divided close to the inferior mesenteric vessels as in Fig. 345. The cuts in the medial leaf of peritoneum and mesocolon are then continued to the bowel at the proximal and distal limits of the resection, and the colon divided here between closely applied pairs of Parker-Kerr clamps. Removal of the carcinomatous segment leaves two colon stumps controlled by clamps for union by end-to-end anastomosis.

The question arises as to whether a proximal decompressive vent in the form of a temporary transverse colostomy or caecostomy should be established at the conclusion of any of these resections. I would say that after elective resections of carcinomas of the colon proper, where a peritoneal-covered stump is available on the proximal and distal side of the anastomosis, it should practically never be necessary at the present time to resort to a temporary transverse colostomy, caecostomy or indwelling rectal tube threaded through the anastomosis at the time of operation. (As will be seen on p. 563 the position is quite different with anterior resections for rectal carcinoma where the distal stump is often devoid of a peritoneal coat and leakage is not uncommon.)

Closure of the Wound

The abdomen is then closed by whatever technique the surgeon prefers. So far as the musculo-aponeurotic layers and anterior parietal peritoneum are concerned, there are in general two main types of abdominal wall suture—mass suture and layer suture.

MASS SUTURE

This has been particularly popular in the USA, but more recently it has found some favour also in Britain. It involves the insertion of wide stitches through the entire musculoaponeurotic layers of the abdominal wall including the peritoneum, but not the subcutaneous fat or skin. A favourite suture for this purpose is the 'far-and-near' stitch of Smead (1940), popularized by Jones et al. (1941) of Cleveland, Ohio. It is usually placed as a series of interrupted stitches, but can take the form of a continuous stitch to diminish the number of knots. As for the choice of material, stainless steel wire has been much used in the past and undoubtedly provides a very secure closure (Jones et al. 1941; Spencer et al. 1963), but wire is rather difficult to work with and in recent years plastic sutures (e.g. monofilament Prolene) have often been used instead (Hermann 1974). A controlled trial by Leaper et al. (1977) of mass suture with wire and Dexon respectively showed a combined incidence of

wound dehiscence and subsequent incisional herniation in non-dehisced cases of 4·2% after the former and 7·4% after the latter, a difference that was not statistically significant in their series. This finding and the remarkably low incidence of dehiscence after mass suture with Dexon reported by Bentley et al. (1978) in a series of 814 cases would suggest that much of the virtue of mass suture resides in the wide and firm application of tissue secured by it rather than in the employment of wire for the stitches, as is usually done.

LAYER SUTURE

This method has been more common in Britain. It involves the insertion of two rows of suture in the musculoaponeurotic layers—one in the posterior rectus sheath (including the anterior parietal peritoneum) and the other in the anterior sheath, the former usually being continuous, the latter continuous or interrupted. Originally chromic catgut was the material most favoured for both rows, but in a controlled trial layer suture with catgut was shown to be followed by many more dehiscences and subsequent incisional hernias than was mass suture with wire (Goligher et al. 1975). The addition of large removable tension sutures of strong silk or monofilament nylon, traversing all layers of the abdominal wall including the skin and anterior parietal peritoneum at intervals of 3 cm throughout the length of the wound, lessened the incidence of dehiscence but not of subsequent herniation (Goligher et al. 1975). More recently it has become fashionable to use continuous non-absorbable material such as monofilament Prolene, for at least the anterior rectus sheath and usually for both posterior and anterior sheaths (Jenkins 1976). Controlled trials by Irvin et al. (1977) and Leaper et al. (1977) have shown roughly the same incidence of dehiscence with this technique as with mass suture with wire. I personally have had a considerable experience with suture by means of two rows of continuous Prolene, and can confirm that it is a quick and effective method of closure. Even in contaminated wounds healing can take place without extrusion of the suture material or development of stitch sinuses, but in a small proportion of such patients sinuses do develop and require the removal of the offending suture before complete healing takes place. Usually the suture and particularly the related knot can be plucked out of the sinus with a sterile domestic crochet hook and cut free without having to re-open the wound, and thereafter the discharge soon ceases even if some suture still remains. In a recent controlled trial (1976) of monofilament Prolene, Dexon and Vicryl as the suture materials used for layer suture Irvin et al. (1976) found no difference in the incidence of dehiscence and herniation with the synthetic absorbable materials, but fewer stitch sinuses. A controlled study by Ellis and Heddle (1978) showed, surprisingly, that suture of the parietal layers with non-absorbable material without suture of the anterior parietal peritoneum was followed by no more frequent wound dehiscence than the same closure combined with suture of the peritoneum.

There has always been controversy as to the relative merits of median and paramedian incisions. In an uncompleted controlled trial which examined this point we found little difference in the frequency of dehiscence and subsequent incisional herniation depending on whether a median or paramedian incision was used—just a very slight advantage for paramedian incisions which however would have required series of 600–800 cases to make it statistically significant (McMahon and Goligher 1977, unpublished material).

SUTURE OR NON-SUTURE OF THE SKIN

In all the various controlled trials mentioned in the foregoing three paragraphs different antibiotic or other antiseptic applications—standardized for each trial—were made to the parietal wounds which were then completely closed, including the skin. The efficacy of such local antiseptic treatment in preventing the development of sepsis in sutured wounds is discussed on p. 442. I personally have no experience of the method of instillation into the parietal wound of an antibiotic solution combined with continuous suction during the postoperative period which was found to be so effective in reducing the incidence of local sepsis by McIlrath et al. (1976). The method of leaving the skin and subcutaneous tissues unsutured in large bowel cases, especially if there has been gross faecal contamination during the operation, has been strongly advocated by Turnbull (1966). The subcutaneous wound is packed open with gauze and delayed suture is practised after seven to eight days, when any infection has subsided. To this end skin sutures may be introduced at the time of the original laparotomy but left untied; alternatively good apposition of the skin can be obtained by using closely placed Steristrip adhesive bands.

The site of the anastomosis is usually drained through a separate incision with a sump suction drain or strand of corrugated rubber (see pp. 437, 443).

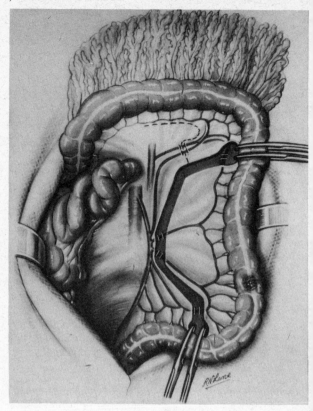

Fig. 345. More restricted left hemicolectomy with preservation of the main inferior mesenteric artery and division of the left colic and first sigmoid arteries close to the main vessels.

POSTOPERATIVE CARE

Postoperative care after colonic resection does not differ materially from that given after any other major abdominal operation involving opening of the alimentary tract. Regarding routine postoperative systemic antibiotics, surgical opinion varies. My practice has been to reserve them for specific infective complications in wound, chest, etc., or for cases with undoubted faecal contamination at operation, though I regularly cover the operation period itself with such therapy. After the effects of the anaesthetic have worn off, the patient is allowed to assume whatever position he finds most comfortable in bed, usually with the head and chest slightly raised. Active movements are encouraged, respiratory exercises are given thrice daily, preceded if necessary by a sedative such as pethidine to minimize the pain which is inseparable from such efforts in the first few days. On the second or third evening he is usually helped out of bed for a few minutes whilst the bed is made; thereafter ambulation is gradually increased. The legs are examined daily for evidence of venous thrombosis, and if calf tenderness or painful limitation of dorsiflexion of the foot is noted anticoagulants are given. As regards the routine administration of prophylactic anticoagulant therapy in the form of low-dosage heparin, this is at present a debatable issue on which each surgeon must make his own policy decision.

Formerly I used to continue the intravenous infusion of $N/5$ saline with 4% dextrose, commenced in the theatre, till intestinal activity was demonstrated to have reasserted itself in a normal way by the detection of vigorous peristaltic sounds on regular auscultation of the abdomen and the passage of flatus per rectum. During this time mouth fluids were severely curtailed and an indwelling nasal gastric tube was usually retained for intermittent suction. I am now convinced that this was an over-cautious attitude, and my present practice is to terminate the 'drip' as soon as it is clear that the patient can manage mouth feeds of 60 or 90 ml hourly without nausea, which is usually within 24 or 36 hours. In the next two or three days the oral feeds are gradually increased and, though they do not at first give the patient a fluid intake comparable to that of a normal healthy adult, they are sufficient to avoid thirst, and serious dehydration does not develop unless paralytic ileus occurs. Gastric suction is no longer employed as a routine, and a nasal gastric or gastroduodenal tube is only passed if the patient should vomit sometime during the postoperative period. Our experience is that such intubation is required in rather less than a quarter of my patients after elective colonic resection. For this reason I have not seen any indication to perform a routine gastrostomy for the purposes of gastric suction, as vehemently advocated by DePeyster and Gilchrist (1958), for all cases undergoing resection of the large bowel.

Flatus is usually passed spontaneously per rectum about the second or third day and the bowels act a day or so later. Their action may be encouraged by the occasional administration of a glycerine suppository, but enemas are obviously contra-indicated, and it is probably wise to avoid aperients, which might damage the suture line in the bowel by vigorous peristalsis. Once the bowels act a light diet is commenced and steadily increased.

Wound drains may be removed on the fourth day but are often required for longer, which has the additional advantage of establishing a definite track down to the anastomosis along which any faecal leak from the bowel may escape to the surface. Skin sutures are removed on the eighth to tenth day, tension sutures on the fourteenth day.

Postoperative Complications

The complications which may follow resection of the colon for carcinoma comprise shock, pulmonary atelectasis and infection, deep leg vein thrombosis and pulmonary embolism, coronary thrombosis, wound sepsis or disruption, paralytic ileus, intestinal obstruction, dehiscence of the anastomosis with leakage, local or general peritonitis, and urinary retention or infection. Most of these conditions are common mishaps after abdominal surgery in general, and will not be further considered in this book. A number, such as shock, paralytic ileus, intestinal obstruction, dehiscence of the anastomosis, peritonitis, faecal fistula, and urinary retention or infection are discussed in connection with operations for rectal cancer (pp. 597–621). But the occurrence of leakage, peritonitis and faecal fistulation in association with colonic resection seem to warrant special comment.

BREAKDOWN OF SUTURE LINE, PERITONITIS AND FAECAL FISTULA

Local, or very rarely diffuse, postoperative peritoneal infection may occasionally be found in the absence of any gross failure of the anastomosis, and is presumably due to contamination at the time of resection, but in the great majority of cases complicated by localized or diffuse peritonitis, an additional finding at re-laparotomy or necropsy is some breakdown of the suture line though whether it is the cause or an effect of the peritonitis is controversial (see p. 425). The dehiscence may vary in extent from a minute leak at one point in the suture line to a wide separation, perhaps with a considerable area of gangrenous bowel. There may have been circumstances at operation predisposing to the subsequent dehiscence—such as excessive tension on the anastomosis, a somewhat impaired blood supply to the bowel ends, or a rough, hasty technique of suture—but sometimes leakage occurs after the most careful operation conducted under ideal conditions. The incidence of anastomotic breakdown is not always clearly stated in reports on the immediate results of resection for carcinoma coli. Hughes (1966a) admits to 14 dehiscences, leading to gross peritonitis or subsequent faecal fistulation in 335 such operations, an incidence of 4·2%. My own experience is similar—and I find, moreover, that separation and leakage are more common in the right colon than the left. But this figure relates to gross dehiscence, detected clinically. If radiological studies are employed, as described on p. 604, the incidence of minor, usually subclinical, dehiscences is much higher.

CLINICAL FEATURES

Local Peritonitis. Though the patient's general condition at first remains good, he develops increasing pain and tenderness in the vicinity of the wound and his temperature is usually elevated. There may be some associated paralytic ileus with a certain amount of abdominal distension. A discharge of pus, and later faecal matter, may occur along the drain and is often followed by a considerable improvement in the patient's condition. But often such discharge is delayed for several days, even when a definite leak has occurred from the anastomosis, and this may confuse the diagnosis.

General Peritonitis. A diffuse peritonitis may manifest itself in several different ways. It may evolve, in a patient who is already believed to have a localized peritonitis, with increasing abdominal distention and a variable amount of tenderness, diminution or absence of peristaltic sounds on auscultation, and a rising pulse rate and temperature. In other cases the onset may be very insidious indeed, with what appears to be paralytic ileus but without any abdominal tenderness or guarding, the general condition being at first well maintained. Occasionally there is just a sudden collapse, the blood pressure falling to a very low level, whilst other signs of peripheral vascular failure develop with dramatic rapidity, and the condition usually proves quickly fatal. Unquestionably postoperative peritonitis may often be very difficult to diagnose, and it should constantly be borne in mind as a cause of ileus or deterioration in the patient's condition after colonic resection.

A plain radiological examination of the abdomen will merely show excessive gaseous distension of the bowel, usually with some fluid levels and rarely evidence of intraperitoneal fluid.

TREATMENT

Localized Peritonitis. If the physical signs are circumscribed and there is no gross distention, and if the patient's bowels are acting and his general condition is good, the treatment should be conservative. A sample of any discharge is sent for bacteriological examination, including determination of sensitivity to various antibiotics, and pending the report the patient is started on a broad-spectrum antibiotic, whilst his progress is observed. The occurrence of a copious spontaneous escape of pus may herald considerable improvement, but occasionally, despite leaving a drain down to the site of the anastomosis at the time of the original operation and maintaining it there for five to seven days, a further limited exploration may later be needed to establish more effective drainage of a pericolic abscess.

If there is some degree of paralytic ileus in association with the local peritonitis it will be necessary also to institute gastric suction by an indwelling nasal tube and to administer intravenous fluids and electrolytes and to note the patient's condition very closely. The important decision to be made is whether the inflammatory process in the region of the anastomosis is being sufficiently contained or whether further surgical intervention is required. For localized peritonitis in relation to the anastomosis after right or transverse colectomy, if it is felt advisable to re-operate, the best plan is to explore the abdomen through the original incision for, if a more limited incision is employed at the site of maximal tenderness, say, in the right iliac region, it is apt to prove inadequate for the intra-abdominal manoeuvres eventually required. If there is peritonitis but no obvious leak from the suture line, it will suffice to provide good drainage to the site of the anastomosis. The establishment of a temporary gastrostomy is a useful addition in saving the patient the discomforts of further prolonged nasal gastric intubation. A day or two later it may be found that faeces are discharging along the new drain. If at the time of the re-laparotomy the anastomosis is discovered to have broken down, it is quite futile to attempt to reconstitute it by suture, for almost inevitably there will be a further dehiscence in due course. The leaking anastomosis should be dismantled and the two ends brought to the surface at separate small incisions as a functioning terminal ileostomy and an inactive colostomy. If the resection was in the distal colon, the choice at re-operation lies between establishment of a right transverse colostomy combined with provision of better drainage of the peritonitis in the left lower abdomen, and separation of the anastomosis to allow the proximal limb of bowel to be fashioned into a terminal colostomy and the distal limb to be either exteriorized or closed by suture, a drain being left down to it.

General Peritonitis. For patients with extensive or generalized peritonitis, re-exploration of the abdomen is required as soon as possible. If the general condition is very poor with gross hypotension, treatment with -plasma infusion, hydrocortisone and, possibly, pressor agents, such as metaraminol (Aramine) or noradrenaline, may be necessary in preparation for laparotomy. At operation the steps to be taken follow the lines already indicated above under Local Peritonitis, but with a greater tendency towards separating the anastomosis and bringing at least the active end to the surface as an ileostomy or colostomy.

In any case with peritonitis, particularly with frank escape of faeces into the peritoneal cavity, an important item in the operation is a thorough peritoneal irrigation with several litres of saline or antiseptic solution such as cephalothin or noxythiolin (see p. 441), and application of antibiotics or providone-iodine to the parietal wound (see p. 442). Equally essential is prompt and vigorous systemic treatment with antibiotics (see p. 443). Simmons (Hau et al. 1978; Hau and Simmons 1978) and Hudspeth (1975) particularly stress the importance of energetic toilet of the peritoneal cavity with removal of fibrinous deposit.

EXTRAPERITONEAL RESECTION

As has already been explained, the place for the Paul–Mikulicz type of resection has now shrunk to quite infinitesimal proportions, but the surgeon may still very occasionally have to resort to it, so that a brief account of the technique of this operation is necessary.

All the steps leading up to the removal of the carcinomatous segment of colon with its related lymphatics are identical with those in a resection with anastomosis. However, for division of the bowel de Martel's (or Cope's) short clamps without handles are preferable, for it is normally better to establish the colostomy at a wound separate from the main incision, and these clamps can be more easily threaded through a small opening than can conventional handled forceps. As a preliminary to exteriorization of the clamped ends, the two limbs of bowel are fastened together for a distance of 7–10 cm to avoid the risk of trapping a loop of small gut when the enterotome is applied postoperatively (Fig. 346A). These stitches of fine silk are inserted preferably along a taenia in each piece of bowel and, when tied, produce a 'double-barrelled' colostomy, the 'barrels' of which are apposed along a line external to the attachment of mesocolon or medial leaf of peritoneum. The cut edges of the latter are finally united by a continuous fine catgut suture taking care to avoid pricking any vessels. The two ends of colon can now be brought out to the surface, either through the main wound, which is closed around them, or preferably through a small separate incision, in order to lessen the risk of wound infection and facilitate the subsequent closure of the colostomy. Thus, in a left hemicolectomy or sigmoid colectomy by the Paul–Mikulicz method, it is an easy matter as a rule to make the colostomy at a small gridiron incision in the left iliac fossa apart from the main left paramedian wound used for the actual resection. Fixation of

the bowel in the wound is perhaps achieved more safely by including conveniently situated appendices epiploicae in sutures in the aponeurosis rather than by direct stitching of the bowel wall to the parietes, which may produce necrosis and subcutaneous fistulas. The skin wound is now sutured snugly round the protruding bowel. Next, the main incision is closed in layers, dressed and covered completely with waterproof Elastoplast. The colostomy wound (or the main wound, if the colostomy emerges through it) is then sealed with a plastic spray. Lastly, dry dressings are placed firmly round the projecting bowel and under the clamps to support them further. If desired, both clamps may be left in position for two or three days as in the Rankin (1945) plan of obstructive resection. But, if the indication for using an extraperitoneal form of resection was at any rate partly the presence of a greater degree of obstruction than would be compatible with a sutured anastomosis, it is preferable to remove the proximal clamp right away and replace it by a Paul's tube, which is tied in position by a ligature of stout braided silk (Fig. 346A).

Postoperative Care

The Paul's tube at first provides a watertight drainage of all discharging faeces but, after five or six days, when the holding ligature cuts through the tube comes out and leakage occurs. About the same time the clamp on the distal limb of bowel separates, and the sooner the enterotome is applied to break down the spur between the two limbs and allow some of the faeces to pass over into the distal bowel, the more comfortable the patient will be.

APPLICATION OF THE ENTEROTOME

There are many different patterns of enterotome available, based on the original instruments of Dupuytren and Mikulicz. Most of them suffer the disadvantage that the end bearing the screw for tightening the clamp projects vertically out of the colostomy for at least 5–7 cm and is liable to be pressed on and moved by the bedclothes, unless they are kept off it by a cage, or, better, by an inverted dressing bowl. My own preference is for the type of enterotome illustrated in Fig. 346B, the blades of which slide on a horizontal bar, which lies against the anterior abdominal wall when in position. This is an altogether more compact arrangement which interferes much less with the patient's movements in bed and his ambulation.

No anaesthetic is needed for the application of an enterotome, but the patient may feel some central abdominal discomfort when the blades are being tightened and it may be necessary to give him a sedative, such as pethidine or morphine, and postpone the final tightening till this has become effective. Before inserting the enterotome the direction of each 'barrel' of the colostomy and the width and depth of the spur should be carefully determined by digital palpation. Some patterns of enterotome can be dismantled so that the two blades may be inserted separately and then the arms are engaged. This is an advantage sometimes when the spur is very wide at its base and the two limbs of bowel do not seem to run closely parallel. But usually it is possible to guide the blades safely into position with the instrument in an assembled condition and widely open. The enterotome is then gradually tightened, the patient's reactions being carefully observed in the process. Even if no pain is experienced it is probably a good plan not to tighten the instrument to its fullest extent in the first instance, but to complete this

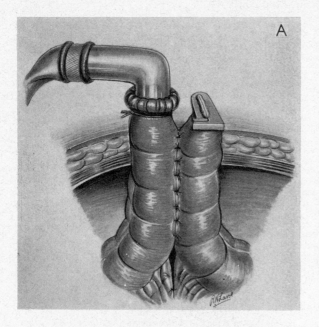

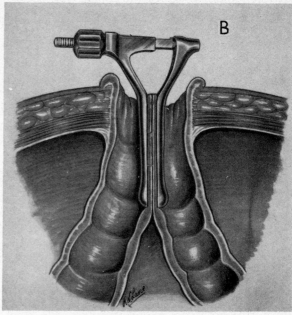

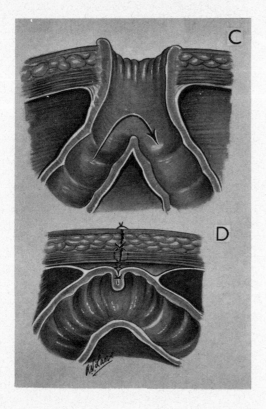

Fig. 346. Paul–Mikulicz type of extraperitoneal resection. (A) Carcinomatous segment has been resected and the two ends of colon have been brought to the surface, a Paul's tube tied into the proximal one, and a Cope's clamp left on the distal one. (B) Application of Lloyd-Davies enterotome. (C) The spur has been largely destroyed so that the faeces can pass mainly into the distal limb of colon. (D) The remaining opening on the abdominal wall has been closed by a small plastic operation.

manoeuvre after 6 or 12 hours so that the blades have time to sink into the tissues of the spur without cutting them through. The projecting part of the enterotome is padded from the abdominal wall by gauze and wool.

Usually an enterotome takes five to six days to cut its way through the spur and become loose. When this happens it should be withdrawn and the spur re-examined with the finger to determine how much remains. If more than one-third persists it is usually well to re-apply the enterotome. Once the spur has been largely destroyed the faeces will pass mainly into the distal bowel and the leakage from the colostomy will diminish markedly (Fig. 346c). In time the colostomy opening will contract, but experience shows that it practically never closes completely, so that there is everything to be said for proceeding to a plastic operation to close the remaining fistula as a routine (Fig. 346D). Immediately after the removal of the enterotome there are still raw areas in the bowel corresponding to the divided spur and associated with these is an inflammatory oedema, which makes operative mobilization and closure of the colostomy difficult and increases the risk of the suture line breaking down and leaking. In my experience it is much better to wait at least four to six weeks before proceeding to final closure of the fistula. The detailed operative technique for closure of the fistula is very similar to that employed in the closure of a transverse colostomy (see p. 484).

Modification of Paul–Mikulicz Operation to Obviate Use of Enterotome

It is customary now to close ordinary loop transverse colostomies by an intraperitoneal operation, without initial 'double-barrelling' of the two limbs of bowel or the application of an enterotome. This technique expedites the process of closure and saves the patient the delay and discomfort associated with the use of an enterotome. The Paul–Mikulicz resection may be similarly modified, omitting the suturing together of the two colon stumps (though bringing together the cut edges of mesocolon or medial leaf of peritoneum) at the first operation, and proceeding after 10 days or so to freeing of the bowel from the abdominal wall and joining the two openings by end-to-end anastomosis, without preliminary application of an enterotome.

RESULTS OF ELECTIVE SURGICAL TREATMENT

Resectability and Operative Mortality

As has been pointed out earlier in this chapter, the last 30 years have seen a progressive lowering of the immediate mortality of radical operations for carcinoma coli; and this achievement has been accomplished despite an increase in the frequency with which resection is being applied to poor-risk patients with advanced lesions, some of them frankly incurable and amenable only to palliative removal. Abundant statistics substantiate this statement.

Thus Allen et al. (1947) reported that during the years 1925–42 when 143 cases of carcinoma of the colon were treated at the Massachusetts General Hospital the resectability rate was 91% and the resection mortality rate 17·5%, most of the operations being two-stage procedures; by contrast during the years 1943–6 105 cases were admitted, and the resectability rate was 95%, the resection mortality rate only 2%, and the majority of the operations were one-stage procedures.

McKittrick (1948) reported that his resection mortality rate in 90 cases of carcinoma coli seen during 1932–41 was 11%, a two-stage operation being often employed; but in 129 cases treated during 1942–7 the resection mortality rate had dropped to 5·4% and in 110 of the patients a one-stage procedure had been adopted with only a 3·6% operative mortality.

Grinnell (1953) in a very illuminating analysis of the experience of the Presbyterian Hospital, New York, in the treatment of 890 cases of carcinoma of the colon found that the resectability rate rose from 50% in 1915–20 to 92·1% in 1945–50, whilst the operative mortality fell from 31·3% to 5·3% for the same periods.

In this country Morgan (1957b) stated that the operative mortality for resection of carcinomas of the left colon at St Mark's Hospital, London, between the years 1928 and 1942 was 14·9% in 87 operations, but between 1943 and 1955 the rate had fallen to 7·4% in 244 operations. This reduction was achieved despite an unspecified increase in the resectability rate.

Our own experiences in Leeds reveal the same trend towards lower operative mortality despite a more frequent application of resection (Table 27). This table brings out another point, namely that the operative mortality of the resections in the distal transverse and left colon was nearly twice that of right-sided colectomies during recent years. Morgan (1957b) mentioned a similar difference in the mortality rates of resections in the left and right colon respectively at St Bartholomew's Hospital, London.

Gilbertsen (1959) reported on the results of operations for cancer of the colon at the Department of Surgery of the University of Minnesota Medical School, Minneapolis, from 1940 to 1955. During this 15-year period 566 patients with colonic carcinoma were seen. The over-all resectability rate was 87%, but 11% were only for palliation. In considering operative mortality Gilbertsen (1959) distinguished between 'regular excisions' and 'enlarged excisions', the latter group including excision of liver, other adherent organs, abdominal wall, etc. The immediate mortality in 393 regular colonic resections was 5·4, but in 80 enlarged resections 27%. It may be noted also that simple colostomy in 41 cases of colon cancer carried an operative mortality of 29%.

TABLE 27. *Resectability Rate and Resection Mortality Rate in the Treatment of Cancer of the Colon at the Leeds General Infirmary between 1938 and 1955*

	1938–43			1947–55		
	Total no. of cases	Resection	Operative deaths	Total no. of cases	Resection	Operative deaths
Right colon growths	36	20 (66%)	4 (20%)	142	79 (55%)	4 (5%)
Distal transverse and left colon growths	151	57 (38%)	12 (21%)	371	204 (55%)	23 (11%)
All growths	187	77 (41%)	16 (21%)	513	283 (55%)	27 (9·5%)

After Smiddy and Goligher (1957).

Hughes (1966*a*, *b*) of Melbourne treated 389 cases of carcinoma of the colon between 1950 and 1964. The resectability rate was 86% (but 17·2% of the cases only had a palliative resection). The operative mortality was 4·8% for all resections or 4·1% for radical resections. Botsford et al. (1970) reported that of 206 patients presenting at the Peter Bent Brigham Hospital, Boston, 70·9% had resection with hope of cure. There were six postoperative deaths, an operative mortality of 4·1%.

Even elderly patients at the present day, despite their general infirmity and frequent associated ailments, seem to stand radical surgery remarkably well, though, not unnaturally, with some increased risks. This is well shown by the analysis made by Jensen et al. (1970*b*) of the fate of 225 patients, aged 70 years or more, with carcinoma of the colon at the Municipal Hospital, Copenhagen from 1950 to 1964. Of these, 150 or 67% proceeded to an ostensibly radical resection, with an operative mortality of 13%.

It must be admitted that most of the figures quoted above relating to operability and operative mortality are derived from major surgical centres, in which it would be reasonable to suppose that the standard of surgical care might be higher than average. An even more important consideration is that the carcinoma coli material dealt with in such centres might not be representative of that encountered in most regional hospitals, particularly in regard to the number of emergency cases with perforation or obstruction. A better idea of the achievements of surgery throughout the country is likely to be obtained from regional statistics, compiled by various cancer registries, which keep records on cancer cases from all hospitals, large and small, in their area. One of the longest established of these is the Connecticut Tumor Registry, which

has records of 12 727 persons (5851 men and 6876 women) with cancer of the colon from 1935 onward (Eisenberg et al. 1967). The operability rate for these growths has risen from 39·5% for males and 38·4% for females in 1935–39 to 60·2% for males 63% for females in 1945–49, whilst in the period 1960–62 it stands at 77% for both males and females. What is not clear is how many palliative excisions and other procedures are included in these percentages in addition to truly radical resections.

The figures from South Western Regional Cancer Bureau in this country (Milnes-Walker 1971) are slightly less favourable. Of 2023 patients registered with carcinoma of the colon from 1962 to 1964 inclusive, 1194 or 59% approximately underwent resection of their growths, but, again, presumably a proportion of these excisions were palliative resections. Finally, the information from the Birming-

TABLE 28. *Carcinoma of Colon (1950–61): Birmingham Cancer Registry. Types of Treatment and Five-year Survival Rates*

Treatment	Total cases	Five-year survival rate (%)	
		Crude	Corrected
Surgery			
Radical	3094 (46·2%)	42·3	52·1
Palliative	1557 (23·3%)	3·1	—
Exploratory	518	0·6	—
Radiotherapy	10	0·0	—
No treatment	1515	0·6	—
Total	6694	20·5	27·0

From Slaney (1971).

ham Cancer Registry (Slaney 1971), which has managed to secure registration of 98% of all cases of malignant disease in the Birmingham (England) region with its population of nearly five million, is even more disappointing (Table 28). Of 6694 cases of cancer of the colon reported in this Registry in the period 1950–61, only 46·2% had radical surgical treatment; another 23·3% received some form of palliative operation. It seems probable, therefore, that, whatever may be the situation for the favoured few, throughout Britain on average rather less than half the patients with cancer of the colon undergo a radical operation for their condition.

Ultimate Survival

SURVIVAL RATE AFTER RESECTION

On the basis of reports from many leading centres and surgeons it has been generally accepted that between 50 and 70% of patients surmounting the immediate hazards of radical resection are likely to be alive and well 5 years later. Thus the crude five-year survival rate for patients who had survived resection was given by Rankin and Olson (1933) as 51%, by Grinnell (1953) as 55·2%, by Gilbertsen (1959) as 60%, by Hughes (1966a) as 62·2% and by Turnbull et al. (1967) as 68·8% in large series of patients followed up by them. But the crude five-year survival rates reported by cancer registries, after what is termed 'resection' or 'surgical treatment', have been less impressive, partly because a proportion of the patients considered in the calculation almost certainly had only palliative excisions performed, and partly because in their statistics those patients alive five years after operation are expressed as a percentage of those submitted to surgical treatment, and not of those surviving that treatment. As a consequence operative deaths are included amongst the non-survivors at five years and make the proportion of five-year survivors correspondingly less. At the Connecticut Tumor Registry Eisenberg et al. (1967) estimated that the corrected* five-year survival rate for 1228 men having surgical treatment for their carcinomas between 1955 and 1959 was 47·4% and for 1434 women surgically treated in the same period it was

* 'Corrected' means corrected from the 'crude' five-year survival rate by means of life tables to exclude deaths due not to carcinoma but to intercurrent conditions. Hence the corrected survival rate is always higher than the crude survival rate, usually by about 10%.

54·8%. At the South Western Regional Cancer Bureau Milnes-Walker (1971) recorded a crude five-year survival rate of only 37% in 1194 patients who underwent resection (sometimes only palliative) in the period 1962–4. Slaney (1971) stated that at the Birmingham Cancer Registry, of 3094 patients having radical resection between 1950 and 1961, 42·3% were alive and well five years later, the corrected five-year survival rate being 52·1% (Table 28).

OVER-ALL OR ABSOLUTE SURVIVAL RATE IN ALL CASES

In some ways a more useful measure of the value of surgical treatment is the overall or absolute survival rate, which expresses the number of patients alive and well after five years as a percentage, not of the immediate survivors of operation, but of the total number of cases presenting to hospital with carcinoma of the colon in the first instance. The absolute survival rate automatically takes into account the resectability and operative mortality rates, as well as the success of the operation in eradicating the growth. Most individual surgeons do not report the absolute survival rates in their series of cases, but a notable exception is Grinnell (1953), who carefully analysed the variations in this rate at different periods from 1916 to 1945 at the Presbyterian Hospital, New York (Table 29). It will be seen that the absolute five-year survival rate over the entire period 1916–45 was 27·4% and that it rose gradually from 5·9% in 1916–20 to a maximum of 32% in 1936–40, thereafter falling to 30·8% in

TABLE 29. *The Absolute Survival Rate of All Cases of Carcinoma of the Colon presenting at the Presbyterian Hospital, New York, from 1916 to 1945 Inclusive*

Years	No. of primary cases admitted	No. of 5-year survivals	5-year survival rate (%)
1916–20	51	3	5·9
1921–5	48	11	22·9
1926–30	75	16	21·3
1931–5	167	42	25·2
1936–40	231	74	32·0
1941–5	318	98	30·8
1916–45	890	244	27·4

From Grinnell (1953).

1941–5. It is difficult to account for this terminal decline for during this last period the resectability rate was at its highest, namely 92·1% (including 16·9% of palliative resections), and the operative mortality at its lowest, namely 5·3%.

The figures for the absolute five-year survival rate at the cancer registries are also interesting. At the Connecticut Tumor Registry, for 1582 male patients registered between 1955 and 1959, the corrected five-year survival rate was 38·4%, and for 1824 female patients during the same period it was 44·8% (Eisenberg et al. 1967); at the South Western Regional Cancer Bureau, for 2036 patients registered during 1962–4, the crude five-year survival rate was 22% (Milnes-Walker 1971); and at the Birmingham Cancer Registry, for the total number of 6694 cases registered between 1950 and 1961, the crude five-year survival rate was 20·5%, the corrected rate 27% (Table 28). The results from the two British registries certainly make depressing reading, for between them these two organizations cover approximately one-sixth of the population of England, and if the findings are representative, they imply that only about a fifth of the patients presenting with cancer of the colon in this country will be alive at the end of five years.

Some interesting data on the 5-year corrected survival rates for carcinoma of the colon for several countries have been compiled from national sources by Cutler and Lourie (1964) and are contained in Table 30.

FACTORS INFLUENCING SURVIVAL RATE

Sex of Patient. As already pointed out (pp. 377, 468), not only is carcinoma of the colon somewhat more frequent in females than males, but the five-year survival rate is slightly higher (Eisenberg et al. 1967).

Age of Patient. It is widely held that the prospects of cure for carcinoma are poorer in *young subjects* than in patients of more usual 'cancer age', because the growths tend to be more active and to have spread more widely by the time they come to operation (see p. 395). In his follow-up studies Gilbertsen (1959) con-

TABLE 30. *Cancers of the Large Intestine Diagnosed 1950–4*[*]: *Survival Experience of Patients under 65 Years of Age at Diagnosis*

Sex and area	No. of patients	5-year corrected survival rate (%)			
		All patients	Confirmed[†] cases		
			Total	Localized tumours	
				All treatments	Treated by surgery
Males					
Denmark	632	30	36	‡	‡
England and Wales	896	33	42	56	56
Finland	186	25	35	53	66
Norway	326	29	36	55	59
U.S. Central‖	1174	41	43	68	71
Connecticut	530	38	41	64	68
Females					
Denmark	779	34	40	‡	‡
England and Wales	1298	33	41	58	59
Finland	258	26	31	53	55
Norway	327	38	44	68	69
U.S. Central	1622	46	48	77	79
Connecticut	770	45	48	76	78

From Cutler and Lourie (1963).

  * Data for England and Wales pertain to cases diagnosed 1952–3; data for Finland and Norway pertain to 1953–6.

  † Diagnosis confirmed by microscopic examination of tissue.

  ‡ Data on patients with localized cancers of the large intestine were not available for Denmark.

  ‖ Combined data from central registries in the states of California, Connecticut, and Massachusetts.

firmed that this is certainly true to some extent, but he emphasized that even patients aged 20–44 years had more than a 40% chance of being alive after having survived a radical operation for cancer of the colon. In this connection the report of Mayo and Pagtalunan (1963) on the experience of the Mayo Clinic is important. They found that no less than 35% of their patients aged less than 30 with carcinoma of the colon (and rectum), unassociated with polyposis or colitis, survived five years after radical surgery (operation deaths excluded). Rosato et al. (1969) also reported favourably on the prognosis of cancer of the colon in young people, but Miller and Liechty (1967) had only 18·2% of five-year survivors in a group of 33 patients with this condition under the age of 30 years.

At the opposite end of the scale in *elderly patients* the prognosis is also somewhat impaired, mainly because of the lower resectability rate and higher operative mortality rate, as pointed out on p. 468. As Jensen et al. (1970*b*) have shown, the crude and corrected five-year survival rates amongst survivors of radical operation for carcinoma coli *over* the age of 70 were 42·3 and 53·8% respectively, which are only slightly inferior to the rates for patients *under* 70 years of age in Denmark after resection for carcinoma coli.

Length of History. Contrary to what might have been expected in some ways, the longer the history of symptoms before the patient comes to operation, the better on average are the prospects of survival, as Copeland et al. (1969) and Slaney (1971) have conclusively demonstrated.

Site of Growth. Some difference of opinion exists as to the influence of the site of the growth in the colon on the ultimate prognosis. Rankin and Olson (1933) and Gilbertsen (1959) found that patients with right-sided growths did rather better than those with lesions in the left colon, and Hughes (1966*b*) and Irvin and Greaney (1977) reported roughly twice as good survival rates for patients with lesions of the right colon as for those with lesions of the left colon. Morgan (1957*b*) and Shepherd and Jones (1971), on the other hand, found the reverse; and Grinnell (1953) and Slaney (1971) noted little difference in the prognosis at different sites, except that the former thought growths at the hepatic flexure had a poorer prognosis and the latter that it was lesions of the splenic flexure that did worst.

Histological Activity and Extent of Spread of Growth. The monumental work of Dukes at St Mark's Hospital, London, in relating the prognosis of patients who have undergone radical surgery for rectal cancer to the extent of spread of the lesion at the time of operation and to its histological type, is referred to elsewhere (p. 402). A similar correlation of pathological findings and prognosis in regard to carcinoma coli has also been undertaken at that hospital, and I am greatly indebted to the consultant staff at St Mark's for kindly allowing me to quote some hitherto unpublished statistics compiled from their cases by Mr Peter Hawley (Table 31).

It will be seen that the influence of the extent of spread on the long-term survival rate is very similar to that noted in connection with carcinoma of the rectum (se Table 43, p. 642), but the proportion of A, B and C cases is rather different, with considerably fewer C cases in the carcinoma coli series. In a study of the outcome in 315 cases of carcinoma coli at the Middlesex Hospital, London, in relation to the extent of spread of the growth as determined by Dukes' dissection; Shepherd and Jones (1971) reached very similar conclusions. These latter authors were also able to demonstrate in B cases that there was a steady worsening of the prognosis with increase in local spread beyond the bowel wall. Surprisingly, peritoneal involvement did not appear very significant unless extensive. Shepherd and Jones (1971) also demonstrated the adverse influence of higher grades of histological activity on the ultimate prognosis.

TECHNIQUE OF RESECTION

As mentioned on p. 442 it has been alleged that an extra-peritoneal type of resection often gives a less adequate removal of a colonic carcinoma than does an intraperitoneal resection with sutured anastomosis, but it is difficult to secure hard comparative data on the subject. More topical has been the claim that attention to certain technical details, designed to lessen the risk of dissemination of malignant cells during the conduct of a resection for cancer of the colon, may improve the results (see p. 443), but again, conclusive information that these precautions do in fact make any difference to the late results is, as yet, lacking. Even the 'no-touch, preliminary isolation' technique, much vaunted by Turnbull et al. (1967), has not in my view been so far adequately evaluated, and I am doubtful whether it will be shown to have a significant effect on the ultimate outcome (see p. 444).

OCCURRENCE OF ACUTE OBSTRUCTION OR PERFORATION

As is explained on pp. 491 and 492, the occurrence of acute obstruction or perforation of the colon in association with colonic carcinoma not only presents many immediate hazards for the patient, but also considerably reduces the prospects of a lasting cure of the disease.

TABLE 31. *Crude and Corrected 5-Year Survival Rates of 308 Patients surviving Radical Operations for Carcinoma Coli at St Mark's Hospital, London between 1948 and 1962*

Dukes' category	No. of cases treated	Crude 5-year survival rate (%)	Corrected 5-year survival rate (%)
A	61	82·0	99·3
B	131	69·0	84·4
C_1	89	59·6	66·3
C_2	19	26·3	35·1

From Hawley (1972).

Diagnosis and Treatment of Recurrent or Inoperable Carcinoma

CLINICAL FEATURES

The detection of recurrence of carcinoma of the colon may be supremely difficult or relatively easy depending on circumstances. The first suspicion of recurrence may be aroused by an insidious failure of general health, with slight loss of weight and energy, and an indifferent appetite; or the patient may have vague discomfort or an actual pain in the abdomen or right lower chest. Rarely bowel symptoms may suggest that something is wrong. At this stage physical examination may be entirely negative. Later signs may manifest themselves which place the diagnosis beyond doubt—the development of a hard irregular enlargement of the liver, the occurrence of a firm mass within the abdomen or pelvis or in the abdominal wall, or the appearance of ascites. When the initial lesion had been in the left colon (or rectum) and the bowel anastomosis after resection lies within reach of the sigmoidoscope, routine examination with this instrument at follow-up may occasionally disclose the presence of residual growth in the vicinity of the suture line.

RADIOLOGICAL INVESTIGATION

X-ray examination may also be helpful. Apart from a routine chest film to exclude pulmonary secondaries, barium enema studies may show recurrence at the site of anastomosis or a fresh primary carcinoma elsewhere in the colon. As Sharpe and Golden (1950), Fleischner and Berenberg (1956), Cronqvist (1957) and Agnew and Cooley (1962) point out, the interpretation of the radiological appearances after an anastomosis may be difficult because artefacts, oedema or spasm may produce filling defects. However, such defects are usually bilateral whilst locally recurrent carcinoma is often more limited in extent, producing only a unilateral defect. But every irregularity, and any mass projecting into the bowel lumen, even the size of a pea, is potentially abnormal, as is also any lack of pliability of the wall or gross irregularity of the mucosal relief at the site of anastomosis. It is a great help to the radiologist if he has a barium enema examination done three to six months after operation; this serves as a base line for assessment of any future changes. Some idea of the value of barium studies in these postoperative cases of colon carcinoma is indicated by Agnew and Cooley's (1962) finding of 12 recurrences and six second primary growths in 111 patients examined.

DIAGNOSIS AND FURTHER OPERATIVE TREATMENT

In very many cases—probably the majority—with recurrent carcinoma the diagnosis is only too evident on clinical examination, with for example gross malignant hepatomegaly, ascites or pleural effusion, and no question of any further operative measures arises. In others, the diagnosis of locally recurrent carcinoma is pretty definitely established on clinical grounds, possibly aided by radiological examination, and there seems some prospect that it might be amenable to further excision. In yet other cases the diagnosis is only strongly suspected. In these latter two groups laparotomy is usually indicated. It seems probable that more regular follow-up examinations conducted in greater detail—including a routine barium enema study—in cases after resection of the colon for carcinoma would result in a greater proportion of patients, doomed to develop recurrence, having it recognized at an earlier stage, when further operative treatment might be possible with more prospect of success. Bacon and Berkley (1959) certainly record some encouraging experiences from the adoption of this policy in the detection and re-resection of 93 recurrent carcinomas of the colon and rectum. In 60 cases the recurrence was in the pelvis, in 25 at a suture line, and in 8 in the abdominal wall. Further excision was possible in 38 of these cases, and 21 patients were alive more than three years afterwards, 15 actually from 5 to 16 years after the second operation.

The usefulness of CEA monitoring in detecting recurrence of colorectal cancer in the liver or elsewhere, possibly at a time when clinical manifestations may be slight or absent, is dis-

cussed on p. 418. It has been suggested that measurement of the plasma enzyme gamma-glutamyl transpeptidase (GGTP) may be of value in diagnosing hepatic metastases, but our studies (Irvin et al. 1973b) and those of Baden et al. (1971) have not substantiated this contention. However, more recently Cooper et al. (1974) have demonstrated that a combination of elevated CEA levels and elevated gamma-glutamyl transpeptidase levels in a patient who has had a previous excision of a colorectal carcinoma strongly suggests the presence of hepatic metastases.

'SECOND LOOK' OPERATION FOR DIAGNOSIS OF RECURRENCE IN ASYMPTOMATIC PATIENTS

In this matter of early detection and further removal of recurrences, Wangensteen (1949) of Minneapolis has gone even further and sought to establish the diagnosis before symptoms or clinical signs have appeared by what he terms 'second look' operation. According to this plan, after excision of cancers in various sites including the colon, if the lymph nodes contain deposits of growth in the operative specimen a further routine laparotomy is carried out six months later to search for and remove any residual growth. If no further growth is found biopsies are made from sites known to be frequently involved by recurrent cancer. If, however, residual tumour is found, all—or a part—of it is excised if possible. Patients who had recurrent cancer removed at a 'second look' operation are subjected to further reoperations at six-monthly intervals, until no residual cancer is found or until the extent of recurrence is overwhelming. Those who have had a final negative look are not submitted to additional operations unless evidence of further recurrence has subsequently been manifested. The second look concept, fundamentally, is one of reoperation on asymptomatic visceral cancer patients. However, Wangensteen has also performed other operations in patients with symptoms suggestive of recurrent tumour; they have been designated 'symptomatic' second look operations to distinguish them from his more usual asymptomatic operations.

A later paper by Gilbertsen and Wangensteen (1962) summarizes their experience with 13 years of the second look programme. It would appear that of the various neoplasms included in this scheme quite the most promising has been cancer of the colon. Approximately half the *asymptomatic* patients submitted to a second look operation are found to have residual growth. Of 43 cases of colon cancer thus demonstrated to have remaining tumour at a second look, nine died in the immediate postoperative period after this intervention or after subsequent review operations, but four patients eventually achieved a negative final look, giving a salvage rate of 11·8%. This may not seem very high—and the price in terms of operative mortality pretty steep—but it must be remembered that all these patients would otherwise have died. The achievement of second look operations in *symptomatic* patients, coming to second look operation after a previous colon resection, were even more impressive. Of 36 such patients six died after the second (or subsequent) look operation, whilst six, or 20%, had a final negative look.

I personally have never practised the second look procedure on asymptomatic patients, but I have done a few re-explorations on patients with known or suspected recurrence and occasionally have found conditions suitable for a further excision. In most of these cases some temporary palliation was achieved, but I have had only two patients (with colonic growths) who did not ultimately recur. Whilst it probably is a good thing for the surgeon to be imbued with a determination to deal radically with recurrences, if at all possible, it is important that this ambition should be tempered by the realization that most patients will not be cured by re-excision and some may be made very much worse if convalescence is prolonged or complications such as a faecal fistula result. Whether significantly earlier detection of recurrence at an asymptomatic stage by serial CEA determinations can provide a more favourable state of affairs for second-look operations, as claimed by Martin et al. (1979), is a matter of some dispute (Moertel et al. 1978). Perhaps CAT scanning for soft tissue swellings due to recurrence may have a role to play in future.

ALTERNATIVE NON-SURGICAL MEASURES IN THE TREATMENT OF RECURRENT OR INOPERABLE GROWTHS

RADIOTHERAPY

It is generally agreed by radiotherapists that carcinomas of the intestinal tract are relatively radio-insensitive. Nonetheless, carcinoma of the rectum sometimes responds to radiotherapy, particularly of megavoltage type (see p. 655). In the treatment of colon carcinomas by X-rays, however, a further difficulty encountered is that the irradiation required inevitably involves a considerable part of the abdominal viscera, which is apt to result in uncomfortable general disturbances for the patient—the so-called 'irradiation sickness'. Though an occasional intestinal growth may appear to be benefited by radiotherapy—especially if combined with chemotherapy (see below)—in most cases the improvement is highly dubious or negligible and is completely outweighed by the inconvenience of the side effects to the patient. In other words, the surgeon will usually look in vain for worthwhile assistance from his colleagues in radiotherapy in the management of recurrent or inoperable cancers of the colon.

CHEMOTHERAPY

Cancer chemotherapy has been tried in cases of advanced, inoperable or recurrent carcinomas of the colon, the drugs being administered systemically or by intra-arterial infusion, and used as the sole form of treatment or given in combination with radio- or antibiotic therapy.

Systemic Chemotherapy with 5-Fluorouracil

From the publications of Hurley and Ellison (1960) and Rochlin et al. (1962, 1965), it seems that the most promising drug to use against intestinal growths is 5-fluorouracil. Rochlin et al. (1965) emphasize two important points in the conduct of chemotherapy: firstly, that it is essential to press the dosage to the stage at which actual toxicity is produced; and secondly, that when some improvement has been achieved the administration should not then be interrupted but on the contrary should be continued, either in the form of repeated courses with the patient being carried to a toxic state each time, as recommended by Curreri et al. (1958), or as a maintenance dose given at regular intervals, as preferred by Rochlin himself. The detailed regimen employed by Rochlin et al. (1962, 1965) for 5-FU was as follows:

An initial loading dose was given, consisting of three to five daily injections, 15 mg/kg of body weight, administered rapidly by the intravenous route, the maximum amount of drug allowed on any one day being 1 g. If no severe toxicity (e.g. nausea, vomiting, diarrhoea or severe stomatitis) occurred, an additional intravenous injection of 7·5 mg/kg of body weight was given every other day until toxic manifestations appeared. The end point of the regimen was determined by a white blood cell count below 4000. Leucopenia was generally preceded by the gastro-intestinal symptoms and stomatitis, so if these symptoms were severe the drug was stopped, since leucopenia inevitably followed. Gastrointestinal symptoms alone, without leucopenia, were never accepted as an indication to terminate the treatment. The leucocyte count was closely observed and, as soon as it returned to a level of 4000, intravenous therapy was resumed at a level of 15 mg/kg of body weight twice a week. The amount of drug administered was gradually decreased to a maintenance dosage of 15 mg/kg of body weight once a week.

Toxicity occurred in all patients treated by Rochlin et al. (1962), since their end point for initial treatment was leucopenia. Stomatitis was usually the first ill-effect noted, and often appeared three to five days after the commencement of therapy. Ulceration of the mouth did not usually occur till between the sixth and tenth days of the regimen. The stomatitis was quite resistant to any form of local treatment. Nausea was very occasionally the earliest sign of toxicity and occurred after the first injection of the drug. It and the associated vomiting and diarrhoea responded in many instances to antiemetics. The combination of severe nausea, vomiting and diarrhoea was sometimes responsible for severe dehydration and electrolyte depletion which necessitated admission to hospital for careful replacement therapy in approximately 10% of the patients. Occasionally patients with diarrhoea showed ulceration on barium enema examination similar to that seen in ulcerative colitis (but Milles et al. (1962) showed that in many cases on systemic 5-FU therapy diarrhoea occurred in the absence of any histological changes in the colonic mucosa). Apart from leucopenia, severe haemotological depression was sometimes revealed by the occurrence of thrombocytopenia. Depilation of the skin and dermatitis were also fairly frequent complications.

In a series of 178 patients with tumours in various sites treated with systemic 5-FU therapy by Rochlin et al. (1962) there were nine deaths whilst under treatment—one due to severe gastro-intestinal bleeding, diarrhoea and shock within eight hours of the start of the injections, four due to dehydration, leucopenia and septicaemia, and four to ill-defined causes in very undernourished, cachectic subjects.

Clinical Response. One of the difficulties has been to assess improvement after chemotherapy. Rochlin et al. (1962) have been guided by the following considerations: (1) disappearance or marked regression in the size of the tumour; (2) weight gain; (3) return to normal activity; and (4) subjective relief of symptoms. Applying these criteria to a group of 144 cases of colon cancer treated by 5-FU, Rochlin et al. (1965) found that 40 obtained a good response and 16 a poor one, whilst 74 patients showed no improvement and 14 could not be properly assessed. The average length of remission in cases showing a favourable response was 7·9 months (range 2–32 months), but several patients were still in remission at the time of writing, so that future analyses of the results should show a larger average period of improvement.

Systemic Chemotherapy with 5-FU, CCNU and Vincristine

Though Giles et al. (1974) did not find that CCNU as the single therapeutic agent was any more effective than say, 5-FU, it had the advantage that it could be taken by mouth. Also it seemed likely that a combination of CCNU with other agents might provide more remissions. Moertel et al. (1975) have reported favourably on triple therapy with 5-FU, methyl CCNU and vincristine with which in a controlled trial they were able to secure a good objective response in 43·5% of patients, compared with 19·5% with 5-FU alone. This combination seems to be the best available for systemic chemotherapy of colorectal cancer at the moment. For details of the dosage schedule employed reference should be made to Moertel et al. (1975).

Systemic Chemotherapy Combined with Supervoltage Radiotherapy

Moertel et al. (1964) have combined systemic treatment with 5-fluorouracil with supervoltage radiotherapy in the management of advanced gastrointestinal cancers, the two forms of therapy being administered simultaneously. Of the 44 patients treated in this way, which included 22 with large bowel carcinomas, some 37% stated that they had obtained complete remission of symptoms and 12% claimed considerable symptomatic relief, the average period of improvement being approximately seven months. More striking was the finding that in four patients with palpable colonic lesions, which could be easily measured to serve as an index of response to therapy, two underwent complete objective remission and a third diminished considerably in size.

Chemotherapy by Intra-arterial Infusion

The technique, introduced by Sullivan et al. (1953), of treating carcinomas of the head and neck by a slow infusion over several days or weeks of cytotoxic drugs into the supplying artery through an indwelling catheter, has been applied to advanced intestinal growths as well by Ariel (1957). The cathether was inserted through the femoral artery, exposed just below the inguinal ligament into the aorta. If the treatment was for cancer of the pelvis or left colon the end of the catheter was manipulated to be 5–7 cm above the bifurcation of the aorta, but if efforts were being made to alleviate hepatic (or gastric) cancer, the catheter was threaded up to the level of the coeliac axis. Once the desired position had been achieved the catheter was fixed in position by stitching it to the femoral artery with a fine catgut suture. Mechlorethamine hydrochloride (nitrogen mustard), 10 mg dissolved in 10 ml of isotonic saline, was injected daily, followed immediately by an injection of oxytetracycline, 0·5–1 g in 100 ml of saline, which was claimed by Barberio et al. (1953) to potentiate the action of the nitrogen mustard. Before each injection tourniquets were applied to each thigh. The treatment usually continued for five days.

Among 60 patients treated by Ariel (1957) for various forms of advanced abdominal cancer were 23 with growths of the large intestine. All died 1–36 months after therapy, the average period of survival being five months. It is claimed that several of them with severe perineal pain obtained some relief of this symptom, which was occasionally assuaged in a dramatic manner. The complications included the usual haemopoietic depression as well as nausea and vomiting and patchy gangrene of the skin.

Lawton (1965) has used 5-fluorouracil by intra-arterial infusion combined with supervoltage radiotherapy. Two techniques were employed for placing the catheter in the artery. By one, the placement was effected at laparotomy, the catheter being inserted into the internal iliacs through the common iliac artery for pelvic growths, or into the hepatic through the gastro-duodenal artery for hepatic metastases. Alternatively, if the opportunity had not been taken at operation to introduce a catheter or no exploration was carried out, insertion was conducted indirectly by the Seldinger technique through the femoral or brachial arteries. Another indirect method of getting a catheter into the internal iliac was through the superior or inferior gluteal artery, exposed by an incision in the buttock. The catheter was then connected via a small portable electric motor pump to a plastic bag containing the infusate. A slow injection could thus be maintained whilst the patient was ambulant over a period of a fortnight or so, the dosage of 5-FU being 5 mg/kg of body weight per day for intrahepatic catheters, often increased to 10 mg/kg of body weight for intrailiac catheters. Simultaneous radiotherapy was given from a cobalt bomb.

Lawton (1965) records several striking examples of complete objective regression of advanced growths under treatment with this regimen, as has Taylor (1978) for perfusion of the liver for colorectal liver metastases.

SIMPLE PALLIATIVE MEASURES

Unfortunately the conduct of chemotherapy for colorectal cancer is gravely handicapped by the lack of a drug that is really effective against this tumour. Till such an agent becomes available the successes of chemotherapy will remain slight, transient and very difficult to predict. Moreover, they are achieved often at the expense of considerable side effects, such as gastrointestinal upsets, anaemia or loss of hair, which largely outweight the benefits, and in many cases the patient experiences only the side-effects and derives no advantage at all from the drug. A dispassionate appraisal would imply that the indications for chemotherapy in this condition ought to be very limited, but such an objective approach is difficult for the clinician to achieve in the management of incurable cancer, whilst he has to contend on the one hand with the anguish and despair of his patients and their relatives, who demand that something should be done, and on the other hand with the persistent propaganda of powerful commercial interests responsible for marketing new chemotherapeutic agents.

For the great majority of cases with recurrent or inoperable lesions simple palliative measures are best, and early recognition of this fact by the surgeon will spare his patient the complications, discomforts and ultimate disappointment often associated with the other forms of therapy outlined above. Such measures comprise modification of diet to suit the patient's reduced appetite, aperients or enemas to assist bowel function, if required, partial or total bed rest, paracentesis for gross ascites, and analgesics culminating finally in opiates. Relatives often ask the probable duration of this terminal phase, but it is extremely difficult to prognosticate in the individual case. In a group of 583 cases at the Mayo Clinic with inoperable or recurrent cancer of the colon and rectum managed along simple palliative lines Pestana et al. (1964) found that 10% lived over two years, and 2% over five years, but the average length of survival was about 10½ months for colon cancer cases and 8½ for cases with rectal cancer. In general, the survival period was related to the grade of malignancy of the growth (11 months with Broders' Grade I cases, but 5½ months with Grade IV cases), and to the location of the metastases (14½ months when these were confined to adjacent organs or nearby nodes, 10 months when extra-abdominal nodes, lungs, etc. were involved, 8½ months when peritoneal carcinomatosis was present, and 9 months when the liver was involved).

Pestana et al. (1964) also compared the survival period in this group of patients having purely expectant treatment and that of a series of 272 inoperable or recurrent cases of rectal or colonic carcinoma receiving radiotherapy. Though a straight comparison of the two groups showed that those having irradiation survived longer, this was accounted for largely by the more advanced state of the majority of the growths in the series not submitted to drug treatment. Restricting the comparison to cases in both groups with lesions confined to adjacent tissue or nodes, the average survival times were almost identical—15 months in 126 patients with radiotherapy, and 14½ months for 88 patients without.

TREATMENT OF CARCINOMA OF THE COLON WITH ACUTE OBSTRUCTION

The treatment of this emergency calls for special consideration for, when a carcinoma has caused acute obstruction, immediate resection is attended by special difficulties and dangers. The patient's general condition may be so affected by the obstruction as to reduce seriously his fitness for a major operation. The highly septic nature of the contents of the obstructed colon, unchecked by any form of intestinal preparation; the oedematous, friable condition of the bowel wall, making it unsuitable for intestinal suture; and the greatly distended state of the colon, which may render operative manipulations in the abdomen unusually difficult—all contrive to increase the hazards of primary resection in these cases.

For these reasons it has become the traditional teaching that in operating upon patients with acutely obstructed carcinomas of the colon the surgeon's prime objective must be to relieve the obstruction by proximal colostomy, caecostomy, or a short-circuiting operation, and that the eradication of the growth and its lymphatic field is a secondary consideration best reserved for a later operation. Though this doctrine is now fairly generally accepted, surgical opinion is still divided as to the ideal emergency measures to be adopted in accordance with it for obstructed growths in different parts of the colon. In addition the whole conception of avoiding primary resection in the presence of acute obstruction has been subjected to increasing criticism in recent years.

Choice of Drainage Operation for Acutely Obstructed Carcinomas in Various Segments of the Colon

CARCINOMA OF SIGMOID OR DESCENDING COLON

Transverse colostomy is now mostly preferred as the initial drainage operation for acute obstructions of the left colon. If the opening is placed in the now classical site at the right end of the transverse colon, as recommended so strongly by Devine (1931, 1948), it is out of the way of any subsequent resection. Further it completely defunctions the distal colon and permits of it being thoroughly cleansed of retained faeces by irrigations and treated by instillations of sulphonamides or antibiotics, so that

it is in a clean, collapsed and relatively sterile condition for the resection. The disadvantage of a transverse colostomy is that it necessitates yet a third operation for its closure after the resection. To obviate this drawback it has been suggested by Waugh (1954) and Brooke (1955) that the colostomy should be placed not in the transverse colon, but a few centimetres proximal to the growth, wherever it may be situated, so that colostomy and carcinoma can be excised together at the subsequent resection operation. There is no denying that it is somewhat inconvenient having the colostomy in the operative field during the latter operation. A more serious objection to an immediately proximal colostomy is that by bringing the bowel to the surface close to the growth one may foster the development of metastases in the wound, as occurred with the old Paul–Mikulicz type of resection, especially when of rather restricted extent, and I do not favour this method of a closely placed colostomy.

Caecostomy used to be the popular operation for obstruction due to growths in the left colon, and it still has its advocates especially among the older generation of surgeons. Like a transverse colostomy it is agreeably remote from the actual growth and does not impede its later removal, but it has the advantage that it may close spontaneously when the tube is removed from the caecum. If necessary, it can be performed under local anaesthesia through a small incision in the right iliac region, which may be useful in very ill late cases. It is also true that in some cases a transverse colostomy is impracticable because of the obesity of the abdominal wall and the fact that the gross distension of the bowel has 'used up' the leaves of the transverse mesocolon, which together make it impossible to bring a loop of colon to the surface. Under these circumstances drainage from the caecum by caecostomy may be the only method of relieving the obstruction.

Caecostomy is criticized on the grounds that it merely decompresses the large bowel and does not provide a total diversion of faeces to the surface, so that the conditions for the subsequent resection are not so satisfactory as after a colostomy. This is true, but a caecostomy can be made reasonably effective in this respect by assiduous attention to postoperative care; by means of really frequent irrigations— say every two or three hours—it is possible over a period of 10–14 days to clean and decompress the colon in a fairly adequate manner, and by the use of locally acting antibiotics to render it suitable for resection with anastomosis. Hughes (1963) stresses the value of manual compression of the colon through the laparotomy wound in securing initial deflation and drainage of faeces through a tube caecostomy, and the importance of frequent wash-outs every few hours subsequently.

Another consideration in regard to the choice of transverse colostomy or caecostomy is the relative safety of the two operations. Our experience in the Leeds General Infirmary is that transverse colostomy is a much safer operation than caecostomy (Goligher and Smiddy 1957). Thus during the years 1938–43 and 1947–53, 47 transverse colostomies were performed for obstructed growths in the left colon with eight deaths, a mortality of 17%, whilst during the same period 74 patients with acute obstruction of carcinomas of the left colon were subjected to caecostomy with 36 deaths, a mortality of 49%. Admittedly the difference in the results may have been due partly to the manner in which patients were chosen for the two operations, for probably caecostomy was selected as a specially suitable minimal procedure in some desperately ill cases, thus loading the scales against it. It is perhaps significant, however, that the cause of death in nearly two-thirds of the fatalities after caecostomy was some form of sepsis, whereas none of the deaths after transverse colostomy could be attributed to infection. This seems to constitute a grave indictment of the former operation. Welch and Donaldson's (1974a) results were also greatly in favour of transverse colostomy as against caecostomy. In fairness, however, it must be mentioned that Campbell et al. (1956), Muir (1956) and Maynard and Turell (1955) found that caecostomy and transverse colostomy employed as emergency procedures for obstructed carcinomas of the left colon carried roughly equal risks. Gerber and Thompson (1965) came to the conclusion that caecostomy was safer than transverse colostomy, and King et al. (1966) strongly recommended caecostomy. Clark and Hubay (1972) also felt that caecostomy was a satisfactory emergency operation for acute large bowel obstruction. Hughes (1963) gave an account of 31 personally conducted tube-caecostomies for carcinoma of the left colon or rectum with only one operative death, which indicates that this can be a very safe operation in experienced hands. But Balslev et al. (1970) reported a 7% operative mortality in 76 patients with acutely obstructed carcinomas of the colon treated by caecostomy. Wound infection occurred in ten cases, and relief of the obstruction was inadequate in eight cases, three of which died from perforation of the colon. In half the cases the caecostomy failed to close spontaneously and required operative closure.

My own preference in the treatment of obstructed left colon growths by drainage is for a subhepatic transverse colostomy; caecostomy is reserved for cases in which for technical reasons a colostomy is found to be impracticable. In the performance of a transverse colostomy it is important to ensure that *the loop of bowel brought to the surface lies to the right of the middle colic artery*, for, if it is desired to carry out a radical left hemicolectomy subsequently with sacrifice of the inferior mesenteric vessels, the proximal colon stump will be dependent on the middle colic branch for its blood supply.

CARCINOMA OF SPLENIC FLEXURE OR DISTAL TWO-THIRDS OF TRANSVERSE COLON

Choice of drainage again rests between transverse colostomy and caecostomy. But the former is certainly liable to interfere with the subsequent resection if it is placed in the Devine position, and if a transverse colostomy is employed it is probably better to site it fairly close to the growth so that it may be deliberately resected with the latter in due course. The alternative of caecostomy has the merit of being well out of the field of the subsequent excision—unless a right hemicolectomy is performed, and then it is easily detached from the anterior abdominal wall—and is the operation I used to favour for obstructions in this site (but in recent years I have preferred where possible to carry out immediate right hemicolectomy extended into the descending or sigmoid colon—see p. 477).

CARCINOMA OF CAECUM, ASCENDING COLON OR RIGHT END OF TRANSVERSE COLON

For an obstructed lesion of the right colon some surgeons used to prefer a side-to-side ileotransverse colostomy, others a caecostomy or even an ileostomy (but there is in my opinion much to be said for immediate right hemicolectomy—see p. 477—and this view is probably shared by the majority of surgeons at the present day).

Immediate Resection for Carcinoma with Acute Obstruction

The principle of eschewing resection in the presence of obstruction has been challenged, notably by Wangensteen (1949), Baronofsky (1950), Wright (1951), Gregg (1955), Smith et al. (1955), Ferguson and Chase (1957), Sames (1960), Gerber et al. (1962), Glashan and John (1965) and Savage (1967), who argue that with attention to technical details a primary excision can often be undertaken with safety and may indeed be the simplest way of relieving the obstruction. It has, too, the great advantage over preliminary drainage with later resection that the patient is spared the discomforts and inconvenience of at least two and usually three abdominal operations before the growth is finally eradicated and intestinal continuity restored. Sometimes after a simple drainage procedure, if the patient has had a particularly troublesome convalescence with several complications, he may refuse to countenance any further operations and is thus left with an unremoved carcinoma. A primary resection avoids this unfortunate state of affairs. Furthermore, it has been suggested by Fielding and Wells (1974) that the long-term prognosis in obstructed cases may be better after primary resections than after staged operations involving preliminary decompression and later resection. However, as Irvin and Greaney (1977) point out, this is possibly a fallacious opinion based on the fact that the majority of Fielding and Wells (1974) cases that were submitted to primary resection had growths in the right colon whilst most of those treated by staged resection had their growths in the left colon. The five-year survival after resection of obstructed (or non-obstructed) carcinomas of the right colon has been shown by Hughes (1966a) and Irvin and Greaney (1977) to be almost twice as high as that of carcinomas of the left colon, which could easily explain the difference in the outcome after primary and staged resection in Fielding and Wells' (1974) study without having to postulate any deleterious effect of staging *per se*.

For obstructed carcinomas of the *right colon* the *a priori* case for primary resection is certainly very strong. A right hemicolectomy involves no greater hazards of anastomosis than does a simple ileotransverse colostomy and may indeed be safer than the latter operation in that it obviates the danger of rupture of the caecum due to continued distension of this organ if the ileocaecal valve remains competent. Actually, when the competence of this valve is maintained, it protects the small bowel from distention, so that the anastomosis with or without hemicolectomy in these cases is often between lower ileum of nearly normal calibre and collapsed transverse colon and thus may not be specially dangerous despite the obstruction. Our experience of right hemicolectomy for obstructed growths of the right colon certainly shows that it can be a safe operation (Goligher and Smiddy 1957).

For obstructed carcinomas of the *left colon* the argument for primary resection has been less persuasive, mainly because in such cases the large bowel can be so easily and satisfactorily decompressed by a proximal transverse colostomy, which

provides such excellent conditions for a later resection. One would be apprehensive, too, that however well the colon might be emptied by suction tubes (such as the decompressor described by Savage (1967)) during a primary segmental resection in the left colon in the presence of acute obstruction, an anastomosis of the remaining stumps of bowel might be specially liable to leak, though Savage (1967) has reported very impressive results with primary resection and anastomosis. Of course, an emergency colectomy of Paul–Mickulicz type avoids the dangers of an intraperitoneal anastomosis, and, for cases with a growth too low in the sigmoid or rectosigmoid for the lower stump to be brought to the surface for a Paul–Mikulicz resection, a Hartmann's operation (see p. 592) may be employed instead, as recommended by Sames (1960), the collapsed distal segment being closed by suture, whilst the proximal segment is brought out as an active colostomy. After six or eight weeks a further laparotomy is carried out to free the colostomy from the abdominal wall and unite it to the blind distal stump, but this step may be deferred indefinitely depending on how the patient took the initial intervention.

Another more audacious way of effecting a primary resection of an obstructed carcinoma of the left colon anywhere down to the lower sigmoid without exposing the patient to the possible dangers of an anastomosis in distended oedematous bowel, is to perform an immediate subtotal or total colectomy with ileosigmoid or ileorectal anastomosis. This method, which has been particularly championed by Hughes (1966a) in suitably selected cases, has the same advantages as right hemicolectomy for obstructed carcinomas of the right colon—namely that it removes all the distended part of the large bowel and provides for a relatively safe union between the normal or nearly normal terminal ileum and the undistended distal colon or upper rectum beyond the site of the lesion. Thus the carcinoma is removed and the obstruction is relieved in one manoeuvre without subjecting the patient to a period of colostomy or caecostomy life and to at least one further operation to complete the surgical treatment.

THE AUTHOR'S PREFERENCES AND RECOMMENDATIONS

I regard right hemicolectomy as the operation of choice for cases with *obstructed carcinomas of the right colon*, unless the patient's condition is poor, or a combination of a very fixed growth and considerable colonic distension is present, which would make resection difficult or dangerous. Under the latter circumstances, a caecostomy or an ileostomy with divided loop—both ends being brought to the surface—or a simple ileotransverse colostomy should be preferred.

For *obstructed carcinomas of the transverse colon, splenic flexure or proximal descending colon*, I personally prefer an extended right hemicolectomy or subtotal colectomy with ileosigmoid anastomosis. However, I would not recommend this practice as a routine to inexperienced surgeons, for in the presence of gross colonic distension the mobilization of the bowel and growth, particularly in the region of the splenic flexure, may be extremely difficult and the colon may be torn in the process. To such surgeons, unless conditions appeared very favourable, I would advise a simple tube caecostomy or a transverse colostomy placed close to the growth, so that it will subsequently be resected with the lesion.

For *obstructed carcinomas of the lower descending or sigmoid colon or the rectosigmoid*, I have until recently been unconvinced that primary resection was as safe in general as a two-stage operation consisting of a loop transverse colostomy in the first instance and an elective resection with simultaneous (or subsequent) closure of the colostomy at the second stage. But in the last few years I have had some impressive experiences with immediate resection, either using the Hartmann procedure or preferably performing a subtotal colectomy with end-to-end or side-to-end ileosigmoid or ileorectal anastomosis. This latter operation has been remarkably well borne even in elderly patients and has usually been followed by a most acceptably swift convalescence, but it is not a procedure for the trainee surgeon.

Clinical Assessment and Preoperative Care

Fortunately the general condition of patients with obstruction due to carcinoma of the colon is often quite good, because vomiting with its resulting dehydration and electrolyte depletion is usually a late phenomenon.

A plain X-ray examination of the abdomen is of the greatest possible value in diagnosis and in determining the exact site of the neoplasm. It will show whether there is gaseous distension of the large or small bowel, and careful observation of the distal extent of the colonic gas shadow will localize the lesion with fair accuracy. Sometimes, however, with obstructing growths of the sigmoid colon, the distension of the descending colon is now well

shown and an erroneous diagnosis of carcinoma of the splenic flexure may be made. In volvulus of the sigmoid, which is an important source of confusion in diagnosis, X-ray examination usually demonstrates clearly the grossly dilated sigmoid loop and avoids error. Generally the plain film gives all the information that is required, but if the appearances are at all difficult to interpret no hesitation should be felt about proceeding to an emergency barium or gastrografin enema examination, which carries no particular dangers, is well tolerated as a rule and may be most revealing.

An attempt may be made in the first instance to relieve the obstruction by one or two soap and water enemas, particularly if the growth is located in the sigmoid and if the patient has recently passed some flatus, suggesting that the blockage may not be quite complete. If this fails arrangements must be made for operation. Certain preoperative measures, however, are necessary. Dehydration and electrolyte deficiency, if present, should be corrected by intravenous therapy, and it is a wise precaution in all cases to have an intravenous infusion commenced before operation. When vomiting is a symptom, or if the X-ray examination reveals gaseous distension of the small gut, it is imperative to pass a Ryle's tube or No. 7 or 8 English gauge oesophageal tube to empty the stomach and avoid regurgitation of gastric contents during induction of the anaesthetic. Long gastrointestinal tubes of the Miller-Abbot or Cantor type are unsuitable in these emergency cases because of the time required to induce them to negotiate the pyloric sphincter and upper intestinal tract. Furthermore, decompression of the small gut usually has no influence on the distension of the large gut and therefore cannot obviate the necessity for operative treatment. Once dehydration and electrolyte depletion have been sufficiently corrected, further delay in submitting the patient to operation is to be deprecated.

Operative Procedure

'BLIND' DRAINAGE OPERATION *versus* ABDOMINAL EXPLORATION

In the past surgeons such as Burgess (1929) and Lockhart-Mummery (1922) advocated an entirely 'blind' caecostomy without exploration of the abdomen, in order to minimize shock and avoid the risk of rupturing the distended colon or the growth by manipulation during laparotomy. But with modern resuscitative measures and the present high standard of general anaesthesia, most patients can be made fit for a gentle exploration to confirm the diagnosis and site of the lesion without any danger of intestinal rupture. Such a laparotomy avoids the risk of a mistake in diagnosis, which may occur despite apparently conclusive clinical and radiological evidence. It is a real tragedy to misdiagnose a volvulus of the sigmoid and treat it by blind caecostomy or transverse colostomy. Consequently, except for patients who are almost moribund and for whom a 'blind' caecostomy may indeed be life-saving, I would always advise a limited exploration.

CHOICE OF APPROACH

1. If the clinical and radiological examinations have definitely located the obstruction in the left colon *a small transverse incision* is made in the right upper abdomen in the situation where the right subhepatic transverse colostomy will be established if the diagnosis is confirmed at exploration. As it is deepened it cuts across the fibres of the rectus muscle and sufficient of the abdominal wall lateral to this to allow of the hand being inserted into the abdomen. The liver is then palpated and the position and state of the primary growth determined. Finally a transverse colostomy is established in the outer part of the wound, the remainder of the incision being closed snugly round it.

2. If the growth has been firmly diagnosed pre-operatively as situated in the right colon, the correct approach will be through a *small right paramedian incision* centred opposite the umbilicus. After exploration this can be enlarged as required to provide sufficient access for the performance of a right hemicolectomy or ileotransverse colostomy, or closed and a separate incision made in the right iliac region for the establishment of a caecostomy.

3. In cases where it is believed that the obstruction lies in the large gut but its precise situation has not been determined before operation, it is often advised that a right paramedian incision should be used for general exploration of the abdomen. Experience shows, however, that the lesion in these cases usually turns out to be in the sigmoid colon, and for its subsequent resection at a second stage a left paramedian incision will often be desirable. But to use such an approach within two or three weeks of a right paramedian incision may result in sloughing of the intermediate strip of abdominal wall, as I know from bitter experience. The surgeon is thus compelled to conduct the resection instead through a right paramedian incision in the line of the old wound or through a left oblique incision, neither of which gives entirely satisfactory access for a modern radical left hemicolectomy. It is better therefore in imperfectly diagnosed cases to carry out the initial exploration through a *left paramedian* or *median approach*. If the obstruction is found after all to be in the right colon it is not a difficult matter as a rule to perform a right hemicolectomy or ileotransverse colostomy through this incision, and if necessary a transverse extension to the right across the right rectus can be added at the upper end.

ASSESSMENT OF RESECTABILITY AND TREATMENT OF UNRESECTABLE CASES

It is difficult to assess with accuracy the fixity of a growth during an emergency laparotomy for acute obstruction, and it is well to err on the side of optimism. Sometimes carcinomas seem to become less fixed after the obstruction has been relieved. It has also to be borne in mind that the emergency operation is often performed by a relatively junior surgeon whose standards of resectability may be much lower than those of the more experienced surgeon who will probably undertake the subsequent resection. A verdict of unresectability at the first operation could only be justified, therefore, by the grossest manifestations of spread, such as extensive peritoneal deposits wide of the growth itself. Under these circumstances it may be taken that the emergency laparotomy is the sole definitive operation and the colostomy should be placed in the optimum position for palliation—namely as close to the growth as possible. Alternatively, a short-circuit between the transverse and sigmoid colon may be considered for an inoperable carcinoma of the left colon, or an ileotransverse colostomy used to bypass an inoperable growth of the caecum or right colon. It is a good working rule, therefore, to assume that all but the exceptional case with extensive peritoneal metastases will proceed to a second laparotomy *à froid*, at which the prospects of resection will be finally assessed.

TECHNIQUE OF RIGHT SUBHEPATIC TRANSVERSE COLOSTOMY

This is most conveniently performed through a small transverse incision dividing the upper right rectus (Fig. 347), but can be placed in the upper end

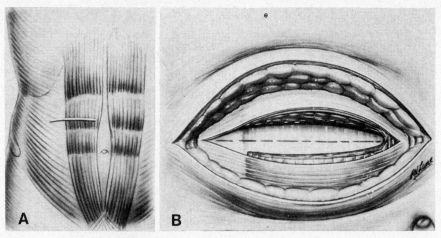

Fig. 347. Incision used for subhepatic right transverse colostomy.

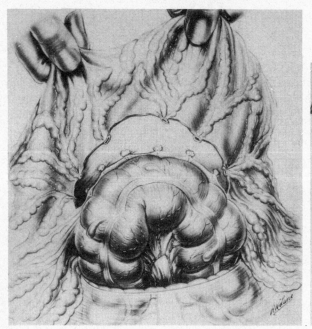

Fig. 348. Loop of transverse colon has been brought out of wound and greater omentum has been separated from it.

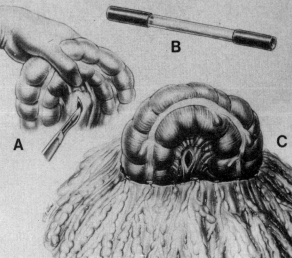

Fig. 349. Freed omentum displaced downwards and forwards exposing loop of colon and mesocolon clearly. (A, C) Making opening in avascular part of mesocolon. (B) Glass rod with segment of rubber tubing at either end, which will be used to support the loop. The rubber is removed from one end whilst the rod is inserted through the hole in the mesocolon and then reapplied where the end emerges on the other side.

of a right paramedian wound. The loop of transverse colon selected should be as near to the hepatic flexure as possible and *well to the right of the middle colic vessels*, the integrity of which must be assured in case the resection at the second stage involves sacrifice of the entire inferior mesenteric artery up to its origin from the abdominal aorta. In cases with gross distension it may be necessary to deflate the bowel with a large-bore needle attached by rubber tubing to a sucker, the puncture hole being afterwards closed by a purse-string suture. The greater

omentum attached to the loop is lightly touched with the scalpel at its attachment to the colon and stripped towards the mesocolon sufficiently to leave the projecting colon bare (Fig. 348). A glass rod is then passed through the mesocolon and superficial to the cut edge of the omentum to support the bowel at the skin level, and portions of rubber tubing are placed over the ends of the rod to prevent it slipping out (Fig. 349). No attempt is made to suture the limbs of the loop together to produce a 'double-barrelled' colostomy, for when it is eventually closed an enterotome is not used, but instead an intraperitoneal technique is preferred. The wound is then sutured round the bowel, and in the process portions of omental fat are included in one or two sutures at either end to prevent the loop from extruding itself (Fig. 350); alternatively stitches may be passed between the bowel wall itself and the parietes, but they should take a very superficial bite of the colon wall. Finally, when the wound has been closed and sealed by dressings, the bowel is opened, and this may be done in either of two ways:

1. Using a Paul's Tube. A purse-string suture of strong linen or cotton thread is inserted on the summit of the loop (Fig. 351). A small cut is then made with diathermy in the area of colon wall encircled by the suture, and a Paul's glass tube is quickly inserted, whilst the suture is tied tightly on it.

2. Without Intubation, Preferably with Primary Mucocutaneous Suture. This method, which is the one I now always use in making a transverse colostomy in an unobstructed case—as for example at the conclusion of an elective low anterior resection of the rectum—is also suitable for patients with obstruction, provided that the sucker is used efficiently to prevent undue contamination with escaping liquid faeces as soon as the bowel is opened. An incision is then made on the convexity of the loop

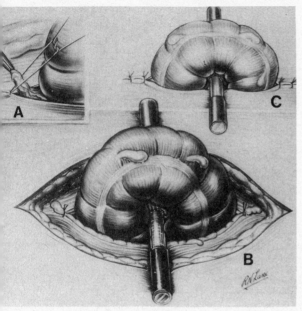

Fig. 350. (A) Fixing the colon by incorporating appendices epiploicae in sutures in the external oblique aponeurosis at end of the wound. (B) Suture of the aponeurosis and fixation of the loop of colon completed. (C) Suture of skin wound.

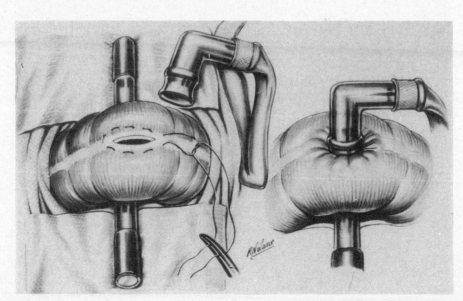

Fig. 351. Method of opening colostomy *if the patient is acutely obstructed.* After placing a purse-string suture of strong silk on the summit of the loop, an incision is made sufficiently large to accommodate a Paul's glass tube. The suture is then tied tightly round the tube, providing a water-tight junction for four or five days and thus avoiding contamination of the wound with liquid faeces.

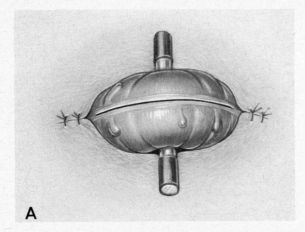

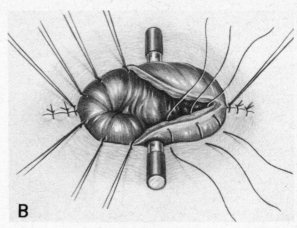

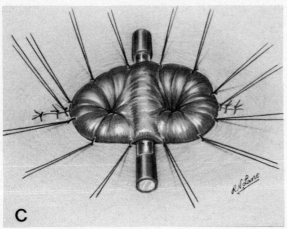

Fig. 352. *Usual method* of opening colostomy loop with immediate mucocutaneous suture. (A) Longitudinal incision in the line of a taenia, extending to within 1 cm of the skin level at either end. (B) Silk sutures are then passed between the edges of the colon wound and those of the skin wound. As these are tied they open up the colostomy and secure mucocutaneous apposition except where the glass rod projects. (C) Final state of affairs.

and in its long axis, extending to within 0·5 cm of the abdominal skin wound at either end (Fig. 352A). I have always used the diathermy knife for this purpose, but one recorded fatal case of explosion resulting from ignition of gas in the colon by diathermy used for opening a caecostomy (Barrkman 1965) suggests that an ordinary scalpel is perhaps safer. Interrupted sutures of silk or catgut are next inserted between the cut edge of the skin on either side of the projecting colon and the edges of the wound in the bowel (Fig. 352B). As these stitches are tied, the effect is to evert the colonic mucosa and produce mucocutaneous apposition all round, except where the glass rod projects on either side (Fig. 352C). The advantage of this technique is that it reduces the amount of granulation tissue and oedema that forms around the colostomy in the postoperative period, if the serosa of the loop is left initially exposed, and this facilitates the subsequent closure. Admittedly some reaction occurs in the vicinity of the glass rod but, in my experience of primarily suturing loop colostomies, unless a rod is used an adequate spur is not maintained. Previously I had employed a vertical mattress stitch between the middle of the two sides of the skin wound, transfixing the mesocolon, but it was not as satisfactory as this method, suggested by Wheatley (1960).

Rickett (1969) has designed a plastic colostomy rod, the ends of which are inserted into the subcutaneous fat of the wound on either side, so that they rest, not on the skin, but directly on the musculoaponeurotic layers of the abdominal wall. A nylon stitch, attached to a perforation on one end of the rod, is brought out through the skin at least 5 cm away from the wound; when the time comes for removal of the rod, say, two weeks later, this stitch is used to pull that end against the skin, whilst, with the aid of local anaesthesia, a tiny incision is made in the latter, allowing the rod to be extracted. The great advantage of this buried rod in making the colostomy is that the cut edge of bowel can be sutured to the skin all round, instead of having to leave a gap superiorly and inferiorly for the ends of the ordinary colostomy rod to project. It would be reasonable to suppose that this

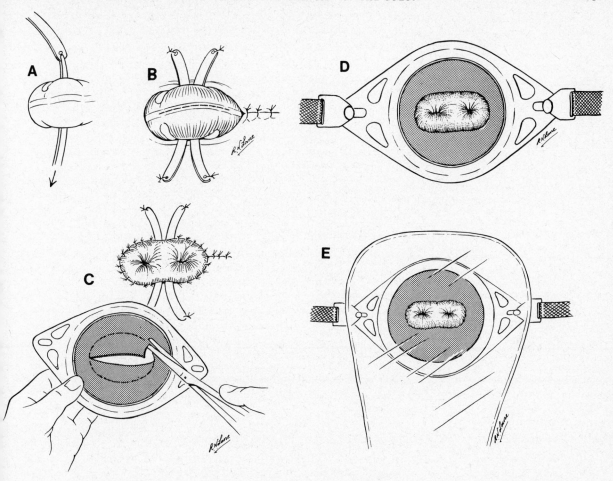

Fig. 353. The Hollister appliance with plastic bridge and large karaya washer, for use on temporary loop colostomies. (A) A loop of transverse colon has been brought out through small transverse incision and is supported by plastic bridge. (B) The method of drawing the bridge, in closed condition, through the transverse mesocolon. (C) Cutting a hole in the karaya washer of a suitable size to fit snugly round the opened up colon sutured to the edges of the skin incision apart from the points where the plastic support emerges above and below. (D) Washer and plastic frame applied to the abdominal wall, overlying and circumscribing the projecting ends of the support. (E) A disposable drainage bag is stuck to the gasket and clipped at its lower end.

might lessen the amount of inflammatory oedema and fibrous reaction, which could facilitate the subsequent colostomy closure. It certainly makes it much easier to change adherent colostomy bags during the immediate postoperative period. My main objection to Rickett's rod is that it does not give a very upstanding spur, so that faecal diversion is not so complete. Also some patients have found its removal a somewhat uncomfortable experience. A rather similar technique described by Schuler and Aliapoulios (1973) allows of easier removal of the rod.

More recently, with the object of facilitating still further the immediate postoperative management of transverse colostomy and in particular of eliminating the need for subsequent formal closure, Rickett (1978) has introduced an obturating balloon technique for construction of the colostomy. In this method no loop of colon is taken through the abdominal wall; instead, the bowel is kept entirely within the abdominal cavity. At the site chosen for the colostomy in the right transverse colon a small incision is made with diathermy on the antimesocolic aspect of the bowel and a purse-string suture of 2/0 chromic catgut is inserted around it. A special rubber tube with a surrounding inflatable balloon is introduced through the incision into the colon in a proximal direction and the purse-string suture is tied. The balloon is then distended with water sufficiently to occlude the lumen of the bowel distal to the internal tip of the tube. A small stab incision is now made through the whole substance of the abdominal wall in the right upper abdomen roughly in the position that would be chosen for a conventional right transverse colostomy, and the other end of the tube plus the small subsidiary tube connected to the balloon is passed through it to the interior. The balloon and colon are drawn snugly up against the anterior parietal peritoneum. A special flange is next slipped over the tube and on to the skin surface, at which level it is fixed to the tube to prevent retraction. The excess of tube projecting beyond the flange is cut off and a conventional drainable colostomy bag is fitted.

When the colostomy has served its purpose and it is considered appropriate to dispense with it, the balloon is deflated and the tube can then easily be withdrawn. The resulting small wound discharges a little faeces for a while, but is said usually to close spontaneously in one to three months; rarely has a small operation been necessary to close it. In 28 cases Rickett (1978) has not had any trouble with necrosis of the colon due to the obturating balloon or of leakage of faeces alongside the tube, which is encouraging, but most surgeons would regard the method as still on trial.

A similar principle is incorporated in a new technique independently elaborated by Sykes (1979). In it the tube for draining the bowel does not have a balloon on it but is instead a large bore de Pezzar catheter, which is passed proximally for 5–6 cm. Temporary obstruction of the colon is achieved by a sling of elastic Penrose drain material holding the part of the colon containing the catheter firmly up against the anterior abdominal wall. It is an easy matter eventually to withdraw the sling and cathether without general anaesthesia, and again it is said that the temporary faecal fistula usually closes soon. Actually Sykes (1979) has not as yet used his method for patients with acute colonic obstruction, but only employed it as a decompressing and defunctioning device instead of conventional transverse colostomy in elective resection of the left colon or rectum.

I have as yet had no personal experience with the techniques of Rickett (1978) or Sykes (1979).

IMMEDIATE POSTOPERATIVE MANAGEMENT OF TRANSVERSE COLOSTOMY

As with terminal iliac colostomies following abdominoperineal excision of the rectum, so with temporary transverse colostomies it is advisable to affix an adherent plastic bag to the abdominal skin around the stoma in order to catch the faecal discharge which at first is often quite liquid. The same range of appliances is available as for permanent iliac colostomies (see p. 625), and the same respective advantages and disadvantages hold. A special problem that arises with transverse loop colostomies relates partly to the larger bulk of the stoma on account of the double opening, but even more so to the supporting glass rod, which has to be negotiated through the cut aperture in the back of the bag in order that the adherent part of the appliance can be stuck to the skin underneath the projecting ends of the rod. This may be quite a tricky manoeuvre. But the difficulty can be overcome if a glass rod not longer than 6·5 cm can be used, for an ordinary Hollister drainage bag with a 7·5 cm flange can be stuck firmly to the skin entirely peripheral to the ends of the rod (see Fig. 353, which shows the use of this arrangement actually in conjunction with a loop ileostomy). Alternatively, a special loop colostomy device introduced by the Hollister firm

may be employed (Poticha 1974). In it the glass rod is replaced by a flat butterfly-shaped polyethylene support 1 mm in thickness, which is folded for passage through the mesocolon (Fig. 353A) and opened up when in position (Fig. 353B). To be used in conjunction with this support is a specially large colostomy appliance. It consists of: (a) a very wide gasket and karaya washer, in which a hole is cut with scissors so that the karaya fits snugly around the protruding loop of bowel and is pressed against the skin and the wings of the butterfly support and is also held by a belt; and (b) disposable plastic drainage bags which are stuck to the gasket surrounding the karaya washer. The karaya washer and gasket usually stay securely in position for four or five days; the bags need to be changed often every two or three days. The firm of Coloplast also make a kit for temporary transverse colostomies comprising a special plastic support rod and a bag with a very large karaya washer. The traditional glass rod is replaced by a rigid plastic support which, after introduction, opens up into two thin flat 'wings', which can be pressed firmly against the skin and are stitched to it at their two ends. A specially large flange consisting of a circle of rigid plastic material and a thick karaya gum washer is then applied firmly to the skin around the colostomy, so as to press the colostomy support against the skin and also make contact with the skin well beyond the ends of the support and thus avoid leakage. The flange is further supported by a belt and usually remains securely in place for six to seven days. To the plastic ring of the flange is stuck a flimsy plastic bag with drainage spout controlled by a clip. These bags usually remain in position for two or three days and can be changed without disturbing the flange.

My own preference is for the method with a short glass rod and large ordinary drainage bag, but sometimes the size of the protruding colostomy loop makes it impracticable and the new Hollister or Coloplast devices are then very useful.

CLOSURE OF THE COLOSTOMY

Though colostomy closure is a relatively small operation, it does involve opening the abdominal cavity. Consequently it *requires full relaxation of the abdominal muscles exactly as for a major laparotomy*. It is important to emphasize this fact, for, unless specifically requested to do so, the anaesthetist, impressed by the smallness of the intervention, is apt to omit relaxant drugs, which will make the operation much more difficult.

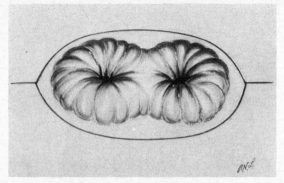

Fig. 354. Closure of transverse colostomy. The skin incision closely surrounds the stoma.

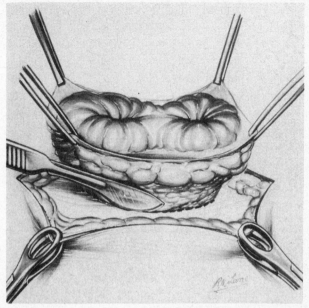

Fig. 355. Freeing the colon from the anterior rectus sheath by sharp dissection whilst strong traction is exerted on the bowel drawing it forcibly out of the abdomen.

After cleansing the colostomy site with a soapy antiseptic such as cetrimide 1%, the abdominal skin is painted with iodine and towels are applied. An incision is made in the skin immediately around the opening, about 1 cm from the edge of the mucosa (Fig. 354). Tissue forceps are applied to the colostomy ring and *strong lifting traction is exerted on the bowel*, whilst the incision is deepened on all aspects through the fat to the aponeurosis, the edge of which is then detached by sharp dissection from the bowel and mesocolon (Fig. 355). This exposes the muscles of the abdominal wall which are similarly separated all round from the bowel wall and mesocolic fat. It is now possible to draw the double tube of colon a considerable distance out of the wound, though it is still attached to the parietal peritoneum of the anterior abdominal wall. It is often possible to mobilize the bowel still further by cautious division of connective tissue bands without opening the peritoneum, but there is no particular virtue in avoiding entry into the peritoneal cavity, and usually the bowel is freely separated from the peritoneum and lifted right out of the wound.

The next step is to remove with scissors the thin rim of skin and subcutaneous fat that surrounds the colostomy opening (Fig. 356), and to mobilize by sharp dissection the mucosal edge which may be fixed by fibrosis in a position of eversion (Fig. 357). Only after the colon wall has been rendered quite free and supple is the suture of the stoma commenced (Fig. 358). For this purpose the margin of the opening is held in fine tissue forceps with its long axis running transversely across the line of the bowel, and a continuous Connell stitch of No. 3/o chromic catgut is inserted, which secures coaptation with excellent inversion of the cut edges (Fig. 359). A further row of interrupted fine catgut or silk

Lembert sutures completes the closure of the bowel (Fig. 359c).

If the closure of the colostomy is being undertaken not eight weeks but two or three weeks after the original operation, the bowel may be found so oedematous at the site of the stoma that it may be extremely difficult to free the mucosa and turn it in in the manner just described. Under these circumstances it will be better to resect the entire loop that was concerned in the colostomy and so make an end-to-end anastomosis between two tubes of pliable colon at a slightly deeper level (Fig. 360). Le Gac has described a method of adding longitudinal incisions for a short distance down both limbs of colon to make the lumen wider at the site of anastomosis (Qvist 1977), but I regard this step as unnecessary as a rule. The moral really is to avoid closing colostomies too soon after operation and the need for resecting the stoma will thereby be completely avoided.

The protruding loop of colon is now pushed back into the abdominal cavity and the edges of the parietal wound held up with forceps. In some instances it is convenient to suture the abdominal wall in layers, but more often these are welded by fibrosis and not easily defined as separate entities. I have therefore usually relied entirely on a single row of closely placed sutures of monofilament

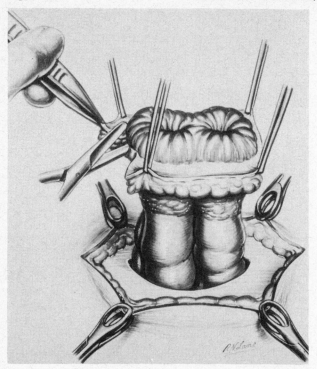

Fig. 356. The colostomy loop has been completely freed from the abdominal wall and lifted well out of the abdomen. The fringe of skin and subcutaneous fat is being removed with scissors.

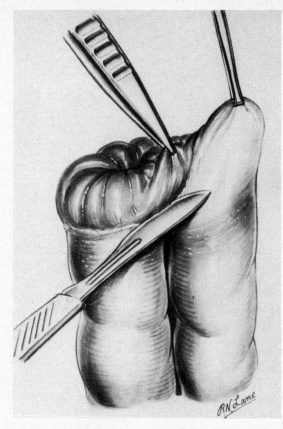

Fig. 357. Mobilizing the everted mucosa at the stoma by sharp dissection, so that it may be more easily turned in during the subsequent closure.

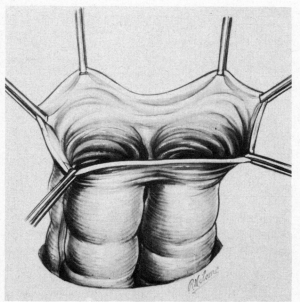

Fig. 358. The pliable edge of the colon is now ready for suture.

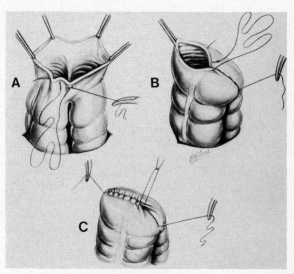

Fig. 359. Suture of the bowel. (A) Commencement of Connell stitch of continuous fine chromic catgut. (B) Connell stitch nearing completion. (C) Burying row of Lembert sutures of interrupted fine serum-proof silk.

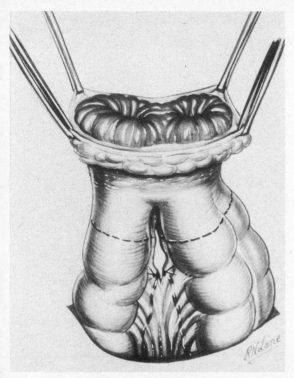

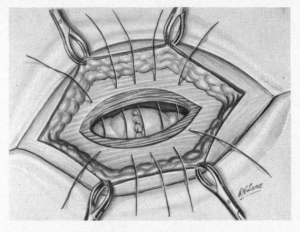

Fig. 361. After replacement of the loop of colon inside the peritoneal cavity, the wound is closed by a series of interrupted Prolene or Dexon sutures embracing the anterior peritoneum and all the musculoaponeurotic structures of the abdominal wall. This is easier than individual layer suture and gives a good closure. A corrugated rubber drain is generally inserted down to the bowel suture line.

Fig. 360. If the region of the colostomy is very oedematous the alternative may be adopted with advantage of resecting the top of the loop after it has been thoroughly freed from the abdominal wall as in Figs 346–8. Limits of resection indicated by dotted lines. Continuity is then restored by end-to-end anastomosis. (*But note that this method need seldom be required.*)

Prolene or Dexon traversing musculoaponeurotic layers (including the peritoneum if it has been opened), and this has given satisfactory results (Fig. 361). It is advisable to place a small corrugated rubber drain down to the suture line in the bowel. The skin wound is closed with interrupted silk sutures or Michel clips.

POSTOPERATIVE COURSE

This operation has a notorious reputation for subsequent breakdown and leakage of faeces, and this is well shown by a recent survey by Knox et al. (1971) of the complications of colostomy closure in 179 patients. Wound infection without faecal discharge was noted in 10% of the cases. Faecal fistulation developed in another 23%—closing spontaneously in 16%, but requiring further operation in 7%. There were four deaths (2·2%) attributable to the closure of the colostomy; in three the cause was breakdown of the intestinal suture and general peritonitis, in the fourth the cause of death was uncer-

tain as no necropsy was performed. Dixon and Benson (1944) also reported a high incidence of faecal fistulation after colostomy closure—some 18%—but Barron and Fallis (1948), Green (1966), Hubbard et al. (1967) and Thomson and Hawley (1972) had many fewer complications. My experience is that, provided care has been taken during the operation to mobilize the bowel wall thoroughly before attempting suture, the complication rate can be kept remarkably low. I reckon that wound infection occurs in about one case in 10 after colostomy closure, and faecal fistulation in one case in 40 or 50 (almost invariably closing of its own accord). I have only twice had to re-operate to reclose a colostomy in several hundreds of cases, most of which have had transverse colostomies in conjunction with low anterior resection, an operation I perform frequently. I agree with Knox et al. (1971) that one of the chief factors contributing to difficulty in colostomy closure is oedema of the tissues, which is most marked in the first few weeks after the colostomy has established. *If the closure can be postponed for, say, at least two months till all oedema has subsided, the incidence of complications will be much reduced.* Patients should therefore be advised strongly to leave hospital with their colostomies and to return later for colostomy closure.

A rare complication of colostomy closure is the development of a tension pneumoperitoneum, which happened in one of my cases (see Hall 1971).

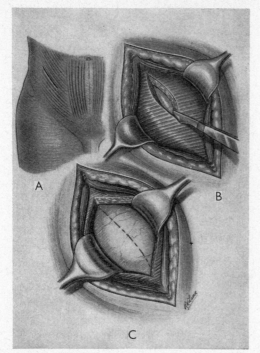

Fig. 362. Oblique muscle-cutting approach used for caecostomy. (A) Incision. (B) After separation of the fibres of the external oblique, the internal oblique and transversus are incised. (C) Exposure and incision of the peritoneum.

The condition has been relieved by paracentesis without peritonitis ensuing, but generally a laparotomy is required.

TECHNIQUE OF CAECOSTOMY

Two main techniques exist for the performance of a caecostomy. In one the exposed anterior caecal wall is sutured all round to the edges of the parietal peritoneal wound; then it is incised and a small glass Paul's tube is tied into its wall. In the other a de Pezzar cathether is buried in the caecal wall by the Kader-Senn method to produce an 'unspillable ink-well' effect and the abdominal wall is sutured round the projecting tube. This latter type of caecostomy is more likely to close spontaneously on withdrawal of the catheter and is the one preferred by me. It is performed as follows:

A muscle-cutting incision is made over the distended caecum and the peritoneum is opened (Fig. 362). Care must be taken that the grossly stretched caecal wall does not burst when deprived of the support of the overlying parietes. After placing packs around the protruding bowel the latter is decompressed by inserting a small-bore trocar and

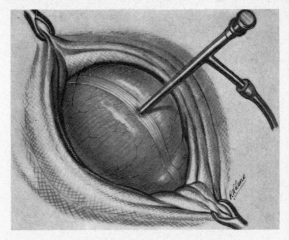

Fig. 363. The distended caecum is deflated by means of a fine trocar and cannula.

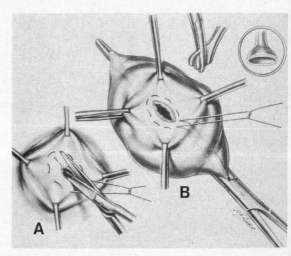

Fig. 364. A spring clamp is placed on the base of the collapsed caecum preparatory to opening it. A purse-string suture is inserted round the cannula and 1·5–2 cm wide of it. On withdrawal of the cannula the opening is enlarged (A) and a de Pezzar catheter with the end cut off is inserted (B).

cannula which is attached by a length of rubber tubing to a suction machine (Fig. 363). The collapsed, deflated bowel is then lifted up with four Allis tissue forceps and an intestinal spring clamp is applied across its base to avoid any faecal leak (Fig. 364). A purse-string suture of No. 1/0 chromic catgut is inserted round the decompressing cannula, which is then removed and the small puncture hole is enlarged sufficiently to admit a self-retaining catheter of the de Pezzar type, about the size of the index finger, with the tip cut off and the 'mush-

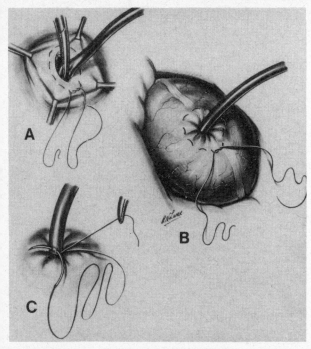

Fig. 365. (A) The purse-string suture is tied tightly round the catheter. (B) A second purse-string suture—and even a third if desired—is then inserted. (C) Finally the stitch takes a bite of the catheter to fix it in position.

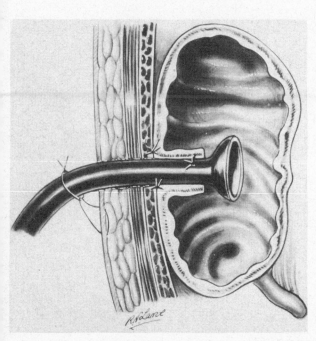

Fig. 366. The caecum is sutured to the anterior parietal peritoneum as the wound is closed round the tube, as shown in this sectional view.

room' folded on itself and held by a long artery forceps (Fig. 365). The purse-string stitch is immediately tied and its end passed through the wall of the catheter to fix it in position. Another purse-string suture is now inserted and drawn tight, whilst the caecal wall is invaginated by pushing the tube towards the lumen. A further purse-string stitch may be used to increase the invagination. The ends of the final suture are passed through the edges of the parietal peritoneum in order to fix the caecum firmly against the parietes (Fig. 366). The abdominal wound is closed in layers and the tube further secured to the skin by tying one of the skin sutures tightly round it. Dressings are applied and the tube is eventually led to a bottle beside the bed.

Results of Operations for Carcinoma Coli with Acute Obstruction

IMMEDIATE MORTALITY

As an indication of the sort of results that may be expected at the present time in the treatment of acute obstruction due to carcinoma of the large intestine, a survey of the experience of the Leeds General Infirmary in the management of these cases during the years 1938–43 and 1947–55 is presented in Table 32.

The nine cases treated expectantly were moribund on admission and never rallied sufficiently for an operation of any kind to be performed before they died. It will be noted also that in 15 other cases the only treatment employed for the obstruction was enemas, which was successful in 14. The remaining patients were subjected to various operations as listed. It is gratifying to note that the overall immediate mortality of acutely obstructed carcinomas has declined from 54% during 1938–43 to 23·4% during 1947–55. Some of this improvement may be attributable to the less frequent use during the latter period of caecostomy, which appears from this analysis to have been a particularly hazardous operation, often followed by fatal sepsis (but selection of this form of drainage as a minimal procedure in particularly ill patients might have been a factor in earning this reputation for it). Other considerations which may have been of importance were the better control of fluid and electrolyte balance and the availability of antibiotics during the second period. But it is clear that acute obstruction due to carcinoma of the large intestine as seen in a busy general hospital still carries a considerable mortality.

A somewhat more favourable impression is gained from reading Hughes' (1966*b*) report on the results obtained by him in a personal series of 127 patients with acute obstruction due to carcinoma coli treated between 1948 and 1964. Two patients died soon after admission before any operation could be performed, and six patients responded to soap-and-water enemas, leaving 119 who had emergency surgical treatment with 14 deaths (=12% operative mortality). Caecostomy was performed in 40 cases with three deaths, colostomy in 31 cases with four deaths, ileotransverse colostomy in 10

is actually quite a high proportion, when it is borne in mind that some of those patients died following the emergency operation for obstruction, and that the resectability rate for 1239 cases presenting with unobstructed carcinomas at the Leeds General Infirmary during the same combined periods was regrettably only 50%. Unfortunately I am unable to give accurate follow-up data on these cases, on which to assess the ultimate rate of cure. However, Gerber et al. (1962) report that, of a series of 168 patients treated between 1950 and 1959 for acutely obstructing carcinomas of the colon, 70 who sur-

TABLE 32. *Immediate Treatment of Acutely Obstructed Carcinoma of Large Intestine*

Forms of treatment employed	1938–43		1947–55	
	No. of cases treated	No. of hospital deaths	No. of cases treated	No. of hospital deaths
Expectant	5	5	4	4
Enemas alone	1	0	14	1
Caecostomy	24	12	54	24
Colostomy, transverse or iliac	14	8	68	11
Ileotransverse colostomy	0	0	31	3
Primary resection:				
Right hemicolectomy with anastomosis	1	0	16	1
Other forms of colectomy with anastomosis	0	0	7	2
By Paul–Mikulicz method	10	3	24	6
Miscellaneous operations	4	4	13	2
All forms of treatment	59	32 (54%)	231	54 (23·4%)

From Smiddy and Goligher (1957).

cases with three deaths and immediate resection in 38 cases with four deaths.

FEASIBILITY OF LATER RESECTION OF GROWTH AND ULTIMATE CURE

There is a fairly widespread impression among surgeons that relatively few of the cases admitted with acute obstruction of colonic carcinomas are ultimately found suitable for radical excision, but this is erroneous. For example, of the entire series of cases with acute obstruction referred to in Table 32, 43% underwent eradication of their growths, which

vived the initial decompression subsequently underwent a resection of the growth. There were 11 operative deaths, and of the 59 survivors only 15 were alive five years later. Thus the absolute five-year survival rate for all cases was only 9%. Hughes (1966*b*) followed up 77 patients who had been treated for acutely obstructed colonic carcinoma at least five years earlier and found that 18% survived for five years or more. Fielding and Wells (1974) reported a 36% five-year survival rate in 50 patients treated for acutely obstructed large bowel cancers and Irvin and Greaney (1977) had a 25% five-year survival rate in 35 cases.

TREATMENT OF CARCINOMA OF THE COLON WITH PERFORATION AND PERITONITIS

Patients with General Peritonitis

Clearly urgent laparotomy is required if life is to be saved after the occurrence of perforation with general peritonitis. Unfortunately some of the cases are already very ill, virtually moribund, on admission and, often in the past, despite resuscitative measures never became fit for an operation. But at the present day with vigorous measures to combat shock this should less often be the case. A central venous catheter is inserted, intravascular volume is restored and broad-spectrum antibiotics administered parenterally in preparation for abdominal exploration.

At laparotomy several possibilities are open to the surgeon depending on the conditions found to be present. *If the perforation lies remote* from the growth, say in the caecum in a case with an obstructed carcinoma of the sigmoid, the correct procedure will be to bring the site of the perforation to the surface as a caecostomy or colostomy and to drain the abdomen or, if this is not possible because of the position of the perforation, the latter should be sutured and a proximal transverse colostomy or caecostomy established. *If the perforation has taken place at or close to the growth*, suture may again be practised, a drain being inserted down to the site of the repair, and a proximal colostomy or caecostomy is made to relieve tension; or alternatively an immediate resection of the bowel containing the growth and the perforation may be performed, either by Paul's (or Hartmann's) method or with anastomosis, as circumstances dictate. It is clear from the accounts given by Mersheimer and Miller (1954), Gregg (1955), Russell and Johnson (1960), Madden and Tan (1961) and Crowder and Cohn (1967) of their experiences in the treatment of perforations of the colon due to carcinoma (or diverticular disease) that primary resection of these lesions at the initial laparotomy may be less hazardous than more conservative measures (see also below).

Apart from the operative manoeuvres to be employed on the bowel it is obviously important to make full use of the various agents now available to counteract faecal contamination and peritonitis—e.g. noxythiolin or saline irrigation, and continued systemic administration of broad-spectrum anti-biotics especially effective against coliform organisms (see pp. 441–3).

Patients with Localized Peritonitis

These patients present much less urgently and tend to be confused with an exacerbation of a diverticulitis of the sigmoid if the growth responsible occurs on the left side, or with acute or subacute appendicitis if, as is usually the case, the carcinoma is in the caecum or ascending colon. In many instances they proceed to operation as examples of appendicitis and the underlying growth may even then elude detection, if simple drainage of the associated abscess is performed (see Patterson 1956). If the true nature of the condition is appreciated an immediate colectomy is probably the best primary treatment despite the local infective condition.

Results of Treatment for Carcinoma of the Colon Complicated by Perforations and Peritonitis

IMMEDIATE MORTALITY

The results of treatment of carcinoma of the colon complicated by perforation and peritonitis make very melancholy reading as seen in Table 33, which records the treatment and results in all such cases admitted to the Leeds General Infirmary during the years 1938–43 and 1947–55.

From these figures and from those quoted by Mersheimer and Miller (1954), Russell and Johnson (1960) and Crowder and Cohn (1967), it appears that perforation of a stercoral ulcer with acutely obstructed growths and the development of faecal peritonitis has been a very lethal complication in the past. It remains to be seen whether the use of intraperitoneal antiseptic solutions, such as noxythiolin, and systemic therapy with newer antibiotics (see p. 441) will lower the mortality in the future. The results so far reported with this regimen by Browne and Stoller (1970) have certainly been encouraging. Perforation of non-obstructed growths with generalized or localized peritonitis is slightly less dangerous, the best results in our experience being obtained in the 21 cases, usually with growths in the right colon, in which it was found possible to carry out a primary colectomy. In the light of these findings it would seem wise always

TABLE 33. *The Methods Employed in the Treatment of Perforation in Association with Carcinoma of the Colon or Rectum and the Resulting Immediate Mortality*

Treatment	Perforation of stercoral ulcer with general peritonitis		Perforation of growth with generalized or localized peritonitis	
	Cases treated	Immediate deaths	Cases treated	Immediate deaths
Expectant	12	12	22	22
Drainage only	2	2	0	0
Suture of perforation combined with caecostomy or colostomy	5	4	52	40
Primary resection (right hemi-colectomy or Paul's operation)	1	0	21	5
All methods	20	18 (90%)	95	67 (70%)

From Goligher and Smiddy (1957).

to give serious consideration to the possibility of performing a primary resection as the emergency procedure in cases with perforated carcinoma coli, where at all practicable.

ULTIMATE RESECTABILITY

Of the 30 patients surviving emergency treatment in the series detailed in Table 33, 16 had been treated by primary colectomy and six of the other 14 subsequently proceeded to radical resection, so that the over-all resectability rate in the 115 patients with perforation was only 19%. The main reason for the low rate of resection was the high initial mortality of this complication. Unfortunately we do not know how many of the 22 patients having a radical resection achieved five-year survival. But Donaldson (1958), reporting on the late results in 132 cases of perforation of the colon in connection with carcinoma coli, stated that of 39 with free perforations only one was alive and well five years later, whilst of 93 with a localized peritonitis and abscess 13 or 14% survived this length of time. But a more recent report from the Massachusetts General Hospital by Welch and Donaldson (1974b) records that of 51 patients with free perforation in the previous 15 years five were alive and well five years later, and that of the patients who underwent an ostensibly curative resection 42% survived five years.

REFERENCES

ADAMS, J. T., SCHWARTZ, S. I., RUBIN, P. and ROB, C. G. (1970) Intralymphatic 5-fluorouracil and radioactive gold as an adjuvant to surgical operation for colorectal carcinoma. *Dis. Colon Rect., 13*, 201.

AGNEW, C. H. and COOLEY, R. N. (1962) Barium-enema study of postoperative recurrences of carcinoma of the colon. *J. Am. med. Ass., 179*, 331.

ALLEN, A. W., WELCH, C. E. and DONALDSON, G. A. (1947) Carcinoma of the colon: effect of recent advances on the surgical management. *Ann. Surg., 126*, 19.

ANDERSEN, B., KORNER, B. and ØSTERGAARD, A. H. (1972) Topical ampicillin against wound infection after colorectal surgery. *Ann. Surg., 176*, 129.

ARIEL, I. M. (1957) Treatment of inoperable cancer by intra-arterial administration of mechlorethamine. *Archs.Surg., Chicago, 74*, 516.

ATIK, M., MASSARI, F. and COHN, I., Jr. (1960) The influence of clorpactin XCB on the spread of tumors of the colon. *Surg. Forum, 11*, 76.

AZAR, H. and DRAPANAS, T. (1968) Relationship of antibiotics to wound infection and enterocolitis in colon surgery. *Am. J. Surg., 115*, 209.

BACON, H. E. and BERKELEY, J. L. (1959) The rationale of re-resection for recurrent cancer of the colon and rectum. *Dis. Colon Rect., 2*, 549.

BACON, H. E. and PEALE, A. R. (1956) Appraisal of adenomatous polyps of the colon, their histopathology and surgical management. *Ann. Surg., 144*, 9.

BADEN, H., ANDERSEN, B., AUGUSTENBORG, G. and HANEL, H. K. (1971) Diagnostic value of gamma-glutamyl transpeptidase and alkaline phosphatase in liver metastases. *Surgery Gynec. Obstet., 133*, 769.

BAKRAN, A., BRADLEY, J. A., BRESNIHAN, E., LINTOTT, D., SIMPKINS, K. C., GOLIGHER, J. C. and HILL, G. L. (1977) Whole gut irrigation: an inadequate preparation for double contrast barium enema examination. *Gastroenterology, 73*, 28.

BALSLEV, I., JENSEN, H. E. and NIELSEN, J. (1970) The place of cecostomy in the relief of obstructive carcinoma of the colon. *Dis. Colon Rect., 13*, 207.

BARBERIO, R., BERRY, N., BATEMAN, J., CROMER, J. K. and KLOPP, C. T. (1953) Combined administration of aureomycin and nitrogen mustard. II. Effects of the intra-arterial administration on human cancer. *Cancer, 6*, 280.

BARKER, K., GRAHAM, N. G., MASON, M. C., DE DOMBAL, F. J. and GOLIGHER, J. C. (1971) The relative significance of preoperative oral antibiotics, mechanical bowel preparation and preoperative peritoneal contamination in the avoidance of sepsis after radical surgery for ulcerative colitis and Crohn's disease of the large bowel. *Br. J. Surg., 58*, 270.

BARONOFSKY, I. D. (1950) Primary resection and aseptic end-to-end anastomosis for acute or subacute large bowel obstructions. *Surgery, St Louis, 27*, 664.

BARRKMAN, M. F. (1965) Intestinal explosion after opening a caecostomy with diathermy. *Br. med. J.*, 1, 1594.

BARRON, J. and FALLIS, L. S. (1958) Colostomy closure by the intraperitoneal method. *Dis. Colon Rect., 1*, 466.

BELL, C. M. A. and LEWIS, C. B. (1968) Effect of neostigmine on integrity of ileorectal anastomoses. *Br. med. J., 3*, 587.

BELSEY, R. (1971) Reconstruction of the oesophagus with left colon. *J. thorac. cardiovasc. Surg., 49*, 33.

BENGMARK, S. (1968) Liver surgery. In *Progress in Surgery*, vol. 6, ed. M. Allgöwer. Basel: Karger.

BENTLEY, P. G., OWEN, W. G., GIROLAMI, P. L. and DAWSON, J. C. (1978) Wound closure with Dexon (polyglycolic acid) mass suture. *Ann. R. Coll. Surg. Engl., 60*, 125.

BIRD, G. G., BUNCH, G. A., CROFT, C. B., HOFFMANN, D. C., HUMPHREY, C. S., RHIND, J. R., ROSENBERG, I. L., WHITTAKER, M., WILKINSON, A. R. and HALL, R. (1971) Topical noxythiolin antisepsis. Report of a controlled trial. *Br. J. Surg., 58*, 447.

BLACK, B. M. (1968) In discussion of paper by Herter and Slanetz (1968).

BLOCH, O. (1894) Extraabdominal resektion af hele colon descendens og et stykke af colon transversum for cancer. (Case of extraabdominal excision of entire colon descendens and of parts of transverse colon for cancer). *Hosp. Tid. Kjøbenh., 4*, pt. ii, 1053.

BOREHAM, P. (1958) Implantation metastases from cancer of the large bowel. *Br. J. Surg., 46*, 103.

BORGSTRÖM, S. and SANDBERG, N. (1960) Healing of colon anastomosis: an experimental study in the rabbit. *Ann. Surg., 151*, 186.

BORNSIDE, G. H. and COHN, I. (1975). Stability of normal human fecal flora during a chemically defined, low residue liquid diet. *Ann. Surg., 181*, 58.

—— CROWDER, V. H., Jr. and COHN, I., Jr. (1969) A bacterial evaluation of surgical scrubbing with disposable iodophor-soap impregnated polyurethane scrub sponges. *Surgery, St Louis, 64*, 743.

BOTSFORD, T. W., ALIAPOULIOS, M. R. and FOGELSON, F. S. (1970) Results of treatment of colorectal cancer at the Peter Bent Brigham Hospital from 1960 to 1965. *Am. J. Surg., 121*, 398.

—— and ZOLLINGER, R. M., Jr. (1969) Diverticulitis of the colon. *Surgery Gynec. Obstet., 128*, 1209.

BROOKE, B. N. (1955) Simplified operative routine for carcinomatous obstruction of the colon. *Lancet, 1*, 945.

BROWNE, M. K. and STOLLER, J. L. (1970) Intraperitoneal noxythiolin in faecal peritonitis. *Br. J. Surg., 57*, 37.

BRUNSCHWIG, A. (1961) Radical surgical management of cancer of the colon spread to tissues and organs beyond the colon. *Dis. Colon Rect., 4*, 83.

BURGESS, A. H. (1929) An address on acute intestinal obstruction. *Lancet, 1*, 857.

BUSSEY, H. J. R., DUKES, C. E. and LOCKHART-MUMMERY, H. E. (1960) Results of the surgical treatment of rectal cancer. In *Cancer of the Rectum*, ed. C. E. Dukes, p. 272. Edinburgh and London: Livingstone.

—— WALLACE, M. H. and MORSON, B. C. (1967) Metachronous carcinoma of the large intestine and intestinal polyps. *Proc. R. Soc. Med., 60*, 208.

BUYERS, R. A. and MEIER, L. A. (1968) Everting suture of the bowel: Experimental and clinical experience in duodenal closure and colorectal anastomosis. *Surgery, St Louis, 63*, 475.

CADY, B., MONSON, D. O. and SWINTON, N. W. (1970) Survival of the patients after colonic resection for carcinoma with simultaneous liver metastases. *Surgery Gynec. Obstet., 131*, 697.

CAMPBELL, J. A., GUNN, A. A. and McLAREN, I. F. (1956) Acute obstruction of the colon. *J. R. Coll. Surg. Edinb., 1*, 231.

CANALIS, F. and RAVITCH, M. M. (1968) Study of healing of inverting and everting intestinal anastomoses. *Surgery Gynec. Obstet., 126*, 109.

CARTER, D. C., JENKINS, D. H. R. and WHITFIELD, H. N. (1972) Omental reinforcement of intestinal anastomoses. *Br. J. Surg., 59*, 10.

CHEEVER, D. (1931) The choice of operation in carcinoma of the colon. *Ann. Surg., 94*, 705.

CLAGETT, O. T., ALLEN, T. H., PAINE, W. S. and WOOLNER, L. B. (1964) The surgical treatment of pulmonary metastases: a 10-year experience. *J. thorac. cardiovasc. Surg., 48*, 39.

CLARK, C. G., WYLLIE, J. H., HAGGIE, S. J. and RENTON, P. (1978) Comparison of catgut and polyglycolic acid sutures in colonic anastomosis. *Wld J. Surg., 1*, 501.

CLARK, D. D. and HUBAY, C. A. (1972) Tube cecostomy: an evaluation of 161 cases. *Ann. Surg., 175*, 55.

COHN, I., Jr. (1960) Dangers of intestinal antisepsis. *Dis. Colon Rect., 3*, 305.

—— (1962) Bacteriologic preparation for colonic operations. *Surg. Clins N. Am., 42*, 1277.

—— and ATIK, M. (1960) Influence of antibiotics on the spread of tumors of the colon: an experimental study. *Ann. Surg., 151*, 917.

—— FLOYD, C. E. and ATIK, M. (1963) Control of tumor implantation during operations on the colon. *Ann. Surg., 157*, 825.

—— and LONGACRE, A. B. (1956/57) Pre-operative sterilization of colon. Comparison of various antibacterial agents. II. *Antibiot. Ann.*, p. 253.

—— and RIVES, J. D. (1956) Protection of colonic anastomoses with antibiotics. *Ann. Surg., 144*, 738.

COLE, W. H., PACKARD, D. and SOUTHWICK, H. W. (1954) Carcinoma of the colon, with special reference to the prevention of recurrence. *J. Am. med. Ass., 155,* 1549.

COLLIS, J. L. (1971) Surgical treatment of carcinoma of the oesophagus and cardia. *Br. J. Surg., 58,* 801.

CONDON, R. E., BARTLETT, J. G. and NICHOLLS, R. L. (1979) Preoperative prophylactic cephalothin fails to control septic complications of colorectal operations: results of controlled clinical trial. *Am. J. Surg., 137,* 68.

CONNELL, M. E. (1893) Intestinal anastomosis—by a new method, without plates and with but two knots—either silk or catgut sutures may be used. *J. Am. med. Ass., 21,* 150.

COOKE, R. V. (1956) Advanced carcinoma of the colon with emphasis on the inflammatory factor. *Ann. R. Coll. Surg. Engl., 18,* 46.

COOPER, E. H., TURNER, R., STEELE, L., NEVILLE, A. M. and MACKAY, A. M. (1974) The contribution of serum enzymes and carcinoembryonic antigen to the early diagnosis of metastatic anorectal cancer. *Br. J. Cancer, 31,* 111.

COPELAND, E. M., MILLER, L. D. and JONES, R. S. (1969) Prognostic factors in carcinoma of the colon and rectum. *Am. J. Surg., 116,* 875.

CRAPP, A. R., TILLOTSON, P., POWIS, S. J. A., COOKE, W. T. and ALEXANDER-WILLIAMS, J. (1975) Preparation of the bowel by whole-gut irrigation. *Lancet, 3,* 1239.

CRONQVIST, S. (1957) Changes in the colon following resection and end-to-end anastomosis. *Acta radiol., 48,* 425.

CROWDER, V. H., Jr. and COHN, I., Jr. (1967) Perforation in cancer of the colon and rectum. *Dis. Colon Rect., 10,* 415.

CRUZ, E. P., McDONALD, G. O. and COLE, W. H. (1956) Prophylactic treatment of cancer: the use of chemotherapeutic agents to prevent tumor metastasis. *Surgery, St Louis, 40,* 291.

CURRERI, A. R., ANSFIELD, F. J., McIVER, F. A., WAISMAN, H. A. and HEIDELBERGER, C. (1958) Clinical studies with 5-fluorouracil. *Cancer Res., 18,* 478.

CUTLER, S. J. and LOURIE, W. I. (1964) End results in cancers of the large intestine and rectum. Presented at the Int. Symp. on End Results of Cancer Therapy, Sandefjord, Norway, Sept. 16–20, 1963, p. 281, *National Cancer Institute Monograph, No. 15.*

DALY, J. M., VARS, H. M. and DUDRICK, S. J. (1970) Correlation of protein depletion with colonic anastomotic strength in rats. *Surg. Forum, 21,* 77.

—— —— (1972) Effect of protein depletion on the strength of colonic anastomoses. *Surgery Gynec. Obstet., 134,* 15.

DAVIES, R. J., VERNON, M. and CROFT, D. N. (1974) Liver snaps and the detection of clinically unsuspected liver metastases. *Lancet, 1,* 279.

DE ALMELDA, A. C. (1971) A modified single layer suture for use in the gastrointestinal tract. *Surgery Gynec. Obstet., 132,* 895.

DEARING, W. H. (1959) Current status of preparation of the intestine for operation: a critical appraisal. *Surg. Clins N. Am., 39,* 1223.

DEDDISH, M. R. and HERTZ, R. E. (1955) Colostomy and coloscopy in the management of mucosal polyps and cancer of the colon. *Am. J. Surg., 90,* 846.

DEPEYSTER, F. A. and GILCHRIST, R. K. (1958) Matching the operative procedure to the patient in carcinoma of the colon, *Surg. Clins N. Am., 38,* 1343.

DEVENEY, K. E. and WAY, L. W. (1976) Effect of different absorbable sutures on healing of gastrointestinal anastomoses. *Am. J. Surg., 133,* 86.

DEVINE, H. B. (1931) Safer colon surgery. *Lancet, 1,* 627.

—— (1935) Carcinoma of the colon. *Br. med. J., 2,* 1245.

—— (1938) Operation on a defunctioned distal colon. *Surgery, St Louis, 3,* 165.

—— (1948) In *British Surgical Practice,* Vol. 3, p. 103, ed. E. Rock Carling and J. Paterson Ross. London: Butterworth.

—— and DEVINE, J. (1948) *Surgery of the Colon and Rectum.* Bristol: John Wright.

DIXON, C. F. and BENSON, R. E. (1944) Closure of colonic stoma: improved results with combined succinylsulfathiazole and sulfathiazole therapy. *Ann. Surg., 120,* 562.

DONALDSON, G. A. (1958) The management of perforative carcinoma of the colon. *New Engl. J. Med., 258,* 201.

DOUGLAS, H. O., Jr. and LE VEEN, H. H. (1971) Tumor recurrence in colon anastomoses: prevention by coagulation and fixation with formalin. *Ann. Surg., 173,* 201.

DWIGHT, R. W., HIGGINS, G. A. and KEEHN, R. J. (1969) Factors influencing survival after resection in cancer of the colon and rectum. *Am. J. Surg., 117,* 512.

EL-DOMEIRI, A. and WHITELEY, H. W. (1970) Prognostic significance of abdominal wall involvement in carcinoma cecum. *Cancer, 26,* 552.

EISENBERG, H., SULLIVAN, P. D. and FOOTE, F. M. (1967) Trends in survival of digestive system cancer patients in Connecticut, 1935 to 1962. *Gastroenterology, 53,* 528.

ELLIS, H. (1971) Curative and palliative surgery in advanced carcinoma of the large bowel. *Br. med. J., 3,* 291.

—— and HEDDLE, R. (1978) Does the peritoneum need to be closed at laparotomy? *Br. J. Surg., 64,* 733.

ENGELL, H. C. (1955) Cancer cells in the circulating blood: a clinical study on the occurrence of cancer cells in the peripheral blood and in venous blood draining the tumor area at operation *Acta chir. scand.,* Suppl. *201.*

EVANS, C. and POLLOCK, A. V. (1973) The reduction of surgical wound infections by prophylactic parenteral cephaloridine. *Br. J. Surg., 60,* 434.

—— —— and ROSENBERG, I. L. (1974) The reduction of surgical wound infections by topical cephaloridine: a controlled clinical trial. *Br. J. Surg., 61,* 133.

EVERETT, M. T., BROGAN, T. D. and NETTLETON, J. (1969) The place of antibiotics in colonic surgery: a clinical study. *Br. J. Surg., 56,* 679.

EVERETT, W. G. (1975) A comparison of one-layer and two-layer techniques for colorectal anastomosis. *Br. J. Surg., 62,* 135.

FAIN, S. N., PATIN, C. S. and MORGENSTERN, L. (1975) Use of a mechanical suturing apparatus in low colorectal anastomosis. *Archs Surg., Chicago, 110,* 1079.

FEATHERS, R. S., SAGOR, G. R., LEWIS, A. A. M., AMIRAK, I. D. and NOONE, P. (1977) Prophylactic systemic antibiotics in colorectal surgery. *Lancet, 2,* 4.

FERGUSON, W. H. and CHASE, W. W. (1957) Emergency definitive one-stage surgery for intestinal obstruction. *Med. Ann. D.C., 26*, 61.

FIELDING, L. P. and WELLS, B. W. (1974) Survival after primary and staged resection for large bowel obstruction caused by cancer. *Br. J. Surg., 61*, 16.

FIROR, W. M. (1942) Intestinal antisepsis with sulfonamides. *Ann. Surg., 115*, 829.

FISHER, E. R. and TURNBULL, R. B., Jr. (1955) The cytologic demonstration and significance of tumor cells in the mesenteric venous blood in patients with colorectal carcinoma. *Surgery Gynec. Obstet., 100*, 102.

FLEISCHNER, F. G. and BERENBERG, A. L. (1956) Recurrent carcinoma of the colon at the site of the anastomosis. *Radiology, 66*, 540.

FRASER, J. and DOTT, N. M. (1924) Aseptic intestinal anastomosis, with special reference to colectomy. *Br. J. Surg., 11*, 439.

GABRIEL, W. B. (1963) *The Principles and Practice of Rectal Surgery*, 5th ed., p. 538. London: H. K. Lewis.

GALLAND, R. B., SAUNDERS J. H. and MOSLEY J. G. (1977) Prevention of wound infection in abdominal operations by peroperative antibiotics or povidone-iodine. *Lancet, 3*, 1043.

GAMBEE, L. P. (1951) Single-layer open intestinal anastomosis applicable to small as well as large intestine. *West. J. Surg., 59*, 1.

—— GARNJOBST, W. and HARDWICK, L. E. (1966) Ten years' experience with a single layer anastomosis in colon surgery. *Am. J. Surg., 92*, 222.

GASTON, E. A. (1966) Liver resection for embolic metastases from cancer of the colon and rectum. *Dis. Colon Rect., 9*, 189.

GERBER, A. and THOMPSON, R. J., Jr. (1965) Use of a tube cecostomy to lower the mortality in acute large intestinal obstruction due to carcinoma. *Am. J. Surg., 110*, 893.

—— —— REISWIG, O. K. and VANNIX, R. S. (1962) Experiences with primary resection for acute obstruction of the large intestine. *Surgery Gynec. Obstet. 115*, 593.

GETZEN, L. C., ROE, R. D. and HOLLOWAY, C. I. (1966) Comparative study of intestinal anastomotic healing in inverted and everted closures. *Surgery Gynec. Obstet., 123*, 1219.

GIBSON, G. R. and STEPHENS, F. O. (1966) Experimental use of cetrimide in the prevention of wound implantation with cancer cells. *Lancet, 2*, 678.

GIBSON, R. M. (1958) Application of antibiotics (Polybactrin) in surgical practice, using the aerosol technique. *Br. med. J., 1*, 1326.

GILBERTSEN, V. A. (1959) Adenocarcinoma of the large bowel: 1,340 cases with 100 per cent follow-up. *Surgery, St Louis, 46*, 1027.

—— and WANGENSTEEN, O. H. (1962) A summary of thirteen years' experience with the second look program. *Surgery Gynec. Obstet., 114*, 438.

GILCHRIST, R. K. and DAVID, V. C. (1947) A consideration of pathological factors influencing five year survival in radical resection of the large bowel and rectum for carcinoma. *Ann. Surg., 126*, 421.

GILES, G. R., BRENNAN, T. G. and WORTHY, T. S. (1974) A trial of 1-(2-chloromethyl)-3-(4-methyl-cyclohexyl)-1-nitrosurea in the treatment of patients with advanced gastro-intestinal cancer. *Br. J. Surg., 61*, 950.

GILL, W., FRASER, J., CARTER, D. C. and HILL, R. (1969) Colonic anastomosis. A clinical and experimental study. *Surgery Gynec. Obstet., 128*, 1297.

GILMORE, O. J. A. and SANDERSON, P. J. (1975) Prophylactic interparietal povedine-iodine in abdominal surgery. *Br. J. Surg., 62*, 792.

GLASHAN, R. W. and JOHN, H. T. (1965) Experience with carcinoma of the large bowel. *Br. J. Surg., 52*, 573.

GLOTZER, D. J., BOYLE, P. L. and SILEN, W. (1973) Preoperative preparation of the colon with an elemental diet. *Surgery, St Louis, 74*, 703.

GOLDRING, J., McNAUGHT, W., SCOTT, A. and GILLESPIE, G. (1975) Prophylactic oral anti-microbial agents in elective colonic surgery: a controlled trial. *Lancet, 3*, 997.

GOLDSMITH, H. S. (1977) Protection of low rectal anastomosis with intact omentum. *Surgery Gynec. Obstet., 144*, 584.

GOLIGHER, J. C. (1976) Visceral and parietal suture in abdominal surgery. *Am. J. Surg., 131*, 130.

—— IRVIN, T. T., JOHNSTON, D., de DOMBAL, F. T., HILL, G. L. and HORROCKS, J. C. (1975) A controlled clinical trial of three methods of closure of laparotomy wounds. *Br. J. Surg., 62*, 823.

—— LEE, P. W. G., SIMPKINS, K. C. and LINTOTT, D. J. (1977) A controlled comparison of one- and two-layer techniques of suture for high and low colorectal anastomoses. *Br. J. Surg., 64*, 49.

—— —— MACFIE, J., SIMPKINS, K. C. and LINTOTT, D. J. (1979) Experiences with the Russian circular suturing device for the construction of colorectal anastomoses. *Surgery Gynec. Obstet.*, (In the Press).

—— MORRIS, C., McADAM, W. A. F., de DOMBAL, F. T. and JOHNSTON, D. (1970) A controlled trial of inverting versus everting intestinal suture in clinical large-bowel surgery. *Br. J. Surg., 57*, 817.

—— and SMIDDY, F. G. (1957) The treatment of acute obstruction or perforation with carcinoma of the colon and rectum. *Br. J. Surg., 45*, 270.

GRAGE, T. B., METTLER, G. E. and CORNELL, G. N. (1976) Adjuvant chemotherapy with 5-fluorouracil after surgical resection of colorectal carcinoma: a preliminary report. *Am. J. Surg., 133*, 59.

GRANT, R. B. and BARBARA, A. C. (1964) Preoperative and postoperative antibiotic therapy in surgery of the colon. *Am. J. Surg., 107*, 810.

GREEN, E. W. (1966) Colostomies and their complications. *Surgery Gynec. Obstet., 122*, 1230.

GREGG, R. O. (1955) The place of emergency resection in the management of obstructing and perforating lesions of the colon. *Surgery, St Louis, 37*, 754.

GRINNELL, R. S. (1953) Results in treatment of carcinoma of the colon and rectum. *Surgery Gynec. Obstet., 96*, 31.

GUBAREFF, N. and SUNTZEFF, V. (1962) Preliminary report on application of iodine in prevention of surgical dissemination of viable malignant cells. *J. surg. Res., 2*, 144.

GURRY, J. F. and ELLIS-PEGLER, R. B. (1976) An elemental diet as preoperative preparation of the colon. *Br. J. Surg., 63*, 969.

HADFIELD, J. I. H. (1965) Preoperative and postoperative intravenous fat therapy. *Br. J. Surg., 52*, 291.

HALL, R. (1971) Delayed tension pneumoperitoneum after colostomy closure. *Br. J. Surg., 58*, 574.

HALSTED, W. S. (1887) Circular suture of the intestine—an experimental study. *Am. J. med. Sci., 94*, 436.

—— (1898) Inflated rubber cylinders for circular suture of the intestine. *Johns Hopk. Hosp. Bull., 9*, 25.

HAMILTON, J. E. (1967) Reappraisal of open intestinal anastomoses. *Ann. Surg., 165,* 917.

HANNINGTON-KIFF, J. G. (1969) Timing of atropine and neostigmine in the reversal of muscle relaxants. *Br. med. J., 1,* 418.

HARGREAVES, A. W. and KEDDIE, N. C. (1968) Colonic anastomosis. A clinical and experimental study. *Br. J. Surg., 55,* 774.

HAU, T., HOFFMANN, R. and SIMMONDS, R. L. (1978) Mechanisms of the adjuvant effect of haemoglobin in experimental peritonitis. *Surgery, St Louis, 83,* 223.

—— and SIMMONDS, R. L. (1978) Heparin in the treatment of experimental peritonitis. *Ann. Surg., 187,* 294.

HAWLEY, P. R. (1972) Personal communication.

—— HUNT, T. K. and DUNPHY, J. E. (1970) The aetiology of colonic anastomotic leaks. *Proc. R. Soc. Med., 63,* 28.

HEALEY, J. E., Jr., McBRIDE, C. M. and GALLAGHER, H. S. (1967) Bowel anastomosis by inverting and everting techniques. *J. surg. Res., 7,* 299.

HERMANN, R. E. (1974) Abdominal wound closure using a new polypropylene monofilament suture. *Surgery Gynec. Obstet., 138,* 84.

HERRINGTON, J. L., Jr. and GRAVES, H. A., Jr. (1968) Emergency and non-planned removal of the left colon. *Surgery Gynec. Obstet., 126,* 1045.

HERTER, F. P. and SBULZ, B. (1966) Inhibition of tumor growth by iodized catgut. *J. surg. Res., 6,* 393.

—— and SLANETZ, C. A. (1967) Influence of antibiotic preparation of the bowel on complications after colon resection. *Am. J. Surg., 113,* 165.

—— —— (1968) Preoperative intestinal preparation in relation to the subsequent development of cancer at the suture line. *Surgery Gynec. Obstet., 127,* 49.

HEWITT, J., REEVE, J., RIGBY, J. and COX, A. G. (1973) Whole gut irrigation in preparation for large-bowel surgery. *Lancet, 2,* 7825.

HIGGINS, G. A., DWIGHT, R. W., SMITH, J. V. and KEEHN, R. J. (1971) Fluorouracil as an adjuvant to surgery in carcinoma of the colon. *Archs Surg., Chicago, 102,* 339.

—— HUMPHREY, E. and JULER, G. L. (1976) Adjuvant chemotherapy in the surgical treatment of large bowel cancer. *Cancer, 38,* 1461.

HOFFMANN, E. (1959) Intraperitoneal and extraperitoneal neomycin as a topical and irrigating agent. *Am. Surg., 25,* 170.

HOLDEN, W. D. and DIXON, W. J. (1962) A study of the use of triethylene-thiophosphoramide as an adjuvant to surgery in the treatment of colorectal cancer. *Cancer Chemother. Rep., 16,* 129.

HUBBARD, T. B., NORICO, A. and HARRIS, R. A. (1967) Two-stage resection of the colon. *Surgery Gynec. Obstet., 124,* 1081.

HUDSPETH, A. S. (1975) Radical surgical debridement in the treatment of generalized bacterial peritonitis. *Archs Surg., Chicago, 110,* 1233.

HUGHES, E. S. R. (1963) Cecostomy: a part of an efficient method of decompressing the colon obstructed by cancer. *Dis. Colon Rect., 6,* 454.

—— (1966a) Carcinoma of the right colon, upper left colon and sigmoid colon. (3 articles). *Aust. N.Z.J. Surg., 35,* 183.

—— (1966b) Mortality of acute large bowel obstruction. *Br. J. Surg., 53,* 593.

—— HARDY, K. J. and CUTHBERTSON, A. M. (1970) Chemoprophylaxis in large bowel surgery. 3. Effect of antibiotics on incidence of local recurrence. *Med. J. Aust., 1,* 369.

HUGHES, L. E. (1977) Personal communication.

HUMMELL, R. P., ALTEMEIER, W. A. and HILL, E. O. (1964) Iatrogenic staphylococcal enterocolitis. *Ann. Surg., 160,* 551.

HURLEY, J. D. and ELLISON, E. H. (1960) Chemotherapy of solid cancer arising from the gastrointestinal tract. *Ann. Surg., 152,* 568.

IRVIN, T. T. and EDWARDS, J. P. (1973) Comparison of single-layer inverting, two-layer inverting, and everting anastomoses in the rabbit colon. *Br. J. Surg., 60,* 453.

—— and GOLIGHER, J. C. (1973) Aetiology of disruption of intestinal anastomosis. *Br. J. Surg., 60,* 461.

—— —— and JOHNSTON, D. (1973a) A randomized prospective clinical trial of single-layer and two-layer inverting intestinal anastomoses. *Br. J. Surg., 60,* 461.

—— and GREANEY, M. G. (1977) The treatment of colonic cancer presenting with intestinal obstruction. *Br. J. Surg., 64,* 741.

—— EDWARDS, J. P. and GOLIGHER, J. C. (1973b) The value of plasma gamma-glutamyl transpeptidase in the detection of hepatic metastases. *Br. J. Surg., 60,* 348.

—— HAYTER, C. J., WARREN, K. E. and GOLIGHER, J. C. (1973c) The effect of intestinal preparation on fluid and electrolyte balance. *Br. J. Surg., 60,* 484.

—— and HUNT, T. K. (1974) Effect of malnutrition on colonic healing. *Ann. Surg., 180,* 765.

—— KOFFMANN, C. G. and DUTHIE, H. L. (1976) Layer closure of laparotomy wounds with absorbable and non-absorbable suture materials. *Br. J. Surg., 63,* 793.

—— STODDARD, C. J., GREANEY, M. G. and DUTHIE, H. L. (1977) Abdominal wound healing: a prospective clinical study. *Br. med. J., 2,* 351.

JAMIESON, C. W. (1972) Inhibition of the growth of tumour cells in culture by noxythiolin. *Br. J. Surg., 59,* 108.

JENKINS, T. P. N. (1976) The burst abdominal wound: a mechanical approach. *Br. J. Surg., 63,* 873.

JENSEN, H. E., BALSLEV, I. and NIELSEN, J. (1970a) Extensive surgery in treatment of carcinoma of the colon. *Acta chir. scand., 136,* 431.

—— NIELSEN, J. and BALSLEV, I. (1970b) Carcinoma of the colon in old age. *Ann. Surg., 171,* 107.

JONES, T. E., NEWELL, E. T. and BRUBAKER, R. E. (1941) The use of alloy steel wire in the closure of abdominal wounds. *Surgery Gynec. Obstet., 71,* 1056.

KEIGHLEY, M. R. B., ARABI, Y. and ALEXANDER-WILLIAMS, J. (1979) Comparison between systemic and oral antimicrobial prophylaxis in colorectal surgery. *Lancet, 1,* 894.

—— CRAPP, A. R., BURDON, D. W., COOKE, W. T. and ALEXANDER-WILLIAMS, J. (1976) Prophylaxis against anaerobic sepsis in bowel surgery. *Br. J. Surg., 63,* 538.

KING, R. D., KAISER, G. C., LEMPKE, R. E. and SHUMACKER, H. B. (1966) An evaluation of catheter cecostomy. *Surgery Gynec. Obstet., 123,* 779.

KLEINFELD, G. and GUMP, F. E. (1960) Complications of colotomy and polypectomy. *Surgery Gynec. Obstet., 111,* 726.

KNOX, A. J. S., BIRKETT, F. D. H. and COLLINS, C. D. (1971) Closure of colostomy. *Br. J. Surg., 58,* 669.

KRATZER, G. L. and ONSANIT, T. (1974) Single layer steel wire anastomosis of the intestine. *Surgery Gynec. Obstet., 139*, 93.

LAHEY, F. H. (1932) Resection of the right colon and anastomosis of the ileum to the transverse colon after the Mikulicz plan. *Surgery Gynec. Obstet., 54*, 923.

—— (1953) A method for segregation of the entire small intestine. *Surgery Gynec. Obstet., 96*, 503.

LARGE, J. M. (1964) Treatment of perforated diverticulitis. *Lancet, 1*, 413.

LAUFMAN, H. and METHOD, H. (1948) Effects of absorbable foreign substance on bowel anastomosis. *Surgery Gynec. Obstet., 86*, 669.

LAWRENCE, W., Jr., JERZ, J. T., HORSLEY, J. S., BROWN, P. W. and ROMERO, C. (1978) Chemotherapy as an adjuvant to surgery for colorectal cancer: a follow-up report. *Archs Surg., Chicago, 113*, 164.

LAWTON, R. L. (1965) Cancer chemotherapy of the gastrointestinal tract with reference to intra-arterial infusion and irradiation. *Am. J. Surg., 109*, 47.

LEAPER, D. J., POLLOCK, A. V. and EVANS, M. (1977) Abdominal wound closure: a trial of nylon, polyglycolic acid and steel sutures. *Br. J. Surg., 64*, 603.

LEMBERT, A. (1826) *Rep. gén. Anzat. Physiol. Path., 2*, 100.

LEONARDO, R. A. (1943) *History of Surgery*, p. 281. New York: Froden.

LILLEHEI, R. C. and WANGENSTEEN, O. H. (1955) Bowel function after colectomy for cancer, polyps and diverticulitis. *J. Am. med. Ass., 159*, 163.

LLOYD-DAVIES, O. V. (1944) Personal communication.

—— (1945) Discussion on the pathology and treatment of carcinoma of the colon. *Proc. R. Soc. Med., 38*, 382.

—— (1947) Carcinoma of the rectum with a single secondary in the liver. Synchronous combined excision and left hepatectomy. *Proc. R. Soc. Med., 40*, 875.

—— and ANGELL, J. (1957) Right hepatic lobectomy. *Br. J. Surg., 45*, 113.

—— MORGAN, C. N. and GOLIGHER, J. C. (1953) The treatment of carcinoma of the colon. In *British Surgical Practice: Progress volume, 1953*, ed. E. Rock Carling and J. Paterson Ross, p. 71. London: Butterworth.

LOCALIO, S. A. (1975) Personal communication.

—— and ENG, K. (1975) Malignant tumours of the rectum. *Current Problems in Surgery, 12*, 1.

LOCKHART-MUMMERY, J. P. (1922) The treatment of acute obstruction from cancer of the colon. *Lancet, 2*, 1117.

—— (1934) *Diseases of Rectum and Colon*, 2nd ed. London: Baillière.

LOEB, M. J. (1967) Comparative strength of inverted, everted and end-on intestinal anastomoses. *Surgery Gynec. Obstet., 125*, 301.

LONG, L., JONASSON, O., ROBERTS, S., McGRATH, R., McGREW, E. and COLE, W. H. (1960) Cancer cells in blood: results of simplified isolation technique. *Archs Surg., Chicago, 80*, 910.

LORTAT-JACOB, J. L. and ROBERT, H. G. (1952) Hepatectomie droite réglée. *Presse méd., 60*, 549.

McADAM, A. J., MEIKLE, A. G. and TAYLOR, J. O. (1970) One layer or two layer anastomoses? *Am. J. Surg., 120*, 546.

—— MEIKLE, G. and MEDINA, R. (1969) An experimental comparison of inversion and eversion colonic anastomoses. *Dis. Colon Rect., 12*, 1.

McCREDIE, J. A. and DE PEYSTER, F. A. (1959) Effects of giving nitrogen mustard by different routes to rats receiving Walker 256 cells intraportally, intraperitoneally, and subcutaneously. *Surgery, St Louis, 45*, 709.

McDONALD, C. T. and WILLIAMSON, A. R. (1960) Dissemination of cancer of the colon and rectum: special reference to four cases of local implantation on perineal wounds. *Dis. Colon Rect., 3*, 117.

McDONALD, G. E., GINES, S. M. and COLE, W. H. (1960) Wound irrigation in cancer surgery. *Archs Surg., Chicago, 80*, 920.

McILRATH, D. C., VAN HEERDEN, J. A., EDIS, A. J. and DOZOIS, R. R. (1976) Closure of abdominal incisions with subcutaneous cathethers. *Surgery, St Louis, 80*, 411.

MACKENZIE, I. and LITTON, A. (1974) *Bacteroides* bacteraemia in surgical patients. *Br. J. Surg., 61*, 288.

McKIBBIN, B. and GAZET, J.-C. (1964) Experimental use of anti-cancer agents in the peritoneal cavity. *Br. J. Surg., 51*, 693.

McLACHLIN, A. D. and DENTON, D. W. (1973) Omental protection of intestinal anastomoses. *Am. J. Surg., 125*, 134.

—— OLSSON, L. S. and PITT, D. F. (1976) Anterior anastomosis of the rectosigmoid colon: an experimental study. *Surgery, St Louis, 80*, 306.

McKITTRICK, L. S. (1948) Principles old and new of resection of the colon for carcinoma. *Surgery Gynec. Obstet., 87*, 15.

—— (1965) Touching all bases. *Am. J. Surg., 109*, 57.

MADDEN, J. L. and TAN, P. Y. (1961) Primary resection and anastomosis in the treatment of perforated lesions of the colon, with abscess or diffusing peritonitis. *Surgery Gynec. Obstet., 113*, 646.

MANZ, C. W., LA TENDRESSE, C. and SAKO, Y. (1970) The detrimental effects of drains on colonic anastomoses: an experimental study. *Dis. Colon Rect., 13*, 17.

MARTI, M.-C. and POURET, J.-P. (1976) La preparation colique rapide. *Chirurgie, 102*, 330.

MARTIN, E. W., COOPERMAN, M. and KING, G. E. (1979) A retrospective and prospective study of serial CEA determination in the early detection of recurrent colon cancer. *Am. J. Surg., 137*, 167.

MATHESON, D. M., ARABI, Y. and BAXTER-SMITH, D. (1978) Randomized multi-centre trial of oral bowel preparation and antimicrobials for elective colorectal operations. *Br. J. Surg., 65*, 47.

MATHESON, N. A. and IRVINE, A. D. (1975) Single layer anastomosis after rectosigmoid resection. *Br. J. Surg., 62*, 239.

MAVLIGIT, G. M., BURGESS, M. A. and SIEBERT, G. B. (1976) Prolongation of postoperative disease-free interval and survival in human colorectal cancer by B.C.G. or B.C.G. plus 5-fluorouracil. *Lancet, 1*, 871.

MAYNARD, A. DE L. and TURELL, R. (1955) Acute left colon obstruction with special reference to cecostomy versus transversostomy. *Surgery Gynec. Obstet., 100*, 667.

MAYO, C. W. and PAGTALUNAN, R. J. G. (1963) Malignancy of colon and rectum in patients under 30 years of age. *Surgery, St Louis, 53*, 711.

MELLISH, R. W., TY, T. C. and KELLER, D. J. (1968) A study of intestinal healing. *J. paediat. Surg., 3*, 286.

MERSHEIMER, W. L. and MILLER, E. M. (1954) Diffuse peritonitis secondary to intestinal perforation complicating malignant lesions of the colon. *Surgery Gynec. Obstet., 99*, 436.

VON MIKULICZ, J. (1903) Small contributions to the surgery of the intestinal tract. *Boston med. surg. J., 148*, 608.

MILANO, G., COOPER, E. H. and GOLIGHER, J. C. (1978) Serum prealbumin, retinol-binding protein, transferrin and albumin levels in patients with large bowel cancer. *J. natn. Cancer Inst., 61*, 687.

MILES, W. E. (1926) *Cancer of the Rectum.* London: Harrison.

MILLER, F. E. and LIECHTY, R. D. (1967) Adenocarcinoma of the colon and rectum in persons under thirty years of age. *Am. J. Surg., 113*, 507.

MILLES, S. S., MUGGIA, A. L. and SPIRO, H. M. (1962) Colonic histologic changes induced by 5-fluorouracil. *Gastroenterology, 43*, 391.

MILNES-WALKER, R. (1971) *Annual Report of South Western Regional Cancer Bureau.* Published by South Western Regional Board, U.T.F. House, King Street, Bristol BS2 8HY.

MOERTEL, C. G., REITEMEIER, R. J., CHILDS, D. S., Jr., COLBY, M. Y. and HOLBROOK, M. A. (1964) Combined 5-fluorouracil and super-voltage radiation therapy in the palliative management of advanced gastrointestinal cancer: a pilot study. *Mayo Clin. Proc., 39*, 767.

—— SHUTT, A. J. and GO, V. L. (1978) Carcinoembryonic antigen test for the detectin of recurrent colorectal carcinoma—inadequacy for early detection. *J. Am. med. Ass., 239*, 1065.

—— —— HAHN, R. G. and REITEMEIER, R. J. (1975) Therapy of advanced colorectal cancer with a combinatin of 5-FU, methyl CCNU and vincristine. *J. natn. Cancer INst., 54*, 69.

MONRO, A. K. (1950) Aseptic intestinal anastomosis. In *Techniques in British Surgery,* ed. R. Maingot, p. 419. Philadelphia and London: W. B. Saunders.

MOORE, G. E. and SAKO, K. (1959) The spread of carcinoma of the colon and rectum: a study of invasion of blood vessels, lymph nodes and the peritoneum bv tumor cells. *Dis. Colon Rect., 2*, 92.

MORGAN, C. N. (1957a) In *Modern Trends in Gastro-enterology,* ed. A. Jones, 2nd ed, p. 340. London: Butterworth.

—— (1957b) Personal communication.

—— (1967) Personal communication, quoted by Muir (1968).

MOUNTAIN, J. C. and SEAL, P. V. (1970) Topical ampicillin in gridiron appendicectomy wounds. *Br. J. clin. Pract., 24*, 111.

MOYNIHAN, B. G. A. (1926) *Abdominal Operations,* 4th ed. Philadelphia and London: Saunders.

MRAZEK, R., ECONOMOU, S., McDONALD, G. O., SLAUGHTER, D. P. and COLE, W. H. (1959) Prophylactic and adjuvant use of nitrogen mustard in the surgical treatment of cancer. *Ann. Surg., 150*, 745.

MUIR, E. G. (1947) Right hemicolectomy. *Proc. R. Soc. Med., 40*, 831.

—— (1956) Results of treatment in carcinoma of colon and rectum. *Br. med. J., 2*, 742.

—— (1968) Safety in colonic resection. *Proc. R. Soc. Med., 61*, 401.

MUKERJEE, P., MEPHAM, J. A., WARNICK, S., DATTA, B. N. and COX, A. G. (1969) The effect of protein deprivation on alimentary healing. *J. surg. Res., 9*, 283.

NASH, A. G. and HUGH, T. B. (1967) Topical ampicillin and wound infection in colon surgery. *Br. med. J., 1*, 471.

NICHOLS, R. L., BROIDO, P., CONDON, R. E., GORBACH, S. L. and NYHUS, L. M. (1973) Effect of preoperative neomycin–erythromycin intestinal preparation on the incidence of infectious complications following colon surgery. *Ann. Surg., 178*, 453.

—— and CONDON, R. E. (1971) Preoperative preparation of the colon: a collective review. *Surgery Gynec. Obstet., 132*, 323.

—— —— (1973) Effect of preoperative neomycin-erythromycin intestinal preparation on the incidence of infectious complications following colon surgery. *Ann. Surg., 178*, 453.

—— —— GORBACH, S. L. and NYHUS, L. M. (1972) Efficacy of preoperative and anti-microbial preparation of bowel. *Ann. Surg., 176*, 227.

O'HARA, M., Jr. (1900) A method of performing anastomosis of hollow viscera by means of a new instrument. *Am. J. Obstet., 42*, 81.

ORR, N. W. M. (1969) A single-layer intestinal anastomosis. *Br. J. Surg., 56*, 771.

PACK, G. T. and BAKER, H. W. (1953) Total right hepatic lobectomy. *Ann. Surg., 138*, 253.

PARKER, E. M. and KERR, H. H. (1908) Intestinal anastomosis without open incisions by means of basting stitches. *Johns Hopk. Hosp. Bull., 19*, 132.

PATTERSON, H. A. (1956) The management of cecal cancer discovered unexpectedly at operation for acute appendicitis. *Ann. Surg., 143*, 670.

PAUL, F. T. (1895) Colectomy. *Br. med. J., 1*, 1136.

—— (1912) Personal experiences in the surgery of the large bowel. *Lancet, 2*, 217.

PEDEN, J. C. and BLALOCK, A. L. (1963) Right hepatic lobectomy for metastatic carcinoma of the large bowel: 5 year survival. *Cancer, 16*, 1133.

PELOSO, O. A., FLOYD, V. T. and WILKINSON, L. H. (1973) Treatment of peritonitis with continuous post-operative peritoneal lavage using cephalothin. *Am. J. Surg., 126*, 742.

PESTANA, C., REITEMEIER, R. J., MOERTEL, C. G., JUDD, E. S. and DOCKERTY, M. B. (1964) The natural history of carcinoma of the colon and rectum. *Am. J. Surg., 108*, 826.

PITTINGER, C. B. and LONG, J. P. (1959) Potential dangers associated with antibiotic administration during anaesthesia and surgery. *Archs Surg., Chicago, 79*, 207.

POLACEK, M. A. and SANFELIPPO, P. (1968) Oral antibiotic bowel preparation and complications in colon surgery. *Archs Surg., Chicago, 97*, 412.

POLK, H. C., Jr. and LOPEZ-MAYOR, J. F. (1969) Postoperative wound infection: a prospective study of determinative factors and prevention. *Surgery, St Louis, 66*, 97.

POLLOCK, A. V., FROOME, K. and EVANS, M. (1978) The bacteriology of primary wound sepsis in potentially contaminated abdominal operations: the effect of irrigation, povidone-iodine and cephaloridine on the sepsis rate assessed in a clinical trial. *Br. J. Surg., 65*, 76.

POLLOCK, T. W., MULLEN, J. L. and TSOU, K. C. (1979) Serum 5′ nucleotide phosphodiesterase as a predictor of hepatic metastases in gastrointestinal cancer. *Am. J. Surg., 137,* 22.

POTH, E. J. (1943) Use of succinylsulfathiazole and phthalysulfathiazole as intestinal antiseptics. *Tex. St. J. Med., 39,* 369.

—— (1953) Intestinal antiseptics in surgery. *J. Am. med. Ass., 153,* 1516.

—— (1954) Symposium on colonic surgery. Intestinal antisepsis. *Am. J. Surg., 88,* 803.

—— (1963) Intestinal antisepsis: interim report. *Dis. Colon Rect., 6,* 45.

—— FROMM, S. M., WISE, R. I. and HSIANG, C. M. (1950) Neomycin, a new intestinal antiseptic. *Tex. Rep. Biol. Med., 8,* 353.

POTH, E. J., ROSS, C. A. and FERNANDEZ, E. B. (1945) An experimental evaluation of sulfasuxidine and sulfathalidine in surgery of the colon. *Surgery, St Louis, 18,* 529.

POTICHA, S. M. (1974) A new technic for loop colostomy with use of a plastic bridge. *Am. J. Surg., 127,* 620.

PRINGLE, A. (1924) Aseptic resection of the intestine. *Br. J. Surg., 12,* 238.

QUATTLEBAUM, J. K. (1962) Hepatic lobectomy for benign and malignant lesions. *Surg. Clins N. Am., 42,* 507.

QVIST, G. (1977) Closure of a loop colostomy by a modified Le Gac's operation. *Br. J. Surg., 64,* 864.

RANKIN, F. W. (1926) *Surgery of the Colon.* New York and London: Appleton.

—— (1928) The technique of anterior resection of the recto-sigmoid. *Surgery Gynec. Obstet., 46,* 537.

—— (1945) In *Cancer of the Colon and Rectum,* ed. F. W. Rankin and A. S. Graham, 2nd ed. Springfield, Ill.: Thomas.

—— BARGEN, J. A. and BUIE, L. A. (1932) *The Colon, Rectum and Anus.* Philadelphia and London: Saunders.

—— and OLSON, P. F. (1933) The hopeful prognosis in cases of carcinoma of the colon. *Surgery Gynec. Obstet., 56,* 366.

RAVEN, R. W. (1957) Liver surgery in relation to diseases of the colon and rectum. *Proc. R. Soc. Med., 50,* 775.

RAVITCH, M. M. (1966) In discussion of paper by Bronwell, A. W., Rutledge, R. and Dalton, M. L., Jr. (1967) Single layer open gastro-intestinal anastomosis. *Ann. Surg., 165,* 925.

—— (1974) Sewing with staples. *Clin. Med., 81,* 17.

—— CANALIS, F., WEINSHELBAUM, A. and McCORMACK, J. (1967a) Studies of intestinal healing. III Observations on everting intestinal anastomosis. *Ann. Surg., 166,* 670.

—— ONG, T. H. and GAZZOLA, L. (1974) A new precise and rapid technique of intestinal resection and anastomosis with staples. *Surgery Gynec. Obstet. 139,* 6.

—— and RIVAROLA, A. (1966) Entero anastomosis with an automatic stapling instrument. *Surgery, St Louis, 59,* 270.

—— —— and VAN GROV, J. (1967b) Studies of intestinal healing. I Preliminary study of the mechanism of healing of the inverting intestinal anastomosis. *Johns Hopk. med. J., 121,* 343.

—— and STEICHEN, F. M. (1972) Techniques of staple suturing in the gastrointestinal tract. *Ann. Surg., 175,* 815.

RICKETT, J. W. S. (1969) A new colostomy rod for subcutaneous implantation. *Br. med. J., 3,* 466.

—— (1978) Obturating balloon colostomy (Torbay colostomy); preliminary communication. *J. R. Soc. Med., 71,* 31.

ROB, C., SCHWARTZ, S. I., MAX, T. C. and RUBIN, P. (1963) A new method of treating lymph node metastasis in potentially curable carcinoma of the large intestine. *Dis. Colon Rect., 6,* 91.

ROCHLIN, D. B., SHINER, J., LANGDON, E. and OTTOMAN, R. (1962) Use of 5-fluorouracil in disseminated solid neoplasms. *Ann. Surg., 156,* 105.

—— SMART, C. R. and SILVA, A. (1965) Chemotherapy of malignancies of the gastrointestinal tract. *Am. J. Surg., 109,* 43.

ROMBEAU, J. L., WILK, P. J, TURNBULL, R. B. and FAZIO, V. W. (1978) Total faecal diversion by the temporary skin level loop transverse colostomy. *Dis. Colon Rect., 21,* 223.

ROSATO, F. E., FRAZIER, T. G., COPELAND, E. M. and MILLER, L. D. (1969) Carcinoma of the colon in young people. *Surgery Gynec. Obstet., 129,* 29.

ROSENBERG, I. L., GRAHAM, N. G., DE DOMBAL, F. T. and GOLIGHER, J. C. (1971) Preparation of the intestine in patients undergoing major large-bowel surgery, mainly for neoplasms of the colon and rectum. *Br. J. Surg., 58,* 266.

ROSENTHAL, I. and BARONOFSKY, I. K. (1960) Prognostic and therapeutic implications of polyps in metachronous colic carcinoma. *J. Am. med. Ass., 172,* 37.

ROUSSELOT, L. M., COLE, D. R., GROSSI, C. E., CONTE, A. J., GONZALEZ, E. M. and PASTERNACK, B. S. (1972) Adjuvant chemotherapy with 5-fluorouracil in surgery for colorectal cancer: eight-year progress report. *Dis. Colon Rect., 15,* 169.

ROWLANDS, R. P. and TURNER, P. (1937) *The Operations of Surgery,* 8th ed., vol. 2, p. 336. London: Churchill.

ROXBURGH, R. A., DAWSON, J. L. and YEO, R. (1968) Emergency resection in treatment of diverticular disease of colon complicated by peritonitis. *Br. med. J., 3,* 465.

RUBBO, S. D., HUGHES, E. S. R., BLAINEY, B. and RUSSELL, I. S. (1965) Role of preoperative chemoprophylaxis in bowel surgery. *Antimicrob. Agents Chemother., 5,* 724.

RUSCA, J. A., BORNSIDE, G. H. and COHN, I. (1969) Everting versus inverting gastrointestinal anastomoses: bacterial leakage and anastomotic disruption. *Ann. Surg., 169,* 343.

RUSSELL, I. and JOHNSON, N. (1960) Perforation of the colon in large bowel obstruction due to carcinoma. *Aust. N.Z. J. Surg., 29,* 332.

RYAN, P. (1958) Emergency resection and anastomosis for perforated sigmoid diverticulitis. *Br. J. Surg., 45,* 611.

—— (1969) An experimental preparation suitable for studying the effect of bacterial contamination and infection upon the healing of colon wounds. *Aust. N.Z. J. Surg., 38,* 364.

—— (1970) The effect of surrounding infection upon the healing of colonic wounds: experimental studies and clinical experiences. *Dis. Colon Rect., 13,* 124.

SAMES, C. P. (1960) Resection of carcinoma of the colon in the presence of obstruction. *Lancet, 2,* 948.

SAVAGE, P. T. (1967) Immediate resection with end-to-end anastomosis for carcinoma of the colon presenting with acute intestinal obstruction. *Proc. R. Soc. Med., 60,* 207.

SCHOEMAKER, J. (1921) Some technical points in abdominal surgery. *Surgery Gynec. Obstet., 33,* 591.

SCHULER, J. G. and ALIAPOULIOS, M. A. (1973) The Cambridge loop colostomy. *Surgery Gynec. Obstet., 137,* 281.

SELWOOD, R. A., BURN, J. I., WATERWORTH, P. A. and WELBOURN, R. D. (1969) A second clinical trial to compare two methods for preoperative preparation of the large bowel. *Br. J. Surg.*, 56, 610.

SHARBAUGH, R. J. and RAMBO, W. M. (1974) Cephalothin and peritoneal lavage in the treatment of experimental peritonitis. *Surg. Gynec. Obstet.*, 139, 211.

SHARPE, M. and GOLDEN, R. (1950) End-to-end anastomosis of the colon following resection: a roentgen study of forty-two cases. *Am. J. Roentgen.*, 64, 769.

SHEPHERD, J. M. and JONES, J. S. P. (1971) Adenocarcinoma of the large bowel. *Br. J. Cancer*, 25, 680.

SILEN, W. (1975) Personal communication.

SIMPSON, B. R., PARKHOUSE, J., MARSHALL, R. and LAMBRECHTS, W. (1962) Extradural anaesthesia and the prevention of postoperative respiratory complications. *Br. J. Anaesth.*, 33, 628.

SINGLETON, A. O., Jr., DAVID, D. and JULIAN, J. (1959) The prevention of wound infection following contamination with colon organisms. *Surgery Gynec. Obstet.*, 108, 389.

—— WHITE, D. and MONTALBO, P. (1968) A comparative study of intestinal anastomoses. *Archs Surg., Chicago*, 96, 563.

SISTRUNK, W. E. (1928) Mikulicz operation for resection of the colon; its advantages and dangers. *Ann. Surg.*, 88, 597.

SLANEY, G. (1971) Results of treatment of carcinoma of the colon and rectum. In *Modern Trends in Surgery* 3, ed. W. T. Irvine. London: Butterworths.

SMEAD, L. (1940) Quoted by Jones et al. (1941).

SMIDDY, F. G. and GOLIGHER, J. C. (1957) Results of surgery in the treatment of cancer of the large intestine. *Br. med. J.*, 1, 793.

SMILEY, D. F. (1966) Perforated sigmoid diverticulitis with spreading peritonitis. *Am. J. Surg.*, 111, 431.

SMITH, G. A., GOTT, V. L., CRISP, N. W. and PERRY, J. F., Jr. (1955) Intestinal obstructions due to primary neoplastic strictures of the bowel. *Surgery, St Louis*, 37, 778.

SORESI, A. L. (1919) Why is end-to-end intestinal anastomosis unsafe? *Ann. Surg.*, 69, 613.

SPENCER, F. C., SHARP, E. H. and JUDE, J. R. (1963) Experiences with wire closure of abdominal incisions in 293 selected patients. *Surgery Gynec. Obstet.*, 117, 235.

STEICHEN, F. M. (1968) The use of staples in anatomical side-to-side and functional end-to-end enteroanastomosis. *Surgery, St Louis*, 64, 948.

—— (1971) Clinical experience with auto suture instruments. *Surgery, St Louis*, 69, 609.

STOKER, T. A. M. and ELLIS, H. (1972) Wound antibiotics in gastro-intestinal surgery. Comparison of ampicillin with penicillin and sulphadiazine. *Br. J. Surg.*, 59, 184.

STOKES, E. J., WATERWORTH, P. M., WATSON, B. and CLARK, C. G. (1974) Short-term routine antibiotic prophylaxis in surgery. *Br. J. Surg.*, 61, 739.

SULLIVAN, R. D., JONES, R., SCHNABEL, T. F., Jr. and SHOREY, J. McC. (1953) The treatment of human cancer with intra-arterial nitrogen mustard (methylbis (2-chloroethyl)amine hydrochloride). *Cancer*, 6, 121.

SYKES, F. R. (1979) Transcutaneous defunctioning tube colostomy. *Br. J. Surg.*, (In the Press).

TAYLOR, I. (1978) Cytotoxic perfusion for colorectal liver metastases. *Br. J. Surg.*, 65, 109.

TAYLOR, S. A. and CAWDERRY, H. M. (1977) The use of metronidazole in the preparation of the bowel for surgery. *Proc. R. Soc. Med.*, 70, 481.

TEICHER, I. and ABRAHAMS, J. I. (1956) The treatment of selected cases of multiple polyps, familial polyposis, and diverticular disease of the colon by subtotal colectomy and ileoproctostomy. *Surgery Gynec. Obstet.*, 103, 136.

THOMPSON, J. P. S. and HAWLEY, P. R. (1972) Results of closure of loop transverse colostomies. *Br. med. J.*, 3, 459.

THORNE, T. C., GALLEY, A. H. and BROMAGE, P. R. (1954) Present position of spinal and extradural anaesthesia. *Proc. R. Soc. Med.*, 47, 301.

TRAVERS, B. (1812) *An Enquiry into the Process of Nature in Repairing Injuries of the Intestine*, p. 129. London: Longman, Rees, Orme, Brown and Green.

TRIMPI, H. D., KHUBCHANDANI, I. T., SHEETS, J. A. and STASIK, J. J. (1976) Advances in intestinal anastomosis: experimental study and an analysis of 984 patients. *Dis. Colon Rectum*, 20, 107.

TROWBRIDGE, P. E. and HOWES, E. L. (1967) Reinforcement of colon anastomoses using polyurethane foam treated with neomycin: an experimental study. *Am. J. Surg.*, 113, 236.

TRUEBLOOD, H. W., NELSON, T. S., KOHATSU, S. and OBERHELMAN, H. A. (1969) Wound healing in the colon: comparison of inverted and everted closures. *Surgery, St Louis*, 65, 919.

TURNBULL, R. B., Jr. (1966) Personal communication.

—— KYLE, K. and WATSON, F. R. (1967) Cancer of the colon: the influence of the no-touch isolation technic on survival rates. *Ann. Surg.*, 166, 420.

TURNER, G. GREY (1955) Operations for intestinal obstruction. *Modern Operative Surgery*. 4th ed., vol. 1, p. 1017. London: Cassell.

TURNER-WARWICK, R. T. (1976) The use of the omental pedicle graft in urinary tract reconstruction. *J. Urol.*, 116, 341.

—— WYNNE, E. J. C. and HANDLEY-ASHKEN, M. (1967) The use of the omental pedicle graft in the repair and reconstruction of the urinary tract. *Br. J. Surg.*, 54, 55.

TYSON, R. R. and SPAULDING, E. H. (1959) Should antibiotics be used in large bowel preparation? *Surgery Gynec. Obstet.*, 108, 623.

VAN PROHASKA, J., GOVOSTIS, M. C. and WASICK, M. (1953) Multiple organ resection for advanced carcinoma of the colon and rectum. *Surgery Gynec. Obstet.*, 97, 177.

VINK, M. (1954) Local recurrence of cancer in the large bowel: the role of implantation metastases and bowel disinfection. *Br. J. Surg.*, 41, 431.

VOGEL, C. M., KINGSBURY, R. J. and BANE, A. E. (1972) Intravenous hyperalimentation. *Archs Surg., Chicago*, 105, 414.

VOITK, A. J., ECHAVE, V., BROWN, R. A., McARDLE, A. H. and GURD, F. N. (1973) Elemental diet in the treatment of fistulas of the alimentary tract. *Surgery Gynec. Obstet.*, 137, 68.

WANEBO, H. J., SEMOGLOU, C., ATTIYEN, F. and STEARNS, M. (1978) Surgical management of patients with primary operable colorectal cancer and synchronous liver metastases. *Am. J. Surg., 135*, 81.

WANGENSTEEN, O. H. (1940) Aseptic gastric resection. *Surgery Gynec. Obstet., 70*, 59.

—— (1949) Quoted by Baronofsky (1950).

—— (1949) Cancer of the colon and rectum. *Wis. med. J., 48*, 591.

—— and GILBERTSON, V. A. (1963) Results of surgery for cancer of colon and rectum at University of Minnesota Medical Center, 1940–54. Presented at Int. Symp. on End Results of Cancer Therapy, Sandefjord, Norway, Sept. 16–20, 1963 *National Cancer Institute Monograph 15*, 325.

WASHINGTON, J. A., DEARING, W. H., JUDD, E. S. and ELVEBACK, L. R. (1974) Effect of preoperative antibiotic regimen on development of infection after intestinal surgery: prospective randomized, double-blind study. *Ann. Surg., 180*, 567.

WAUGH, J. M. (1954) Discussion on acute intestinal obstruction. *Lancet, 1*, 1125.

WELCH, J. P. and DONALDSON, G. A. (1974a) Management of severe obstruction of the large bowel due to malignant disease. *Am. J. Surg., 127*, 492.

—— —— (1974b) Perforative carcinoma of colon and rectum. *Ann. Surg., 180*, 734.

WHEATLEY, A. E. (1960) Skin level loop colostomy. *Proc. R. Soc. Med., 53*, 654.

WHIPPLE, A. O. (1931) Advantages of cecostomy preliminary to resections of colon and rectum. *J. Am. med. Ass., 97*, 1962.

WILKIE, D. P. D. (1934) Cancer of the colon: its surgical treatment. *Lancet, 1*, 65.

WILKINS, J. L., HARDCASTLE, J. D., MANN, C. V. and KAUFMAN, L. (1970) Effects of neostigmine and atropine on motor activity of ileum, colon and rectum of anaesthetized subjects. *Br. med. J., 1*, 793.

WILLIS, A. T., FERGUSON, I. R. and JONES, P. H. (1977) Metronidazole in prevention and treatment of *Bacteroides* infections in elective colon surgery. *Br. med. J., 1*, 607.

WILSON, H. and WOLF, R. Y. (1966) Hepatic lobectomy: indications, technique and results. *Surgery, St Louis, 59*, 472.

WILSON, S. M. and ADSON, M. A. (1976) Surgical treatment of hepatic metastases from colorectal causes. *Archs Surg., Chicago, 111*, 329.

WINITZ, M., ADAMS, R. F. and SEEDMAN, D. A. (1970) Studies in metabolic nutrition employing chemically define diets: II. Effect on gut microflora populations. *Am. J. clin. Nutr., 23*, 546.

—— GRAFF, J. and GALLAGHER, N. (1965) Evaluation of chemical diets as nutrition for man in space. *Nature, Lond., 205*, 741.

WOODWARD, S. C., HERRMANN, J. B., SHADOMY, S. and PULASKI, E. J. (1964) Oral neomycin and the healing of colonic anastomoses in the rat. *Surgery Gynec. Obstet., 119*, 799.

WRIGHT, A. D. (1951) Personal communication.

18

Treatment of Carcinoma of the Rectum

Only two forms of treatment are capable of offering any prospects of complete cure of rectal carcinoma, namely surgery and radiotherapy. The former has been the method hitherto mainly employed, and though advances in radiotherapy in recent years have undoubtedly increased its value in this situation as elsewhere, surgical excision still remains our principal mode of treatment for rectal cancer. Many different techniques have been devised for removal of the rectum for malignant disease, and the more important of these will now be briefly surveyed to indicate their advantages and disadvantages, before discussing present-day practice.

EVOLUTION OF EXCISION OF THE RECTUM

Perineal Excision

A very limited, entirely extraperitoneal excision of the rectum by this route had been practised by Faget (1739), Lisfranc (1826), Verneuil (1873) and Allingham and Allingham (1901), but it was J. P. Lockhart-Mummery (1907, 1920) who was mainly responsible for developing this very inadequate method into a worthwhile cancer operation. Like Allingham, with whom he worked at St Mark's Hospital, he also employed a preliminary loop iliac colostomy, the opportunity being taken at this stage to perform an exploratory laparotomy to assess the operability of the growth from the abdominal aspect and to determine the presence of hepatic or peritoneal deposits. The perineal operation was performed two weeks or so later; during the interval the distal bowel was washed out daily from colostomy to anus. For the excision the patient was placed on the left side with the knees drawn up and a wide elliptical incision made round the anus and prolonged backwards to the coccyx, which was excised. The levatores ani were divided some distance from their attachment to the bowel, and the plane of cleavage between the front of the rectum and the prostate and vesicles followed by careful dissection till the pelvic peritoneum was encountered. This was opened and the cut prolonged upwards with scissors on either side of the rectum. The lateral ligaments were then divided, completing the mobilization. The rectum could now be drawn down strongly whilst the superior haemorrhoidal vessels were isolated posteriorly and ligated as high as possible. Lastly the bowel itself was severed between crushing clamps in the upper part of the wound and the blind stump closed by an inverting stitch of Moynihan–Mikulicz type, as used to close the duodenal stump after a Polya gastrectomy. The wound was sutured loosely around a large rubber drain.

By this extended perineal excision it was possible to remove on the average about 22–25 cm of rectum and distal sigmoid, and Lockhart-Mummery (1926) used it for practically all rectal growths but admitted that it was unsuitable for lesions of the upper end of the rectum or rectosigmoid. As regards upward lymphatic spread, however, it was a relatively restricted operation even for carcinomas of the rectum proper, for, as Gabriel (1948) has pointed out, through a purely perineal wound the highest possible point of ligation of the superior haemorrhoidal vessels was 5–7.5 cm below the promontory of the sacrum (which is 11–13.5 cm below the bifurcation of the abdominal aorta and 15–17.5 cm below the origin of the inferior mesenteric artery—see Fig. 20). Another disadvantage was the mechanically unsatisfactory arrangement of a blind end of bowel distal to the colostomy, which might leak and give rise to a mucous fistula through the perineal wound, or even to a discharge of faeces if, as sometimes happened in time, the colostomy spur receded allowing bowel contents to pass into the distal limb. But Lockhart-Mummery (1926) was able to show that despite these objections, the method could be very satisfactory in actual practice. This was amply confirmed by the collective experience of St Mark's Hospital where, up to the early 1930s, this technique of preliminary laparotomy and colostomy followed by extended perineal excision was almost the routine operation for excisable carcinoma of the rectum. From 1910 to 1931, during which time the operability rate for rectal cancer was 50%, 370 cases were treated by perineal excision with an 11.6% immediate mortality, and 40% of five-year survivals (Gabriel 1932).

The chief virtue of this operation was that, in the days before blood transfusion and other ancillaries of modern surgery were readily available, it was a relatively safe and simple operation even in the hands of the average surgeon. For that reason during the period up to World War II it became quite the most popular method in this country and in America, where it was known

TABLE 34. *Five-Year Survival Rate after Excision of the Rectum (Operation Deaths Excluded)*

Group	Perineal excision (%)	Combined excision (%)
A	82·2	83·9
B	61·7	62·3
C	17·9	31·0
Total	44·9	47·1

St Mark's Hospital Statistics: Dukes, quoted by Gabriel (1948).

either as Lockhart-Mummery's operation or as posterior excision. The main inadequacy of the perineal route was in dealing with the important superior zone of lymphatic spread, and this was well demonstrated by Dukes (quoted by Gabriel 1948) in a comparative study of the late results of perineal and combined abdominoperineal excision (Table 34). It will be noted that there was no significant difference in the five-year survival rates for the two operations in cases without lymphatic metastases (A and B cases), but that when lymphatic spread had occurred (C cases) perineal excision was notably less efficient than the combined operation. With the increasing safety of surgery in recent years most surgeons have preferred more radical methods than perineal excision, which has accordingly been largely abandoned, but it certainly played a most valuable role in the management of rectal cancer during the inter-war years and many patients owed their lives to it.

Sacral Excision

Though this method had been employed by Kocher in 1875, its introduction into surgical practice was due to Kraske, who described the technique in detail to the Fourteenth Congress of the German Association of Surgeons in 1885, and with his name it has ever since been associated. With the patient lying on the left or right side an incision was made from behind the anus over the lower sacrum, usually inclining to one or other side of the midline. By removal of the coccyx and the lowermost two pieces of the sacrum good access was obtained to the back of the rectum above the levator muscles. The peritoneum was opened on one side of the bowel, which was then drawn downwards as far as possible and the superior haemorrhoidal vessels divided. Inferiorly the dissection was carried as far as necessary, the operation being completed either by excising the entire rectum and anal canal and establishing a sacral anus at the posterior end of the wound—the so-called *amputation of the rectum*—or by removing a sleeve of bowel containing the growth and restoring continuity by end-to-end anastomosis—the so-called *resection of the rectum.*

Sacral excision rapidly became the most popular method in Germany and Austria and various modifications of Kraske's original technique were introduced by Bardenheuer, Rose, Hochenegg, Billroth, Rehn, Heinecke and Rydygier (see Rankin et al. 1932). These were mostly concerned with the disposition of the incision and the amount of sacrum that should be removed or temporarily resected as an osteo-integumentary flap. Other innovations related to the method of restoring continuity if a resection were performed, for it had soon become apparent that end-to-end anastomosis by simple circular suture was very prone to be followed by breakdown and the formation of a faecal fistula, which was extremely difficult to close. To try to avoid this complication Hochenegg (1888, 1889) developed two alternative techniques for effecting union:

The invagination method in which the upper edge of the distal stump of bowel was turned into the lumen and out through the anus, whilst the proximal stump was drawn down through it, so that the cut edges of the two tubes of the bowel could be united by suture outside the anus. The effect was that when the anastomosis was subsequently returned through the anal canal the actual suture line was well inverted into the lumen. (Looked at from the point of view of the surgeon working through a sacral wound, the anorectal stump was certainly *in*vaginated into the distal bowel lumen, but in relation to the anal canal it would be more appropriately regarded as *e*vaginated.)

The Durchzug method, in which the distal stump was again turned temporarily inside out through the anus but in this technique the exposed mucosa was completely excised from it; it was then returned to the pelvis and the proximal stump drawn down through it to the anal orifice, where its cut lower edge was sutured to the skin. It was hoped thereby to effect a broad union between the serous surface of the colon and the raw inner aspect of the lower rectum and anal canal, but it is not at all clear that this was in fact often achieved (see Mandl 1922). Küttner (1910, 1916), recognizing the inevitability of frequent dehiscence of the bowel suture line if primary anastomosis were attempted in these cases, developed a type of Mikulicz–Paul exteriorization resection through the sacral wound with subsequent staged closure. Surprisingly enough a proximal colostomy as a temporary defunctioning manoeuvre was not often employed by Continental surgeons in conjunction with sacral resection.

The best exposition of the results of these sacral operations is perhaps that of Mandl (1922, 1929) who conducted a careful statistical analysis of the clinical material at Hochenegg's Clinic in Vienna. In his second report he refers to a total of 1704 patients with rectal cancer seen at that clinic, of whom 984 or some 58% were subjected to sacral excision (a few others were treated by combined excision) with an immediate mortality of 11·6%. The five-year survival rate was 30%. Approximately half the operations were conducted as amputations with establishment of a sacral anus, and half as resections with restoration of continuity. In fact sacral excision had much the same advantages and disadvantages as perineal excision; in other words it was a fairly safe operation at a time when abdominoperineal excision carried a high mortality and it gave fairly good late results, but its limited upper extent made it a somewhat inadequate operation in cases with lymphatic spread. In an endeavour to increase the upward scope of sacral excision, Westhues (1933) developed the use of the prone or 'hanging-belly' position for this operation. This certainly improved access to the upper pelvis, and by employing this method and adopting an extrafascial, presacral, approach to the vascular pedicle, Goetze (1931) claimed to be able to tie the inferior mesenteric vessels almost at the promontory of the sacrum. But even this fell short of what could be achieved by operations including an abdominal phase, and for that reason, as the latter operations became safer in practice, they have largely displaced sacral excisions on the Continent.

The sacral operation never enjoyed much vogue in this country or America, despite its strong advocacy by Harrison Cripps (1907), Swinford Edwards (1908) and Grey Turner (1931).

Combined Abdominoperineal or Perineo-Abdominal Excision

A combined operation involving abdominal and perineal phases for excision of the rectum was first performed by Czerny (1883) not as a premeditated plan but as a means of finishing a sacral excision which he had found himself unable to complete from below. In carrying out combined excision as a deliberate procedure most surgeons have preferred to perform the abdominal phase first. It is difficult to discover who originated this method but it was early associated on the Continent with the name of Quénu (quoted by Kocher 1907). However, it was undoubtedly the work of Ernest Miles (1908) that established the abdominoperineal operation in favour in England and America. Following his researches into the mode of spread of rectal cancer (see p. 391), he concluded that a radical excision for this condition, wherever situated in the rectum, ought to embrace the following structures: the entire rectum including the anal canal and sphincters, considerable parts of the levator ani muscles and ischiorectal fat, practically all the sigmoid colon and mesocolon including the superior haemorrhoidal and inferior mesenteric vessels and glands lying in its base, and a portion of the pelvic peritoneum adjacent to the rectum. Obviously nothing short of an extensive abdominoperineal operation, inevitably involving the creation of an iliac colostomy, would satisfy these criteria, and his consistent advocacy of this form of operation and beautifully designed technique for executing it have very fittingly resulted in the abdominoperineal excision being referred to as the Miles operation.

The great drawback to this operation when first introduced was that it was an extremely shocking procedure with a high initial mortality. Thus in Miles' first 61 cases, treated during the period up to 1914, there were 22 immediate deaths, a mortality of 36·2%. As a consequence abdominoperineal excision was only very slowly adopted by surgeons in general, and not till the late 1930s was it at all widely used. But since then, as surgery has become safer and it has been possible to carry out combined excision with a steadily decreasing mortality, the method has become the most commonly accepted operation for rectal cancer in Britain and America.

The technique of the Miles operation will be described in detail later (see p. 525), but certain modifications of this technique which were introduced with the object of simplifying its performance or making it safer will now be mentioned.

TWO-STAGE COMBINED EXCISION

Some surgeons thought that if the operation were divided into two stages it might be better borne by the patient. The first stage consisted of the establishment of a colostomy alone or involved a variable amount of abdominal dissection of the rectum and division of its superior vascular pedicle. Several techniques were described by Coffey (1915), Fiske Jones and McKittrick (1922), Rankin (1929) and Lahey (1930), all of which were at one time believed to be valuable. But it is fair to say that these methods of performing two-stage combined excision have been abandoned in favour of the one-stage operation.

PERINEO-ABDOMINAL EXCISION

The original technique of Czerny (1883) was apparently allowed to lapse till Grey Turner revived it as a two-stage operation in 1920. Gabriel (1934*b*) subsequently developed this method as a single-stage procedure and became its chief advocate. He considered it to be a less shocking operation than abdominoperineal excision and, for a surgeon familiar with perineal dissections, much simpler to perform than the Miles operation. In fact it is really a perineal excision finished through the abdomen to give a higher division of the main vessels, a greater removal of bowel, and a terminal colostomy rather than a loop colostomy with a distal blind end. With the patient in the left lateral position the rectum is freed from below exactly as in a perineal excision but, instead of dividing the superior haemorrhoidal vessels and bowel in the perineal wound, the mobilized segment is pushed up into the abdominal cavity through the cut in the pelvic peritoneum. The latter may then be partly sutured from below, and the perineal wound loosely closed round a stout rubber drain. The patient is now turned on to his back, the abdomen opened and the freed stump of bowel drawn up whilst the inferior mesenteric vessels are defined and divided. A small incision is next made in the abdominal wall of the left iliac region and the intact tube of rectum and sigmoid threaded through it. The suture of the pelvic peritoneum is now completed and the abdominal wound closed and dressed. Lastly the protruding bowel is amputated 5–8 cm beyond the skin level leaving a well-projecting iliac colostomy, which may be trimmed later in the postoperative period as required.

Gabriel's (1957) unique experience demonstrated beyond question that this method could be very safe. But to the average surgeon, who has not had the benefit of the long apprenticeship in perineal excision that Gabriel enjoyed with P. Lockhart-Mummery, the abdominoperineal method, in which the bulk of the dissection is done from above, seems to make better use of his general abdominal experience than does the perineo-abdominal operation. Also, though the latter is termed perineo-abdominal, it is in fact abdominoperineo-abdominal, for the initial step in the operation is exploration of the abdomen, which is then closed temporarily whilst the patient is turned on to his side for the perineal phase. This may strike many as a rather circuitous way of removing the rectum. It is probably for these reasons that this operation has never become popular.

SYNCHRONOUS COMBINED EXCISION

Bloodgood (1906) and Clogg (1923) both suggested that, with a suitable arrangement of the patient the abdominal and perineal phases of a combined excision might be performed simultaneously, and both of them essayed such operations. But it was Kirschner of Heidelberg (1934) who demonstrated conclusively that this was a practicable procedure. Devine (1937) introduced the method afresh to the English-speaking world, and Lloyd-Davies (1939), by devising special adjustable leg rests to support the patient in the lithotomy–Trendelenburg position necessary for a synchronous approach to abdomen and perineum, and elaborating various other refinements of technique, greatly assisted the development of the operation. The advantages claimed for this method are that it saves a considerable amount of operating time; that it makes the removal of very advanced fixed growths easier because their dissection can proceed from above and below simultaneously, and that it greatly facilitates suture of the pelvic peritoneum because this takes place over an empty pelvis and not on top of the divided sigmoid colon, mesocolon, and rectum, waiting to be removed from below.

Certain criticisms have been levelled at the synchronous technique. First of all it is said that the lithotomy–Trendelenburg position offers a poor approach for both the abdominal and the perineal dissections. It certainly is something of a compromise but, with attention to the details of the initial positioning of the patient and the arrangement of instrument tables and towelling etc., satisfactory access can always be obtained for both operators. Secondly, the synchronous operation is said to be more shocking than an ordinary abdominoperineal or perineo-abdominal excision because the total trauma is inflicted in a shorter space of time from two fields simultaneously. I doubt if there is any validity in this charge. And thirdly, it is complained that for this operation two surgeons are required instead of one, and that this may be inconvenient. This is certainly true and I would emphasize that it is not sufficient to detail a junior assistant to carry out the perineal part of the excision; indeed nothing is more likely to discredit the method, because the anterior dissection from below is quite the most difficult part of the whole operation as a rule. Even if an experienced colleague is available it must be admitted that some surgeons are by temperament unable to bring themselves to delegate responsibility for a considerable portion of the operation to an associate. But a lone operator may use the lithotomy–Trendelenburg position to perform an abdominoperineal, or perineo-abdominal, excision in sequence rather than synchronously, though this means losing some of the advantage of the position.

These points may be disputed but the fact is that, due in large measure to the convincing demonstration of the feasibility and advantages of the synchronous operation by Lloyd-Davies and his colleagues at St Mark's Hospital, this method has now become the favourite technique for combined excision of the rectum throughout the British Commonwealth. In America this method, which often goes by the name of the 'two-team technique', has enjoyed apparently only a very limited vogue, and the same is true in Germany and other Continental countries.

EXTENDED COMBINED EXCISION

Attempts have been made to increase the scope of combined excision still farther in various ways:

HIGHER LIGATION OF THE INFERIOR MESENTERIC VESSELS WITH OR WITHOUT EXTENDED LEFT COLECTOMY

Miles (1926) recommended that in the performance of his operation the main ligature should be placed opposite the bifurcation of the abdominal aorta. This tie usually lies just below the origin of the left colic or first sigmoid artery, so that whilst it permitted of a fairly high division of the inferior mesenteric vessels, it also ensured a good direct blood supply to the portion of the colon selected for the establishment of the colostomy (Fig. 19A). However, the inferior mesenteric artery arises from the aorta 3·75 cm above this point, and this technique therefore leaves a small portion of vessel with related lymph glands which might have been excised making the operation slightly more radical. Moynihan (1908), Deddish (1950), State (1951), Ault et al. (1952) and Grinnell and Hiatt (1952) have recommended tying the inferior mesenteric artery at its origin from the abdominal aorta to avoid leaving this remnant of artery and associated lymphatics, and Grinnell and Hiatt (1952) and McElwain et al. (1954) describe specimens showing involved lymph glands at the upper end of the inferior mesenteric chain, which were removed by high ligation but would undoubtedly have been left *in situ* if the vessels had been divided at the level of the aortic bifurcation.

However, the evidence as to whether the higher ligation does in fact confer any practical benefit on the patient is somewhat equivocal. Morgan and Griffiths (1959) reported that, in a series of 220 cases of cancer of the rectum or distal colon treated by radical excisions of various kinds (but all incorporating a high ligation of the inferior mesenteric vessels) dissection of the operative specimens revealed a C_2 state of spread of the lesion—that is, lymph nodes involved up to the ligature on the main vessels—in 8%. In a comparable series of 206 patients operated on before the practice of high ligation was introduced, the proportion of C_2 cases was significantly greater—namely 16%. But in a similar survey of dissected operation specimens Grinnell (1965) found 13% of C_2 cases in 193 cancers removed without high ligation, and nearly as many—11·8%—in 161 cancers treated with high ligation. More important perhaps are the findings on follow-up. Grinnell (1965) has worked out the five-year survival rates in two fairly similar groups of patients with cancers of the rectum or distal colon treated by radical excision, respectively with and without high inferior mesenteric ligation. There was a 5·7% advantage in favour of high ligation, a difference that was not considered to be statistically significant. Most impressive of all is the information given by Grinnell (1965) on the ultimate fate of the 19 individual patients who all had high-lying lymph node metastases that would not have been removed if high ligation had not been practised. None of this small group survived free of disease, so that the salvage rate of the higher ligation was nil. These findings suggest that, when the highest inferior mesenteric nodes are implicated, cancer cells have usually spread elsewhere beyond the reach of radical surgery.

An obvious consequence of ligation of the inferior mesenteric artery at its origin is that the left colic branch is sacrificed. This means that the only blood supply remaining to the descending and iliac colon is that derived from the middle colic artery and conveyed by the marginal artery (see Fig. 19B). Some surgeons practising high ligation during rectal excision have taken the view that this supply would be adequate only for the survival of a limited amount of colon and have therefore recommended extending the resection almost up to the splenic flexure or into the transverse colon in order to diminish the amount of bowel nourished solely by the marginal vessels. But observations by myself (Goligher 1954) and by Griffiths (1956) and Morgan (1956) show quite conclusively that these fears are without foundation, and that in the vast majority of cases this marginal supply from the middle colic artery is perfectly adequate to maintain the viability of all the left colon down to an iliac colostomy. From the patient's point of view colostomy in this site probably has advantages over the less easily regulated transverse colostomy.

An additional argument for resecting the left colon in conjunction with high ligation of the inferior mesenteric vessels is that the paracolic glands alongside the iliac and descending colon may contain metastases and that their removal by extended colectomy may make the operation more radical (State 1951). However, most researches into the spread of rectal cancer in recent years, such as those of Dukes (1930), have shown that upward lymphatic extension is confined with remarkable constancy to the glands intimately related to the main superior haemorrhoidal and inferior mesenteric vessels. Only in very advanced, probably quite incurable, cases in which these main glands have undergone extensive blockage by metastases, would the paracolic glands be likely to contain growth, and their removal would probably make little difference to the ultimate prognosis.

A further reason for resecting the left colon after high inferior mesenteric ligation is the possibly increased malignant potential of the mucosa of the entire large intestine, particularly in its distal half, in cases of carcinoma coli or recti. Excision of the left colon in addition to the rectum might thus be regarded as a sound prophylactic measure against the development of further primary growths. The precise value of this more extensive removal of large bowel in actual practice is extremely difficult to judge (see p. 431).

EXCISION OF LYMPH-GLANDS FROM PELVIC SIDE-WALLS

Deddish (1950) and Sauer and Bacon (1952) have attempted to broaden the scope of radical excisions for cancer of the rectum by dissection of the internal iliac lymph glands. These glands lie external to the parietal pelvic fascia and are quite untouched by an orthodox abdominoperineal excision, even when the lateral ligaments are divided close to the pelvic side-wall. For their proper demonstration and removal the parietal pelvic fascia must be divided at the pelvic brim and dissected downwards, exposing the glands as they lie on the iliac vessels and obturator muscle. In 11 cases with *intra*peritoneal growths Sauer and Bacon (1952) found that the excised internal iliac glands were all free from deposits, but in 21 cases with *extra*peritoneal growths they noted metastases in the internal iliac glands in six. They concluded that pelvic adenectomy should be reserved for low-lying growths. My own impression is that when glands on the pelvic side-wall are implicated the condition is really incurable, for dissection of these glands can never be complete; it is, moreover, liable to be attended by considerable haemorrhage and operative difficulty which prolongs the operation, thus possibly increasing the immediate mortality and morbidity. Deddish (1952) has commented on the increased incidence of post-operative bladder complications after pelvic adenectomy, and a long-term report on the results of the manoeuvre by Stearns and Deddish (1959) failed to disclose any significant advantage in this form of extended excision over orthodox combined excision.

MULTIVISCERAL RESECTIONS, COMPLETE PELVIC CLEARANCE, AND TRANSLUMBAR AMPUTATION

Multivisceral Resections

Not infrequently carcinoma of the rectum has become adherent to other organs anteriorly by the time the patient comes to hospital, and if removal of the growth is to be accomplished these adherent viscera must be excised in part or *in toto*. Removal of a loop of small intestine is a very simple addition to a combined excision of the rectum, as is excision of the posterior vaginal wall, which is often advisable. Ablation of an adherent uterus and uterine appendages by total hysterectomy is a more serious extension of rectal excision, but, when required, can now be performed without inordinate risk. Adherence to the prostate, seminal vesicles or bladder in the male patient is a more difficult problem. It may sometimes be dealt with by removal of a thin shaving of tissue from the posterior aspect of the prostate and by excision of the vesicles and possibly an area of the bladder wall—in which case the main hope of successful eradication probably depends on finding that the portions of tissue removed from these organs were not after all invaded by growth.

Complete Pelvic Clearance

Alternatively the drastic step may be taken of performing a total cystoprostatectomy *en bloc* with the rectal excision, as has been urged particularly by Brunschwig (1948, 1961), Deddish (1950) and Appleby (1950). If this is done the surgeon is faced with the problem of how to dispose of the ureters. Originally the favourite plan was to implant them into the sigmoid colon or the caecum. The result was a 'wet' colostomy, but it was claimed by Appleby (1950) that the colostomy actions were less liquid after caecal than sigmoid implants. However, as the patient had to wear an adhesive type of ileostomy bag on his colostomy after either form of ureteric implant into the large intestine, it did not seem to matter whether the colostomy actions were rather more or less liquid. One respect in which the caecal implant was probably less satisfactory than a ureterosigmoid anastomosis was in regard to absorption of chloride and urea from the urine in the colon leading possibly to hyperchloraemic acidosis and uraemia. But from this point of view neither method was satisfactory and a better arrangement designed to eliminate the risk of hyperchloraemia and also to minimize the danger of ascending urinary infection is that of Bricker (1950). He has advised that the ureters should be implanted into an isolated short segment of lower ileum, the distal end of which is brought to the surface as a urinary ileostomy (Fig. 367). This piece of ileum acts not as a substitute bladder, but as a short conduit to the surface, conveying the urine immediately into an ileostomy bag. For that reason it is superior to the technique suggested by Gilchrist et al. (1950) of constructing a substitute urinary bladder from caecum into which the ureters are implanted, the exit being provided by the attached segment of terminal ileum which is brought to the surface as an ileostomy but, owing to the ileocaecal valve and the direction of peristalsis, does not empty except when a catheter is passed through it into the caecum. Clearly this latter arrangement provides opportunities for considerable re-absorption of urinary electrolytes in the intervals between emptying of the 'bladder'. A report on the encouraging results can be obtained by the Bricker manoeuvre has been given by Bricker et al. (1960).

Diversion of urine into an ileal loop has been extensively practised in connection with total cystectomy for carcinoma of the bladder by urological surgeons in recent years, and Pyrah and Raper (1955) gave a good account of the technique and results of this manoeuvre. A sutured uretero-enteric anastomosis, as advised by Cordonnier (1950), Nesbit (1948) and Leadbetter (1951) to secure apposition of the ureteric and ileal mucosa, is recommended instead of the simpler 'pull-through' method of Coffey (1931), which usually led to stenosis and hydronephrosis (Fig. 368A, B). Another method of accomplishing a sutured uretero-enteric anastomosis is that of Goodwin et al. (1953). The bowel is opened through a lengthy incision on the antimesenteric border to expose its interior. Each ureter in turn is then drawn through an oblique stab wound in the intestinal wall (Fig. 368c) and its end is sutured to the ileal mucosa *within the lumen of the bowel*, thus securing good inversion. Finally the longitudinal cut in the ileum is closed with an inverting Connell stitch.

Yet another plan for providing a piece of intestine as a urinary conduit from the ureters to the surface in the operation of pelvic clearance is that of Turner-Warwick (1959). Here the upper part of the sigmoid loop nourished by the left colic artery is isolated for the purpose, the ureters being implanted into the proximal end, which is closed, whilst the distal end is brought out as a urinary colostomy on the right side of the abdomen. The faecal colostomy is established on the left side of the abdomen at the lower end of the descending colon, which is nourished by the middle colic artery through the descending marginal vessels. Symmonds and Gibbs (1970) have also used this method.

It should be borne in mind that the operative steps required to construct a separate urinary ileostomy or colostomy may represent a critical addition to the already formidable procedure of complete pelvic clearance, which is a good deal more severe than a total cystoprostatectomy alone. The tendency to acidosis after conventional ureterosigmoid anastomoses can be combated to some extent by prescribing large doses of sodium bicarbonate by mouth as emphasized by Ferris and Odel (1950), but this still leaves the patient exposed to the risk of ascending urinary infection which, if he survives for a long period after his operation, will probably lead to considerable impairment of urinary function.

An alternative to any form of uretero-intestinal anastomosis after pelvic clearance is to bring the ureters to the surface as cutaneous ureterostomies, but these are usually more difficult to fit with a satisfactory appliance than is an ileostomy or wet colostomy. Fish and Stevenson (1949), however, have described what they term 'a pedicle graft cutaneous ureterostomy' of an abdominal flap of skin and subcutaneous tissue. The fitting of a ureterostomy cup is thus said to be facilitated.

Translumbar Amputation

It is in the highest degree debatable whether the operation of translumbar amputation for locally inoperable malignant disease in the pelvis without obvious distant metastases—as practised successfully by Aust and Absolon (1962) and Miller et al. (1966b)—should ever be contemplated, because of the manifold psychological, social and economic problems involved. Very few patients would have the courage to accept such an operation—comprising, as it does, removal of the lower half of the body, and leaving them without lower limbs or pelvis and creating urinary and faecal stomas—even if the necessary social and economic resources were available to make an attempt at subsequent rehabilitation possible. Moreover, there must always be a risk that remote metastases in liver or elsewhere are not really absent but merely latent, and may tragically manifest themselves some months or a year or so after the patient has managed to survive the formidable immediate hazards and psychological strain of this most ruthless operation, as in the case reported by Miller et al. (1966a). But, if hemicorporectomy is ever to be considered an ethical procedure, conceivably there could be occasional patients with carcinoma of the rectum on which it might justifiably be performed. I doubt if I personally would ever feel inclined to undertake this operation.

Prophylactic Oöphorectomy in Conjunction with Excision of Rectal Carcinoma

Apart from removal of ovaries, tubes and uterus, adherent to a rectal carcinoma, it has been suggested by Burt (1960), originally in 1951, that routine oöphorectomy might be a useful addition to rectal or colonic excision, because of the occasional presence of secondary deposits in the ovaries, even when the latter appear macroscopically normal and there are no obvious deposits elsewhere in the peritoneal cavity. This practice has also been adopted by Rendleman and Gilchrist (1959), Deddish and Stearns (1960), Barr et al. (1962) and Sherman et al. (1965). No less than 8% of the cases with apparently normal ovaries removed in this way by Deddish and Stearns (1960) were found to contain occult deposits of growth. From the published material it is impossible to say whether prophylactic oöphorectomy has contributed significantly to the cure of patients with carcinoma

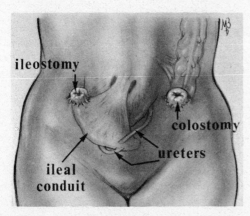

Fig. 367. A plan of the Bricker manoeuvre of implanting the ureters into an isolated loop of lower ileum which drains to the surface as a urinary ileostomy, whilst the colon discharges through a terminal left iliac colostomy.

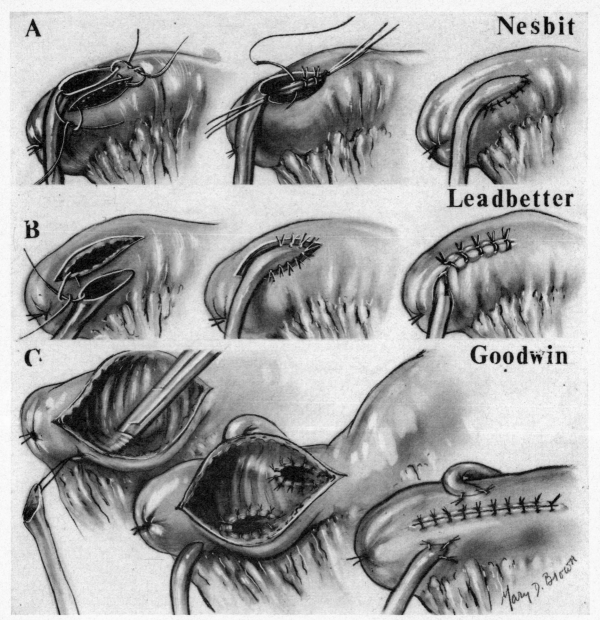

Fig. 368. Modern methods of ureterointestinal implantation providing for mucomucosal apposition. (A) The *Nesbit technique*, in which the obliquely cut end of the ureter is united by direct suture to the whole thickness of the edge of a slit in the bowel wall. (B) The *Leadbetter method*, which is similar, but the ureter is sutured to the intestinal mucosa only, and subsequent seromuscular sutures unite the bowel wall over the ureter. (C) The *Goodwin technique*, which provides for intraluminal suturing of the ureters to the bowel mucosa. A longitudinal incision is made along the antimesenteric edge of the gut. An oblique tunnel is made in the intestinal wall for each ureter which is then drawn into the bowel lumen and its obliquely cut end is sutured to the gut mucosa. Finally, the intestinal wound is closed with inverting sutures. A few stitches may be applied externally also to fix each ureter to the serosa. I use No. 4/o silk for ureteric suturing.

of the rectum or colon. Most patients with these growths have passed the menopause, so that hormonal effects from the ovarian ablation would not be a problem, but in younger patients the disadvantages of inducing an artificial menopause by oöphorectomy would have to be considered.

Sphincter-Saving Resections

Following the work of Westhues (1930, 1934), Dukes (1930, 1940) and other investigators, which showed that the lymphatic spread of rectal cancer is mainly in an upward direction, there was a resurgence of interest in Britain and America in the possibility of sphincter preservation in the radical excision of carcinomas of the upper rectum and rectosigmoid, and various forms of sphincter-saving resection were revived or developed:

SACRAL RESECTION

Though many hundreds of resections with restoration of continuity by the sacral route have been performed in Continental clinics since the close of the last century, as explained on p. 503, this method suffered two disadvantages: first there was a considerable tendency for the anastomosis to break down and give rise to an intractable sacral fistula; and secondly by modern standards it could only be regarded as a grossly inadequate operation so far as removal of the tissues of the upward zone of lymphatic spread was concerned. In the recent revival of sphincter-saving resections, therefore, it was natural to turn rather to methods incorporating an abdominal phase, which permitted of really high ligation of the inferior mesenteric vessels as in an orthodox combined abdominoperineal excision, with which of course these operations would now have to compete. However some of the techniques of anastomosis developed in connection with sacral resection have been embodied in these newer methods.

ABDOMINOSACRAL RESECTION

This operation, which overcomes the second objection to the purely sacral type of resection, was extensively practised many years ago by Finsterer (1941), Goetze (1944) and above all by d'Allaines (1956). It was also the first method employed by Pannett (1935), one of the earliest pioneers of sphincter-saving resection in this country. In this technique the main vessels are tied and the sigmoid colon and rectum mobilized as in the abdominal phase of Miles' operation, but the bowel is not divided. Instead it is pushed down into the pelvis and the pelvic peritoneum sutured over and around it or left unsutured. The abdomen is then closed and the patient placed on one side or in a prone position and a sacral incision made, through which the appropriate amount of bowel is resected and union effected by end-to-end anastomosis.

Unfortunately the risk of formation of a persistent faecal fistula through the posterior wound still remains as in sacral resection, as Goetze (1944) and d'Allaines (1956) clearly recognized. In addition, the patient is exposed to all the ordinary discomforts of a sacral wound which, apart from faecal fistulation, is particularly liable to give rise to trouble from haematoma formation and sepsis. The abdominosacral operation has never been much used in Britain and it is, I think, particularly significant that Pannett (1951) eventually gave it up in favour of anterior resection when the latter became popular in the late 1940s. However, more recently Donaldson et al. (1966) of Boston, and Localio of New York (Localio and Stahl 1969; Localio and Baron 1973; Localio and Eng 1975; Localio et al. 1978) have turned to abdominosacral resection again, not as a substitute for anterior resection, but for use in patients with growths too low for this latter operation but suitable for a sphincter-saving type of resection. Localio has unrivalled experience with the abdominosacral procedure and is now its chief advocate. He has developed a special technique whereby the entire operation is conducted with the patient lying on the right side and has demonstrated conclusively its ready feasibility and the excellent immediate results, with an immediate mortality of only 2% and a clinical anastomotic dehiscence rate of only 12%, despite the fact that most of the anastomoses lie 4–5 cm from the anal verge and he seldom uses a covering colostomy. One-third of the cases with anastomotic dehiscence required re-laparotomy for faecal peritonitis, with one death. It is to be noted that using the same criteria of assessement, Localio et al. (1978) had a clinical anastomotic dehiscence rate of under 1% after anterior resection. As regards anorectal function, most of the patients experience severe diarrhoea, sometimes with a little incontinence for some weeks after the operation, but eventually control becomes normal in the great majority of cases. The late results reported by him are certainly very good, but difficult to evaluate.

My own experience of 18 abdominosacral resections in the last three and a half years confirms in a small way Localio's findings, but I have been impressed by the inconvenience of the posterior wound in terms of discomfort, infection and haematoma formation; one persistent faecal fistula developed through it. (For technical details of abdominosacral resection, see p. 584).

ABDOMINOTRANSSPHINCTERIC

Mason has developed a modification of the abdominosacral resection in which the posterior wound involving removal of the coccyx is replaced by one in which the *external* anal sphincter and levator are divided, exposing the lower rectum which can then be freed in continuity with the previous abdominal dissection, and a resection performed down to the top of the *intact internal* anal sphincter. A colorectal anastomosis at this level

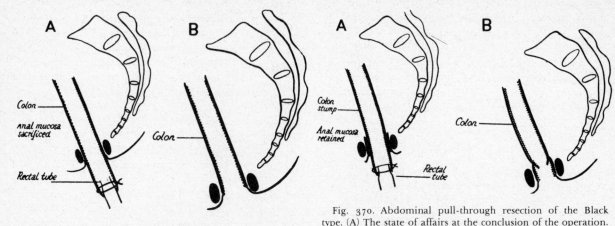

Fig. 369. Abdominoanal pull-through resection of the Bacon type. (A) The state of affairs at the conclusion of the operation. Both sphincters have been divided in the midline and resutured around the colon. (B) The final condition two or three weeks later after diathermy excision of the excess colon. (*After Goligher 1951b*)

Fig. 370. Abdominal pull-through resection of the Black type. (A) The state of affairs at the conclusion of the operation. Both the anal canal lining and the sphincters have been preserved scrupulously in an intact condition, though the canal has been stretched. (B) The final condition. (*After Goligher 1951b*)

through this kind of approach is not unduly difficult. The levator and external sphincter muscles are then reconstituted by suture. (For technical details of Mason's operation, see p. 588.)

My experience leaves me in no doubt about the technical feasibility of this operation. But very few surgeons have as yet done more than a few cases by this method, so that the main source of information about immediate functional results is Mason (1976, 1977a, b) himself, who writes enthusiastically on these scores. Clearly, further more extensive appraisal is needed.

ABDOMINOANAL PULL-THROUGH RESECTION

THE BACON–BABCOCK–BLACK OPERATION

In this operation, developed by Sebrechts (1935), Rayner (1935), Babcock (1939, 1947), Bacon (1945) and Black (1952), the rectum and sigmoid are mobilized from the abdominal aspect down to a level just above the anal sphincters. In the Bacon (1945) version, which was at one stage moderately popular, the lining of the anal canal from just below the pectinate line is then cored out to just above the sphincters, after which the plane of dissection is taken externally all round through the muscle coat of the rectal wall to reach the plane of the abdominal dissection. To facilitate this dissection the sphincters are usually divided in the mid line posteriorly. Next the mobilized rectum and sigmoid are drawn through the bared anal canal (Fig. 369A). Most of the bowel is amputated leaving a 5 cm stump into which a stout tube is tied. The sphincters are sutured with catgut around the emerging colon. When union has taken place between the outer aspect of the colon and the broad circumferential raw area in the anal

canal after 10 days or so, the excess of the colon projecting from the anus is removed by diathermy leaving the state of affairs shown in Fig. 369B.

In view of the trauma to the sphincters and the sacrifice of the anal canal lining it is not surprising that continence was frequently grossly impaired after this operation. Bacon (1945) and Waugh et al. (1954), who used this technique extensively, admitted that most of their patients were not properly continent after it, but claimed that about a third of them enjoyed something akin to normal function. My experience of 8 patients on whom I performed the Bacon operation—taking special care, however, to preserve both anal sphincters in an undamaged condition—was that even they were all incontinent and had little better than anal colostomies. Four of them were subsequently converted to abdominal colostomies with much more satisfactory results.

In *Black's (1952) version* of this operation both the sphincters and the lining of the anal canal are preserved intact. Consequently, when the colon stump is drawn through the canal, union can only take place between the cut upper edge of the anorectal remnant and the serosal surface of the colon (Fig. 370A). There apparently is a real risk that this slender basis of healing may be inadequate to prevent the colon stump from pulling up into the pelvis, particularly if the part in and beyond the anal canal underwent necrosis, but in a series of 59 cases operated on by this technique Black (1961) had no more trouble with sloughing or slipping of the colon than had Waugh and Turner (1958), using the Bacon technique. At a later stage, when sound union has taken place, the colon projecting beyond the site of healing with the upper end of the anal canal is excised by diathermy (Fig. 370B).

THE MAUNSELL–WEIR OPERATION

This method of abdominal resection was suggested by Maunsell (1892) and first practised by Weir (1901). A similar technique was elaborated quite independently by Lloyd-Davies (1950).

After an entirely abdominal dissection, the rectum is resected, leaving a long colon stump and a short anorectal one (Fig. 371). The anastomosis is then completed in a manner very similar to Hochenegg's (1888) invagination technique for union after sacral resection, the anorectal stump being turned inside out through

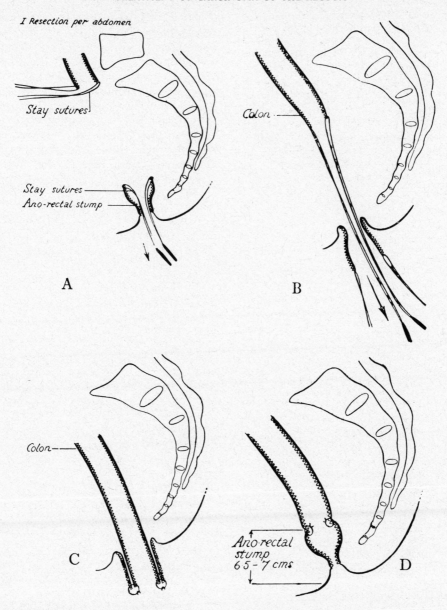

I Resection per abdomen

Stay sutures

Stay sutures
Ano-rectal stump

A

Colon

B

Colon

C

Ano-rectal
stump
6·5 - 7 cms

D

Fig. 371. Abdominoanal resection of Maunsell–Weir type. (A) Excision of carcinomatous segment completed through the abdomen leaving colonic and short anorectal stumps. (B) Anorectal stump everted; colon being drawn through. (C) Suture of anorectal and colon stumps outside anus. (D) Replacement of anastomosis in pelvis. (*From Goligher 1951b*)

the anus so that its cut upper edge becomes the projecting lower margin, and the colon stump is drawn down through it so that the free edges of both stumps lie opposite one another and can be sutured together outside the anus. The anastomosis is then pushed back through the anus into the pelvis (Fig. 371B, C, D). This method—which embodies the same principal as the later-introduced Swenson operation for Hirschsprung's disease (see pp. 291–3)—enables one to achieve a very low colorectal anastomosis without a sacral or perineal wound and without sacrificing the mucosa of the anal canal or rectum, or damaging

the anal sphincters. Accordingly the functional results might be expected to be better than after the Bacon–Babcock operation (but not the Black modification of this operation), and the majority of patients eventually attain normal continence after it (Goligher 1951b), though many of them pass through a rather uncomfortable phase at first when they are troubled by frequent small motions, and their control for flatus and liquid faeces may be somewhat impaired. It is in fact usually four to six months before rectal function becomes really worthwhile. It must be admitted also that complications referable to breakdown of the anastomosis are particularly common after this operation, and a proximal transverse colostomy should always be established at the time of the resection. This method used to be popular with my colleagues and myself at St Mark's Hospital (see Mann 1972 for a report of results), but was then completely supplanted by low anterior resection.

THE TURNBULL–CUTAIT OPERATION

This technique, which was devised separately by Turnbull of Cleveland, Ohio (Turnbull and Cuthbertson 1961) and Cutait of Sao Paolo, Brazil (Cutait and Figlioni 1961), is in essence a two-stage Maunsell–Weir operation. The *first stage* differs in no important respect from the steps of the latter operation up to the point where the anorectal stump is everted through the anus (Fig. 371A, B). After stretching the everted anal canal with the fingers for a few minutes to reduce sphincter tone, the colon stump is drawn through to project 10 or 12·5 cm beyond the cut edge of the anorectal remnant (Fig. 372A). The excess of colon is not amputated then; instead, the two protruding

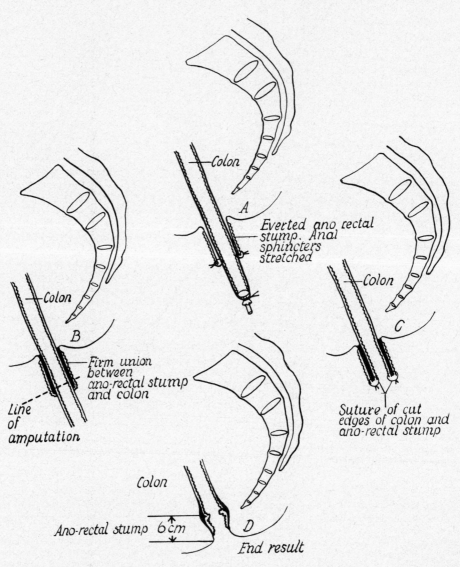

Fig. 372. The Turnbull–Cutait form of pull-through abdominoanal excision. (A) State of affairs *at conclusion of first stage*, the colon stump having been drawn through the everted anorectal stump and left in that position. (B) *Second stage*, carried out after 10–14 days, when the two stumps have become gummed together, and consisting of amputation of the excess of colon and the extreme edge of the rectal remnant. (C) The amputation has been completed by suture together of the rectal and colonic mucosae. (D) *The final state* reached after spontaneous recession of the stumps into the pelvis.

stumps are left in this position for 10–14 days, during which time they become gummed together and firmly united (Fig. 372B). At the *second stage* the projecting bowel is amputated through the edge of the anorectal remnant (Fig. 372B), and the freshly cut rectal and colonic mucosae are sutured together with fine interrupted chromic catgut or silk stitches (Fig. 372C). Gradually during the next 7–10 days—sometimes more quickly—the stumps recede through the anus into the pelvis, and final condition being similar to that after the single-stage Maunsell–Weir operation (Fig. 372D). A detailed description of the technique of the operation is given on pp. 574–7.

One of the attractions of this operation as originally propounded was that a covering transverse colostomy did not seem to be necessary, as the patient had in fact a perineal colostomy till union had taken place between the colon and rectal stumps outside the body, and there was no intrapelvic suture-line to leak. But some surgeons, including more recently Turnbull (1964), have preferred to establish a temporary loop transverse colostomy at the end of the first stage. Cutait and Figlioni (1961) and Turnbull and Cuthbertson (1961) have not encountered any serious postoperative complications referable to the choice of this particular technique of operation, but Hughes et al. (1962) have reported several rectovaginal fistulae following its use, and I myself have had to contend with major necrosis of the colon stump in no less than 9 of some 50 cases treated by the Turnbull–Cutait method (Goligher et al. 1965). Fortunately it was possible to rescue all these patients so complicated without mortality by early re-intervention to carry out excision of the remnant of anorectum and the necrotic colon and establish an iliac colostomy by an abdominoperineal operation. There is some evidence to suggest that a proximal transverse colostomy at the first stage helps to lessen the risk of subsequent sloughing of the colon stump.

The functional results of the Turnbull–Cutait operation in our hands (Goligher et al. 1965) have varied greatly from case to case, depending apparently largely upon the length of the anorectal remnant. Stumps of less than 7 cm from the anal verge were associated with indifferent control, sometimes amounting to complete incontinence, but with stumps of greater length function was usually very good. Patients may take many months to adapt to the new state of affairs, so that the length of the follow-up is very important in determining the results (Kennedy et al. 1970). Also it is unlikely that a patient undergoing a palliative excision will live long enough to make this adap-

tation fully, so that this type of operation is unsuitable for palliative cases.

ABDOMINOTRANSANAL RESECTION WITH
SUTURED COLO-ANAL SLEEVE ANASTOMOSIS

Parks (1972, 1977*a*, *b*), has described a modification of abdomino-anal resection in which the anorectal stump is not everted through the anus and the colon stump drawn through it, but instead the end of the colon is attached to the anorectal stump by sutures passed from below through a widely opened bivalve speculum. The anastomosis can be done to the top of the anorectal remnant, but this is technically very difficult and it is easier and more secure first of all to dissect off some of the anorectal mucosa and have the lowermost 3–4 cm or so of the colon stump in contact with the resulting raw area whilst its lower edge is sutured to the lower part of the anorectal mucosa as in the Soave procedure for Hirschsprung's disease. (For full technical details see p. 577.)

It might be thought that so far as the final anatomical effect of the operation is concerned it would not differ materially from that after the Bacon pull-through operation (see p. 510) but in fact the internal sphincter is zealously guarded against injury in the abdomino-transanal operation, as is also the anal canal lining up *to 0·5–1 cm above the pectinate line*. The immediate and functional results of this operation are still being accumulated, but seem quite encouraging (Lane and Parks 1977; Parks 1977*a*, *b*). Though most patients pass through a disturbing period of several weeks of great frequency of calls to stool with some leakage, many—perhaps the majority—eventually obtain satisfactory function. Lane and Parks (1977) postulate—not entirely convincingly to my mind—that the return of normal continence after this operation is due to 'rectal' sensation being provided in the colonic stump by pressure on nerve endings in the levator muscles and other pelvic structures when it is distended. The functional results are often impaired if there is prolonged sepsis or haematoma formation in the pelvis, either of which complications might lessen the close contact of the colon stump with adjacent structures. In my series of eleven cases treated by this operation, six healed their anastomoses by first intention and all eventually got good continence; five had some degree of anastomotic dehiscence or sepsis, gross in one and resulting in a tight stenosis and permanent colostomy, less severe in the other four, of whom one has satisfactory control and the other three are still only partly continent.

Abdominal or Anterior Resection

WITHOUT ANASTOMOSIS—HARTMANN'S OPERATION

At a time when anastomosis of the colon to the rectum after abdominal resection of carcinomas of the upper rectum or rectosigmoid was particularly difficult and dangerous, Hartmann (1923) employed the method of terminating such a resection by closing the upper end of the rectal stump and establishing a terminal iliac colostomy. Rankin (1928), Muir (1939) and Gabriel (1948) reported favourably on the method, but commented, as did Lloyd-Davies (1950), on the possibility of a second carcinoma arising in the retained rectal stump. Most surgeons using Hartmann's technique have employed it as an entirely intraperitoneal operation with the retention of a fairly long segment of rectum and suture of its upper end. For such cases at the present day an anterior resection with colorectal anastomosis would undoubtedly always be preferred, and indeed I have converted several cases from the state of affairs resulting from a Hartmann's operation to a sutured anastomosis between the iliac colon and the rectal stump, with very gratifying results. It is possible also to perform what may be termed an *extended Hartmann's operation*, in which the entire rectum down almost to the anorectal ring is removed, leaving merely the anal canal. No attempt is made to suture the upper end of the latter, but instead the pelvic peritoneum is closed over the pelvic cavity, and the anus is used to transmit the drainage tube. This method may be useful occasionally as a means of terminating a rectal excision rapidly without the trauma of a perineal dissection in a patient whose condition during operation has suddenly deteriorated. (For technical details see p. 592.)

WITH ANASTOMOSIS

In this connection there are two techniques to be considered:

Anterior Resection with Restoration of Continuity by Telescopic or Tube Technique

In the early years of this century operations had been devised independently by Rutherford Morison (see Grey Turner 1943), Lockhart-Mummery (1934) and Balfour (1910) for the resection of carcinomas of the rectosigmoid region by an entirely abdominal approach, with subsequent restoration of continuity by a telescopic or tube technique. This involved tying a long stout rubber or metal tube into the proximal stump of bowel and passing it into the distal stump and through the anus. By traction on the tube the bowel could be drawn into the upper part of the rectal lumen whilst sutures were inserted between the outer surface of the colon and the cut edge of the rectum. When this

row was completed, further traction on the tube produced an infolding of the upper rectal margin and facilitated the insertion of yet another layer of sutures between the walls of the colon and rectum. It is difficult to discover any accurate reports of the results of these operations but they were apparently followed by a considerable mortality and were soon discarded. But it is to be noted that d'Allaines (1956) occasionally used such a technique in more recent times.

Modern Anterior Resection with Sutured Anastomosis

This procedure has nothing whatever to do with the tube technique and is completed entirely by suture. It might be termed the 'Mayo Clinic operation' or 'Dixon's operation', for the credit for popularizing it undoubtedly lies with C. F. Dixon, C. W. Mayo, J. M. Waugh, B. M. Black and E. S. Judd of the Mayo Clinic. Wangensteen (1943, 1945) was once another very influential advocate of this operation. Certainly by this method it is possible to deal with practically all growths of the intraperitoneal part of the rectum and the rectosigmoid without having to resort to an abdominosacral or -anal technique to complete the anastomosis. It is undoubtedly an advantage to be able to avoid these latter methods, because after anterior resection healing of the anastomosis is usually more certain, and, due to the larger rectal stump retained, the functional result is generally much better. In both these respects, however, it is important to distinguish between high and low versions of this operation. *High* anterior resection, which is applicable to growths of the extreme upper end of the rectum or of the rectosigmoid, can be conducted without disturbing the pelvic peritoneum or mobilizing the rectum from the concavity of the sacrum, and the final anastomosis is between colon and a rectal stump with a short cuff of peritoneum surrounding its anterior two-thirds or three-quarters. This type of operation is usually thought to be followed by uneventful healing of the suture line in the bowel (but see p. 604), and rectal function afterwards is nearly always perfect. *Low* anterior resection involves opening the pelvic peritoneum, dividing the lateral ligaments and freeing the rectum from its sacral bed often right down to the anorectal ring. The anastomosis is then between colon and a rectal stump devoid of peritoneal covering. There is a considerable risk of partial breakdown of the suture line, particularly with very low anastomosis (see p. 604). Rectal function may be entirely satisfactory with normal control for faeces and flatus, but with very short rectal stumps 6 cm or less from the anal verge, there may be some temporary incontinence, especially for flatus (Goligher et al. 1965). It will be appreciated

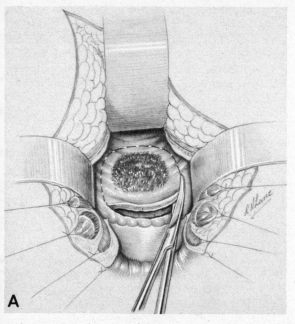
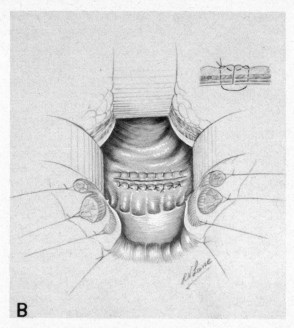

Fig. 373. Posterior transsphincteric exposure of localized relatively favourable carcinoma of the anterior rectal wall for local removal. (A) A circumcision is made with diathermy or scissors through the whole thickness of the rectal wall 1 cm from the margin of the growth. (B) When the disc of wall including the lesion has been removed the gap is closed by a single layer of vertical mattress sutures.

that this distinction into high and low resections is a little arbitrary and that in some cases the operation is a compromise between these two techniques.

The technical aspects of anterior resection are dealt with in detail on pp. 563–74, but it may be mentioned here that several variations in the method of suture and choice of suture material are available. It is also possible to achieve the anastomosis by means of mechanical devices. The earliest of these incorporated the principle of the Murphy button (Hallenbeck et al. 1963; Brummelkamp 1965), whereby the two segments of bowel are held together till union takes place and then the device comes away. The more recent devices appose the ends of the bowel taking part in the anastomosis and at the same time insert metal staples which remain in position indefinitely (see pp. 435–6). One model of the latter type is the United States Surgical Corporation TA instrument, which, if used for an end-to-end union, necessitates that the anastomosis should be triangulated. Unfortunately the suture clamp can only be applied to one side of the triangle from within the bowel lumen—that is, in inversion. To the other two sides it has to be applied in turn from the outside with the edges in eversion. There could be theoretical objections to this technique, though Ferguson and Houston

(1975) and Weakley (1978) claim very satisfactory results. A further more practical criticism of this device for anterior resection is that with it it would be more difficult to carry out a really low anastomosis.

Unquestionably a more effective suture apparatus for this purpose, and especially for low anterior resections, is the recently introduced Russian SPTU circular stapling machine*—the so-called Russian 'stapling gun'—which provides an end-to-end anastomosis with inversion of all parts of the suture line (Fain et al. 1975; Goligher et al. 1978). (For technical details see pp. 570–4.) We have found in 35 patients that anastomoses made with this device were at least as secure as those effected with hand-placed sutures. Furthermore we have convinced ourselves that it is possible with it to construct anastomoses at a lower level in some cases than would be feasible with conventional suture—for example, at 4 or 4·5 cm from the anal verge. The morbidity rate has been negligible compared with that of most other methods of exceptionally low anastomosis and the functional results have also been very satisfactory, though as with other low

* Or its American equivalent, the E-E-A, made by the United States Surgical Corporation of New York City.

anastomoses there has been great frequency of motions for the first few weeks after the covering colostomy was closed.

Methods of Local Removal or Destruction of the Primary Growth

When rectal carcinomas take the form of a well-defined polyp with a stalk on a narrow base making it easy to create a short pseudo-stalk by traction on the lesion, removal by diathermy snaring or other means, as described in dealing with benign polyps on p. 341, is probably the most generally accepted method of treatment. Indeed with this sort of small polypoid tumour the treatment by total excision in this way for the purposes of thorough histological examination often precedes the diagnosis of carcinoma and presents the surgeon with the problem of deciding whether any further surgical measures are required for a small carcinoma that was removed by snaring on the erroneous initial diagnosis of a benign polyp (see p 358).

But sometimes in the management of frank ulcerating carcinomas of a relatively localized apparently favourable kind in the lowermost 8–10 cm of rectum, particularly in poor-risk patients or in those who have refused rectal excision because of their abhorrence of a colostomy, treatment by purely local destruction or excision may be considered, though this is a highly debatable issue. Three or four methods are available:

ELECTROCOAGULATION

This technique was introduced by Strauss et al. (1935) and has been strongly advocated by Wittoesch and Jackman (1958), Madden and Kandalaft (1967, 1971a, b) and Crile and Turnbull (1972). Under general, caudal or low spinal anaesthesia, the lesion is exposed either by an operating sigmoidoscope (see Fig. 215A) with the patient in the left lateral position, or by a bivalve or trivalve anal speculum (see Fig. 37) with the patient in the lithotomy, left lateral or prone position, depending on the site of the growth of the rectal wall. With the current set at medium strength for coagulation, the entire surface of the growth is diathermized using a needle point electrode in preference to one of button point or disc type. During this process it is important to have the suction tube of the sigmoidoscope in action (see Fig. 251B) to remove smoke and allow a clear view to be obtained. When the coagulation has been completed a sharp spoon

or uterine curette is used to scrape off the superficial coagulum and expose the underlying untreated parts of the tumour. The same sequence of coagulation and curettage is then repeated once or several times to destroy the tumour more deeply, digital palpation after such curettage being a most important manoeuvre in detecting residual portions of growth. Though Madden and Kandalaft (1967) are prepared to do up to five or six fulgurations and scrapings at one session in an effort to destroy the entire tumour on that occasion, I prefer to proceed with great caution and to leave some tumour for treatment at a subsequent session.

In any event two weeks after the initial fulguration session the patient should again be taken to the theatre for a repeat examination under anaesthetic. Any areas of induration detected on digital palpation are biopsied for frozen section examination and, if positive or doubtful, are treated by further coagulation and curettage. The patient is allowed to return home a few days later but he reports at monthly intervals for six months for a careful rectal examination including digital palpation and endoscopy. If any residual growth is found, it is treated as described. After six months the patient is seen at three- to six-monthly intervals. If there is still growth present 12 months after the first session of electrocoagulation, it is best to abandon this form of treatment in favour of abdominoperineal excision.

Complications. Crile and Turnbull (1972) admit to no morbidity or mortality in their 62 patients treated by electrocoagulation, but in 77 patients similarly managed by Madden and Kandalaft (1971a, b) complications are reported in 22 (28·5%), the most frequent being haemorrhage, which was noted in 17 cases. In 10 patients the bleeding stopped spontaneously, whilst in seven operative haemostasis was required, usually by further electrocoagulation, rarely by suture ligature. Perforation into the peritoneal cavity occurred in two patients and non-fatal pulmonary embolism in colostomy, the other by abdominoperineal excision. Rectovaginal fistula also developed in two patients and non-fatal pulmonary embolism in another patient.

Eventual Results. The earliest report of a really large series of patients treated by electro-coagulation appears to be that of Wittoesch and Jackman (1958) from the Mayo Clinic. During the five-year period 1945–9 inclusive, approximately 2028 patients were treated in the Clinic for carcinoma of the rectum; 1900 underwent some form of rectal excision, but in 128 cases, because of some associated debilitating condition or the rejection by the patient of a major operation, only conservative treatment was employed, consisting usually of electrocoagulation, rarely of irradiation or local excision. It is emphasized that the patients included in this group were suffering, not just from pedunculated or sessile adenomatous lesions with carcinomatous change, but from invasive carcinoma. A follow-up survey showed that no less than 54 of these patients survived for more than five years after their initial conservative treatment, and that six were still living more than ten years later! Of the 75 patients who died in less than five years after treatment, 24 apparently succumbed from causes unrelated to the rectal carcinoma.

Similar testimony is provided by Madden and Kandalaft (1971a), who stated that of 77 patients subjected by them to electrocoagulation between 1954 and 1971, 42 had been treated for 4–17 years and of these 20 (47%) approximately were alive and well. Crile and Turnbull (1972), too, found that of 62 patients having electrocoagulation between 1952 and 1965, 42 (68%) lived at least five years. There can be no doubt, therefore, that for certain growths—presumably the very early localized ones —this method can be definitely curative, the main problem being to select the right cases for it. Strauss (1969) has postulated that in addition to the direct destruction of some of the carcinoma by electrocoagulation there may be an immunological response to the presence of dead tumour leading to rejection of remaining living tumour, but this is highly speculative.

ENDOCAVITARY CONTACT IRRADIATION

This method of treatment is dealt with on pp. 657–8.

LOCAL EXCISION

The tumour may be excised locally, the approach being either through the anus by means of a bivalve anal speculum (see p. 37) or through a posterior wound dividing the anal sphincters, levators and posterior rectal wall (see p. 355) as for benign tumours, except that the dissection of the actual lesion is not in the submucous plane but instead involves excision of a disc of the full thickness of the rectal wall (Fig. 373A) with a 1 cm margin of clearance all round. The gap in the wall of the rectum is closed with a single row of vertical mattress sutures of 2/0 chromic catgut or Dexon (Fig. 373B).

A very important step in the conduct of local excision of a rectal carcinoma in this way is the *processing of the operative specimen*. The disc of tissue removed should be pinned out on a cork square which is then floated upside down in a fixative solution. In this way the pathologist is enabled to prepare more accurately his histological sections to show the extent of the spread of the growth through the rectal wall. Clearly, if the lesion has extended completely through the wall of the bowel to reach the perirectal tissues and become at least a Dukes B growth, the desirability of proceeding to a formal rectal excision has immediately to be considered.

Bevan (1917), Mason (1976, 1977a), Parks (1977b) and Morson et al. (1977) have written strongly in favour of local excision for certain cases of rectal cancer, but the five-year results reported for this treatment of 22 *non-peduculated* small carcinomas at St Mark's Hospital by Lock et al. (1978) are a little discouraging. Five patients underwent early reoperation for suspected incomplete removal, though residual tumour was found in only two. Two other patients developed recurrence. By contrast, of 88 patients with *pedunculated* rectal carcinomas, 68 required no further operation, although one died with widespread metastases. Twenty patients underwent further operation, 16 for suspected residual tumour and four later for recurrent disease.

PRESENT-DAY CHOICE OF RADICAL OPERATION FOR RECTAL CANCER

All researches into the mode of spread of carcinoma of the rectum are agreed in emphasizing the paramount importance of upward lymphatic spread along the superior haemorrhoidal and inferior mesenteric vessels in the dissemination of this disease. In its radical removal therefore it is essential to excise these vessels with their accompanying lymphatics to as high a level as possible, which in turn implies the necessity for opening the abdomen, for only through an abdominal approach can ligation of this vascular pedicle be effected at any point above the sacral promontory. There are other advantages too in incorporating an abdominal phase in the operation. The surgeon can assess more accurately the extent of spread of the growth and the prognosis, and can undertake simultaneously resection of adherent viscera which would be impossible from below.

Clearly the only operations that satisfy these requirements are a *combined excision* and *certain forms of sphincter-saving resection conducted wholly or partly through the abdomen*, and at the present time the choice of radical operation lies essentially between these two alternatives. Theoretically there ought perhaps still to be a place for purely perineal or sacral excision as procedures of less radical scope—and lesser severity—for certain poor-risk subjects, but in actual practice, unless a surgeon is doing an operation fairly frequently, he is not really in a position to exploit its safety to maximum advantage, and I doubt if the occasional perineal excision in the hands of a man who habitually employs combined excision is any safer than his well-polished performance of the latter operation. In fact I have not found it necessary to use perineal excision even once during the last 20 years.

For the occasional cases with what are judged clinically to be very localized favourable carcinomas in the lower rectum, particularly if the general condition is poor, making a formal rectal excision specially hazardous, or if the patient adamantly refuses such an operation, local destruction or removal of the primary growth by electrocoagulation, endocavitary contact irradiation or local excision is a method that requires to be considered.

Combined Excision

For the average surgeon this may now be regarded as the standard operation for most cases of rectal cancer. The choice of technique for its performance from amongst the three main methods available —the Miles operation, the perineo-abdominal excision, and the synchronous combined excision —is a very personal matter, in which the surgeon's training, experience, and natural bent must play a big part. For the reasons indicated on p. 504, few surgeons have felt attracted to the perineo-abdominal method of effecting a combined removal of the rectum. Surgical preference has thus usually lain with the classical abdominoperineal technique of Miles or with the synchronous combined operation, either of which utilizes to greater advantage the average surgeon's general abdominal experience. I would say that the choice between these two techniques must depend largely on the organization that the surgeon can command. I have no doubt, however, that, where the synchronous technique is feasible, it has very definite advantages

over the classical abdominoperineal operation done by a single operator, and I am certain that few surgeons who have ever had the opportunity of practising the synchronous method *under good conditions* will want to return to the Miles technique. For the lone surgeon who has no colleague with whom he feels willing to cooperate to achieve a synchronous combined removal, the lithotomy–Trendelenburg position may still be useful for the performance of an ordinary abdominoperineal excision in sequence without moving the patient between the abdominal and perineal phases, but probably the majority of surgeons under these circumstances will prefer to practise the classical Miles technique. In the detailed account of operative technique that follows, therefore, both the synchronous combined excision and the Miles operation will be described.

EXTENDED COMBINED EXCISION

The value of *ligation of the inferior mesenteric vessels at the level of the origin of the artery* from the abdominal aorta, instead of opposite the aortic bifurcation, is probably quite minimal, but it is a rational extension to combined excision, which my own experience and that of others (Griffiths 1956; Grinnell 1965) has shown to be quite innocuous as a rule. My practice, therefore, is to tie the vessels at this level whenever it is easily possible to do so, but to accept a lower ligation in obese subjects or other patients in whom the additional exposure necessary for a high tie is difficult to secure and might add to the immediate hazards of the operation.

On the other hand, I have never been convinced of the value of *dissection of the internal iliac glands* on the pelvic side-wall and am impressed by the increased haemorrhage and additional morbidity possibly resulting from this step. I have no hesitation in advising strongly against the adoption of this extension of combined excision as any sort of routine manoeuvre, a condemnation substantiated by the report of Stearns and Deddish (1959).

Resection of adherent small gut, uterus, vagina, seminal vesicles or ureter is employed freely as required, but I must admit that I have been very guarded in my indications for *complete pelvic clearance*. In fact in my series of just over 1100 rectal excisions there have been only 19 pelvic clearances, with five immediate deaths and no long-term survivors, though two patients lived for five years and two for three and a half years before manifesting recurrence. But Brunschwig (1961) had six five-year survivors in 19 patients treated by pelvic exenteration for large bowel cancer, and Bricker et al. (1960) eight in 31 cases similarly treated. In more recent cases subjected to pelvic exenteration I have adopted the Bricker (1950) method of implanting the ureters into an isolated short loop of ileum draining to the surface as a urinary ileostomy, except in two cases where I employed, instead, Turner-Warwick's (1959) method of isolating a segment of sigmoid for this purpose. As regards the actual implantation into the bowel, my preferred technique at present is that of Goodwin et al. (1953) (see Fig. 368c).

In female patients beyond the menopause, *prophylactic oöphorectomy* is certainly a reasonable routine addition to rectal excision.

Resection with Restoration of Continuity

During the past two and a half decades sphincter-saving resections have been subjected to intensive clinical trial. In addition a number of very careful follow-up studies of the immediate and long-term results of these operations have been reported (Waugh et al. 1955; Morgan 1955, 1965; Mayo and Fly 1956; Mayo et al. 1958; Mayo and Cullen 1960;

Deddish and Stearns 1961; Cullen and Mayo 1963), which, though open to some criticism on the score of their comparative data (Goligher 1962), have convinced most surgeons that modern sphincter-saving resections can offer as good a chance of cure as abdominoperineal excision for many growths in the rectosigmoid or upper half (or possibly two-thirds) of the rectum. They may, therefore, now be regarded as established surgical procedures in the treatment of growths in these situations. However, if disappointments are to be avoided in their application, the utmost care must be exercised in regard to the scope of the resection and the selection of patients for it.

AMOUNT OF TISSUE TO BE REMOVED IN SPHINCTER-SAVING RESECTION

Perhaps the best way to illustrate the extent of a modern conservative resection is to compare the respective scopes of this operation and an orthodox combined excision as in Fig. 374. It will be seen that so far as *upward extent* is concerned the two operations are in all essential respects similar, and this includes ligation of the inferior mesenteric

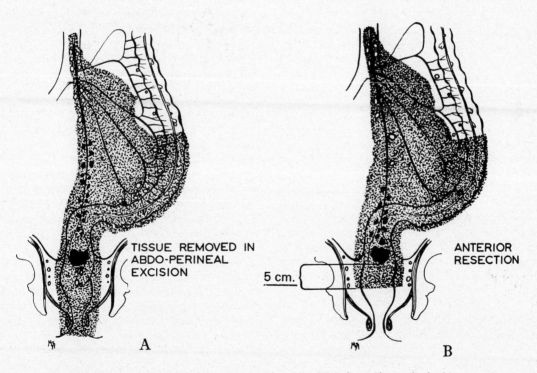

Fig. 374. The respective scopes of combined abdominoperineal excision (A) and a modern radical sphincter-saving resection (B). Stippled areas indicate the tissues to be removed.

artery at its origin if desired; perhaps a little more colon may be retained in anterior resection but the difference is slight. As for the *width of tissue removed*, that also is exactly the same in the two operations. Great importance attaches to *the precise situation of the lower limit of the resection* relative to the growth. Originally Westhues (1934), Pannett (1935) and Wangensteen (1945) stated that a 2·5 cm margin of macroscopically normal bowel wall distal to the lower edge of the growth would suffice for adequate clearance in this direction. Re-investigation of this point by Goligher et al. (1951a), Quer et al. (1953) and Grinnell (1954), following some disappointing local recurrences after anterior resection, suggested that a 5 *cm margin of bowel and perirectal fat, vessels and lymphatics beyond the carcinoma* should always be secured in resection specimens (see p. 387). An alternative policy favoured by some surgeons is to aim for a smaller margin of clearance, say 2–3 cm, and to subject this fringe of apparently normal tissue to immediate frozen section histological examination at several points to make sure that it is not infiltrated with growth. Depending on the pathological findings a further short segment may have to be removed from the top of the rectal stump before the anastomosis is performed.

CRITERIA FOR SELECTION OF PATIENTS FOR RESECTION WITH RESTORATION OF CONTINUITY

HEIGHT OF GROWTH AND SEX AND OBESITY OF PATIENT

These are the most important considerations determining the suitability of a case for a sphincter-saving excision, and also influence greatly the type of resection to be chosen.

Carcinomas of Anal Canal and Lower Third of Rectum. Growths in this part, i.e. with their lower margins anywhere up to 7 cm from the anal verge on sigmoidoscopy (Fig. 375A), are obviously unsuitable for sphincter conservation in radical treatment, and the correct operation is an abdominoperineal excision.

Carcinomas of the Upper Third of Rectum and Recto-sigmoid. For lesions that lie with their inferior edges between 12 and 16·5 cm from the anal margin (Fig. 375A), the operative indications are almost completely reversed, for with few exceptions these growths are eminently suited for sphincter-saving

excision. Moreover, it can usually be conducted by an anterior resection—and often indeed by the high intraperitoneal version of this operation, the convalescence from which is usually smooth and uneventful and function perfect. Unquestionably this is one of the most gratifying operations of major abdominal surgery.

Carcinomas of the Middle Third of Rectum. It is in regard to growths with their lower margins situated between 7·5 and 11·5 cm from the anal verge (Fig. 375A), that controversy still exists. At first sight it would seem that, if on sigmoidoscopy the inferior edge of the lesion lies at 7·5 cm and the top of the anal canal is at 3·5 cm, it would be impossible to secure a 4–5 cm margin of clearance below the growth in a resection operation without encroaching on the sphincters. However, when the lateral ligaments are divided at operation and the rectum is thoroughly mobilized, 7·5 cm may rise to 12·5 cm or higher (Fig. 375B), and a sphincter-saving resection becomes theoretically possible. But whether such a resection will be feasible and by what means depends on the sex and obesity of the patient as well as on the skill of the surgeon, and the *final decision can usually not be reached till the rectum and growth have been fully mobilized at operation.*

Most surgeons of considerable experience in the treatment of rectal cancer will generally find it quite possible in a thin female patient to treat a carcinoma with its lower edge at 7·5–8·0 cm by *anterior resection*. But in an obese female or even in a thin male, they would consider themselves fortunate to be able to apply this operation to a growth at, say, 10 cm, and in an obese male the lower limit for use of anterior resection even in the most highly skilled hands might well be 12 cm.

They will, in fact, treat about 40–45% of their cases with rectal cancer by this method, but it will be appreciated that, if anterior resection is the only method available for sphincter-saving resection, a few other patients (perhaps 10 in every 100 coming to rectal excision, two or three women and seven or eight men) with carcinomas in the middle third of the rectum pathologically suitable for radical surgery with conservation of the sphincters, will be denied the opportunity to have this type of operation and will instead be relegated to abdominoperineal excision with permanent iliac colostomy. It must be admitted, however, that most of the alternative methods of sphincter-saving resection to anterior resection have associated with them various technical difficulties, complications, and uncertainties of result, which have deterred

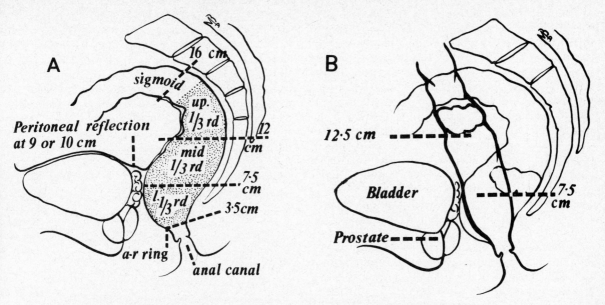

Fig. 375. (A) Diagrammatic representation of thirds of rectum as defined by sigmoidoscopic distances from the anal verge. (B) When the lateral ligaments are divided and the rectum is thoroughly mobilized from the sacral concavity, a growth lying at 7·5 cm from the anal verge may rise to 12·5 cm or higher.

very many surgeons from using them. Instead they prefer just to rely on anterior resection, to the limit of technical feasibility and to treat virtually all growths beyond the reach of this operation by abdominoperineal excision. This has been the policy of such an experienced rectal surgeon as Beahrs (1975) and many of his colleagues at the Mayo Clinic, and, after a number of disappointing experiences with the alternative procedures in the late 1950s and early 1960s, my own therapeutic philosophy was similar till a few years ago. But more recently there has been a great revival of interest, in which we have shared, in the use of other forms of sphincter-saving resection for lower lesions of the middle third of the rectum. The methods available are *anterior resection using the SPTU or E-E-A stapling guns, abdominoanal pull-through resection (and abdominotransanal resection) and abdominosacral resection (and the Mason 1972 version of this operation).*

These different procedures have their respective advantages and disadvantages, as outlined on pp. 508–16, and different surgeons will undoubtedly weigh these up differently. As regards subsequent function it might be held on theoretical grounds that downward extension of anterior resection with the SPTU or E-E-A stapling guns or the classical abdominosacral resection ought to have the advantage that in neither of them is the anal

canal in any way damaged, unlike the state of affairs in the abdominoanal pull-through resection, the abdominotransanal resection or the Mason modification of the abdominosacral resection, in all of which the anal canal is considerably traumatized by dissection of its lining or by vigorous stretching or division of the sphincters. But from the practical point of view it seems to me that a very important consideration in determining the use that is made of these methods in Britain is the fact that most surgeons in this country use the synchronous combined technique for abdominoperineal excision. This means putting the patient in the modified lithotomy–Trendelenburg position (see p. 526), which is very convenient not only for abdominoperineal excision but also for anterior resection and for all forms of abdominoanal resection. But this position is not suitable for abdominosacral resection or the Mason modification of it. For these operations the flat supine position (or right lateral position; Localio and Stahl 1969) is required for the abdominal dissection, and the patient is then turned to the right lateral or prone position for the sacral or perineal phase. But it may be found at laparotomy that the lesion is unsuitable for a sphincter-saving resection and an abdominoperineal excision may be required. If the surgeon has started the operation with the patient flat (or on the right side), he must complete the abdominoperineal excision as a classical Miles operation (see p. 504), a technique with which few British surgeons are now familiar. It seems likely, therefore, that in their resort to alternative forms of sphincter-saving excision to ordinary anterior resection, most surgeons in this country will prefer methods that can be applied with the patient in the modified lithotomy–Trendelenburg position. Their choice will then be restricted to downward extension of the reach of anterior resection by the use of the SPTU stapling gun and to some variant of abdominoanal excision, of which the most popular in Britain at the moment is the abdominotransanal resection with sutured coloanal anastomosis. If the early promise of the stapling gun is maintained and no serious drawbacks to it emerge with increased experience, I think that it could considerably reduce the need for the abdominotransanal or abdomino-anal pull-through procedure, but I cannot believe that it will dispense with them entirely. In America, where most surgeons use the classical Miles operation for abdominoperineal excision, there may be a greater willingness to consider abdomino-sacral resection or the Mason variant of it as alternative types of sphincter-saving excision in certain cases, but here again the need for them might be considerably diminished by the availability of the stapling guns (see Goligher 1979a for further discussion).

By a combination of low anterior resection and other sphincter-saving methods in suitable cases I believe it should be possible for a surgeon specially experienced in the management of rectal carcinoma to practise sphincter-conservation in the radical treatment of the majority of middle-third growths. But to the less experienced surgeon I would not recommend these technically somewhat demanding procedures. For him I think the better plan is to use anterior resection for as many of the growths in the upper part of the middle third as can be *easily* dealt with by this operation; for the rest, a straight-forward abdominoperineal excision will be found to give the best overall results.

If any form of very low rectal anastomosis is undertaken, I would urge that a right transverse loop colostomy should be established at the conclusion of the operation, as has been my practice for many years, though some leading authorities would regard this precaution as unnecessary (Turnbull 1975; Beahrs 1975). Another additional operative manoeuvre that may have some protective value in regard specially to these somewhat precarious low rectal anastomoses is the preparation of a pedicle graft of greater omentum for wrapping round the

bowel at the anastomotic site, as urged by McLachlin and Denton (1973), McLachlin et al. (1976), Localio and Baron (1973), Silen (1975), Turner-Warwick (1976) and Goldsmith (1977). Though there is no good objective clinical evidence to confirm the value of using an omental tail in this way, perhaps for an outlay of 10 minutes of operative time, it is worth taking this relatively simple and innocuous step. (For operative details see p. 438.)

THE STATE OF THE GROWTH

In the earlier days of sphincter-saving resections, when their value was *sub judice*, attempts were often made to select for them cases with specially early growths. But now that these operations have been shown to be thoroughly radical for suitably placed lesions, such efforts at selection are now less important. The only step I take towards choosing cases for anterior resection according to the state of their growths, is to carry out routine preoperative sigmoidoscopic biopsy. Any case showing a highly active anaplastic type of growth on histological section is usually rejected for a low sphincter-saving resection, because of the risk of unusually wide spread in the bowel wall with such lesions (Goligher et al. 1951a; Quer et al. 1953). However, with poorly differentiated growths at a higher level in the bowel I have been prepared to use sphincter-saving resection, employing a low anterior resection technique in order to give a distal margin of clearance of 7–8 cm.

THE PRESENCE OF HEPATIC METASTASES

Special mention should be made of cases with hepatic deposits. Obviously the palliative value of excision for these patients is greatly enhanced if it can be carried out as a resection without sacrifice of the sphincters. When therefore liver metastases are present it is tempting to make every effort to perform a resection rather than an ordinary excision, the indication being sometimes stretched to include rather lower growths than would normally be accepted for resections with a view to cure. Bitter experience has shown me, however, that there is a high complication rate after difficult anterior resections performed in accordance with this policy, and the palliative value of the operation is often lost by having to prolong the patient's postoperative stay in hospital. Contrary to previous advice by me (Goligher 1951a), I would warn strongly against any relaxation of the normal criteria of selection for anterior resection in such cases.

The contribution which sphincter-saving resections can legitimately make to the management of rectal carcinoma as a whole clearly depends in large measure on the extent to which they are employed for middle-third growths and, as already pointed out, this will vary greatly according to the surgeon's expertise. In the hands of specialists in this branch of surgery, who are prepared to make the fullest possible use of them compatible with the requirements of adequate excision and satisfactory post-operative function, as many as 50–55% of all patients with carcinomas in the rectum and recto-sigmoid may be treated by these operations. In the hands of those less experienced in this field, however, the proportion of cases likely to be deemed suitable for resection with sphincter conservation is unlikely to be more than 25–30%.

Methods Providing for Purely Local Destruction or Excision of Primary Growth

It could be argued that the great weakness of the Dukes' (1930, 1940) system of categorization of rectal carcinomas according to the extent of spread is that it is not available till after the growth has been removed! Clearly, if one knew in advance of operation whether the carcinoma was a Dukes A (or even an early B) lesion it would be possible legitimately to treat it by purely local removal or destruction without having to submit the patient to a formal rectal excision in order to remove the related uninvolved lymph nodes. Unfortunately such precise pathologically based preoperative information is not available. But it has been claimed by a number of surgeons and radio-therapists that by means of careful clinical examination it is possible to gauge the extent of spread with a fair degree of accuracy (Crile and Turnbull 1972; Turnbull 1975; Papillon 1973; Mason 1970, 1976, 1977a, b), sufficient to justify the selection of certain patients with specially favourable growths for purely local forms of therapy.

Certainly if 100 consecutive patients with carcinoma of the rectum presenting to a rectal clinic are submitted to radical rectal excision, it is well known that approximately 50 of them will be found on Dukes' processing of the operative specimens to have C lesions with involved lymph nodes (see p. 401). By contrast, if 100 consecutive patients with

small, mainly polypoid or not deeply ulcerating, rather mobile rectal carcinomas, which on biopsy are found to be well differentiated or of average differentiation, are similarly submitted to rectal excision only nine or ten will turn out to be C lesions (Morson 1966). If these 100 patients with such favourable growths had been treated by purely local measures, there would probably be no operative deaths, but the nine or ten cases with C lesions would not be cured by this treatment—though some of them might be salvaged by a subsequent rectal excision. If, on the other hand, we consider the probable fate of these 100 patients with favourable lesions following radical rectal excision, we have to allow for an operative mortality of say, 3 or 4%, and of the nine or 10 cases with C lesions probably five or six will not be cured by the operation. In terms of overall cure, therefore, there would not be much difference in the achievements of the two methods of treatment, though it must be remembered that many of those submitted to formal rectal excision would be left with a permanent colostomy. Also, obviously if the patients happened to be poor operative risks because of cardiac or pulmonary disease, making the operative mortality of rectal excision perhaps 10 or 12% or higher, the relative advantages of local forms of treatment would be further enhanced.

Surgeons and radiotherapists such as Jackman (1961), Madden and Kandalaft 1971a, b), Papillon (1973), Mason (1970, 1976, 1977a, b) and Parks (1972, 1977a, b) are prepared to employ purely local forms of therapy to small favourable carcinomas in the lower rectum—and I am referring not to polyps which on snaring turn out to be carcinomas, but to frank sessile cancers—even in patients who are otherwise fit and well able to stand the alternative of a rectal excision. Crile and Turnbull (1972) even go so far as to claim that most small low-lying rectal carcinomas of up to 5 cm in diameter should be treated by diathermy fulguration in the first instance. They maintain that, if it fails, there is no special difficulty about proceeding subsequently to rectal excision. I must confess that I myself have nearly always restricted local forms of treatment to patients who, apart from having small early lesions, were also poor risks for a major operation. Wilson (1973) and Kratzer and Onsanit (1972) give good accounts of the place of local therapy in the management of rectal carcinoma.

It may be helpful to summarize the clinical characteristics of rectal carcinomas that may be regarded as possibly suitable for purely local methods of treatment. They should be situated in the lowermost 8–10 cm of the rectum, should be small in size (not more than 4 or 5 cm in diameter and preferably smaller), should tend to project into the lumen rather than ulcerate deeply, and should be mobile on the underlying muscle coat of the rectum and unassociated with any indurated lymph nodes palpable through the rectal wall. Biopsy should show a well-differentiated growth as a rule.

As for the relative merits of the different forms of local therapy the surgeon's view will be very much coloured by his personal predilections. Electro-coagulation is the method that has hitherto been most frequently used and is the one which I myself have till recently usually favoured. Contact ir-radiation is very simple and does not necessitate an anaesthetic but good cooperation with a radio-therapist specially interested in this problem is essential. Local excision peranally or—more easily—through a posterior transsphincteric approach is technically more demanding, but it has the great advantage that it provides a specimen of the tumour for the pathologist to dissect, so that he can give to the surgeon an assessment of the extent of spread in the rectal wall (Morson et al. 1977) and enable him to decide at the outset whether the local treatment is likely to be enough (if the growth is a Dukes A or possibly minimal B lesion), or should be immediately succeeded—say in 7–10 days' time—by a formal rectal excision (if the growth had exten-sively penetrated the bowel wall or proved to be poorly differentiated on more thorough histo-logical examination, contrary to the result of the initial piece biopsy finding).

DETAILED SURGICAL MANAGEMENT OF PATIENTS WITH CARCINOMA OF THE RECTUM

Clinical Assessment of Operability

In considering whether a rectal carcinoma can be excised or not, the surgeon will bear in mind that the main hope, not only of cure but of effective palliation, rests on removal of the primary growth. Experience has shown that a simple colostomy without excision of the growth seldom affords any real palliation and all too frequently its only effect is to add the inconveniences of an artifical anus to the patient's existing discomforts. Though it over-comes any obstructive element, it does little to allay

the other distressing features of an inoperable growth—the incessant spurious diarrhoea with discharge of slime and blood, the occasional profuse and alarming haemorrhages, the severe sacral and sciatic pain, and the development of fistulas externally or into other organs. This is not surprising, for these symptoms all spring directly from the continued presence of the growth in the bowel and can only be obviated by its surgical removal or its destruction by X-rays. It is only in recent years, as more powerful sources of ir-radiation have come into use, that radiotherapy has been able to offer any assistance in the treatment of these relatively non-radiosensitive carcinomas, and even now the response in any particular case is most unpredictable. It is also true that, in selected cases with localized early carcinomas, diathermy ful-guration or endocavitary low-voltage contact ir-radiation may sometimes be curative or capable of useful palliation. But the most reliable method is still surgical excision, and it is clearly desirable, therefore, in treating cancer of the rectum to excise the primary growth whenever possible for palliative purposes alone quite apart from any question of cure.

As with carcinoma coli (see p. 446), so with rectal carcinoma the assessment of operability depends partly on the patient's general condition and partly on the state of the growth. Though the sufferers from colorectal cancer include many elderly, frail individuals, who not infrequently have chronic bronchopulmonary or circulatory lesions as well, it is only rarely that they cannot be made justifiable risks for an excision operation. For example in the last 100 cases of rectal cancer seen by me there were only three patients who were thought to be unfit to stand an excision. As for the state of the growth itself, it is important to appreciate the difficulty of assessing the extent of spread on clinical exa-mination alone. The patient may occasionally have obvious clinical signs, such as a hard nodular enlargement of the liver, free fluid in the peritoneal cavity, or gross abnormalities on examination of the chest, which indicate the presence of distant metastases, and usually though not invariably put operation out of court. More often no such manifestations are evident, and the surgeon has to be guided as regards the state of the growth by his findings on rectal examination. In the past great significance was attached to the detection of fixation of the growth on digital palpation in the assessment of its resectability, and many patients were con-demned as inoperable because their lesions were held to be too fixed to be removed. It cannot be stated too strongly that local fixation as elicited on clinical examination is an unreliable sign on which to base a verdict of unresectability. Nearly always in such cases it is found possible at operation to dissect the growth free and carry out an excision, which in not a few instances is rewarded by a lasting cure. The moral is that, however fixed the growth may seem clinically, it is wise to proceed to laparotomy before making a decision regarding the feasibility of its excision.

Preoperative Care

The preparation of the patient for operative treatment of a rectal carcinoma follows the lines already indicated for the preoperative care of patients with carcinoma coli (see p. 447), but three points require special attention *immediately before* pelvic operations.

The Intravenous Drip Infusion should be placed in the *right* forearm so that attention to it during the operation will interfere less with the surgeon, who usually stands on the left side. Suitably long plastic tubing is used to enable the arm to be *maintained at the side of the trunk throughout the operation.*

Insertion of an Indwelling Urethal Catheter and Emptying of the Bladder by Compression. This is an essential preliminary to any operation in the pelvis, for only thus can the surgeon be sure that the bladder has been completely emptied. Once the Foley catheter has been inserted and has been connected by sterile tubing to the plastic container, the closed fist is applied to the suprapubic region and pressed firmly backwards and downwards towards the sacrum (Fig. 376). In this way the bladder is entirely emptied of any residual urine.

Stitching the Anus. In cases intended for combined excision, the anus should be closed securely by one or two purse-string sutures of stout braided silk, whilst the patient is still in the anaesthetic room. As an additional precaution against leakage it is wise to commence by inserting a gauze swab into the anal canal and lower rectum and then to include its tail in the grip of the first suture so that it helps to plug the opening. A further circular suture, inserted a little more widely, buries the first one and completes the closure. If the operation planned is a sphincter-saving resection, obviously closure of the anus is not required but if there is doubt as to whether a combined excision or resection will be performed, as there sometimes is till the abdomen

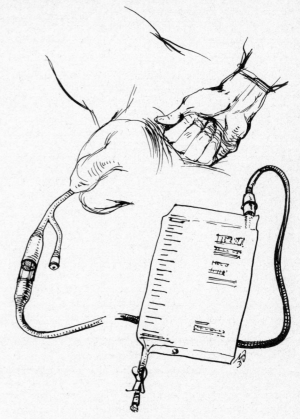

Fig. 376. Emptying the bladder by forcible compresion of the suprapubic region with the clenched fist.

is explored, it is better that the anus should be sutured in the first instance. If it is finally elected to carry out a resection, the anal suture can be easily removed; in my experience no septic complications or other harm seem to result from its temporary insertion.

Abdominoperineal Excision

ANAESTHETIC

This is discussed in relation to operations for carcinoma coli, on p. 452.

POSITION OF THE PATIENT

For the Miles operation a steep Trendelenburg tilt is often recommended for the abdominal phase of the dissection partly to displace the small gut into the

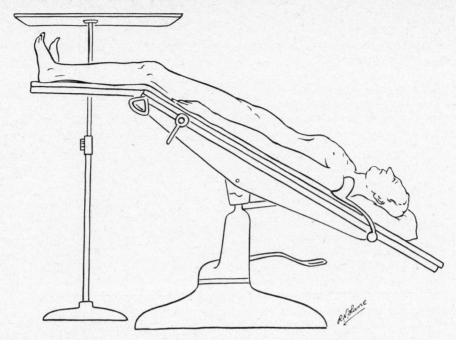

Fig. 377. Moderate Trendelenburg position with 15–20° of head-down tilt, used for the Miles operation. Note the position of the instrument table overlying the slightly flexed legs.

upper abdomen out of the pelvis, but at the present time, when the loops of intestine are usually confined within a plastic bag or held in the upper abdomen by packs and a reliable pattern of self-retaining retractor, such extreme depression of the head-end of the table is no longer necessary and is probably better avoided on general grounds. A 15–20° tilt gives the most convenient operating position for pelvic dissection. To prevent the patient sliding headwards off the table his legs and the terminal part of the table are flexed to a right angle and in addition shoulder rests are fitted (Fig. 377). There is a risk of producing brachial plexus palsies by such rests, as Ewing (1950) has warned, particularly if the arm is abducted at the shoulder, as for the setting up of an intravenous drip infusion. It is essential therefore that the arms should be maintained at the sides of the body throughout and that the 'drip' tubing should be sufficiently long for it to extend from the container, under the sterile towelling, to the forearm in this position. In addition it is important to see that the shoulder rests are applied to the outer extremity of the shoulder tip on the acromion process itself and are not allowed to slide inwards against the brachial plexus. The Frankis Evans shoulder rests, which form a cup over the shoulder-tip and cannot become displaced medially, are an advantage from this point of view.

An alternative to shoulder rests is to use a Hewer's transversely corrugated rubber mattress on the top of the table; this is most effective in preventing slipping of the patient even with a steep tilt, and I can commend it strongly. The most convenient place for the instrument tray when the patient is in the Trendelenburg position is at the foot of the table overlying the flexed legs (Fig. 377).

For the perineal phase of the Miles operation the patient is placed on his side, either the left or the right, with the buttocks projecting slightly over the edge of the table, the knees well drawn up and the shoulders slightly forwards. A slight head-down tilt improves the view of the pelvic cavity during the perineal dissection. Some surgeons, such as d'Allaines (1956), use an exaggerated lithotomy position, but I think this is less satisfactory than a side position.

For the synchronous combined excision the legs must be supported in such a way as to afford simultaneous access to the perineum and the abdomen, and the adjustable leg rests designed by Lloyd-Davies (1939) are ideal for this purpose (Fig. 378A, B). This arrangement of the patient has been termed the lithotomy–Trendelenburg position, but that is not an accurate description, for it implies that the trunk is tilted head-down whilst the thighs are flexed to a right angle at the hips. Such a posture, whilst very

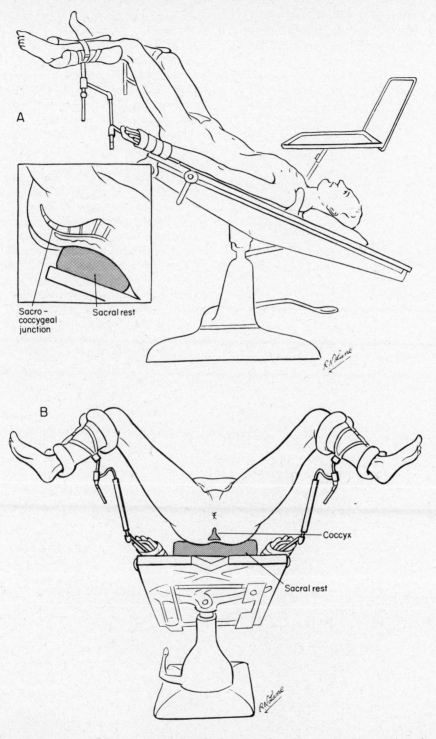

Fig. 378. Patient in position for synchronous combined abdominoperineal excision with legs supported on Lloyd-Davies leg rests and sacrum on a special padded sacral rest. (A) Lateral view: note that there is almost no flexion of the hips to embarrass the abdominal operator, the front of the thighs and the anterior abdominal wall being in almost the same plane. The instrument table for the abdominal surgeon is situated immediately above the patient's head. (B) Perineal view: note position of coccyx marked by stippled triangle, relative to edge of sacral rest. The access to the perineum is obtained by wide separation of the thighs.

satisfactory for the perineal operator, would
seriously inconvenience the abdominal operator
for, as the Trendelenburg tilt is steepened, the left

thigh would impinge to an increasing extent on his
left forearm. Actually access to the perineum is
secured not by flexing the thighs so much as by
separating them, and in most cases it is possible to
have the *fronts of the thighs almost in the same plane as the
anterior abdominal wall.* The position used in fact
would be more correctly described as an abducted
thighs-Trendelenburg position.

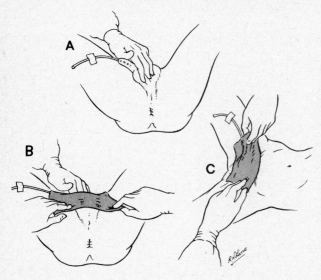

Fig. 379. Fixing the genitalia and urethral catheter to the thigh with adhesive plaster strapping.

The relationship of the sacrococcygeal region to
the end of the table is also of great importance in
positioning the patient for the synchronous
operation. It is useful to have a special sacral rest,
such as my own pattern (see Fig. 378B) at the end of
the table. The sacrum is placed on this in such a
position that the sacrococcygeal articulation projects about 2·5–3 cm beyond the distal edge of the
rest. The shoulder supports are then adjusted
tightly so that there can be no slipping of the body
headwards when the Trendelenburg position is
assumed. It is always wise to test for a slip by trying
the patient in a moderate tilt before towelling-up,
and, as it is the surgeon working at the lower end
who will suffer if the perineum recedes up the table,
a good working rule is to make him responsible for

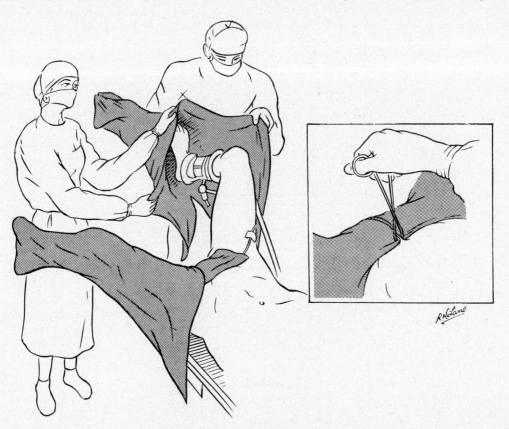

Fig. 380. Covering the legs and leg rests with sterile leggings. *Inset:* Fixing leggings together in the pubic region.

the positioning of the patient! Actually, so far as the abdominal operator is concerned a tilt of 15° would suffice, but the perineal dissection is facilitated if a slightly steeper tilt can be secured without embarrassment to the patient.

The arms are supported at the sides of the trunk by bandaging the hands and forearms to the horizontal parts of the leg rests. The external genitalia in male patients require to be supported out of the way of the perianal operator. This is accomplished, after the bladder has been emptied by compression, by strapping them and the end of the indwelling catheter with broad strips of Elastoplast against the front of one thigh (Fig. 379).

Two other matters require to be mentioned in connection with the general arrangements for synchronous combined excision—the use of special sterile leggings for the projecting lower limbs, and the placing of instrument tables. It is a great convenience in towelling these patients for operation to have sterile leggings, triangular in shape, 130 cm long, and 75 cm wide at the base, for enclosing the lower limbs (Fig. 380). The instrument table for the abdominal operator is placed over the patient's head and has a wire frame for supporting a mackintosh and towel to shut off the anaesthetist from the sterile field (Fig. 378). The perineal operator, who sits to the operation, has a low instrument table over his knees (Fig. 381).

Lighting

Good illumination is of course essential, and for the perineal phase of both the Miles and the synchronous operations mobile lights are needed to give a horizontal beam. Alternatively a head-light may be used, but most surgeons find it irksome.

Special Instruments

Much of the pelvic dissection in rectal excision is conducted at considerable depth and, if the surgeon is to do himself justice, he must have suitably long instruments. Self-retaining retractors to hold open the abdominal and perineal wounds are also desirable. The following is a list of the more

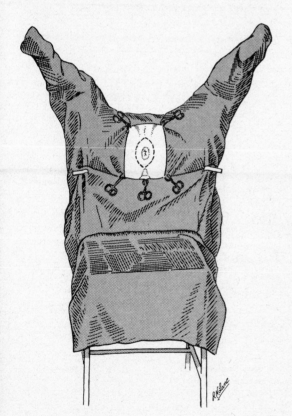

Fig. 381. Perineal view of towelled patient ready for synchronous combined excision. Note the instrument table overlying the perineal operator's knees. Position of coccyx outlined on skin.

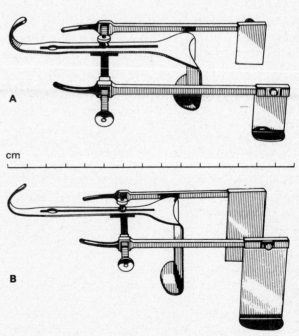

Fig. 382. Goligher's modification of the Berkeley–Bonney self-retaining three-bladed abdominal retractor with interchangeable blades of two sizes, 5 cm and 10 cm deep, so that it can be made suitable for both average and obese subjects.

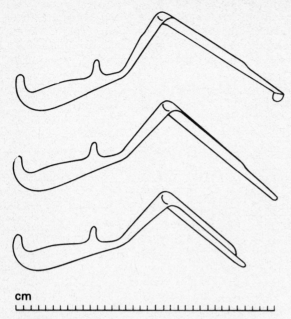

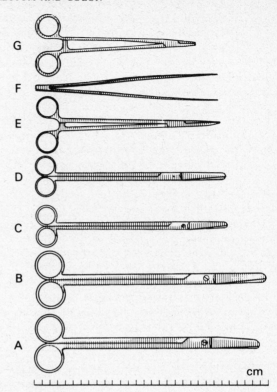

Fig. 383. St Mark's Hospital pattern of deep pelvic retractors with blades 12·5 and 17·5 cm long respectively. The model with the turned-back distal edge is preferable as it secures a better grip on the tissues.

important special instruments that I myself use in rectal excision:

1. A three-bladed abdominal retractor with detachable blades of two sizes so that it can be made suitable for both average and obese subjects (Fig. 382).

2. Long deep pelvic retractors with blades 12·5 cm and 17·5 cm long, their distal edges being turned back to give them a better grip of the tissues during retraction (Fig. 383).

3. Two pairs of heavier long scissors, such as the 29·5 cm pattern used by myself for cutting indurated tissues, one straight, the other curved on the flat (Fig. 384A, B).

4. Two pairs of Lloyd-Davies scissors 26 cm long, one straight, the other curved on the flat (Fig. 384C, D).

5. 25 cm long, slightly curved, artery forceps (Fig. 384E).

6. Dissecting forceps 25 cm (Fig. 384F).

7. A 22·5 cm long Mayo's needle-holder (Fig. 384G).

8. Swab-holders 25 cm long.

9. Parker–Kerr intestinal clamps slightly curved on the flat, preferably with metal caps.

10. Cope's modification of Martel's intestinal clamp (Fig. 385).

Fig. 384. Some long instruments of special value during rectal excision. (A) Goligher's strong 29·5 cm rectal scissors, curved on the flat. (B) Goligher's strong 29·5 cm rectal scissors, straight on the flat. (C) Lloyd-Davies' finer 26 cm scissors, curved on the flat. (D) Lloyd-Davies' finer 26 cm scissors, straight. (E) Lloyd-Davies' 25 cm curved artery forceps. (F) Non-toothed dissecting forceps, 25 cm long. (G) 22·5 cm needle-holder, Mayo pattern.

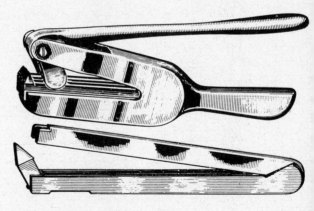

Fig. 385. Zachary Cope's modification of Martel's crushing intestinal clamp.

11. St Mark's Hospital pattern of perineal rectractor (Fig. 386).

In the category of well-nigh indispensable equipment I would place the surgical diathermy, for it is

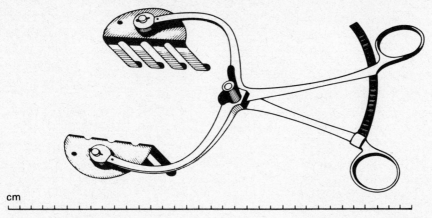

cm

Fig. 386. St Mark's Hospital pattern of perineal retractor. Note the small perforation on each of the blades for clipping to the skin with towel clips when in position.

an enormous convenience in dealing with bleeding at a depth and in expediting the ordinary process of haemostasis throughout the operation.

ABDOMINAL INCISION

For the abdominal incision and initial phases of the abdominal dissection in either the synchronous combined excision or the classical Miles operation, *the patient should be in a horizontal position without any head-down tilt.*

Several surgeons, such as Bacon (1945) and d'Allaines (1956), have recommended an oblique muscle-cutting incision in the left iliac region for the abdominal phase of operations for rectal excision, the colostomy being established in this main wound. In my experience, however, this approach is frequently unsatisfactory, for it is impossible with it to use a self-retaining retractor, and access to the depths of the pelvis for a difficult dissection is often inadequate. I have no doubt that the best approach is a long left paramedian (or median) incision which extends from the pubis to a point at least 5 or 7·5 cm above the level of the umbilicus, and often almost to the costal margin (Fig. 387). The anterior rectus sheath is incised, its inner flap dissected up and the rectus muscle retracted laterally throughout the length of the incision, the pyramidalis at the lower end being taken to the medial or lateral side as desired (Fig. 388). The posterior rectus sheath and peritoneum are then opened, the obliterated umbilical artery being divided low down in the process.

EXPLORATION OF ABDOMEN AND ASSESSMENT OF EXCISABILITY

The general plan of abdominal exploration to be followed in these cases and the points to which attention should be particularly directed are described in relation to operations for carcinoma of the colon on p. 452. In dealing with rectal cancer a matter that requires even more special consideration is *fixation of the primary growth.* In some cases, though the growth is adherent on some aspect, it is possible to impart slight movement to it, and the surgeon can feel quite confident about the prospects of excising it. In other cases, in which it is rigidly fixed and it is tempting to consider it irremovable, a trial dissection should always be attempted on the more adherent aspects before reaching a final verdict. In the great majority of cases this is successful in freeing the rectum, or alternatively it is possible to resect the organ to which the growth is adherent, and indeed in the female the decision to carry out a hysterectomy *en bloc* with the rectum resolves many problems with fixed rectal carcinomas. The surgeon's success in dealing with adherent lesions will obviously be influenced by his experience in this field, but one who is operating frequently in the pelvis will seldom be baulked in his efforts to perform an excision by local fixation, except with a so-called 'frozen' pelvis.

The bearing of associated hepatic, peritoneal or obvious lymph node metastases on decision about operative procedure is discussed on p. 427, whilst the management of synchronous adenomatous polyps and carcinomas and the possible prevention of metachronous tumours is considered on p. 431.

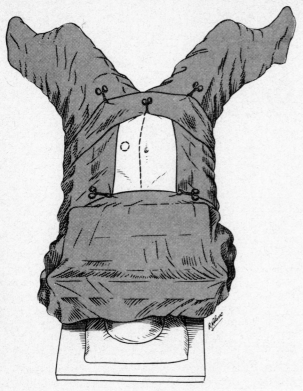

Fig. 387. Towelled-up patient seen from the head end. The main left paramedian incision is outlined: note that it extends from the pubis below to the upper epigastrum above. The position for the circular or 'trephine' colostomy wound is shown in the left iliac fossa just lateral to the outer edge of the rectus muscle.

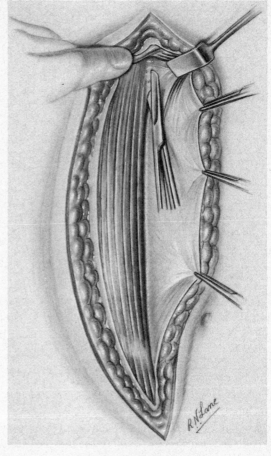

Fig. 388. The left rectus muscle is displaced laterally. At the lower end the pyramidalis muscle has to be retracted medially to allow the inner border of the rectus to be freed down to the pubis.

INSERTION OF SELF-RETAINING RETRACTOR AND PACKING-OFF SMALL INTESTINE

The first step in the actual excision consists of inserting a self-retaining retractor to hold the edges of the wound apart. The next step is to displace the loops of small bowel into the upper abdomen and retain them there by the application over the intestines of two or three large moist packs, which in turn are held in position by the adjustable third blade of the self-retaining retractor. Alternatively, the coils of intestine may be turned out of the abdominal cavity on to the front of the upper part of the anterior abdominal wall, where they are covered with warm moist packs and towelling or accommodated in a plastic or rubber bag, as recommended by Lahey (1953).* The latter

* A plastic version, the Aldon Intestinal bag, is made by Aldington Laboratories, Mersham, Ashford, Kent, UK.

manoeuvre is the one I have favoured in recent years, because it affords better access to the upper reaches of the inferior mesenteric vessels and to the front of the abdominal aorta.

APPLICATION OF LIGATURE OF SILK OR TAPE TO RECTUM ABOVE GROWTH

The next step is the application of a ligature of stout braided silk to the bowel 5 cm or so above the growth to prevent malignant cells, that may be exfoliated into the lumen of the gut during the subsequent manipulations, from extending into the sigmoid loop, which is going to be used for establishing the colostomy, or forming an anastomosis with the lower rectum after resection of the growth. This silk ligature is not shown in the illustrations that follow, for they were prepared before this plan became an integral part of my operative technique.

SEPARATION OF DEVELOPMENTAL ADHESIONS TO ILIAC MESOCOLON

The sigmoid loop is grasped by the assistant with both hands and drawn strongly to the right to display the adhesions, which are present in at least 75% of subjects, between the posterior peritoneum of the left iliac fossa and the outer surface of the iliac mesocolon and colon. By snipping with scissors *just to the right of the dentate edge of this raised parietal peritoneum*, the latter can be gradually detached from the mesocolon and pushed back intact into its proper place in the iliac fossa (Fig. 389). At the same time the iliac colon has restored to it a free mesocolon like the rest of the sigmoid loop. If the surgeon unwittingly cuts across the actual folds of peritoneum, he will find that he has divided the posterior parietal peritoneum of the left iliac region, leaving some of it attached to the specimen, which is eventually removed; this is unfortunate for he may badly need all the available peritoneum for closure of the pelvic peritoneal floor at the end of the operation.

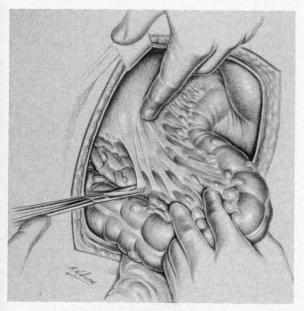

Fig. 389. Separation of developmental adhesions on the outer side of the iliac colon and mesocolon.

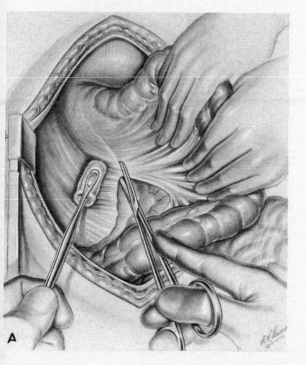

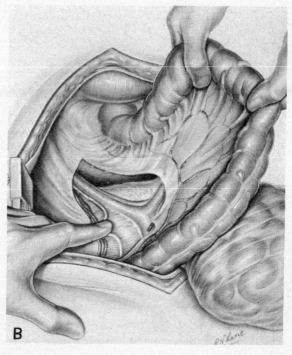

Fig. 390. (A) Scissor cut in the peritoneum on the left side of the base of the mesosigmoid. (B) As this cut is opened up and deepened the left ureter is displayed and can be pushed laterally with the finger.

INCISION OF LEFT LEAF OF SIGMOID MESOCOLON

The assistant renders the peritoneum of the left side of the sigmoid mesocolon and mesorectum taut by drawing the rectum and sigmoid strongly upwards and to the patient's right. A snick is made in this peritoneal leaf where it joins the peritoneum of the posterior abdominal wall at a point corresponding to the apex of the former intersigmoid fossa, which usually accurately overlies the left ureter. This cut is extended up and down for 10–12 cm (Fig. 390A, B), and when opened up it exposes the left ureter where it lies on the common iliac artery at its bifurcation into external and internal iliacs and for a short distance above and below that point. The ureter can be distinguished from the more laterally lying spermatic vessels by the characteristic vermicular movement which it gives on touching. In certain cases pathological adhesions may draw the ureter medially towards the growth, if it is situated high in the rectum or rectosigmoid, so that a careful sharp dissection may be required to free it; in some instances it may be so implicated as to necessitate division of the ureter above and below, leaving the adherent portion still attached to the lesion. At the upper end the ureter should be firmly displaced laterally to obviate any risk of it being caught up during ligation of the inferior mesenteric vessels at a later stage of the operation.

LIGATION OF INTERNAL ILIAC ARTERY

At this stage ligation of the internal iliac artery is easily carried out, if desired. The artery is traced down from the common iliac stem on to the pelvic side-wall. In some cases it is possible to display the anterior and posterior terminal divisions of the internal iliac and to ligate the former alone, but in other instances it may be difficult to carry the dissection far enough to do so, and then the tie has to be applied to the whole internal iliac. The practice of bilateral internal iliac ligation was recommended by Quénu (quoted by Thomson and Miles 1920) as a means of reducing haemorrhage during abdominoperineal excision, but in my experience it has been very variable in its results, even when combined with ligation of the middle sacral artery (p. 24), and I have given it up.

INCISION OF PERITONEUM OF RIGHT LEAF OF SIGMOID MESCOLON, DEFINITION OF INFERIOR MESENTERIC VESSELS AND PREPARATION OF COLON STUMP FOR COLOSTOMY

HIGH LIGATION

The peritoneum on the right side of the sigmoid mesocolon and upper mesorectum is now made taut by the surgeon drawing the rectum and sigmoid upwards and to the left with his left hand, whilst he makes a scissor cut at the junction of this peritoneal leaf with the peritoneum of the posterior abdominal wall just to the right of the uppermost 7–10 cm of the inferior mesenteric artery and extending upwards to the lower border of the third part of the duodenum. The cut is deepened and opened up to expose the front of the right common iliac artery and aorta and the tips of the surgeon's left index and middle finger can then be passed to the patient's left between the inferior mesenteric vessels and the front of the aorta to enter the space previously created on that side by division of the left peritoneal leaf. Sometimes the central root of the presacral nerve is stripped up with the inferior mesenteric pedicle, but the nerve is actually quite closely applied to the aorta and, if a little care is exercised, it is usually possible to leave it behind without obviously rendering the excision any less

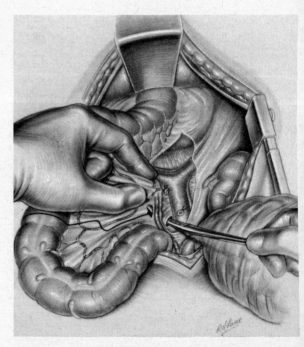

Fig. 391. A scissor cut has been made in peritoneum on the right side of the base of the sigmoid mesocolon and prolonged upwards almost to the lower border of the third part of the duodenum and then transversely across the front of the inferior mesenteric vessels. The artery has been tied flush with the aorta and divided, and the vein is about to be treated in the same way. The heavy black line on the mesocolon extending from the site of ligation of the inferior mesenteric vessels to the iliac colon indicates the intended line of mesocolic division in preparing the colon stump for the colostomy.

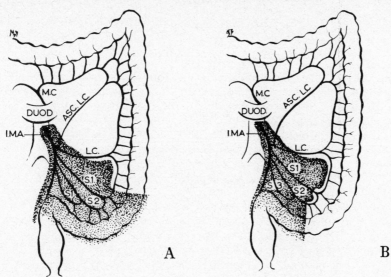

Fig. 392. The plan of division of the inferior mesenteric vessels and their branches in the average case undergoing a high tie. (*From Goligher 1958*)

radical. A transverse cut is now made in the peritoneum overlying the inferior mesenteric vessels at a point corresponding roughly to the origin of the artery from the aorta. The vessels are next defined, ligated and divided either separately or together at this level (Fig. 391), *care being taken first of all to throw the sigmoid colon and mesocolon temporarily to the right again to re-identify the left ureter and push it out of harm's way.* (The right ureter lies farther away more under cover of the right leaf of peritoneum and, except when drawn medially by an adherent growth, is not normally in jeopardy and does not need to be clearly defined.)

Finally the sigmoid mesocolon is divided obliquely from the point of ligation of the inferior mesenteric vessels to the site on the iliac colon chosen for the colostomy. This cut crosses three vessels—the ascending left colic running to the splenic flexure, the left colic proper, and the marginal artery between the left colic and the first sigmoid vessels (Fig. 392A) or between individual sigmoid branches (Fig. 392B)—and these have to be secured and divided. Finally the colon is divided between Cope's crushing clamps (Fig. 393).

The effect of division of the inferior mesenteric vessels at this site is to leave the entire left colon down to the iliac colostomy dependent on the marginal artery descending from the middle colic for its blood supply (Fig. 392). Usually this is quite adequate, as shown by the retention of its normal pink colour, confirmed if necessary by cutting one

of the small mural arteries on the colon at the point intended for the colostomy and noting whether this gives rise to arterial bleeding or not. Only excessively rarely, in my experience, is it ever necessary because of insufficient blood supply to the colon after high ligation of the inferior mesenteric vessels, to carry the proximal limit of the excision of bowel to a higher level. This is accomplished by dividing the peritoneum on the outer side of the descending colon and splenic flexure and mobilizing the entire left colon (Fig. 394). A convenient point is then chosen on the descending or distal transverse colon for division of the bowel, and the posterior parietal peritoneum, and if necessary the transverse mesocolon, are severed from the point of ligation of the inferior mesenteric vessels to this site on the bowel, the marginal artery being divided in the process. Finally the Cope's clamps are applied and the colon sectioned between them as before.

LOW LIGATION

In some cases a high ligation is clearly inadvisable, as for example in very obese subjects, in whom the additional dissection might be technically difficult, in poor-risk patients, in whom a rapid smooth operation is particularly desirable, or in patients undergoing palliative excision in the presence of hepatic metastases. In these cases the ligature may be conveniently applied to the inferior mesenteric vessels just below the origin of the left colic artery

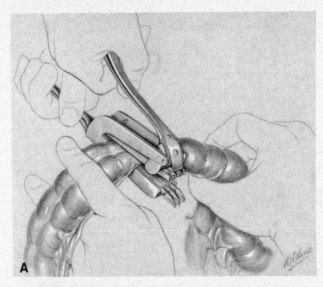

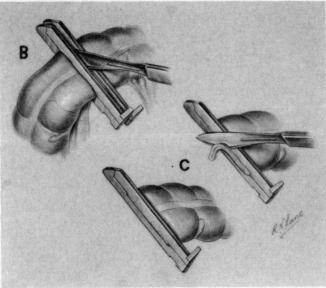

Fig. 393. (A) Application of Cope's clamp to sigmoid colon. (B) After removal of the middle clamp the crushed bowel is divided by the scalpel. (C) Shaving off the projecting fringe of crushed colon.

proper or the first sigmoid branch, which is usually about the level of the aortic bifurcation (Fig. 395). The index finger is worked under the pedicle as before, separating it from the presacral nerve, and the peritoneum is incised over the vessels. Finally the ligature is placed with the aid of cholecystectomy forceps, care being taken to avoid the left ureter which is again in danger. Finally the sigmoid mesocolon is cut with scissors parallel and about 1 cm distal to the left colic or first sigmoid

artery, as the case may be, till the marginal vessels are reached close to the bowel. They are ligated and divided, and the colon severed between Cope's clamps.

THE POSTERIOR PELVIC DISSECTION

The tongue of tissue represented by the ligated superior vascular pedicle is now stripped down off

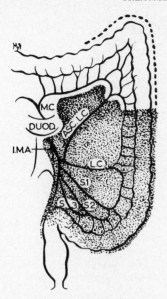

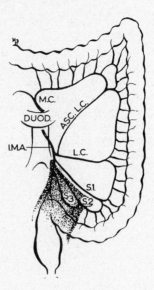

Fig. 394. Method of mobilizing the entire left colon by dividing the peritoneum on the outer side of the descending colon and splenic flexure. (*From Goligher 1958*)

Fig. 395. Site of a low tie of the inferior mesenteric vessels at or below the level of the aortic bifurcation and the left colic or first sigmoid artery. (*From Goligher 1958*)

the front of the lower aorta, the right common iliac vein and the fifth lumbar vertebra to the promontory of the sacrum. If the central root of the presacral nerve was included in the main ligature, this nerve will now be lifted forwards with the pedicle, but if the root was avoided the presacral nerve will often be fairly clearly distinguishable lying on the iliac vein and dividing below into its two branches. These latter cling close to the rectum as they separate to run towards the sides of the pelvis and, if not brushed downwards off the back of the bowel, are liable to be divided or torn during the next step of the operation. This consists of inserting a pair of long scissors into the soft presacral connective tissue between the sacrum and the rectum and opening the blades slightly (Fig. 396). Into the space thus created the fingers, and then the whole hand are gradually introduced lifting the rectum out of the sacral concavity (Fig. 397). In this way the rectum is mobilized posteriorly as far as the tip of the coccyx. Usually this is an entirely bloodless manoeuvre, but sometimes small veins extending from the rectum into the middle sacral veins are torn and bleed or, if the growth was adherent posteriorly, its separation, which may involve scissor dissection, may lead to tearing of the middle sacral vessels themselves. Such bleeding can usually be controlled by diathermy coagulation; rarely underruning with a catgut suture is required or pressure with Surgicel may be employed.

THE ANTERIOR PELVIC DISSECTION

In preparation for this step the *table is tilted 20° or so head down and the top light is adjusted to shine from above the patient's (or anaesthetist's) head downwards obliquely into the pelvis*. A deep pelvic retractor is inserted anteriorly to lift the bladder forwards. The scissor cuts that were made in the peritoneum on either side of the base of the mesosigmoid and upper mesorectum are now prolonged downwards around the brim of the pelvis on either side to meet in midline anteriorly, not in the bottom of the recto-vesical pouch but on the base of the bladder 2–3 cm higher up (Fig. 398). The posterior edge of the peritoneal cut on the bladder base is caught with three long artery forceps for traction (Fig. 399). By cautious scissor dissection the cut is gradually deepened in the plane immediately behind the vasa and the seminal vesicles, so that the latter are laid quite bare and the fascia of Denonvillier falls back with the rectum (Fig. 399, *inset*). When the dissection has proceeded in this plane as far as the base of the prostate it is necessary to incise the fascia with scissors (Fig. 400A, B, C) to allow the index and middle fingers to be inserted between the rectum and the back of the prostate as far as its apex. Bleeding is often quite troublesome during the anterior dissection, especially when the vesicles are being defined, and it is best checked by diathermy coagulation.

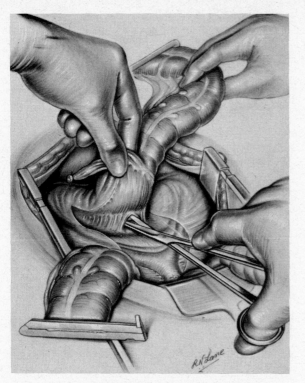

Fig. 396. Freeing the ligated mesosigmoid pedicle and meso-rectum from the aorta and sacrum. (In this case the presacral nerve was sacrificed but often it can be preserved.)

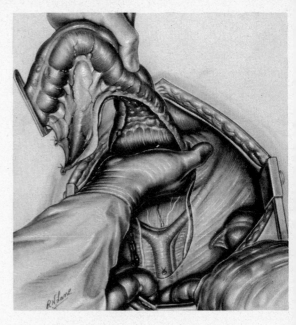

Fig. 397. Lifting the rectum out of the sacral concavity with the whole hand.

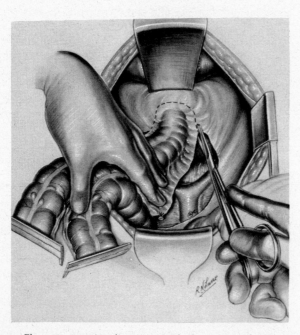

Fig. 398. Anterior dissection. With the patient tilted head-down the pelvic peritoneum is divided with long scissors.

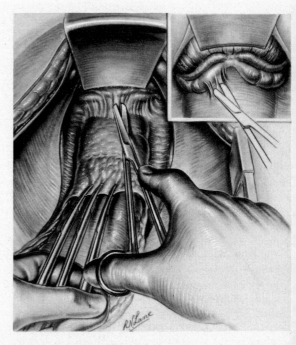

Fig. 399. Anterior dissection. Striking the plane behind the vasa and seminal vesicles. *Inset:* Exposure of the vasa and vesicles.

Taking the Lateral Ligaments

The rectum has been freed posteriorly and anteriorly and it only remains attached on either side by the lateral ligaments, which have now to be divided. Note that the right ureter lies well lateral to the junction of the ligament with the pelvic side wall. If necessary it should be specially freed and retracted. As the ligament is divided with scissors bleeding points are dealt with by diathermy. The ligaments are rendered taut by drawing the rectum firmly upwards. The right hand is then passed down behind the rectum into the lower part of the pelvis and the index finger is burrowed forwards through the connective tissue at one side of the rectum, below the essential part of the lateral ligament, to emerge in front, thus creating a hole in this band of connective tissues. The lateral ligament is now engaged between the middle and index fingers of the left hand, whilst the rectum is pressed strongly to the opposite side (Fig. 401). Before the ligament is divided, however, it is essential to be sure that the ureter lies well lateral; if necessary it should be freed and retracted with another laterally placed deep retractor. Division of the ligament is now accomplished by means of long straight or slightly curved scissors (preferably a heavier pattern than shown in Fig. 400) close to the pelvic side wall. As the middle haemorrhoidal artery (or arteries) is contained in the ligament, it is liable to bleed briskly when it is severed and it is thus better to conduct the division piecemeal and to deal with bleeding points as they arise by diathermy coagulation. Alternatively in thin subjects with a roomy pelvis the ligament may be doubly clamped by curved Parker–Kerr clamps close to the pelvic side-wall and divided between them, the clamped tissue being subsequently ligated. But this latter method is open to the objection—perhaps theoretical more than practical—that it might result in a less radical removal of the lesion than would simple division as far laterally as possible. The opposite ligament is then dealt with in the same way.

In the classical Miles operation the lateral ligaments have to be divided entirely from the abdominal aspect by one or other of the methods just described. In the synchronous operation this is not entirely essential, for a variable amount of the division may be conducted by the perineal dissector, depending on the relative *tempi* of the synchronously occurring abdominal and perineal dissections. If the abdominal operator is delayed, as for example by the dissection of the ureters from an adherent growth, the lateral ligament is divided entirely by the perineal operator.

Removal or Displacement into the Pelvis of the Mobilized Rectum and Sigmoid Colon and Closure of the Pelvic Peritoneal Floor

At this stage obviously a divergence of procedure develops depending on whether the classical Miles technique or the synchronous method of operating is being followed. In the former case the clamped sigmoid end of the mobilized bowel is pushed down as far as possible into the presacral space behind the rectum, to be readily available for pulling out from below when the coccyx is disarticulated during the subsequent perineal dissection (Fig. 402). The lateral flaps of pelvic peritoneum, which were freed and thinned out to some extent during the initial stages of the abdominal dissection, are now sutured over this displaced bowel. In a thin subject this is usually quite easy, but in stout patients, in whom the sigmoid mesocolon and the mesorectum may be laden with fat, a veritable mountain of tissue may bulge out of the pelvis. Under these circumstances the pelvic peritoneum will usually require to be teased out a great deal more in order to cover the pelvic contents; it may sometimes be found easier to mobilize peritoneum from the top of the bladder as well and to close the pelvic peritoneal floor from before backwards, as favoured by Miles, rather than from side to side (Fig. 403). Alternatively, if such efforts to make the peritoneum meet are unsuccessful, a considerable part of the sigmoidorectal segment of bowel may be resected, thus reducing the amount of tissue remaining to be buried; it is indeed always wise to have an additional set of Cope's clamps available for dividing the bowel at a lower level in this way.

It is one of the great virtues of the synchronous combined technique that these difficulties with suture of the pelvic peritoneum do not arise, for by the time the abdominal dissection is complete the rectum has been freed from its perineal attachments and the operative specimen can be immediately removed. Closure of the pelvic peritoneal floor thus takes place over an empty pelvis and is very rapidly and simply accomplished, at any rate as far as the upper end of the gap (Fig. 404A). Above the level of the bifurcation of the aorta the right edge of peritoneum has to be stitched to the edge of the piece of mesocolon or posterior parietal peritoneum going to the sigmoid stump forming the colostomy (Fig. 404B). The left leaf of pelvic

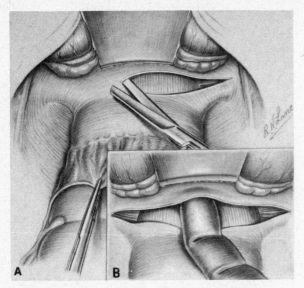

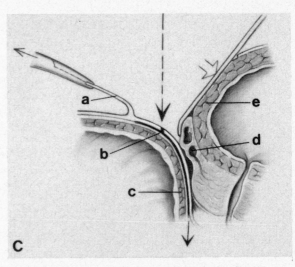

Fig. 400. Anterior dissection. (A) Whilst the seminal vesicles and vasa deferentia are held forwards by the deep pelvic retractor the fascia of Denonvillier is divided with scissors across the front of the rectum and lateral ligaments. (B) A finger is then passed down between the rectum posteriorly and the fascia and prostate anteriorly. (C) A diagrammatic representation of the plane of this finger dissection. *a* = posterior clipped edge of pelvic peritoneum; *b* = fascia of Denonvillier; *c* = rectal wall; *d* = seminal vesicle; *e* = bladder wall.

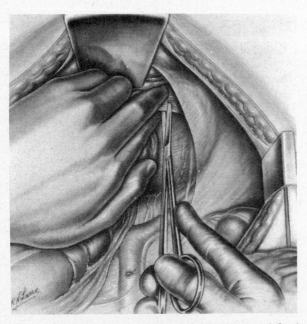

Fig. 401. Taking the lateral ligament: the ligament is defined between the second and third fingers of the left hand as the rectum is held upwards and to the opposite side of the pelvis. Note that the right ureter lies well lateral to the junction of the ligament with the pelvic side wall. If necessary, it should be specially freed and retracted. As the ligament is divided with scissors, bleeding points are dealt with by diathermy.

peritoneum recedes markedly to the left at this level over the psoas muscle into the left iliac fossa; It may or may not be sutured to the back of the sigmoid stump to close the raw area revealed in this situation.

(See p. 557 also for discussion of whether pelvic peritoneum needs to be sutured or not.)

Making the Iliac Colostomy

ORDINARY TECHNIQUE

The self-retaining abdominal retractor is removed, and the cut edges of the peritoneum, rectus sheath, and subcutaneous fat revealed in the left wound margin are caught with artery forceps a little below the level of the umbilicus. Traction on these forceps by the assistant draws all layers of the left half of the anterior abdominal wall strongly to the right in preparation for the making of the separate wound in the iliac region for the colostomy. This should be centred roughly on or just above the line between the anterior superior iliac spine and the umbilicus and not closer than 6 cm to the former. To make this point on the parietes prominent during the incision, the assistant presses the end of a proctoscope or his finger with a thimble on it against the anterior abdominal wall from inside the abdomen. At the prominence thus created the skin is lifted up

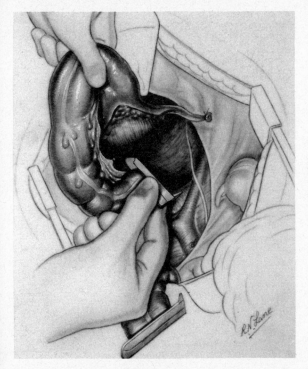

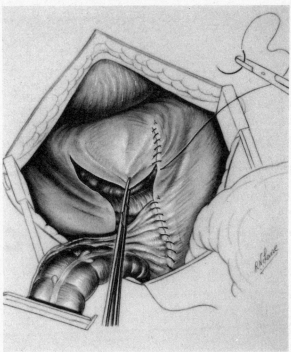

Fig. 402. Miles' operation: displacement of the mobilized sigmoid colon and rectum into the pelvis preparatory to suture of the pelvic peritoneum. The clamped end of bowel is placed near the tip of the coccyx.

Fig. 403. Miles' operation: suture of the pelvic peritoneum.

with toothed dissecting forceps and the raised disc of skin and subcutaneous tissue amputated with the scalpel, leaving a circular wound (Fig. 405A). If the patient is at all obese, it will be necessary to excise a disc of subcutaneous fat in the same manner before the aponeurosis is completely bared. The external oblique is then opened either by removal of a disc of it or by a cruciate incision (Fig. 405B). The fibres of the internal oblique and transversus muscles are next divided and separated and the peritoneum opened (Fig. 405C). When the wound is completed it should be tested for size; it is a good working rule that, if it is not to constrict the bowel too much, it should take two fingers comfortably, though obviously in fat patients with a very bulky sigmoid mesocolon the opening should be appropriately larger.

The colon is not immediately drawn through the opening. Instead *the lateral paracolostomy gutter is first of all closed*, and this is most conveniently done through the main paramedian wound in the following way. A large pair of scissors is threaded through the stab wound into the peritoneal cavity and then out again through the main wound. If the surgeon holds the point of this pair of scissors strongly forwards with his left hand, and draws the sigmoid stump medially with his right, the lateral space is very clearly displayed. The assistant now inserts a purse-string suture in the parietal peritoneum from the inner end of the colostomy wound to the lateral edge of the sigmoid stump, but not actually entering the bowel wall (Fig. 406). When this is tied it effectively obliterates the paracolostomy gutter (Fig. 407); only at this stage is the sigmoid stump, controlled by the Cope clamp, drawn through the colostomy wound, for to do so earlier would obscure the view of the space for closure. It is advisable to use non-absorbable suture material for closing the lateral space, for there are cases on record where the gap has reformed following its closure with catgut (Goligher et al. 1951*b*; Bliss 1963).

A further advantage of this lateral space stitch is that it holds the colon firmly up to the colostomy wound, so that usually no other fixation of the colon stump to the wound is required. If it is felt that further anchorage is advisable, this may be very simply achieved by incorporating two or three of the appendices epiploicae in the knots of sutures

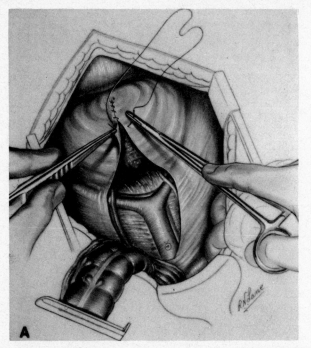

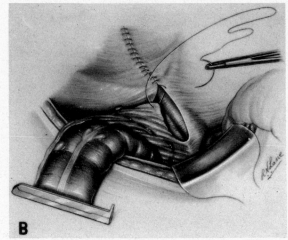

Fig. 404. Synchronous combined excision. (A) The specimen has been removed from below and the pelvic peritoneum is now being sutured over the empty pelvis with a 2/0 continuous chromic catgut stitch on a small, half-circle, atraumatic needle. (B) The edge of the iliac mesocolon is taken up in the suture.

placed on the edge of the external oblique aponeurosis. This is generally held to be preferable to stitching the actual colon wall, for such sutures may produce spots of necrosis and leakage from the bowel, with the production of a troublesome subcutaneous faecal fistula. However, I have found stitches to be quite safe provided that very fine needles and suture material are used and very superficial bites of bowel wall are taken.

EXTRAPERITONEAL TECHNIQUE

Instead of bringing the sigmoid stump forwards to the anterior abdominal wall *through* the peritoneal cavity it may be taken extraperitoneally *round its left edge*; in this way the creation of a lateral space is avoided. When the extraperitoneal colostomy technique is being used, the *pelvic peritoneum should not be sutured till after the colostomy has been established*. The upper part of its left leaf is now seized with long artery forceps, and by scissor and finger dissection an extraperitoneal space is formed, which circumvents the lateral recess of the peritoneal cavity to reach the extraperitoneal tissues of the anterior abdominal wall at the site selected for the separate

colostomy wound (Fig. 408A). The tunnel thus fashioned is well stretched with the fingers to make sure that it will accommodate the colon stump without undue constriction. The assistant passes a proctoscope or his finger with a thimble through the space to impinge firmly against the musculo-aponeurotic layers of the anterior abdominal parietes, whilst the colostomy wound is made as shown in Fig. 404, except that it eventually opens into the extraperitoneal space instead of the peritoneal cavity. The colon stump is then passed forwards to the exterior (Fig. 408B). A few suture-ligatures are used to fix the appendices epiploicae to the external oblique aponeurosis in the colostomy wound. The peritoneum is finally sutured as depicted in Fig. 408C.

INCORPORATION OF MAGNETIC CLOSING DEVICE IN COLOSTOMY

For technical details of the method of implanting a magnetic ring in the abdominal wall round the emerging colon stump and an assessment of the value of the magnetic closing device see p. 633.

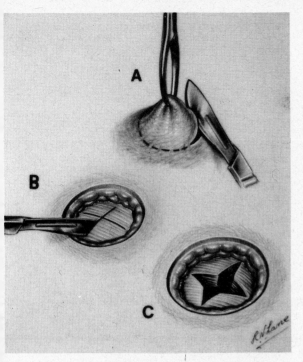

Fig. 405. Making a separate wound for the colostomy. Whilst the layers of the abdominal wall are held taut by traction to the right on artery forceps attached to the left edge of the paramedian wound and the assistant pushes his finger forward from inside the abdomen to indicate the site for the colostomy, a disc of skin and subcutaneous fat is raised by forceps and amputated (A). After some further excision of subcutaneous fat the bared external oblique aponeurosis and underlying layers are incised in cruciate fashion (B), to produce an opening through to the peritoneal cavity (C).

CLOSURE OF THE ABDOMINAL WOUND

The greater omentum is drawn down into the lower abdomen to provide a covering for the small intestine and be readily available to deal with any local infective complications in the postoperative period. The paramedian wound is then closed in layers according to the surgeon's particular preference in regard to suture of abdominal wounds (see p. 461).

COMPLETION OF THE COLOSTOMY

After the main wound has been towelled off, attention is turned to completion of the colostomy. It used to be the practice with the majority of surgeons many years ago to leave the clamp on the colon stump for 24 or 36 hours to avoid contamination of the colostomy wound before the colon had become adherent to the parietes to seal off the peritoneal cavity. However, an extensive experience with opening the colostomy in the theatre at the conclusion of the operation has shown that these fears about wound infection are quite unfounded. As a matter of fact very little other than flatus usually escapes from the colostomy for 36–48 hours. Immediate opening of the colostomy is more comfortable for the patient and for a long time now I have adopted no other method.

The technique formerly employed by many surgeons for finishing the colostomy was to apply dressings around the projecting bowel, and then to remove the clamp, leaving the colon stump protruding, with its serous surface in contact with the dressings. In the course of time granulations formed on the peritoneal aspect of the bowel, and as they became converted into fibrous tissue which contracted, the mucosa was gradually everted and drawn down to the skin surface. Unfortunately the shrinkage of this fibrous tissue also frequently led to constriction of the bowel, with the formation of a troublesome, tight stenosis at skin level (Fig. 540, p. 735). To avoid the development of granulation tissue in this manner with the risk of a subsequent stricture, I have followed the lead of Patey (1951) and Butler (1952) in the construction of colostomies (and ileostomies) and practised immediate suture of the end of the bowel to the edges of the skin wound (Fig. 409). It is remarkable how frequently these sutured colostomies heal *per primam* and, even if some slight infection should occur, separation usually affects only a small part of the circumference of the stoma. The final result with this method is a very soft pliable opening which generally shows no tendency to stenose. I can recommend this technique unreservedly for routine use.

In carrying out the method of primary suture of the end of the colon to the edges of the skin wound, it is important first of all to see that there is an adequate amount of bowel projecting beyond the skin level. I think the ideal projection is about 2 cm; more than that makes rather a bulky colostomy bud, and much less than that might be dangerous in that subsequent slight indrawing of the colon stump might result in the end of the bowel scarcely reaching to the surface. During the intraperitoneal part of the operation it is wise to err in the direction of leaving the colon stump too long; at the stage of completion of the colostomy any excess of bowel and mesosigmoid can be amputated as required at an appropriate distance from the skin surface. Three to four stay sutures are inserted between the

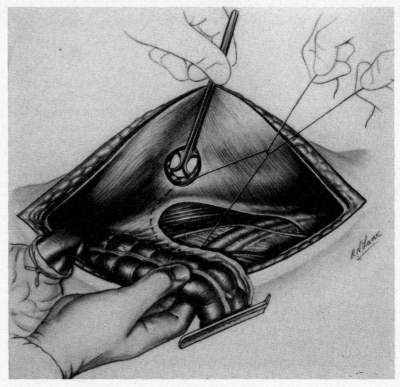

Fig. 406. Closing the paracolostomy space by purse-string suture. View of the inside of the left iliac region as seen from the right side. Whilst the left edge of the main paramedian wound is elevated by scissors threaded through the separate colostomy wound, a purse-string suture of linen thread is placed round the lateral space. Note that at the colostomy wound the purse-string stitch takes a bite of muscle of the abdominal wall as well as the parietal peritoneum.

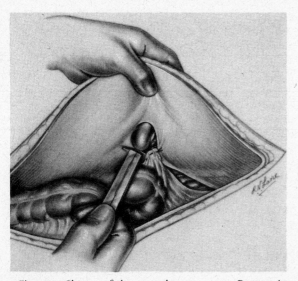

Fig. 407. Closure of the paracolostomy space. Purse-string suture tied.

edges of the circular skin wound and the open end of bowel; these stitches penetrate not merely the mucosa but the whole thickness of the colon wall (Fig. 409). Further sutures are then placed between the stays to secure a close and accurate apposition of the two epithelial surfaces. I generally use fine serum-proof silk on fine straight cutting needles for the stitches between the skin and bowel, but fine chromic catgut is probably equally satisfactory and saves the nursing staff the trouble of removing the sutures subsequently—and perhaps inadvertently missing one or two!

If desired, the colon stump may be irrigated or injected with a cytotoxic agent before the colostomy is established but it is rather difficult to devise a convenient and satisfactory technique for so doing. One method is that outlined in Fig. 322A, to be applied before the colon stump is drawn through the abdominal wall, or indeed even before the lateral space is closed by purse-string suture, though the presence of an occlusion clamp is a considerable inconvenience during the subsequent manoeuvres. An easier method, which is a modification of that shown in Fig. 323, is simply to swab out the colon stump with the drug, as soon

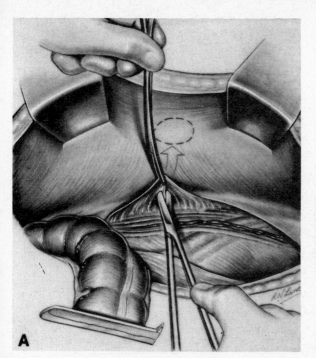
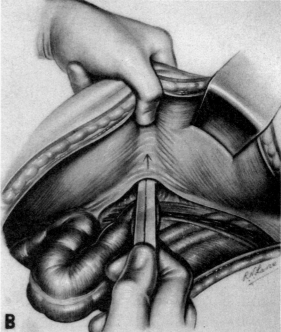
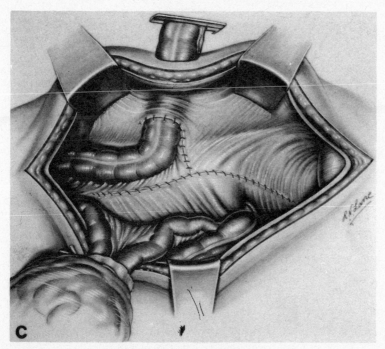

Fig. 408. Extraperitoneal colostomy technique. View of the inside of the left iliac region as seen from the right side. (A) Making the extraperitoneal tunnel. (B) Passing the clamped colon stump through the tunnel. (C) The iliac colon in position and retroperitonealization completed.

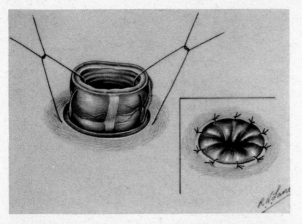

Fig. 409. Completion of colostomy by immediate muco-cutaneous suture. Insertion of stay sutures. Usually three or four are required. They transfix *all layers* of the bowel wall and may be of fine non-absorbable material or chromic catgut. *Inset:* Finished colostomy.

as the clamp is taken off the end of the colon, prior to stitching the bowel to the edges of the skin. However, I personally have not used anti-cancer applications in this connection and have never seen carcinomatous deposits arising in relation to the colostomy in such a way as to suggest that they were due to implantation of malignant cells on the mucocutaneous suture line. It is significant that Boreham (1958) in a survey of very many hundreds of colostomy cases at St Mark's Hospital was able to discover only two examples of what he deemed to be metastases by implantation.

Excision of the Vasa Deferentia and Seminal Vesicles with the Rectum

In this modification of the abdominal phase, the lateral peritoneal incisions meet anteriorly on the top of the back of the bladder as in an ordinary abdominoperineal excision. As the plane of dissection is deepened in front, the vasa deferentia and the superior aspects of the seminal vesicles are exposed. The vasa are divided and tied on either side, care being taken to avoid the ureters, and the forceps controlling the inner cut end of either vasa are drawn backwards, so that the plane of dissection then proceeds between the bladder in front and the vasa and vesicles behind. When the base of the prostate is reached the lower ends of the vasa are divided and the prostatorectal plane entered. The dissection of the rectum on the posterior and lateral aspects is then carried out as in an ordinary abdominoperineal excision.

Excision of the Urinary Bladder with the Rectum—Complete Pelvic Clearance

Sometimes when a carcinoma of the upper rectum or recto-sigmoid has fallen on to the top of the bladder and become adherent to it, it may be possible, if this extension lies well in front of the ureteric orifices, to deal with it by removal of a disc of bladder wall along with the rectum and by subsequent closure of the vesical gap by suture, an indwelling urethral catheter being left in for 7–10 days. More usually, however, it is the trigonal region or the part of the bladder immediately above it that is apt to be affected by forward spread of a rectal carcinoma, and if the growth has actually infiltrated the bladder wall, the only prospect of eradication lies with the excision of the bladder, prostate, vesicles, vasa and fistula along with the rectum. This operation of complete pelvic clearance is certainly a formidable undertaking with a high initial mortality, and it is particularly galling if, when the operative specimen secured by it is examined pathologically, it is found that the bladder wall was not actually invaded by growth! Brunschwig and Barber (1969) have even applied the operation to some patients with extension of their carcinomas also to the pelvis, so that they have had to resect a segment of bone, but none of these cases has achieved complete cure, though a few survived for a surprisingly long time. Personally, I have always reserved pelvic clearance for patients with growths extending exclusively forwards, apparently to involve the bladder, seminal vesicles and prostate deeply, and *have regarded any serious adherence posteriorly or laterally to the walls of the pelvis or evidence of involvement of lymph nodes on the pelvic side walls as strong contraindications to its use.* I am sure there is a small but definite place for this very radical operation in the management of rectal carcinoma. The procedure is, of course, merely a combination of total cystoprostatectomy, as for carcinoma of the bladder, with an abdominoperineal excision, and the surgeon should therefore familiarize himself with the technique of the former operation, as described so clearly by Millin and Masina (1949). The method of dealing with the ureters is preferably that of Bricker (1950), in which they are implanted into an isolated loop of ileum, brought out as a urinary ileostomy (see Pyrah and Raper 1955 and p. 506).

In the performance of complete pelvic clearance the lateral incisions in the pelvic peritoneum are carried forwards to meet, not on the top of the base of the bladder, but near the front of its superior surface. The resulting wound is opened up on either side to display the ureters and the vasa deferentia. Both these structures are tied and divided fairly close to the bladder. The plane between the bladder and the side-wall of the pelvis is then cautiously opened up on one side as far forwards as the back of the pubis and down to the side of the prostate, the obliterated hypogastric artery with its superior vesical branch and the inferior vesical artery being ligated and divided in the process. The bladder is then similarly freed on the opposite side. These two lateral planes of separation meet anteriorly, where the median umbilical ligament, which is attached to the apex of the bladder, is now divided. It only remains to divide the lateral and median prostatic ligaments and the apex of the prostatic urethra to free the bladder and prostate except for their attachment to the rectum, but these steps are better carried out from the perineal aspect, for haemorrhage, which is common, can be more easily dealt with from below.

The ligation of the inferior mesenteric vessels and the mobilization of the rectum on its posterior and lateral aspects now proceed as in a straightforward abdominoperineal excision. Due to the great sacrifice of pelvic peritoneum in complete pelvic clearance, suture of the pelvic peritoneal floor after this operation is generally impossible, even when the synchronous technique is being used and the rectum, bladder, and prostate are removed from below before any attempt is made to close the peritoneum. The best plan is to leave the peritoneum quite unsutured and to allow the loops of small intestine to fall down into the pelvis, either into the empty pelvis or on to a large gauze pack introduced inside a plastic Lahey bag (see p. 532), through

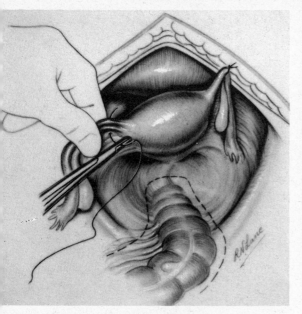

Fig. 410. Anterior dissection in the female. Hitching up the uterus with stay sutures under the uterine tubes.

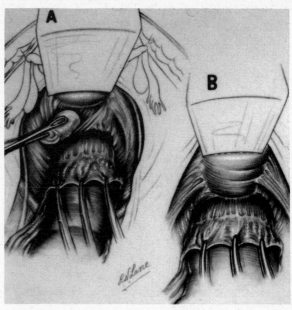

Fig. 411. Separation of the rectum from the uterus and vagina.

the perineal wound. As Trimpi and Bacon (1952) have shown experimentally and clinically, a new pelvic peritoneal floor rapidly forms under these circumstances.

RESECTION OF A LOOP OF SMALL GUT WITH THE RECTUM

One of the lower loops of ileum may become adherent to a growth of the intraperitoneal rectum or rectosigmoid and require to be resected along with the growth. But it is important not to embark on the resection of the ileal loop till the surgeon has satisfied himself by trial dissection that he can in fact mobilize and remove the rectum, otherwise he may land himself in the awkward predicament of having an isolated loop of small intestine attached to an unresectable growth. Once a firm decision has been reached on the feasibility of removing the growth, the ileal mesentery is divided between forceps and the afferent and efferent limbs of the loop divided between crushing clamps. The isolated loop is drawn forwards and to the side with the growth, whilst the continuity of the small intestine is restored by end-to-end anastomosis. The excision of the rectum then proceeds as ordinarily.

ABDOMINAL DISSECTION IN THE FEMALE

The dissection in the female naturally differs from that in the male on the anterior and, to some extent, the lateral aspects. Incidentally, to facilitate the dissection on these aspects, it is a good plan to commence the operation by *hitching up the uterus*

with stay sutures passed under the inner ends of the uterine tubes and affixing them to the anterior rectus sheath at the lower angle of the parietal wound (Fig. 410). The rectum is then drawn upwards and backwards and the uterus is retracted strongly forwards with a deep pelvic retractor, whilst the peritoneal scissor cuts on either side of the base of the mesosigmoid and upper mesorectum are extended round the brim of the pelvis to meet anteriorly just below the cervix uteri (making a considerably wider sweep than is indicated in Fig. 410). The posterior edge of the peritoneal cut behind the cervix uteri is then caught with long artery forceps and drawn upwards and backwards whilst the cervix is retracted forwards (Fig. 411A). A few snips with scissors and a little blunt dissection with a swab on a sponge-holder suffices to strike the plane between the posterior vaginal wall and the rectum. These structures are then rapidly separated by further gauze dissection, any small bleeding points on the vaginal wall being checked by diathermy coagulation (Fig. 411B). The fascia of Denonvillier, which remains on the front of the rectum and the lateral ligaments as they are displaced backwards, is finally incised low down, transversely, with scissors, and the lateral ligaments are then defined and divided.

The remainder of the abdominal phase is similar to that in male patients, except that the closure of the pelvic peritoneal floor is usually easier because peritoneum can be 'borrowed' from the posterior leaf of the broad ligaments as required.

REMOVAL OF THE POSTERIOR VAGINAL WALL WITH THE RECTUM

If it is decided to remove the posterior vaginal wall *en bloc* with the rectum, as is usually my practice, the separation of these two structures is halted as soon as the uppermost 2 cm of vagina has been exposed. A transverse incision is made in the vaginal wall just below the cervix uteri, and extended to either side, the ureters being carefully retracted out of the way (Fig. 412A). Longitudinal scissor cuts are then started on either side running downwards from each end of the transverse incision to be met by similar incisions coming up from the perineal dissection in due course (Fig. 412B).

REMOVAL OF UTERUS, UTERINE APPENDAGES AND POSTERIOR VAGINAL WALL WITH THE RECTUM

A simultaneous total hysterectomy together with rectal excision is not infrequently required for anteriorly situated growths in the female, and every surgeon undertaking the treatment of rectal cancer should have in his repertoire a well rehearsed technique for this extended operation.

After separation of the developmental adhesions on the outer side of the sigmoid colon and mesocolon, it is best then to proceed with the uterine part of the operation. A long straight artery forceps is applied to the right uterine appendages close to the body of the uterus, and, by drawing it strongly upwards and to the opposite side, the round ligament and the ovarian ligament are rendered taut and prominent. Each of these ligaments is clipped and divided between forceps (Fig. 413). The intact peritoneum between these sites of division is then severed and the peritoneal cut prolonged forwards to the midline between the uterus and the bladder, and backwards on to the right side of the sigmoid mesocolon roughly as far as the bifurcation of the abdominal aorta. The artery forceps are replaced by ligatures and the long wound in the peritoneum opened up to display the right ureter. Usually it is found *closely applied to the medial leaf of peritoneum*. It is traced downwards and forwards to where it enters the 'ureteric canal' (MacLeod and Howkins 1964), which is formed by the uterine artery crossing above the ureter on its

way to the side of the uterus (Fig. 414A). The further exposure of the ureter necessitates the division of the uterine vessels between ligatures or forceps, care being taken not to miss any of the veins that accompany the artery (Fig. 414B). The ureter can now be traced forwards at the side of the upper end of the vagina to its termination in the bladder. By exactly the same manoeuvres the uterus is freed on the left side and the left ureter displayed throughout its length down to its entry into the bladder.

The bladder is then brushed down off the front of the upper part of the vagina and a transverse incision made with scalpel or scissors in the anterior vaginal wall just below the cervix uteri, the ureters being protected from damage in the process (Fig. 415A). From the ends of this incision longitudinal cuts are carried out down either side-wall of the vagina with scissors as far as can conveniently be reached (Fig. 415B). (In this connection it may be mentioned that, if hysterectomy is being performed in conjunction with anterior resection, the vagina is now cut right across at a suitable distance below the growth (Fig. 416A). The rectum is then mobilized and, after division of the lateral ligaments, the cut upper end of the vagina is closed by suture (Fig. 416B).)

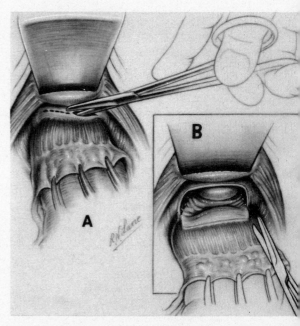

Fig. 412. Taking the posterior vaginal wall with the rectum. (A) Opening the posterior fornix of the vagina. (B) Extending the scissor cuts downwards.

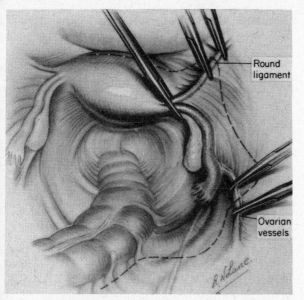

Fig. 413. Combined total hysterectomy and rectal excision. Uterine appendages on one side have been seized with artery forceps and drawn upwards and to the opposite side. The round ligament and ovarian ligament have been clipped and the line of peritoneal incision is indicated.

So far the rectum has not been mobilized in any way, and the surgeon next turns to this part of the operation. The inferior mesenteric vessels are ligated and divided high or low depending on circumstances and the sigmoid mesocolon and colon divided. The presacral space is then opened up, freeing the rectum posteriorly as far as the tip of the coccyx, and finally the lateral ligaments are divided in turn either with or without preliminary clamping.

This completes the dissection of the uterus, vagina and rectum from the abdominal aspect. If the operation is being conducted as a synchronous abdominoperineal excision, the perineal operator will have finished his phase of the dissection by now, so that the operative specimen can be removed, which greatly facilitates the suture of the pelvic peritoneum. If on the other hand the Miles technique is being followed, it will be found extremely difficult to bury the mobilized viscera beneath the pelvic peritoneum even after amputation of the sigmoid and mesosigmoid from the specimen. It may be indeed that the peritoneum will have to be left unsutured at this stage.

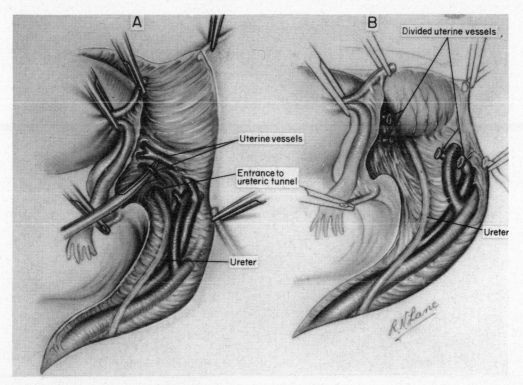

Fig. 414. Combined total hysterectomy and rectal excision. Exposing the ureter and uterine artery. (A) The round ligament and ovarian vessels are divided and the tissue spaces are opened up to display the ureter and the uterine artery as it crosses the ureter in the ureteric canal. (B) Complete exposure of the ureter down to the bladder after division of the uterine vessels.

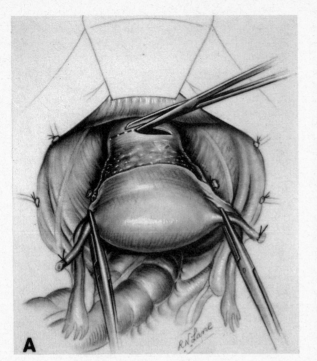

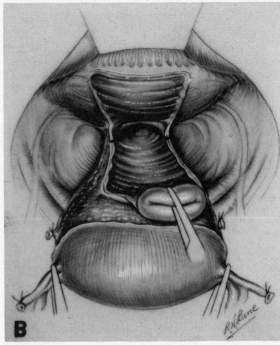

Fig. 415. Combined total hysterectomy and rectal excision. (A) Opening the vagina from the front. (B) Extending the cuts dividing the vagina into anterior and posterior halves.

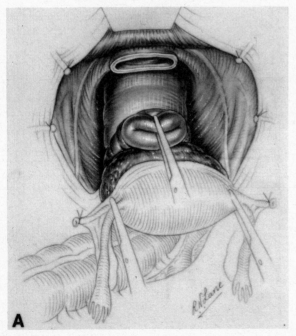

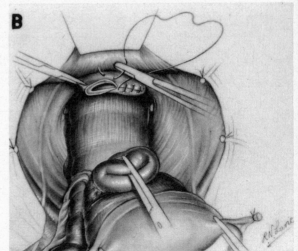

Fig. 416. Combined total hysterectomy and anterior resection. (A) Vaginal tube cut across, fascia of Denonvillier incised. (B) Rectum mobilized, vagina being closed.

THE PERINEAL DISSECTION IN THE SYNCHRONOUS OPERATION

INCISION

Miles (1926) at one stage favoured the incision shown in Fig. 417A, with transverse cuts in the front and behind for the perineal dissection, and many surgeons have followed him, using it also for the synchronous type of combined excision. My own preference is for a wide elliptical circumcision of the anus, which is prolonged backwards as a simple linear incision over the sacrococcygeal junction (Fig. 417B). The slackness of the perianal skin makes it difficult to incise neatly, and it is an advantage to render it taut by grasping the anal orifice, closed by the preliminary purse-string suture, with a pair of stout tissue forceps and drawing it to each side in turn, whilst the skin of the buttock is retracted by pressure of the hand to the opposite side as each half of the elliptical incision is made.

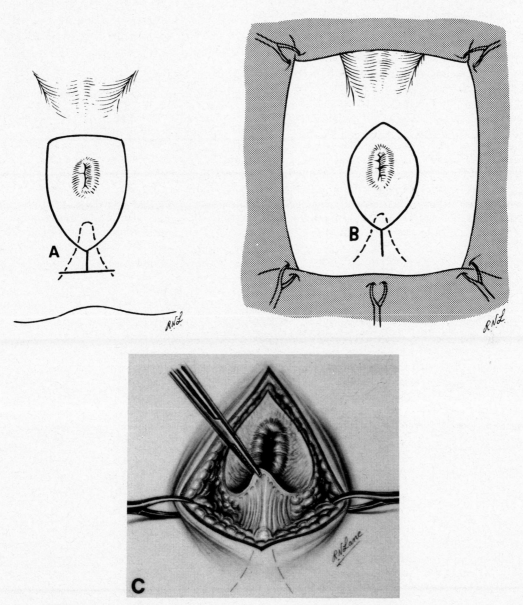

Fig. 417. (A, B) Alternative incisions for perineal dissection of synchronous combined excision in the male. (C) Opening up the posterior part of the wound to expose the coccyx.

DISARTICULATION OF THE COCCYX

The posterior part of the incision alone is deepened in the first instance and the edges of the resulting wound are retracted laterally, whilst the coccyx is defined by scalpel dissection (Fig. 417C). Finally, when the surface and edges of the bone have been fairly clearly exposed, the sacrococcygeal and inter-coccygeal articulations are flexed strongly forwards by pressure on the tip of the coccyx with the thumb of the left hand. One of these joints—generally an intercoccygeal one—is sought with the point of the scalpel, and, when it is found, the coccyx is completely divided across at the line of the articulation (Fig. 418). The terminal piece of bone is then either displaced forward, or preferably excised from its muscular attachments by traction on it with a pair of tissue forceps, whilst the scalpel cuts round its edges and tip, most conveniently from the deep aspect. Not infrequently the middle or lateral sacral vessels are divided during the disarticulation of the coccyx and cause sharp bleeding till checked by diathermy coagulation or a stitch. Occasionally in older subjects the coccyx cannot be separated in this manner by the scalpel because the joints have become fused and rigid. It is then necessary to use an osteotome or chisel and mallet to remove it, and these instruments should always be available in case of need.

But there is no special virtue in removing the coccyx and, instead, the anococcygeal raphe may be incised just in front of the tip of the bone, thus giving access to the pelvis (Fig. 419, *inset*). The retention of the bone does not usually hamper the surgeon in his subsequent dissection, and the patient is possibly more comfortable during the postoperative period if the coccyx is not removed. It is also true that coccygectomy in no way contributes to the actual eradication of the growth itself. Indeed the only argument for removing the coccyx during abdominoperineal rectal excision is that this provides a readier method for entering the pelvis than does division of the more yielding anococcygeal raphe.

DIVISION OF THE PERIANAL AND ISCHIORECTAL FAT AND LEVATORES ANI

The edges of the perianal ellipse of skin are clipped together over the anus with three or four pairs of tissue forceps, and the outer margin of the elliptical wound on either side is also caught with forceps for retraction. The left half of the wound is now opened up by the assistant exerting counter traction on the anal forceps and on those holding the left skin edge, whilst the surgeon inserts the extended index and middle fingers of his left hand through the bed of the coccyx into the pelvis above

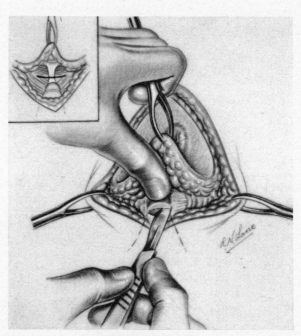

Fig. 418. Dissection of the terminal part of the coccyx. *Inset:* An alternative, now more common, method of cutting across the anococcygeal raphe.

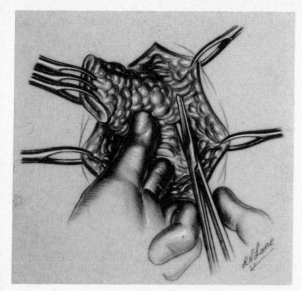

Fig. 419. Insertion of two fingers of the left hand into the pelvis through the hole created by the removal of the coccyx. The fingers are pressed forwards on the left side of the rectum above the levator muscle, and the perianal and ischiorectal fat is divided with scissors down to the muscle.

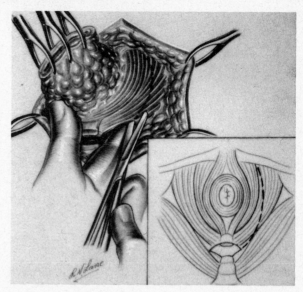

Fig. 420. Dividing the ileococcygeus part of the levator ani. *Inset:* The line of division of the muscle shown more diagrammatically.

the levator muscle on the left side of the rectum (Fig. 419). Using scissors he then cuts through the fine-lobulated perianal and coarser-lobulated ischiorectal fat on to the levator muscle, branches of the inferior haemorrhoidal vessels being encountered and divided in the process especially as the muscle itself is approached. Finally the ileococcygeus part of the levator muscle is exposed; it is divided with scissors from behind forwards and usually it is a relatively avascular structure, so that not much bleeding results (Fig. 420).

The fingers of the left hand are then reinserted on the right side of the rectum above the right levator ani and this muscle, together with the overlying fatty tissues, is divided in the same way as on the left side.

INSERTION OF SELF-RETAINING PERINEAL RETRACTOR

A St Mark's Hospital pattern of self-retaining retractor is now inserted to hold the sides of the wound strongly apart (Fig. 421). (To prevent the retractor from sliding down in the wound the blades may be clipped to the skin edges with towel clips through special small perforations in one version of this instrument; see Fig. 386.)

DIVISION OF FASCIA OF WALDEYER AND POSTERIOR MOBILIZATION OF RECTUM

If the tissue forceps attached to the anal skin are lifted forcibly forwards, the back of the mobilized rectum is clearly exposed. It is still covered by the thick tough white fascia of Waldeyer, which is now incised with scissors or scalpel just distal to the cut end of the sacrum or coccyx and round either side of the rectum (Fig. 421). When this has been done, fat usually bulges through the gap, indicating that the perirectal space has been entered. The fingers, and then the whole hand, can be gradually insinuated through this fascial opening and the rectum lifted forwards off the front of the sacrum (Fig. 421, *inset*). The abdominal operator has usually mobilized the rectum from behind by this stage also; the plane of separation effected by him, however, does not usually coincide with that of the perineal operator, but generally lies slightly in front of it, and a certain amount of blunt dissection is necessary to bring the perineal and abdominal fields into continuity.

ANTERIOR DISSECTION

The rectum is now drawn downwards and the anterior part of the incision deepened by scissor dissection on to the central point of the perineum. The superficial and deep transverse perineal

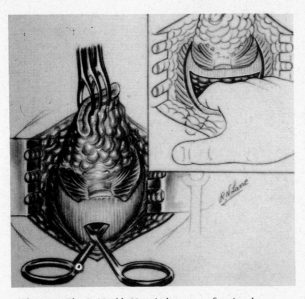

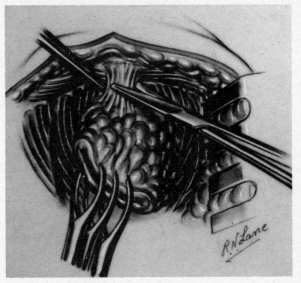

Fig. 421. The St Mark's Hospital pattern of perineal retractor has been inserted. The anal canal is lifted up to expose the stout white 'fascia of Waldeyer', which is divided transversely with scissors distal to the cut surface of the coccyx or sacrum. *Inset:* The surgeon's hand being passed into the pelvis to separate the rectum from the sacrum.

Fig. 422. Commencement of anterior dissection by separating the superficial transverse perineal muscle from the front of the anal canal.

muscles are then separated from the front of the external anal sphincter (Fig. 422). This carries the dissection on to a layer of muscle with fibres running roughly in the anteroposterior plane, which comprises the pubococcygeus and puborectalis parts of the levator ani muscle on either side and the rectourethralis muscle in the centre. These muscular attachments have to be divided and this is done first from one side and then from the other. The rectum is drawn downwards and to the patient's right by the assistant, whilst the surgeon defines the lateral (or upper) edge of the left pubococcygeus as it crosses the white homogeneous surface of the rectum from behind forwards. Slipping the tips of his left index and middle fingers above and below the muscle edge he snips it gradually with scissors (Fig. 423). As the division proceeds it is found that the muscle mass is much more substantial than it at first appeared. The cut is terminated above 1·5 cm from the midline, when clearly some further muscle remains to be severed on that side. The rectum is then drawn downwards and to the patient's left whilst the right pubococcygeus and puborectalis are divided in a similar manner.

The effect of these divisions is to leave the rectum tethered in front at the level of the anorectal junction by a narrow bundle of muscle about 1·5–2 cm wide, and this must now be divided. Undoubtedly this is the most difficult step in the perineal dissection, or indeed in the whole operation, for a slight error of judgement in the division of this band of tissue may result in opening the rectum or the membranous urethra. It is important to appreciate that *the rectum is sharply angulated at this point* (Fig. 423B). Due to the downward traction on on the forceps attached to the perianal skin, the axis of the anal canal is directed upwards towards the pubic region as well as headwards; above the anorectal junction and the attachment of the rectourethrales and the remnants of the puborectales, the rectum inclines backwards as well as in a headward direction as it runs closely applied to the posterior surface of the prostate. Its axis at this stage can be more readily visualized if the firm lateral edges of the prostate are felt by the tips of the index finger and thumb passed upwards on either side of the rectum. When the slope of the prostate has been gauged in this way, the blades of the scissors are applied to the anterior muscle band with the long axis of the instrument held in the midline and *in the same plane as the posterior surface of the prostate* (Fig. 424). As the muscle is divided, the tissue plane between the rectum and prostate is opened up, disclosing the back of the latter.

The danger of injury to the rectum or urinary tract arises usually from holding the scissors in too

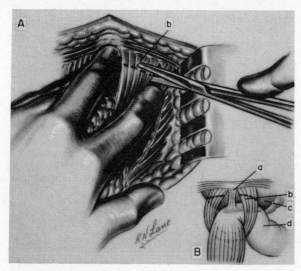

Fig. 423. (A) Division of the pubococcygeus and puborectales muscles whilst they are defined between the index and middle fingers. (B) Semidiagrammatic view of relative positions of prostate, rectum, anal canal, puborectalis sling and recto-urethralis during this step of the operation. *a* = rectourethralis; *b* = pubococcygeus and puborectalis; *c* = prostate; *d* = rectum.

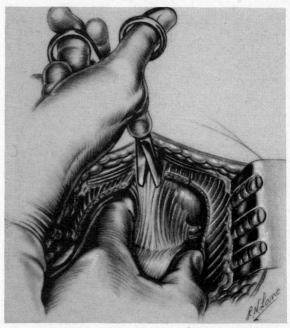

Fig. 424. Division of the rectourethralis and remnants of puborectales. Note that the scissors are held in the same plane as the posterior surface of the prostate in order to lessen the risk of opening the rectum or cutting into the membranous or prostatic urethra.

horizontal a direction when making the initial muscle cut. Then there is obviously a real risk of cutting off the point of the angulated anterior anorectal wall, or of opening into the membranous urethra or back to the prostate.

An alternative method of completing the division of the anterior muscular attachment of the anorectal junction is to approach it not from the midline below, but from above and from the side, after the plane between the prostate and rectum has been found on the lateral aspect and traced downwards (a good idea of this approach is conveyed by Fig. 423B). In this technique the rectum is displaced somewhat to one side to allow of a view being obtained of the groove between the lateral edge of the prostate and the front of the rectal ampulla. By cautious scissor dissection the plane between these viscera is struck, and this separation is continued down to the anorectal junction, where the upper edge of the muscular attachment is defined. It is now an easy matter to sever this muscle from the side allowing the rectum to fall backwards.

Whichever method has been employed to enter the tissue plane between the rectum and prostate, it is found that as the separation proceeds upwards a band of connective tissue connects these two organs at their lateral margins and has to be divided as the dissection is carried to the upper border of the prostate and the seminal vesicles (Fig. 425A). The latter are still covered by the thin fascia of Denonvillier and for that reason are not as clearly seen as during the abdominal dissection, in which they are bared of this fascia. At this stage the planes of the abdominal and perineal operators can be made to meet by simply tearing this fascial partition.

TAKING THE LATERAL LIGAMENTS

The only structures holding the rectum are now the lateral ligaments, unless these have already been divided by the abdominal operator; even if he has taken them, a small amount of tissue of the lower parts of the ligaments generally remains to be divided from below. To display the ligament from the perineal aspect the rectum is drawn strongly to the opposite side, and any remnant of the fascia of Waldeyer on this aspect divided with scissors. This allows the rectum to descend another 2 or 3 cm and displays the fat of the lower part of the lateral ligament. The middle and index fingers of the left hand are passed upwards in front of and behind the ligament respectively, to define it more accurately and to displace the rectum still further with the palm of the hand to the opposite side of the pelvis

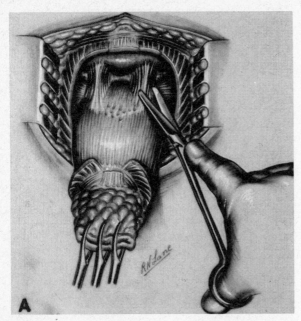 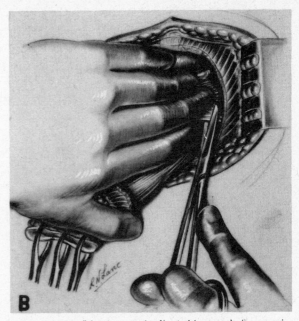

Fig. 425. (A) The prostatorectal plane has been entered from below after division of the rectourethralis. A thin strand of connective tissue is encountered on either side, extending backwards from the edges of the prostate to the front of the rectum, and has to be cut. (B) Defining the lateral ligament preparatory to its division.

(Fig. 425B). The ligament can now be divided with scissors as close as possible to the pelvic side-wall. The same performance is repeated for the other lateral ligament and the rectum will then be found to be completely free. If the abdominal operator has already divided the sigmoid colon and mesocolon, the operative specimen is passed down into the pelvis and delivered through the perineal wound. Alternatively, if the specimen is still attached at its upper end, the perineal operator encloses the anal end in a rubber glove which is tied in position, and the rectum is passed up into the abdomen to be brought out through the abdominal wound on to the front of the abdomen by the abdominal operator.

HAEMOSTASIS AND SUTURE OF PERINEAL WOUND

The empty pelvic cavity is carefully scrutinized for bleeding points. These are found principally in the situation of the divided lateral ligaments, and on the back of the prostate and the membranous urethra. They are controlled by diathermy or ligature. The final arrangement of the perineal wound may then follow one of four or five lines:

Partial Suture and Packing. Ernest Miles (1926) recommended packing the pelvic cavity after abdominoperineal excision with two objects—to support the delicate pelvic peritoneal floor, and to assist in haemostasis. In order to prevent the pack becoming adherent to the peritoneum and tearing it on withdrawal, he always lined the cavity with a square of oiled silk and packed the roll of gauze inside this material, the perineal wound being partly closed round the projecting edges of the square and the end of the pack. Actually the pelvic floor usually does not need support, and despite the thinness of the peritoneum it heals very readily as a rule without disruption. As for haemostasis, it is usually possible to control bleeding sufficiently at the time of the operation to be able to dispense with any form of pack. If packing should be required, my experience is that a pack inside a square of oiled silk or a plastic bag is less effective than a naked pack, and I have not had trouble with the former becoming adherent to the peritoneum, though its removal has sometimes necessitated a brief general anaesthetic.

Partial Suture and 'Open' Drainage. If a pack can be avoided, as is feasible in many cases, the patient is possibly more comfortable. One substitute for packing is simply to drain the pelvic cavity with a piece of corrugated rubber or a stout rubber tube, brought out through the middle third of the

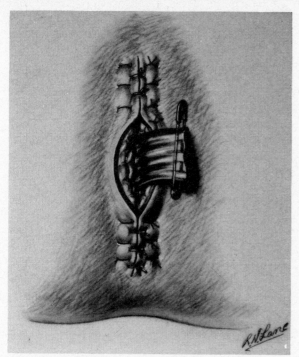

Fig. 426. Final closure of the perineal wound, the middle third being left open for a corrugated rubber drain.

perineal wound, whilst its front and back thirds alone are sutured (Fig. 426). This unsutured gap allows plenty of room for subsequent irrigations and remains open sufficiently long to permit the pelvic cavity to fill with granulations from the depths before epithelialization is complete.

Complete Suture of Skin and Fat and Suction Drainage. A third plan of management for the perineal wound, which is now much favoured, is to close it completely with two rows of catgut stitches for the fat and one row of silk stitches for the skin, and to drain the pelvic cavity by means of suction drainage. The latter may be effected by 'closed suction' drains of Zimmer or Redivac type, or preferably, I think, by sump suction drains. The tube or tubes—for it is an advantage to use two or three to lessen the risk of blockage with clot, if closed drainage is used—may be passed through the perineum, either at the perineal wound itself or at separate stab wounds to one or other side of the main wound, or through a suprapubic stab wound, from which they reach the pelvic cavity by an extraperitoneal route over the brim of the pelvis. It is hoped by this method to prevent any substantial accumulation of fluid in the

pelvic cavity, so that, after the tube is removed in four or more days, healing *per primam* will ensue, without there being any open wound requiring irrigations. However, in some cases haematoma formation or infection occurs necessitating laying the wound open, or a persistent sinus or recurrent abscess develops.

A further modification of the technique of complete suture with suction drainage is that advocated by Kelly (Schwab and Kelly 1974; Kelly 1977), in which irrigation is combined with suction in the hope of maintaining better evacuation of material from the pelvic cavity. In this method two large-bore tubes are inserted into the sub-peritoneal pelvis through stab wounds lateral to the main perineal wound. Through one catheter a constant infusion of normal saline is administered at a rate of 50 ml per hour, whilst suction is applied continuously to the other catheter, usually for four or five days. More recently antibiotics have been added to the irrigating fluid (Kelly 1977).

Complete Suture of Skin and Fat, but not of Pelvic Peritoneum, combined with Suction Drainage. The perineal wound may be completely closed by suture of the skin and fat, whilst the pelvic peritoneum is left unsutured by the abdominal operator, with the object of encouraging the small bowel and greater omentum to fall down into the pelvis and help to fill it and even perhaps of allowing any fluid that exudes into the pelvic cavity to escape upwards into the general peritoneum, where it might be more easily absorbed. One might fear with this method that the extraperitoneal position of part of the small intestine would predispose to paralytic ileus in the immediate postoperative period or to mechanical intestinal obstruction or sacral herniation at a later stage. Though quite a number of surgeons claim to use this plan of management of the perineal wound after abdominoperineal excision with very satisfactory results (e.g. Haxton 1970), precise information has till recently been lacking as to the proportion of cases in which primary healing was secured and the incidence of complications. When I have used this technique, as a precaution I have usually left in a suprapubic suction drain for three or four days.

A modification of this method is that advocated by Ruckley et al. (1970), in which *an omental tail, manufactured by detaching this structure from part of the greater curvature of the stomach* (see p. 438), *is swung down into the empty pelvis after the rectum has been removed.* It is stitched in position there by the perineal operator with catgut sutures to the sub-cutaneous fat of the perineum. The perineal wound is then closed completely in two layers, a closed suction drain having been inserted into it through a separate stab wound in the perineal skin on either side of the perineal suture line. The abdominal operator sutures the pelvic peritoneum around the omental pedicle.

Surgeons are divided in their opinions regarding the merits of these various methods of managing the perineal wound. The only thing that is absolutely certain in this matter is *the necessity for packing in any patient in whom it has not been found possible to achieve complete control of bleeding by diathermy, ligature and suture*. My own preference in such cases is for naked gauze packs, and I have no hesitation about using them when I am unhappy about haemostasis. The postoperative management after packing is described on p. 556, but, in my experience and contrary to popular belief, there is little difference in the amount of discomfort to the patient or the course of the convalescence, if the perineum is packed or is treated by open corrugated rubber drainage. There has been no

trouble with tearing of the pelvic peritoneum when the pack is removed three days later.

In cases *with good control of bleeding and no gross faecal contamination* the choice between partial suture with open drainage and subsequent irrigations and complete closure of the perineal wound with or without peritoneal suture and omental tamponade is, in the present state of our knowledge, extremely controversial. The open method is safe and sure, but rather tedious for the patient and certainly extravagant in the use of nursing time—an important consideration in these days of shortage of nurses. If primary healing can be obtained even in a proportion of the patients treated by the various forms of complete suture with suction drainage, this is a substantial achievement. Oates and Williams (1970) claim primary healing in 67 of 84 patients managed in this way with closed suprapubic suction drainage; Hultén et al. (1971) had the same ideal result in 27 of 36 patients similarly managed except that a sump drain was sometimes used instead of closed suction though more recently he has had

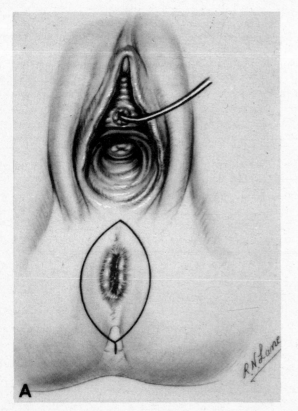
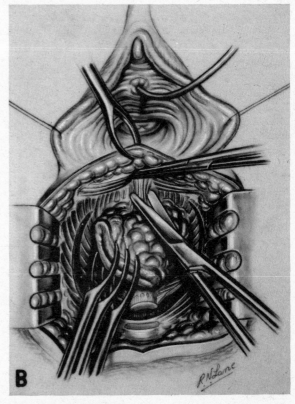

Fig. 427. (A) Outline of incision for perineal dissection in the female with conservation of the posterior vaginal wall. (B) Separation of anal canal and rectum from vagina.

much less satisfactory results (Hultén (1977). Encouraging results have also been reported by Dencker et al. (1973), Broader et al. (1974), Walton and Mallik (1974) and Kelly (1977). In all these series the original conditions for which the operation was performed in quite a number of the patients were ulcerative colitis or Crohn's disease, which usually present even greater problems in regard to perineal wound healing. The results obtained, therefore, are all the more creditable. My own personal experience with complete suture of the perineum combined with perineal or supra-pubic suction drainage (and systemic broad-spectrum antibiotic cover) has been rather less impressive than that just quoted (Irvin and Goligher 1975). About half my patients have obtained total primary healing. In another quarter, or slightly more, though haematoma formation or sepsis necessitated removal of some sutures, the eventual healing time was probably less than if the wound had been left partly open *ab initio* for irrigation treatment. In the rest it was difficult to discern any clear advantage from the use of this method—indeed in a few of them it seemed as if the

patient may have suffered slightly from the pent-up haematoma or infection, either systemically or from possible pressure on the vagina with subsequent fistulation.

As for the value of leaving the pelvic peritoneum unsutured in association with primary closure of the perineal wound, in our trial (Irvin and Goligher 1975) a comparison was made between two series, one with the peritoneum closed and the other with it left unsutured. There was no obvious difference in the healing of the perineal wound in these two groups. It must be added, too, that paralytic ileus and mechanical intestinal obstruction were *not* more frequent in the unsutured cases. It thus seems immaterial whether the pelvic peritoneum is closed or not. My own preference is to close it where possible, which means nearly always. Ruckley et al. (1970) in their original report of the use of a pedicle graft of greater omentum to fill the pelvic cavity claimed primary healing in only 50% of their cases, results which scarcely differ from those obtained by us (Irvin and Goligher 1975) with primary suture with suction drainage (with or without pelvic peritoneal suture).

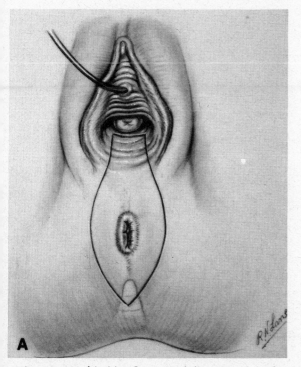

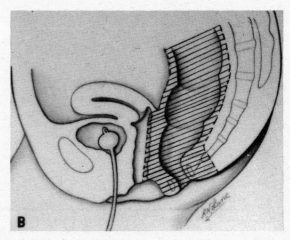

Fig. 428. Usual incision for perineal dissection in the female with removal of the entire posterior vaginal wall. (A) Outline of incision as seen from perineal aspect. (B) Side view showing the vaginal extension of the incision.

THE PERINEAL DISSECTION IN CASES HAVING COMPLETE PELVIC CLEARANCE

The only particular in which this differs from the perineal phase in an ordinary synchronous combined excision is in regard to the anterior dissection. This proceeds as usual up to the point where

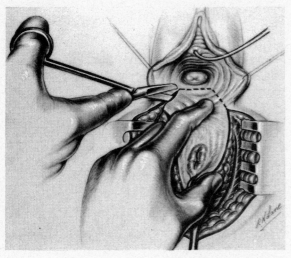

Fig. 429. After freeing the rectum posteriorly and laterally the vaginal wall is divided longitudinally on one side and then on the other.

the puborectalis is divided on either side and the rectourethralis is cut in the midline exposing the apical part of the prostate. Instead of continuing the dissection up in the plane between the rectum and prostate, the urethra is divided just below the prostate, and the anterior plane of the abdominal dissection is entered. The excision then proceeds up to delivery of the specimen. In these cases, as the pelvic peritoneum cannot be sutured, the coils of small gut fall down into the pelvis. The perineal wound can be either closed completely by skin suture with or without suction drainage, or it may be partly sutured round a pack inserted into the pelvis inside a plastic square, as recommended by Trimpi and Bacon (1952), or plastic bag such as we use to enclose the loops of small bowel temporarily during rectal excision (see p. 532).

THE PERINEAL DISSECTION IN THE FEMALE

This differs from the dissection in the male only in front where the rectum has to be separated from the posterior vaginal wall, and care is needed to avoid buttonholing the latter (Fig. 427A and B). In cases with growths lying in relation to the vaginal wall or adherent to it, it is preferable to excise this structure *en bloc* with the rectum (Figs 428–431); the perineal wound is then completely sutured and the pelvic cavity is drained into the vagina and through the

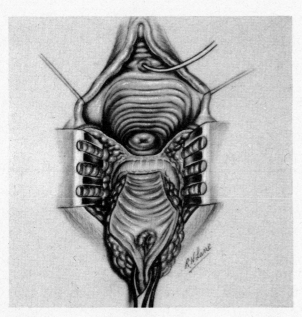

Fig. 430. State of affairs after completion of the longitudinal and transverse vaginal incisions. The rectum has still to be separated from the back of the cervix uteri.

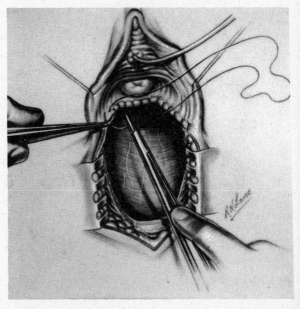

Fig. 431. After removal of the rectum, bleeding from the cut edges of the vagina is best checked by a continuous haemostatic stitch of strong catgut on a cutting needle.

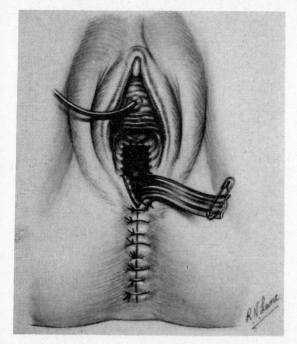

Fig. 432. Perineal wound finally sutured up to a point 2·5 cm or so behind the introitus to the vulva. Corrugated rubber drain passes through the vulva and the defect in posterior vaginal wall to reach the pelvic cavity.

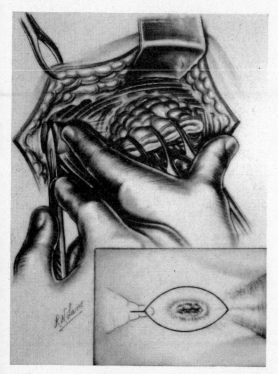

Fig. 433. Perineal dissection in Miles operation. Forward flexion and disarticulation of coccyx. *Inset:* Outline of incision.

vulva to the exterior (Fig. 432). Experience shows that this gives a very smooth convalescence and that the posterior vaginal wall rapidly regenerates, so that it is eventually almost indistinguishable from normal. I have been so impressed with the effectiveness of this method of conducting the perineal wound in the female that I now excise the posterior vaginal wall almost as a routine in operating for carcinoma of the rectum wherever situated in female patients.

THE PERINEAL DISSECTION IN THE MILES OPERATION

I prefer to have the patient lying on his left side for this phase of the Miles operation.

INCISION AND DISARTICULATION OF COCCYX

A wide elliptical incision with a posterior linear prolongation is used as in the synchronous operation. The posterior part of the wound is opened up first of all to expose the coccyx and allow of its disarticulation and excision (Fig. 433).

DIVISION OF THE ISCHIORECTAL FAT AND LEVATORES ANI, AND DELIVERY OF THE SIGMOID COLON AND UPPER RECTUM

Two fingers of the left hand are inserted into the pelvis, first deep to one levator and then to the other, whilst the overlying fat and muscles are rapidly divided with the scalpel (Fig. 434A). The fascia of Waldeyer is then incised transversely in front of the end of the sacrum and forwards on either side from this, and the clamped sigmoid end of the operative specimen is seized and drawn out through the posterior end of the wound till the sigmoid colon and upper two-thirds of the rectum have been thus delivered out of the pelvic cavity (Fig. 434B).

CONTINUATION OF ANTERIOR DISSECTION

The back of the seminal vesicles and prostate is now exposed, and the anterior dissection, which had been carried down to the apex of the prostate during the abdominal phase, is continued downwards by dividing the pubococcygei, puborectales and rectourethrales muscles from the right side and separating the anal canal from the back of the transverse perineal muscles and the urethral bulb (Fig. 435). By further dissection these muscles are severed on the left side as well. This only takes a few moments to do, and the operative specimen is then

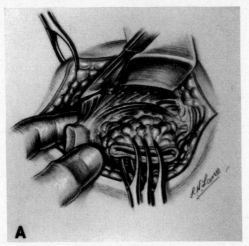

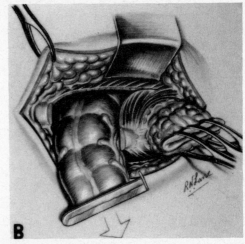

Fig. 434. (A) Finger introduced under right levator ani whilst the latter is incised. (B) After division of both levators and forward displacement of the anal canal and coccyx, the clamped upper end of the specimen is pulled out of the pelvis.

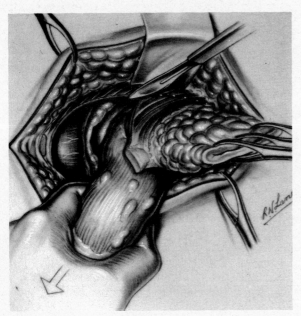

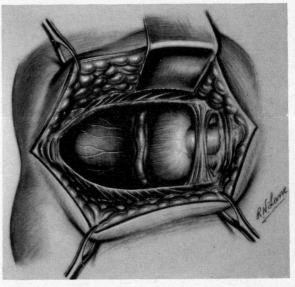

Fig. 435. The rectum is drawn strongly downwards, exposing the lower limit of the anterior plane of dissection between the rectum and prostate reached during the abdominal phase. Scalpel dissection continues this plane of separation perineal-wards, the pubococcygeus and puborectalis being divided in the process and the anal canal separated from the back of the membranous urethra and urethral bulb.

Fig. 436. Wide view obtained of the empty pelvis after removal of the rectum, showing very clearly the back of the prostate and seminal vesicles and the front of the sacrum.

completely freed (Fig. 436). Indeed the whole perineal phase in the Miles operation can be carried out with astonishing rapidity, and may take no more than four or five minutes.

HAEMOSTASIS AND SUTURE OF PERINEAL WOUND

After securing bleeding points, which is particularly easy with the patient in the lateral semi-prone position used for this operation, the wound is treated by suture and suction drainage as described on p. 557.

THE PERINEAL DISSECTION IN THE FEMALE

Here, as in the synchronous operation, the posterior vaginal wall may be preserved or, more usually, removed, and in the latter case the perineal wound is completely closed and drainage is instituted through the vulva.

Anterior Resection, Low and High

PRELIMINARY OR SIMULTANEOUS TRANSVERSE COLOSTOMY

In the earlier days of anterior resection, when the influence of Devine's (1937) teaching was still strong, it was quite unthinkable to do this operation without a *preliminary* transverse colostomy. This was placed well to the right, close to the hepatic flexure, so as to leave the left half of the abdomen and the left colon undisturbed for the subsequent resection two or three weeks later. During the interval between the two stages the colon was cleansed and sterilized by irrigations from the colostomy to the anus and *vice versa*, and by insertion into the colostomy of suppositories containing phthalylsulphathiazole.

However, as confidence was gained in the efficacy of non-absorbable sulphonamides and antibiotics in bowel preparation, a preliminary colostomy was gradually discarded except when the patient was admitted with acute or subacute obstruction. Instead, for a time *simultaneous* transverse colostomy was freely employed, the colostomy being established *at the conclusion* of the main resection operation, with the object of reducing somewhat the strain on the anastomosis. But even that came to be dispensed with usually, and simultaneous colostomy was restricted to those cases where the anastomosis had proved exceptionally difficult or the colon had been unduly loaded. In this connection an important distinction would seem to be that between *high*, usually entirely intraperitoneal, anterior resection and *low* anterior resection. Healing of the colorectal anastomosis after the former operation appears clinically uneventful as a rule (but see p. 604), and a covering colostomy is usually quite unnecessary. After the latter, however, partial breakdown is not infrequent (p. 604). Whilst it is not clear whether a proximal colostomy made at the time of the resection—and leaving a column of faeces between the colostomy, and the anastomosis—helps to prevent anastomotic dehiscence, certainly the subsequent care of patients suffering from this complication is facilitated by the presence of such an opening. For a number of years now it has been my practice to perform transverse colostomy almost as a routine at the time of all *really low* anterior resections, but I am perhaps unduly cautious in this respect for many very experienced colorectal surgeons, such as Beahrs (1975) and several of his colleagues at the Mayo Clinic, very seldom employ transverse colostomy in conjunction with low anterior resection. In making these colostomies the limbs of the loop are not 'double-barrelled', for in the subsequent closure an enterotome is not used, but instead an entirely intraperitoneal technique is employed (p. 484).

The local and general preparation of the patient for anterior resection differs in no essential respect from that employed for abdominoperineal excision, but naturally the more efficient the mechanical emptying of the colon by mild aperients and enemas and wash-outs, the more satisfactory the conditions for anastomosis. If, despite preparation, the colon is found to be very loaded at operation, the surgeon has four options—to be content simply to establish a transverse colostomy at this intervention, leaving the resection for a subsequent operation; to empty the colon on the table (see p. 440) and then proceed with the resection; to milk as much faeces as possible into the segment of bowel that is to be resected and to press on with resection; or to abandon the idea of an anterior resection and perform instead an abdominoperineal excision with terminal iliac colostomy.

TECHNIQUE OF RESECTION

It is convenient to consider either form of anterior resection as consisting of three fairly distinct phases: *the first* is concerned with the definition of the upper limits of the resection and includes ligation of the upper part of the inferior mesenteric vessels and the preparation of the colon stump; *the second* phase comprises mobilization of the rectum, division of the mesorectum and lower end of the superior haemorrhoidal vessels and preparation of the rectal stump; and *the third phase* is the actual anastomosis.

Ligation of Inferior Mesenteric Vessels and Preparation of Colon Stump for Low *and* High *Resection*
Like all the preliminary parts of the operation —namely the positioning of the patient on the table, the emptying of the bladder, and the incision and exploration of the abdomen—the steps of the dissection leading up to the exposure and division of the stem of the inferior mesenteric vessels and the

preparation of the colon stump are *absolutely identical with those of an abdominoperineal excision* as described on p. 534. Finally the colon is clamped not by Cope's clamps but by two closely applied Parker–Kerr clamps placed obliquely across the bowel, and divided between them, leaving the colon stump for use in the anastomosis controlled by the proximal clamp (Fig. 437). Many people imagine that for anterior resection a specially long piece of bowel is required in order to reach down into the pelvis. This is quite incorrect. As a rule one needs little more colon for this purpose than for establishing an ordinary left iliac colostomy in connection with an abdominoperineal excision. If, exceptionally, a greater length of bowel is needed it can be obtained either by preserving more of the sigmoid colon, nourished by the intersigmoidal marginal arcades, or preferably by dividing the peritoneum on the outer side of the descending colon and splenic flexure and mobilizing the entire left colon (see Figs 392A, B, 394).

With any of these preparations of the colon stump it is of course essential, as in abdomino-perineal excision, to satisfy oneself as to the adequacy of the blood supply to the bowel by the retention of its normal pink colour and if necessary by the occurrence of *arterial* bleeding from a divided mural artery.

Preparation of Rectal Stump *for* Low *Anterior Resection*

In this operation the freeing of the rectum from the sacrum posteriorly, and from the bladder, vesicles, and prostate or uterus and vagina anteriorly, and the definition and division of the lateral ligaments on either side are all carried out *exactly as in an abdominoperineal excision*. The result is that the rectum is completely mobilized as far as the anorectal junction.

The next step is to divide between artery forceps any obvious vessels on the wall of the rectum, especially posteriorly in the fanned out mesorectum, at the level chosen for future division of the bowel below the growth, which should be not less

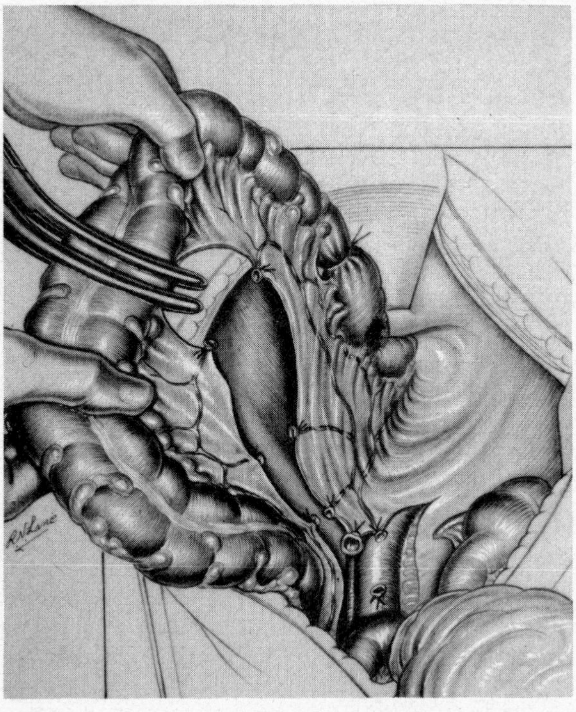

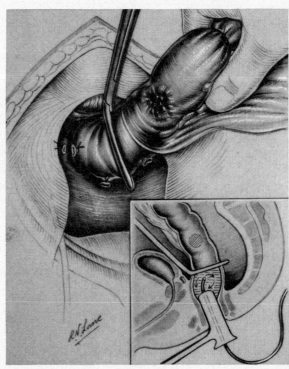

Fig. 437. Anterior resection. Inferior mesenteric vessels have been ligated and severed, the iliac mesocolon divided and the colon doubly clamped with Parker–Kerr clamps at the point chosen as the distal extremity of the colon stump for the subsequent anastomosis.

Fig. 438. Preparation of the rectal stump for low anterior resection. A slightly angled version of the Parker–Kerr intestinal clamp is applied across the bowel exactly in the sagittal plane 4–5 cm below the palpable lower edge of the primary growth. *Inset:* Subsequently a proctoscope is passed per anum to allow the rectum below the clamp to be irrigated with cetrimide and mustine solutions.

than 4–5 cm from its inferior border. These forceps are then tied off or touched with diathermy.

The bowel is now clamped 5 cm below the lower margin of the growth (there is some dispute as to how wide this margin of clearance should be and whether 5 cm is necessary, see p. 387) to prevent further faeces descending into the rectum whilst it is irrigated from below. Many surgeons employ a right-angled clamp for this purpose, but I prefer to use an ordinary curved Parker–Kerr, or a slightly angled version of this clamp (Fig. 438), applied *exactly in the anteroposterior or sagittal plane*, with its handles just above the pubis and its concavity uppermost. An assistant now passes a proctoscope per anum (Fig. 438, *inset*)—and one of the great advantages of the modified lithotomy–Trendelenburg position for anterior resection is that it facilitates this manoeuvre—and through a rubber catheter irrigates the rectum up to the clamp with 1 litre of a 1% solution of cetrimide to cleanse it thoroughly, followed by 1 litre of 1–2% nitrogen mustard in isotonic saline, for its possible cancericidal effect on any remaining exfoliated malignant cells (see p. 399). Finally, the rectal stump is swabbed dry.

The Anastomosis in Low Anterior Resection

There has been a good deal of controversy in recent years as to the relative merits of one and two layers of suture, of different suture materials and of stapling devices for this particular anastomosis as for large bowel anastomoses in general (see also p. 432). Everett's (1975) controlled trial and uncontrolled experience favoured a one-layer inverting technique for *low* anterior resection instead of the more conventional two-layer inverting method. Our controlled trial (Goligher et al. 1977*b*) suggested that in our hands a two-layer technique was safer, but the advantage over the one-layer technique was not statistically significant. Clearly the choice of suture technique—as also of different suture materials—for this operation is still an open question and both methods will therefore be here described. As for anastomosis by stapling, our experience with the SPTU or E-E-A suture gun would lead me to conclude tentatively that it provides rectal anastomoses just as secure as, or more so than, those made by hand suture, and in addition sometimes permits an anastomosis to be effected at a lower level than would be technically feasible with hand-placed sutures in a low anterior

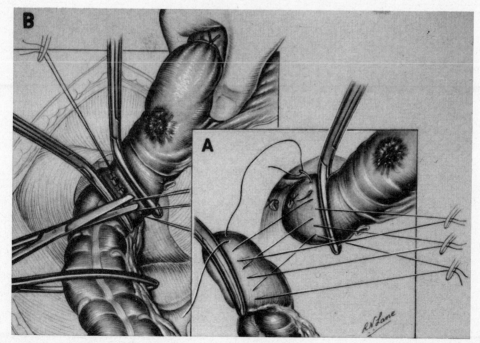

Fig. 439. The anastomosis in low anterior resection. (A) Left lateral row of Lembert sutures being inserted. Note that the colon and rectal stumps are 10 or 12·5 cm apart, with their mesenteric borders directed posteriorly, and that the sutures are placed as mattress stitches. They are left untied till all have been inserted. (B) Colon stump has been slid down on the Lembert sutures to come in contact with the rectum, and these stitches are then tied. The front and back sutures are retained as stays, the remainder being cut.

resection. Accordingly, the technique of use of these new stapling devices will also be detailed.

Two-Layer Inverting Technique. In preparation for the anastomosis the sigmoid and rectum above the Parker–Kerr clamp are drawn vertically upwards to lift the lower rectum as far as possible out of the pelvis and facilitate the insertion of sutures into it, in the same way that traction exerted on the body of the stomach is useful during gastrectomy. If it is desired to introduce a cytotoxic chemical into the colon stump, this should now be done, using the technique illustrated in Figs 322, 323, in which 20 ml of a 2% nitrogen mustard solution in saline are injected by syringe into the terminal 10 cm of bowel, isolated by application of a spring clamp. The Parker–Kerr clamp controlling the end of the colon stump is then rested on the left edge of the abdominal wound, with its mesenteric border directed posteriorly, and separated by a distance of 10 or 12·5 cm from the rectum. A series of mattress Lembert sutures of fine serum-proof silk, No. 3/0, is now inserted between the left lateral aspect of the rectum and the adjacent surface of the colon, 1 cm distant from the controlling clamps in either case, and left untied till all have been placed (Fig. 439A). The colon is then slid down on these sutures to come into apposition with the rectum, and the stitches are tied, the tails of the first and last being retained for traction, all the others being cut (Fig. 439B). The crushing clamps are now excised with a scalpel, and in the case of the rectum this means also removal of the entire operative specimen (Fig.

440A). This rectal stump is nourished only by the inferior haemorrhoidal arteries, the middle haemorrhoidals having been divided in the lateral ligaments, but bleeding from the cut upper edge of the rectum usually gives reassuring evidence of an adequate blood supply.

A continuous No. 3/0 chromic catgut suture on a fine curved Kelly atraumatic needle is what I prefer to use to unite cut edges of the colon and rectum, but it has been suggested recently by Deveney and Way (1977) on the basis of experimental work and by Clark et al. (1977) on the strength of a controlled clinical trial that polyglycolic acid should give better results. Also some surgeons favour interrupted sutures of silk or other non-absorbable material for this layer. If a continuous stitch is used it proceeds from front to back (Fig. 440B) and when the mesenteric poles are reached posteriorly it changes from a simple over-and-over stitch to a Connell or 'loop on the mucosa' stitch to give good inversion of the right lateral edges (Fig. 441A). The Connell stitch is then continued forward (Fig. 441B) eventually to reach the anterior poles of the bowel lumina.

Finally, the right lateral row of Lembert stitches is inserted. These sutures of serum-proof silk are, like the left lateral row, placed mattress-wise, for as such they secure a better grip of the longitudinally running muscle fibres of the rectum, and are actually much easier to insert in the depths of the pelvis than are simple cross stitches (Fig. 442A).

As regards *drainage* of the pelvic cavity and site of anastomosis, I have had experience with several

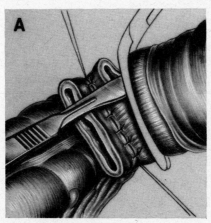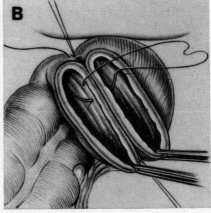

Fig. 440. The two-layer anastomosis in low anterior resection. (A) The colon stump is slid down on the Lembert sutures to come into apposition with the rectum, and the stitches are tied. The clamps are then excised, removing any crushed tissue with them. (B) The continuous through-and-through suture of 3/0 chromic catgut on a fine atraumatic Kelly needle. This commences at the anterior or antimesenteric borders of the colon and rectum.

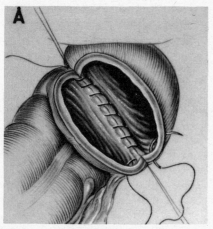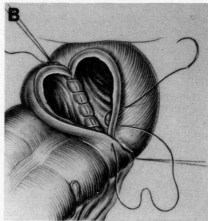

Fig. 441. The two-layer anastomosis in low anterior resection. (A) The continuous through-and-through suture. A simple over-and-over stitch is used for the left lateral edges, but this changes to a Connell or loop on the mucosa stitch at the posterior poles. (B) The Connell stitch is continued forwards on the right lateral edges.

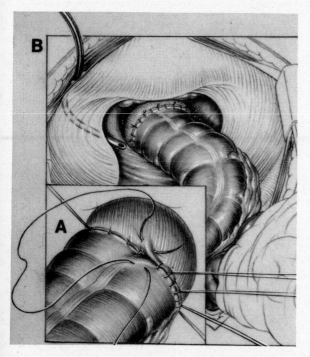

Fig. 442. The two-layer anastomosis in low anterior resection. (A) The right lateral row of mattress Lembert sutures of 3/0 silk is being inserted. (B) The completed anastomosis, with a sump suction drain placed extraperitoneally down to the anastomotic site. It is usual now for the pelvic peritoneum to be left unsutured as here.

different methods over the years. Originally a simple corrugated rubber drain or rubber tube was brought out from the region of the anastomosis, underneath the pelvic peritoneum at the side of the bladder, to emerge through the lower end of the main paramedian wound or through a separate stab wound in the left iliac fossa (Fig. 442B). Then for a while a paracoccygeal drain of rubber tubing, connected to an underwater seal or suction machine, was used instead in the hope that, aided by gravity, it would remove more effectively any effusion into the low pelvis and better protect the anastomosis from being possibly disrupted by the fluid bursting into the bowel through the suture line. I doubt if this form of drainage proved any more efficient or lessened the frequency of anastomotic dehiscence. I am glad to say that we did not have any persistent faecal fistulas through the drain wounds, as used to occur after abdominosacral resections (see p. 509). But patients found the tube in the coccygeal region for four or five days irksome. In the past few years, therefore, I have gone back to suprapubic drainage, using either a closed suction system (Zimmer or Redivac) or more recently sump drains, two or three being brought out to the iliac region. I have no experience of the combination of irrigation with saline and sump suction which is popular at the Cleveland Clinic (Fazio 1978).

There is also some difference of opinion as to *how to deal with the pelvic peritoneum* at the conclusion of the operation. It used to be the common practice to extraperitonealize the completed anastomosis by suturing the pelvic peritoneum over it. But most surgeons now leave the pelvic peritoneal flaps unsutured, with the intention of allowing the omentum and lower loops of small intestine to gravitate into the pelvis around the anastomosis, which is held by some (p. 436) to assist in the healing of the intestinal suture line and to minimize the risk of anastomotic dehiscence. I have left the pelvic peritoneum unsutured in my cases of low anterior resection in the last 3 years but have not noticed any marked difference in the incidence or severity of suture line dehiscence since doing so. A topical question at the moment is whether a pedicle graft of greater omentum should be formally prepared (see Fig. 318), for accurately wrapping round the anastomosis, but, as explained on p. 438, insufficient evidence is available at present to give a firm answer.

At the conclusion of the operation, some surgeons, such as Wangensteen (1945), like to have a stout rectal or stomach tube passed per anum by an assistant during the operation, the point being negotiated through the anastomosis by the surgeon to lie in the colon 7–10 cm above it. The tube is extracted 1 cm or so each day, and removed completely after four or five days. It is hoped thereby to decompress the large intestine and protect the suture line. Other surgeons, such as Mayo (1952), prefer simply to stretch the anal sphincters vigorously at the conclusion of the operation to paralyse them temporarily and prevent accumulation of flatus in the rectum under tension. I have used both these tactics in the past but gave them up, with no apparent alteration in the results. My present practice, moreover, of establishing a temporary transverse colostomy in most cases having low anterior resection naturally reduces their relevance.

One-Layer Inverting Technique. If a one-layer technique is being used most surgeons prefer a non-absorbable suture material—silk, linen, cotton, Ethiflex, Supramid or wire. But, for all we know, absorbable sutures of catgut or polyglycolic might do as well. I have generally employed No. 3/0 silk, slightly waxed to make it slide through the tissues more easily, and inserted as vertical mattress sutures as follows:

The Parker–Kerr clamp that controls the end of the colon stump is excised by a scalpel from the bowel leaving an open end of colon, bleeding from the cut edge being checked by diathermy coagulation as required. Then, also with a scalpel, the rectum is divided immediately below the sagittally placed Parker–Kerr clamp shown in Fig. 438, bleeding from the top edge of the rectal

remnant again being controlled by diathermy. In anastomosing these two open stumps of bowel by the one-layer technique it is easier to keep them 12–15 cm apart till the posterior two-thirds of the sutures have all been inserted ready for tying. The first suture is placed at the mesenteric poles of the two stumps (Fig. 443A, B). It is passed from the mucosal aspect of the colon 5 mm from the end of the bowel to emerge from the serosal surface. It is then inserted through the rectal wall from without inwards a similar distance from its cut edge. On its way back from the rectum the needle takes a fine bite of the rectal mucosal edge from within outwards, and of the colonic mucosal edge from without inwards (Fig. 443B). The suture is left untied, the ends being clipped with an artery forceps.

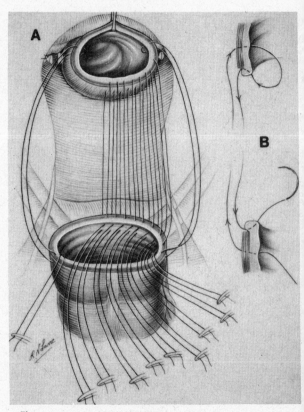

Fig. 443. The one-layer anastomosis for low anterior resection. (A) With open colon and rectal stumps separated by 12–15 cm interrupted vertical mattress sutures of 3/0 silk are placed in the posterior two-thirds of the bowel circumference: the first one in the midline posteriorly, the next two on either side one-third of the circumference from the posterior midline, and the remainder at intervals of 4 mm to fill these two gaps. (B) The exact course of the vertical mattress suture, which starts and finishes at the colonic mucosa.

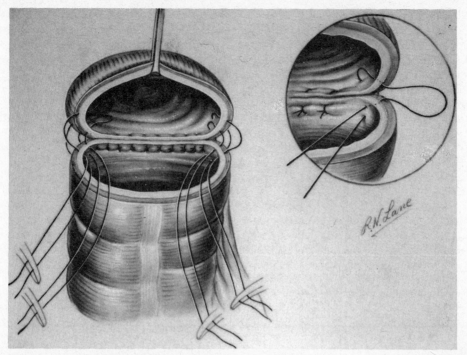

Fig. 444. The one-layer anastomosis for low anterior resection. The colonic stump has been slid down on the tautly held untied silk sutures to make contact with the rectal stump and the silks are then tied with their knots on the colonic mucosa. *Inset:* When the lateralmost sutures are tied they coapt and turn in the lateral corners very effectively.

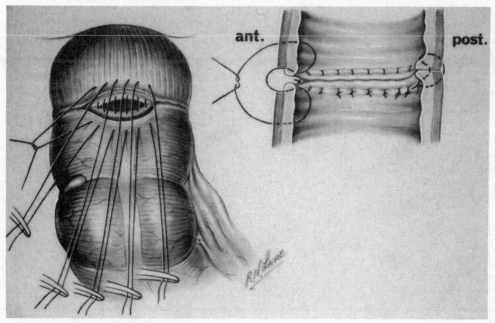

Fig. 445. The one-layer anastomosis for low anterior resection. The anterior third of the bowel circumference which remains unsutured can be closed by a small series of Gambee sutures of 3/0 silk, if the anastomosis is not too low in the pelvis for this type of stitch to be feasible. *Inset:* The course of the anterior Gambee sutures compared with that of the posterior vertical mattress stitches.

The next two sutures are placed in exactly the same way as markers on either side of the bowel, each of them one-third of the way round the circumference from the posterior midline. They are also left long and clipped with forceps. The two gaps between the marker sutures and the suture at the mesenteric poles are now filled in with a close series of other vertical mattress sutures loosely placed every 4–5 mm. Fig. 443A shows how this has been done in relation to the right posterior third. When the left posterior gap has been similarly dealt with, the colon stump is slid down on the tautly held silk strands, till the colonic and rectal stumps make contact at their posterior edges. The sutures are then tied starting in the middle posteriorly and proceeding laterally on either side (Fig. 444). As the most lateral sutures are tied they oppose and slightly inturn the two side 'corners' of bowel (Fig. 444, *inset*), leaving only a small gap in front, corresponding to about one-third of the circumference, still to be sutured. A series of vertical mattress sutures inserted from outside the bowel on the Gambee principle (see p. 432) may be employed for this remaining segment (Fig. 445), but, working in the depths of the pelvis, it may be difficult to place

these sutures in the longitudinal axis of the bowel. For a really low anastomosis it is therefore easier to use Lembert sutures of horizontal mattress type (Fig. 446). Finally the suture line is rotated slightly for inspection of the posterior aspect to see if any re-inforcing sutures are required (Fig. 447).

The disposal of the pelvic peritoneum, the possible placement of omentum and small gut around the anastomosis and the establishment of pelvic drainage are naturally as for two-layer anastomoses.

Automatic Stapling Technique. It is possible to do an end-to-end anastomosis after anterior resection with the aid of the TA stapler, using the tri-angulation technique described on p. 435, as Ferguson and Houston (1975) have done, but the use of this device for a really low anastomosis is in my view difficult. Alternatively a lateral colorectal anastomosis may be constructed using the GIA stapler, the ends of the colonic and rectal stumps being closed by the TA stapler or by hand suture (Weakley 1978) but I imagine that this method would also have limitations in regard to very low resections leaving but a tiny rectal remnant, and it certainly seems rather cumbersome, though Weakley (1978) manages very low resection with it. Undoubtedly the most convenient and promising

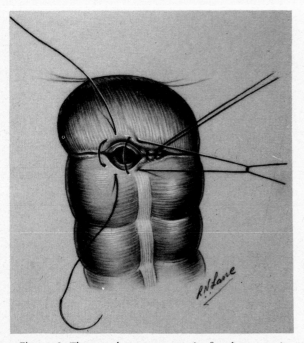

Fig. 446. The one-layer anastomosis for low anterior resection. Alternative plan of completing anterior third of anastomosis with horizontally placed Lembert sutures of 3/0 silk, which are easier to insert in the depths of the pelvis.

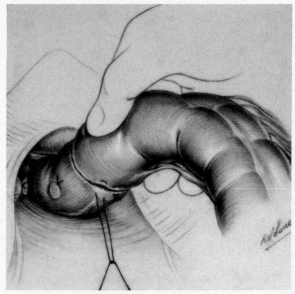

Fig. 447. The one-layer anastomosis for low anterior resection. Completed anastomosis being inspected posteriorly from outside to see if any re-inforcing sutures are required.

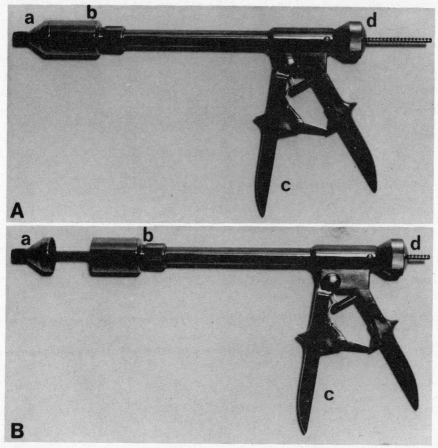

Fig. 448. The SPTU suture gun (A) in closed condition ready for introduction into the rectum through the anus, and (B) opened to separate the head (*a*) from the shoulder piece (*b*) by rotating the wheel (*d*) on the central shaft. Approximation of the two limbs of the handle of the instrument (*c*) 'fires' the staples and projects a circular knife contained within the shoulder segment. (*From Goligher et al. 1979*)

stapling instrument for low anterior resection is the SPTU style of circular suturing device (Fig. 448), which is inserted from below through the anus to the anastomotic site and achieves an *end-to-end anastomosis with inversion of all parts of the bowel circumference* (Fain et al. 1975; Goligher et al. 1978).

In general appearance the SPTU rather resembles a submachine gun, hence the somewhat irreverent description of it as the 'Russian suture gun' (Fig. 448A). The expanded portion at the tip of the 'barrel' consists of a conical shaped head with a terminal knob (*a*), resting on a shoulder segment (*b*). The head is attached to the rest of the instrument by a fine central metal shaft, which projects at the other end of the barrel and has a rotating wheel (*d*) on it, anticlockwise rotation of which causes the head to separate from the shoulder piece (Fig. 448B). When the head and shoulder

segment are thus separated and the limbs of the handle (c) of the instrument are approximated, it will be seen on close-up view (Fig. 449) that the ends of the ⊔ shaped stainless steel staples emerge from a circumferential series of slots in the rim of the shoulder segment and at the same time a circular knife or trephine is advanced from within the lumen of this segment. Normally, of course, the staples and knife are not protruded except when the instrument is 'closed', i.e. when the head and shoulderpiece are in contact, separated only by a thin layer of rectal and colonic wall. When advancement occurs under these circumstances the two ends of each staple transfix the tissues and strike a corresponding shallow groove in the base of the head, the impact forcing them towards one another and then backwards to convert the ⊔ into a capital ⌒⌒ lying on its side. It is claimed that the

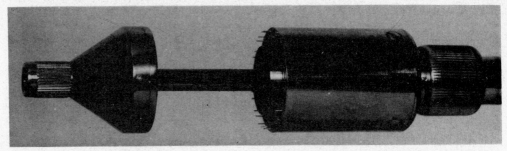

Fig. 449. Close-up view of the head and shoulder segment when the instrument is opened-up, showing the central metal shaft on which the head is mounted. By slightly compressing the limbs of the handle the metal staples and circular knife have been partially projected from the shoulder-piece. (*From Goligher et al. 1979*)

closed staples do not sufficiently compress the tissues to prevent blood proceeding along fine vessels through the holes of the ⌒⌒. In the original Russian instrument, here illustrated, the staples, which are 5·5 mm long, have to be inserted individually into the slots in the shoulderpiece by hand and special forceps each time before use, which takes about 5–7 minutes to do. (In a version of the instrument made under patent rights in America by the USS Corporation there is a double circumferential row of staples and they are loaded in a disposable shoulderpiece and head, which is quickly and simply clipped in position but these disposable parts are quite expensive.) The SPTU gun can be separated into its various parts for purposes of cleaning. It is sterilized by autoclaving. Four sizes of head and shoulder-piece, of diameters of 21, 26, 29 and 32 mm respectively, are provided with each instrument for use according to the calibre of the bowel being anastomosed.

The first practical point when considering the use of the SPTU device is that in order to be able to introduce the instrument conveniently through the anus from below during the course of the resection, *it is essential that the patient should have been put up in the modified lithotomy–Trendelenburg position* for the operation. When the excision of the segment of bowel containing the growth has been completed leaving an open colonic and open rectal stump (as described above in connection with the one layer technique of hand suture for low anterior resection) bleeding from the cut edges of these stumps being controlled by diathermy coagulation as required, the next step is to place purse-string sutures round the ends of both stumps. The importance of accurate insertion of these two sutures for the success of this method of anastomosis cannot be too strongly emphasized. The stitch commences at the antimesenteric border, being passed from the

outside to inside 3–4 mm from the cut edge. In the case of the rather thicker-walled rectal stump it need not necessarily include the muscle coat but should take a good bite of the mucosa and submucosa. Having entered the lumen it is passed immediately out again through the left lateral wall again and is continued circumferentially round the bowel as a series of bites at intervals of 4 mm and passed in the same direction from within outwards, each of them 3–4 mm from the cut edge, till the anterior pole is again reached (Fig. 450). The two ends of the suture are then temporarily clipped with artery forceps. (When the stitch is in due course tied

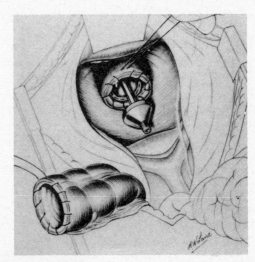

Fig. 450. Introduction of the SPTU gun into the pelvis from below through the anus and anorectal stump remaining after anterior resection for rectal cancer. Note that purse-string sutures of 2/0 monofilament prolene have been inserted along the cut edges of the rectal and colonic stumps. The head of the instrument has been separated from the shoulder-piece. (*From Goligher et al. 1979*)

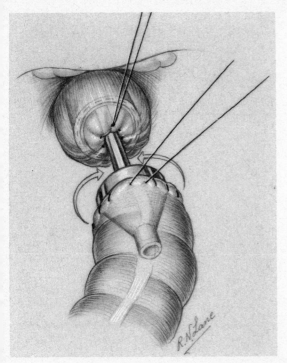

Fig. 451. The purse-string suture in the top of the anorectal remnant has been tied to the central metal shaft just above the shoulder-piece. The colonic stump is in the process of being fitted on to the head of the gun (*From Goligher et al. 1979*)

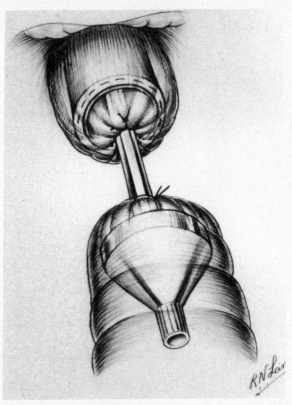

Fig. 452. The purse-string suture in the end of the colonic stump has also been tied to the metal shaft, preparatory to closing the gun. (*From Goligher et al. 1979*)

on the central shaft of the suture gun all parts of the cut edge of bowel are securely held against the shaft, but the mucosa is inverted into the lumen of the bowel and very little tissue projects beyond the stitch to make a bulky swelling which the circular knife might have difficulty in enclosing.) We find that the best suture material for the purse-string sutures is 3/o monofilament Prolene on an atraumatic needle, because it slides easily through the tissues and readily puckers them up when the knot is tied.

Next an appropriate size of head and shoulder-piece is chosen depending on the calibre of the bowel—particularly of the colon stump. (The size that we have found most generally useful has been the 29 mm.) It is fitted to the instrument, loaded with staples and the head and shoulder-piece are then firmly approximated. After lubrication the tip of the barrel is introduced by an assistant from below into the anal canal and anorectal remnant. When the knob on the head starts to emerge at the top of the rectal stump, the wheel on the shaft is rotated to separate the head 4–5 cm from the shoulder-piece (Fig. 450). The surgeon then ties the rectal purse-string suture on the central shaft

immediately above the shoulder-piece and starts to slide the colon stump over the head of the gun (Fig. 451). When the colonic purse-string suture has also been tied on the shaft (Fig. 452), the wheel is rotated to bring the head and shoulder segment together, separated only by the compressed tissues of the rectal and colonic 'hoods' (Fig. 453). The wheel should be rotated sufficiently to narrow the gap between the head and shoulder-piece to between 1 and 2 mm. The next step is for the assistant to 'fire' the gun by a sudden strong compression of the limbs of the handle. The effect of this move is indicated diagrammatically in Fig. 454A. Finally the wheel is rotated anticlockwise to separate slightly the head and shoulder-piece and allow the flange of stapled tissue to be released from the grip of the gun, and, whilst the surgeon holds the anastomosis in his hand, the instrument is extricated from the bowel by a combination of rotation and gentle traction. Though this manoeuvre often seems somewhat traumatic to the anastomosis, no harm appears to result as a rule. If desired a few Lembert sutures of silk can be inserted to reinforce the anastomosis,

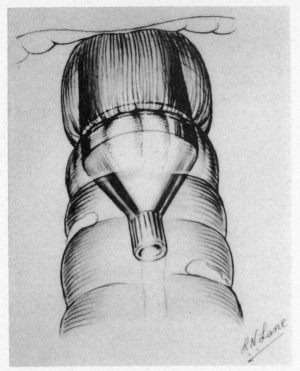

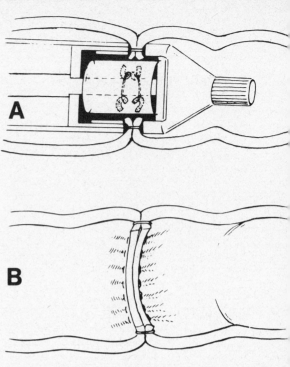

Fig. 453. By rotating the controlling wheel the head and shoulder-piece of the gun are now approximated, compressing the tissues of the colonic and rectal stumps firmly between them. The gap remaining between the head and shoulder-piece to accommodate these tissues varies depending on the thickness of the intestinal walls, but is usually not more than 0·5 mm. (*From Goligher et al. 1979*)

Fig. 454. (A) The next step is to 'fire' the metal staples into the contiguous rectal and colonic walls by approximating the limbs of the handle of the instrument, which at the same time advances the circular knife to cut the bowel free from the central metal shaft as shown here diagrammatically. (B) State of affairs when the gun has subsequently been extracted. (*From Goligher 1979*)

but we have seldom done so. The final state after removal of the gun is shown diagrammatically in Fig. 454B.

The pelvic peritoneum is left unsutured and the pelvic cavity is drained by at least two sump suction drains as after the other form of anastomosis.

The appearance of the staples two weeks after operation on a Gastrografin enema study is shown in Fig. 455A, B, and the fact that an exceptionally low anastomosis after anterior resection can be made with the suture gun is convincingly demonstrated by Fig. 455C. The staple line in this latter case lay 4·5 cm from the anal verge on sigmoidoscopy, and we have a number of other patients with equally low anastomoses by this technique (Goligher et al. 1978). It is also possible to place the purse-string suture in the top of a very low anorectal stump not from above but from below through a trivalve anal speculum (see p. 583), and to obtain even lower anastomoses. This alternative technique is helpful particularly in obese or solidly built male patients and in effect amounts to doing an abdomino-

transanal resection using a suture gun instead of placing sutures by hand.

Preparation of Rectal Stump for High *Anterior Resection*

If the carcinoma is situated in the rectosigmoid region 7–10 cm above the peritoneal reflection it is not necessary to mobilize the rectum on all aspects down to the anorectal ring. The cuts on either side of the mesorectum are not extended round the brim of the pelvis but instead run to the back of the rectum 5 cm below the growth (Figs 456, 457). The superior rectal vessels can then be divided at this level (Fig. 457, *inset*), leaving a rectal stump which projects up to 5 cm above the peritoneal reflection and has a surrounding cuff of peritoneum. One sometimes passes a hand down between the rectum and the sacrum to mobilize the rectum somewhat posteriorly, but the lateral ligaments are not divided and there is no anterior dissection. A Parker–Kerr clamp or angled clamp is then placed across the bowel in the anteroposterior plane just above the intended site of section (Fig. 458). The rectum is irrigated from below through the anus with cetrimide and nitrogen mustard, as indicated.

The Anastomosis in High Anterior Resection

The anastomosis of the colon to the rectal stump in high anterior resection follows the same lines as those outlined for low resections. Any one of the three techniques there described may be used also for high anterior resection except that the higher the anastomosis in the rectum the more difficult it is to employ the SPTU suture gun introduced through the anus. It can of course be passed from above, through a cut in the colon stump which is later sutured, but this seems more trouble than it is worth. The completed union is depicted in Fig. 459. I usually leave a corrugated rubber drain or sump suction drain down to the anastomosis through the peritoneal cavity, the other end being brought out through the lower extremity of the main paramedian wound or through a separate stab wound in the left iliac region.

Abdomino-Anal Pull Through Excision (Turnbull–Cutait Technique)

FIRST STAGE

This operation is most conveniently performed with the patient in the lithotomy–Trendelenburg position used for the synchronous combined excision (Fig. 378A, B). The abdominal phase follows the lines of a low anterior resection except that a much longer colon stump is required and, if a high ligation of the inferior mesenteric vessels is practised, it will be necessary to mobilize the splenic flexure as indicated in Fig. 394, in order to obtain enough bowel to extend some 12–15 cm through the anus. For this reason the abdominal incision should extend almost up to the left costal margin. In gauging where to clamp and divide the mobilized bowel in preparing the colon stump, a rough guide is to lift the sigmoid and descending colon out of the wound and draw them downwards in front of the pubis. If the moderately taut bowel is then divided between Cope's clamps 5 *cm beyond the pubic crest*—which will usually correspond to a point on the lower descending colon—a proximal stump of sufficient length for a pull-through excision will be obtained. Needless to add, it is essential to verify that the blood supply to the bowel is adequate by observing closely its colour and the state of the mural vessels at its lower end.

The rectum is freed down to the anorectal junction as in low anterior resection, but the upper surface of the levator muscles and the angle between them and the lower rectum are even more carefully defined, as in the Roscoe Graham operation for rectal prolapse (Fig. 174). An angled clamp is then applied to the bowel in the sagittal plane 5 cm below the growth, which, with lesions at the levels normally accepted for pull-through excision, will mean that it lies just above the top of the anal canal—that is about 4–5 cm above the anal verge. The small anorectal stump can now be irrigated with cetrimide followed by nitrogen mustard solution, if desired.

Insertion of Stay Sutures and Division of Rectum. After the irrigation has been completed, two stay sutures of silk are inserted into the rectal stump in front and behind, and the bowel is divided between the sutures and the clamp, removing the operative specimen and leaving a very small remnant of rectum low in the pelvis (Fig. 460A).

Eversion of Anorectal Stump and Stretching of Sphincters. A scrubbed-up assistant towels the perineal region and passes a long pair of sponge-holding forceps through the anal canal into the pelvis. The stay sutures on the rectum are fed to these forceps and carried down through the anus as the forceps are withdrawn (Fig. 460B). In some cases with a rather longer anorectal stump, traction on these sutures may suffice to draw the cut edge of rectum easily through the anus, where it can be grasped by fine tissue forceps. With the more usual length of stump the process of eversion has to be assisted by a certain amount of finger dissection (Fig. 460C). Finally, with the anal canal partially or completely everted, the sphincters are subjected to steady, firm stretching with four fingers for four minutes (Fig. 460D) to produce a relaxed opening through which the colon may subsequently be drawn without risk of injurious constriction.

Pulling the Colon through the Anus. The Cope's clamp on the end of the colon stump is now passed through the everted anorectal remnant to the perineal operator, who then draws the colon down till it is just taut, care being taken to avoid axial rotation in the process. If the length of the colon stump was correctly judged at the abdominal phase of the dissection, the colon should now project about 10–12·5 cm beyond the cut edge of the rectum. A series of very fine interrupted catgut sutures is passed between the end of the rectum and the serosa of the colon (Fig. 460E). Finally, the Cope's clamp is removed and a wide de Pezzer catheter, with part of its expanded portion cut off, is inserted into the end of the colon and tied in

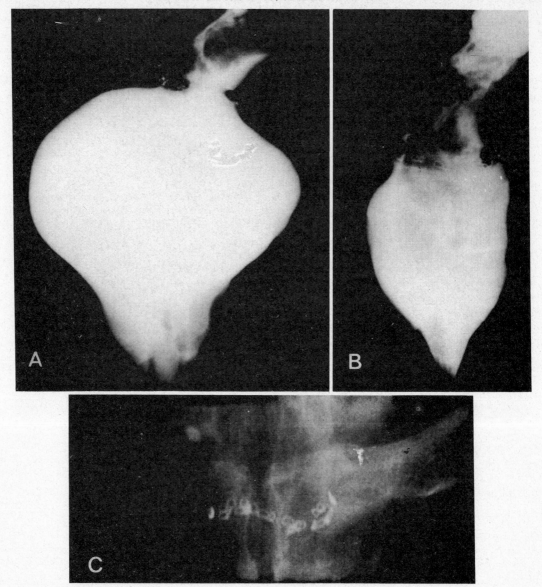

Fig. 455. (A, B) Radiographs taken after Gastrographin enemas given 14 days after low anterior resection using the SPTU suture gun. (C) Plain X-ray some months after low anterior resection using the SPTU device, showing the ring of staples. (*From Goligher et al. 1979*)

position with a strong silk ligature. Dressings are applied to the projecting stumps and the drain site.

Establishment of a Temporary Transverse Colostomy. Though this operation was designed to be done without a covering colostomy, my experience suggests that it is a wise precaution to establish a loop colostomy in the right transverse at the time of the resection in order to diminish faecal loading of the colon stump, which might predispose to necrosis in

the postoperative period. This is currently also Turnbull's (1975) practice.

Institution of Pelvic Drainage and Closure of Abdomen. The final step before closing the abdomen is to institute drainage of the pelvic cavity. As explained in connection with anterior resection (p. 566), this may be effected in various ways, but is probably best accomplished by two or three sump suction drains, introduced through stab incisions in either

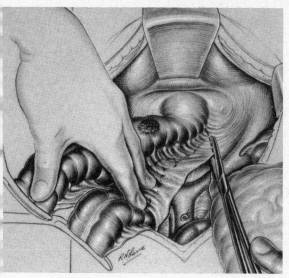

Fig. 456. Preparation of rectal stump in *high* anterior resection. Peritoneum is not divided round the pelvic brim, but instead cuts are made in the peritoneal leaves of the mesorectum up to the bowel. Here the right leaf is being divided with scissors.

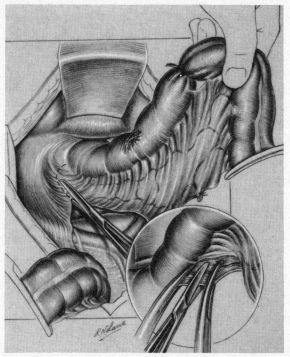

Fig. 457. Preparation of rectal stump in *high* anterior resection. Division of left leaf of mesorectum by curved scissors cut. *Inset:* The superior haemorrhoidal vessels in the mesorectum have now been doubly clamped and are being divided.

iliac fossa and taken to the pelvis extraperitoneally alongside the bladder. The pelvic peritoneum is probably preferably left unsutured, allowing the greater omentum and coils of small intestine to fall down into the pelvis. The abdominal wound is then closed in the usual way.

SECOND STAGE

This is performed 10–14 days after the first stage, if the convalescence from the latter has been uncomplicated. It consists simply of an amputation through the extreme edge of the anorectal stump and the underlying colon (Fig. 461A). Quite sharp bleeding ensues, particularly on the side of the mesocolon, and usually requires two or three catgut stitches to control it. Thereafter the freshly cut edges of rectum and colon are united by a circumferential series of fine chromic catgut or silk sutures (Fig. 461B). In some cases the sutured stumps slip back through the anus as soon as the tails of the sutures are cut. In other cases they remain projecting and only gradually recede over a period of several days. Occasionally, when the anorectal stump has been exceptionally long, it may be necessary eventually to reduce the protrusion under another short general anaesthetic. The final low colorectal anastomosis, lying in the pelvis, is shown in Fig. 461C.

The transverse colostomy may conveniently be closed at the second stage, thus avoiding any further operative intervention.

Abdominotransanal Resection with Sutured Coloanal or Colorectal Sleeve Anastomosis (Parks' Technique)

For this operation also the patient should be in the lithotomy–Trendelenburg position which provides ideal conditions for the abdominal and anal phases, either consecutively or to some extent simultaneously as desired. Indeed it would be very difficult, if not impossible, to practice this technique except in this position.

ABDOMINAL DISSECTION AND RESECTION OF BOWEL

This phase is identical with that of the abdominoanal pull-through resection (see p. 574) up to the

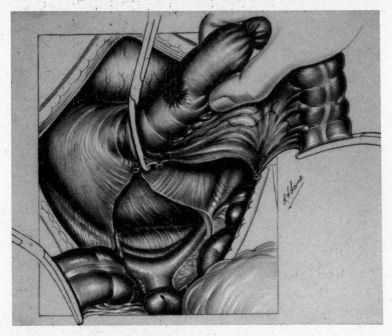

Fig. 458. Preparation of rectal stump in *high* anterior resection. The superior haemorrhoidal vessels have been divided and tied, and the bowel is being severed between two angled crushing clamps applied in the sagittal plane.

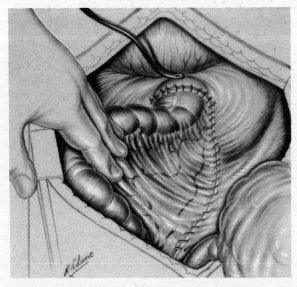

Fig. 459. Completed *high* anterior resection, showing the colon united to a rectal stump which projects about 2·5–4 cm above the peritoneal reflection anteriorly.

point where the actual resection of the segment of bowel containing the carcinoma is completed by clamping the rectum by a sagittally placed angled Parker–Kerr clamp 4 to 5 cm below the lesion and

(after irrigation per anum with cetrimide and nitrogen mustard solutions) the bowel is divided with a scalpel from before backwards immediately below the clamp. Bleeding from the cut upper edge of the piece of rectum being left is controlled with diathermy coagulation as the rectal division proceeds cautiously from front to back (Fig. 462). Note that no stay sutures have been inserted in the upper end of the anorectal stump. A moist pack is now placed in the pelvis whilst attention is turned to the anal region for preparation of the anorectal remnant from below for the coloanal anastomosis.

PREPARATION OF ANORECTAL REMNANT FOR ANASTOMOSIS

A bivalve anal speculum (Fig. 38) is placed in the anal canal and opened to its maximum extent, a third blade also being inserted to increase the exposure. (A useful alternative, at any rate for some stages of the preparation and subsequent coloanal anastomosis, is a Sims vaginal speculum.) Through this speculum it is possible to get a complete view of one wall of the anorectal remnant at a time up to its cut upper edge; in Fig. 463 it is the posterior sector that is thus exposed. An injection of saline with 1 in 200 000 adrenaline is now made into the submucosa to balloon it up and 'float' the entire

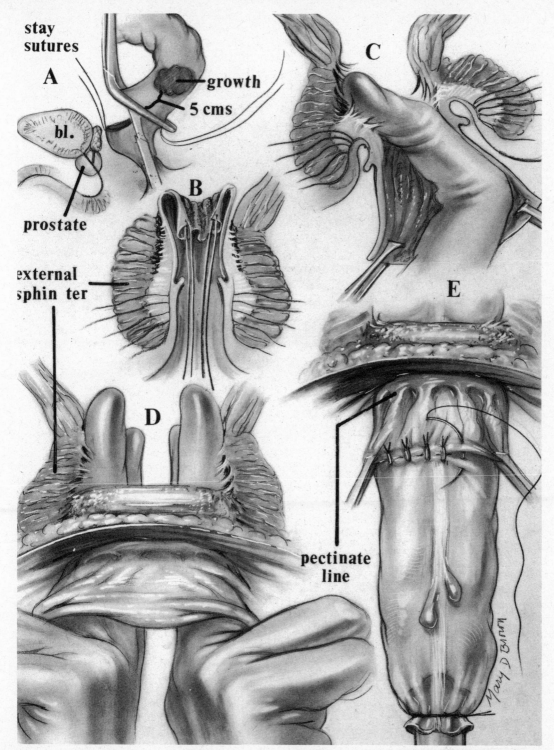

Fig. 460. Turnbull–Cutait pull-through abdominoanal excision, *first stage*. (A) The mobilized rectum has been clamped with an angled clamp and is being divided below it. Note the stay sutures in the anorectal remnant. (B) Anorectal remnant being everted by drawing stay sutures through the anus. (C) Assisting the process of eversion with finger dissection. (D) Stretching the anal sphincters. (E) Colon stump drawn through and cut edge of everted rectal remnant being lightly sutured to it.

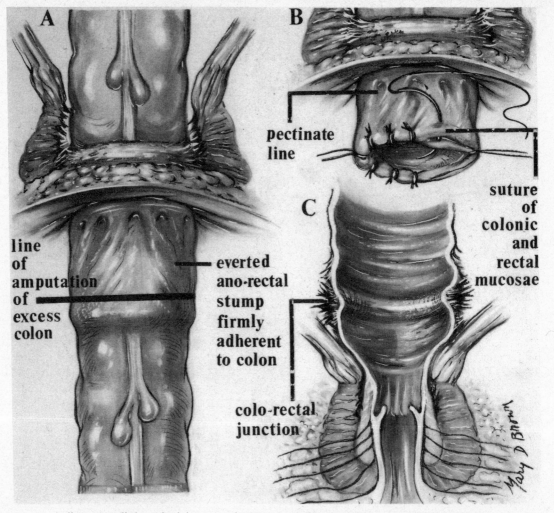

Fig. 461. Turnbull–Cutait pull-through abdominoanal excision, *second stage*. (A) Line of amputation of stumps. (B) Suture of freshly cut edges of stumps. (C) Final state on return of sutured stumps to pelvis.

exposed mucosa off the underlying internal anal sphincter and circular muscle coat of the remaining fringe of rectum. Using Metzenbaum's scissors (with sharp points and slightly curved on the flat), a cut is made in the mucosa about 1 cm above the pectinate line (Fig. 464). Working upwards in the artificially oedematous submucosa a broad strip of mucosa with some submucosa is dissected off the muscle coat up to the top of the anorectal remnant (Fig. 465). The trivalve speculum is now rotated round to expose the right lateral wall, the anterior wall and the left lateral wall in succession, and the same procedure of submucous infiltration with saline and adrenaline and mucosal excision is carried out on each in turn, till finally the anorectal remnant has been completely circumferentially denuded of its

lining from 1 cm above the pectinate line to its cut upper edge. It is important to re-survey all parts of the interior of the remnant to make sure no strands of mucosa remain and to complete haemostasis by further diathermy coagulation as required. A gauze swab is tucked in the anal canal and the anal speculum is removed.

FINAL PREPARATION OF THE COLON STUMP

The colon stump, prepared as described on p. 575 to ensure that it would be of sufficient length to extend to the anal region whilst leaving a considerable 'slack' in the pelvis, has till now been controlled by a Cope's clamp or other form of crushing clamp. During the time taken to prepare the

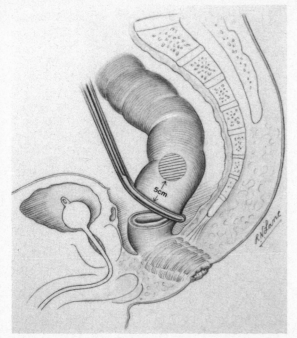

Fig. 462. Abdominotransanal resection. From the abdominal aspect the rectum is clamped with an angled Parker–Kerr clamp in the sagittal plane a short distance above the top of the anal canal and 4–5 cm below the growth. The bowel is then divided from before backwards with a scalpel just below the clamp, bleeding from the distal cut edge being checked by diathermy coagulation.

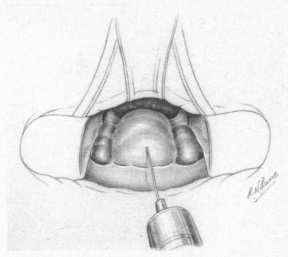

Fig. 463. Abdominotransanal resection. A trivalve anal retractor has been placed in the anal canal and opened up to display the posterior wall up to the top of the anorectal remnant. A weak adrenaline solution is being injected into the submucosa.

anorectal remnant, a fair amount of faeces often accumulates in the colon above this clamp. Accordingly when the clamp is removed—preferably by excision with the scalpel to sacrifice any crushed tissue between the blades of the clamp, followed by light coagulation of any bleeding points in the cut edge—an important consideration is to remove these faeces by a suction tube inserted as far as possible into the colon stump or by milking them out into a kidney dish. Having thoroughly emptied the colon stump in this way, it is now ready to be passed down to the pelvis for the anastomosis. There are several ways of delivering it to the anal region. One is to close the open end of bowel with a temporary running suture of catgut or silk, the tails of which are left long to be passed down to the anal operator for traction (the suture subsequently being removed just before the anastomosis commences). An alternative plan, which is what I personally prefer, is to leave the end of the colon open and simply to insert a couple of long silk stay sutures in the cut edge at the mesenteric and antimesenteric borders respectively. The ends of these sutures are

then delivered through the anus for traction from below.

THE PERANAL COLOANORECTAL ANASTOMOSIS

The gauze swab in the anus is removed, the bivalve anal speculum re-introduced and opened up, and the third blade fitted. A long curved artery forceps or sponge-holding forceps is passed up through the anal canal into the upper pelvis and opened to receive the ends of the stay sutures attached to the colon stump which are caught and drawn down to the anal region. As further traction is exerted on these sutures, the abdominal operator or assistant at the abdominal end guides the colon stump down into the pelvis with his hand to make sure that it does not get rotated or caught on any prominence of tissue. Gradually the open end of the colon stump appears in lumen of the anal canal *within the three blades of the anal speculum*. The existing two stay sutures are supplemented by two more in the lateral quadrants to display clearly all parts of the cut edge of colon preparatory to commencing the anastomosis (Fig. 466).

At this point Parks (1977a) likes to place in each of the four quadrants a suture of Dexon or silk between the exposed muscle coat of the upper part of the anorectal remnant and the serosal surface of the colon stump 4 or 5 cm above its cut lower end. But the access for inserting these stitches is often very poor and I have usually abandoned the

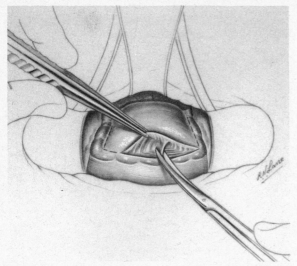

Fig. 464. Abdominotransanal resection. Using Metzenbaum's sharp-pointed slightly curved scissors the mucosa is being dissected off the muscle coat.

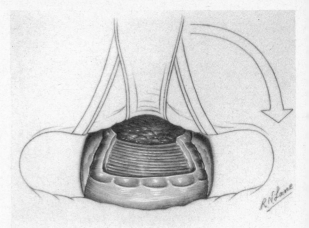

Fig. 465. Abdominotransanal resection. The mucosal excision has been completed on the posterior wall. The retractor is now rotated to display in turn the right lateral, anterior, and left lateral walls for similar treatment.

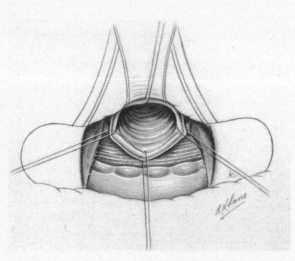

Fig. 466. Abdominotransanal resection. Whilst the anal retractor stretches the anorectal remnant, the colon stump is drawn down into the denuded anal canal *inside the blades of the retractor*.

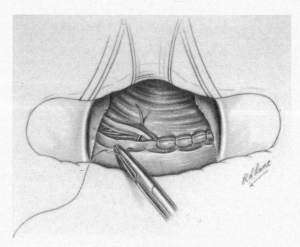

Fig. 467. Abdominotransanal resection. The cut end of the colon stump is sutured to the anal mucosal edge just above the pectinate line with interrupted 2/o Dexon sutures, some of the internal sphincter being included in the bite of each stitch.

attempt to secure this approximation from below. (Instead, at the completion of the anastomosis I have sutured the cut upper edge of the anorectal remnant to the outer aspect of the colon stump as it passes through the remnant, but this is also technically quite a difficult manoeuvre.)

In suturing the cut end of the colon stump to the anal canal deep sutures of No. 1/o or 2/o Dexon or chromic catgut are used, being passed through the remnant of anal mucosa above the pectinate line *and the internal sphincter* before transfixing the colon wall. Three or four such stitches are inserted and tied in the posterior sector with the anal retractor in position as shown in Fig. 467. Then, after removing the third blade of the retractor but keeping the other two blades as they are, a further three or four similar stitches can be placed in the anterior sector. Now the bivalve speculum is removed and reintroduced in a different axis, with its blades lying not laterally but *anteriorly and posteriorly* and with their upper ends not outside the colon stump but *within the colonic lumen*. This exposes the two lateral sectors for coloanal suture. The insertion of a complete circumferential row of sutures in this way can be difficult at times, but, with rotation of the anal speculum and periodic palpation of the suture line to detect any obvious defects in the suture line, a satisfactory anastomosis can normally be achieved (Fig. 468).

COMPLETION OF ABDOMINAL PHASE

If suture of the upper part of the anorectal remnant to the serosal aspect of the colon stump from below was not possible, an attempt is now made to approximate the cut upper edge of the remnant to the outer aspect of the emerging colon with a few sutures of No. 3/0 silk (Fig. 468).

It is probably wise to close the gap between the long colon stump and the posterior abdominal wall especially in its upper part, to prevent the loops of small intestine (temporarily contained in a plastic Lahey bag during the operation, as shown in Fig. 468) from being subsequently obstructed in it. An attempt should therefore be made to suture the cut edge of the mesocolon to the peritoneum and other tissues of the abdominal wall as available by a running stitch of No. 3/0 chromic catgut, starting above and extending downwards as far as possible.

As with low anterior resection and abdomino-anal pull-through resection a covering loop transverse colostomy is established at the conclusion of this operation.

The pelvic peritoneum is left unsutured and the loops of small gut, released from the Lahey bag, are tumbled down into the pelvis along with any available pendulous portion of the greater omentum. (Whether a pedicle graft of omentum should be formally prepared, as described on p. 438, for wrapping more accurately round the anastomotic area, is more debatable.) Finally two sump suction drains are left down to the pelvis from separate stab wounds in the iliac fossa and the laparotomy wound is closed.

Use of SPTU or EEA Stapling Devices for the Coloanal Anastomosis. Recently I have used the SPTU suture

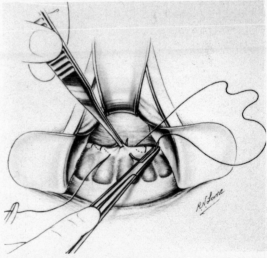

Fig. 469. The view obtained of the interior or the anorectal remnant with the anal speculum in position. The 2/0 monofilament Prolene suture has been inserted along the top of the remnant, starting in the midline posteriorly and continuing as an over-and-over stitch from inside the lumen 4 mm or so from the cut edge, the retractor having been rotated to expose each sector of the bowel in turn. The stitch has reached the posterior sector again and is approaching the starting point. (*From Goligher 1979b*)

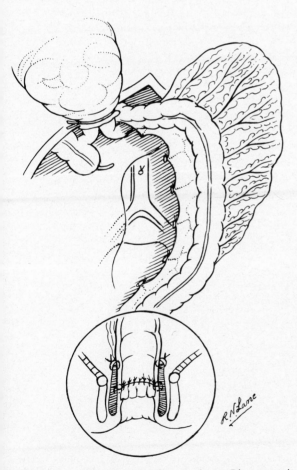

Fig. 468. Abdominotransanal resection. Diagrammatic representation of completed coloanal anastomosis.

gun for effecting the anastomosis in three cases with very satisfactory results (Goligher 1979a, b). The technique of using the gun is as described on p. 570, except that the purse-string suture of 3/0 monofilament Prolene in the top of the small anorectal remnant is inserted not from above in the depths of the pelvis but from below through a trivalve anal speculum as shown in Fig. 469. This step is certainly easier than placing sutures between the end of the colon stump and the anorectum through the anal canal. The opened gun is then introduced till its head is above the top of the anorectal remnant and the purse-string suture in the latter is tied on the central shaft of the instrument from below (Fig. 470). Alternatively, and perhaps preferably, before the gun is inserted the tails of the purse-string suture are passed up through the anal canal to the abdominal operator. The gun is then introduced from below and opened, and the abdominal operator ties the purse-string suture on the shaft (Fig. 471). Thereafter the colon stump is slipped over the head of the gun from above and its purse-string suture tied (Fig. 472). Then the head and shoulder segment are approximated in the usual way and the gun 'fired'. The resulting anastomosis, after extraction of the gun, usually lies about 3·5 cm from the anal verge (Fig. 473). The use of this stapling device for the anastomosis makes the operation of abdominotransanal resection very much easier and is now my preferred method for doing this operation.

Abdominosacral Resection

POSITION OF THE PATIENT

In the classical method of performing this operation the patient is placed in an ordinary supine position with a Trendelenburg tilt for the abdominal phase and is then turned on to his right (or left) side and slightly prone for the sacral phase. But Localio and Stahl (1969) have developed a technique for doing both phases with the patient in the same position throughout—namely on his right side with the left shoulder and upper chest slightly thrown backwards and using an oblique incision for the abdominal dissection (Fig. 474). There are certainly some advantages in having the abdominal and sacral wounds both open at the same time. For one thing it facilitates the passage of the mobilized colon out of the sacral wound if the sigmoid loop can be guided down into the pelvis to the sacral wound by the abdominal operator rather than the latter having to pluck the colon out of the pelvic cavity through a relatively small posterior wound. For another, if a sphincter-saving resection proves impossible it is a simple matter to proceed with a Miles type of operation, whereas, if the abdomen has

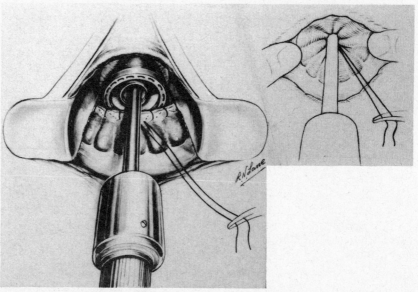

Fig. 470. The third blade of the anal retractor has been removed and the separation of the other two blades reduced somewhat, whilst the head end of the suture gun is inserted through the anal canal to beyond the top of the anorectal remnant. *Inset:* The anal retractor has been removed and the anorectal purse-string suture has been tied from below on the central shaft. (*From Goligher 1979b*)

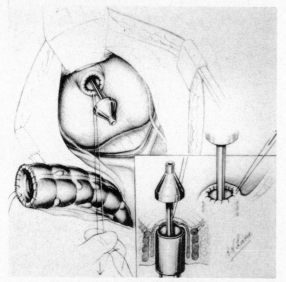

Fig. 471. An alternative method of tying the purse-string suture from above. The tails of the suture have been passed up through the anal canal to the abdominal operator. Whilst the bladder and prostate are retracted strongly forwards to expose the top of the anorectal remnant held up by the purse-string suture, the suture gun is inserted from below by an assistant and opened to carry the head into the pelvis beyond the edge of the anorectal stump, whilst the distal edge of the shoulder-piece still lies in the remnant. *Inset:* The purse-string suture is then tied on the central shaft just above the shoulder-piece. (*From Goligher 1979b*)

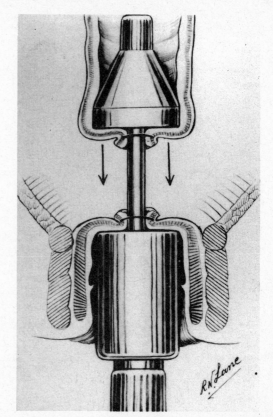

Fig. 472. The 'opened' suture gun in position with the purse-string suture in both anorectal and colonic stumps tied and the instrument about to be 'closed' preparatory to 'firing' the staples. (*From Goligher 1979b*)

already been closed and the patient been turned on his side before this decision is reached, it means re-opening the abdomen (and usually undoing a transverse colostomy) before this alternative procedure can be performed. The only argument against the Localio method is that most surgeons are accustomed to a vertical incision and a supine position of the patient for the abdominal dissection for rectal excision and to standing on the left side of the patient for this part of the operation, and are a little reluctant to train themselves to doing this dissection with the patient on his side and working through an oblique incision whilst standing or sitting on the right side. In the following account of the operation the patient is in the supine position for the abdominal phase and in the right lateral position for the sacral phase.

It should be emphasized that unfortunately *abdominosacral resection cannot be conveniently performed in the lithotomy–Trendelenburg position*.

ABDOMINAL PHASE

With the patient in a supine position and moderately head-down tilted the abdomen is

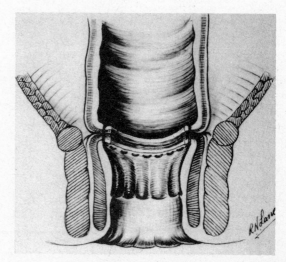

Fig. 473. The stapled anastomosis at or just above the anorectal ring after withdrawal of the gun. (*From Goligher 1979b*)

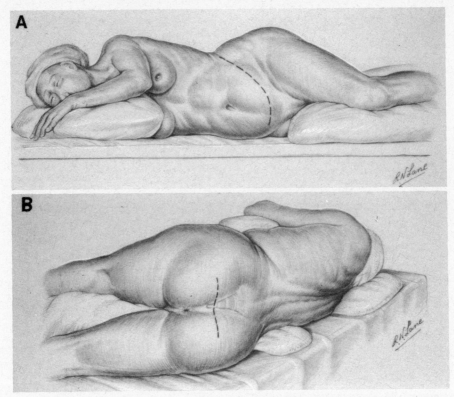

Fig. 474. Abdominosacral resection. The right lateral position used by Localio for both phases of this operation. (A) Access to the abdomen in this synchrous combined abdominosacral technique is provided by a long oblique muscle-cutting incision extending from the suprapubic region to the left loin, which gives very good exposure, particularly of the splenic flexure. (B) The sacral approach: note that the left shoulder and upper chest are thrown slightly backwards. A transverse incision at the sacrococcygeal junction is used for this phase.

opened through a long left paramedian incision. If the lesion is operable and deemed suitable for resection, the dissection proceeds as already described for low anterior resection (p. 563) or for abdominoanal pull-through incision (p. 574) or abdominotransanal resection (p. 577) up to the completion of mobilization of the left colon, sigmoid and rectum down to the anorectal junction. The splenic flexure usually needs to be freed to mobilize a long enough colon stump to extend to the low pelvis. A suitable length of colon stump is one that is found to reach to 5 cm or so beyond the pubes (Fig. 475). The distal end of this intended stump is marked by tying a piece of gauze to it with a stout silk ligature. A loop of intact colon with this ligature and gauze at its summit is tucked deeply into the pelvis behind the rectum, with the swab resting near the sacrococcygeal junction (Fig. 476). The gap between the edge of the mescolon to the colon stump and the posterior abdominal wall is closed as far as possible by suture, but no attempt is made to try to close the pelvic peritoneum. I have always made a covering transverse colostomy at this

stage of the operation but Localio and Eng (1975) have avoided it except in a few heavily built male patients where anastomosis proved specially difficult. The loops of small gut are then released from the Lahey bag and they and the more dependent part of the greater omentum are allowed to gravitate towards the pelvis. Finally the abdomen is closed.

SACRAL PHASE

The arrangement of the patient on his right side for the sacral phase is shown in Fig. 477. A double-channel irrigating tube is tied in the anus for irrigation of the anorectum with cetrimide and nitrogen mustard after a crushing clamp has been applied to the rectum below the growth during the sacral phase. (As soon as the irrigation has been given it is a convenience to remove the irrigating tube before carrying out the anastomosis, hence it is useful to tie the perianal purse-string suture holding the tube with a bow so that it may be easily undone under the sterile towelling during the operation.)

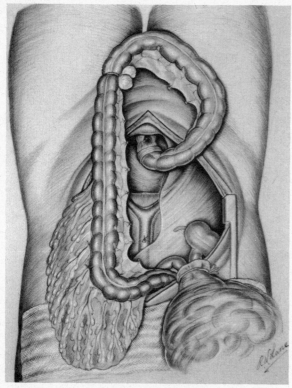

Fig. 475. Abdominosacral resection. View from the head end of the table of the completion of the mobilization of the left colon and rectum. Note the loops of small bowel confined in a Lahey bag. The lower limit of the proposed colon stump is marked by a strong silk ligature with an included gauze swab.

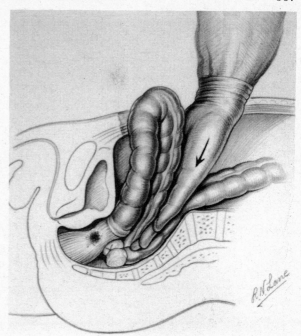

Fig. 476. Abdominosacral resection. Diagrammatic representation showing how the colon loop is tucked into the pelvis behind the rectum with the marking gauze swab placed near the sacrococcygeal junction, so that it should be easily found and extracted when the sacral wound is made.

After sterilizing the skin and applying sterile towels around the operation site, an adhesive Steri-drape is fixed to the exposed skin and towelling particularly to seal off the anal region and irrigating tube from the operative field (Fig. 478A). The transverse incision is then made and deepened on to and through the sacrococcygeal junction or the joint between the basal two segments of coccyx. The latter is then excised (Fig. 478B). After enlargement of the gap thus created by cutting into the muscles for a short distance on either side, the so-called fascia of Waldeyer is exposed. When it is incised or broken with the finger, the gauze swab tied to the loop of colon comes into view (Fig. 479A). It is 'fished' out of the pelvis with forceps and drags the mobilized sigmoid and rectum with it, including the carcinomatous segment (Fig. 479B). The loop is doubly clamped proximally just above the ligature and gauze swab and distally 2 cm or so above the intended site of division of the rectum. The colon is immediately divided proximally between the Parker–Kerr clamps, but the rectum is kept intact and the stump of bowel containing the growth and attached to the anal canal is used for traction to

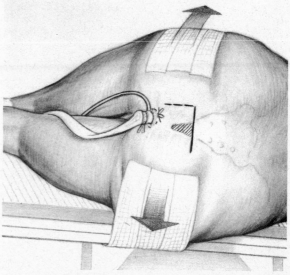

Fig. 477. Abdominosacral resection. Approach for the sacral phase. Note how the buttocks project slightly over the edge of the table and are both retracted laterally by adhesive strapping. A double-channel irrigating tube (e.g. Muir's, see p. 440) has been secured in the anal canal by means of purse-string suture, tied with a bow so that it can be undone under the sterile towels during the operation and the tube extracted before the anastomosis is completed. The line of the incision is indicated. Usually a simple transverse cut at the sacrococcygeal junction suffices, but sometimes it is helpful to make an angled extension at one end of it.

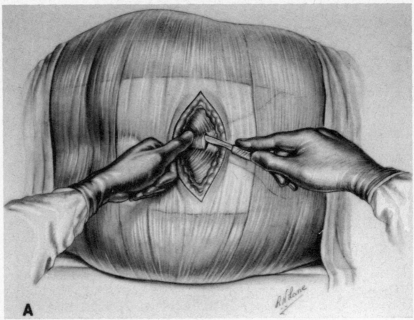

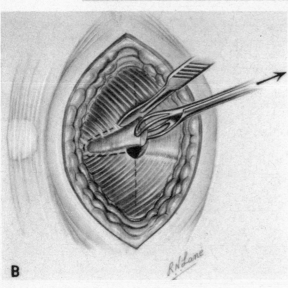

Fig. 478. Abdominosacral resection. Sacral phase. Note sealing off of operation site with adhesive Steridrape. (A) Transverse incision deepened to expose the coccyx and open the sacrococcygeal junction. (B) The coccyx then dissected out mainly from the deeper aspect.

bring the rectum below the clamp more to the surface for the purposes of the anastomosis. But before commencing the latter, the small part of the anorectum below the rectal clamp is irrigated through the double channel and tube with cetrimide and nitrogen mustard solutions, and when this has been completed the tube is released and removed from the anus by a non-sterile assistant working under the towelling (Fig. 480).

The steps of the subsequent colorectal anastomosis, using a single layer of interrupted silk sutures, are clearly depicted in Fig. 481. But a two-layer technique is at least as convenient and satisfactory.

The pelvic cavity is drained by a couple of sump suction drains brought out through the buttocks away from the main sacral wound, and the latter is closed by continuous and interrupted chromic catgut sutures for the musculoaponeurotic layers and silk sutures for the skin. The wound area is sealed with a plastic spray and dressings are applied.

Abdominotranssphincteric Resection (Mason Technique)

This operation is identical with the abdominosacral resection just described up to the posterior

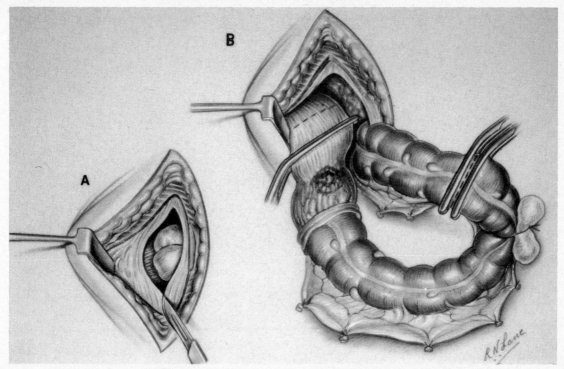

Fig. 479. Abdominosacral resection, sacral phase. (A) Deepening the incision exposes the fascia of Waldeyer, and, after its division, the gauze swab tied to the colon is revealed. (B) Traction on the gauze draws the mobilized loop of colon and rectum, including the carcinoma, out of the pelvis for clamping above and below preparatory to resection.

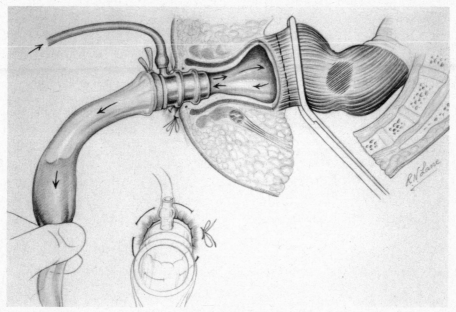

Fig. 480. Abdominosacral resection, sacral phase. The plan of irrigation below the clamp on the rectum.

phase, access for which is obtained, not by a transverse incision removing the coccyx, but by an oblique one extending headwards from the pos-terior anal margin and dividing the *external* sphincter the levator muscle as in the purely posterior transsphincteric approach developed by

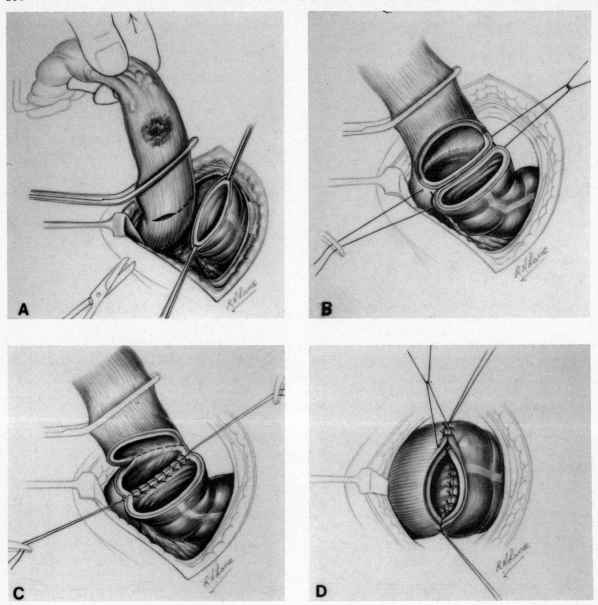

Fig. 481. Abdominosacral resection, sacral phase. Successive steps in the colorectal anastomosis using a one-layer technique with interrupted 3/0 silk.

Mason (1970) for dealing with benign villous papillomas of the rectum and with prostatorectal fistulae (see p. 355). This posterior phase can be done with the patient on his side as in the ordinary abdominosacral resection, but the system of marking with stay sutures the muscular structures as they are encountered during the transsphincteric incision is much easier practised if the patient is in a symmetrical prone position. Accordingly, in the abdominotranssphincteric operation it is better to have the patient on his face for the second phase.

The incision is carried out as described on p. 355 down to the point where the external sphincter and levator muscle have been divided exposing the internal sphincter and rectal wall. It is to be noted that *the internal sphincter is not divided*. Instead the

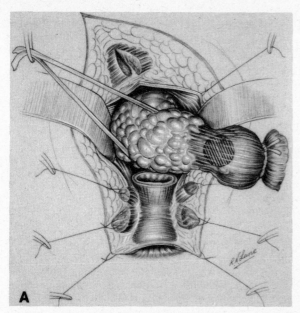

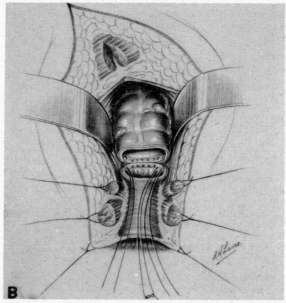

Fig. 482. The abdominotranssphincteric resection. Transsphincteric phases with patient prone. Though the levator and external sphincter have been divided to expose the lower rectum and anal canal, the internal sphincter and lining of the anal canal are preserved intact. (A) The rectal tube has been divided transversely close to the top of the internal sphincter and the colon is being drawn down. (B) The segment of rectum containing the growth and the distal part of the left colon have been resected and an end-to-end colorectal anastomosis in one layer is being made.

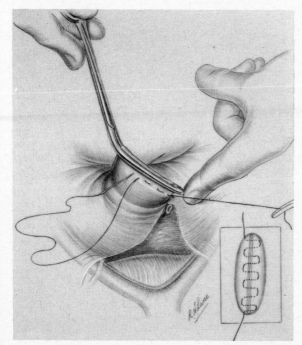

Fig. 483. Hartmann's operation. A continuous mattress suture of 2/0 chromic catgut on a straight needle is being inserted below the sagittally placed Parker clamp, whilst the assistant places a finger on the tip of the clamp to prevent the suture catching on the clamp.

plane of separation already established around the rectum down to the anorectal junction during the abdominal phase is now entered and opened up still further. Next the tube of rectum is divided an adequate distance below the growth and usually just above the internal sphincter (Fig. 482A). (Note that with this technique of resection an irrigation of the distal anorectum before the bowel is divided is not readily feasible without a great deal of contamination.) The divided rectum and colon are then drawn down till the site marked on the colon at the abdominal phase as the distal limit of the colon stump is reached. The bowel is divided just above this point and an end-to-end anastomosis is established between the colon and the distal rectum, using most conveniently a one-layer suture technique (Fig. 482B).

A couple of sump suction drains are brought out from the anastomotic site through the muscle and skin lateral to the posterior wound. The external anal sphincter and levator musculature are then reconstituted as described on p. 356, and the skin wound is finally closed, sealed with a plastic spray and dressed. (*A covering transverse colostomy at the conclusion of the abdominal phase is always advisable in this operation.*)

Hartmann's Operation

As explained on p. 514, this operation, in which a variable amount of the sigmoid colon and upper rectum is excised, the rectal stump closed by suture and the colon stump brought out as a terminal iliac colostomy, is only very occasionally practised at the present day in the treatment of carcinoma. It is in fact more often used in the management of acute episodes of diverticular disease calling for urgent surgical intervention. Also the closure of a rectal or rectosigmoid stump, as in a Hartmann's operation, is not infrequently required in cases submitted to an ileostomy and total or subtotal colectomy for inflammatory bowel disease.

The opening and exploration of the abdomen and the steps of the dissection leading up to resection of the carcinomatous segment of rectum and sigmoid are exactly the same as in a high anterior resection. The bowel at the upper limit of the resection is divided between Cope's (Martel's) clamps, and that at the lower limit between sagittally placed slightly angled Parker–Kerr clamps, the handles of which lie over the pubes. With the proximal colon stump a terminal iliac colostomy is fashioned at a separate small wound in the left lower quadrant of the anterior abdominal wall in precisely the same way as in an abdominoperineal excision (see pp. 540–6). As for the closure of the top of the rectal stump, there are a number of methods of effecting such a closure by suture and it can also be done by a TA stapler. My own

preference is for the suture technique illustrated in Figs 483–5, which is very simple and quick. I usually leave a sump suction drain down to the sutured stump (for three or four days or longer depending on the amount of fluid withdrawn), but perhaps this is unnecessary. The abdomen is then closed in the usual way.

Extended Hartmann's Operation

In this variant of the operation the rectum is mobilized as in the dissection for a low anterior resection with cutting of the pelvic peritoneum and division of the lateral ligaments (see p. 564). The lower limit of the resection traverses the *extra*-peritoneal rectum and the resulting rectal stump has no peritoneal coat. It can be closed by suture as described above for classical Hartmann's resection or, if this is difficult, a simple and satisfactory alternative is to leave the top of the rectal stump open and to pass a drain through this stump and the anal canal to the exterior to drain the pelvic cavity, whilst the pelvic peritoneum is reconstituted by suture over the stump. The peranal drain is retained for five to seven days as a rule.

Local Excision or Destruction of Small Favourable Rectal Carcinomas

The techniques for practising local excision by the peranal or transsphincteric routes are sufficiently

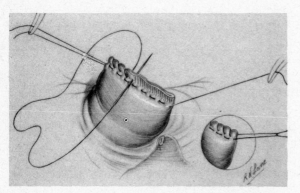

Fig. 484. Hartmann's operation. The Parker–Kerr clamp is removed on completion of the mattress suture, and after tying the suture it is continued as a simple over-and-over stitch backwards along the crushed end of the bowel. *Inset:* The suture has now reached the starting point of the mattress suture at the mesenteric border of the bowel and the two tails are being tied.

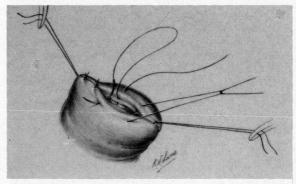

Fig. 485. Hartmann's operation. The line of the catgut suture is being buried by a series of interrupted Lembert sutures of 3/0 silk. It is best to start with a suture at either end, as shown, and then to fill in the interval between these two sutures with four or five other sutures.

described on p. 517, and accounts of the methods of local destruction by diathermy coagulation or contact irradiation are given on pp. 516 and 657.

Postoperative Management

The postoperative care of patients after rectal excision follows the general lines of treatment adopted after any major abdominal operation, but the presence of a colostomy and a perineal wound, or of a rectal anastomosis, naturally calls for special consideration. The following are some of the more relevant points in the management of these cases:

POSITION OF THE PATIENT IN BED

After anterior resection the most comfortable posture for the patient, as soon as he has recovered from the anaesthetic and shock, is a low sitting position. *After abdominoperineal or abdominosacral excision* the sitting position is less satisfactory, for it means that the patient is resting on the posterior end of the perineal wound where it overlies the tip of the sacrum or coccyx, and this probably predisposes to wound separation. This objection applies less to a flat supine position, but in my opinion the best position for these cases is a lateral one, the patient being changed from one side to the other every four or six hours. *After pull-through excision* the sitting position is even more strongly contraindicated, for it could seriously damage the protruding stump of colon and lead to the development of necrosis of the bowel. Instead, alternating right and left lateral positions should be used, the greatest care being taken to avoid injurious pressure on the projecting 'tail' of bowel.

ANTIBIOTICS

The systemic administration of antibiotics as a prophylactic measure during the postoperative period is a debatable matter, which each surgeon must settle according to his views on this subject in general (see pp. 443, 449). My own practice in recent years in all cases of rectal excision—abdominoperineal excision or relatively clean resections with anastomosis—has been to use 'antibiotic cover' consisting of two intramuscular doses of gentamicin 80 mg and lincomycin 600 mg, one given with the anaesthetic premedication, the other

six to eight hours later. But in patients with a greater degree of contamination at the time of anastomosis or where the bowel was torn during abdominoperineal excision the gentamicin and lincomycin have been continued for a full five-day course, whilst in patients who for some reason have had very gross faecal contamination an even more intensive antibiotic regimen may be employed.

FLUID AND ELECTROLYTE ADMINISTRATION AND DIET

It is usually convenient to continue the intravenous 'drip' used for the administration of blood during and immediately after operation as an infusion of $N/5$ saline for the first 48–72 hours. If at the end of that time the patient is able to cope with 90 ml or so of fluid hourly by mouth without nausea or vomiting or abdominal distension, and flatus has escaped freely per colostomy or per anum, as the case may be, the drip may be dismantled and the oral fluids gradually increased and varied. Once a motion has been passed, a light diet may be started and is progressively increased according to the patient's desire for food.

IMMEDIATE CARE OF THE COLOSTOMY

It is usually two or three days before the colostomy discharges faeces, though flatus may escape before then, and exceptionally there may be a faecal action soon after return to the ward. Failure of the colostomy to act after three or four days need occasion no alarm provided that the patient is able to take fluids by mouth without nausea or vomiting and particularly also if flatus is escaping freely. It is useful to pass a finger into the stoma to make sure that the bowel is not being unduly constricted by the abdominal wall. Sometimes indeed as the finger is withdrawn it is followed by a burst of flatus or a gush of faeces. A bisacodyl suppository may be inserted into the colostomy, and repeated once or twice, or a colostomy wash-out may be given. Of course, if the failure of the colostomy to act is associated with abdominal distension and vomiting, it will be necessary, in addition to any local attentions to the colostomy itself, to institute a regimen of intravenous fluid administration and gastric suction as described on p. 463.

The most convenient way to manage the colostomy during the early postoperative period is to apply to the stoma at the conclusion of the operation one of the several patterns of adherent drainable plastic ileostomy bag now available (see Figs 562–4). When the colostomy begins to act, the faeces are at first very fluid and abundant, and the bag needs to be emptied or changed frequently, but after 10–14 days, as a rule, the motions have become firmer in consistency and less irregular and unpredictable in their timing. At this stage the patient is usually in a condition to take some interest in the care of his colostomy, and a decision can be reached as to which type of appliance and which routine should be adopted for its ultimate management (see p. 625).

If the technique of immediate suture of the end of the colon to the skin edges with silk stitches has been employed, these sutures should be removed on the seventh to tenth day. If, on the other hand, the older method of leaving the end of the colon simply projecting 7–10 cm beyond the skin of the abdominal wall has been adopted, it will usually be advisable, when the colostomy has become firmly fixed in position after 10–14 days, to trim it by amputating all but the proximal 2 cm. This little operation can, if desired, be done without a general anaesthetic, after infiltration of the bowel wall with a local anaesthetic solution.

Care of the Perineal Wound after Abdominoperineal Excision

When primary suture has been practised and suction drainage established, either suprapubic or perineal, as much as 250–300 ml of blood-stained fluid may be removed during the first 24 hours. This usually diminishes to 100 ml or less daily over the next two or three days and has practically ceased by the fourth or fifth day, when the tube or tubes should be completely withdrawn and a small dry dressing applied to the drain site. Just occasionally the amount of discharge warrants keeping the suction going for as long as seven to eight days. Usually the perineal stitches are removed on the eight day. Unfortunately, in my experience the management of the perineal wound has not infrequently to depart from this routine, because of haematoma formation or the development of infection. The presence of a haematoma may be suspected from the occurrence of considerable diffuse swelling, induration and tenderness in the perineal area, and is confirmed by the escape of some blood-stained fluid between the stitches of the perineal wound. The development of sepsis may be suggested by the

appearance of signs of inflammation in the perineum, but, because the infection lies deep, such local inflammatory changes may be absent, and the diagnosis may depend on the occurrence of a considerable pyrexia, which is not explained by signs of sepsis elsewhere. It will be appreciated that haematoma and infection often exist together in the perineal wound. If suspicion of either complication is sufficiently strong, and particularly if the patient is pyrexial, the best plan is to remove one stitch and try the insertion of a pair of sinus forceps, which is usually possible without a general anaesthetic and merely under the influence of an injection of morphine. Depending on the findings, however, it may be necessary to proceed to general anaesthesia and opening up of the wound sufficiently to insert a finger and explore the pelvic cavity, evacuating blood clot and pus. Finally a corrugated rubber drain or tail of gauze dressing soaked in Milton is introduced, and thereafter the patient has irrigations and dressings as in the 'open' management described below.

When open drainage has been adopted, during the first 12–24 hours the outer dressing on the perineal wound may require to be renewed two or three times because of further bleeding. After that bleeding usually lessens considerably but a change of outer dressing is advisable morning and evening to make sure that the wound is well covered. On the morning of the third postoperative day, counting the day of operation as the first, the first complete redressing is done, with removal of the rubber drain or pack and irrigation of the wound cavity with 1 litre of dilute hydrogen peroxide solution followed by 1 or 2 litres of Eusol or 2.5% Milton solution. This irrigation and dressing are best carried out with the patient lying on the left side with the buttocks projecting slightly over the edge of the bed and with a square of mackintosh tucked under the lower hip and extending down into a bucket as described on p. 91. In this way large quantities of irrigating fluid may be used in a vigorous manner without wetting the bedclothes. Finally, when the irrigation has been completed, any remaining fluid in the wound is removed by gentle swabbing with gauze, and a single gauze swab soaked in Milton is opened out and tucked into the cavity with its end projecting out of the perineum to keep the skin edges apart. Further external dressings of Milton gauze, dry gauze and wool are then applied and kept in place with a firm bandage.

This regimen of irrigations and dressings is

repeated evening and morning. For the first one or two dressings it is wise to sedate the patient with a preliminary injection of 100 mg of pethidine or 15 mg of morphine. Though the dressings are normally carried out by the nursing staff it is imperative that the surgeon should personally review the wound every four or five days to satisfy himself that healing is proceeding in an orderly fashion. The large pelvic cavity left at the end of the operation closes partly by the descent of the pelvic peritoneum, but mainly by filling up with granulation tissue from the apex of the cavity high up on the front of the sacrum down to its base at the level of the perineal skin wound. There is a tendency for a constriction to develop in the middle of the cavity shutting off an attic which thus escapes irrigation and tends to accumulate pus. To guard against this development the surgeon should explore the cavity with his finger at each review and should gently break down any incipient narrowing.

The perineal skin sutures are removed generally on the eighth day, but may be taken out a little sooner with advantage if there is slight infection around the stitches. As soon as the abdominal wound has healed completely and the patient has become fairly steady on his feet when ambulant, which is usually about the fourteenth day or later, he should have a bath once or twice a day, so timed as to precede his irrigations and dressings. By the end of three or four weeks, healing of the perineal wound has usually proceeded sufficiently to be able to allow the patient to leave hospital, to go either to a convalescent home or to his own home if suitable arrangements can be made for a continuation by a district nurse of the irrigations and dressings to his wound at least once daily.

In the management of the open perineal wound a method on trial at the moment is that of using foam elastomer packs (for details see p. 91) instead of gauze packs, which may have the advantage of greater convenience for the patient insofar as he can insert the pack himself (Wood and Hughes 1975). A switch is made to foam elastomer about 10–14 days after operation. Thereafter a new elastomer mould is made for the wound cavity each week. The patient can take the mould out himself before bathing and re-introduce it afterwards and this is perhaps the main attraction of the method rather than any improvement in the quality of healing (Wood et al. 1977).

In female cases, *where the posterior vaginal wall has been preserved*, it is important to be on the alert during the convalescence for the development of a perforation in this structure. Even though the perineal operator may be emphatic that he did not breach the posterior vaginal wall during the dissection, experience shows that sometimes a small or large vaginal perforation develops subsequently, presumably due to necrosis following operative trauma or diathermy coagulation. A vaginal perforation of this kind in association with the perineal wound following excision of the rectum considerably delays healing and invariably results in the ultimate development of a vaginoperineal fistula when the wound finally heals. Usually much quicker healing is secured if, as soon as the vaginal perforation is detected, the posterior vaginal wall from the level of the perforation downwards and the related remnant of perineum are divided, thus producing a common cavity composed of the lower part of the vagina and the perineal wound. The end result is very satisfactory as a rule, but occasionally the consequences of a wide vaginal introitus, as described below, accrue.

In female cases, *where the posterior vaginal wall has been excised along with the rectum*, the healing of the back wound is particularly straightforward as a rule, but the same periodic digital examination of the pelvic cavity per vaginam is required. Usually within three weeks the cavity has completely filled up with granulations and these rapidly acquire an epithelial covering in front, as the posterior vaginal wall is regenerated. The final result is very satisfactory, and it may be extremely difficult a few months after the operation to discern that any part of the vagina has been removed. The functional result in younger patients also seems to be excellent. These remarks apply in cases where the posterior vaginal wall has been removed if the sutured perineal wound itself heals *per primam* throughout its length. But in some cases the perineal wound may break down to a greater or lesser extent, either at the anterior end, enlarging the introitus to the vagina or in its middle, creating a fistula from the vagina to the perineum, to deal with which it is necessary to split open the perineal wound as far back as the fistulous opening in its central part. In either event the patient is left with a very wide introitus to the vagina which exposes the anterior vaginal wall. Under the circumstances there is some predisposition to the development of a cystocele, and sexual function may be unsatisfactory. In a few cases where this has happened I have had the opening narrowed by a secondary plastic operation by gynaecological colleagues with considerable improvement.

When a pack has been used instead of a drain in the perineal wound, this is quite easily extracted if it has been encased in a plastic or oiled silk covering, and this is best done on the third day after operation. A naked pack, however, sometimes requires a short general anaesthetic for its removal, because it becomes adherent to the walls of the cavity; it is also well to have available facilities for a blood transfusion in case the separation of the pack should lead to further haemorrhage.

CARE OF THE SACRAL WOUND AFTER ABDOMINOSACRAL RESECTION

In a sense the sacral wound following abdomino-sacral resection—of classical type or Mason version—requires no particular attention beyond the exercise of care to keep pressure off it by having the patient lie largely on alternative sides rather than on his back. In addition a periodic scrutiny should be conducted of the wound area to look for signs of developing infection or of haematoma formation. The suction drains employed in connection with these operations may be brought out supra-pubically or may emerge through the skin of the buttocks. The time of removal of these drains will depend on the amount of fluid being withdrawn, but is seldom sooner than the fifth day.

CARE OF THE BLADDER

The self-retaining urethral catheter introduced immediately before operation should be left *in situ* for four or five days because experience has shown that its early removal is frequently followed by retention needing further catheterization. Whilst the indwelling catheter is in position it is connected by tubing to a container beside the bed and drains into it continuously. On removing the catheter after the fourth day, normal micturition may be immediately re-established, or it may be necessary to give a subcutaneous injection of carbachol, 0·25 mg, to assist spontaneous emptying of the bladder. This may have to be repeated occasionally if micturition continues to prove difficult. It is also important to make sure that the bladder is emptying itself completely during these first few days of spontaneous micturition and not developing chronic retention with overflow; if there is any doubt on

that score a catheter should be passed each evening for two or three days. If the patient's efforts at natural micturition after withdrawal of the catheter are unavailing or inadequate, the Foley catheter will have to be reintroduced for another few days. Sometimes the patient is able to make a better attempt when his general condition has improved as his convalescence proceeds, but if this is not so he should be referred for expert urological opinion as to the cause of his retention (see p. 613).

RESPIRATORY AND GENERAL EXERCISES AND AMBULATION

Respiratory and leg exercises are an integral part of the postoperative care and are particularly important because there is a considerable tendency to chest complications, thrombophlebitis and pulmonary embolism in these cases. Though I favour early ambulation after abdominal surgery in general and this policy is applied to my patients after rectal excision, I must admit that, because of the discomfort of the perineal wound and their encumbrance with a urethral catheter and urinary drainage bag as well as an intravenous 'drip', it is quite a performance getting them out of bed during the first two or three days after operation.

CARE OF THE ANASTOMOSIS AND PELVIC DRAIN AFTER ANTERIOR RESECTION AND OTHER ANASTOMOTIC OPERATIONS

Sometimes the bowels act per anum within a few hours of the operation, but more usually it is two or three days before a bowel action occurs. To assist the passage of flatus or, later, faeces, a bisacodyl suppository may be used if the anastomosis is in the upper rectum, but is better avoided with low-lying anastomoses, which might conceivably be damaged by the suppository. Enemas at this stage are *contra*-indicated in all cases with a rectal suture line, high or low. The suprapubic suction drain now usually employed in cases with a rectal anastomosis generally produces 150–300 ml of blood-stained fluid during the first 24 hours and diminishing amounts daily thereafter, so that by the fourth or fifth postoperative day there is negligible drainage as a rule and the tube (or tubes) should then be removed. Rarely the drain may continue to withdraw quantities of serous fluid of the order of 70–100 ml each day for a week or more, and, if so, it should be left *in situ* for as long as necessary. If a suprapubic corrugated rubber drain has been used, it is customarily left in position for at least five or six days.

If proximal transverse colostomy has been established as it often is at the conclusion of a low anterior, abdominoanal abdominosacral resection, it may be closed by an intraperitoneal technique 21 days or so after the resection, *provided that the patient is then apyrexial and digital examination of the rectum or sigmoidoscopy (and possibly a very gentle gastrografin enema examination) reveals that the anastomosis has healed satisfactorily.* If some breakdown of the suture line has taken place, the colostomy may have to be retained for much longer, and in any event colostomy closure is technically much easier after an interval of six to eight weeks to allow oedema to subside. Accordingly my present practice is to discharge the patient temporarily and readmit him for delayed closure of the colostomy when conditions are optimal for this operation.

Care of Protruding Stumps and Pelvic Drain between First and Second Stages of Pull-Through Excision (Turnbull–Cutait Technique)

As stressed on p. 593, the patient is nursed on his side to avoid injurious pressure on the protruding rectal and colonic stumps. The dressing on the latter is changed daily or oftener as required, and the state of the colon wall is carefully observed each time as regards viability. The catheter conducting the faeces away from the end of the colon usually becomes loose about the fourth or fifth day and is then removed. If a covering transverse colostomy has not been established, there will usually be a profuse fluid faecal discharge from the stump by this time. It is a good plan, therefore, to fit a colostomy type of plastic bag on the protruding 'tail' of bowel and to change it as required. The suprapubic suction drain (or drains) to the pelvis is withdrawn on the fifth or sixth day, or sooner if the aspiration has ceased to withdraw any fluid for 24 hours or so.

Complications and Sequelae

Rectal excision may be followed by any of the complications and sequelae of major abdominal surgery in general, such as shock, paralytic ileus and intestinal obstruction, wound infection, disruption or herniation, bronchitis, pulmonary collapse or pneumonia, leg thrombosis or pulmonary embolism, and coronary thrombosis or cerebrovascular accidents, but in this section only shock and paralytic ileus and intestinal obstruction—which are quite common after this operation—and certain other complications more specifically related to the nature of the operation will be considered.

Shock

Early. Arterial hypotension occurring in the first 24–48 hours or so after operation usually results from *inadequately replaced blood loss* from the pelvic cavity. Though the raw surfaces of this cavity may have appeared perfectly dry immediately before the conclusion of the operation, a fair amount of oozing of serosanguinous fluid from it is not uncommon during the next two or three days, and occasionally quite a brisk reactionary haemorrhage takes place. It may be difficult to gauge accurately the severity of this loss because, if suction drainage is used, the suction may not be entirely effective, or, if open drainage is in force, the amount of soakage of the external dressings may be underestimated. Consquently there is a tendency to undertransfuse these cases. Monitoring of the central venous pressure with a radiopaque catheter, such as the E-Z Cath (Deseret Pharmaceutical Company) introduced percutaneously into the superior vena cava and connected to a saline manometer, is helpful in management, although absolute pressure values should not be used as a guide to volume replacement. Actually, in many patients undergoing major rectal or colonic operations at the present time the anaesthetist will have initiated central venous pressure recording to guide him as to the amount of blood to be transfused during operation. It will thus be convenient usually to maintain the central venous line for 48 hours or so to assist in postoperative care. I must add, however, that I have considerable misgivings about the retention of these long catheters for prolonged periods, for I have the impression that they predispose to the development of septicaemia.

In the treatment of arterial hypotension due to haemorrhage the important initial step is transfusion of an appropriate amount of blood. In many cases this is all that is required, but, if on investigation it seems that the bleeding is continuing at a considerable rate, the perineal wound will need to be re-explored (see Haemorrhage, below).

Occasionally hypotension in the early post-operative period is due to other causes than bleeding, such as *pulmonary insufficiency* or *myocardial infarction*, or very rarely the action of analgesics particularly in elderly subjects. Thus evaluation of the difficult case may include radiological examination of the chest, electrocardiography and arterial blood gas analysis.

Late. An exceptionally rare cause of hypotension developing suddenly some days or a week or so after operation is a *secondary haemorrhage* from a septic perineal wound. This may produce rapid exsanguination and call for the most energetic management with massive blood transfusions and immediate exploration of the perineum to discover the bleeding point. But nearly always shock arising at this stage is due, not to blood loss, but to *cardiorespiratory causes* or to *severe sepsis*. In my experience septic shock is most liable to be due to fulminating peritonitis, such as occurs with dehiscence of anastomoses. However, sometimes rigors, fever and hypotension precede the appearance of significant abdominal signs by some hours or days, and such cases are liable to be labelled as suffering from unexplained *bacteraemic shock*. Blood cultures seldom produce any bacterial growth, and in the fullness of time the source of the sepsis becomes evident. The urgent requirements in treatment of septic shock are blood volume replacement—which necessitates the use of plasma, perhaps up to 1000–1500 ml, rather than blood—and massive therapy with antibiotics possessing a broad spectrum of activity and particular efficacy against coliform organisms—such as ampicillin, cephaloridine, kanamycin, gentamicin and lincomycin—preferably using two agents simultaneously. Occasionally digitalization is required and large doses of hydrocortisone may be indicated in desperate cases. After the blood pressure has been adequately restored, due consideration must be given to the cause of the sepsis, for, if a spreading peritonitis resulting from a leaking anastomosis is present, antibiotic and supportive therapy alone will most assuredly fail.

COMPLICATIONS RELATING TO THE PERINEAL WOUND

HAEMORRHAGE

As mentioned above a variable amount of bleeding may take place from the perineal wound but usually ceases after 36–48 hours. All that is needed is full sedation with morphine, further transfusion and changes of the outer dressing as required, if open drainage has been used. If, on the other hand, primary suture has been practised with suprapubic or perineal suction drainage, it will be necessary to keep a close eye on excessive amounts of blood being aspirated and also to bear in mind the possibility that blood may be accumulating partly in clotted form in the pelvic cavity (see also p. 597). Occasionally the bleeding is more severe and necessitates a return to the operating theatre for re-examination of the wound cavity under general anaesthesia. With the patient either in the lithotomy position with a moderate degree of Trendelenburg tilt or on his side with the upper buttock elevated by the assistant, some or all the skin sutures are removed, fluid and clotted blood is evacuated with the aid of an irrigation, and a self-retaining retractor is inserted. A careful search is now made for any bleeding point or points and these are controlled by ligature, stitch, or diathermy. If any obvious source for the haemorrhage has thus been discovered, the wound may be re-closed loosely around a corrugated rubber drain, but if the bleeding seems to have occurred as a more diffuse ooze or from several points, it will be wiser to pack the cavity with a naked gauze roll which is left *in situ* for three or four days. It goes without saying that, in addition to the attentions to the site of the bleeding, these patients require immediate blood transfusion to compensate for their blood loss.

RUPTURE OF THE PELVIC PERITONEUM

Considering the thinness of the teased-out pelvic peritoneum at the conclusion of an abdominoperineal excision and the strain to which it is subjected during respiration and coughing etc., it is surprising that the suture line in it does not more often give way during the postoperative period.

Actually this is an excessively rare complication which I have only seen happen five times in many hundreds of cases submitted to rectal excision. In its more usual form it consists of a very limited breakdown, through which a single loop of small gut prolapses and becomes obstructed, or possibly strangulated, with the insidious development of obstructive symptoms. The separation, however, may be extensive, allowing many coils of small intestine to descend into the pelvic cavity; in one of my cases in which this occurred the onset was associated with sudden severe lower abdominal pain and a sensation of something 'giving way'.

There is apt to be considerable delay in the recognition of this complication and it may only be accurately diagnosed at laparotomy undertaken for postoperative obstruction. If the affected loop is non-viable, it will have to be resected. It may be possible to close the gap in the peritoneum by suture alone or assisted by an omental graft. The pelvic peritoneum should be well supported by a gauze pack inside a plastic bag inserted into the pelvic cavity from below for four or five days. If fortunately the condition has been recognized by noticing the projection of bowel into the pelvic cavity on digital or sigmoidoscopic examination of the perineal wound, it may be possible under anaesthesia to reduce the loop of intestine from below, if it is viable, and to retain it in the peritoneal cavity by suturing the pelvic peritoneum through the perineum and supporting it with a generous pack inside a plastic covering.

INFECTION

When the perineal wound is managed along 'open' lines, some degree of infection is not uncommon, either around the stitch holes or in the wound cavity, but it is seldom a serious complication. Sepsis round the stitches is an indication for their earlier removal if possible, say on the fifth or sixth day, following which the infection quickly subsides as a rule. Infection in the pelvic cavity leading to an abundant discharge of pus usually responds to the ordinary regimen of irrigations and dressings twice daily. Occasionally it is necessary to open the wound a little more, if the existing unsutured gap is inadequate for drainage. It is also important to remember that persistent sepsis in the perineal wound may be due to a gauze swab having slipped inside and been overlooked, so that the wound cavity should be thoroughly explored with the finger. Bacterio-logical examination of a sample of the pus should be undertaken to determine the predominant organisms and their sensitivity to antibiotics, but usually the condition responds to the simple measures outlined above without having to resort to treatment with antibiotics. In some cases with a particularly septic perineal wound it may be useful to employ noxythiolin as the solution for irrigation instead of hydrogen peroxide and Milton.

When the perineal wound has been completely sutured and is being drained with suprapubic or perineal suction drains, in my experience infection is quite frequent, despite the administration of covering systemic antibiotic therapy in most of these cases (see p. 593). It apparently often arises on the basis of haematoma formation in the wound. The diagnosis of sepsis in the perineum may initially be difficult and should always be thought of when patients, whose perineal wounds have been closed, develop a pyrexia, which cannot be plausibly explained on the basis of infection elsewhere. If suspicion persists, a cautious exploration of the wound may be necessary (see p. 594), leading on possibly to more or less opening up of the perineum, with subsequent 'open' management as detailed above.

NECROSIS AND SEPARATION

Despite the avoidance of pressure on the perineal wound by not allowing the patient to sit on the sacral region during the early postoperative period, necrosis of the perineal skin or separation of the wound edges may still sometimes take place, particularly in elderly debilitated subjects. If a perforation should develop in the line of the wound due to partial separation, it is usually best to open the wound from the central drainage site back to the perforation.

STENOSIS

When the perineal wound is being managed on the 'open' regimen, narrowing may be found to develop either as an hour-glass constriction of the wound cavity or as a stenosis at the skin level. It has been customary to correct these tendencies—by stretching the former with the finger or incising the latter—because many experienced surgeons have encountered cases where pocketing of pus occurred proximal to such strictures, and the infection only resolved after treatment directed to the narrowing.

PERSISTENT OR RECURRENT SINUS

This is most often due to faulty healing resulting from the sort of mechanism referred to above, but may rarely be due to other factors—to the retention of foreign material such as a swab in the wound, to infection of the sacrum with sequestrum formation, or to recurrence of the growth in the pelvic cavity.

PERINEAL OR SACRAL HERNIA

It is remarkable how soundly the perineal region heals after rectal excision, and though there is often a slight impulse and bulge on coughing this seldom amounts to very much. Exceptionally, however, there may be a more definite swelling, justifying the title of 'perineal or sacral hernia'. This is found less rarely in females than in males, and is particularly liable to occur in cases where the pelvic peritoneum has been left unsutured as in extended excisions and pelvic clearance operations. The condition may be symptomless or may give rise to a dragging sensation in the perineum on standing or walking. The bulge may be supported with a variable degree of success by a firm pad and T-bandage or by a special broad perineal band attached to the back of the colostomy belt. If the hernia is very big, operative repair may rarely be required and several methods are available. Yeomans (1939) described an operation to deal with the condition from the abdominal aspect, with obliteration of the pelvic peritoneal sac with purse-string sutures of linen thread, and Gabriel (1948) has employed a perineal repair on a number of these cases. In this latter method the perineal sac is exposed from below and removed up to its 'neck', which is closed with mattress sutures of catgut. Sutures of floss-silk, fascial strips, or stainless steel wire are then passed between the margins of the gluteus maximus muscles to form a lattice work to support the pelvic floor, and the skin wound is closed. Gabriel reports fairly satisfactory results. Ego-Aguirre et al. (1964) also describe the successful perineal repair, using fascia lata grafts or Marlex mesh, of the large sacral hernias often seen after complete pelvic clearance. Cawkwell (1963) advocated a synchronous abdominal and perineal approach in the repair of large perineal hernias, using a nylon mesh implant to reconstitute the pelvic peritoneal floor, and I myself have employed a similar implant by the abdominal route in one case. Bach-Nielsen (1967) has described the successful repair of a sacral hernia

by a perineal approach, turning back the uterus and stitching the fundus to the sacrum and side walls of the pelvis; but in three cases, in which I used this device through an abdominal incision, the hernia recurred in one.

LOCAL RECURRENCE (see also p. 648)

Recurrence of the growth in the perineal wound or pelvis may show itself in a variety of ways, usually by causing pain in the perineum or the sacral or sciatic regions, less commonly by producing a local swelling or induration, an abscess or discharging fistula, oedema of the lower limbs, or urinary symptoms. *Persistent perineal pain* after an abdominoperineal excision may be due to other causes, such as a tender scar or lower end of sacrum, but is *always highly suggestive of local recurrence*. The diagnosis may sometimes be confirmed by radiological examination showing destruction of the sacrum, or by biopsy, but often the surgeon has to rely on his clinical suspicions. As a rule nothing is to be gained from exploration of the perineum or attempts at excision of the recurrence; such efforts are usually unsuccessful and may result in injury to the bladder or urethra with the formation of a urinary fistula, which adds greatly to the patient's discomfort. It remains to be seen whether computerized axial tomography will prove helpful in the diagnosis of such local recurrences. I have certainly seen one case where it was successful in demonstrating a soft tissue shadow due to this cause. The best hope of alleviation lies with some form of *supervoltage radiotherapy*, which should be used as soon as recurrence is suspected and without waiting till the diagnosis is beyond doubt.

PHANTOM RECTUM

Every now and again patients who have had the rectum excised mention that they have had the sensation since the operation that the bowel is still there, as indicated by the occasional feeling that they wanted to pass faeces or flatus by the normal route. Sometimes the 'rectal' sensation seems to be experienced just before the colostomy acts. I would off-hand have reckoned that about 10% of patients might have these symptoms of 'phantom rectum', but, in a special enquiry amongst 50 persons who had complete rectal excision between six months and 14 years previously, Farley and Smith (1968) found that no less than 34 (68%) admitted to such symptoms. However Farley and Smith (1968) emphasize that the sensation is *not one of actual pain* (c.f. Local Recurrence, above); only one of their patients was at all upset by it, and, after reassurance as to the innocent nature of the complaint, he rapidly improved. In another survey Devlin et al. (1971) put the incidence of phantom rectum at 50% of patients after rectal excision. The cause of the condition is unknown. In some cases the symptoms improve spontaneously over the years, in others there is no change. No treatment seems indicated beyond firm reassurance.

COMPLICATIONS RELATING TO THE COLOSTOMY

NECROSIS AND RETRACTION

Necrosis of the terminal part of the colon may occur, due to faulty judgement at the time of the operation as to the adequacy of its blood supply, or to too tight a compression of the bowel by the opening in the anterior abdominal wall. It can, however, usually be avoided by scrupulous attention to operative technique. If necrosis should develop, it may be confined to that part of the bowel which projects beyond the level of the skin or at least of the peritoneum, as shown by a careful inspection of the mucosa at the colostomy and more proximally by a cautious sigmoidoscopy; in this case an expectant attitude may be adopted, waiting for the necrotic portion to separate in due course. If, on the other hand, the process seems to extend more deeply, the colostomy wound should be explored and the colon drawn out till obviously viable bowel is reached; if this proves impossible because of the extent of the gangrene, the main wound will have to be re-opened to allow of more careful inspection of the left colon from the abdominal aspect and resection of as much intestine as is required, with the establishment of a new terminal colostomy, probably in the transverse colon.

INFECTION AND SEPARATION

It is remarkable how consistently uneventful primary healing results from the application of the technique of immediate mucocutaneous suture described on p. 543. But in a small proportion of cases some infection and cellulitis occurs; this usually settles down rapidly with or without the discharge of pus and with a variable amount of separation of the end of the colon from the skin edge. The raw area thus created heals by granulation in due course.

FISTULA FORMATION

With the method described above (p. 543) for the formation of a colostomy, which eschews the use of buried sutures to fix the emerging colon stump to the parietes, it is hard to see how a subcutaneous fistula could develop between the bowel lumen and the pericolostomic skin, and in fact I have never seen this complication in any of my own patients. But I have seen fistulas of this kind in two cases operated on by other surgeons. It may be possible to lay the fistula open along the same lines as followed in the treatment of an anal fistula, but, if the track lies very deeply, it may be better to re-fashion the entire colostomy as in the treatment of colostomy stenosis (see below). This was the procedure adopted by me in both of the cases mentioned above.

STENOSIS

This is largely a complication of the older technique of making a colostomy by simply leaving the colon stump projecting beyond the skin of the anterior abdominal wall. The granulations which form on the exposed serosal surface of the bowel become converted into fibrous tissue, and, as this contracts, it everts and draws the mucosa down to the skin level and at the same time may cause a tight stenosis (see Fig. 540); this is liable to occur even if a disc of skin has been removed from the colostomy wound. This tendency to contract is to some extent counteracted by the dilating effect of passing a semi-solid motion each day; but this regular dilatation is not secured by the liquid motion resulting from a colostomy wash-out, so that if this regimen is adopted there is an increased predisposition to stenosis. Some surgeons advise that a finger should be passed into the colostomy each day to prevent a stricture forming, but the best way to eliminate colostomy stenosis is to make it by a sutured technique in the first instance. This results in a soft supple mucocutaneous junction which shows no tendency to undergo narrowing with the passage of time and requires no regular digitation. Only if there were severe infection around the colostomy

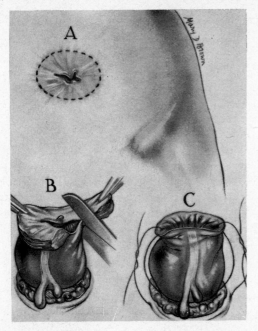

Fig. 486. Refashioning of terminal iliac colostomy for stenosis. (A) Circular incision with removal of a disc of skin and subcutaneous fat around the stenosed opening. (B) Colon freed from the layers of the abdominal wall and drawn out of the abdomen. Rim of skin and fat at the distal end excised leaving a soft pliable edge of bowel. (C) Suture of end of colon to skin.

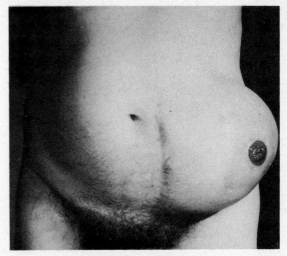

Fig. 487. Large colostomy hernia in connection with a terminal iliac colostomy.

with separation of the bowel and skin, would stenosis be likely to occur after this technique.

In dealing with an established colostomy stenosis the best plan is to re-fashion the colostomy. This little operation can, if necessary, be done under local infiltration anaesthesia, though a general anaesthetic is normally preferable. A circumcision is made round the stoma 6–12 mm from the mucosa (Fig. 486A). Four forceps are then applied in the rim of skin attached to the bowel and, whilst traction is exerted on these to lift the bowel out of the wound, the incision is deepened on to the aponeurosis. Further sharp dissection between the colon wall and the edge of the hole in the parietes frees the colon stump, so that it can be lifted 3·5–5 cm out of the abdomen, sometimes entering the peritoneal cavity in the process, at other times not opening the peritoneum (Fig. 486B). The ring of skin and under-lying fibrous tissue is then excised with scissors leaving a fresh pliable cut edge of colon, which can be sutured by a series of interrupted stitches to the margin of the skin all round, as in making a fresh colostomy (Fig. 486c).

HERNIATION

Some degree of herniation around the colostomy is so common that this complication may be regarded as virtually inevitable. It may amount to only a slight bulging on coughing, or may be very large, with the colostomy perched on top of the swelling. These grosser forms of the condition are found almost exclusively in cases where the colon has been brought out in the line of the main paramedian or oblique iliac wound used for the excision (Fig. 487). If a separate stab wound has been employed for making the colostomy, the resulting hernia is usually less, and if this wound is kept small so that the abdominal parietes fit snugly around the protruding colon, any large herniation can usually be avoided, but there is still almost invariably some slight bulging. I know of no certain preventive of this complication. In my experience, even if the colon is stitched all round to the peritoneum as it passes through the anterior abdominal wall, hernia still usually occurs. I had hoped that one of the advantages of the extraperitoneal technique for making iliac colostomies (see p. 542) might be that it would lessen the incidence of herniation, because of the oblique manner in which the colon stump then emerges from the abdominal cavity, but this has not been so. It is interesting that ileostomy, which in its formation is practically identical with a colostomy, is seldom followed by peri-ileostomic herniation. The only treatment required for a colostomy hernia as a rule is firm support of the colostomy site by a well-made colostomy belt, preferably one incorporating a plastic disc over the stoma. If the hernia is very troublesome, an operation to re-site the colostomy and repair the abdominal weakness may be indicated, though I myself have encountered only two cases where I thought this was worth advising. In such patients there is always a risk of further herniation at the new site, which might lead to considerable disappointment. Thorlakson (1965) has described a technique for repair of a colostomy hernia leaving the bowel in the same site, but I would fear a much greater risk of troublesome recurrence of the herniation than if the colostomy were transplanted.

PROLAPSE

A minor degree of prolapse of the colostomy involving a very slight increase over the years in the amount of protrusion of the bowel on standing or coughing, is not infrequent, but it represents no inconvenience to the patient and requires no treatment. By contrast a major degree of prolapse, in which the bowel projects anything from 5 to 12·5 or 15 cm, is most uncommon—I have only seen five or six examples in many hundreds of patients with terminal iliac colostomies after abdominoperineal excision of the rectum. (Incidentally, it may be pointed out that gross prolapse occurs more readily with loop iliac or transverse colostomies, especially in children and if the precaution has not been taken to site the stoma as close to the lower end of the descending colon or to the hepatic flexure as is technically possible.) When a major prolapse does occur, it is quite a nuisance to the patient and surgical treatment is frequently requested. In my hands, this has usually taken the form of a resection

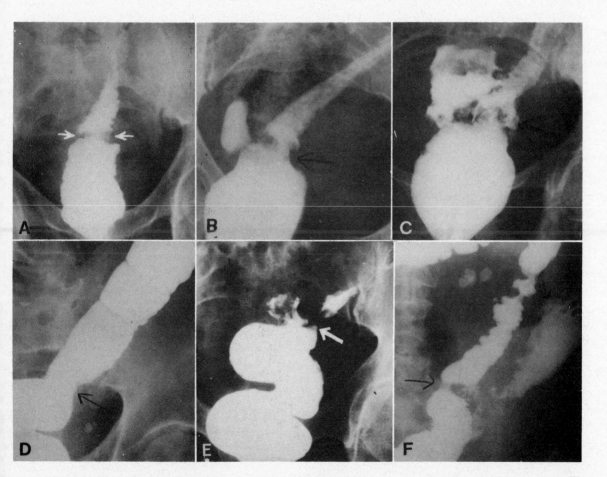

Fig. 488. Barium enema studies made 14 days after anterior resection. (A) Normal well healed anastomosis (indicated by arrow) after *low* resection, showing turned-in flange of tissue. (B) Small leak after *low* resection. (C) Gross leakage after *low* resection. (D) Normal completely healed anastomosis after *high* resection. (E) Small leak after *high* resection showing as a protruding knuckle of barium on right side. (F) Gross leakage after *high* anterior resection. (*From Goligher et al. 1970*)

of the terminal prolapsing portion of the colon through the original separate small wound in the parietes for the colostomy. With the colostomy in a prolapsed state, a circumcision is made at its base accurately on the mucocutaneous junction. The cut is deepened through the outer tube of bowel on to the inner tube and the mesocolon; they can then be drawn down through the hole in the parietal peritoneum and musculoaponeurotic layers till all slack colon has been brought to the exterior. A point on the colon 12–18 mm beyond the level of the anterior abdominal skin is chosen as the site for division of the bowel; the mesocolon is doubly clamped, divided and tied up to this point; the colon is then transected. The size of the hole in the musculoaponeurosis is gauged with the fingers. If it takes more than two with ease, it should be narrowed to this size by insertion of interrupted No. 1 or 2 chromic catgut stitches as required. The cut end of the colon is then sutured circumferentially to the skin edge of the small circular cutaneous wound with fine silk or chromic catgut sutures, and finally an adherent plastic colostomy bag is applied. The immediate results of this operation have invariably been excellent, but one patient returned after two years with a recurrence of the prolapse and had a further resection of another 17·5 cm of colon by the same technique.

COMPLICATIONS RELATING TO THE ANASTOMOSIS AFTER ANTERIOR RESECTION

SEPARATION OF THE SUTURE LINE WITH OR WITHOUT THE FORMATION OF A FAECAL FISTULA

Incidence and Severity
A partial dehiscence of the anastomosis is not at all uncommon after this operation, but the exact frequency is not appreciated unless a careful rectal examination with the finger, the sigmoidoscope and a barium (or gastrografin) enema is carried out as a routine during the postoperative period. Thus, in a group of 135 of my patients recently treated by anterior resection mainly for carcinoma or diverticular disease (84 by high resection, 51 by low resection), assessment of the state of the anastomosis along these lines (Goligher et al. 1977a) showed evidence of dehiscence in roughly 35·6% (6·6% clinical; 27% radiological). The great frequency of breakdown after *low* resection —amounting to 49% of the cases submitted to

this type of operation—accorded well with my previous impression (Goligher 1951b, 1958, 1962; Goligher et al. 1970), though the incidence was even higher than I had imagined. 16% of these breakdowns were of a major kind and were detected on simple digital or sigmoidoscopic examination, being *nearly always located in the posterior part of the bowel circumference*. Radiological study in these cases was superfluous as a rule in making a diagnosis of dehiscence, but it provided a useful permanent record of the severity of the leak (Fig. 488) and in addition showed another 33% of patients had sub-clinical leaks. The surprising finding in this study was that dehiscence, usually of a less extensive kind, occurred not infrequently also after *high* resection (Fig. 488)—actually in 20% of the patients so treated (1·2% clinical; 18·8% radiological). I had hitherto believed that after this type of resection uneventful healing of the anastomosis was well nigh inevitable (Goligher 1962). This opinion had been based on simple clinical observations, supplemented by some sporadic sigmoidoscopic examinations, which usually failed to demonstrate any definite breach of the suture line. What was mainly responsible for securing the full measure of dehiscence after high resection in this inquiry was the routine use of radiological examination after an opaque enema. However, it could well be argued that, because most of these smaller dehiscences were detected radio-logically and not clinically, they were of little practical significance.

Aetiology and Prevention
It would be reasonable to wonder whether the *technique of suture* might not influence the frequency of anastomotic breakdown. Till fairly recently most surgeons probably preferred a conventional two-layer inverting technique of suture, but in recent years a one-layer inverting technique has been strongly recommended by several authors. Everett (1975) reported the results of a well controlled trial of one- and two-layer methods of suture for anterior resection. This confirmed the findings of an earlier controlled trial (Irvin and Goligher 1975) that, so far as *high* anterior resection is concerned, there was virtually no difference in the incidence of anastomotic leakage according to whether a one- or two-layer technique had been employed. But with *low* anterior resection, there was a significant difference in favour of one-layer suture, with a dehiscence rate of 18·2% for this technique as against 50% for the two-layer technique, most of the dehiscences after either method being detected only on radiological study. At about the same time Matheson and Irvin (1975) recorded their uncontrolled experience with a one-layer technique of anastomosis in 52 consecutive cases of anterior resection, using radiological assessment of the results, with a dehiscence rate of only 5–7%. Admittedly their series included a large number of high anterior resections which might be partly responsible for these relatively more favourable results. Another point to mention is that Matheson and Irving's (1975) technique of one-layer suture was different from Everett's (1975) in that the

sutures were placed from outside, they did not include the mucosa and the knots were tied on the serosal aspect, whilst in Everett's (1975) technique—and ours—the sutures included all coats, and were inserted from inside the lumen with the knots tied on the mucosal aspect.

But still more recently the results of our controlled trial of one-layer and two-layer suture for high and low anterior resection have become available (Goligher et al. 1977b). They surprisingly show a slight advantage for the two-layer technique for both high and low resection. Why there should be this partial conflict of findings with those of Everett (1975) is difficult to understand but, on the evidence available, it would seem reasonable for the average surgeon to adopt either one- or two-layer suture technique for anterior resection according to his personal preference.

When a two-layer technique is chosen, many surgeons favour a continuous inner all-coats suture of catgut and an outer row of interrupted non-absorbable sutures (see Figs 311–316). But in this connection a recent controlled trial by Clark et al. (1977) is of interest. They compared catgut and Dexon for the inner layer of the anastomosis and found a significantly lower incidence of anastomotic dehiscence in the Dexon group. When a single-layer technique of suture is employed many different non-absorbable suture materials have been used. Kratzer and Onsanit (1974) and Trimpi et al. (1976) make strong claims for interrupted stainless steel wire inserted in the way that Matheson and Irving (1975) placed the braided nylon sutures in their anastomoses (see above) but their clinical comparison of dehiscence rates with other materials is uncontrolled.

It is also appropriate to mention that our incidence of dehiscence after using the suture gun (see p. 570) was nil in 38 cases done by high resection and six in 24 cases given low resections—results which seem to contrast quite favourably with ours for hand suture for these operations, though of course the number of cases is as yet small and the comparison is not based on a controlled trial (Goligher et al. 1979).

Apart from the differences in the suture of the anorectal stump in high and low resections, other factors have been incriminated by various authors to account for the greater incidence of dehiscence after the low operation. Boxall et al. 1963) suggested that the *blood supply to the rectal stump* is poorer after low resection than after high resection, because in the former operation the lateral ligaments with their contained middle haemorrhoidal vessels are sacrificed. Frankly, I am not convinced that ischaemia of the rectal stump can often have been the cause of dehiscence in my cases of low resection, for usually when the rectum was being divided its cut edge bled freely, sometimes embarrassingly so.

As a consequence of the thorough mobilization of the rectum from its sacral bed in low anterior resection—something which is avoided in high anterior resection—extensive raw areas are created in the pelvis, from which an abundant exudate is likely to accumulate in the pelvis, especially if the pelvic peritoneum has been sutured. Previously (Goligher 1962), I thought that *bursting of the pelvic exudate through the suture line* into the rectal lumen might be an additional cause of dehiscence after low anterior resection. But in all the patients in the study quoted (Goligher et al 1977b) the pelvic peritoneum was not sutured and suprapubic suction drainage was maintained for four or five days, with-drawing considerable quantities of serosanguineous fluid. It seems hard to believe, therefore, that accumulation of exudate in the pelvis and its rupturing through the suture line played a significant part in the production of dehiscence.

Another factor that may also predispose to the occurrence of dehiscence after either low or high anterior resection is the presence of a substantial degree of *faecal loading* at the time of operation (Goligher et al. 1970). If such faecal accumulation can be avoided by preoperative mechanical preparation (p. 447), this should help to lessen the incidence of major dehiscence. But it should be noted that even when a *preliminary* transverse colostomy has been established and anterior resection is per-formed in a completely empty 'defunctioned' distal colon and rectum, anastomotic dehiscence sometimes occurs (Goligher et al. 1970). As for *simultaneous* transverse colostomy, performed at the conclusion of the resection, obviously there may be a fair amount of faeces in the left colon between it and the anasto-mosis. Though the colostomy will obviate further entry of flatus and faeces into this distal segment, it cannot prevent the passage through the anastomosis in due course of the initial faecal column. Thus the possible protection for the suture line pro-vided by a simultaneous colostomy ought theoretically to be less than that afforded by a preliminary colostomy, and it is to be noted that the high incidence of dehiscence after low resection in our study (Goligher et al. 1977b) occurred despite the fact that a simultaneous transverse colostomy was established in most of these patients. Perhaps the main value of a colostomy at the conclusion of an anterior resection is not so much to prevent dehiscence, as to facilitate its management, if it should occur. If a gross degree of faecal loading is encountered at laparotomy in a patient otherwise suitable for anterior resection, the best plan is to perform only a right transverse colostomy and to reserve the resection for a subsequent occasion, or to abandon resection entirely in favour of a one-stage abdominoperineal excision with terminal iliac colostomy (but see p. 440).

The evidence as to the influence of *preoperative preparation with bowel antiseptics* on the incidence of anastomotic dehiscence is complicating. Herter and Slanetz (1967) thought from a retro-spective study that preparation by these agents had little effect on the incidence of septic complications—presumed to be due to anastomotic leaks—after high resection, but did seem to diminish their frequency after low resection. But in our study (Goligher et al. 1970) the incidence of objectively demonstrated dehiscences after high resection was significantly less when intestinal antiseptics had been employed, whilst the incidence in low resection cases was unaffected by their use.

The possible bearing of *postoperative drainage* of the anastomotic site and of *administration of neostigmine* by the anaesthetist at the conclusion of the operation to reverse the action of relaxant drugs is discussed on p. 437.

Management

In the treatment of separation of the suture line no active measures are required as a rule, if there has been no suprapubic leakage of faeces along the drain track. Indeed, it is remarkable how innocuous this complication often seems to be. The presacral cavity slowly fills with granulation tissue, so that after three weeks or so the only indication that there has been a breakdown is a deep puckering on the posterior part of the anastomotic line. If a faecal fistula is present, this may close spontaneously after a week or so if the discharge is slight, but if much faeces is escaping or if the gap in the suture line is large, it will be necessary to proceed to a transverse colostomy (if this was not established at the time of the resection) in order to induce the fistula to close. In fact it is *probably quickest in every case complicated by faecal fistulation to carry out a transverse colostomy without further delay.* After diversion of the faeces has thus been achieved, the further care resolves itself essentially into daily irrigations of the left colon from the colostomy to the anus and vice versa. A useful manoeuvre for the latter is to pass a narrow-bore sigmoidoscope per anum into the presacral cavity—and it often lies exactly in the axis of instrumentation—and to irrigate directly into the cavity through it. It may take three to six weeks at least before it is considerd safe to close the colostomy. It is not necessary to wait till the cavity has completely closed; it suffices that the cavity should have acquired a firm lining of granulations and that a wash through from colostomy to anus and in the reverse direction should not leak suprapubically.

PELVIC ABSCESS AND PERITONITIS

A pelvic abscess may form and, if so, it is usually found in association with some separation of the suture line, though which of these occurrences is the primary event is difficult to be sure (see p. 436). The treatment is as for breakdown of the anastomosis in general (see above). Sometimes, however, the abscess bursts into the vagina. When this happens, a transverse colostomy should be established without delay and irrigations started from the colostomy and the anus to secure speedy healing and avoid the development of a permanent rectovaginal fistula. I have had three temporary rectovaginal fistulas, all of which closed spontaneously on this regimen; Cullen and Mayo (1963) report a similar incidence of this complication.

A great deal of separation of the suture line with resulting leakage and sepsis in the pelvis may occur without general peritoneal infection. But occasionally peritonitis results and may be fatal as it was in 6 of my 553 cases treated by anterior resection, and in 12 of Mayo's 424 cases submitted to this operation (Cullen and Mayo 1963). The condition may be overlooked clinically or misdiagnosed as one of paralytic ileus, but, if recognized, it should be treated by further laparotomy and drainage, as well as transverse colostomy, if one is not already present. Occasionally the more drastic manoeuvre of completing the separation of the anastomosis and bringing the iliac colon out as a terminal colostomy, in the manner of a Hartmann's operation, may be preferred (see also pp. 514, 592).

STRICTURE

During the first few weeks after anterior resection there is almost invariably some narrowing at the site of anastomosis, which is easily appreciated by the examining finger. In the course of time, due to the dilating effect of the motions, this stenosis gradually disappears in the majority of cases, so that after six months or a year it may be very difficult on digital and sigmoidoscopic examination to determine the exact site of the anastomosis. A fine white fibrous line can usually be seen and felt with the end of the sigmoidoscope but there is no actual constriction. In some cases, however, the initial stenosis, instead of dilating fully, persists or becomes more marked. These are mostly patients who have had some breakdown of the anastomosis and have had to have a temporary transverse colostomy. But even they, in my experience, eventually undergo spontaneous dilatation of their strictures in time unless the breakdown has been completely or almost completely circumferential. It is only in this latter group that instrumental dilatation with double-ended Hegar's dilators is usually required. I have had 6 such patients in my group of 553 cases treated by anterior resection. The need for caution in performing dilatation is indicated by the fact that, in doing so in one case, I split the stricture and opened the rectum into the peritoneal cavity. Though an immediate laparotomy was carried out to close the rent and drain the site, a series of complications occurred from which he eventually died. In two other cases I was unable to keep the stricture dilated by regular instrumentation and had eventually to perform an abdominoperineal excision with establishment of a permanent iliac colostomy.

LOCAL RECURRENCE (see also p. 399)

In the earlier days of anterior resection local recurrence was found to be not an uncommon complication of this operation. The recurrent growths were located sometimes in the tissues of the pelvis entirely outside the bowel, sometimes in the bowel wall itself, usually in the region of the suture line, and sometimes in both situations. However, local recurrences now seem to be much less common than formerly, possibly due to the more radical type of resection now in vogue and also to the precautions that are now usually taken to guard against implantation of malignant cells on the suture line at the time of operation (pp. 444, 564). In order to recognize such recurrences as early as possible it is desirable that every patient treated by resection should be subjected to regular review including *sigmoidoscopy at three-monthly intervals* for the first two or three years. Any doubtful thickening or ulceration of the anastomotic line should be biopsied. In the majority of cases this will show only inflammatory changes, due to a granulomatous reaction around a non-absorbable suture.

In the treatment of local recurrence after anastomotic operations it is occasionally possible to carry out a further excision by the abdomino-perineal technique—albeit with considerable difficulty because of fixation—with some prospect of lasting cure, but more usually the condition is quite inoperable on account of local fixity and other evidences of spread. Thus in my group of 16 patients with known local recurrence after anterior resection four were treated by further excision with one five-year cure. Black and Kelly (1955) and Lofgren et al. (1957) of the Mayo Clinic have examined the therapeutic problems of local recurrence after anterior resection. The latter authors mention that of a group of 108 patients with recurrent sigmoidal and rectal cancer, only 37 underwent further excision, often with the utmost technical difficulty, and with many early deaths. Radiotherapy was frequently used in the inoperable cases with some improvement. Vandertoll and Beahrs (1965) point out that more than 80% of the patients developing anastomotic recurrences after anterior resection at the Mayo Clinic have died of their disease.

INCONTINENCE

As mentioned on pp. 312 and 514, a crucial consideration in regard to the quality of continence after anterior resection would appear to be the length of the remaining stump of anorectum (Goligher 1951*b*; Goligher et al. 1965). If it is *7 cm or more*, as measured postoperatively, from the anal verge—and most anterior resections, even under the most favourable technical circumstances, leave a distal stump of 8–10 cm—function is well-nigh perfect in most cases. However, owing to the loss of the sigmoid reservoir for faeces, motions are passed more frequently, usually after every meal at first, but this gradually corrects itself in time so that eventually the frequency is reduced to once or twice per day or the patient may even be constipated. Just occasionally in very old infirm subjects anterior resection is followed by some degree of incontinence which is probably due to the effects of senility aggravated by the operation. A daily enema to clear the bowel regularly may be useful in diminishing leakage. If the anorectal remnant is *6 cm or less*—and this is more apt to be the case after particularly low resections using the stapling gun—there is often initially considerable frequency of

defaecation and some impairment of control for flatus and liquid faeces. But in three to six months time this usually rectifies itself, though a few patients may suffer some permanent incontinence (Goligher et al. 1979).

COMPLICATIONS RELATING TO THE CARE OF THE COLON STUMP AFTER PULL-THROUGH ABDOMINOANAL EXCISION

There are five main complications peculiar to the particular form of rectal excision, though there are considerable variations in their relative frequencies in the hands of different surgeons, as is shown by the detailed reports of Bacon (1956), Waugh and Turner (1958), Black and Botham (1958), Hughes et al. (1962), Goligher et al. (1965), Kratzer (1967, 1969), Kennedy et al. (1970) and Wenckert (1970).

NECROSIS OR RETRACTION OF COLON

It is not uncommon to find some sloughing occurring in the terminal 1–2 cm of the colon stump (even proximal to the ligature holding the Malecot catheter in position), but this need not occasion any alarm provided there is a good projection of viable bowel beyond the edge of the everted anorectal stump. Unfortunately, sometimes necrosis is more extensive and stretches upwards to involve the colon as it lies within the grip of the anorectal remnant or even more proximally. Needless to say, this is a potentially serious state of affairs, for it introduces the risk of pelvic infection or even peritonitis. Unquestionably, major necrosis of the colon stump has been the major problem after the pull-through operation in my experience and occurred in roughly 20% of my 59 patients. What has made it such a disturbing and perplexing complication is that we have not been able to predict with any reliability the patients who might be thus affected. In some cases colon stumps which were clearly viable at the time of operation, as shown by their colour and the presence of pulsation in the intramural vessels or of brisk arterial bleeding from them on incision, have subsequently developed necrosis; whilst in other patients colon which has given rise to a little anxiety at the time of operation, because of its somewhat dubious blood supply, has subsequently survived without incident. It would be natural to wonder whether constriction of the colon stump by the anal sphincters might not be responsible for the latter necrosis. It is to be noted, however, that in our patients the sphincters were very thoroughly stretched at the operation, and further, that in most instances the gangrene extended a variable distance into the pelvis—up to but never above the pelvic peritoneal floor.

A factor that may be important in the aetiology of stump necrosis is the amount of faecal content in the colon at the time of operation, for in retrospect it is notable that a high proportion of our patients who later developed major necrosis had had pronounced faecal loading at the time of operation (Goligher et al. 1965). Admittedly, it is difficult to understand how such distension with faeces could operate to impair viability of the colon stump, except by compressing the gut wall against the sphincter ring or the aperture in the pelvic peritoneum; but, as already pointed out, the area of major gangrene usually extended *above* the sphincters but only occasionally reached to the level of the peritoneum. However, as a precaution against this possible causal factor, I have in recent cases established a covering right transverse colostomy at the conclusion of a pull-through excision unless the colon is particularly empty, and this is now also Turnbull's (1964) practice.

Apparently I have been unusually unfortunate in regard to the occurrence of stump necrosis, for other surgeons have had a much lower incidence. Thus Bacon (1956) states that in only six of his series of 660 pull-through operations did high necrosis occur, Black and Botham (1958) had some sloughing in 21 of 114 cases, but in only four did it extend high enough to disrupt the continuity of the bowel. Waugh and Turner (1958) report some measure of gangrene of the transplanted colon with retraction into the pelvis in 36 of their 268 patients treated by pull-through excision, but the complication was apparently minimal in all except two cases. Kratzer (1967) appears to have had only one major colonic necrosis—which was fatal—in 80 patients and Kirwan et al (1978) also only one in 84 cases. But Kennedy et al. (1970) noted major sloughing of the colon stump in seven of their 158 cases. It would seem also that most of these authors have been more fortunate as regards treatment of the complication, for in no instance did Bacon (1956) find it necessary to undertake any emergency operation such as proximal colostomy, Black and Botham (1958) had to establish colostomy in three of their cases, and Waugh and Turner (1958) resorted to a permanent colostomy in two patients. But in three of Kennedy et al.'s (1970) cases with colonic necrosis a fatal peritonitis developed. In our first case with this complication we contented ourselves with the formation of a proximal loop transverse colostomy, but there was prolonged pelvic sepsis, and the subsequent conversion to a terminal left iliac colostomy was a very difficult manoeuvre, which was followed by the development of a small bowel faecal fistula for a time. In subsequent cases with major stump necrosis we have preferred to re-intervene, as soon as a confident diagnosis of gangrene could be made, to carry out what is in effect a second-stage abdomino-perineal excision. In the abdominal phase the colon is divided flush with the reconstituted pelvic peritoneal floor and a terminal left iliac colostomy is established. The bowel below the pelvic floor is removed from the perineum after the anus and rectal stump have been circumcised. Pelvic sepsis was frequent following this procedure; it usually cleared in three to four weeks, but lasted several months in one case. Fortunately we have lost only two of our 10 patients with this complication.

One of the difficulties, incidentally, in managing colon necrosis is to recognize the onset of gangrene from the colour changes evident on the serosal aspect of the colon stump. Usually the bowel presents a slightly oedematous, dull, brick-red appearance for two or three days, after which it may slowly exhibit frank changes of necrosis, or may continue to survive. In a few cases sigmoidoscopy was used, in the hope that the appearances of gangrene might be more distinctive on the mucosal aspect and their proximal extent more easily judged, but the findings did not prove very reliable.

PELVIC (PRESACRAL) INFECTION

This is the complication most frequently recorded after pull-through excision and occurred in 5% of Bacon's (1956) cases, in about 12% of Black and Botham's (1958), in 20·9% of Waugh and Turner's (1958), and in some 17% of Hughes et al.'s (1962). It usually responds to conservative management (unless there is necrosis of the colon extending up into the pelvis), but occasionally a temporary transverse colostomy is necessary. In my own cases pelvic infection was confined almost entirely to patients with extensive gangrene of the colon, and *if the bowel remained viable the convalescence was astonishingly smooth and uneventful, as a rule.*

FAECAL FISTULAS

Various types of fistula are liable to develop after pull-through excision and are reported in 0·5% of Bacon's (1956) series, in 3% of Waugh and Turner's (1958), in 4% of Kennedy et al.'s (1970), in 1% of Kratzer's (1967) and in 1·5% of mine. The most frequent type is a rectovaginal fistula, which may close spontaneously or may require the provision of a temporary right transverse colostomy to secure its healing.

STRICTURE

Though this sequel has been glossed over by some of the authors quoted above, it is in fact a not infrequent occurrence after the pull-through operation, especially when done by the technique favoured by Bacon (1945) and Waugh and Turner (1958), with coring out of the mucocutaneous lining of the anal canal before the colon is drawn through. Black and Botham (1958) reported the late development of stricturing in three patients in their series. Kennedy et al. (1970) admit to 28 strictures in 158 cases treated by the Turnbull–Cutait method, and we had six strictures in 59 patients treated by the same method. All the narrowings in my cases have been satisfactorily corrected by periodic dilatation.

INCONTINENCE

It is very difficult to compare our findings (Goligher et al. 1965) in regard to rectal function after the pull-through operation with those reported by other surgeons because of differences in the criteria of assessment and mode of expression of the degree of control obtained. Turnbull and Cuthbertson (1961) do not comment at all on the functional results. We find it impossible to interpret the results reported by Bacon (1956) and Hughes et al. (1962) in terms similar to those applied to our cases. Black and Botham (1958), whose operative technique preserved the lining of the anal canal, claimed *full* continence for 92% of their patients and Wenckert (1970) roughly similar results for his very much smaller series of cases treated by the same technique. Waugh and Turner (1958), who mostly used the Bacon (1945) method of denuding the canal of its lining, found only 9% of their patients to be completely continent, but Kratzer (1967, 1969) reported that 34% of his patients managed by this method had normal control. Kennedy et al. (1970) found that 29% of their patients had reasonable control but some defects, and 23% were quite unsatisfactory from the point of view of function. They stressed, as do Bennett et al. (1972), the tendency towards improvement in continence up to two or more years after operation. Kirwan et al. (1978) report good if not quite perfect continence in about 60% of their 84 patients one year or more after the Turnbull–Cutait operation. We have to report that only 25% of our patients, after pull-through excision of this type, are fully continent for flatus, and only 39% have perfect continence for faeces at all times. As regards the 61% of patients who could not always control faeces, and mostly wore a perineal pad, we were surprised to discover that the majority were reasonably satisfied with the result of their operation. They may have what amounts to little more than a perineal colostomy, but most of them seem to be able to regulate it fairly well either with dietetic management or with irrigations. However, a few of these persons have found it extremely difficult to organize their bowel actions in this way, and may spend up to $1\frac{1}{2}$ hours daily cleaning up after four to six motions have escaped on to their pad; two of them experienced such trouble that they were eventually converted to abdominal colostomies, which they found much more manageable and satisfactory.

Analysis of the causes of indifferent function after this operation in our cases (Goligher et al. 1965) revealed that most of the poor functional results occurred in patients with short anorectal stumps—usually less than 6 or 7 cm postoperatively from the anal verge. Patients with longer stumps than this generally had a satisfactory degree of continence. In the light of this experience, we came to the conclusion that if a stump of at least 6–7 cm could not be preserved in a pull-through excision (or a low anterior resection) the patient would, apart from psychological considerations, be better treated by abdomino-perineal excision. However, this may be an oversimplification because more recent experience with abdominotransanal and abdominosacral resections (see pp. 509, 513) shows that good control can often be obtained with anorectal stumps as short as 4 cm or less.

COMPLICATIONS RELATING TO THE ANASTOMOSIS AFTER ABDOMINOTRANSANAL RESECTION

Our information regarding the complications arising in connection with the anastomosis after this technique of resection is relatively limited at the moment and has already been briefly outlined on p. 513.

COMPLICATIONS RELATING TO THE ANASTOMOSIS AFTER ABDOMINOSACRAL RESECTION

These are sufficiently indicated on p. 509.

INTESTINAL OBSTRUCTION

PARALYTIC ILEUS

This is the usual cause of small gut obstruction after rectal excision. Formerly very common, it is now much less frequent. It is to be suspected when the patient develops nausea, vomiting and abdominal distension during the first two or three days after operation, and the colostomy fails to act or to pass flatus. The treatment now usually favoured follows well recognized conservative lines, consisting of the passage of a nasal gastric tube and institution of intermittent or continuous suction, the administration of intravenous fluids, and the use of small doses of sedatives such as morphine or pethidine as frequently as required. Small amounts of fluid may be allowed by mouth for psychological reasons and to moisten the tongue. The basic intravenous fluid should be $N/5$ saline, of which 2–5.5 litres may be given in the 24 hours. In addition losses by vomiting or gastric suction should be made good by administration of equal quantities of N saline in the intravenous 'drip'.

Once a free diuresis has been secured 2–4 g of potassium chloride should be added to the infusing fluid per day. An accurate record must be kept of fluid and electrolytes administered and fluids passed or withdrawn, and it is useful though not essential to have daily estimations of the plasma electrolytes as a guide in determining the composition and amount of the intravenous infusate. Attempts may be made to stimulate the colon to activity by enemas, wash-outs or bisacodyl suppositories given into the colostomy, but the consensus of surgical opinion is against the use of drugs such as prostigmine to provoke peristalsis, for though they may produce vigorous peristalic activity temporarily, as revealed by ausculation or by the escape of flatus or faeces from the colostomy, this is apt to be followed by further ileus. I must admit, however, that I have occasionally used stimulant tactics when the period of ileus has been very prolonged and sometimes had quite dramatic and sustained good results with them. But probably the best policy, as a rule, is to refrain from such efforts at stimulation and continue with a strictly passive regimen. The cessation of the ileus is indicated by the great diminution in the quantities of aspirate removed from the upper alimentary tract. More fluids may then be allowed by mouth and the frequency of aspirations reduced. Shortly afterwards the colostomy may act spontaneously or in response to a suppository or wash-out.

More recently Catchpole's (1969) work has revived interest in the stimulant mode of management of paralytic ileus. He has suggested that if the use of parasympatheticomimetic drugs, such as neostigmine, is preceded by the administration of sympathetic blocking drugs, such as guanethidine or phenotolamine, a much more prolonged restoration of peristalsis is obtained. In the routine recommended by him 20 mg of guanethidine (or 20 mg of phentolamine) are injected intravenously in a saline infusion over a period of 40 minutes. When bowel sounds are well established, the neostigmine is given intravenously in a dose of 0.05 mg every three to four minutes up to a total of 0.5 mg. A careful watch is kept on the blood pressure and pulse rate and the patient is confined to bed for 24 hours. Catchpole (1969) has claimed good results with this method of treating established paralytic ileus and has even suggested that it might be extended to patients who are slow to develop normal bowel activity after laparotomy. But Heimbach and Crout (1971), who conducted a controlled trial of the Catchpole regimen (using bethanidine sulphate 30 mg in 150 ml of dextrose water instead of guanethidine, which is unavailable in the U.S.A.) could not demonstrate that it had any advantages over neostigmine alone.

MECHANICAL OBSTRUCTION

A true mechanical obstruction occurs as a post-operative complication or later sequel of combined excision of the rectum far more often than after most other abdominal operations. Thus Goligher et al. (1951b) reported an incidence of mechanical intestinal obstruction of approximately 3% in a series of 1302 cases followed up after combined excision of the rectum at St Mark's Hospital. The particular predisposition to obstruction after combined excision is due to the fact that, in addition to the ordinary risks of developing adhesions to the anterior parietal wound or between adjacent coils of gut, special hazards exist in regard to the suture line in the pelvic peritoneal floor, the colostomy site and the terminal ileum. A loop of small gut may become adherent to the pelvic peritoneum at the site of suture, usually at its upper end, and very occasionally a knuckle of bowel may be herniated through the peritoneal floor. In the vicinity of the colostomy a coil of gut may become adherent to the parietes or to the edge of the mesocolon as it runs forwards with the colon stump; in addition small bowel may become strangulated in the paracolic gutter or lateral space on the outer side of the colostomy (Fig. 489), if this has not been securely closed by a non-absorbable suture or otherwise obliterated at the original operation. Lastly, the terminal ileum may be kinked by the drag on an ileal band during suture of the pelvic peritoneal floor, with resulting obstruction (Fig. 490). Some of these dangers can possibly be lessened by attention to the initial operative technique—as by closure of the lateral space or complete extra-peritonealization of the colon stump, by care in the suture of the pelvic peritoneum to bring the upper surfaces into apposition and turn the free edges downwards towards the pelvis, and by division of any taut ileal band—but some risk of post-operative obstruction presumably remains.

Diagnosis

Recognition of *late obstructions*, arising after the patient has been discharged from hospital, is usually straightforward. The sudden onset and persistence of abdominal pain and vomiting, and the cessation of colostomy actions at this stage admit of no other explanation than that of a mechanical obstruction, and the patient is usually transferred to hospital without delay for further operative treatment. However, I have known of cases where it was assumed that the obstruction was probably due to malignant deposits in the peritoneum to which a loop of small bowel had become adherent and kinked, and operation was withheld. At autopsy the obstructing lesion was shown to be a

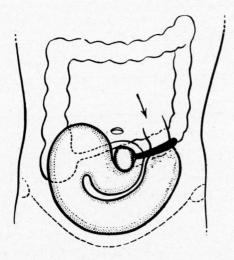

Fig. 489. Mechanism of strangulation of a loop of small gut in the lateral or paracolostomy space. (*From Goligher et al. 1951b*)

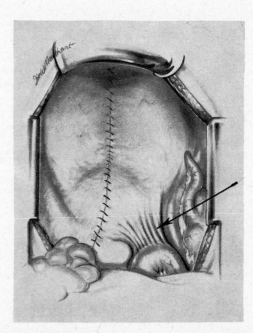

Fig. 490. Kinking of terminal ileum by the drag on an ileal band (arrowed) during suture of the pelvic peritoneum after combined excision. (*From Goligher et al. 1951b*)

simple fibrous adhesion, which could easily have been divided at laparotomy, and there was no evidence of local recurrence or remote metastases!

The diagnosis and management of *obstructions in the immediate postoperative period* after combined excision is much more difficult because of the confusion that often exists at this stage with paralytic ileus. Classically, cases with mechanical obstruction differ from those with adynamic ileus in that they have intestinal colic and the symptoms originate not immediately after operation but some days later after the patient has already had one or more bowel actions. In my experience, however, such a clear distinction is not always possible. Some patients with mechanical obstruction do not have colicky pains and on auscultation of their abdomens no exaggerated peristalsis can be detected but only faint tinkling sounds such as are often present in cases of paralytic ileus. Further, it often happens that the obstructive symptoms commence soon after operation without any latent interval, presumably because the mechanical obstruction has supervened on a pre-existing ileus. A striking feature of obstruction cases, however, is that with gastric suction and intravenous fluids the symptoms may subside and the colostomy even act slightly for a time, only to be followed in a day or two by further obstructive symptoms. These in turn may also respond temporarily to conservative measures only to recur later. This intermittency of symptoms is always very suggestive of a mechanical obstruction. Radiological examination of the abdomen is not usually very helpful in distinguishing between a mechanical obstruction and paralytic ileus, for both conditions give gaseous distension of the small intestine with fluid levels, but sometimes when a strangulation obstruction is present the strangulated loop may be recognizable radiologically as a specially distended loop. In doubtful cases the rare possibility of prolapse and strangulation of a knuckle of bowel through the pelvic peritoneal floor should be borne in mind; it can sometimes be excluded by passing a sterile sigmoidoscope into the perineal wound and inspecting the suture line.

Treatment

Management is along conservative lines in the first instance, with gastric suction and intravenous fluids, till a definite decision is reached as to the presence of a mechanical obstruction. Once this diagnosis is made the abdomen should be opened, preferably through the previous left paramedian incision, and the various lesions encountered dealt with appropriately, adhesions being divided, hernias reduced and kinkings corrected.

In cases with strangulation in the paracolostomy or lateral space it might be anticipated that in order to secure reduction of the strangulated ileal coils it would sometimes be necessary to break the constricting ring by dividing the iliac colon between clamps applied close to the anterior parietal peritoneum. But despite considerable intestinal distension, reduction of the gut has always been achieved in my experience without resorting to this manoeuvre (Goligher et al. 1951*b*). The space which then remains is very large, much larger than that present normally because of the stretching of the iliac colon on its inner side, but it is usually possible to close the gap by a suitable suture technique.

URINARY RETENTION AND INCONTINENCE

Retention of urine is a common complication after rectal excision. As Watson (1951) has shown, about 50% of male patients undergoing abdominoperineal excision of the rectum have difficulty in re-establishing normal micturition following the removal of the indwelling urethral catheter on the third or fourth postoperative day. In some cases the delay in achieving a normal urinary flow is very transient and lasts for only a few days; in others it is more prolonged. Retention is less frequent but by no means uncommon after anterior resection, particularly after really low resections involving a deep pelvic dissection. It also occurs less often in women than men after either abdominoperineal excision or anterior resection.

Several factors may be responsible for the urinary retention in these postoperative cases, often more than one factor being present in any particular patient. They may be considered as follows:

POSTURAL DIFFICULTIES CONSEQUENT UPON ALTERATION IN THE ANATOMY OF THE PELVIS

After excision of the rectum the bladder and prostatic urethra drop backwards towards the sacrum from the fixed point of the membraneous urethra in the urogenital diaphragm. There is nothing in this alteration of anatomy to constitute a hindrance to the outflow of urine in the erect position, but it obviously puts the recumbent patient at a distinct disadvantage in that he has to eject urine almost vertically upwards from the bladder. This doubtless accounts in part for the marked improvement in micturition that often results when the patient becomes ambulant.

POOR PHYSIQUE AND POOR GENERAL CONDITION IN OLDER PATIENTS

The postural difficulties mentioned above call for a greater intravesical pressure than is usually required during micturition. This can be achieved either by reserves of bladder muscle power, which are absent in the elderly, or by voluntary abdominal straining, which old and ill patients may be unable to manage or disinclined to attempt.

PROSTATIC ENLARGEMENT

Some enlargement of the prostate is frequently found in older men presenting with carcinoma of the rectum, but it is often difficult to assess the part played by it in producing postoperative retention. Slight degrees of prostatic obstruction, for which the patient has completely compensated in the ordinary way, may obviously contribute to the postural and general factors, already described, in causing postoperative urinary difficulty, but once these other factors are overcome micturition as a rule rapidly returns to normal. With greater enlargement of the prostate, however, severe and prolonged retention is very liable to occur. Watson (1951) considered that prostatic obstruction was a major factor in the production of postoperative retention in seven of the 50 consecutive male patients carefully investigated by him (Watson and Williams 1952) from the urological point of view before and after combined excision of the rectum; five of these seven patients, however, eventually achieved normal micturition, and only two required prostatectomy or transurethral prostatic resection.

PELVIC NERVE INJURY

The function of micturition may be impaired by operative injury to the nerves supplying the bladder during rectal excision. It might be expected that division of the sympathetic supply—which is motor to the bladder neck and internal sphincter, and inhibitory to the detrusor muscle—might lead to frequent micturition or even actual incontinence. But after presacral neurectomy, which I have performed as a deliberate manoeuvre on several occasions during abdominoperineal excision of the rectum, and which completely interrupts the sympathetic innervation of the bladder, there are no consistent subjective disturbances of micturition

and no objective alteration of bladder function as determined by cystometry. It is injury to the parasympathetic supply—which is normally responsible for contraction of the detrusor muscle and relaxation of the bladder neck and conveys the sensation of bladder distension—that is held to be responsible for the impairment of micturition in these cases of neurogenic bladder dysfunction.

The effect of this injury is to produce a fairly characteristic clinical picture. In the first stage there is complete retention when the catheter is withdrawn after operation. No urine is passed, the bladder becomes progressively distended and in time, if the condition is allowed to continue untreated, overflow incontinence occurs. After a variable period the second stage is reached, when micturition is re-established by straining with the abdominal muscles. The residual urine is now large and usually heavily infected, and the patient is incontinent by day and night. In the course of months the quantity of residual urine diminishes till eventually it becomes negligible. The incontinence remains but is then chiefly nocturnal; this is the third stage of the condition.

The *diagnosis* is suggested by the painlessness of the distension and can be readily confirmed by cystometry, which shows that the bladder is of moderate or large capacity and the pressure within it rises steadily with increasing volume, unaccompanied by any true sensation of bladder distension. The phase of isotonic filling seen in the normal bladder is either absent or very short.

The *mechanism* of the retention–incontinence in neurogenic bladder disorders is readily explicable on the basis of a parasympathetic nerve injury. It may be that there is a concomitant injury to the sympathetic as well as to the parasympathetic supply, as a result of which the internal sphincter undergoes relaxation, though, as pointed out previously, an isolated injury of the sympathetic leaves sphincter function unaffected. But even if the internal sphincter were thus paralysed, it is remarkable that the external sphincter, the supply to which from the pudendal nerve is most unlikely to be damaged during a rectal excision operation, however extensive, does not suffice to maintain continence as it does after prostatectomy. We must suppose that its efficiency is somehow impaired by the altered disposition of the bladder and posterior urethra. It seems likely that the gradual recovery of control in these cases is due to voluntary effort and that the persistence of nocturnal incontinence may be attributed to relaxation of the voluntary muscles during sleep.

Equally unsettled is the site and mechanism of injury to the parasympathetic nerves responsible for the pelvic nerve syndrome. The nerves in question are the three nervi erigentes arising from the second, third and fourth sacral nerves on either side and running laterally and forwards to join the corresponding branch of the presacral nerve to form the pelvic plexus on the side-wall of the pelvis. From this plexus mixed sympathetic and parasympathetic fibres proceed medially to the various pelvic organs including the bladder and seminal vesicles. Once the parasympathetic filaments reach the pelvic side-wall it is a little difficult to see how they can be completely divided during rectal excision, except by the most radical dissection involving a very wide removal of both lateral ligaments and a bilateral dissection of the internal iliac lymph glands. With any less extensive operation it would seem that some of the parasympathetic innervation to the bladder must escape injury and, as Watson (1951) has pointed out, *many of the patients who develop neurogenic bladder disorders have not had specially difficult or wide dissections.* He suggests that the site of the injury to the parasympathetic may be posteriorly, at the stems of the nervi erigentes close to their origin from the sacral nerves. According to Ashley and Anson (1946), these nerves penetrate the fascia of Waldeyer very soon after their commencement, so that, if the perineal operator were to strike a faulty plane of dissection from below and instead of dividing the fascia of Waldeyer at the tip of the coccyx were to proceed upwards in the plane between the sacrum and the fascia, avulsion of the nervi erigentes would appear inevitable. I am not satisfied that this is the usual mechanism of injury, for I have seen the pelvic nerve syndrome arise in cases where I had personally performed the perineal dissection and taken care to divide the fascia correctly, and also in some cases treated by low anterior resection where of course there was no perineal dissection at all.

There is some difference of opinion as to the frequency of pelvic nerve injury as a cause of urinary disorder after rectal excision. Watson (1951) and Watson and Williams (1952) in their consecutive series of 50 cases treated by abdominoperineal excision, and specially investigated by cystometry, found only two examples of the characteristic syndrome, though Watson (1951) wondered whether partial parasympathetic denervation might not be a factor in some other cases with postoperative urinary retention in this group of patients. By contrast, on the basis of cystometric and urethral flow measurements, Rankin (1969) was able to demonstrate evidence of pelvic nerve damage on cystometry in some 25 of 96 patients and Fowler (1973) in eight of 28 patients in the immediate postoperative period after this operation.

MANAGEMENT OF URINARY RETENTION

If there is complete retention on removal of the indwelling catheter on the fourth day, the patient may be well enough to stand out of bed in order to assist micturition, or he may manage to kneel in bed, which may be helpful. One or two injections of 500 μg of distigmine may be effective, but, if these measures do not succeed, there should be no further delay in reinserting a Foley catheter before the bladder becomes unduly distended. This is best left *in situ* for a further four or five days, by which time the patient may be ambulant and is then likely to micturate without difficulty. Repeated removal and reinsertion of the catheter at short intervals is pointless; it causes considerable urethral trauma and the recurring failure to void naturally is bad for the patient's morale.

If urine is passed after withdrawing the catheter, it is advisable to estimate the residual urine 12–24 hours later, however satisfactory micturition seems to be. A large and increasing residuum may cause no symptoms until there is gross distension or even overflow. If the residual urine is more than 150 ml, it should be removed once or twice per day according to its volume. And, if there is no improvement within two or three days, a further period of continuous drainage is indicated.

Persistent retention is rarely worth investigating whilst the patient is still in bed, for it so frequently clears up once the patient is ambulant. But if complete retention or a large volume of residual urine persists after the patient has been up for several days, investigation will be required by cystoscopy and cystometry to determine the presence of prostatic enlargement or pelvic nerve injury. It is usually best at this stage to invite a urological colleague to take over the management of these patients from the urinary aspect. If *enlargement of the prostate* is considered to be a factor, it may very conveniently be treated by transurethral resection, or a formal prostatectomy may be advised. There need, however, be no urgency about the latter, and, if desired on general grounds, the operation may be postponed for several weeks, the patient meanwhile being maintained on an indwelling Foley catheter. *With pelvic nerve* disruption considerable spontaneous improvement takes place as the patient learns to empty the bladder by straining. Distigmine 5 mg given orally three times a day may also be helpful. Whilst incontinence is occurring, an appliance may have to be worn on the penis to keep the patient dry. Patients with a *combination of prostatic enlargement and pelvic nerve injury* present a difficult urological problem. In some of them a judicious transurethral resection may be beneficial, but if it is overdone their incontinence may be aggravated.

PRELIMINARY OR SIMULTANEOUS PROSTATECTOMY

From the foregoing remarks it will be seen that most patients with associated prostatic enlargement can be successfully managed from the urological point of view during rectal excision and eventually returned to their normal preoperative urinary condition. Occasionally, however, when the patient is having severe difficulty with micturition before operation, it may be wise to undertake a *preliminary prostatectomy or transurethral resection*. I doubt if the delay of three weeks or so imposed on the eradication of the rectal carcinoma will often make any significant difference to the prognosis. It is quite possible, however, in such cases to carry out *simultaneous prostatectomy and rectal excision*, the prostate being removed by the Millin retropubic technique, as I have occasionally done, with very satisfactory results—though I must admit in retrospect that such a combined manoeuvre smacks of *bravura*.

URINARY RETENTION AS A FACTOR IN THE PRODUCTION OF ABDOMINAL WOUND DISRUPTION

Before leaving the subject of postoperative urinary retention, it may be well to mention the frequent association of urinary retention and wound disruption after rectal excision. I have seen at least five cases in which gross, unrecognized, distension of the bladder up to the umbilicus was found in conjunction with bursting of the abdominal wound. One can see how the elevation of the peritoneum of the lower anterior abdominal wall might lead to dehiscence of the peritoneal suture line and thus initiate a complete disruption.

URINARY INFECTION

From the report of Watson (1951) it would seem that the majority of patients undergoing rectal excision and having an indwelling urethral catheter for four or five days develop a urinary infection as determined by bacteriological examination, but this only rarely causes symptoms. Moreover, it usually dies out without treatment in the cases without serious urinary obstruction. It is only in patients with gross stasis that serious and troublesome bladder infection is likely to occur. Occasionally in cases treated by prolonged catheterization an epididymitis develops, and rarely an acute pyelonephritis.

The treatment of urinary tract infection resolves itself essentially into the management of any obstruction present, and the use of antibiotics to which the causal organisms have been found to be sensitive. In cases without gross obstruction the infection may be relied upon to clear up in due course without active treatment, but antibiotic therapy may assist the process.

INJURIES TO THE URINARY TRACT AND THE DEVELOPMENT OF URINARY FISTULAS

The ureters, bladder and prostatic or membraneous urethra are all exposed to the risk of accidental injury during rectal excision. This occurs usually in dealing with difficult adherent growths, but sometimes may happen in removing a mobile lesion due to errors of technique. In addition, part of the urinary tract may be deliberately resected *en bloc* with the rectum as a means of completing the eradication of certain advanced, fixed carcinomas.

URETERIC INJURIES

Frequency of Injury
This naturally varies with the experience of the surgeon, for by careful dissection of these structures at vulnerable points damage can usually be avoided. But even in expert hands there still remains a small risk of injury, as shown by the report of Graham and Goligher (1954) who found that the ureter was accidentally divided in 14 of 1605 patients undergoing rectal excision at St Mark's Hospital—an incidence of 0·93 or just under 1%. In one case both ureters were divided.

Sites of Injury
These are indicated in Table 35, and it would appear that the ureter is equally liable to be divided on either side below the brim of the pelvis, usually in taking the lateral ligament. Above the pelvic brim, an additional hazard for the left ureter is

TABLE 35. *Sites of Accidental Ureteric Injury During Excision of Rectum*

Sites of injury	No. of injuries	
	Left ureter	Right ureter
At level of ligature on inferior mesenteric vessels	2	–
At or just above the level of lateral ligament of rectum	7	6
All sites	9	6

Graham and Goligher (1954).

represented by the main ligature on the inferior mesenteric vessels, for in two cases in this series the left ureter was caught up in this ligature and divided. The right ureter lies farther away from the mesenteric vessels, which incline somewhat to the left of the midline, as shown in Fig. 21, and this accounts for the immunity which the right ureter apparently enjoys from injury at this level.

Incidence of Injury Relative to Type of Operation

A variety of operative techniques was used in the series analysed by Graham and Goligher (1954) but most of the operations were synchronous combined or perineo-abdominal excisions. The incidence of ureteric injury seemed to be much lower—indeed almost non-existent—with the latter technique; this is probably explained by the fact that in this method the greater part of the dissection is carried out from the perineum, and ureteric injury is essentially a complication of the abdominal phase of combined excision.

Prevention of Accidental Injuries

In the light of the foregoing remarks, an obvious safeguard for the ureters during rectal excision would be to employ the perineo-abdominal technique to the exclusion of the abdominoperineal or synchronous combined operations! But, for the reasons mentioned on p. 504, it is probable that the majority of operations for carcinoma of the rectum will continue to be other than perineo-abdominal excisions. In operations in which the dissection is conducted largely or entirely through the abdomen, such as the Miles operation, the synchronous combined excision or anterior resection, the following precautions are strongly advised:

1. Before attempting to pass the ligature round the inferior mesenteric vessels, it is essential to define the left ureter at this level and to push it firmly laterally for 8 or 10 cm to displace it well away from the main mesenteric vessels (see Fig. 390B.

2. During division of each lateral ligament the ureter must be retracted lateral to the point of proposed section by a broad deep retractor. In a case with a non-adherent growth it may be possible to do so blindly by retraction of the peritoneum and underlying connective tissues in this region, but the only absolutely reliable method is to expose the ureter from the brim of the pelvis down to the bladder to ensure that it is accurately hooked aside under vision by the retractor. Though I regularly adopt this tactic in regard to the left ureter, I must confess that, except when dealing with an adherent carcinoma of the upper rectum or rectosigmoid, I seldom use it on the right side, where the ureter always seems to lie further laterally, more under the peritoneum and out of the way of the dissection than on the left side. When the growth is extensive, it may be found that the ureter is drawn medially by adhesions and that a determined dissection is necessary to separate it. In some cases it will be found that the ureter is so stuck to the neoplasm that it may be considered to be invaded by it and the decision taken to resect 5 or 7·5 cm of it along with the rectum.

3. Routine preliminary cystoscopy and introduction of ureteric catheters has been recommended as a means of rendering the ureters more easily identifiable and avoidable during the operation. I am not convinced that this rather cumbersome step would be of any real assistance, at any rate to an experienced pelvic surgeon, in demonstrating the ureters, and I have never incorporated it in my practice, but I have to allow that it might conceivably be a useful aid to those who operate less frequently in the pelvis. On the other hand, I am very much in favour of the extremely simple manoeuvre of preoperative intravenous pyelography, perhaps as a routine and certainly in all cases with growths situated at a level at which they might if adherent implicate the ureter, i.e. in the upper rectum or rectosigmoid. The pyelograms may provide the surgeon with useful advance information about ureteric distortion, dilatation of the ureter or renal pelvis or the absence of a functioning kidney on one side.

Treatment of Accidental Injuries and Deliberate Resections of Ureter

A number of methods have been employed for dealing with the ureter after accidental or deliberate division during excision or other operations:

1. *Double ligation of both cut ends*. When the kidney on the opposite side can be felt to be normal—or, better still, has been shown by preoperative intravenous pyelography to be functioning normally—the treatment frequently recommended in the past for the divided ureter was that of double ligation of both cut ends, thus sacrificing renal function on that side. It has often been claimed that, if the ureter is doubly tied with non-absorbable material such as silk or cotton, there is usually no trouble from urinary leakage subsequently and the kidney undergoes symptomless atrophy. That was not the experience in our survey (Graham and Goligher 1954), for six of eight cases treated in this way had later complications, such as urinary fistula, hydronephrosis or infection, and subsequent nephrectomy was frequently necessary. The only virtue of the method is its extreme simplicity, which enables the surgeon speedily to get out of his immediate difficulties, a point that may be important because injuries or resections of the ureter are more apt to take place in cases in which the excision of the rectum has been difficult and prolonged. If removal of the kidney is required later, the necessity for this step normally does not arise till some time after the main operation, when the patient may perhaps be better able to stand a nephrectomy. My own feeling is that this method, involving as it does the deliberate sacrifice of an important organ, should be avoided at almost all costs in favour of some one of the conservative measures (listed below), more in keeping with the spirit of modern surgery.

2. *End-to-end ureteric anastomosis*. This might be regarded as the ideal conservative operation and good results have been recorded after its use in clinical practice by Newell (1939), Moore (1948), Millin (1949) and Ogilvie (1954) and in experimental work by Dempster (1954). But our survey (Graham and Goligher 1954) of cases so treated at St Mark's Hospital was bitterly disappointing: of six patients given uretero-ureteral anastomoses none was really successful, persistent urinary fistulas, hydronephrosis, infection and failure of renal function on that side being the rule. Charles (1967) in his report on a large series of ureteric injuries during gynaecological operations stated that three were treated by ureteric anastomosis with only one success. However, I should add that in four more recent personal cases using a more careful technique of suture I obtained excellent results in three instances.

In the performance of a uretero-ureteral anastomosis the terminal 2 cm of each segment of ureter is cleared of all adventitious fatty tissue and then divided obliquely or slit up on one side for 12 mm to provide a wider lumen at the site of the anastomosis. The two cut ends are apposed by means of interrupted or continuous sutures of 4/o chromic catgut on fine half-circle atraumatic needles. The resulting anastomosis is splinted by a ureteric catheter, which is introduced upwards and downwards in the ureter when the posterior half of the circumference of the suture line has been constructed; the anterior half is completed with the catheter *in situ*. A small anterior cystotomy allows the lower end of the catheter, which is coiled up in the bladder, to be passed through the eye of the indwelling Foley urethral catheter to the exterior. Care is taken to push the ureteric catheter upwards to the maximum extent towards the kidney and then it is fixed to the vesical mucosa by an encircling chromic catgut suture as it emerges from the ureteric orifice into the bladder to prevent it gradually slipping down out of the ureter during the early postoperative period. The cystotomy wound is then closed by two rows of 2/o catgut sutures. It is probably a good plan to wrap a tail of greater omentum around the ureteric anastomosis, if this is technically possible (see p. 438), and certainly to lay a corrugated rubber or sump suction drain down to the site. The ureteric catheter is retained till the integrity of the ureteric suture line has been confirmed by an IVP 14 days after operation. (An alternative to an ordinary ureteric catheter as a splint for the anastomosis is a fine ureterostomy T-tube, with the transverse section of the tube passing through the anastomosis and the stem of the tube being brought out through a side hole in the ureter at least 4 or 5 cm below or above the uretero-ureterostomy. The main advantage of the T-tube is that it cannot slip out of place; it should be retained for three or four weeks.)

3. *Implantation of the proximal cut end into the bladder*. This is a well established method with an excellent record of success. Thus in Graham and Goligher's (1954) survey it was employed in four instances, all with satisfactory results; in Charles' (1967) series it was used in 16 cases with a successful outcome in 13, and I personally have adopted this method in five patients, all with good results. In the conduct of a neo-ureterocystotomy the cut end of the ureter to be implanted is cleared of fatty and connective tissue for 2 cm and divided obliquely or slit up for 12 mm. Two stay sutures are then inserted at opposite poles of the elliptical cut edge. Next the bladder is opened anteriorly by a short incision and through the resulting wound the

mucosa of the posterosuperior part of the dome of the bladder on the side of the affected ureter is exposed so that a cut 10 mm long can be made in it with diathermy or scissors. A curved artery forceps is then inserted from within outwards through the mucosal slit and along the submucosa for 2 cm before being forced through the muscle coat. The hole in the bladder muscle is stretched slightly by opening the blades of the forceps a trifle to make sure that it will accommodate the ureter without undue constriction. The stay sutures on the lower end of the ureter are fed to the artery forceps which is then withdrawn into the bladder, dragging the sutures and ureter into the vesical lumen. The cut end of the ureter is stitched to the edges of the small slit in the bladder mucosa by interrupted or continuous sutures of 4/0 chromic catgut inserted from inside the bladder. Two or three catgut sutures may also be placed from outside the bladder between the ureter and the vesical muscle coat at the point of entry of the former into the bladder. A ureteric catheter is inserted upwards through the new ureteric orifice, stitched in place and passed to the exterior via the Foley catheter as described in connection with uretero-ureterostomy (see p. 616). Finally, the cystotomy wound is closed with two rows of 2/0 chromic catgut. The submucous course of the terminal 2 cm of ureter confers a valvular action on the neo-ureterocystotomy preventing reflex up the ureter.

Neo-ureterocystotomy is easy to perform when the division of the ureter lies not more than 5 cm above the bladder. When the injury is situated at a slightly higher level implantation of the ureter into the bladder may still be possible with the aid of one or other of two special technical devices—the 'psoas hitch' suture of the bladder (Turner-Warwick and Worth 1969) and the Boari flap (Casati and Boari 1894; Spies et al. 1933; Ockerblad 1947; Blandy and Anderson 1977). In the *psoas hitch* technique the bladder is thoroughly mobilized, particularly on the opposite side to that of the ureteric injury, with division of the superior vesical vessels and the contralateral peritoneal attachment, and the vesical dome is then drawn strongly upwards and towards the affected side whilst three or four 2/0 chromic catgut sutures are inserted between its muscle and outer coat and the psoas muscle (Fig. 491). When these are tied they keep this part of the bladder elevated enabling a ureterocystotomy to be effected 2·5–3 cm higher than would otherwise have been possible in the ordinary way. In the *Boari flap* method a pedicled rectangular flap of the superior wall of the bladder 4 or 5 cm wide and 10 cm long is turned up and fashioned into a tube, the upper end of which is available for anastomosis over a splintering catheter to the ureter 7–10 cm higher than would be possible in conventional uretero-

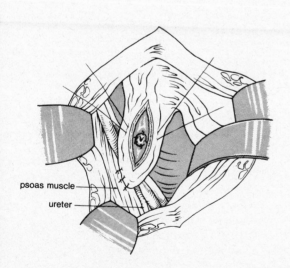

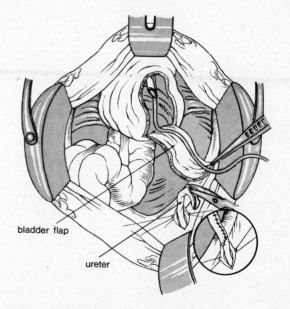

Fig. 491. Neo-ureterocystostomy, the end of the ureter being drawn through a submucosal vesicle tunnel to prevent reflux and the bladder wall stitched to the psoas muscle—the so-called psoas hitch—to avoid tension on the anastomosis. (*From Hendry 1977*)

Fig. 492. The Boari flap method ureterocystostomy, in which a rectangular flap of the dome of the bladder with the base posteriorly is turned up to form a tube extending up to the cut end of the ureter. (*From Hendry 1977*)

cystotomy (Fig. 492). Though excellent results have been reported with the Boari flap by Blandy and Anderson (1977), in a survey of the literature Smith and Smith (1975) found that only 45% of these operations were successful. As the latter authors emphasize this is a demanding technique which requires a good deal of practice to yield satisfactory results.

4. *Implantation of the proximal cut end into the bowel.* It used to be common practice in the performance of complete pelvic clearance to implant the ends of the ureters into the iliac colon or caecum (see p. 506). In the same way the proximal end of the ureter, accidentally or deliberately divided during rectal excision, can be implanted into the large bowel, which means that, if the patient is given a colostomy, it will be a 'wet' colostomy and he will have to wear an adherent applicance on it.

More recently ureterocolic anastomoses have fallen out of favour because of the frequent sequels of ascending infection, hydronephrosis and biochemical disturbance (Jacobs 1953). Instead the Bricker (1950) manoeuvre of implanting the ureters end-to-side into an isolated 25–30 cm segment of lower ileum is now generally preferred, the distal extremity of the loop being brought to the surface as a urinary ileostomy. A unilateral implant following injury or resection of one ureter during rectal excision could be performed in the same way, but this would mean inflicting on the patient an ileostomy in addition to the colostomy (if he is having a complete rectal excision). A more attractive alternative, therefore, is not to bring the distal end of the ileal loop to the surface, but to anastomose it to the top of the urinary bladder. Annis (1952) and Davids and Lesnick (1953) performed successful uretero-ileocystotomies in dogs and my colleagues L. N. Pyrah and the late F. P. Raper (1959) employed this operation clinically with satisfactory results. In my own limited experience with this technique, persistent urinary infection and discharge of mucus has sometimes been a problem, occasionally necessitating the ultimate removal of the kidney and ileal implant.

5. *Implantation of the proximal end into the opposite ureter—cross uretero-ureterostomy.* This method, which was first tried experimentally by Casati and Boari (1894) and Monari (1896) and first used clinically by Higgins (1934), involves implantation of the upper end of the divided ureter into the side of the opposite intact ureter. The procedure has been warmly recommended by Hodges and his colleagues (Anderson et al. 1959; Udall et al. 1973), who report 76 personal cases in which it was almost invariably successful, by Madden et al. (1967), who have conducted extensive experimental and clinical studies on the subject, and by Smith (1969) and Smith and Smith (1975), who have been the chief advocates in Britain and have recorded good results in 52 of 56 cases subjected to cross uretero-ureterostomy. But the operation has evoked mixed feelings amongst surgeons, as Smith and Smith (1975) have demonstrated by an enquiry amongst members of the British Association of Urological Surgeons. The majority were strongly opposed to cross uretero-ureterostomy on the grounds that it jeopardizes the uninjured side, but others maintained that despite this theoretical objection, in practice the method gives excellent results and does not lead to the development of urinary fistula from the normal ureter.

The technique of cross uretero-ureterostomy is relatively simple. The peritoneum over each ureter is freely incised and 5–10 cm of both ureters are mobilized medially. The divided ureter is tunnelled behind the peritoneum in front of the aorta and inferior vena cava, either below or above the inferior mesenteric artery. Its end is cut obliquely and a longitudinal incision to match is made on the medial aspect of the other ureter. The two openings are anastomosed by means of interrupted or continuous sutures of 4/0 chromic catgut. In most of the published cases no ureteric catheter or ureterostomy T-tube has been used to splint the anastomosis, but a drain has usually been left down to the site.

6. *Establishment of a cutaneous ureterostomy.* The proximal end of the cut ureter may be brought to the surface as a ureterostomy, but it is especially difficult to keep ureterostomy patients dry with any form of applicance, so that this is an even less attractive alternative than a urinary ileostomy.

7. *Disconnection of the renal vessels from the aorta and vena cava and transplantation of the kidney to the iliac fossa.* A theoretical possibility when only a short segment of the upper ureter remains would be to divide the renal vessels to allow the kidney to be moved downwards to the appropriate iliac fossa where the vessels could be anastomosed to the iliac vessels and the ureter implanted in the bladder.

Recommended Plan of Action in Cases with Damaged Ureters

A practical classification of these injuries is into those situated low down in the pelvis, those occurring at or just below the pelvic brim, and those involving the ureter well out of the pelvis.

Low pelvic injuries. There is absolutely no problem about their treatment, for the upper end of the ureter can always be relatively quickly implanted into the bladder with excellent prospects of a perfect result.

High pelvic or abdominal injuries. It is around the management of these lesions that the difficulties and controversies are centred. *If the patient's condition is good* I believe that an attempt should always be made to preserve renal function on that side, the actual methods to be employed depending on the actual height of the injury and the surgeon's own predilections. For the higher pelvic lesions neo-ureterocystotomy, using the 'psoas hitch' technique or a Boari flap, should be considered, the best alternatives being an end-to-end ureteric anastomosis or a cross uretero-ureterostomy. For injuries out of the pelvis the choice will lie between the latter two alternatives. *Only if the patient's condition is extremely poor, making precipitate termination of the operation essential* (and the opposite kidney can be demonstrated by palpation at laparotomy—and ideally by preoperative IVP—to be normal), should double ligation of both cut ends of the ureter with linen or cotton be countenanced. Though the majority of the patients so treated will develop urinary complications necessitating subsequent nephrectomy on that side, the need for this step will not arise till some time after the main operation when the patient will usually be better able to stand it.

BLADDER INJURIES

In reasonably skilful hands injury to the bladder is only likely to occur when freeing a fixed growth adherent in front in a male patient. Sometimes the bladder is inadvertently opened during the anterior dissection in such cases. If the bladder wall seems to be actually invaded by growth or if a fistula is known to be present between the bladder and the bowel, it will be necessary to carry out a partial or total cystectomy. Though the latter is undoubtedly preferable so far as eradication of the growth is concerned, it carries a high operative mortality and morbidity and imposes the hardship of a urinary ileostomy on the patient, so that I have always tried to avoid it whenever possible. In several cases, when the vesical dome was the part mainly implicated, it has been found possible to resect the top of the bladder with a sufficient margin of clearance without encroaching on the trigonal region. In one case I have even sacrificed one of the ureteric orifices and re-implanted the ureter into the bladder with a satisfactory immediate result and no subsequent recurrence in the bladder, but I have never had occasion to resect the upper part of the trigone on both sides and re-implant both ureters in this way, for a growth of this extent has always seemed to me to demand pelvic clearance if operable.

If the bladder has been opened or part of its wall has been resected, the resulting rent or gap is sutured by two rows of continuous 2/0 or 3/0 plain or chromic catgut stitches. Usually an indwelling urethral catheter suffices to drain the bladder and it should be retained for 10–14 days; only rarely, if bleeding has not been well controlled, should a suprapubic cystostomy with a small Malecot catheter be necessary. But a corrugated rubber drain should be laid down suprapubically to the vesical suture line for four or five days. There may be slight urinary leakage along the drain track or through the perineal wound in some cases but this usually rapidly ceases; it may require reintroduction of the urethral catheter for a few days. If a considerable part of the bladder wall has been removed and bladder capacity accordingly reduced, there may at first be greatly increased frequency of micturition for several weeks or months; this improves in time.

INJURIES TO THE MEMBRANOUS OR
PROSTATIC URETHRA

Injury to the membranous or prostatic urethra may arise during the anterior dissection of the perineal phase of the operation, due to striking a faulty plane in the region of the rectourethrales muscles, or to attempts being made to shave off part of the back of the prostate together with the rectum in cases with extensive growths fixed anteriorly. I have had two urethral injuries in a series of over 620 personally-conducted perineal dissections. In one the membranous urethra was almost completely divided across at the apex of the prostate, due to the former mistake. This was treated by end-to-end suture with fine plain catgut stitches over an indwelling Foley catheter, a suprapubic cystostomy also being performed for suction drainage of the bladder to divert the urinary stream temporarily. Primary healing without leakage was obtained, the eventual result being excellent.

In the other case the prostatic urethra was opened almost throughout its length in endeavouring to excise the posterior capsule and posterior part of the prostate substance in an advanced case. By suturing the two lateral lobes of the prostate backwards over an indwelling catheter it was possible to secure a very firm repair; temporary urinary diversion was established by suprapubic cystostomy. This patient was apparently obtaining satisfactory healing of his prostatic wound when he died of a pulmonary embolism on the sixteenth day. Obviously owing to the presence of the large wound cavity after rectal excision, which deprives the urethra of its normal support behind, there must always be a considerable risk of urethral repairs of this kind breaking down and forming fistulas, especially if some degree of infection occurs in the perineal wound. But these two cases serve to illustrate what can sometimes be accomplished.

POSTOPERATIVE URINARY FISTULA

This may arise as a sequel to an injury to a ureter, to the bladder or to the urethra, that has been recognized to have taken place and has been appropriately dealt with at the original operation, or it may be the first unwelcome indication that any part of the urinary tract has been injured, as when a ureter has been unconsciously clamped, cut and ligated. As a rule the resulting escape of urine from the perineal wound is easily recognized for what it is, but sometimes doubt may exist as to whether the fluid is in fact urine or an unusually profuse serous discharge from the raw surfaces of the perineal or abdominal wound cavity. The *urinary nature* of any such discharge *can always be established* beyond equivocation by sending a sample for estimation of its urea content; no other body fluid has nearly so high a concentration of urea as has urine. Alternatively an intravenous injection of methylene blue or indigocarmine may be given. These dyes stain the urine deeply, so that the discoloration or otherwise of the perineal fluid will afford a clear indication as to whether it has originated in the urinary tract or not.

Determination of the Site of the Fistula. This may be easy or may require special investigations. In *ureteric fistulas* the escape of urine is continuous and occurs independently of micturition. The passage of a urethral catheter and filling the bladder causes no fluid discharge from the perineum. Intravenous pyelography and ureterography may actually show the site of the fistula and may reveal the presence of hydronephrosis on that side. Cystoscopy and intravenous injection of indigocarmine will establish that there is no urinary efflux on one side; the arrest in the passage of a ureteric catheter on that side will give some idea of the level of the ureteric injury. *Fistulas of the bladder and posterior urethra* may sometimes be evident if the anterior wall of the pelvic cavity is carefully inspected through the perineal wound. With urethral fistulas the discharge takes place chiefly or entirely during the act of micturition, but with bladder fistulas it is a continuous process. The passage of a catheter may sometimes be difficult in cases with a fistula of the urethra, or indeed the tip of the catheter may emerge through the fistula into the perineal wound. When the fistula is situated in the bladder, catheterization and filling of the bladder results in the fluid escaping from the perineum. Urethroscopy and cystoscopy will establish the precise situation of the opening relative to the internal sphincter.

Treatment of Urinary Fistulas. The treatment of a *ureteric fistula* depends on whether the causal injury of the ureter has divided it partially or completely. If the intravenous pyelogram and ureterogram indicate that the ureter is partly intact, and in particular if a ureteric catheter can be negotiated past the site of injury up to the kidney, an expectant approach is indicated in the hope that the hole in the ureter will eventually heal. Perhaps this healing process will be facilitated if an indwelling ureteric catheter can be left in position draining the kidney on the affected side. It is reasonable to persist with this regimen for several weeks, but, if spontaneous closure is not achieved with partial injuries or if the division was shown initially to be complete, a resort must be made to operative treatment along the lines indicated on p. 618. If possible the cut upper end should be implanted into the bladder or into an upward extension of the bladder in the form of a Boari (Casati and Boari 1894) flap. If this is impossible a uretero-ureteral anastomosis may be attempted over an indwelling ureteric catheter, or a crossed uretero-ureterostomy may be considered. But if these methods are considered to be impracticable or too uncertain in their results, or if they have been tried and failed, a lumbar nephrectomy will be required—presuming that the intravenous pyelogram shows a normal kidney on the contralateral side. Another factor influencing the decision towards nephrectomy would be an advanced state of spread of the growth for which rectal excision had been performed, making the ultimate prognosis very poor. *Bladder fistulas*, unless the hole in the bladder wall is very wide, should close with conservative treatment—that is with continuous suction through an indwelling urethral catheter—though this regimen may have to be maintained for several weeks. The closure is assisted by the gradual filling in of the perineal wound cavity with granulations. Sometimes it may be an advantage to have the patient in the prone position to encourage the urine to gravitate into the anterior part of the bladder and away from the fistula on the posterior wall, but this is irksome for the patient to maintain for any length of time. *Urethral fistulas* should also be managed conservatively in the first instance with an indwelling urethral catheter or urinary diversion by means of a suprapubic cystostomy. If the fistula persists, an attempt at a plastic repair will have to be undertaken, preferably by a urological surgeon specially versed in the treatment of these lesions. My former urological colleague, the late Mr. F. P. Raper, told me that he had operated on four cases for the closure of such urethal fistulas resulting from rectal excision, with eventual complete success in all instances, though in one of the cases there was some breakdown after the first attempt and the repair had to be repeated.

DISORDERS OF SEXUAL FUNCTION

It is well known that sexual function is sometimes seriously disturbed or completely abolished in male patients due to autonomic nerve injury during excision of the rectum, and in younger patients this may on occasions prove a disastrous consequence of operation. The general impression amongst surgeons is that these complications are extremely common, but it seems usually to be forgotten that the majority of patients undergoing rectal excision for carcinoma are already elderly at the time of operation, and with them sexual function has often abated years previously, or was so much on the wane that the general effect of a major operation might perhaps be sufficient to bring about its total cessation, quite apart from any damage to pelvic nerves. In an investigation which I conducted into the frequency of disorders of sexual function after excision of the rectum at St Mark's Hospital in 1951, I was at some pains to avoid this source of error, and therefore confined my enquiries to male patients under the age of 60 who had been enjoying an active sex life up to or shortly before the time of operation. The manner in which patients were selected for this study is shown in Table 36.

It should be explained that, when the patients were written to, no indication was given as to why they were being asked to report to hospital. Further,

TABLE 36. *Selection of Rectal Excision Cases for Investigation of Sexual Function*

No. of male patients who had excision of rectum at St Mark's Hospital 1933–49	1024
No. who were 60 years of age or under at time of operation	522
No. who were still alive and well at time of investigation	280
No. who were living sufficiently near hospital to be interviewed	176
No. who actually attended in response to call-up letters	121
No. of these who had been enjoying active sex life up to the time of operation	95

After Goligher (1951*c*).

it is unlikely that any patient's decision whether to attend or not was influenced by the effect of the operation on his sexual function. The 95 patients eventually chosen for investigation regarding their postoperative sexual function may thus be regarded as a fair sample of the younger group of cases. The findings of the enquiry in regard to them may be summarized briefly as follows:

1. Roughly two-thirds of the patients retained normal potency after operation.

2. Though most of these potent patients achieved a more or less normal sensation of orgasm during the sexual act, only about a half of them apparently were capable of ejaculation.

3. These disorders of function occurred after synchronous combined excision, perineo-abdominal excision and sphincter-saving resections (mostly anterior resections) respectively; the incidence seemed rather lower with the latter two operations but the difference was not significant.

4. No striking difference could be demonstrated in the frequency of these disorders according to the extent of spread of the growth; they were certainly not confined to cases with adherent lesions.

MECHANISM OF DISTURBANCES OF SEXUAL FUNCTION

Impotence. This is presumably due to injury to the parasympathetic innervation, though the same uncertainty exists, as with neurogenic bladder disorders, as to where exactly the parasympathetic pathway is usually damaged in rectal excision (see p. 612). The fact that impotence has sometimes followed sphincter-saving types of resection without a perineal phase indicates that avulsion of the stems of the six nervi erigentes themselves by stripping the fascia of Waldeyer off the front of the sacrum is certainly not the only mechanism of injury in these cases.

Failure of Ejaculation. It appears from the work of Learmonth (1931) that the seminal vesicles and trigonal region of the bladder are both innervated by the sympathetic nerves. An injury to the sympathetic supply could result in failure of ejaculation either from abolition of seminal vesicular contraction or alternatively from paralysis of the internal sphincter allowing seminal fluid to regurgitate back into the bladder as in post-prostatectomy cases. In the latter event one would expect that at the next micturition the urine would be intermixed with semen. 33 of the St Mark's Hospital cases investigated by me were questioned on this point, and they were all emphatic that the urine passed after intercourse appeared perfectly normal, but this statement was not confirmed by microscopical examination of the urine. In this connection it is to be noted that, despite the absence of an ejaculate, practically all these patients experienced a satisfactory sensation of orgasm. Presumably therefore the orgasm is not due, as is often imagined, to the contraction of the seminal vesicles, but is an entirely sensory phenomenon.

The Site of Injury to the Sympathetic. The places where the sympathetic fibres to the seminal vesicles (and bladder) are liable to be injured without damage to the parasympathetic nerves during rectal excision are where they are running in the roots, trunk or branches of the presacral nerve. In my experience of dissections in the cadaver and at operation, the roots of the presacral nerve are very closely applied to the front of the aorta and the common iliac arteries so that, even if a high ligation of the inferior mesenteric artery is practised, these nerve roots may well remain undisturbed unless the arteries are very cleanly dissected. The presacral nerve trunk itself is more likely to be lifted up with the inferior mesenteric vessels during low ligation between the level of the aortic bifurcation and the sacral promontory, but the most vulnerable part of the sympathetic pathway is the two main branches of the presacral nerve which, as they separate to run to either side of the pelvis, lie closely against the back and sides of the rectum. At these points they are very liable to be torn as the presacral space behind the rectum is being opened up by scissor and hand dissection.

The sympathetic innervation might also be interrupted by injury to the pelvic plexuses on either side of the pelvis during division of the base of the lateral ligament, but in this situation one would expect a concomitant interruption of the parasympathetic supply with resulting impotence. It is probable that in most patients rendered impotent by rectal excision a sympathetic lesion coexists, but we have no means of knowing for certain. We are here only considering the patients who have managed to avoid a parasympathetic injury.

The Management of a Permanent Iliac Colostomy

For the management of a temporary loop transverse colostomy see p. 484.

The importance of this subject cannot be overestimated, for the full success of surgical treatment of rectal cancer so often depends on the establishment of a satisfactory mode of life for the patient left with a colostomy. It is the surgeon's responsibility to see that the patient is properly instructed in the care of his colostomy; this duty should not devolve—as it unfortunately sometimes does—on the general practitioner, who does not have adequate experience to enable him to advise confidently about colostomy management. The aim of the surgeon and his staff should be to teach and equip the patient so that he is able to look after his colostomy entirely by himself by the time he is discharged from hospital. The programme necessary to achieve this end may be considered under the following headings:

ALLAYING THE PATIENT'S FEARS AND MISAPPREHENSIONS

This is the first step and commences before the operation, for it is necessary to explain to the patient preoperatively that rectal excision will often involve the creation of a permanent colostomy and to reassure him on his score. The average lay person is naturally repelled by the thought of an artificial anus and it may sometimes require considerable feats of persuasion to induce him to accept an operation carrying this implication. Surprisingly enough women are often less dismayed than men by the prospect of a colostomy, probably because of their earlier experiences in looking after babies and young children, and because much housework is dirty and unpleasant. Sometimes a talk with another patient who has a well-established colostomy may be more convincing than any amount of eloquence by the surgeon, and may help a reluctant patient decide in favour of operation.

It is also wise, as a rule, to tell the patient that a firm decision as to whether a colostomy will be necessary or the condition can be treated by a sphincter-saving type of operation can only be made at laparotomy, and that naturally every effort will be made to avoid an artificial anus, if this proves compatible with the requirements of thorough treatment. It can be explained, however, that if a colostomy should be required, this is a well-tried operation which has been performed hundreds of thousands of times now, and that countless people in all walks of life are enjoying splendid health and leading full normal lives despite the fact that they have such an opening. It may be emphasized further that very many of the patients have been able to return to their previous occupations and activities even though these may have involved manual work. Similarly they have not been debarred from recreation and social life; those who desire it have been able to take part in meetings, dancing, golf, cricket, tennis and even swimming, in accordance, of course, with their age and general condition.

CARE OF THE COLOSTOMY IN THE IMMEDIATE POSTOPERATIVE PERIOD

This phase of colostomy management has been referred to on p. 593 and will not be further discussed here. In this section we are concerned rather with the ultimate care by the patient himself before and after he leaves hospital.

ULTIMATE REGULATION AND CARE OF COLOSTOMY ACTIONS

Patients with well-functioning colostomies sometimes talk about having 'acquired control' of their colostomy, and the same expression is occasionally used in surgical parlance. But this merely means that the patient has been fortunate, in that his colostomy only acts once or twice a day and at the same time every day. It certainly does not imply the development of control in the sense that the normal anus is controlled by the anal sphincters, for a colostomy is devoid of a proper sphincter. Admittedly it is surrounded by the strong muscular bellies of the internal oblique and transversus abdominis, and it might perhaps be thought that in the course of time the patient could learn to contract these muscles so as to grip the colostomy sufficiently to exercise control. But even when a 'gridiron' principle has been strictly followed in making the colostomy wound, and muscle fibres have not been divided but merely separated so that they fit snugly round the bowel, it is found that no effective muscular control is ever possible.

In this connection it may be mentioned that in the early days of the development of colostomy as a surgical operation, this idea of securing local control was pursued in several techniques. In them the bowel was brought obliquely through the abdominal wall so that it lay for some centimetres between, say, the internal and external oblique muscles, or in the subcutaneous tissues (Tuttle 1903; Kirschner 1937). In this position it was hoped that it would be more susceptible to compression by the contractions of the muscles or by the colostomy belt pressing against the abdominal wall. Another technique consisted of rotating the colon stump axially through 180° or so. But these and similar methods were found to be unsuccessful and have long since been relegated to the limbo of failed operations. Recently Kock (Säuberli et al. 1974) has tried to make ordinary colostomies continent in dogs with 'nipple valves' of the type used in reservoir ileostomies (see p. 798), but this work awaits clinical application. Ceulemans (1977) has claimed that by a combination of parasympathetic denervation of the distal left colon and siting of the colostomy high in the abdominal wall just below the left costal margin, some degree of continence is obtained, but I find this unconvincing. Schmidt et al. (1979) have attempted to secure sphincter control in animals (and a few patients), by surrounding the end of the colon leading to the colostomy with a free transplant of the entire seromuscular coat dissected out of a previously resected short segment of terminal colon.

There is another reason why attempts to fashion a viable sphincter for colostomies seem to me doomed to failure, and that is the lack of a sensory component to act as a trigger for the mechanism. However long a patient may possess a colostomy, he never develops any sensation from it comparable to the very specific feeling of rectal distension that heralds defaecation in a normal individual (Goligher and Hughes 1951). He will undoubtedly find that, when his colostomy has been properly regulated, it will act at a nearly constant time each day, and he may indeed experience some vague warning, in the form of slight central abdominal colic, that peristalsis is taking place and an action may be expected shortly, but this is very different from the urgent and immediate sensation of rectal distension in normal individuals that indicates the need for defaecation or passage of flatus—and incidentally distinguishes very accurately between these two requirements. Without such accurate sensory information an efficient sphincter mechanism to control a colostomy would clearly be impossible.

Accepting that a colostomy is a sphincterless opening, the aim of colostomy management is to enable the patient to cope with this incontinent anus with the minimum of soiling and inconvenience. There are three ways of attempting to secure this end—(a) *by allowing spontaneous colon activity to occur normally and arranging to catch the motions in a suitable colostomy bag; (b) by emptying the colon forcibly at a set time each day by means of a colostomy wash-out or enema regimen; and (c) by the use of a magnetic closing device to confer an artificial sort of continence on the colostomy.*

SPONTANEOUS COLOSTOMY ACTIONS AND
EFFECTS OF DIET AND DRUGS

Within a month or so of the operation the patient usually finds that, whilst he is on an ordinary diet, the motions passed by his colostomy have become more formed in character and are discharged much less frequently and irregularly than in the early postoperative days. A few patients are exceptionally fortunate in that the colostomy action occurs only once or at most twice in the 24 hours. The commonest time for this to happen is before breakfast, often after an early morning cup of tea. Sometimes a subsidiary action, or the main action, takes place after breakfast. Other patients find that the chief stimulus is the evening meal, or there may be a motion after every meal or oftener. It is the experience of perhaps the majority of patients after a while that, whether the motions are frequent or infrequent, their timing is roughly the same each day, so that a definite pattern of colostomy actions emerges. But in some patients such a rhythm never develops, and they are quite unable to predict when their colostomy will work. Over the succeeding months there may be some tendency for the motions to become rather less frequent and more constant in their pattern of occurrence, but the change after the first few weeks, in my experience, is usually slight. A more precise assessment of the final state as regards spontaneous colostomy actions was made by Grier et al. (1964), who conducted a careful review of a group of colostomy cases—including a number of my own patients. They found that only 38% of these patients achieved the ideal of one to two motions daily, 30% had three to four motions and 32% experienced a continuous discharge or at least five motions per day.

These findings are considerably at variance with the rosy reports of Lockhart-Mummery (1934), Gabriel (1945, 1963) and Dukes (1947) as to the infrequency and reliability of spontaneous colostomy activity. The latter authors, indeed, considered that as a rule colostomy patients had their colostomy actions so regulated they could anticipate with accuracy when the motion would occur and could thus repair to the toilet (or preferably to a combined toilet and bathroom) five minutes or so before this event was due to take place. They would then remove their colostomy appliances and set themselves down with a kidney dish tucked under the stoma and with dressing material within easy reach for cleansing afterwards. For most of my patients, however, this plan would be quite impracticable, either because the timing of their colostomy actions is insufficiently precise, or because the motions occur too frequently. Also, the modern trend towards using disposable plastic colostomy bags, rather than dressing materials and a simple colostomy belt, fortunately makes anticipation of the colostomy actions no longer important, for the bag will accommodate the faeces till it is convenient to deal with them.

Effect of Diet
Items of diet, which in excess are liable to produce rather loose motions or even frank diarrhoea in normal people, will have the same effect, only slightly more severely, on patients with colostomies. For example, large quantities of fruit and vegetables—especially if uncooked—cereals, wholemeal bread, beer, stout and some wines cause considerable looseness and some increased frequency of the colostomy actions. In addition, normal individuals are sometimes aware of particular dishes to which they seem to have a special idiosyncracy, with resulting diarrhoea, and this will equally apply to colostomy patients. Clearly persons with a colostomy are well advised, in the interests of the regular behaviour of their bowel, to avoid excessive ingestion of any of the substances mentioned, if this has the effect described. But most people manage to take a moderate amount of the majority of foods without any very pronounced consequences as regards the activity of their colostomy.

Whether it is possible for patients, whose misfortune is to have several, perhaps quite unpredictable, motions a day, or a more or less continuous discharge of faeces from the colostomy, to change this pattern of behaviour to one or two well regulated colostomy actions daily by major alterations to their diet, is much more debatable. Dukes (1947) and Gabriel (1945, 1963) implied that it is, but I must confess that I have not been impressed by the achievements of dieting in this respect. Another consideration bearing on this matter is that patients often find it more trouble than it is worth to stick to a special diet, rather than to take the ordinary meals that are served in the home and elsewhere.

Effect of Drugs
In patients whose colostomy motions remain unduly soft and frequent, help may sometimes be derived from taking hydrophilic *methylcellulose preparations* to make the faeces firmer. Examples of

these are Isogel (Allen and Hanbury), Normacol (H. R. Napp), and Celevac (Harker Stagg), the dosage of all of which is 1 to 2 teaspoonfuls taken in a very small amount of water each evening or morning and evening. Unfortunately the efficacy of this medication in colostomy management usually falls far short of what one might be led to expect from commercial propaganda. Some patients find that *kaolin powder* in doses of 1 to 2 heaped tea-spoonfuls twice or thrice a day is fairly effective in rendering the motions more solid. Other classical drugs in this connection are *codeine phosphate* in a dose of 30–60 mg thrice daily, *diphenoxylate* (Lomotil) two tablets four times daily and *loperamide* one or two capsules thrice daily.

If, on the contrary, there is any tendency to constipation, this can usually be corrected by taking more fruit or vegetables in the meals, but, if this does not prove effective, a small dose of liquid paraffin or a stool softener (e.g. Normax) will generally put matters right. As a rule stronger aperients are better avoided.

DISPOSABLE ADHERENT COLOSTOMY APPLIANCES

As mentioned on p. 593, during the immediate postoperative period when the initial colostomy motions are usually liquid and profuse, it is convenient to use an *adherent bag with a drainage vent*, as employed in the regular care of an *ileostomy* (see p. 768), such as the Hollister, Coloplast, Simpla-Sassco or Surgicare System 2. This appliance is kept in position for four or five days at a time as a rule and emptied as required. Some patients, indeed, persist with this routine indefinitely, but more usually, when after a few weeks the motions become semi-solid and are difficult to evacuate from a bag in situ, the patient prefers to employ a blind pouch which is discarded every time it fills with faeces.

The earliest patterns of *non-drainage adherent bags* were the Chiron (Down Bros.) and the Meredith (Eschmann Bros. and Walsh), which were stuck to the skin around the colostomy by a square or circle of double-sided adhesive plaster. A slightly more sophisticated variant is the Simpla-Sassco bag (Fig.

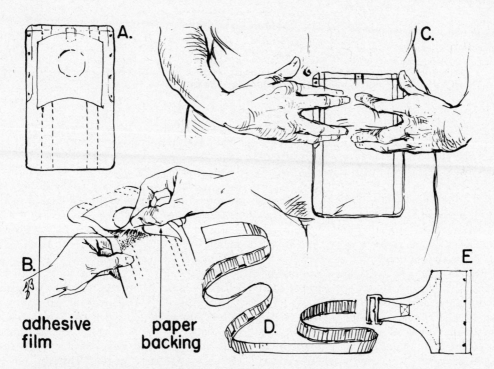

adhesive film   paper backing

Fig. 493. The Simpla-Sassco appliance. It is made in soft, blue-tinted plastic material which is somewhat opaque to the colour of faeces. (A) Back view, showing the hole near upper end into which the colostomy fits, surrounded by an adherent area covered by paper backing till the bag is about to be used. (B) Removing the paper cover immediately preparatory to use. (C) The bag has been applied to the abdomen, firm pressure being exerted to make the adherent area around the stoma stick to the skin. (D) The belt that provides additional support for the appliance. (E) The broad attachments that clip on to either side of the bag and have a buckle to which the belt is fixed.

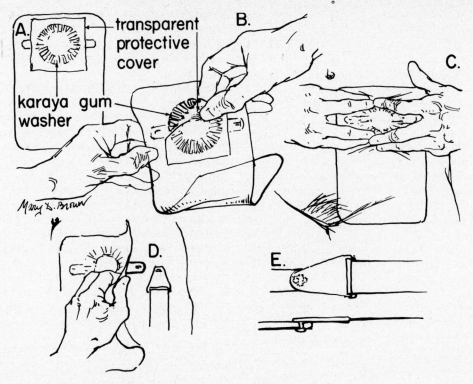

Fig. 494. The Hollister non-drainable adherent colostomy bag. (A) Back view, showing the opening into which the colostomy fits surrounded by karaya gum washer, covered with waterproof paper backing. (B) The paper cover being removed from the karaya ring just before use. (C) The bag has been placed in position, the karaya gum washer being pressed firmly against the skin around the stoma. (D, E) The edge of the bag is being turned forwards to expose the rigid plastic arm to which the belt is attached.

493), in which an adhesive substance is incorporated in the back of the bag adjacent to the opening for the stoma. One other useful feature of the Simpla-Sassco appliance is that it has a small air vent near its top in front to allow flatus to escape and avoid flatulent distension of the bag. (If such distension is a troublesome occurrence with other appliances, it can be prevented by routine puncture of the bag on the front near its upper end with a pin.) The main snag to the regular use of non-drainable adherent bags of the sort just described is that it is not long before the peristomal skin becomes irritated and sore from the frequent changes of plaster, as the appliance is taken off say two or three times a day. One way of avoiding this trouble is to use less irritating plasters made from low sensitizing porous non-woven fabric such as Stoma Squares (C. F. Thackray), or to employ appliances which rely on karaya washers instead of ordinary adhesive plasters to stick the bag in position. Popular examples of this sort of appliance are the Hollister (Fig. 494), Coloplast, Salt, New Simpla and Eschmann. Karaya gum is a very good

adhesive which, so far from irritating the skin, has even a soothing effect on a sore skin surface (see p. 735).

Another way of obviating soreness of the skin around the stoma, when wearing a non-drainable adherent bag, has been to use a *two-piece* non-drainable appliance, the first of which was the Translet (Fig. 495). It consists of (*a*) a more rigid plastic flange which is stuck to the skin by a double-sided adhesive plaster and usually is left in position for two or three days at a time; and (*b*) a thin pliable plastic disposable bag, the opening at the upper end of which is contracted by means of an elastic rubber band, and is fixed on to a groove on the flange. This is a very neat and convenient appliance, but occasionally leakage occurs between the bag and the flange. A very recent addition to the two-piece appliances available has been the *Surgicare System 2* (E. R. Squibb) (Fig. 496) which consists of: (*a*) a thin plastic flange incorporated in a square of Stomahesive, giving very good non-irritating adhesion to the skin for several days at least as a rule; and (*b*) a blind

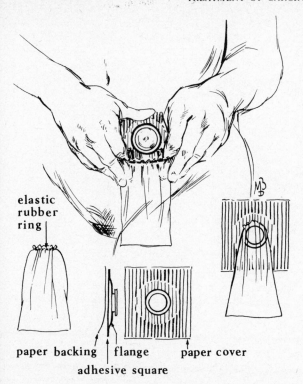

elastic
rubber
ring

paper backing | flange   paper cover
        adhesive square

Fig. 495. The Translet adherent colostomy bag. It consists of a very light rigid plastic flange, which is stuck to the abdominal skin around the colostomy with an adhesive square, and a plastic bag with an elastic rubber ring at its top. The appliance is usually also supported by a belt or corset.

bag or pouch made of transparent or opaque, white laminated plastic material and possessing on its posterior surface near the top an aperture in the edges of which is incorporated a rigid plastic gasket. This gasket has a groove on its exposed edge which clips on to the free edge of the flange to provide a gas-proof and liquid-proof junction. The gasket also has a perforated projection on either side for attachment of a belt to afford additional support. Two-piece appliances are made by other firms as well, such as Down Bros.

Routine of Emptying, Changing and Disposing of Plastic Colostomy Bags

The time at which the patient chooses to empty and/or change his colostomy bag will vary depending on the type of appliance he is wearing, as well as on the frequency of the colostomy actions and on his fastidiousness and personal preference. If a drainable bag is being used, it will usually be kept attached to the skin for at least 24 hours and emptied as required in that time. There is no immediate urgency about emptying the bag as soon as a motion occurs, but most patients will prefer not to have the bag in a heavily loaded condition longer than necessary, and so they will choose to empty it as soon as convenient after a major colostomy action, whenever that may be. As for when the bag itself should be removed and changed, this is something for the patient to decide, depending on his routine of life.

If a non-drainable bag is used, which necessitates complete removal of the bag to empty it, the time of changing the bag will probably be soon after any considerable escape of faeces from the colostomy. This usually means one change after breakfast and possibly others throughout the day depending on how active the colostomy is.

When a loaded bag is removed, the faeces are milked out of it into the lavatory, care being taken to squeeze out any air at the same time, before it is discarded into the lavatory, otherwise difficulty may be experienced in getting it to sink. An additional precaution to prevent it floating is to snick it with scissors in two or three places before putting it in the lavatory bowl. An alternative disposal of emptied colostomy bags is to roll them up and wrap them in paper or place them in sanitary-style envelopes, so that they may be taken and burnt in an Aga or similar type of kitchen stove or in a garden incinerator. They are not easily burnt in an ordinary domestic hearth. If necessary they may be disposed of with the household rubbish.

At the time of changing the bag the skin around the colostomy is cleansed, and, if convenient, washed with plain white soap and water and dried. (For all cleansing activities in connection with the colostomy it is better to use *paper tissues* or *cellulose wadding* rather than cotton wool or gauze, for they can safely be discarded into the lavatory, whilst wool, if got rid of in this way, is liable to block the drains.) Before re-applying a bag fixed with adhesive plaster (not karaya or Stomahesive) it is important to ensure that the skin is absolutely dry and free from grease by swabbing it with carbon tetrachloride. If there is any soreness of the skin, it is a good plan to apply a little barrier cream, such as Kerodex or Siopel.

Further Supply of Colostomy Bags and Belts and Related Materials

Most of the items of equipment for dealing with the colostomy, such as bags and belts, are in Britain available to patients free on the National Health Service, either through the Appliance Department of the hospital or from a chemist's shop or the

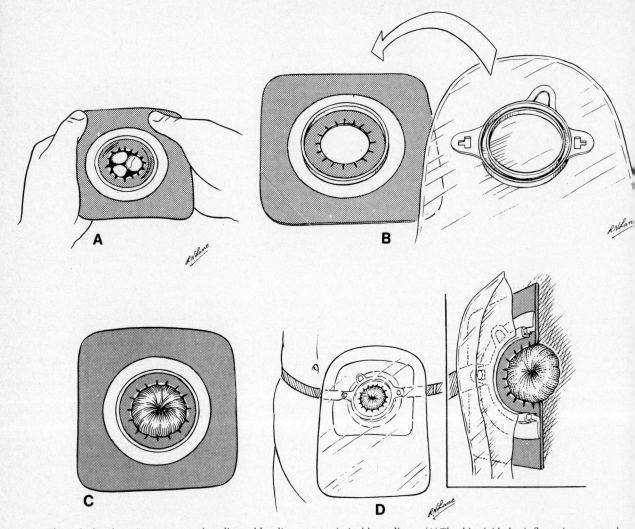

Fig. 496. Surgicare System 2 two-piece disposable adherent non-drainable appliance. (A) The thin rigid plastic flange incorporated in a Stomahesive square, the opening in which has been enlarged by cutting with scissors and the cut edges snicked and stretched slightly with the fingers to fit accurately the size of the colostomy. (B) The opaque plastic bag (back view) alongside the prepared flange and square. (C) The flange has been fitted to the skin around the stoma. (D) The bag has been clipped onto the flange (see inset for the method of clipping them together) and the belt has been attached and is in position.

manufacturer on the family doctor's prescription. Unfortunately, because these appliances are free, most NHS patients and many of the general medical practitioners have little idea of how much they cost and of the implications in terms of national expenditure. One of the more sophisticated plastic non-drainable bags with incorporated karaya washer costs at the present time (1979) approximately 72p. The average patient with a fairly well regulated colostomy will use two or three bags daily, which represents a cost per day of £1.44 to £2.16 or per year of £525 to £788. I have

known patients use as many as six or seven bags a day, quite unaware of the fact that they were costing the taxpayers £1600 to £1850 per year!

COLOSTOMY WASH-OUTS

The alternative regimen involves a regular daily wash-out to empty the colon thoroughly every 24 hours. By this means it is hoped to concentrate the colostomy action into one major daily evacuation and to avoid further small troublesome motions throughout the day. It probably does give a greater degree of assurance against unwanted actions at inconvenient times than does the system of spontaneous natural colostomy evacuations, but several disadvantages attach to it. (*a*) Unless the patient allows a good deal of time—up to nearly an hour for the wash-out to be returned completely—some fluid may remain and give rise to an action 30–60 minutes later. (*b*) It involves rather a lot of impedimenta in the way of douche can, tubing, and catheter, so that it is difficult to organize except in a combined bathroom and lavatory and in the privacy of the patient's own home. For that reason the patient on this routine is apt to be apprehensive about travelling or staying with friends, in case circumstances are unfavourable for the administration of his wash-out. He is thus more restricted in his activities than is the patient on the simple dietetic regimen. (*c*) The liquid action resulting from wash-outs deprives the colostomy of the dilating effect of normal semi-solid motions so that in the long run the stoma may undergo stenosis. This is probably unlikely to happen with the modern colostomy made by the technique of mucocutaneous suture, but with old-style colostomies it was an undoubted disadvantage of the wash-out regimen. (*d*) It is possible to perforate the colon by the catheter which is introduced to give the colostomy wash-out. I have seen four cases in which this happened, in three with fatal results due to delay in recognition of the calamity. Gabriel (1948), Spiro and Hertz (1966) and Seargeant (1966) also report examples of this accident. Considering the large number of wash-outs that are given, the incidence of injury is probably very small, but when it occurs it is a serious accident with a fairly high mortality. For that reason it must be regarded as a major drawback to the use of the wash-out regimen—at least by certain techniques.

Opinion on the value of the wash-out system in the regular management of colostomies is sharply divided. It is virtually the routine method in North America, where Binkley (1952) has given a good account of its technique and advantages. In this country it has been strongly advocated by Miles (1926, 1945) and his followers at the Gordon Hospital, London, and Seargeant (1966) has reported a postal inquiry on the results of this regimen in 216 patients who were believed still to be living after abdominoperineal excision and colostomy at that hospital. Three patients were found to have died and 48 could not be traced, leaving 165 who replied to a questionnaire. Of these, 34 had entirely ceased giving themselves wash-outs and another 15 used them only infrequently, but 116 (or 70%) still adhered to the routine of a daily or fairly frequent wash-out, as taught to them in hospital; 64% of these 116 patients took between one and two hours for their wash-outs (including subsequent cleansing of equipment), 27% required three-quarters of an hour, and 9% managed it in half an hour. As regards the risk of perforating the colon during the wash-out, this accident occurred in three or some 2% of the 165 patients who replied, but all three cases survived after further operative treatment. Finally, though it is frequently claimed that the wash-out regimen enables the patients to lead a freer life than does the alternative regimen (because they do not have to cope with unexpected colostomy actions at other times of the day and can thus dispense with the wearing of a bag or belt), 52 of the patients questioned admitted that they occasionally wore some form of colostomy appliance as a precaution.

Most British surgeons have, like myself, reserved the wash-out regimen for those patients who fail to achieve a satisfactory routine of spontaneous evacuations. A further consideration militating against its popularity in Britain as compared with America is the lower standard of domestic sanitation to be found in this country, with relatively many fewer combined toilets and bathrooms found in the homes. Some years ago I decided to adopt, for a limited period as a trial, the wash-out regimen as my routine management for patients currently coming to colostomy. But when these patients reported to the out-patient clinics, they would get into conversation with other colostomy patients, who were having spontaneous colostomy actions managed with plastic colostomy bags. Within a short space of time, practically all my patients on irrigations asked to try the alternative method and expressed their preference for it. But with some of the lighter, more convenient and probably safer equipment now available for administering colostomy wash-outs (see Technique II below) the opinion of surgeons and patients in regard to the usefulness of this routine in Britain could change.

Two methods will be described for administering a colostomy wash-out:

Technique I
This might be termed the conventional or old-style method which has been in use for very many years. The equipment required for it comprises the following:

A 1 litre douche can with hook for fastening to the wall

2 m of 1 cm bore rubber or plastic tubing with glass connection

A No. 19 English gauge Jacques rubber or plastic catheter

A spring clip for compressing the tubing

Catheter lubricant

A plastic colostomy cup with rubber or plastic chute and belt

Cellulose tissues

When preparing for a colostomy wash-out the douche can, tubing and catheter are connected, and the spring clip is applied to the tube. The can is then suspended from the nail or hook on the wall at what will be shoulder height level when the patient is sitting, and filled with 1 litre of lukewarm tap water. The fluid is gently run through to expel any air from the tube. The patient then seats himself on the toilet or a stool, with the colostomy site exposed. It is usually advised that the colostomy cup should now be applied to the abdominal wall over the

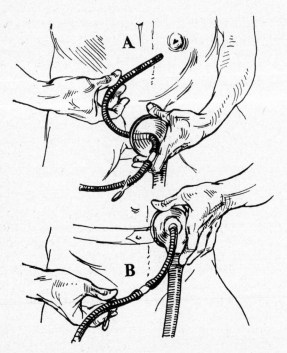

Fig. 497. Technique I for a colostomy wash-out. (A) The well lubricated catheter has been passed through the hole on the dome of the colostomy cup and is being inserted into the colostomy; it will finally be passed 10–15 cm into the bowel, with the utmost gentleness and with any forcing being avoided. (B) The colostomy cup is now fixed in position and the stop-cock is being released to allow fluid into the colon. After the wash-out has all been administered, the catheter is withdrawn and the perforation on the colostomy cup is corked with a rubber bung to prevent leakage during subsequent further actions.

stoma and fastened firmly in place with the belt, whilst the chute hangs down into the toilet bowl or other receptacle. The rubber bung is removed from the hole on the summit of the cup and the lubricated catheter is inserted through it and into the colostomy. However, the catheter has to fit the aperture in the appliance quite snugly to avoid subsequent leakage of fluid during the administration of the wash-out, and this produces some frictional resistance which in turn detracts from the sensitivity of the concomitant catheterization of the colostomy. I think that a safer, less traumatic technique is to pass the catheter for 15 cm or so through the perforation on the cup before the latter is applied to the abdominal wall. The protruding catheter is then passed into the colon as shown in Fig. 497A, and in due course the cup itself is applied to the skin and firmly fastened in position by tightening, and clipping the belt (Fig. 497B). The stop-cock is released, allowing the fluid to flow; though most of it runs upwards into the colon, some gravitates immediately alongside the catheter into the colostomy cup and chute. When the contents of the douche can have all passed in, the catheter is withdrawn and the hole on the colostomy cup is bunged. The cup and chute are maintained in position for as long as experience has taught the patient it is necessary to wait till the colostomy action has completed itself and all fluid has been returned. Incidentally, though the wash-out is usually done with simple tap water, if this proves consistently ineffective in producing a good colostomy action, soft soap may be added to the water at a rate of 25 g to the litre.

Technique II

More recently variants of the basic equipment for colostomy wash-outs have been proposed (e.g. Laird 1969; Mazier et al. 1976), which are probably somewhat more convenient for the patient. The firm of Hollister manufactures a very neat kit for the purpose (Fig. 498), as does also the firm of Coloplast. Instead of a rigid douche can there is a soft plastic container. The rigid colostomy cup and chute are replaced by what is in essence a specially long Hollister drainage bag but without karaya washer. The fluid may be conveyed into the colostomy via tubing and an ordinary plastic catheter which is passed through a small opening on the upper part of the front of the drainage bag. This opening is surrounded by a valve to prevent leakage of fluid when the catheter is removed after the wash-out has been given. But a more popular alternative is to have the catheter terminating in a

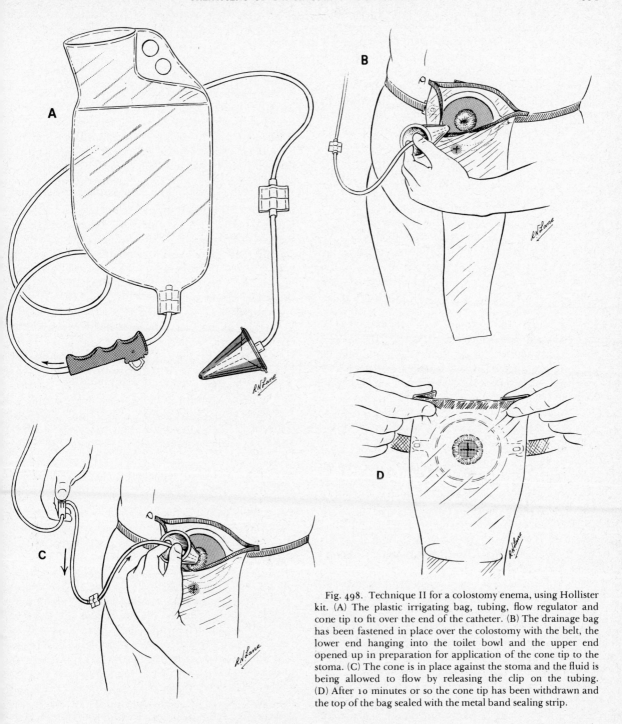

Fig. 498. Technique II for a colostomy enema, using Hollister kit. (A) The plastic irrigating bag, tubing, flow regulator and cone tip to fit over the end of the catheter. (B) The drainage bag has been fastened in place over the colostomy with the belt, the lower end hanging into the toilet bowl and the upper end opened up in preparation for application of the cone tip to the stoma. (C) The cone is in place against the stoma and the fluid is being allowed to flow by releasing the clip on the tubing. (D) After 10 minutes or so the cone tip has been withdrawn and the top of the bag sealed with the metal band sealing strip.

cone-shaped expansion (as originally proposed by Laird 1969), which is pressed against the colostomy with the point of the cone entered into the stoma. To make this possible a special drainage bag is used, the upper part of which in front can be torn down a short distance to expose the stoma (and subsequently re-sealed when the wash-out has been given and the cone is removed). One effect of the cone ending is that it obviates all risk of perforating the bowel. Another is that it makes the wash-out really an enema, in so far as no fluid can escape till all has been delivered into the bowel and the cone is removed, usually after ten minutes or so.

After the first burst of colonic activity following the administration of the wash-out, the lower end of the drainage bag may be closed with a Hollister clip, making it possible for the patient to walk around or sit elsewhere than on the toilet for another half-hour or more till all the fluid has been returned.

Covering of Colostomy between Wash-outs

The covering worn over the colostomy in the intervals between wash-outs varies from patient to patient, depending in considerable measure on how successful the wash-out regimen is in avoiding faecal leakage at other times. If this ideal has been attained, it suffices to cover the colostomy with a small piece of gauze and strapping or with strapping alone. If the regulation of colostomy action has not been so effective, the patient will feel safer wearing a plastic bag over the stoma as a safeguard. A convenient covering if leakage is slight is the Hollister adherent colostomy cap, which is very neat and contains absorbent tissue; it has an air vent to allow flatus to escape.

ESCAPE OF FLATUS AND USE OF DEODORANTS

A worry for many colostomy patients is that the involuntary passage of flatus may occasion embarrassment by causing impolite noises or malodour. The best that can be done for them is to advise the elimination from their diet of items which they have found to contribute greatly to intestinal flatulence and to prescribe deodorants to be taken by mouth or applied to the vicinity of the colostomy. Oral drugs that have been recommended are chlorophyll, powdered charcoal and bismuth subgallate, given in a dosage of 20 mg, 1–2 g, and 400 mg respectively, four times daily. Patients differ greatly in their opinions as to the effectiveness of such preparations. Examples of locally applied deodorants are Dor (made by Simpla-Sassco) and Stomogel or Stomosol (made by C. F. Thackeray); a drop or two is smeared with the finger on the inside of the plastic bag immediately before application. Unless used in strict moderation, the deodorant, which has a sweet sickly smell, may be more objectionable than the normal odour of the faeces. Naturally, after changing the appliance, it is an advantage to use one of the many brands of air

spray freshner available to counteract residual malodour in the room in which the change took place.

COLOSTOMY BOOKLETS

A very useful plan, which has been adopted by several hospitals and clinics, including my own, is to have a small booklet written on the care of a colostomy for the guidance of colostomy patients (Goligher and Pollard 1978). This contains information rather similar to that conveyed by the foregoing pages of this section but written in a more colloquial style suitable for lay readers. It supplements very nicely the practical instruction that the patient receives in the ward before his discharge from hospital, and is always available for reference. Similar pamphlets are also available from several of the leading manufacturers of enterostomal appliances and equipment. They are usually far more elegantly produced than is possible with a non-commercially sponsored booklet, but they are open to the charge of bias, however subtly exercised, in favour of the products of the particular firm concerned. Further advice about colostomy management may be obtained from the Colostomy Welfare Group, 38–9 Eccleston Square, London SW1V 1PB. In addition, good texts dealing with all aspects of stomal care are those of Todd (1978) and Walker (1975), more suitable for surgeons, doctors and enterostomal therapists than for patients.

MEDICAL AND SOCIAL CARE AFTER LEAVING HOSPITAL

After discharge the patient will be seen periodically at the out-patient department on routine 'follow-up'. At these attendances it is important that the surgeon should take time to enquire about the effectiveness of the patient's colostomy management and any problems that he may have encountered, because, unless he is asked, the patient may be reluctant to mention his difficulties. Actually, in my clinics in Leeds, which have been attended by very many patients after colostomy (and ileostomy) operations, all cases with an artificial anus have also been seen at each visit by my enterostomal therapist, Mrs Muriel Pollard. She has not only checked that they have an adequate supply of bags, adhesives, etc., but also advised them about other problems in regard to their stoma and its management, such as skin soreness, and I am deeply indebted to her for her invaluable assistance over the years. I have no doubt at all that the cooperation of a person like her, specially versed in the care of ileal and colonic stomas, is indispensible in providing a really high-grade service to patients after major colorectal surgery.

The social conditions of patients who have had a colostomy operation, particularly those of advanced years and in impoverished circumstances, often leave a great deal to be desired, as Devlin et al. (1971) have stressed, and there may be much for the medical social worker to do for them. To start with, she has usually to arrange convalescence in a suitable convalescent home, which may be quite difficult to organize, as not all such homes are willing to accept patients who have a colostomy. The conditions in the patient's home require to be investigated, for, as pointed out on p. 629, a fair proportion of houses in Britain lack good sanitary facilities. Such circumstances are hard enough for fit individuals to bear, but for colostomy patients they are well-nigh intolerable and constitute particularly strong grounds for rehousing. A major problem with older patients with a colostomy is their tendency to feel isolated and depressed and to lose all interest in feeding and looking after themselves. This needs to be combatted as far as possible by relatives, friendly neighbours or the community social services.

MAGNETIC CLOSING DEVICE TO CONFER ARTIFICIAL CONTINENCE

Remaining to be considered is the most controversial current major issue concerning colostomy care—namely the use of the magnetic closing device introduced by Feustel and Hennig of Erlangen in 1975 to attempt to provide some patients with an artificial sort of continence at their colostomies. This device consists of a ring and cap, both magnetized (Fig. 499). The ring is composed of samarium–cobalt with a coating of Palacos (a medically approved acrylate) or tantalum, which is implanted in the abdominal wall around the emerging colon. The cap is a plastic disc with a central protruding spigot or core, both the disc and core also containing samarium–cobalt. The spigot fits into the stoma and the cap rests on the skin around the opening with an adherent charcoal-containing filter-washer interposed between them (Fig. 500). The washer helps to fix the cap securely in place, yet by virtue of its charcoal content sometimes allows flatus to escape in a gradual and relatively non-odorous fashion without the patient having to lift off the cap. Feustel and Hennig (1975) found that a cap without a magnetized core was not sufficiently attracted to the buried ring to provide a firm sealing of the stoma. But a cap with a cobalt-containing spigot 30 mm long did experience a nearly constant force of attraction at a distance of the disc from the ring of between 10 and 30 mm. At a distance of more than 30 mm (as would be the case in an obese patient) the magnetic attraction would be much reduced and probably inadequate for continence in a colostomy, and when the distance is less than 10 mm (as would happen in a very thin patient) the force of attraction might be so great as to damage the tissues. Magnets made of samarium–cobalt are not influenced by external magnetic fields and maintain their magnetization much

longer than any patient is likely to live. The manufacture of the Erlangen magnetic equipment has been entrusted to the colostomy appliance firm of Coloplast-International of 3060 Espergaerde, Denmark, and is now marketed by them under the trade name of the Maclet system. The rings are issued pre-sterilized in sterile plastic containers.

Selection of Patients for Magnetic Ring Colostomies

Experience in Erlangen (Hager et al. 1976), and in several centres in Britian (Alexander-Williams et al. 1977; Goligher et al. 1977a) has shown clearly that *not every patient is suitable for a magnetic ring colostomy*. The chief contraindications to the use of the magnetic device are:

1. The existence of a greater thickness of subcutaneous fat in the abdominal wall than 2·5–3 cm.
2. The presence at or close to the proposed site of the colostomy of unusual rolls of skin and fat or of scars that would mar the flatness of the skin surface around the stoma, making it difficult subsequently to fit a magnetic cap securely.
3. Impaired mental faculties due to cerebral arteriosclerosis or old age, which would prevent the patient learning to cope with the magnetic device.

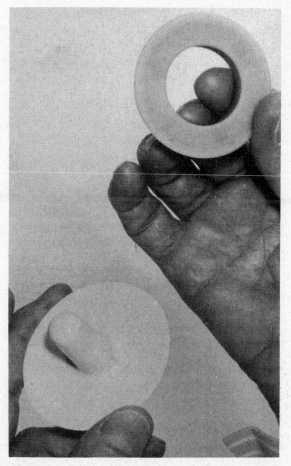

Fig. 499. The Erlangen magnetic colostomy ring and cap with spigot.

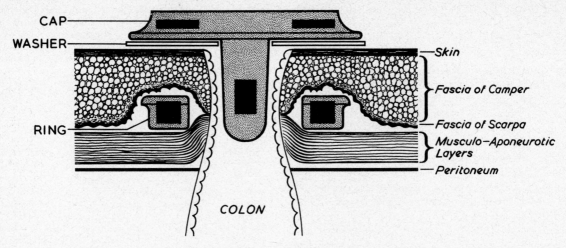

CAP
WASHER
RING

Skin

Fascia of Camper

Fascia of Scarpa
Musculo–Aponeurotic Layers
Peritoneum

COLON

Fig. 510. Loop iliac colostomy. (A) Incision. (B) Closing the lateral space by purse-string suture. (C) Suture of wound round the

4. Advanced malignant disease allowing a limited period of survival.

Operative Technique (Goligher et al. 1977a)

Selection of Site for Colostomy. An important principle in making a magnetic ring colostomy is that the colon stump should come *straight forward* through the substance of the abdominal wall and through the magnetic ring for suture *absolutely at right angles to the skin*; so that ultimately the cap and spigot will lie exactly superficial to the ring at all times. Obviously if, when the patient stands, the skin and subcutaneous fat drop down, the relationship between the cap and the ring will be disturbed. It is generally easier to make a colostomy that satisfies these require-

ments at all times during the various ambulant activities of the patient if it is placed, not in the usual site in the left iliac fossa, but rather higher up, where the abdominal wall has less subcutaneous fat and the stoma is above any 'spare tyre' of skin and fat. It is wise to choose and mark the site preoperatively after observing the patient in the supine and erect positions

Primary Implantation of Ring into Colostomy Wound from the Front. The steps involved in introducing the ring from the front are illustrated in Figs 501–4.

Primary Implantation Laterally from the Main Laparotomy Wound. An alternative way of inserting the rings is by creating a subcutaneous pocket extending from the main laparotomy

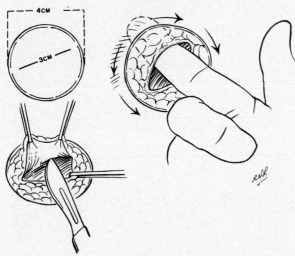

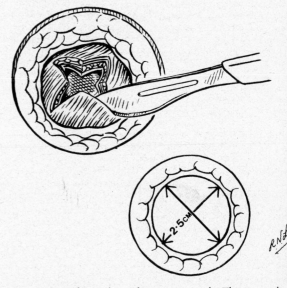

Fig. 501. Making the colostomy wound. A disc of skin 4 cm in diameter has been excised with as little subcutaneous fat as possible. The latter is then incised down to the external oblique aponeurosis and the fascia of Scarpa with overlying fat is elevated all round with a mixture of scalpel and finger dissection to create a bed for the ring.

Fig. 502. Making the colostomy wound. The musculo-aponeurotic layers and peritoneum are incised crucially through to the peritoneal cavity.

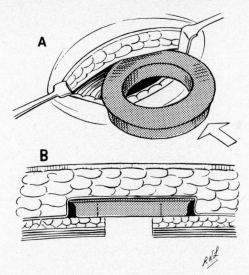

Fig. 503. Insertion of the magnetic ring. (A) Whilst the skin wound (diameter 4 cm) is stretched slightly, the ring (diameter roughly 5 cm) is slipped into the prepared bed. (B) The ring in place between the fascia of Scarpa and the external oblique aponeurosis. Note that the surface of the ring that has a slight flange is placed anteriorly.

wound to the colostomy wound (Fig. 507). The theoretical disadvantage of this route is that, if sepsis occurs in the laparotomy wound, as is not too uncommon, it might spread to the colostomy site. The advantage of lateral insertion is that it enables one to keep the colostomy wound smaller—say 2·5 cm in diameter—which may be helpful in securing continence. My more recent preference has been for this method.

Secondary Implantations. The first essential in considering implantation of a magnetic ring as a secondary procedure is to assess whether the patient has the necessary mental agility to manage a magnetic colostomy, and the second essential is to decide whether the site and structure of the existing stoma are

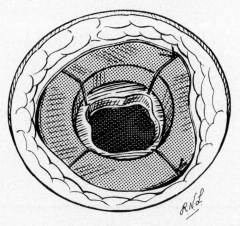

Fig. 504. Fixing the ring to the musculoaponeurosis layers with sutures of monofilament prolene No. 1/0.

such that it would suffice merely to introduce a magnetic ring around the bowel in that situation. If there are serious doubts on this latter score, the colostomy should be re-sited, preferably at a higher point in the abdominal wall well clear of the previous site. To do so will require a re-laparotomy through the scar of the original paramedian or median laparotomy wound, at which the colon stump is freed from the abdominal wall at the colostomy, and, after the small wound at the old colostomy site has been closed, a new colostomy is fashioned with a magnetic ring being implanted by either of the methods described above for primary operations.

If, however, the site and structure of the existing colostomy are deemed to be satisfactory for it to be converted into a magnetically controlled stoma where it lies, a purely local operation suffices. A convenient technique is that of Heald (1977) in which the colostomy is circumcised, not at the mucocutaneous junction, but 1 cm or slightly more wide of the mucosal edge. A neat way to make this circumcision of the right size is to place a Maclet ring accurately over the colostomy and adjacent skin and to carry the scalpel blade circumferentially round it with the blade running along the peripheral edge of the ring (Schellerer 1978). The ring is then laid aside and the incision is deepened down to the aponeurosis. With a little dissection a sufficient space is developed in the subcutaneous tissues to accommodate the ring which is threaded over the colon stump and its fringe of attached skin and fat. A few sutures of fine Dexon are then used to approximate the fat superficial to the ring and finally the skin wound is closed with silk sutures with careful apposition of the cutaneous edges. It might be feared that the rim of skin left attached to the separated stoma in this method of circumcision would sometimes have an inadequate blood supply and undergo necrosis. But apparently provided 6–12 months have elapsed since the original colostomy operation, no complication of this kind has occurred.

Stomal Care in Patients with Magnetic Ring Colostomies

It is customary to allow the colostomy wound four to six weeks to heal soundly before fitting the magnetic cap, and during that interval the stoma is managed along conventional lines with adherent plastic bags.

When the use of the cap is commenced (Fig. 508) the routine for employing it varies. Some patients keep—or try to keep—it in position throughout the 24 hours except for an hour or so once or twice a day for evacuation of the colon, which is allowed to take place into the kidney dish or temporarily applied adherent bag. Many more prefer to wear a bag during the night and for the first two or three hours of the day till the colostomy acts after breakfast. Thereafter the bag is removed and the cap is worn ideally till bedtime.

Results

The immediate hazards of magnetic ring implantation are apparently slight (Feustel and Hennig 1975; Hager et al. 1976; Alexander-Williams et al. 1977; Goligher et al. 1977a). Contrary to what might have been expected, sepsis in the colostomy wound is quite rare, at any rate after primary implantations, though not so uncommon after secondary implantations, and may necessitate removal of the ring.

As regards *functional results*, evidence has been conflicting. The initial impression from Erlangen (Feustel and Hennig 1975) was very favourable, but the subsequent report from that centre by Hager et al. (1976) showed that only approximately 30% of the patients given rings obtained worthwhile continence, and the results collected by Alexander-Williams et al. (1977) from various

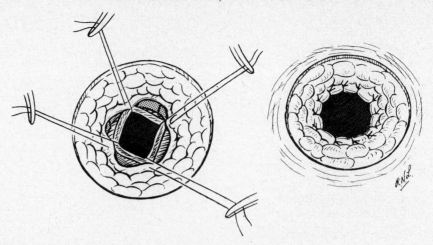

Fig. 505. Suture of the cut edge of the fascia of Scarpa and the fat to the edge of the hole in the musculoaponeurotic layers with 2/0 Dexon to bury the magnetic ring completely.

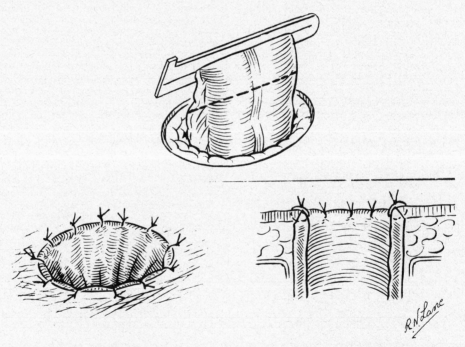

Fig. 506. After the colon stump, controlled by a Cope's clamp (or closed by suture or staples), is delivered through the abdominal wall and magnetic ring, it is amputated accurately at the skin level or immediately beyond, so that on suture of the cut end of the colon to the skin a right angled junction is secured.

British centres and those obtained by us in Leeds (Goligher et al. 1977a) were of roughly the same order. It is clear, however, that many failures were due to poor selection of patients or the construction of stomas that were far from perfect for the purposes of a magnetic closing device; for example, the course of the terminal colon to the colostomy being oblique rather than at right angles to the skin surface. There are good grounds for believing that a stricter choice of cases, with perhaps rejection of as many as half the patients coming to abdominoperineal excision, and a more meticulous operative technique might provide good results in at least 50% of the cases given rings. Incidentally for patients with obliquely placed colostomies special magnetic caps with spigots at an oblique angle are available, but in our hands they have proved less helpful than had been hoped. The magnetic colostomy closing device must be regarded as still being on trial and it will be interesting to see how much favour it finds with surgeons in general during the next few years. I must confess that to date my own results with

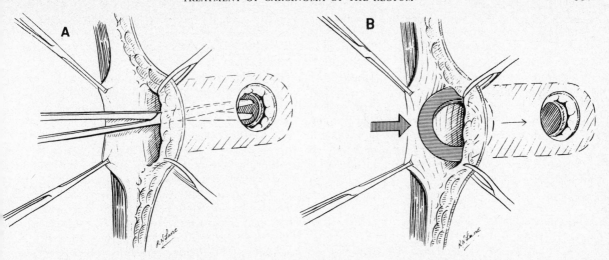

Fig. 507. Inserting the magnetic ring into the colostomy site sideways from the main laparotomy wound. (A) After dissecting up the cut edge of the fascia of Scarpa and fat from the underlying anterior rectus sheath in the left margin of the laparotomy wound, a pocket is created extending to the colostomy wound. (B) The ring is now slipped through this pocket to the colostomy wound where it is fixed as described in Figs 504 and 505.

the device have been rather disappointing. But at least it can be argued that, if it does not work well, no great harm has been done, for in most instances the ring may simply be left *in situ*, the use of the cap discontinued and a regimen of bags or wash-outs employed instead. Another possible routine that remains to be tried is a combination of the magnetic closing device with regular colostomy wash-outs.

The Results of Radical Surgical Treatment

IMMEDIATE MORTALITY

AFTER COMBINED EXCISION

Due to improvements in anaesthesia and in the pre- and postoperative care of patients in recent years, there has been a remarkable decline in the operative morbidity and mortality of the once formidable combined excision, and several large series of cases treated by this operation have now been published with astonishingly low mortality rates. Mayo et al. (1951) reported an immediate mortality of 4·1% in 689 consecutive Miles operations at the Mayo Clinic, and Abel (1957) using the same technique had a mortality of 5·3% in 188 cases at the Royal Marsden Hospital, London. In a personal series of 1223 perineo-abdominal operations Gabriel's (1957) mortality was 9·2% but in 422 consecutive cases done more recently at St Mark's Hospital it fell to 2·6%, and at one time he had a run of 168 cases without a single death—a truly splendid achievement. Lloyd-Davies (1957) reported a collective series of 1090 synchronous combined excisions from St Mark's Hospital with an operative mortality of 8·6% and in the later years this had declined to 4·4%. In a personal series of 615 synchronous

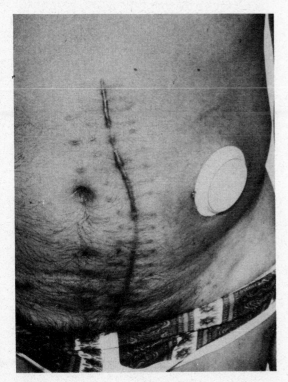

Fig. 508. A patient with a magnetic ring colostomy wearing the magnetic cap.

combined excisions Morgan (1965) had an immediate fatality rate of only 3·1%. The immediate mortality in my own personal series of 876 combined excisions, some done by the Miles method, the majority by the synchronous operation, is rather higher than these figures, namely 6·7%, due in large measure to the fact that in about 25% of the cases the operation was purely palliative. The causes of death are listed in Table 37 from which it will be seen that most of the deaths were due to cardiovascular or pulmonary complications beyond the control of the surgeon.

Factors Influencing the Operative Mortality of Combined Excision

The Operability (Excisability) Rate. As with any other major operation the operative mortality of combined excision can be considerably influenced by the selection of cases for it. If only patients in excellent general condition and with readily operable growths were accepted for excision, it would be easily possible to keep the immediate mortality at a very low level indeed. What makes the excellent mortality figures that have just been quoted above so creditable is that they have been achieved in the face of high operability (excisability) rates, which have steadily increased each year during the period of accumulation of the series. This fall in operative mortality, despite an increasing acceptance of patients for radical operation, is well shown in the collective statistics relating to rectal excision for cancer at St Mark's Hospital as reported by Dukes (1957) and Lockhart-Mummery et al. (1976) (Table 38).

It is important moreover to appreciate that the figures in Table 38 and apparently in all the other statistics of mortality so far quoted, include a number of purely palliative excisions as well as potentially curative ones, which has increased especially in the latter years to approximately 20%. This has a further adverse influence on the overall mortality rate, for the patients undergoing excision for palliation are generally poor operative risks. Thus in my own series of 876 combined excisions, 695 were performed with a chance of cure with an operative mortality of 3%, whilst 181 were solely for palliation with a mortality of 21%. Even amongst the cases having potentially curative excisions the immediate mortality can be shown to be somewhat affected by the extent of spread of the growth, being higher in cases with very advanced growths, which have undermined the patient's general health and call for more difficult excisions (see Gabriel 1948).

The Age and Sex of the Patients. It is a matter of common experience that the immediate risks are much less in younger patients, but it is not always appreciated that the sex of the patient also exerts an influence, the mortality at all ages being lower in women than in men. This is well demonstrated in Gabriel's (1948) statistics.

The Skill and Experience of the Surgeon and his Staff. It would be reasonable to suppose that the mortality of any major operation such as rectal excision will vary with the skill and experience of the surgeon and his assistants, the anaesthetist and the nursing staff, but it is difficult to assess these factors. Gabriel (1957) points out that his mortality was 26% in his

TABLE 37. *Causes of 59 Operative Deaths after 876 Combined Excisions of the Rectum for Cancer*

Cause of death	No of cases
Shock and circulatory failure	12
Pulmonary embolism	11
Intestinal obstruction or ileus	9
Coronary thrombosis	9
Bronchopneumonia	7
Cerebrovascular accidents	8
Difficult to determine	3
All causes	59

TABLE 38. *Excisability Rate and Operative Mortality of Rectal Cancer at St Mark's Hospital 1928–72*

Period	Percentage of patients seen accepted for excision (includes palliative excisions)	Operative mortality (%)
1928–32	46·5	12·8
1933–37	57·6	11·0
1938–42	69·4	11·1
1943–47	79·0	7·9
1948–52	92·7	6·8
1953–57		4·0
1958–62	93·2	3·1
1963–67		2·3
1968–72		2·1

After Dukes (1957) and Lockhart-Mummery et al. (1976).

first 81 perineo-abdominal excisions (1932–6), 11% in his next 517 (1937–46), and 5·3% in his last 625 (1947–56). But, whilst the steadily diminishing mortality may have been due in part to the greater familiarity of the surgeon and his staff with the special requirements of this operation, it was probably also in part attributable to the greatly increased safety of surgery in general in the later periods under review.

AFTER ANTERIOR RESECTION

Numerous statistics published in recent years attest to the fact that anterior resection with restoration of continuity can also be carried out with a low operative mortality. Thus Vandertoll and Beahrs (1965) have reported that in a series of 1766 cases treated by anterior resection at the Mayo Clinic between 1946 and 1957, the operative mortality was 4·2%. Rather more than a third of the 74 deaths were due to complications associated with leaks from the anastomosis. Deddish and Stearns (1961) commented on their experiences with 189 anterior resections, 19 of which were considered to be palliative because of distant metastases. There were 10 operative deaths, a mortality of approximately 5%. In the patients whose growths lay within 6–10 cm from the anal verge the mortality was 9%. Morgan (1965) had an immediate mortality of 4·4% in 251 anterior resections, mostly for growths in the upper third of the rectum and in the rectosigmoid and Lockhart-Mummery et al. (1976) report a mortality of 4·2% in 751 anterior resections at St Mark's Hospital 1948–72. In my own series of 535 cases treated by anterior resection—roughly three-fifths being high resections and slightly less than two-fifths low resections—there were 39 deaths (7·3%),

TABLE 39. *Causes of 39 Operative Deaths after 553 Anterior Resections for Cancer of the Rectum or Rectosigmoid*

Cause of death	No. of cases
Peritonitis	7
Pulmonary embolism	9
Coronary occlusion	10
Bronchopneumonia	7
Pelvic abscess	2
Shock	1
Not clearly determined	3
All causes	39

which occurred mostly in the cases undergoing palliative excisions. The causes of death are listed in Table 39 from which it will be seen that sepsis was responsible for some of the mortality.

AFTER ABDOMINOANAL PULL-THROUGH EXCISION

This form of sphincter-saving resection carries a notorious reputation for the frequency of post-operative complications following its use, particularly those resulting from necrosis of colon or infection in the presacral space. But it is clear from some of the published results achieved with it that it can be performed with an immediate mortality not exceeding that of anterior resection or abdomino-perineal excision. Thus Black and Botham (1958) had six deaths (5·7%) in 106 cases, only one death being referable to sepsis; in Waugh and Turner's (1958) series of 268 patients there were nine hospital fatalities, a mortality of 3·4%, again only one death being caused by bowel necrosis and infection; in Bacon's (1960) large series of 673 cases the immediate mortality was 4·3%. Turnbull and Cuthbertson (1961) had no deaths in 25 cases with carcinoma or villous papilloma. Hughes et al. (1962) reported one death in 44 cases, and Kennedy et al. (1970) seven in 158 cases (4·5%), three of the deaths being attributable to sloughing of the colon stump. My own experience comprises 59 abdominoanal pull-through excisions, most of them done by the Turnbull–Cutait method and usually for growths of the mid-third of the rectum; there were six deaths, two of them due to sloughing of the colon and infection.

AFTER ABDOMINOTRANSANAL RESECTION

There are no large well-documented published series of cases treated by this operation as yet, but it is likely that it will be on a par with abdominoanal pull-through resection as regards immediate mortality and morbidity. In eight cases treated by the abdominotransanal method I had no deaths but some morbidity from pelvic sepsis in three cases.

AFTER ABDOMINOSACRAL RESECTION

The largest modern series of patients treated by this operation is that of Localio et al. (1978) which comprised 100 cases; there were only two operative deaths.

AFTER PERINEAL OR SACRAL EXCISION

The immediate results of these operations, which

are now seldom performed, are described on pp. 502–3.

ULTIMATE SURVIVAL

IN GENERAL

With few other forms of malignant disease do we possess such detailed information relating to the late results of operative treatment as we do in regard to carcinoma of the rectum. Thanks particularly to the painstaking analyses and reports of Gabriel, Dukes, Morgan, Lloyd-Davies, Bussey, Lockhart-Mummery, Jean Ritchie and Hawley from St Mark's Hospital, London, of Grinnell from the Presbyterian Hospital, New York, and of Waugh, Mayo, Beahrs and their associates from the Mayo Clinic, a vast fund of accurate data has been amassed regarding the prospects of survival after rectal excision for cancer. In this section only the more salient points of this material will be outlined.

The yard-stick by which the curative value of surgical treatment is generally assessed is the five-year survival rate, and it is important to distinguish between the 'crude' and 'corrected' five-year survival rates. The crude rate is calculated by determining the number of patients still alive after five years and expressing it as a percentage of the original series. Some of the patients who have not survived have died of their cancer, but others have succumbed to other conditions; yet the crude five-year survival rate makes no distinction between these two forms of death. Obviously, the chances of developing an intercurrent fatal illness are much greater in an older group of patients than they are in a younger one. The crude five-year survival rate is thus a more reliable index of the effectiveness of surgical treatment of cancer in young or middle-aged persons than in elderly people.

To overcome the confusion introduced by deaths from intercurrent diseases, an effort might be made to discover the exact cause of death in each fatal case, but in practice this is extremely difficult to do. It is, therefore, more satisfactory to make allowance for intercurrent deaths by means of life tables, which indicate the normal expectancy of life of the general population of both sexes in different age groups. When this correction has been made the term 'corrected five-year survival rate' is used, and this rate gives a much more accurate picture of the curative value of surgical treatment.

Before considering the application of this criterion to various surgical procedures, it may be helpful to indicate some of the factors that may influence the five-year survival rate in general and require to be taken into account in making comparisons.

The Influence of a Rise in the Excision Rate and a Fall in the Operative Mortality Rate

Obviously, if the operability rate rises, the proportion of patients with particularly unfavourable growths being accepted for operation will be increased, so that the operation survivors will be diluted by a number of cases with slight prospects of achieving a lasting cure. Consequently, other things being equal, the five-year survival rate of the whole group of operation survivors ought to diminish. Similarly, if the operative mortality is reduced, a certain number of patients with very extensive lesions which have considerably undermined the patient's general health may manage to surmount the hazards of operation which, if the operative mortality had been higher, they might not have survived. Their inclusion amongst the operation survivors will likewise tend to lower the five-year survival rate of these patients. As has been mentioned earlier, one of the remarkable features of surgical treatment for cancer of the rectum over the past two decades has been the steady rise in the operability rate and the fall in the operative mortality (Table 38). It might be expected that this would result in a progressive decline in the five-year survival rate after surgical treatment. But this has not been so, for, as Dukes (1957) has shown, the crude five-year survival rate after rectal excision at St Mark's Hospital has been maintained at a fairly constant level of just at or below 50% over this period (and corrected five-year survival rate of around 56%), due presumably to the increasing effectiveness of the operative methods in vogue, as for example by the gradual displacement of the less radical perineal excision by the combined abdominoperineal operation and by other refinements of technique.

A better way of assessing the over-all benefits of surgical treatment, so as to take into account the wider application of radical surgery and its lower mortality in recent years, is to express the number of five-year survivors as a percentage, not of the immediate operation survivors but *of all patients presenting for treatment*; this is the absolute five-year survival rate. It has been calculated by Grinnell (1953) for the 1026 cases of rectal cancer reporting to the Presbyterian Hospital, New York from 1916 to 1945. During that time the resectability rate (excluding palliative resection) rose steadily from 57·5% in 1916–20 to 68·3% in 1946–50 and the

TABLE 40. *The Absolute Survival Rate of All Cases of Carcinoma of the Rectum Presenting for Treatment at the Presbyterian Hospital, New York, from 1916 to 1945 Inclusive*

Years	No. of primary cases admitted	No. of five-year survivals	Five-year survival rate (%)
1916–1920	40	7	17·5
1921–1925	39	7	17·9
1926–1930	89	11	12·4
1931–1935	164	38	23·2
1936–1940	214	70	32·7
1941–1945	231	66	28·6
1916–1945	777	199	25·6

After Grinnell (1953).

TABLE 41. *Corrected Five-year Survival Rate for Male Patients with Carcinoma of the Rectum in the Connecticut Tumor Registry*

Period of diagnosis	Total cases	Operability rate (%)	Corrected five-year survival rate (%)	
			Absolute	Surgically treated cases
1935–39	443	30·7	12·4	33·6
1940–44	628	40·9	17·8	37·3
1945–49	834	60·3	27·0	40·9
1950–54	980	73·0	37·6	48·8
1955–59	1058	71·1	36·1	48·7

After Eisenberg et al. (1967).

TABLE 42. *Corrected Five-year Survival Rate for Female Patients with Carcinoma of the Rectum in the Connecticut Tumor Registry*

Period of diagnosis	Total cases	Operability rate (%)	Corrected five-year survival rate (%)	
			Absolute	Surgically treated cases
1935–39	323	37·5	13·4	30·1
1940–44	467	46·0	26·2	49·3
1945–49	598	61·5	30·9	46·0
1950–54	765	71·9	39·6	52·0
1955–59	880	73·9	38·1	48·9

After Eisenberg et al. (1967).

operative mortality declined from 40·9% to 6·7%. The alteration in the absolute five-year survival rate over these 30 years is shown in Table 40 which indicates that there has been a progressive gain in the over-all achievements of surgery from 17·5% of five-year survivors in 1916–20 up to 32·7% in 1936–40, but a slight fall in 1941–5 to 28·6%.

The information from cancer registries is also interesting in this connection. Data from the Connecticut Tumor Registry (Eisenberg et al. 1967) are given in Tables 41 and 42 for male and female patients during the period 1935 to 1959. It will be seen that there was a very considerable rise in the absolute five-year survival rate during the first 10–15 years of the existence of the Registry, apparently due mainly to the considerable increase in operability rate during these early years. In comparing these survival rates with those reported by Grinnell (1953) (Table 40), it must be remembered that the former are corrected rates, the latter crude rates. But a comparison of the Connecticut Tumor Registry figures for surgically treated cases with the corrected five-year survival rate of approximately 56% recorded by Dukes (1957) from St Mark's Hospital shows that the Registry results fall somewhat short of the achievements of St Mark's Hospital. This is not, perhaps, surprising, considering the specialized nature of the latter institution and the fact that the Tumor Registry includes cases from many different types of hospital in Connecticut. Another factor contributing slightly to the difference is that the Registry figures apparently include operative deaths, whilst the St Mark's Hospital statistics are based on the immediate survivors of operation.

A comparison with the findings of cancer registries in Britain is particularly relevant and chastening. The Birmingham Regional Cancer Registry has records of 5800 cases of rectal cancer treated between the years 1950 and 1961 inclusive (Slaney 1971); 3005 or 52% underwent radical resection. The crude and corrected five-year survival rates for resected cases were 39·8% and 48·6% respectively, and the crude and corrected five-year survival rates for all cases registered were 21·9% and 29·2% respectively. During the years 1962–64 inclusive the South Western Regional Cancer Bureau (Walker 1971) registered 1346 patients with cancer of the rectum; 923 or 68·6% had excision, but this figure presumably includes also palliative resections. The crude five-year survival rate in resected cases was 34·1%, and for all cases registered 23·5%. These reports show what a discrepancy there is between the results that are possible under specially favourable circumstances and those regularly obtained in various regions of the country, including the small and large hospitals in these areas. Probably the main factor responsible for the poorer results in the regions is the lower operability rate there, which in turn may largely reflect differences in the clinical material presenting.

The Effect of the Extent of Spread of the Growth on the Survival Rate

The bearing of the extent of spread of the growth on the ultimate prognosis has been very clearly and conclusively demonstrated by Dukes (1957). The operative specimens in 2256 cases of rectal cancer subjected to excision of the rectum were classified by him into categories A, B and C (see p. 401), and, on the basis of a meticulous follow-up of the patients, the five-year survival rate was calculated for each category (Table 43). The excellent prospects afforded by surgical treatment for patients with A and B growths are evident, but it is noteworthy that about a third of the patients with C growths also secured a cure of their lesion. Very similar figures are produced by many other writers more recently, such as Corman et al. (1973) and Lockhart-Mummery et al. (1976).

The Bearing of Certain Operative Findings Relating to the Spread of the Growth on the Five-Year Survival Rate after Rectal Excision

So much interest has attached to the prognostic significance of the Dukes' system of categorization of the extent of spread of the tumour as revealed in the operative specimen, that relatively little attention has been devoted to determining the bearing on prognosis of certain features of the growth that can best be assessed by the surgeon himself when he examines the lesion at laparotomy. Among these characteristics are such findings as whether the tumour had extended through the wall to involve the peritoneal coat or to produce peritoneal plaques, or had become very fixed to surrounding structures. We have tried to establish more accurately the significance of these various operative findings in regard to ultimate outcome (Whittaker and Goligher 1976). It appeared that involvement of the overlying peritoneum or the presence of discrete peritoneal nodules did not carry quite such grave prognostic import as has usually been imagined, and that the significance of local fixation is very variable.

The Effect of Age on the Survival Rate

As already explained, the age of the patient is important in trying to assess the results of operation, because of the increased incidence of *deaths due to intercurrent disease in the upper age groups*. However, age is also important because of *its influence on the rate of growth* of the actual tumour. It has been established by Dukes (1957) that rectal carcinomas tend to be more active in younger patients, as shown by the greatly increased incidence of lymphatic metastases in such patients. As a consequence the prognosis as regards ultimate survival in young patients is poor, and it has often been stated, for example, that a patient under 30 years of age with a rectal cancer has a negligible chance of cure even with the most radical operation. But some patients below this age have in fact survived for five years and more, and this is well emphasized in a report by Mayo and Pagtalunan (1963) that 35% of patients aged less than 30 years with carcinoma of the colon (and rectum), unassociated with polyposis or colitis, survived five years after radical surgery (operation deaths excluded).

The Influence of Sex on the Survival Rate

As Dukes (1957) has pointed out, the crude five-year survival rate varies in the two sexes but tends to be higher in women than in men, due to a number of factors, which are partly controlled in the corrected five-year survival rate (see Table 43). The way in which the results are slightly more favourable for female patients in crude survival statistics is shown in the Mayo Clinic series of 1146 cases of carcinoma of the rectum followed up by Mayo and Fly (1956). They found that the five-year survival rate was 5% better for women than men for growths in each of the various sites in the rectum and for each of the types of operation used in treatment.

TABLE 43. *Cancer of Rectum. Five-Year Survival for A, B and C Cases (Operation Deaths Excluded)*

No. of cases	Stage	Crude five-year survival rate (%)	Corrected five-year survival rate (%)
Men			
206	A	80·4	99·9
565	B	61·3	76·0
717	C	26·1	31·3
Women			
129	A	81·8	93·8
206	B	71·6	82·0
433	C	29·1	32·7

After Dukes (1957).

The Influence of the Site of the Growth on the Survival Rate

The suggestion that the prognosis might be affected by the level of the growth was first made by Gilchrist and David (1947) of the Presbyterian Hospital, Chicago. They conducted a follow-up survey on 200 patients with carcinomas in different parts of the rectum treated by combined excision and found that the crude five-year survival rate for cases with lesions in the intraperitoneal part of the rectum was 65·4%, but for extraperitoneal growths only 51·8%. Waugh and Kirklin (1949) of the Mayo Clinic have also found that the prognosis varied with the height of the growth in the rectum. In 388 cases of rectal cancer treated by the Miles operation they related the crude five-year survival rate to the site of the growth, the site being determined by the distance of its lower edge from the anal verge on sigmoidoscopy before operation. Cases having purely palliative excisions were excluded. For growths lying between 0 and 5 cm inclusive there were 46·2% of five-year survivors, for growths between 6 and 10 cm, 51·1%, and for growths between 11 and 15 cm, 53·8%. Their detailed analysis of the survival rate in these cases according to the site of the growth and the presence or absence of lymphatic metastases is given in Table 44. Stearns and Binkley (1953) noted a similar but more marked difference in a follow-up survey of 369 patients surviving the operative risks of abdominoperineal excision for rectal cancer at the Memorial Hospital, New York. According to the level of the growth the five-year survival rate was:

0–6 cm, 52·8%; 6–11 cm, 61·8%; above 11 cm, 72·5%. Gilbertsen (1960b, 1962) of Minneapolis reported an overall five-year survival rate of 46·8% for 359 patients submitted to ostensibly curative excision for carcinoma of the rectum; in the 118 cases with lesions lying 11–17 cm from the anal verge the rate was 52·5%, but in 241 cases with growths situated within 11 cm of the anal margin it was only 44%.

Survival Beyond Five Years

The follow-up department at St Mark's Hospital now includes so many patients treated for much longer periods than five years that it has been possible to calculate survival rates for 10, 15 and 20 years (Bussey 1963). These are shown in Fig. 509, from which it will be seen that the corrected survival-rate for all cases falls from 57·5% at five years to 49·8% at 20 years. The effect of subdivision of the cases into Dukes' A, B, and C classification is also shown in Fig. 509. Those cases limited to the bowel wall (A cases) maintain over the entire 20-year period a high level of survival in the region of 95%. The cure rate of B cases (with spread to the perirectal tissues but no lymphatic metastases) falls to 77% at the end of five years and then flattens out to a final figure of about 70%, whilst C cases (with lymphatic metastases) decline steeply at first and achieve only a 25% survival after ten years. It may be concluded therefore that the great majority of patients who are going to die from recurrence do so before five years, and only relatively few between five and ten years. After ten years recurrence has a

TABLE 44. *Survival Rate of Patients having Carcinoma of the Rectum and Rectosigmoid Treated by Abdominoperineal Resection*

Level of lower edge of lesion above anal margin	Lymphatic metastases	No. of patients treated		No. of patients traced	Lived five or more years after operation	
					Number	Percentage of traced patients
0–5 cm	All cases	100		93	43	46·2
	without		56	50	33	66·0
	with		44	43	10	23·3
6–10 cm	All cases	201		182	93	51·1
	without		105	94	71	75·5
	with		96	88	22	25·0
11 cm or more	All cases	87		80	43	53·8
	without		54	47	32	68·1
	with		33	33	11	33·3

After Waugh and Kirklin (1949).

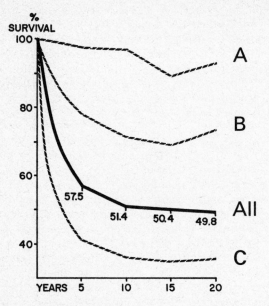

Fig. 509. Corrected survival-rate or 'cure-rate' of 2083 patients treated surgically for cancer of the rectum at St Mark's Hospital between 1928 and 1952 (data of Bussey 1963). Results shown separately for *all* cases and for A, B and C cases.

negligible effect on the cure rate, which by then is stabilized at approximately 50% for all cases.

Survival Rates for Patients with Carcinoma of the Rectum in Different Countries

Cutler and Lourie (1964) have compared the survival experience of patients with rectal cancer in five countries and shown some differences, but to what extent these are determined by geographical and social factors and not the method of collection of the data is uncertain.

AFTER PARTICULAR OPERATIONS

After Combined Excision

The report of Waugh and Kirklin (1949) on the late results in 388 cases treated by the Miles operation at the Mayo Clinic has already been referred to in Table 44. They found that the crude five-year survival rate (operation deaths excluded) for the entire series was 50·4%. In a later paper dealing with 625 cases treated by abdomino-perineal excision the crude five-year survival rate was given as 51·6% (Waugh et al. 1955). Abel (1957) of the Royal Marsden Hospital recorded a crude five-year survival rate after the Miles operation of

53% in a series of 280 cases treated between 1947 and 1951. Gilbertsen (1960b) found the crude five-year survival rate after 147 Miles operations in Wangensteen's department in Minneapolis to be 52%. Many other follow-up studies have given very similar results, namely a crude five-year survival rate of approximately 50% or slightly better, probably depending on the selection of cases for the operation. In this connection the late results worked out at St Mark's Hospital are particularly valuable because of their great accuracy (Bussey et al. 1960). They are recorded separately for the perineo-abdominal and synchronous combined operations, which are the two techniques for combined excision that have been used at that hospital:

Perineo-abdominal Excision. The total number of cases treated up to 1952 by this method was 993 (642 males, 351 females). The average age of the men was 59·6 years, of the women 58·1 years. The operative mortality was 8·2%. 14·2% proved to be A cases, 32·1% B cases and 53·7% C cases. The crude five-year survival rate after *radical* perineo-abdominal excision (operation deaths excluded) was 55·5% and the corrected five-year survival rate 65·8%.

Synchronous Combined Excision. 1214 patients were submitted to this operation (814 males and 400 females). The average age was roughly one year older for each sex than those treated by perineo-abdominal excision. The operative mortality was 7·9%. 12·7% were A cases, 35·1% B cases and 52·2% C cases. The crude five-year survival rate after *radical* synchronous combined excision (operation deaths excluded) was 55·8%, and the corrected five-year survival rate 67·2%. A more recent report by Lockhart-Mummery et al. (1976) dealing with cases treated by *radical* synchronous combined excision up to 1967 gives a crude five-year survival rate of 52·7% and a corrected rate of 63·8%.

A matter to be considered is whether the enlargement of the scope of combined excision achieved by *high ligation of the inferior mesenteric vessels or the dissection of the internal iliac glands* on the pelvic side-walls has had any demonstrable effect on the long-term survival. Stearns and Deddish (1959) came to the conclusion on follow-up that these manoeuvres had not improved the prospects of survival, but had added to the immediate morbidity. Bacon (1960), on the other hand, claimed that there was virtually no increase in operative mortality or morbidity following the use of these extensions to the operation but that the five-year survival rate was improved by 3·9% (a difference that would not seem to be significant in the context of his data). Grinnell (1965), in a typically thorough study of the effects of incorporating high ligation of the inferior mesenteric vessels in the technique of radical excision for rectal and rectosigmoid cancer (including some sphincter-saving resections as well as combined excisions), found that the immediate mortality was essentially unchanged but that the five-year survival rate was raised by about 5%. However, he comments on the difficulties of securing identical series for comparison and emphasizes that the difference elicited was not statistically significant (see also p. 505). The usefulness of this extension of the operation must be regarded as still *sub judice*.

The value of *multivisceral excisions* also warrants comment. The St Mark's Hospital results quoted above include some cases in which a part or all of an adherent related organ such as the posterior vaginal wall, uterus or small bowel was removed *en bloc* at the time of a combined excision. Unfortunately there has been no separate analysis of the outcome after these more extensive operations. However, Gilbertsen (1960b) has provided data on this point. Of 23 patients who had extended combined excisions at Minneapolis, 18 survived the immediate hazards of the operation, and 17% of the survivors lived five or more years subsequently. Cooke (1956) of Bristol and van Prohaska et al. (1953) of Chicago have also recorded a number of five-year survivals after multivisceral excisions for rectal cancer. As regards the most extreme form of this type of operation, namely complete pelvic clearance, Brunschwig and Daniel (1960) report that, of 21 cases of carcinoma of the rectum treated by this operation, one died in the immediate postoperative period and six, or 33%, survived for five yeras or longer; whilst Bricker et al. (1960) had six immediate deaths in 31 cases of rectal cancer submitted to pelvic exenteration with 31% of five-year survivors, which is distinctly encouraging.

After Anterior Resection

As already emphasized in discussing the immediate results of rectal excision, the patients treated by anterior resection are in several ways a specially favourable group. Their growths are mostly in the upper third or half of the rectum above the peritoneal reflection, and there may also have been some selection according to the extent of the spread, the more advanced lesions being rejected for this operation. Usually a higher proportion of female patients is included, because the wide female pelvis is conducive to the performance of anterior resection for certain growths for which in male patients it would not be readily feasible. One would therefore expect the late results of anterior resection to be better than those of combined excision in general, for this latter operation is used for carcinomas in all parts of the rectum; indeed, if it is the surgeon's practice to employ anterior resection for lesions of the upper rectum and rectosigmoid, there will be a disproportionately large percentage of lower rectal growths in the group treated by combined excision, and the only higher lesions submitted to this operation will be the unfavourable, difficult or advanced ones. Various published reports confirm these expectations. Thus, Dixon (1948), who used anterior resection mainly for very high rectal or rectosigmoid growths, found that the five-year survival rate in 272 cases treated by this operation at the Mayo Clinic was 67·7%, which contrasts with the five-year survival rates of 50% or slightly better for combined excision quoted on p. 644 from various sources including the Mayo Clinic itself.

Lockhart-Mummery et al. (1976) report on the use of anterior resection at St Mark's Hospital between 1948 and 1972. Due to changes in staff the proportion of patients undergoing radical surgery for rectal carcinoma who were given anterior resection as contrasted with combined excision increased from 16·9% during 1948–52 to 41·1% during 1968–72. The overall operative mortality for anterior resection from 1948 to 1972 was 4·2%, the crude five-year survival rate 66·7%, the corrected five-year survival rate 79·4%. (The corresponding figures of crude and corrected five-year survival rate for synchronous combined excision during that same period were 52·7% and 63·8% respectively.)

At the Mayo Clinic anterior resection has long been used by many of the surgeons for middle third growths as well as those in the upper rectum and rectosigmoid. Mayo et al. (1958) give an account of the results obtained in 507 cases treated by this operation during the years 1945–51. Excluding operative deaths and palliative cases crude five-year survival rate was 60·1%, compared with 51·7% for 580 patients treated by abdominoperineal excision during the same period. Cullen and Mayo (1963) report a crude five-year survival rate of 61·4% and a ten-year survival rate of 49·7% in Mayo's personal series of 424 cases submitted to anterior resection.

In order to secure a fair comparison between the results of anterior resection and combined excision it is clearly necessary to contrast similar series of cases treated by the two operations—namely series of similar age and sex composition with growths in the same segment of the rectum and not deliberately selected to exclude the more advanced lesions. A number of studies satisfying some or all of these criteria have been undertaken by Waugh et al. (1955), Mayo and Fly (1956) and Mayo et al. (1958) at the Mayo Clinic, by Deddish and Stearns (1961) at the Memorial Hospital, New York, and by Morgan (1955, 1965) at St Mark's Hospital. One of the most comprehensive of these enquiries is that of Mayo et al. (1958). They compared the five-year survivals following all anterior resections and combined excisions performed at the Mayo Clinic between 1945 and 1951 for growths the lower edges of which lay between 7·5 and 15·5 cm from the anal verge on sigmoidoscopy. Operation deaths and palliative excisions were excluded. The results are shown in Table 45, which is a slight modification of that in the original paper.

The five-year survival rate after anterior resection is 7% better than after combined excision. This would suggest that there must have been some selection of cases for the former operation for, whilst it might be hoped that anterior resection would give as good a chance of survival as combined excision for an upper rectal growth, it would be illogical to suppose that it might offer a better prospect of cure! It is stated that there was no significant difference in the two series as regards the age distribution or proportion of growths with and without lymphatic metastases, but that there were relatively more women treated by anterior resection. Also, although over-all siting of the lesions in the two series is the same—that is, between 7·5 and 15·5 cm—if the two subdivisions of this area, one between 7·5 and 10·5 cm and the other between 11·5 and 15·5 cm, are separately examined in Table 45 it will be seen that there is a notable difference in the distribution of the carcinomas treated by anterior resection and those subjected to combined excision. The bulk of the growths having anterior resection were in the upper portion, whilst the greater number of the lesions in the combined excision series were in the lower segment. The survival rate after anterior resection is better with growths in the 11·5–15·5 cm region than with those in the 7·5–10·5 cm area, and the prognosis with the latter might have been poorer still if more cases in this situation—and not, presumably, only the hand-picked, specially a favourable few—had been submitted to anterior resection, instead of being relegated to combined excision.

TABLE 45. *Five-year Survivals after Anterior Resection and Combined Excision for Carcinoma between 7·5 and 15·5 cm from the Anal Verge*

Distance of lower edge of growth from anal verge (cm)	Anterior resection		Combined excision	
	No. of cases treated and traced	Five-year survivors (%)	No. of cases treated and traced	Five-year survivors (%)
7·5–10·5	95	53	219	55
11·5–15·5	333	61	98	48
7·5–15·5	428	60	317	53

After Mayo et al. (1958).

The difference in the survival rate after combined excision, depending on whether the growth was in the middle or upper part of the rectum, makes interesting reading, for it is the exact reverse of what was found by Waugh and Kirklin (1949) from the Mayo Clinic 10 years earlier (see Table 44). The reason for the relatively poorer prognosis with cancers of the upper third treated by combined excision in the series reported by Mayo et al. (1958) is presumably that anterior resection has now become the procedure of choice at that clinic for growths of the upper third unless they are advanced or otherwise unfavourable, when they are treated by combined excision.

Deddish and Stearns (1961) compared the late results of 189 anterior resections and 301 abdominoperineal excisions for rectal and rectosigmoid cancer at the Memorial Hospital, New York, during the years 1947–54. Operation deaths, palliative cases and a few cases that could not be traced were all excluded, and the five-year survival rate was worked out for the two procedures for growths of the middle and upper thirds respectively (Table 46). At both levels the results after anterior resection were as good as those after combined excision. It is admitted that there were relatively more women in the group treated by anterior resection than in the series having combined excision, but the distribution of Dukes' A, B and C lesions is said to be the same in the two groups. It would be reasonable to suppose, however, that there was a considerable measure of selection of cases for anterior resection.

Morgan (1965), in reporting the five-year survival rate of his personal series of 251 anterior resections done for growths above the peritoneal reflection, has compared it with that which might be expected in a 'made-up' series of cases with supraperitoneal

TABLE 46. *Comparative Five-Year Survival Rate after Abdominoperineal Excision and Anterior Resection according to Height of Lesions*

Height of lesion above anal verge (cm)	Abdominoperineal excision		Anterior resection	
	No. of cases treated	Five-year survival	No. of cases treated	Five-year survival
6–10	172	106 (62%)	51	33 (65%)
11–16	76	55 (72%)	99	70 (70%)

After Deddish and Stearns (1961).

growths, adjusted to have the same proportion of men and women and of A, B and C lesions, and treated by combined excision. This synthetic series was compiled from the follow-up records of St Mark's Hospital relating to the period prior to 1943, when combined excision was the only radical operation available for carcinoma at this level, anterior resection not yet having been adopted. The corrected five-year survival rate for the cases treated by anterior resection was 76·3%, and for the control cases treated by combined excision 78·5%.

Gilbertsen (1960b), in his survey of the results of operations for rectal and rectosigmoid cancer in Minneapolis, found that the crude five-year survival rate for growths lying between 11 and 17 cm from the anal verge was slightly greater after anterior resection than after abdominoperineal excision (Table 47) but for lesions below 11 cm the latter operation gave better results. However, the number of cases treated by anterior resection below 11 cm was very small.

It will be apparent that a great deal of information is now available regarding the late results of anterior resection for cancer of the rectosigmoid and upper two-thirds of the rectum. But unfortunately much of it is open to criticism, for the crucial

point with all these retrospective studies comparing the outcome after two types of operation is whether the series being contrasted are in fact absolutely similar. Uncertainty on this score means that some doubt will remain regarding the relative curative values of anterior resection and combined excision till a properly controlled trial has been conducted in which a group of cases with suitably selected growths has been split in random fashion into two sub-series for treatment by these two operations. Meanwhile the most that can fairly be concluded is that for the average carcinoma in the rectosigmoid or upper half or two-thirds of the rectum a well executed radical anterior resection *probably* offers as good a chance of cure as does a combined excision and this is now generally accepted surgical philosophy.

After Abdominoanal Pull-Through Excision
As has been emphasized in connection with anterior resection, so with abdominoanal pull-through excision the quality of the long-term results may be to some extent favourably influenced by the selection of patients for this operation. Clearly the outcome should be compared with that after combined excision, used as far as possible under identical conditions. Unfortunately the nearest approach to such an assessment has been to contrast the results of the two operations when employed for growths at similar levels in the bowel, but usually without correction for discrepancies in sex incidence and in the amount of spread. Bacon (1960), who has used the pull-through operation for carcinomas of the rectosigmoid and upper two-thirds of the rectum, reports a crude five-year survival rate of 55·1% in his personal series of 673 cases treated by this operation. However, his comparison of this result with a five-year survival rate of 52·6% for 439 combined excisions done for growths in the lower third of the rectum or anal canal is not valid.

TABLE 47. *Crude Five-year Survival Rate after Abdominoperineal Excision and Anterior Resection according to Level of Growth*

Distance of lesion from anal verge (cm)	Abdominoperineal excision		Anterior resection		Pull-through excision	
	No. of cases treated	Five-year survivors	No. of cases treated	Five-year survivors	No. of cases treated	Five-year survivors
0–11	117	55 (47·0%)	17	6 (35·3%)	17	9 (53%)
11–17	24	12 (50%)	42	23 (57·1%)	0	0

After Gilbertsen (1960b). Operative deaths and palliative operations excluded.

J. M. Waugh generally reserved pull-through excision for middle third lesions. He reported (Waugh and Turner 1958) a crude five-year survival rate with it of 52·7%, which contrasts with a figure of 51·1% for combined excision used for growths at the same level (Waugh and Kirklin 1949). Operation deaths and palliative operations were excluded in calculating both these statistics. The proportion of patients with lymphatic metastases was roughly similar in the two series (Table 44) but the proportion of male and female patients and different age groups in the two series are not mentioned.

B. M. Black has also employed pull-through excision mainly for middle third growths, and in a series of 114 cases so treated found (Black and Botham 1958) that the crude five-year survival rate (operation deaths and palliative cases excluded) was 53%.

Gilbertsen (1960b) has reported the comparative crude five-year survival rates for a small series of pull-through excisions for growths between 0 and 11 cm from the anal verge and for abdominoperineal excisions for lesions at the same level (Table 47). It will be seen that the pull-through cases fared slightly better, but the numbers are small.

Altogether, the information on the curative value of pull-through excision for growths in the region in which it is most useful—namely between 7 and 11 cm—is still somewhat meagre.

After Abdominotransanal or Abdominosacral Resection

As yet there are no extensive long-term results available for analysis after these relatively recently popular operations, though Localio et al. (1978) report that, in 36 patients followed up for at least five years after abdominosacral resection, the survival rate lay somewhere between that obtained after abdominoperineal excision and that after anterior resection.

After Diathermy Destruction or Local Excision of Growth

The results following this form of treatment are adequately described on pp. 516, 517.

After Perineal or Sacral Excision

The late results of these operations are discussed on pp. 502 and 503.

RECURRENCE

Another way of assessing the efficacy of operations designed to eradicate cancer of the rectum, as of operations for growths in other organs, is to determine the frequency of recurrence of the disease. In addition, the actual sites of recurrence might give an indication of the particular deficiencies of the operative method being studied and of the directions in which it might usefully be extended. Indeed Ernest Miles' (1908) formulation of the standard abdominoperineal excision was based in no small measure on an examination of the patterns of recurrence after lesser operations for rectal cancer.

But there are obvious difficulties in detecting local or distant recurrences on clinical examination, for many recurrent lesions may be symptomless or completely overshadowed symptomatically by simultaneous recurrences at other sites. Similarly, radiological studies are of only limited value. Thus it is all too easy to overlook further manifestations of growth. Consequently, even in patients who are obviously dying of recurrence, it is usually difficult to be sure of the complete distribution of recurrent lesions. In fact the only way to be certain of not missing some recurrences is to undertake routine necropsy. But there are often considerable practical difficulties about securing a post-mortem examination, and in most studies of the incidence of recurrence after operations for rectal cancer the information has been derived from this source in only a proportion of the patients. In many cases the decision about recurrent growth was based on the clinical and radiological findings elicited at the follow-up clinic or on similar even more limited information provided by the patient's own general practitioner. It is thus easy to understand the discrepancies in the results reported from different studies, and it is fair to assume that all these estimates tend to underrate the incidence of recurrence. Some of the more important published work

TABLE 48. *Survival Rates after Pull-through Excision and Ordinary Combined Excision*

| Type of operation | Level of lesion above anal verge (cm) | Nodal metastases traced patients | | Lived five or more years after operation |
		Condition	No. of cases	
Pull-through	5–10 (in 81% of lesions)	Without	73	53 (72·6%)
		With	58	16 (27·6%)
		Total	131	69 (52·7%)
A–P excision	6–10	Without	94	71 (75·5%)
		With	88	22 (25·0%)
		Total	182	93 (51·1%)

After Waugh and Turner (1958). Hospital deaths and palliative cases excluded.

on the subject will now be briefly reviewed in relation to the three main operations.

AFTER COMBINED EXCISION

One of the first careful investigations was that of Gilchrist and David (1947) who followed up 112 patients after radical operations for rectal carcinoma lying *partly or completely below the peritoneal reflection*. 16·1% developed local recurrence, 11·6% metastases in the liver, and 3·6% secondary deposits in the skeleton or elsewhere. The incidence of local recurrence was five times as high in the cases that had had lymphatic metastases demonstrated on the operative specimen as in those in which the nodes were negative. Of 55 patients with entirely *intraperitoneal* growths, only 3·6% were found to produce local recurrence, but 11% had recurrence in the liver and 3·6% in the lungs or generally.

Stearns and Binkley (1953) reported the incidence of recurrence revealed in a follow-up study of 369 patients treated by abdominoperineal excision at the Memorial Hospital, New York, during the years 1928–45. 21·9% produced local recurrences and 19% distant recurrences. The frequency of local recurrence varied inversely with the height of the primary lesion, being 30% for growths lying 0–6 cm from the anal verge, 20% for those at 6–11 cm, and 14·5% for growths above 11 cm. The incidence of distant metastases also varied somewhat, but not consistently, depending on the position of the growth. Another factor influencing the number of local and distant recurrences was the extent of spread of the growth as determined by dissection of the operative specimen. Thus the local recurrence rate in A cases was 6·1%, in B cases 24%, and in C cases 31%. The highest incidence of local recurrence was with C growths situated in the lower or middle thirds of the rectum.

Gilbertsen (1960a, 1962), in the course of his meticulous analysis of the results of operations for rectal cancer at the University Hospital, Minneapolis, during 1940–50, found that, of 117 immediate survivors of 'curative' abdominoperineal excision for growths within 11 cm of the anal verge, 24% developed local recurrence and 19·7% distant recurrences. He also noted that the incidence of recurrence was affected by the extent of spread of the growth—in A cases being 9·1% local and 13·6% distant, in B cases 16·7% local and 29% distant, and in C cases 40·8% local and 28·5% distant.

Morson et al. (1963) have examined the frequency of local recurrence after 1596 radical sphincter-sacrificing operations (combined or perineal excisions mostly) performed at St Mark's Hospital up to 1952, and report an incidence a good deal lower than in the American studies just quoted—namely 9·7%. They find also that the incidence is influenced by the site of the growth, being 14·5% with cancers of the lower third, 8·3% with lesions of the middle third, and 5·2% with upper third growths. Similarly the frequency was considerably affected by the extent of spread, being 0·8% in A cases, 5·2% in B cases and 16% in C cases, or—to consider only the extent of *local* spread and not also lymph node metastases—the incidence of recurrence was 0·9% in cases with no demonstrable local extension, 5·9% in cases with slight spread, and 16·8% in cases with extensive spread.

It will be seen that there is general agreement regarding the influence of the extent of spread of the growth and its site on the tendency to local recurrence. Whilst the higher figures recorded for carcinomas of the lower and middle thirds may be attributable to the readier spread of growths in these segments and the greater difficulty of eradicating them, it may also conceivably reflect in part the easier detection of local recurrences at these levels than in the peritoneal cavity.

The *sites* of local recurrence were examined in detail by Gilbertsen (1960a), with particular reference to extraperitoneal growths treated by abdominoperineal excision. He found that in the female the commonest sites are the posterior vaginal wall and the pelvic peritoneum, whilst in the male some recurrences were also found anteriorly on the back of the prostate, vesicles and bladder and in the rectovesical pouch of peritoneum, but for some reason difficult to understand the majority occurred posteriorly in the perineum or on the front of the sacrum.

The *mechanism* of local recurrence is presumably inadequate excision in most instances, but it is surprising to note that no less than 6% of Stearn's and Binkley's (1953) A cases, 9·1% of Gilbertsen's (1960a) A cases and 0·8% of Morson et al.'s (1963) A cases developed local recurrence. An alternative explanation of some recurrences is that of implantation of loose cancer cells in raw areas in the pelvis at the time of operation. Morson et al. (1963) considered that the local recurrence in 105 of their cases was due to incomplete removal and in 45 to surgical implantation.

AFTER ANTERIOR RESECTION

The development of local recurrences in the vicinity of the anastomosis and in the pelvis after anterior resection has attracted much attention. According to some of the earlier enquiries this was a common occurrence. Thus Garlock and Ginsburg (1950) reported a local recurrence rate in the bowel of 35·7% in a small series of cases treated by anterior resection at the Mount Sinai Hospital, New York. In addition 7·1% of the patients developed pelvic recurrence entirely outside the bowel. They emphasized that this was a complication of anterior resections for middle or lower rectal growths, and that for lesions above 12·7 cm (i.e. in the upper rectum or rectosigmoid) the local recurrence rate was only 3·3% and the extrarectal pelvic recurrence rate 1·6%. Similarly Judd and Bellegie (1952), in a review of 282 patients who had survived radical anterior resection for rectal or rectosigmoid cancer at the Mayo Clinic during the years 1936–45, found that no less than 25% had recurrence within the bowel. The incidence was greatest when the original growth lay less than 11 cm from the anal verge, and on the strength of this finding Judd and Bellegie (1952) recommended that anterior resection should be reserved for cancers of the upper third of the rectum or the rectosigmoid.

Other workers have reported a lower incidence of local recurrence. Goligher et al. (1951a) gave the local recurrence rate in a series of 162 cases treated by sphincter-saving operations (105 anterior resections, 31 Hartmann operations and 26 abdomino-anal excisions) as 10%, and Warren Cole (1952) had a similar incidence at the University of Illinois Medical Center. Deddish and Stearns (1961), in a group of 150 cases followed up after anterior resection, noted 11 anastomotic or pelvic recurrences, an incidence of 7·3% (Table 49). In the 51 patients whose initial lesions were situated between 6 and 10 cm from the anal verge the recurrence rate was 11·7%, but in 99 patients with lesions between 11 and 16 cm from the anus the recurrences amounted to 5%. The incidence of local recurrence also varied with the extent of spread of the original growth, being nil in 35 A cases, 3·4% in 59 B cases, and 10% in 55 C cases. It is to be noted, however, that both Goligher et al. (1951a) and Lofgren et al. (1957) observed that anastomotic recurrences sometimes developed in cases with A lesions, whilst Vandertoll and Beahrs (1965) in a follow-up study of 1741 patients surviving anterior resection at the Mayo Clinic found that 11·5% developed local recurrence, but that the incidence in Dukes' A and B cases combined was 11·2% and in Dukes' C cases virtually the same, namely 12·6%. Cullen and Mayo (1963) examined in detail the local recurrence rate in relation to the site of the growth in a follow-up of Mayo's personal series of 309 cases treated by anterior resection (Table 50).

Finally, Morson et al. (1963) have reported on some experiences at St Mark's Hospital in regard to local recurrence after anterior resection. 217 patients survived this operation during the period 1947–52 and 177 of these were deemed to have had radical operations with a chance of cure; 14, or 7·9%, subsequently developed local recurrence, four on the suture line, 10 in the pelvis. 40 had palliative operations (five on account of incomplete local removal, the rest mainly because of hepatic metastases); six of these later produced pelvic recurrences, an incidence of 15%, three being on the suture line.

Mechanism of Local Recurrence after Anterior Resection. There are four ways in which such further manifestations of growth might arise: (a) By the

TABLE 49. *Incidence of Local Recurrence after Abdominoperineal Excision and Anterior Resection according to Height of Original Lesion*

Distance of growth from and verge	No. of patients traced	Local recurrences		
		Anastomotic	Pelvic	Total
6–10 cm				
A-P excision	172	—	34	34 (19·8%)
Anterior resection	51	2	4	6 (11·7%)
11–16 cm				
A-P excision	76	—	11	11 (14·5%)
Anterior resection	99	4	1	5 (5·0%)
Total				
A-P excision	248	—	45	45 (18·1%)
Anterior resection	150	6	5	11 (7·3%)

After Deddish and Stearns (1961). Operative deaths and palliative cases excluded.

TABLE 50. *Three-year Local Recurrence Rate according to the Height of the Original Carcinoma*

Distance from anal margin (cm)	No. of cases treated	Intraluminal recurrences	Intraluminal + pelvic recurrences
10	81	12 (14·8%)	19 (23·5%)
10–14	158	14 (8·9%)	20 (12·7%)
15–19	55	4 (7·3%)	5 (9·1%)
20–24	15	0	0
Total	309	30 (9·7%)	44 (14·2%)

After Cullen and Mayo (1963). Hospital deaths and palliative cases excluded.

development of a fresh primary growth in the mucosa of the remaining large bowel mucosa. (*b*) As a consequence of incomplete excision of the ramifications of the original tumour in the pelvis. (*c*) Due to inadequate removal of apparently normal rectal wall distal to the primary lesion, so that microscopic intramural extension of the growth remains in the upper end of the retained rectal stump. (*d*) By surgical implantation of exfoliated malignant cells on the suture line or other raw surfaces created during the operation.

In our earlier enquiries into this problem (Goligher et al. 1951*a*) we accepted that some 'recurrences' might be due to mechanisms (*a*), (*b*) or (*c*), but we were impressed by the fact that the further development of growth was often mainly or entirely intramural and intraluminal; that it frequently appeared in places where a raw area had existed at the time of operation, as for example on the suture line; that in many cases there was an apparently adequate distal margin of normal bowel in the resection specimen; and that *in a few instances the initial growth was a Dukes' A lesion, and sometimes the recurrent growth was in the same category.* It seemed to us probable that in many cases the causal mechanism was that of surgical implantation, as earlier suggested by Lloyd-Davies (1948, 1950) and Morgan (1950). This also seemed a plausible explanation of many of the cases reported by Cole (1952), Cole et al. (1954), McGrew et al. (1954), Lofgren et al. (1957), Boreham (1958) and Keynes (1961). A recent study by Rosenberg et al. (1978), however, casts considerable doubt on the viability of exfoliated carcinoma cells in the lumen of the bowel in cases of carcinoma coli and therefore on their capacity to successfully ingraft themselves on a suture line or other raw surface (see also p. 399).

What we had not fully appreciated at that stage—though we ought to have from the work of Gilchrist and David (1947)—was that local recurrence in the pelvic cavity is also common after abdomino-perineal excision and occurs sometimes even after removal of A growths, as the researches of Stearns and Binkley (1953), Gilbertsen (1960*a*, 1962), Deddish and Stearns (1961) and Morson et al. (1963) clearly show. Indeed, if allowance is made for the fact that local recurrences are probably detected more readily after sphincter-saving resection than after abdominoperineal excision because the presence of the rectum allows palpation of the pelvis and endoscopy, there is probably little real difference in the incidence of local recurrences after the two types of operation according to the latest statistics. For example, there is a close similarity in

the frequency of local recurrence found by Cullen and Mayo (1963) after anterior resection and that reported by Stearns and Binkley (1953) after combined excision, and the differences in the local recurrence rate reported for the two operations by Deddish and Stearns (1961) and Morson et al. (1963) are slight. Perhaps many of the recurrences in the region of the anastomosis after anterior resection are simply pelvic recurrences, which have extended centripetally into the rectal wall and lumen, as postulated by Deddish and Stearns (1961) and Morson et al. (1963). Compared with some of the earlier estimates of the frequency of local recurrences after anterior resection the present incidence is apparently a good deal lower. It would be tempting to attribute this reduction to the adoption of precautions against implantation (see pp. 444 and 564), but the issue is confused by the fact that most surgeons are probably now more careful to obtain a margin of at least 5 cm of normal rectum distal to the carcinoma in performing anterior resection. Certainly the incidence of local recurrence after anterior resection, even when used for middle third growths, does not seem seriously out of proportion to that after combined excision for lesions at the same level when the readier detection of such recurrences after a sphincter-saving operation is borne in mind.

AFTER ABDOMINOANAL PULL-THROUGH EXCISION

So far as I can discover there is little reliable information available on the incidence of recurrence after this operation. Bacon (1956) mentions that of 346 patients traced for up to five years after surviving radical pull-through excision, 70 or 22·8% developed local recurrence.

AFTER ABDOMINOTRANSANAL OR ABDOMINOSACRAL RESECTION

I am not aware of any really comprehensive published study of the frequency and form of recurrence after these operations, though Localio et al. (1978) provide some interesting data in regard to the abdominosacral operation.

AFTER LOCAL DESTRUCTION OR LOCAL EXCISION

One of the serious possibilities after these more limited forms of treatment is obviously local recurrence but sufficient has been written about it on p. 517.

AFTER PERINEAL OR SACRAL EXCISION

Some information will be found in the literature referred to on p. 502; it is not proposed to consider these little-used operations further in this section.

PALLIATIVE TREATMENT OF INCURABLE RECTAL CANCER

The following measures are available for the palliation of incurable rectal growths:

Palliative Excision

As already emphasized in discussing radical surgical treatment, a palliative excision is the procedure of choice for growths that are still locally removable, and in fact there are few incurable carcinomas of the rectum that cannot be thus excised. For example, of the last 100 cases with cancer of the rectum seen by me, 95 proceeded to an excision of their growth, in 68 with a view to cure, and in 29 purely for palliation. This is a higher proportion of palliative excisions than that recorded by most surgeons, due to the poor condition and advanced disease of many of the patients admitted to the general wards of the Leeds General Infirmary; but in most published series at the present time, though the operability or excisability rate is usually of the order of 90–95%, at least 20% of the excisions are undertaken solely for palliation.

Radiotherapy

The place of radiotherapy as a palliative measure is discussed on p. 655.

Chemotherapy

The use of cytotoxic drugs in the treatment of inoperable or recurrent colorectal carcinomas is considered on p. 473.

Palliative Colostomy

In former years when the operability rate of rectal cancer was low it was customary to treat the inoperable cases almost as a routine by a proximal loop iliac colostomy. It was hoped that this operation, by relieving any obstructive element, would lead to an improvement in the patient's general health and comfort, and such claims were strongly argued by Gabriel and Lloyd-Davies (1935). It has to be admitted, however, that in many cases, perhaps the majority, the operation afforded no worthwhile palliation, and indeed made the patients a good deal less comfortable by simply adding the burden of an artificial anus to their existing discomforts. For unfortunately these latter, especially the incessant, spurious diarrhoea with passage of blood and slime, are directly attributable to the primary growth itself and can only be eliminated by its removal (or destruction by other means). Realization of this fact has had two effects: firstly, it has induced the surgeon to undertake excision whenever possible, and secondly, it has restrained him from performing a proximal colostomy unless the patient is in fact verging on acute obstruction. In those cases without complete or nearly complete obstruction it is better to leave the patient without a colostomy in the first instance. If acute obstructive symptoms develop later, an emergency colostomy may be required, but, with the very advanced lesions for which colostomy alone is now reserved, this eventuality seldom arises; more usually the patient dies of the general effects of his growth before this can happen. The infrequency with which so-called palliative colostomy is now practised is shown by the fact that in the last 100 cases of carcinoma of the rectum coming under my care a colostomy alone as the final definitive treatment was employed on only two occasions.

TECHNIQUE OF LEFT ILIAC COLOSTOMY FOR IRREMOVABLE RECTAL CANCER

From the foregoing remarks it will be appreciated that this operation is now only likely to be performed either at the conclusion of a laparotomy at which the growth has been demonstrated to be quite irremovable and verging on complete obstruction, or less commonly at a separate emergency intervention for acute obstruction in a patient known to have an irremovable rectal carcinoma. A separate small oblique muscle splitting incision should be made in the left iliac region with its centre about the junction of the middle and outer thirds of the line joining the anterior superior iliac spine and the umbilicus (Fig. 510A). The iliac

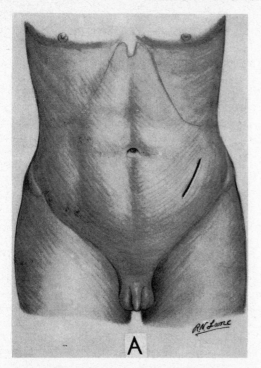
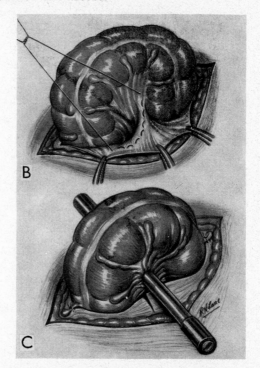

Fig. 510. Loop iliac colostomy. (A) Incision. (B) Closing the lateral space by purse-string suture. (C) Suture of wound round the loop of colon which is prevented from receding by the glass rod and from extending farther by incorporating two or three appendices epiploicae in sutures placed in the external oblique aponeurosis. Note that the sharp edges of the latter are snicked to avoid injurious constriction of the bowel. The skin remains to be sutured, dressings applied, and the loop opened by a transverse or cruciate incision on its summit.

colon is identified and drawn out of the wound, the aim being to establish the colostomy *as far proximally as possible in this piece of the bowel*. The lateral space or paracolic gutter is closed by a purse-string suture of fine linen (Fig. 510B) and a glass rod is passed through the mesocolon to hold the loop out of the abdomen. The wound is then closed in layers with catgut sutures snugly round the protruding loop (Fig. 510C). In the suture of the external oblique aponeurosis there are two points to be mentioned:

1. Care should be taken not to constrict the bowel too tightly, and it is a good plan to cut the edge of the aponeurosis transversely to the axis of its fibres for 1–1·5 cm on either side at the position of the glass rod.

2. To prevent the loop being further extruded during the immediate postoperative period, it is useful to incorporate several appendices epiploicae in stitches in the aponeurosis. Finally the skin is approximated with interrupted silk sutures.

If a main paramedian wound is present as well, it is now closed in the usual way, dressed and covered with waterproof strapping. Attention is then turned to the colostomy loop, the bowel being opened longitudinally, as shown in Fig. 352A, and the edges of the resulting wound being immediately sutured to the margins of the skin wound (Fig. 352B, C), except where the glass rod projects. If the colostomy is being performed in the presence of acute or subacute obstruction, this method of opening the colostomy is still practicable if the sucker is used to take up escaping liquid faeces and subsequently empty the proximal limb of bowel to some extent before starting the suturing. Alternatively, a Paul's tube may be inserted, as described in Fig. 351.

Postoperative Care. If a Paul's tube has been used, it usually becomes loose about the fifth day and is then removed. If immediate mucocutaneous suture was practised, the stitches should be removed on the eighth to tenth day at the same time as the ordinary skin sutures. The glass rod should be retained for at least two weeks and on its removal a rubber tube should be substituted, the ends being turned back after its introduction and tied to

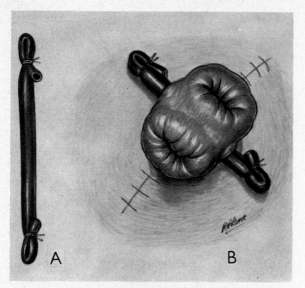

Fig. 511. (A) Method of preparing a stout rubber tube as a support to the spur of a loop colostomy after removal of the glass rod. (B) Rubber tube in use.

prevent it sliding out (Fig. 511). This relatively softer support may be worn without discomfort by the patient for several weeks, during which time the spur of the colostomy becomes consolidated so that after removal of the tube subsequent recession is unlikely to occur. Without this precaution, the spur not infrequently recedes below the surface and allows faeces to pass over into the distal bowel. The management of the colostomy actions and provision of colostomy appliances is as described for a permanent colostomy in connection with abdominoperineal excision (see p. 622). If discharge from the rectum is troublesome, occasional washes-through from the colostomy to the anus may be helpful, using plain water to which has been added 15 g of soft soap to the litre.

ALTERNATIVE TECHNIQUES

Many alternative techniques exist for making a palliative iliac colostomy. To support the loop more securely and avoid subsequent spur retraction a bridge formed by a strip of external oblique aponeurosis or of skin may be taken across from the middle of one side of the wound to a corresponding point on the opposite side. Or the loop of colon and mesocolon may be completely divided across, the two ends being separately implanted in the abdominal wall, the active one at the upper corner of the iliac wound, the inactive one at the lower

corner of this wound or of the paramedian wound. But all these methods are a little more complicated than the very simple technique with a glass rod just described. They may have had their advantages in cases where the colostomy was part of a perineal or sacral excision and the patient might live for many years to develop colostomy complications such as recession, but in the type of case for which a palliative iliac colostomy is now performed the period of survival is seldom more than a few months, and the simpler the operative technique the better.

Curettage: Diathermy Fulguration: Cryosurgery

Sometimes patients who have an irremovable carcinoma of the rectum may be made more comfortable by curettage of a considerable part of the tumour with a large Volkmann's spoon per anum. This treatment, which naturally requires general anaesthesia, is more readily applicable to projecting growths which form a big intraluminal mass, for this may be steadily scraped away, often with a considerable, though temporary, reduction in the amount of discharge and bleeding. There is obviously a danger of perforating the bowel if the curettage is continued too far, and the surgeon should be satisfied with modest gains at any one session. This palliative treatment may be used to supplement a proximal colostomy or as the sole form of therapy.

Diathermy fulguration per anum is another method of achieving the same effect. The growth is extensively destroyed *in situ* with the coagulating current of an ordinary surgical diathermy machine applied with a disc electrode or malleable blade under general anaesthesia. If desired, curettage and diathermy fulguration may be combined, most of the obvious projecting tissue being first of all scraped away and then the remaining bared portion being coagulated with the diathermy. For a period of seven to ten days after fulguration charred tissue sloughs away leaving a flat ulcer which sometimes heals completely. Some astonishing results have been reported with this method of treatment (see p. 516).

More recently cryosurgery has been used by some surgeons instead of diathermy for inoperable growths of this kind (Osborne et al. 1978), employing the sort of equipment described in connection with cryosurgery for haemorrhoids (see p. 126).

Intrathecal Injection of Alcohol or Phenol

One of the unpleasant developments with an inoperable carcinoma of the rectum is extension of the lesion to involve surrounding, more sensitive parts such as the sacral plexus or the pelvis, with resulting severe sacral, perineal or sciatic pain. An attempt may be made to relieve this pain by intrathecal injection of alcohol to destroy the relevant posterior nerve roots. The principle of the method is that the alcohol is lighter than the cerebrospinal fluid so that after the lumbar puncture needle has been introduced, preferably through the first lumbar interspace, the patient is so positioned that the posterior sacral roots transmitting the pain lie above the point of the needle. For full details of the method the reader is referred to Ottley (1938) or to standard neurosurgical texts. In practice it is best to enlist the aid of a neurosurgical colleague in selecting patients for this form of treatment and in carrying it out. Errors in technique may result in loss of control of the bladder sphincter.

More recently phenol has been introduced as a substitute for alcohol for intrathecal injection by Nathan and Scott (1958) and Brown (1958). It has the advantage that it seems to have a selective affinity for sensory nerve fibres so that the risk of motor nerve lesions with resulting paralysis is largely reduced. A good account of the achievements of this form of palliation is given by Robbie (1969).

Chordotomy

As an alternative to intrathecal injections for intractable pain, chordotomy may be employed, and it will be for the neurosurgeon consulted to decide which, if either, of these operations is to be advised, the tendency at the moment apparently being to try the more minor procedure of phenol injection in the first instance and to reserve the chordotomy for the cases that remain unrelieved by it (see O'Connell 1969).

Sedatives and Other Symptomatic Measures

In the long run the majority of cases with inoperable or recurrent rectal carcinomas require sedation and other symptomatic treatment for pain, fistulous discharges and other complications of the disease as they arise.

THE PLACE OF RADIOTHERAPY IN THE TREATMENT OF CARCINOMA OF THE RECTUM

In the 1920s when radium was being extensively tried in the treatment of various carcinomas, efforts were made to treat rectal cancer by the same means. The radium was sometimes applied to the luminal surface by the medium of a surface applicator, which consisted essentially of a rubber catheter into which the radium was loaded. More usually, however, the technique employed was that of interstitial irradiation, radium needles being inserted as a barrage around the growth from inside the lumen, through a posterior surgical approach, or through the perianal skin or vagina. Despite very occasional successes the results of this treatment were bitterly disappointing, as the report of Gordon-Watson (1930a, b) made abundantly clear. Not only did it usually fail to arrest the growth, but it frequently made the patients worse from the development of sepsis, fistulation and even second primary growths. The consequence was that, as in so many other situations, interstitial radium treatment was completely abandoned, and for many years the only form of irradiation considered was teleradiation with X-rays.

In the management of cases with inoperable rectal carcinomas, or with more favourable lesions for which the patient refused to accept operation, *conventional radiotherapy* with 200–250 kV X-rays sometimes yielded a good palliative result, and even a very occasional apparent cure (see Roberts 1942). But much more often it failed to produce any substantial improvement and in some instances it undoubtedly aggravated the patient's discomfort by producing severe skin irritation or irradiation cystitis. Altogether the impression left with surgeons referring cases for treatment was not very encouraging. What has aroused fresh interest in the possibilities of radiotherapy in recent years has been the introduction of more powerful sources of irradiation, such as the million volt apparatus, or the cobalt bomb. Phillips (1942), working with the million volt machine at St Bartholomew's Hospital, London, was the first to draw attention to the special advantages of *supervoltage radiotherapy* for carcinoma of the rectum. He reported a series of 65 cases of rectal carcinoma treated by this means. They included 22 recurrent cases after previous radical operation, 36 patients with locally inoperable primary growths, and seven who had locally operable lesions but were unfit for operation because of their general conditions. In 19 of the whole group the carcinoma disappeared after treatment, this effect being obtained in six of the seven operable cases. Unfortunately the period of follow-up was not more than four years and often much less, so that the precise curative value of the therapy could not be reliably assessed on Phillips' (1942) report. However, Williams, who continued this work at St Bartholomew's Hospital, recorded (Williams and Horwitz 1959) that between 1937 and 1949 165 cases with carcinoma of the rectum were treated primarily by radiotherapy. Many of these patients had very advanced growths and 24 would obviously have been incurable by surgery because of the presence of distant metastases. Of the other 141, nine or 6·4% survived for five years or more. Even in the group of 26 relatively favourable cases there were only two five-year survivors. Williams emphasized also some of the disadvantages and complications of radiotherapy. Nearly all patients developed an early or late reaction in the neighbouring tissues. Included among the immediate effects were diarrhoea, cystitis, vaginitis and dermatitis. In some 50% of the patients they were so severe as to curtail or modify treatment. The late irradiation reactions were more serious, but fortunately less frequent. Fistulas, mainly rectovaginal, developed in 6% of the cases, but failure to control the primary malignant process might have been a factor in their production in some instances.

Fibrosis at the site of the neoplasm leading to rectal stenosis occurred in 17%; many of these patients required a colostomy, if they did not already have one. In some cases a more diffuse fibrosis developed in the bowel wall, leading to the formation of a long tubular stricture involving most of the rectum. It will be seen that these results of attempted cure by supervoltage radiotherapy, unlike the earlier favourable impressions of Phillips (1942), are distinctly discouraging. However, by contrast with Phillips (1942), Williams has been impressed by the palliative value of supervoltage therapy in cases of recurrent carcinoma recti (Williams et al. 1957), as have Schulz and Wang (1962) and Stearns and Whiteley (1970).

Preoperative Radiotherapy for Cancer of the Rectum

A retrospective survey of the patients treated for carcinoma of the rectum and rectosigmoid at the Memorial Hospital, New York City, during the years 1939–51 showed that those having preoperative radiotherapy—and merely conventional radiotherapy at that—prior to radical operation achieved a significantly better five-year survival rate than did those treated solely by operation (Stearns et al. 1959). Analysis of these results in regard to the extent of spread of the growths revealed that the improvement related mainly to cases with lymphatic metastases, the five-year survival rate in 195 patients who had had X-ray therapy before radical operation being 72%, as contrasted with only 46% in 201 who had had radical surgery alone. As a consequence of these findings the members of the rectum and colon service at the Memorial Hospital in 1957 agreed to resume

TABLE 51. *Survival of Patients with Carcinoma of the Rectum after Radical Excision, with or without Preoperative Radiotherapy, at the Memorial Hospital, New York City*

	1939–51 (uncontrolled)		1957–62 (controlled)	
	No radiotherapy	Radiotherapy	No radiotherapy	Radiotherapy
Nodes negative				
Number of patients	241	264	163	127
Indeterminate	20	27	21	17
Five-year survivors	161	179	113	80
Five-year survival rate				
Overall	62%	68%	70%	63%
Determinate	73%	75%	80%	73%
Nodes positive				
Number of patients	201	195	105	67
Indeterminate	10	14	6	8
Five-year survivors	46	72	43	23
Five-year survival rate				
Overall	23%	37%	41%	34%
Determinate	27%	43%	44%	39%

After Stearns et al. (1968).

the use of preoperative radiotherapy as an adjuvant measure in connection with radical surgical treatment of cancer of the rectum and rectosigmoid, but *to use it on a random basis* in order to secure a control untreated group, against which to measure the results. Only patients who underwent an ostensibly curative operation, who had no obvious evidence of residual or metastatic cancer in distant sites were included. In 1968 Stearns et al. gave a report on the five-year survival rates of the first 459 cases entered in this trial between 1957 and 1962, and in addition made some comparisons with the results in their 1939–51 cases (Table 51).

Contrary to the experience in the 1939–51 series of cases, in their controlled trial adjuvant radiotherapy was found not to have improved the five-year survival rates, either of the entire group irradiated or more specifically of those patients with lymphatic metastases. Comparison of the survival rates of the combined irradiated and non-irradiated patients in the 1939–51 and 1957–62 series shows an improved overall survival rate in the latter series. The improvement occurred in the group of patients in this series who had had lymphatic metastases and were treated by radical operation without radiotherapy. It is a matter for speculation whether this improvement in results in the more recently treated cases has been due to refinements of surgical technique.

But rather more encouraging results from preoperative radiotherapy in conjunction with radical surgery for rectal carcinoma have been reported by Dwight et al. (1972), who conducted a controlled trial on 700 patients treated in a group of hospitals belonging to the Veterans Administration in USA. Roughly half of the cases were randomly allocated to preoperative radiotherapy (2000–2500 rad), the other half being exempted from this treatment. Subsequently both groups proceeded to laparotomy and 613 patients underwent removal of their growths (183 by anterior resection, 414 by abdominoperineal excision, and 16 by other methods), the operability rate being roughly the same in the cases treated by X-rays and in those not so treated. Initially the operative mortality was higher in the patients treated by X-rays, later this difference diminished. A subsequent report on the Veterans Hospitals trial by Higgins (1974) and Higgins et al. (1974) showed that when only patients who had had ostensibly curative excisions are considered the five-year survival rate in 229 treated patients is 49% as against 39% in 224 non-treated patients. When only 'curative' abdominoperineal excisions are considered the five-year survival rate for 162 patients receiving preoperative radiotherapy is 47%, compared with 34% for 143 control patients, a statistically significant difference ($P = 0.02$). An interesting point made by Higgins (1974) relates to the reduced frequency of lymph node mestastases in the irradiated patients: only 27% of them had positive nodes as contrasted with 45% of the patients who proceeded to rectal excision without radiotherapy.

Clearly there is a contradiction between the findings of these two controlled trials of preoperative irradiation in USA, and to try to discover whether radiotherapy in this connection is beneficial the Medical Research Council in Britain embarked in early 1976 on a multicentre trial in the British Isles. The patients were randomized to three groups, one having simply rectal excision, the second having rectal excision preceded by a single dose of 500 rads of irradiation, and the third having rectal excision preceded by 2000–2500 rads of irradiation over a ten-day period. By the end of 1978 approximately 800 patients had been included in the trial. Of course the follow-up will have to continue for another four or five years to give a proper measure of the effect of the radiotherapy. All that can be said at this stage is that there was no significant increase in the postoperative morbidity or mortality in the treated groups,

and no significant difference in medium-term survival has yet emerged between the treated and non-treated patients (Duncan 1979).

With regard to the current treatment of patients with operable carcinomas of the rectum coming to operation, my feeling is that, until we have a decision from the MRC trial, it would be better to withhold preoperative radiotherapy.

Recent Experiences with Endocavitary Contact Irradiation and Interstitial Radiation Implantation for Rectal Carcinoma

One of the most exciting innovations in the therapy of carcinoma of the rectum in recent years has been the development by Papillon (1973) of Lyon and other French radiotherapists of the method of treating certain lower rectal growths by *contact irradiation.* For this purpose the Philips Contact X-ray machine is used, which has a low voltage (50 V), a short focal distance (4 cm) and a high output (2000 rad per minute in the air). The rays are delivered through a narrow tube capable of being inserted via a special proctoscope of 3 cm diameter. By varying the position of the proctoscope and X-ray tube, contact therapy can be applied to different parts of the surface of the tumour, each area irradiated being 3 cm in diameter. The treatment is on an out-patient basis, the patients attending for three, four or five treatments over a period of four to six weeks, the total dose at the surface of the lesion being between 9000 and 15 000 rad. The effect of treatment is to produce a rapid shrinkage of the part of the tumour projecting into the lumen of the bowel, so that at subsequent attendances the growth presents with a greatly reduced volume compared with its initial size. The dose at each visit, the size of the field and the intervals between each treatment are calculated in relation to the spread or shrinkage of the tumour. The last application usually takes place when the growth has clinically disappeared.

It may well be asked how rectal cancer, which is well known to be relatively radioresistant as a rule to external irradiation, becomes radiosensitive and radiocurable when treated by endocavitary contact X-ray therapy. The explanation lies with the important differences in the time–dose and volume–dose relationships in the two methods of treatment. In external irradiation a dose of 4000 rad is given over four weeks to a very large volume of *normal* tissue as well as tumour. In contact X-ray therapy the same dose of 4000 rad is delivered in three minutes to a very small volume of mainly *tumour* tissue.

But the possibilities of endocavitary contact X-ray therapy are strictly limited. It is only applicable to very carefully selected tumours which satisfy the following criteria: (*a*) there must be perfect accessibility to all parts of the surface of the tumour and this means in effect that the lesion must be in the lowermost 10–12 cm of rectum; (*b*) the tumour must not be too large, as each field of irradiation is only 3 cm in diameter. It is possible to use two overlapping fields for cancers of 5 cm in length and 3 cm in width; (*c*) tumours projecting into the lumen of the bowel are better adapted to this treatment than infiltrating growths, because of the rapid absorption of the X-ray beam; and (*d*) poorly differentiated tumours are quite unsuitable for intracavitary irradiation because of the high incidence of lymphatic spread with such growths.

Interstitial radium implantation has also been revived by Papillon (1973) in the treatment of certain rectal carcinomas, often in conjunction with contact X-ray therapy. After the projecting part of the tumour has been destroyed by X-rays, radium needles are applied six weeks later to the bed of the tumour, which is still indurated, to 'sterilize' the infiltrated area of the rectal wall. The needles are not sutured to the wall of the bowel but are kept in place for two to three days by a rubber tube inserted into the rectum through the anus and stitched to the anal verge.

The results reported by Papillon (1973) are certainly impressive. Of 106 patients mostly with polypoid cancers treated by these methods between 1951 and 1966 and all followed up for more than five years, 75 or 70% are still alive and well and free from disease (71 having been treated by irradiation alone, four having required subsequent radical surgery for failure, these being the only four of the 75 to have a colostomy). It is clear from this experience that for small, well differentiated mainly projecting or exophytic carcinomas of the lower rectum which are unlikely to be associated with lymphatic metastases, endocavitary contact irradiation may often be very effective. For unfit subjects for whom a major rectal excision would be particularly hazardous, the treatment of choice for lesions of this kind may well be irradiation by this technique (or electrocoagulation or local excision, see pp. 516 and 517).

Present Indications for Radiotherapy

Assuming that some form of supervoltage therapy is available, I would consider the indications for irradiation in the treatment of rectal cancer at the present time to be as follows:

1. For inoperable growths, either recurrent after a previous radical excision, or primarily inoperable. There will be very few of the latter in experienced surgical hands. As for the former, further surgical treatment is usually impossible, and, though I have not been impressed by the results of radiotherapy myself in this group, in view of Williams et al. (1957) report I would not feel justified in withholding this treatment.

2. For operable growths where operation is refused by the patient or his general condition is likely to render any attempt at radical excision exceptionally hazardous. For relatively small growths of mainly projecting type in the lowermost 10 cm of rectum, endocavitary contact radiotherapy is the ideal method and may offer an excellent prospect of lasting cure—though it has to be considered in competition with purely local excision or diathermy fulguration (see p. 654). The really debatable case for radiotherapy is the patient who has a carcinoma of dubious operability, which will probably involve a very difficult excision, and whose general condition is poor due to a cardiac lesion or chest condition. Such a lesion will be unsuitable for contact irradiation and will require external irradiation if radiotherapy is to be undertaken. The operative mortality in this selected group is undoubtedly very high and often the prospects of lasting cure slight, but the palliative value of the operation may be considerable and is generally more reliable than that of irradiation. My own feeling, therefore, would usually be in favour of surgical excision, unless the patient's general state made him a very poor risk indeed, when I might invoke radiotherapeutic aid instead of operation. It is important to bear in mind that a full course of irradiation is often found by the patient to be an extremely uncomfortable experience.

Another indication in operable cases, urged by Williams et al. (1957), is the use of *radiotherapy as a supplement to radical excision* in cases where it has seemed at operation that the growth had probably not been completely removed. In this situation radiotherapy would be in competition with chemotherapy, which many surgeons would prefer as supplementary treatment.

REFERENCES

ABEL, A. L. (1957) Discussion on major surgery in carcinoma of the rectum, with or without colostomy excluding anal canal and including the rectosigmoid. *Proc. R. Soc. Med., 50*, 1035.

ALEXANDER-WILLIAMS, J., AMERY, A. H. and DEVLIN, H. B. (1977) Magnetic continent colostomy device. *Br. med. J., 1*, 1269.

ALLINGHAM, W. and ALLINGHAM, H. W. (1901) *The Diagnosis and Treatment of Diseases of the Rectum*, 7th ed. London: Baillière.

ANDERSON, H. U., HODGES, C. U., BENHAM, A. M. and OCKER, J. M. (1959) Transuretero-ureterostomy (contralateral uretero-ureterostomy): experimental and clinical experiences. *Trans. W. Sect. Am. urol. Ass.*, 27, 99.

ANNIS, D. (1952) Replacement of the ureter by small intestine. An experimental study. *Proc. R. Soc. Med.*, 45, 483.

APPLEBY, L. H. (1950) Discussion on the treatment of advanced cancer of the rectum. *Proc. R. Soc. Med.*, 43, 1071.

ASHLEY, F. L. and ANSON, B. J. (1946) The pelvic autonomic nerves in the male. *Surgery Gynec. Obstet.*, 82, 598.

AULT, G. W., CASTRO, A. F. and SMITH, R. S. (1952) Clinical study of ligation of the inferior mesenteric artery in left colon resections. *Surgery Gynec. Obstet.*, 94, 223.

AUST, J. B. and ABSOLON, K. B. (1962) A successful lumbosacral amputation, hemicorporectomy. *Surgery, St Louis*, 52, 756.

BABCOCK, W. W. (1939) Experiences with resection of the colon and the elimination of colostomy. *Am. J. Surg.*, 46, 186.

—— (1947) Radical single-stage extirpation for cancer of the large bowel, with retained functional anus. *Surgery Gynec. Obstet.*, 85, 1.

BACH-NIELSEN, P. (1967) New surgical method of repairing sacral hernia following abdomino-perineal excision of the rectum. *Acta chir. scand.*, 133, 67.

BACON, H. E. (1945) Evolution of sphincter muscle preservation and re-establishment of continuity in the operative treatment of rectal and sigmoidal cancer. *Surgery Gynec. Obstet.*, 81, 113.

—— (1956) Abdominoperineal proctosigmoidectomy with sphincter preservation. Five-year and ten-year survival after pull-through operation for cancer of the rectum. *J. Am. med. Ass.*, 160, 628.

—— (1960) Major surgery of the colon and rectum: rehabilitation and survival rate in 2,457 patients. *Dis. Colon Rect.*, 3, 393.

BALFOUR, D. C. (1910) A method of anastomosis between sigmoid and rectum. *Ann. Surg.*, 51, 239.

BARR, S. S., VALIENTE, M. A. and BACON, H. E. (1962) Rationale of bilateral oophorectomy concomitant with resection for carcinoma of the rectum and colon. *Dis. Colon Rect.*, 5, 450.

BEAHRS, O. H. (1975) Personal communication.

BENNETT, R. C., HUGHES, E. S. R. and CUTHBERTSON, A. M. (1972) Long-term review of function following pull-through operations of the rectum. *Br. J. Surg.*, 59, 723.

BEVAN, A. D. (1917) Carcinoma of the rectum: treatment by local excision. *Surg. Clins N. Am.*, 1, 1233.

BINKLEY, G. E. (1952) Construction and care of abdominal colostomy. *Am. J. Surg.*, 83, 807.

BLACK, B. M. (1952) Combined abdomino-endo-rectal resection: technical aspects and indications. *Archs Surg., Chicago*, 65, 406.

—— (1961) Symposium on surgery of the colon. Pull through procedures. *Proc. Mayo Clin.*, 36, 476.

—— and BOTHAM, R. J. (1958) Combined abdominoendorectal resections for lesions of the mid and upper parts of the rectum. *Archs Surg., Chicago*, 76, 688.

—— and KELLY, A. H. (1955) Recurrent carcinoma of the rectum and rectosigmoid; results of treatment after continence-preserving procedures. *Archs Surg., Chicago*, 71, 538.

BLANDY, J. P. and ANDERSON, J. D. (1977) Management of the injured ureter. *Proc. R. Soc. Med.*, 70, 137.

BLISS, B. P. (1963) Dehiscence of the lateral space following its closure in colostomy and ileostomy. *Br. J. Surg.*, 50, 730.

BLOODGOOD, J. C. (1906) Surgery of carcinoma of the upper portion of the rectum and sigmoid colon: combined sacral and abdominal operations. *Surgery Gynec. Obstet.*, 3, 284.

BOREHAM, P. (1958) Implantation metastases from cancer of the large bowel. *Br. J. Surg.*, 46, 103.

BOXALL, T. A., SMART, P. J. G. and GRIFFITHS, J. D. (1963) The blood supply of the distal segment of the rectum in anterior resection. *Br. J. Surg.*, 50, 399.

BRICKER, E. M. (1950) Bladder substitution after pelvic evisceration. *Surg. Clins N. Am.*, 30, 1511.

—— BUTCHER, H. R., Jr., LAWLER, W. H., Jr. and McAFEE, C. A. (1960) Surgical treatment of advanced and recurrent carcinoma of the pelvic viscera; an evaluation of 10 years experience. *Ann. Surg.*, 152, 388.

BROADER, J. H., MASSELINK, B. A., OAKES, G. D. and ALEXANDER-WILLIAMS, J. (1974) Management of the pelvic space after proctectomy. *Br. J. Surg.*, 61, 94.

BROWN, A. S. (1958) Treatment of intractable pain by subarachnoid injection of carbolic acid. *Lancet*, 2, 975.

BRUMMELKAMP, R. (1965) The Rectoresector: a new instrument for resection of the rectum and colorectal anastomosis without sutures. *Dis. Colon Rect.*, 8, 49.

BRUNSCHWIG, A. (1948) Complete excision of pelvic viscera for advanced carcinoma: one stage abdominoperineal operation with end colostomy and bilateral ureteral implantation into colon above colostomy. *Cancer*, 1, 177.

—— (1961) Radical surgical management of cancer of the colon spread in tissues and organs beyond the colon. *Dis. Colon Rect.*, 4, 83.

—— and BARBER, H. K. (1969) Pelvic exenteration combined with resection of segments of bony pelvis. *Surgery, St Louis*, 65, 41

—— and DANIEL, W. D. (1960) Pelvic exenteration operations: with summary of sixty-six cases surviving more than five years. *Ann. Surg.*, 151, 571.

BURT, C. A. V. (1960) Carcinoma of ovaries secondary to cancer of the colon and rectum. *Dis. Colon Rect.*, 3, 352.

BUSSEY, H. J. R. (1963) The long term results of surgical treatment of cancer of the rectum. *Proc. R. Soc. Med.*, 56, 494.

—— DUKES, C. E. and LOCKHART-MUMMERY, H. E. (1960) Results of the surgical treatment of rectal cancer. In *Cancer of the Rectum*, ed. C. E. Dukes, p. 267. London: Livingstone.

BUTLER, C. (1952) Some observations on the treatment of carcinoma of the rectum. *Proc. R. Soc. Med.*, 45, 41.

CASATI, E. and BOARI, A. (1894) Contributo serpimentale alla plastica dell'uretere. *Atti Acad. Sci. Med. Nat. Ferrara*, 68, 149 (quoted by Spies et al. 1933).

CATCHPOLE, B. W. (1969) Ileus: use of sympathetic blocking agents in its treatment. *Surgery, St Louis*, 66, 811.

CAWKWELL, W. I. (1963) Perineal hernia complicating abdominoperineal excision of the rectum. *Br. J. Surg.*, 50, 431.

CEULEMANS, G. (1977) Colostomie continente. *Chirurgie*, 103, 491.

CHARLES, A. H. (1967) Some hazards of pelvic surgery. *Proc. R. Soc. Med.*, 60, 565.

CLARK, C. G., WYLLIE, J. H., HAGGIE, S. J. and RENTON, P. (1977) Comparison of catgut and polyglycolic acid sutures in colonic anastomoses. *Wld J. Surg.*, 1, 501.

CLOGG, H. S. (1923) In *A System of Surgery*, ed. C. C. Choyce and J. M. Beattie, 2nd ed., vol. 2, p. 739. London: Cassell.

COFFEY, R. C. (1915) The major procedure first in the two-stage operation for relief of cancer of the rectum. *Ann. Surg.*, 61, 446.

COFFEY, R. C. (1931) Transplantation of ureters into large intestine. *Br. J. Urol., 3*, 353.

COLE, W. H. (1952) Recurrence in carcinoma of colon and proximal rectum following resection for carcinoma. *Archs Surg., Chicago, 65*, 264.

—— PACKARD, D. and SOUTHWICK, H. W. (1954) Carcinoma of the colon with special reference to prevention of recurrence. *J. Am. med. Ass., 155*, 1549.

COOKE, R. V. (1956) Advanced carcinoma of the colon with emphasis on the inflammatory factor. *Ann. R. Coll. Surg. Engl., 18*, 46.

CORDONNIER, J. J. (1950) Ureterosigmoid anastomosis. *J. Urol., 63*, 276.

CORMAN, M. L., SWINTON, N. W., O'KEEFE, D. D. and VERDENHEIMER, M. C. (1973) Colorectal carcinoma at the Lahey Clinic 1962 to 1966. *Am. J. Surg., 125*, 424.

CRILE, G., Jr. and TURNBULL, R. B., Jr. (1972) The role of electrocoagulation in the treatment of carcinoma of the rectum. *Surgery Gynec. Obstet., 135*, 391.

CRIPPS, W. H. (1907) *On Diseases of the Rectum and Anus*, 3rd ed. London: Churchill.

CULLEN, P. K., Jr. and MAYO, C. W. (1963) A further evaluation of the one-stage low anterior resection. *Dis Colon Rect., 6*, 415.

CUTAIT, D. E. and FIGLIONI, F. J. (1961) A new method of colorectal anastomosis in abdominoperineal resection. *Dis. Colon Rect., 4*, 335.

CUTLER, S. J. and LOURIE, W. I. (1964) End results in cancers of the large intestine and rectum. Presented at the International Symposium on End Results of Cancer Therapy, Sandefjord, Norway, September 16–20, 1963, *National Cancer Institute Monograph, 15*, 281.

CZERNY (1883) Quoted by Rankin et al. (1932).

D'ALLAINES, F. (1956) *Die Chirurgische Behandlung des Rektumkarzinoms*. Leipzig: Barth.

DAVIDS, A. M. and LESNICK, G. J. (1953) Experimental reconstruction of ureters by substitution of small bowel segments. *Ann. Surg., 137*, 389.

DEDDISH, M. R. (1950) Discussion on the treatment of advanced cancer of the rectum. *Proc. R. Soc. Med., 43*, 1075.

—— (1952) Personal communication.

—— and STEARNS, M. W., Jr. (1960) Surgical procedures for carcinoma of the left colon and rectum with five year results following abdominopelvic dissection of lymph nodes. *Am. J. Surg., 99*, 188.

—— —— (1961) Anterior resection for carcinoma of the rectum and rectosigmoid area. *Ann. Surg., 154*, 961.

DEMPTSTER, W. J. (1954) Quoted in Graham and Goligher (1954).

DENCKER, H., NORRYD, C. and TRANBERG, K. G. (1973) Management of the perineal wound after rectal excision. *Acta chir. scand., 139*, 568.

DEVENEY, K. E. and WAY, L. R. (1976) Effect of different absorbable sutures on healing of gastrointestinal anastomoses. *Am. J. Surg., 133*, 86.

DEVINE, SIR HUGH (1937) Excision of the rectum. *Br. J. Surg., 25*, 351.

DEVLIN, H. B., PLANT, J. A. and GRIFFIN, M. (1971) Aftermath of surgery for anorectal cancer. *Br. med. J., 2*, 413.

DIXON, C. F. (1948) Anterior resection for malignant lesions of the upper part of the rectum and lower part of the sigmoid. *Trans. Am. surg. Ass., 66*, 175.

DONALDSON, G. A. RODKEY, G. V. and BEHRINGER, G. E. (1966) Resection of the rectum with anal preservation. *Surgery Gynec. Obstet., 123*, 571.

DUKES, C. E. (1930) The spread of cancer of the rectum. *Br. J. Surg., 17*, 643.

—— (1940) Cancer of the rectum: an analysis of 1000 cases. *J. Path. Bact., 50*, 527.

—— (1947) Management of a permanent colostomy. *Lancet, 2*, 12.

—— (1957) Discussion on major surgery in carcinoma of the rectum with or without colostomy, excluding the anal canal and including the rectosigmoid. *Proc. R. Soc. Med., 50*, 1031.

DUNCAN, W. (1979) Personal communication.

DWIGHT, R. W., HIGGINS, G. A., ROSWIT, B., LE VEEN, H. H. and KEEHN, R. J. (1972) Preoperative radiation and surgery for cancer of the sigmoid colon and rectum. *Am. J. Surg., 123*, 93.

EDWARDS, F. SWINFORD (1908) *Diseases of the Rectum, Anus and Sigmoid Colon*, p. 293. London: Churchill.

EGO-AGUIRRE, E., SPRATT, J. S., Jr., BUTCHER, H. R., Jr. and BRICKER, E. M. (1964) Repair of perineal hernias developing subsequent to pelvic exenteration. *Ann. Surg., 159*, 66.

EISENBERG, H., SULLIVAN, P. D. and FOOTE, F. M. (1967) Trends in survival of digestive system cancer patients in Connecticut, 1935 to 1962. *Gastroenterology, 53*, 528.

EVERETT, W. G. (1975) A comparison of one layer and two layer techniques for colorectal anastomoses. *Br. J. Surg., 62*, 135.

EWING, M. R. (1950) Post-operative paralysis in the upper extremity. *Lancet, 1*, 99.

FAGET (1739) Quoted by Rankin et al. (1932).

FAIN, S. N., PATIN, C. S. and MORGENSTERN, L. (1975) Use of a mechanical suturing apparatus in low colorectal anastomosis. *Archs Surg., Chicago, 110*, 1079.

FARLEY, D. and SMITH, I. (1968) Phantom rectum after complete rectal excision. *Br. J. Surg., 55*, 40.

FAZIO, V. W. (1978) Sump suction and irrigation of the presacral space. *Dis. Colon Rect., 21*, 401.

FERGUSON, E. F. and HOUSTON, C. H. (1975) Simplified anterior resection using the TA stapler. *Dis. Colon Rect., 18*, 311.

FERRIS, D. O. and ODEL, H. M. (1950) Electrolyte pattern of blood after bilateral uretero-sigmoidostomy. *J. Am. med. Ass., 142*, 634.

FEUSTEL, H. and HENNIG, G. (1975) Kontinente Kolostomie durch Magnet-Verschluss. *Dt. med. Wschr., 100*, 1063.

FINSTERER, H. (1941) Zur chirurgischen Behandlung des Rektumkarzinoms. *Arch. klin. Chir., 202*, 15.

FISH, G. W. and STEVENSON, T. W. (1949) Pedicle graft cutaneous ureterostomy. *J. Urol., 16*, 749.

FOWLER, J. W. (1973) Bladder function following abdominoperineal excision of the rectum for carcinoma. *Br. J. Surg., 60*, 574.

GABRIEL, W. B. (1932) The end-results of perineal excision and of radium in the treatment of cancer of the rectum. *Br. J. Surg., 20*, 234.

—— (1934a) In discussion on treatment of carcinoma of the rectum. *Proc. R. Soc. Med., 50*, 1041.

GABRIEL, W. B. (1934b) Perineo-abdominal excision of the rectum in one stage. *Lancet, 2*, 69.

—— (1945) Discussion of the management of permanent colostomy. *Proc. R. Soc. Med., 38*, 692.

—— (1948) *Principles and Practice of Rectal Surgery*, 4th ed. London: H. K. Lewis.

—— (1957) Discussion on major surgery in carcinoma of the rectum, with or without colostomy, excluding the anal canal and including the rectosigmoid. *Proc. R. Soc. Med., 50*, 1041.

—— (1963) *The Principles and Practice of Rectal Surgery*, 5th ed. London: H. K. Lewis.

—— and LLOYD-DAVIES, O. V. (1935) Colostomy. *Br. J. Surg., 22*, 520.

GARLOCK, J. H. and GINSBURG, L. (1950) An appraisal of the operation of anterior resection for carcinoma of the rectum and rectosigmoid. *Surgery Gynec. Obstet., 90*, 525.

GILBERTSEN, V. A. (1960a) Adenocarcinoma of the rectum. Incidence and locations of recurrent tumor following present day operations performed for carcinoma. *Ann. Surg., 151*, 340.

—— (1960b) Adenocarcinoma of the rectum. A fifteen year study with evaluation of the results of curative therapy. *Archs Surg., Chicago, 80*, 135.

—— (1962) The results of the surgical treatment of cancer of the rectum. *Surgery Gynec Obstet., 114*, 313.

GILCHRIST, R. K. and DAVID, V. C. (1947) A consideration of pathological factors influencing five year survival in radical resection of the large bowel and rectum for carcinoma. *Ann. Surg., 126*, 421.

—— MERRICKS, J. W., HAMLIN, H. H. and RIEGER, I. T. (1950) Construction of substitute bladder and urethra. *Surgery Gynec. Obstet., 90*, 752.

GOETZE, O. (1931) Das Rektumkarzinom als Exstirpationsobjekt, Vorschläge zur sakralen und abdominosakralen Operation. *Zbl. Chir., 58*, 1746.

—— (1944) Die abdominosakrale Resektion des Mastdarms mit Wiederherstellung der natürlichen Kontinenz. *Arch. klin. Chir., 206*, 293.

GOLDSMITH, H. S. (1977) Protection of low rectal anastomosis with intact omentum. *Surgery Gynec. Obstet., 144*, 584.

GOLIGHER, J. C. (1951a) Resection with restoration of continuity in the treatment of carcinoma of the rectum and rectosigmoid. *Postgrad. med. J., 27*, 568.

—— (1951b) The functional results after sphincter-saving resections of the rectum. *Ann. R. Coll. Surg. Eng., 8*, 421.

—— (1951c) Sexual function after excision of the rectum. *Proc. R. Soc. Med., 44*, 824.

—— (1954) The adequacy of the marginal blood supply to the left colon after high ligation of the inferior mesenteric artery during excision of the rectum. *Br. J. Surg., 41*, 351.

—— (1958) Preservation of the anal sphincters in the radical treatment of rectal cancer. *Ann. R. Coll. Surg. Engl., 22*, 311.

—— (1962) Further reflections on sphincter conservation in the radical treatment of rectal cancer. *Proc. R. Soc. Med., 55*, 341.

—— (1979a) Recent trends in the practice of sphincter-saving excision for rectal cancer. *Ann. R. Coll. Surg. Engl., 61*, 169.

—— (1979b) Use of circular stapling device for the construction of the anastomosis in abdomino-transanal resection. *Br. J. Surg.*, in the press.

—— DUKES, C. E. and BUSSEY, H. J. R. (1951a) Local recurrences after sphincter-saving excision for carcinoma of the rectum and rectosigmoid. *Br. J. Surg., 39*, 199.

—— DUTHIE, H. L., DE DOMBAL, F. T. and WATTS, J. M. (1965) The pull-through abdominoanal excision for carcinoma of the middle third of the rectum: a comparison with low anterior resection. *Br. J. Surg., 52*, 323.

—— GRAHAM, N. G. and DE DOMBAL, F. T. (1970) Anastomotic dehiscence after anterior resection of rectum and sigmoid. *Br. J. Surg., 57*, 9.

—— and HUGHES, E. S. R. (1951) Sensibility of the rectum and colon. *Lancet, 1*, 543.

—— LEE, P. W. R., McMAHON, M. J. and POLLARD, M. (1977a) The Erlangen magnetic colostomy control device: technique of use and results in 22 patients. *Br. J. Surg., 64*, 501.

—— —— SIMPKINS, K. C. and LINTOTT, D. J. (1977b) A controlled comparison of one- and two-layer techniques of suture for high and low colorectal anastomoses. *Br. J. Surg., 64*, 609.

—— —— McFIE, J., SIMPKINS, K. C. and LINTOTT, D. J. (1979) Experience with the Russian suture gun for rectal anastomoses. *Surgery Gynec. Obstet., 148*, 517.

—— LLOYD-DAVIES, O. V. and ROBERTSON, C. T. (1951b) Small-gut obstruction following combined excision of the rectum, with special reference to strangulation round the colostomy. *Br. J. Surg., 38*, 467.

—— and POLLARD, M. (1978) *The Care of Your Colostomy*, 3rd ed. London: Baillière Tindall.

GOODWIN, W. E., HARRIS, A. P., KAUFMAN, J. J. and BEAL, J. M. (1953) Open transcolonic ureterointestinal anastomosis. *Surgery Gynec. Obstet., 97*, 295.

GORDON-WATSON, SIR CHARLES (1930a) Discussion on radium in the treatment of carcinoma of the rectum and colon. *Proc. R. Soc. Med., 23*, 1465.

—— (1930b) Treatment of carcinoma of the rectum with radium. *Br. J. Surg., 17*, 643.

GRAHAM, J.W. and GOLIGHER, J. C. (1954) The management of accidental injuries and deliberate resections of the ureter during excision of the rectum. *Br. J. Surg., 42*, 151.

GRIER, W. R., POSTEL, A. H., SYARSE, A. and LOCALIO, S. A. (1964) An evaluation of colonic stoma management without irrigations. *Surgery Gynec. Obstet., 118*, 1234.

GRIFFITHS, J. D. (1956) Surgical anatomy of the blood supply of the distal colon. *Ann. R. Coll. Surg. Engl., 19*, 241.

GRINNELL, R. S. (1953) Results in the treatment of carcinoma of the colon and rectum. *Surgery Gynec. Obstet., 96*, 31.

—— (1954) Distal intramural spread of carcinoma of the rectum and rectosigmoid. *Surgery Gynec. Obstet., 99*, 421.

—— (1965) Results of ligation of inferior mesenteric artery at the aorta in resections of carcinoma of the descending and sigmoid colon and rectum. *Surgery Gynec. Obstet., 120*, 1031.

—— and HIATT, R. B. (1952) Ligation of the inferior mesenteric artery at the aorta in resections for carcinoma of the sigmoid and rectum. *Surgery Gynec. Obstet., 94*, 526.

HAGER, T., SCHWEIGER, M. and BOTTICHER, D. (1976). The Erlangen magnetic closure system for colostomies and ileostomies. Paper presented to the International Society of University Colon and Rectal Surgeons, 6th International Congress, Salzburg, Sept. 1976.

HALLENBECK, G. A., JUDD, E. S. and DAVID, C. (1963) An instrument for colorectal anastomosis without suture. *Dis. Colon Rect.*, *6*, 98.

HARTMANN, H. (1923) *Congr. fr. Chir.*, *30*, 411.

—— (1931) *Chirurgie du Rectum*. Paris: Masson.

HAXTON, H. (1970) *Surgical Techniques*. Bristol: John Wright.

HEIMBACH, D. M. and CROUT, J. R. (1971) Treatment of paralytic ileus with adrenergic neuronal blocking drugs. *Surgery, St Louis, 69*, 582.

HEALD, R. J. (1977) Personal communication.

HENDRY, W. F. (1977) Injuries to the pelvic ureter. *Proc. R. Soc. Med.*, *70*, 183.

HERTER, F. P. and SLANETZ, C. A. (1967) Influence of antibiotic preparation of bowel on complications after colonic surgery. *Am. J. Surg.*, *113*, 165.

HIGGINS, C. C. (1934) Transuretero-ureteral anastomosis. *Trans. Am. Ass. genitour. Surg.*, *27*, 279.

HIGGINS, G. A., Jr. (1974) Carcinoma of the rectum: preoperative radiation therapy as an adjunct to surgery. *Dis. Colon Rect.*, *17*, 598.

—— CONN, J. H. and JORDAN, P. H., Jr. (1974) Prospective radiotherapy for colorectal cancer. *Ann. Surg., 181*, 624.

HOCHENEGG, J. (1888) Die sakrale Methode der Exstirpation von Mastdarmkrebsen nach Prof. Kraske. *Wien. klin. Wschr.*, *1*, 254, 272, 290, 309, 324, 348.

—— (1889) Beiträge zur Chirurgie des Rektums und der Beckenorgane. *Wien. klin. Wschr.*, *2*, 578.

HUGHES, E. S. R., CUTHBERTSON, A. M. and CARDEN, A. B. G. (1962) Pull-through operations for carcinoma of the rectum. *Med. J. Aust.*, *2*, 907.

HULTÉN, L. (1977) Personal communication.

—— KEWENTER, J., KNUTSSON, U. and OLBE, L. (1971) Primary closure of perineal wound after proctocolectomy or rectal excision. *Acta chir. scand.*, *137*, 467.

IRVIN, T. T. and GOLIGHER, J. C. (1975) A controlled trial of three methods of managing the perineal wound after abdomino-perineal excision of the rectum. *Br. J. Surg.*, *62*, 287.

JACKMAN, R. J. (1961) Conservative management of selected patients with carcinoma of the rectum. *Dis Colon Rect.*, *4*, 429.

JACOBS, A. (1953) Transplantation of the ureters: results and effects. In *Modern Trends in Urology*, ed. E. W. Riches, p. 175. London: Butterworth.

JONES, D. F. and MCKITTRICK, L. S. (1922) End results of operations for carcinoma of the rectum. *Ann. Surg.*, *76*, 386.

JUDD, E. S. and BELLEGIE, N. J. (1952) Carcinoma of rectosigmoid and upper part of rectum. (Recurrence following low anterior resection). *Archs Surg., Chicago, 64*, 697.

KELLY, K. A. (1977) Personal communication.

KENNEDY, J. T., MCOMISH, D., BENNETT, R. C., HUGHES, E. S. R. and CUTHBERTSON, A. M. (1970) Abdomino-anal pull-through resection of the rectum. *Br. J. Surg.*, *57*, 589.

KEYNES, W. M. (1961) Implantation from the bowel lumen in cancer of the large intestine. *Ann. Surg.*, *153*, 357.

KIRSCHNER, M. (1934) Das synchrone kombinierte Verfahren bei der Radikalbehandlung des Mastdarmkrebses. *Arch. klin. Chir.*, *180*, 296.

—— (1937) *Operative Surgery*, trans. I. S. Ravdin. Philadelphia: Lippincott.

KIRWAN, W. O., TURNBULL, R. B., Jr., FAZIO, V. W. and WEAKLEY, F. L. (1978) Pull-through operation and delayed anastomosis for rectal cancer. *Br. J. Surg., 65*, 695.

KOCHER, T. (1875) Quoted by Rankin, Bargen and Buie.

—— (1907) *Chirurgische Operationslehre*, 5th ed., p. 981. Jena: Fischer.

KRASKE, P. (1885) Zur Exstirpation hochsitzender Mastdarmkrebse. *Verh. dt. ges. Chir.*, *14*, 464.

KRATZER, G. L. (1967) The pull-through operation. *Dis. Colon Rect.*, *10*, 112.

—— (1969) Deductions regarding the pull-through operation, based on subjective reactions described by the patients. *Dis. Colon Rect.*, *12*, 386.

—— and ONSANIT, T. (1972) Fulguration of selected cancers of the rectum. *Dis. Colon Rect.*, *15*, 431.

—— —— (1974) Single layer steel wire anastomosis of the intestine. *Surgery Gynec. Obstet.*, *139*, 93.

KÜTTNER, H. (1910) Die sakrale Vorlagerungsmethode beim hochsitzenden Rektumkarzinom. *Dt. med. Wschr.*, *36*, 606.

—— (1916) Zur Technik meiner sakralen Vorlagerungsmethode beim hochsitzenden Rektumkarzinom. *Zbl. Chir.*, *43*, 905.

LAHEY, F. H. (1930) Two-stage abdomino-perineal removal of cancer of the rectum. *Surgery Gynec. Obstet.*, *51*, 692.

—— (1953) A method for segregation of the entire small intestine. *Surgery Gynec. Obstet.*, *96*, 503.

LAIRD, D. R. (1969) A colostomy safety tip. *Dis Colon Rect., 12*, 59.

LANE, R. H. S. and PARKS, A. G. (1977) Function of the anal sphincters following colo-anal anastomosis. *Br. J. Surg., 64*, 596.

LEADBETTER, W. F. (1951) Consideration of problems incident to performance of uretero-enterostomy: report of a technique. *J. Urol.*, *65*, 818.

LEARMONTH, J. R. (1931) A contribution to the neurophysiology of the urinary bladder in man. *Brain*, *54*, 147.

LISFRANC (1826) Quoted by Rankin, Bargen and Buie (1932).

LLOYD-DAVIES, O. V. (1939) Lithotomy–Trendelenburg position for resection of rectum and lower pelvic colon. *Lancet, 2, 74*.

—— (1948) Radical excision of carcinoma of the rectum with conservation of the sphincters. *Proc. R. Soc. Med.*, *41*, 822.

—— (1950) Discussion on conservative resection in carcinoma of the rectum. *Proc. R. Soc. Med.*, *43*, 706.

—— (1957) Discussion on major surgery in carcinoma of the rectum with or without colostomy, excluding the anal canal and including the rectosigmoid. *Proc. R. Soc. Med.*, *50*, 1047.

LOCALIO, S. A. and BARON, B. (1973) Abdomino-sacral resection and anastomosis for mid-rectal cancer. *Ann. Surg., 178*, 540.

—— and ENG, K. (1975) Malignant tumours of the rectum. *Current Prob. Surg.*, *12*, 1.

—— —— GOUGE, T. H. and RANSOME, J. H. C. (1978) Abdomino-sacral resection for carcinoma of the midrectum: 10 years experience. *Ann. Surg., 188*, 745.

LOCALIO, S. A. and STAHL, W. M. (1969) Simultaneous abdomino-transsacral resection and anastomosis for midrectal cancer. *Am. J. Surg., 117*, 282.

LOCK, M. R., CAIRNS, D. W., RITCHIE, J. K. and LOCKHART-MUMMERY, H. E. (1978) Results of local excisions for early colorectal cancer. *Br. J. Surg., 65*, 346.

LOCKHART-MUMMERY, H. E., RITCHIE, J. K. and HAWLEY, P. R. (1976) The results of surgical treatment for carcinoma of the rectum at St. Mark's Hospital from 1948 to 1972. *Br. J. Surg., 63*, 673.

LOCKHART-MUMMERY, J. P. (1907) *Diseases of the Rectum*, 7th ed. London: Baillière.

—— (1920) Resection of the rectum for cancer. *Lancet, 1*, 20.

—— (1926) Two hundred cases of cancer of the rectum treated by perineal excision. *Br. J. Surg., 14*, 110.

—— (1934) *Diseases of the Rectum and Colon*, 2nd ed. London: Baillière.

LOFGREN, E. P., WAUGH, J. M. AND LOCKERTY, M. B. (1957) Local recurrence of carcinoma after anterior resection of the rectum and the sigmoid. *Archs Surg., Chicago, 74*, 825.

McELWAIN, J. W., BACON, H. E. and TRIMPI, H. D. (1954) Lymph node metastases: experience with aortic ligation of inferior mesentery artery in cancer of the rectum. *Surgery, St. Louis, 35*, 513.

McGREW, E. A., LAWS, J. F. and COLE, W. H. (1954) Free malignant cells in relation to recurrence of carcinoma of the colon. *J. Am. med. Ass., 154*, 1251.

McLACHLIN, A. D. and DENTON, D. W. (1973) Omental protection of intestinal anastomoses. *Am. J. Surg., 125*, 134.

—— OLSSON, L. S. and PITT, D. F. (1976) Anterior anastomosis of the rectosigmoid colon: an experimental study. *Surgery, St Louis, 80*, 306.

MACLEOD, D. H. and HOWKINS, J. (1964) *Bonney's Gynaecological Surgery*, 7th ed. London: Cassell.

MADDEN, J. L. and KANDALAFT, S. (1967) Electrocoagulation: a primary and preferred method of treatment for cancer of the rectum. *Ann. Surg., 166*, 413.

—— —— (1971a) Clinical evaluation of electrocoagulation in the treatment of cancer of the rectum. *Am. J. Surg., 122*, 347.

—— —— (1971b) Electrocoagulation in the treatment of cancer of the rectum: a continuing study. *Ann. Surg., 174*, 530.

—— —— (1967) Electrocoagulation: a primary and preferred method of treatment for cancer of the rectum. *Ann. Surg., 166*, 413.

—— TAN, P. Y. and McCANN, W. J. (1967) An experimental and clinical study of cross uretero-ureterostomy. *Surgery Gynec. Obstet., 124*, 483.

MANDL, F. (1922) Über den Mastdarmkrebs. *Dt. Z. Chir., 168*, 145.

—— (1929) Über 1000 sakrale Mastdarmkrebsexstirpationen. (Aus dem Hocheneggschen Material). *Dt. Z. Chir., 219*, 3.

MANN, C. V. (1972) Late results of abdomino-anal pull-through resection. *Proc. R. Soc. Med., 65*, 976.

MASON, A. Y. (1970) Surgical access to the rectum—a transsphincteric approach. *Proc. R. Soc. Med., 63*, 91.

—— (1972) Transsphincteric exposure of the rectum. *Ann. R. Coll. Surg. Engl., 51*, 320.

—— (1976) Selective surgery for carcinoma of the rectum. *Aust. N.Z. J. Surg., 46*, 322.

—— (1977a) In *Surgical Techniques Illustrated*, ed. R. Malt and F. Robinson, Vol. 2, no. 2, p. 71. Boston: Little Brown.

—— (1977b) Personal communication.

MATHESON, N. A. and IRVING, A. D. (1975) Single layer anastomosis after rectosigmoid resection. *Br. J. Surg., 62*, 239.

MAUNSELL, H. W. (1892) A new method of excising the two upper portions of the rectum and the lower segment of the sigmoid flexure of the colon. *Lancet, 2*, 473.

MAYO, C. W. (1952) Personal communication.

—— and CULLEN, P. K., Jr. (1960) An evaluation of one stage low anterior resection. *Surgery Gynec. Obstet., 111*, 82.

—— and FLY, O. A. (1956) Analysis of five-year survival in carcinoma of the rectum and rectosigmoid. *Surgery Gynec. Obstet., 103*, 94.

—— LABERGE, M. Y. and HARDY, W. M. (1958) Five-year survival after anterior resection for carcinoma of the rectum and rectosigmoid. *Surgery Gynec. Obstet., 106*, 695.

—— LEE, M. J. and DAVIS, R. M. (1951) A comparative study of operations for carcinoma of the rectum and rectosigmoid. *Surgery Gynec. Obstet., 92*, 360.

—— and PAGTALUNAN, R. J. G. (1963) Malignancy of colon and rectum in patients under 30 years of age. *Surgery, St Louis, 53*, 711.

MAZIER, W. P., DIGNAN, R. D., CAPEHART, R. J. and SMITH, B. C. (1976) Effective colostomy irrigation. *Surgery Gynec. Obstet., 142*, 905.

MILES, W. E. (1908) A method of performing abdominoperineal excision for carcinoma of the rectum and of the terminal portion of the pelvic colon. *Lancet, 2*, 1812.

—— (1926) *Cancer of the Rectum*. London: Harrison.

—— (1945) Discussion on the management of permanent colostomy. *Proc. R. Soc. Med., 38*, 692.

MILLER, J. R., MACKENZIE, A. R. and KARASEWICH, E. G. (1966a) Translumbar amputation for carcinoma of the vagina. *Archs Surg., Chicago, 93*, 502.

—— RANDALL, H. T. and TIGNER, S. P. (1966b) Hemicorporectomy. *Surgery, St Louis, 59*, 988.

MILLIN, T. J. (1949) The ureter, the gynaecologist and the urologist. *J. Urol., 59*, 712.

—— and MASINA, F. (1949) Total cystectomy: consideration of technique. *Br. J. Urol., 21*, 108.

MONARI, U. (1896) Über Ureter-anastomosen: experimentelle Untersuchungen. *Bruns Beitr. klin. Chir., 15*, 720.

MOORE, T. D. (1948) Management of surgically traumatized ureter. *J. Urol., 59*, 712.

MORGAN, C. N. (1950) Discussion on conservative resection in carcinoma of the rectum. *Proc. R. Soc. Med., 43*, 701.

—— (1955) Trends in the treatment of tumours of the rectum, rectosigmoid and left colon. *J. R. Coll. Surg. Edinb., 1*, 112.

—— (1956) Quoted in Griffiths (1956).

—— (1965) Carcinoma of the rectum. *Ann. R. Coll. Surg. Engl., 36*, 73.

—— and GRIFFITHS, J. D. (1959) High ligation of the inferior mesenteric artery during operations for carcinoma of the distal colon and rectum. *Surgery Gynec. Obstet., 108*, 641.

MORSON, B. C. (1966) Factors influencing the prognosis of early cancer of the rectum. *Proc. R. Soc. Med., 59*, 607.

—— BUSSEY, H. J. R. and SAMOURIAN, S. (1977) A policy of local excision for early cancer of the colorectum. *Gut, 18*, 1045.

—— VAUGHAN, E. G. and BUSSEY, H. J. R. (1963) Pelvic recurrence after excision of rectum for carcinoma. *Br. med. J., 2*, 13.

MOYNIHAN, B. G. A. (1908) Cancer of the sigmoid flexure and rectum. *Surgery Gynec. Obstet., 6*, 463.

MUIR, E. G. (1939) Abdominal resection for rectal cancer. *Lancet, 1*, 1094.

NATHAN, P. W. and SCOTT, T. G. (1958) Intrathecal phenol for intractable pain. *Lancet, 1*, 76.

NESBIT, R. M. (1948) Ureterosigmoid anastomosis by direct elliptical connection; preliminary report. *Univ. Hosp. Bull., Mich., 14*, 45.

NEWELL, Q. U. (1939) Injury to ureters during pelvic operations. *Ann. Surg., 109*, 981.

OATES, G. D. and WILLIAMS, J. A. (1970) Primary closure of the perineal wound in excision of the rectum. *Proc. R. Soc. Med., 63*, 128.

OCKERBLAD, N. F. (1947) Reimplantation of the ureter into the bladder by a flap method. *J. Urol., 37*, 845.

O'CONNELL, J. E. A. (1969) Anterolateral chordotomy for intractable pain in carcinoma of the rectum. *Proc. R. Soc. Med., 62*, 1223.

OGILVIE, SIR HENEAGE (1954) Quoted in Graham and Goligher (1954).

OSBORNE, D. R., HIGGINS, A. F. and HOBBS, K. E. F. (1978) Cryosurgery in the management of rectal tumours. *Br. J. Surg., 65*, 859.

OTTLEY, C. (1938) Intrathecal alcohol for relief of pain: review. *Br. med. J., 1*, 510.

PANNETT, C. A. (1935) Resection of the rectum with restoration of continuity. *Lancet, 2*, 423.

—— (1951) Personal communication.

PAPILLON, J. (1973) Endocavitary irradiation of early rectal cancer for cure: a series of 123 cases. *Proc. R. Soc. Med., 66*, 1179.

PARKS, A. G. (1972) Transanal technique in low rectal anastomosis. *Proc. R. Soc. Med., 65*, 975.

—— (1977a) Personal communication.

—— (1977b) In *Surgical Techniques Illustrated*, ed. R. Malt and F. Robinson, vol. 2, no. 2, p. 65. Boston: Little Brown.

PATEY, D. H. (1951) Primary epithelial apposition in colostomy. *Proc. R. Soc. Med., 44*, 423.

PHILLIPS, R. (1942) Discussion on the treatment of inoperable carcinoma of the rectum. *Proc. R. Soc. Med., 35*, 768.

PYRAH, L. H. and RAPER, F. P. (1955) Some uses of an isolated loop of ileum in genito-urinary surgery. *Br. J. Surg., 42*, 337.

QUER, E. A., DAHLIN, D. C. and MAYO, C. W. (1953) Retrograde intramural spread of carcinoma of the rectum and rectosigmoid: a microscopic study. *Surgery Gynec. Obstet., 96*, 24.

RANKIN, F. W. (1928) The technique of anterior resection of the rectosigmoid. *Surgery Gynec. Obstet., 46*, 537.

—— (1929) The technique of combined abdomino-perineal resection of the rectum. *Surgery Gynec. Obstet., 49*, 193.

—— BARGEN, J. A. and BUIE, L. A. (1932) *The Colon, Rectum and Anus*. Philadelphia: Saunders.

RANKIN, J. T. (1969) Urological complications of rectal surgery. *Br. J. Urol., 41*, 655.

RAYNER, H. H. (1935) Discussion on the conservative surgery of carcinoma of the rectum. *Proc. R. Soc. Med., 28*, 1563.

RENDLEMAN, D. F. and GILCHRIST, R. K. (1959) Indications for oophorectomy in cancer of the gastrointestinal tract. *Surgery Gynec. Obstet., 109*, 364.

ROBBIE, D. S. (1969) General management of intractable pain in advanced carcinoma of the rectum. *Proc. R. Soc. Med., 62*, 1225.

ROBERTS, F. (1942) Discussion on the treatment of inoperable carcinoma of the rectum. *Proc. R. Soc. Med., 35*, 771.

ROSENBERG, I. L., RUSSELL, C. W. and GILES, G. R. (1978) Cell viability studies on the exfoliated colonic cancer cell. *Br. J. Surg., 65*, 188.

RUCKLEY, C. V., SMITH, A. N. and BALFOUR, T. W. (1970). Perineal closure by omental graft. *Surgery Gynec. Obstet., 131*, 300.

SÄUBERLI, H., GEROULANOS, S., HAHNLOSER, P., SCHAUWECKER, H. and KOCK, N. G. (1974) Studies of the dynamics of the 'nipple valve' in dogs with continent colostomies. *Dis. Colon Rect., 17*, 735.

SAUER, I. and BACON, H. E. (1952) A new approach for excision of carcinoma of the lower portion of the rectum and anal canal. *Surgery Gynec. Obstet., 95*, 229.

SCHELLERER, W. (1978) Personal communication.

SCHMIDT, E., BRUCH, H.-P. and GREULICH, M. (1979) Kontinente Colostomie durch freie Transplantation autologer Dickdarmmuskulatur. *Chirurg, 50*, 96.

SCHULTZ, M. D. and WANG, C. C. (1962) The role of radiation therapy in the management of carcinoma of the sigmoid, rectosigmoid and rectum. *Radiology, 79*, 1.

SCHWAB, P. M. and KELLY, K. A. (1974) Primary closure of the perineal wound after protectomy: a new technique. *Mayo Clin. Proc., 49*, 176.

SEARGEANT, P. W. (1966) Colostomy management by the irrigation technique: review of 165 cases. *Br. med. J., 2*, 25.

SEBRECHTS (1935) Quoted by Rayner (1935).

SHERMAN, L. E., TENNER, R. J. and CHADBOURN, W. A. (1965) Prophylactic oophorectomy with carcinoma of the rectum and colon. *Dis. Colon Rect., 7*, 521.

SILEN, W. (1975) Personal communication.

SLANEY, G. (1971) Results of treatment of carcinoma of the colon and rectum. In *Modern Trends in Surgery, 3*, ed. W. T. Irvine. London: Butterworth.

SMITH, I. B. (1969) Trans-uretero-ureterostomy. *Br. J. Urol., 41*, 14.

—— and SMITH, J. C. (1975) Trans-utero-ureterostomy: British experience. *Br. J. Urol., 47*, 519.

SPIES, J. W., JOHNSON, C. E. and WILSON, C. S. (1933) Reconstruction of the ureter by means of bladder flaps. *Proc. Soc. exp. Biol. Med., 30*, 425.

SPIRO, R. H. and HERTZ, R. E. (1966) Colostomy perforation. *Surgery, St Louis, 60*, 590.

STATE, D. (1951) Combined abdomino-perineal excision of the rectum—a plan for standardization of the proximal extent of dissection. *Surgery, St Louis, 30*, 349.

STEARNS, M. W., Jr. and BINKLEY, G. E. (1953) The influence of location on prognosis in operable rectal cancer. *Surgery Gynec. Obstet., 96*, 368.

—— and DEDDISH, M. R. (1959) Five year results of abdomino-pelvic lymph node dissection for carcinoma of the rectum. *Dis. Colon Rect., 2*, 169.

STEARNS, M. J., Jr., QUAN, S. H. Q. and QUAN, S. H. Q. (1959) Preoperative roentgen therapy for cancer of the rectum. *Surgery Gynec. Obstet., 109*, 225.

—— —— —— (1968) Preoperative irradiation for cancer of the rectum and rectosigmoid: preliminary review of recent experience (1957–1962). *Dis. Colon Rect., 11*, 281.

—— and WHITELEY, H. W., Jr. (1970) Palliative radiation therapy in patients with localized cancer of the colon and rectum. *Dis. Colon Rect.*, *13*, 112.

STRAUSS, A. A. (1969) *Immunologic Resistance to Carcinoma Produced by Electrocoagulation Based on 5–7 Years of Experimental and Clinical Results.* Springfield, Ill.: Charles C. Thomas.

—— STRAUSS, S. F., CRAWFORD, R. A. and STRAUSS, H. A. (1935) Surgical diathermy of carcinoma of rectum: its clinical end results. *J. Am. med. Ass.*, *104*, 1480.

SYMMONDS, R. E. and GIBBS, C. P. (1970) Urinary diversion by way of sigmoid conduit. *Surgery Gynec. Obstet.*, *131*, 687.

THOMSON, A. and MILES, A. (1920) *Operative Surgery*, 3rd ed., p. 383. Oxford: University Press.

THORLAKSON, R. H. (1965) Technique of repair of herniations associated with colonic stomas. *Surgery Gynec. Obstet.*, *120*, 347.

TODD, I. P. (1978) *Intestinal Stomas.* London: Heinemann Medical.

TRIMPI, H. D. and BACON, H. E. (1952) Clinical and experimental study of denuded surfaces in extensive surgery of the colon and rectum. *Am. J. Surg.*, *84*, 596.

—— KHUBCHANDANI, I. T., SHEETS, J. A. and STASIK, J. J. (1976) Advances in intestinal anastomoses: experimental study and an analysis of 984 patients. *Dis. Colon Rect.*, *20*, 107.

TURNBULL, R. B. Jr. (1964) Personal communication.

—— (1975) Personal communication.

—— and CUTHBERTSON, A. M. (1961) Abdomino-rectal pull-through resection for cancer and for Hirschsprung's disease. *Cleveland clin. Quart.*, *28*, 109.

TURNER, G. GREY (1931) Ideals and the art of surgery. *Surg. Gynec. Obstet.*, *52*, 273.

—— (1943) In *Modern Operative Surgery*, 3rd ed., vol. I, p. 960. London: Cassell.

TURNER-WARWICK, R. (1959) Technique for the separate diversion of urine and faeces. *Lancet*, *1*, 1021.

—— (1976) The use of the omental pedicle graft in urinary tract reconstruction. *J. Urol.*, *116*, 341.

—— and WORTH, P. H. L. (1969) The psoas bladder-hitch procedure for the replacement of the lower third of the ureter. *Br. J. Urol.*, *41*, 701.

TUTTLE, J. P. (1903) *A Treatise on the Diseases of the Anus, Rectum and Pelvic Colon.* New York: Appleton.

UDALL, D. A., HODGES, C. V., PEARSE, H. M. and BURNS, A. B. (1973) Transuretero-ureterostomy: a neglected procedure. *J. Urol.*, *109*, 817.

VANDERTOLL, D. J. and BEAHRS, O. H. (1965). Carcinoma of rectum and low sigmoid. Evaluation of anterior resection of 1766 favourable lesions. *Archs Surg., Chicago, 90*, 793.

VAN PROHASKA, J., GOVOSTIS, M. C. and WASICK, M. (1953) Multiple organ resection for advanced carcinoma of the colon and rectum. *Surgery Gynec. Obstet.*, *97*, 177.

VERNEUIL (1873) Quoted by Rankin et al. (1932).

WALKER, R. M. (1971) *Annual Report of South Western Regional Cancer Bureau.* U.T.F. House, King Square, Bristol BS2 8HY.

WALKER, F. C. (1975) *Stomal Care.* London: MacMillan.

WALTON, P. and MALLIK, M. K. (1974) Management of the perineal wound after rectal excision. *J. R. Coll. Surg., Edinb.*, *19*, 251.

WANGENSTEEN, O. H. (1943) Symposium on surgical management of malignancy of the colon. Primary resection (closed anastomosis) of colon and rectosigmoid including description of abdomino-anal methods for restoration of continuity accompanying excision of carcinoma of rectal ampulla. *Surgery, St Louis, 14*, 403.

—— (1945) Primary resection (closed anastomosis) of rectal ampulla for malignancy with preservation of sphincteric function. *Surgery Gynec. Obstet.*, *81*, 1.

WARWICK, R. (1959) Technique for the separate diversion of urine and faeces. *Lancet*, *1*, 1021.

WATSON, P. C. (1951) Discussion on urological complications of excision of the rectum. *Proc. R. Soc. Med.*, *44*, 820.

—— and WILLIAMS, D. I. (1952) The urological complications of excision of the rectum. *Br. J. Surg.*, *40*, 19.

WAUGH, J. M., BLOCK, M. A. and GAGE, R. P. (1955) Three and five-year survivals following combined abdominoperineal resection, abdominoperineal resection with sphincter preservation, and anterior resection for carcinoma of the rectum and lower part of the sigmoid colon. *Ann. Surg.*, *142*, 752.

—— and KIRKLIN, J. W. (1949) The importance of the level of the lesion in the prognosis and treatment of carcinoma of the rectum and low sigmoid colon. *Ann. Surg.*, *129*, 22.

—— MILLER, E. M. and KURZWEG, F. T. (1954) Abdomino-perineal resection with sphincter-preservation for carcinoma of the midrectum. *Archs Surg., Chicago, 68*, 469.

—— and TURNER, J. C., Jr. (1958) Abdominoperineal resection with preservation of the anal sphincter for carcinoma of the midrectum. *Surgery Gynec. Obstet.*, *107*, 777.

WEAKLEY, F. L. (1978) Anterior resection and anastomosis. *Surg. Rounds*, *1*, 10.

WEIR, R. F. (1901) An improved method of treating high-seated cancers of the rectum. *J. Am. med. Ass.*, *37*, 801.

WENCKERT, A. (1970) Endorectal (pull-through) resection for tumours of the rectum. *Acta chir. scand.*, *136*, 337.

WESTHUES, H. (1930) Über die Entstehung und Vermeidung des lokalen Rektumkarzinom-Rezidivs. *Arch. klin. Chir.*, *161*, 582.

—— (1933) Quoted by Bier, Braun and Kümmell. *Operative Surgery*, 2nd ed. Leipzig: Barth.

—— (1934) *Die Pathologisch-anatomischen Grundlagen der Chirurgie des Rektumkarzinoms.* Leipzig: Thieme.

WHITTAKER, M. and GOLIGHER, J. C. (1976) The prognosis after surgical treatment for carcinoma of the rectum. *Br. J. Surg.*, *63*, 384.

WILLIAMS, I. G. and HORWITZ, H. (1959) Radiotherapy in carcinoma of the rectum and anal canal. In *Diseases of the Colon and Anorectum*, ed. R. Turell, p. 537. Philadelphia and London: Saunders.

WILLIAMS, I. G., SHULMAN, I. M. and TODD, I. P. (1957) The treatment of recurrent carcinoma of the rectum by supervoltage X-ray therapy. *Br. J. Surg.*, *44*, 506.

WILSON, E. (1973) Local treatment of cancer of the rectum. *Dis. Colon Rect.*, *16*, 194.

WITTOESCH, J. H. and JACKMAN, R. J. (1958) Results of conservative management of cancer of the rectum in poor risk patients. *Surgery Gynec. Obstet.*, *107*, 648.

Wood, R. A. B. and Hughes, L. E. (1975) Silicone foam sponge for pilonidal sinus: a new technique for dressing open granulating wounds. *Br. med. J.*, *3*, 131.

—— Williams, R. H. P. and Hughes, L. E. (1977) Foam elastomer dressings in the management of open granulating wounds: experience with 250 patients. *Br. J. Surg.*, *64*, 554.

Yeomans, F. C. (1939) Levator hernia, perineal and pudendal. *Am. J. Surg.*, *43*, 695.

19

Carcinoma of the Anal Canal and Anus

Malignant epithelial growths in the anal region may be of five types:

1. Adenocarcinoma of the rectum descending into the anal canal.
2. Squamous cell carcinoma.
3. Basal cell carcinoma.
4. Malignant melanoma.
5. Primary adenocarcinoma of the anal canal and perianal tissues.

ADENOCARCINOMA DESCENDING FROM RECTUM

Low rectal carcinomas may spread downwards and invade the anal canal, sometimes even projecting through the anal orifice. This occurs not uncommonly and from my experience I would say that, when a growth presents at the anus, there is an even chance that it will turn out to be an adenocarcinoma rather than any other sort of tumour. Digital examination of the rectum, if that is possible—or vaginal examination, if the growth does not transmit a finger—may reveal that the lesion extends well up into the rectal ampulla and suggest that it probably is a primary rectal carcinoma. It must be remembered, however, that a squamous cell anal lesion may spread extensively in a proximal direction. A very hard lesion is perhaps more likely to be squamous, whilst a softer lesion, especially if it exudes colloid material on digital examination, is more probably an adenocarcinoma. But the precise histological diagnosis can only be established by biopsy. The treatment is by combined excision, if possible, exactly as for any other lower rectal carcinoma, but the involvement of the skin of the anal canal and anus opens the avenue of lymphatic spread to the inguinal glands, which, therefore, require to be carefully examined. Their management follows the lines adopted in cases of squamous cell carcinoma (see p. 669). Actually, metastases in the inguinal nodes are rare with adenocarcinoma, unless the skin of the anal orifice and perianal region is implicated.

SQUAMOUS CELL CARCINOMA

Incidence

As already mentioned, squamous cell epithelioma probably accounts for about half the malignant epithelial growths of the anus and anal canal. Compared with the total incidence of adenocarcinoma of the rectum it is a rare disease. Thus Morson (1959) found that only 157 or 3·5% of 4396 cases of carcinoma of the rectum, anal canal and anus seen at St Mark's Hospital between 1928 and 1956 had squamous cell growths. Sweet (1947) of the Massachusetts General Hospital put the incidence at 4·7% of all rectal carcinomas, whilst Cattell and Williams (1943) of the Lahey Clinic have estimated it at 1·7%, Bacon (1949) of Philadelphia at 6% and Richards et al. (1962) of the Mayo Clinic at 1% approximately.

SEX AND SITE INCIDENCE

Gabriel (1941) in his classical paper on the subject found that, by contrast with the marked preponderance of adenocarcinoma of the rectum in males, there was an almost equal distribution of squamous cell epithelioma in men and women, a finding with which Morson (1959) and McQuarrie and Buie (1950) agreed. However, on separating the cases of squamous cell carcinoma into those commencing in the anal canal and those arising at the anal margin, a very striking difference in the sex incidence is revealed. This is well shown in Morson's (1959) collective series of 157 cases in which *carcinoma of the anus* occurred chiefly in males (31 males to 7 females), whilst *carcinoma of the anal canal* was commoner in females (59 females to 44 males); in 16 cases the site of the growth was indeterminate. The very much higher incidence of carcinoma of the anus in men may be attributable to a number of factors. Anal pruritus is certainly commoner in this sex and may be a predisposing cause, though, considering its great frequency and the relative rarity of anal carcinoma, it cannot be regarded as a definitely precancerous condition. The dangers of indiscriminate, repeated radiotherapy, however, in the treatment of pruritus ani need no emphasis in this condition. Fistula-in-ano is also much commoner in men than women, and, though the carcinomas which arise in connection with long-standing fistulas are usually adenocarcinomas, they sometimes assume a squamous form (Rosser 1931). Another factor that may be important is the repeated effect of rough underclothing and trousers on the anal and perianal skin in men of labouring class. No plausible explanation suggests itself for the higher incidence of squamous cell carcinoma of the anal canal in women than men.

In terms of the anal circumference Gabriel (1941) found a much *greater incidence* of squamous cell carcinomas *in the anterior quadrants*, but in the larger series reported by Morson (1959) no particular quadrant of the anal canal or sector of the anal circumference seemed to be specially prone to develop these growths.

Pathology

Histologically squamous cell carcinomas of the anal region vary considerably from well-differentiated tumours with much keratinization and well-marked cell nests to entirely cellular, completely undifferentiated growths. Gabriel (1941) found that when the growths in his series of 55 cases were classified into three grades of malignancy according to Broders' (1925) criteria, an interesting difference was revealed between the two sexes: the lesions in men were much more frequently of low-grade malignancy, whilst those in women were usually of high grade. Owing to the difference in the distribution of the growths in men and women (see above) this

means in turn that carcinoma of the anal margin and perianal region is usually a well-differentiated lesion of low malignancy, whilst squamous cell carcinoma of the anal canal is generally poorly differentiated and much more malignant in character. In addition, as Morson (1960a) has shown, other intermediate types of growth may occur in the anal canal, such as basisquamous, mucoepidermoid and transitional-cell tumours—also known as cloacogenic carcinomas (Grinvalsky and Helwig 1956; Kheir et al. 1972) or basaloid carcinomas (Grodsky 1969).

Clinical Appearances

A squamous cell carcinoma of the anal region may present a variety of clinical appearances. A very early lesion may produce a localized ulcer or a raised warty growth with an irregular ulcerated surface, usually on the anterior aspect of the anus. At this stage the lesion can be lifted off the underlying structures but it is indurated. At a later stage a more extensive hard projecting or ulcerating lesion may be present, perhaps completely surrounding the anus and firmly fixed to the deeper tissues. In some cases an indurated edge may be palpable through the intact skin some distance beyond the more obvious lesion.

To determine the proximal extent of the lesion digital examination of the anal canal and rectum should be carried out, but, if a completely annular growth is present, it may be impossible to pass a finger, at any rate without a general anaesthetic. In such cases a vaginal examination is often very helpful in indicating the upper limit of the growth; it is also important to note whether the posterior vaginal wall is involved, as indicated by fixation, ulceration or the presence of a rectovaginal fistula, which is not uncommon.

The inguinal lymph glands require to be examined carefully for evidence of involvement. The superficial inguinal group in one or both groins may be enlarged due to septic absorption from the ulcerated surface of the growth or to the presence of metastases. Septic glands are soft or firm, glands containing malignant deposits hard and, in the later stages, fixed. In advanced cases the external iliac glands may also be enlarged and palpable above the inguinal ligament. Unfortunately, many patients with squamous cell carcinomas are found to have massive fixed primary growths and extensive involvement of glands by the time they present for treatment.

Symptoms

These are also very variable. Probably the majority of patients present with the complaint of a lump in the anal region or bleeding, diagnosed as due to 'haemorrhoids'. In other cases pain at defaecation is the main complaint. Another symptom often mentioned is discharge from the anal region or incontinence due to malignant infiltration and destruction of the sphincters; and in female patients in whom a rectovaginal fistula has developed, a discharge of faeces or flatus from the vagina may be noted. Lastly, some patients complain mainly of difficulty with defaecation, or spurious diarrhoea and other disturbances of bowel habits as with a low rectal carcinoma.

Diagnosis

When the lesion is advanced and forms a large ulcerating tumour with a characteristically raised indurated edge, it usually presents no problem in diagnosis. But at an earlier stage, when strictly localized, it may be confused with other conditions, such as a simple papilloma or cluster of warts, anal condylomas, a primary chancre, an anal fissure or a prolapsed thrombosed internal haemorrhoid. Another source of confusion is anal ulceration due to Crohn's disease (p. 833; Plate V). The frequency of a wrong initial diagnosis is emphasized by Binkley (1950), who noted that in a series of 125 cases with squamous cell carcinoma of the anus seen at the Memorial Hospital, New York, no less than 36 had already been treated by 'haemorrhoidectomy' or excision of an 'anal fissure or fistula' before reporting to him! The feature that should raise the suspicion of carcinoma even with the most atypical lesions is *induration*. The assessment and diagnosis of these cases is often impeded by pain and spasm of the sphincters or actual organic narrowing of the anus, and re-examination under general anaesthesia is often required. The diagnosis should always be confirmed by *biopsy*, which will establish whether a growth is present and will distinguish between a squamous cell lesion and an adenocarcinoma or other rarer tumours.

Treatment

There has been much divergence of opinion as to the relative merits of some form of irradiation and surgical treatment in the treatment of squamous cell carcinomas of the anal region.

IRRADIATION

Irradiation by implanted radium needles, teleradium or X-rays has frequently been employed in the past and was at one stage perhaps the favourite treatment for these lesions. As Gordon-Watson (1930) and Gabriel (1932, 1941) showed, excellent results could sometimes be obtained by interstitial radium in the treatment of localized carcinomas of the anal margin, a most attractive feature of this management, of course, being the hope it offered of preserving the anal sphincters and avoiding a colostomy. Roux-Berger and Ennuyer (1948) have reported the late results in 51 consecutive cases of squamous cell carcinoma of the anus treated by radium or radiotherapy at the Curie Foundation, Paris, between 1921 and 1940; 18 patients or 35% were alive and well after five years. Of 11 cases with primary lesions which 'did not extend beyond the limits of the anal canal' seven achieved five-year cures. On the other hand, they mention that seven of their 18 successful cases developed a complete or partial fibrous stenosis of the anus necessitating the establishment of an iliac colostomy, so that the functional results often fell short of expectations. To avoid this complication, which was almost exclusively one of interstitial radium, they, like most other radiotherapists in recent years, have abandoned radium in favour of radiotherapy, either short-distance low-voltage therapy for early superficial lesions or supervoltage therapy for advanced and extensive growths.

It must be admitted however that most reports on the results of irradiation for anal carcinomas have been a good deal less encouraging. Thus Sweet (1947) of Boston had only one five-year survival out of 19 cases treated by radium or X-rays, and though these included a number of patients with very advanced lesions there were some with early growths. Raven's (1941) report from the Royal Cancer Hospital, London, is almost equally depressing. Gabriel (1941, 1960) also emphasized the unreliability of irradiation, which he felt was much less certain in its effects than surgical excision. But it must be borne in mind that there have been considerable advances in radiotherapeutic technique since most of these experiences were recorded. Possibly modern radiotherapy may have more to offer. On theoretical grounds it would seem reasonable to suppose that one ought to be able to treat a localized squamous cell epithelioma of the *perianal region* as effectively by X-rays as by simple local excision, which is the usual surgical alternative for such a growth in this situation. With supervoltage radiotherapy it should be possible to avoid radionecrosis of the sensitive perineal tissues (Williams 1962). Unfortunately, no really large series of cases of anal carcinoma so treated and followed up for a lengthy period of time has yet been reported, but Williams' (1962) results are encouraging (see below). It remains to be seen whether the recently introduced method of irradiation with fast neutrons, which has been an advance in the treatment of carcinoma in the head and neck, offers any improvement in the radiotherapy of anal cancer (Franklyn and Parks 1979).

For squamous cell carcinoma of the *anal canal* the prospects with radiotherapy are obviously less promising, for with lesions in this situation spread to the superior haemorrhoidal and inferior mesenteric lymph nodes is possible, just as with an ordinary adenocarcinoma of the rectum (see below). The question whether X-ray treatment can deal effectively with such metastases is similar to that which arises in connection with the treatment of adenocarcinoma by supervoltage radiotherapy (see p. 669), except that squamous cell lesions are possibly more radiosensitive so that the prognosis might be better. As in the management of adenocarcinomas, the consensus of surgical opinion now strongly favours combined excision as the method of first choice for squamous cell carcinomas of the anal canal, but for patients with locally inoperable growths or whose general condition would make major surgery particularly hazardous radiotherapy can often usefully be employed. This is well shown by the experience of Williams (1962), who treated 32 patients with such lesions by supervoltage radiotherapy five or more years prior to the time of his report; 12 (37.5%) secured five-year cures and there were no instances of troublesome radionecrosis.

SURGICAL EXCISION

Due to the strenuous advocacy of Gilchrist and David (1938), Gabriel (1941, 1963), Cattell and Williams (1943), Harvey (1946) and Sweet (1947), surgical excision has largely replaced irradiation in the practice of the majority of surgeons at the present day, including myself, in the treatment of anal carcinoma (Stearns 1955; Richards et al. 1962; Dillard et al. 1963; Stearns and Quan 1970).

This may consist of a strictly local excision of the growth leaving the rectum and greater part of the anal canal, or may include rectal excision by perineal or abdominoperineal route, depending on the site and extent of the lesion and on the personal predilection of the surgeon concerned.

In planning surgical treatment of these lesions a most important consideration is whether the growth extends upwards to involve the rectal mucosa proper, or is confined to the anal and perianal skin:

GROWTHS EXTENDING ABOVE THE PECTINATE LINE

As Gilchrist and David (1938) and Gabriel (1941, 1960) have convincingly shown in dissected rectal excision specimens of squamous cell carcinomas extending up to the rectal mucosa above the pectinate line, spread is liable to occur in the rectal lymphatics and give rise to metastases in the glands on the back of the rectum and alongside the superior haemorrhoidal or inferior mesenteric vessels. Thus, in the series of 67 cases of squamous cell carcinoma of the anal canal reported by Gabriel (1960) in which combined rectal excision was performed, 43.3% had involvement of these glands. Similarly extension may take place via the middle haemorrhoidal lymphatics to the internal iliac glands, as emphasized by Sauer and Bacon (1952). There can be no doubt therefore that a *radical excision of the rectum, preferably by the abdominoperineal method*, is required exactly as in the treatment of a low rectal adenocarcinoma. In the performance of this operation a specially wide margin of perianal skin, fat and muscle should be secured in the perineal dissection and in women the posterior vaginal wall should always be removed. It has been recommended by Stearns (1955) that an effort should also be made to deal with possible spread to the internal iliac lymph glands by carrying out a pelvic adenectomy as part of abdominoperineal excision for carcinoma of the anal canal. Though it might seem a forlorn hope to be able to deal effectively in this way with metastases in these nodes (see p. 506), Stearns and Quan (1970) have been able to report a few five-year survivors after dissection of involved internal iliac nodes.

With these growths lymphatic spread may also take place to the inguinal glands from the skin-lined part of the anal canal or the perianal skin so that excision of these glands may also have to be considered as described below.

GROWTHS OF THE ANUS AND PERIANAL REGION

It is generally believed that the lymphatic drainage from the perianal skin and the skin-lined part of the anal canal below the pectinate line is exclusively to the inguinal glands and that proximal spread to the lymphatics of the rectum does not occur. Consequently rectal excision is not usually considered necessary in the treatment of squamous cell growths that are confined to the skin of the anus and perianal region well below the pectinate line, and surgical treatment of these lesions has usually consisted of a wide local excision with sacrifice of some of the lower part of the anal sphincters but without removal of the rectum. Morson (1960a) mentions that nine of the 38 cases with squamous cell carcinomas of the anal margin at St Mark's Hospital, London, were treated by combined rectal excision and all these operative specimens were dissected for lymph glandular metastases. In no instance were any of the superior haemorrhoidal or inferior mesenteric glands involved. One could wish for more extensive confirmation of this finding, but, so far as it goes, it supports conventional practice in not removing the rectum in treating subpectinate growths. In the performance of local excision it is customary to use the cutting diathermy and to aim at a margin of clearance of at least 2·5 cm on all aspects of the growth. As a rule this is easily enough obtained except possibly at the most proximal pole of the lesion which projects towards the anal canal. *Unless an adequate margin can be secured between the growth and the pectinate line, it is unwise to persist with a purely local removal*; instead, a rectal excision should be carried out together with wide dissection of the tissues of the perianal region on that side.

Treatment of the Inguinal Glands

The frequency with which the inguinal lymph glands are implicated in carcinoma of the anus or anal canal has varied widely in different reported series: 8% (Grinnell 1954), 42% (Stearns 1955), 35% (Morson 1959), 24·2% (Dillard et al. 1963), 39% (Wolfe and Bussey 1968) and 40% (Stearns and Quan 1970). In Wolfe and Bussey's (1968) collective series of 70 cases at St Marks' Hospital, the incidence of inguinal metastases was slightly higher (42%) with carcinomas of the anal margin than with carcinomas of the anal canal (37%). There is general agreement that the occurrence of deposits in the inguinal glands is a development of grave prognostic significance, but it would appear from the surveys of Wolfe and Bussey (1968) and Stearns and Quan (1970) that the outlook for patients with inguinal metastases is not quite as black as it once appeared to be. In the treatment of involved inguinal lymph glands, supervoltage radiotherapy,

teleradium or cobalt rays are favoured by some authorities, but a block dissection is probably preferable, as it is for the cervical lymph nodes in cases of carcinoma of the lip or tongue. I personally have reserved radiotherapy for cases with fixed inoperable glands.

INDICATIONS FOR BLOCK DISSECTION

1. If on clinical examination *the glands are obviously involved*—that is to say if they are enlarged and hard rather than firm—a block dissection should be done on one or both groins as required. This operation is best postponed till the patient is thoroughly convalescent from the rectal or local excision of the primary growth, or its radiotherapeutic treatment, which usually imposes a delay of five or six weeks.

2. If *the inguinal glands do not appear clinically implicated*, there are two possible courses of management, as in the treatment of clinically negative cervical nodes in cases of cancer of the lip or tongue. According to one, a conservative attitude is adopted in the first instance, and this is combined with a vigilant 'follow-up' to detect clinical signs of gland involvement at the earliest possible moment. This implies frequent attendances by the patient for re-examination of the groins, for of course postal information from the patient or his doctor is quite unreliable. He should report every month for the first six months, and then every two months for another 2½ years or so. If longer intervals are allowed to elapse, it may be found that wide infiltration of the glands has occurred since the last visit, even up to the extent of inoperability. If it seems likely that the patient will not be able to attend regularly for interview, this expectant regimen should not be embarked upon. At the first clinical evidence of lymphatic metastases a unilateral or bilateral block dissection is performed, according to the indications.

The alternative course is to carry out a prophylactic gland dissection in all cases, to ensure removing all minute inconspicuous metastases that might later blossom into clinically obvious deposits. The disadvantage of this policy is that it subjects a considerable number of patients to an unnecessary operation. This operation does not carry a serious risk to life; it does, however, expose the patient to the possibility of quite considerable postoperative morbidity. The immediate convalescence after block dissection of the groin glands may be prolonged by necrosis of the skin flaps and infection, and there may be very considerable disability subsequently due to lymphoedema and gross elephantiasis of the leg and external genitalia. I think that these disadvantages considerably outweigh the possible gain for, provided the follow-up on the waiting regimen is carefully conducted, glandular involvement will still be detected at a relatively early stage and I doubt if the prognosis will be adversely affected by the slight delay entailed, as compared with that after an immediate gland dissection. This has certainly been the plan followed by me in such cases with the exception of three patients who were clearly not going to be able to guarantee regular follow-up attendances, and on whom I therefore advised prophylactic block dissection, with positive glands in one instance.

Removal of a single gland or two or three glands for diagnostic purposes is not likely to be helpful. If clinical suspicions of glandular metastases are roused, it is better to proceed to a formal dissection.

TECHNIQUE OF BLOCK DISSECTION OF
INGUINAL GLANDS

Two variants of this operation are available—a superficial gland dissection without dividing the inguinal ligament or entering the pelvis, which is the operation usually favoured, and a more radical dissection which involves division of the inguinal ligament and removal of the glands along the external and common iliac vessels as well as the superficial inguinal nodes.

Superficial Inguinal Gland Dissection. An oblique incision parallel to and 2·5 cm below the inguinal ligament throughout its length may suffice, though more usually it is necessary to make a vertical addition downwards for 10 cm or so from the inner end of this incision, depending on the difficulties of the dissection. The skin flaps are raised so as to display the lowermost 5 cm of the related part of the anterior abdominal wall and the uppermost 10 or 12·5 cm of the front of the thigh. The deep fascia is then incised circumferentially at the periphery of the operative field thus exposed, and this incision will traverse the main trunk or trunks of the internal saphenous vein in the lower part of the wound, and the tributaries of the vein and accompanying branches of the femoral artery at its medial, lateral and upper margins; these should all be doubly secured and divided. The fascia is then dissected off the underlying muscles and femoral nerve and vessels towards the saphenofemoral venous junction, the subcutaneous fat, fascia and glands being removed *en masse.* Finally, the great saphenous vein is ligated and divided near its junction with the

femoral, and this completes the removal of tissue. After meticulous haemostasis it only remains to close the skin wound, a step that raises certain problems discussed in relation to *deep inguinal gland dissection* (p. 673).

Deeper Inguinal Gland Dissection. Good accounts of the more radical inguinal dissection are given by Milton et al. (1968) and Gupta (1969). The initial part of this operation is similar to that just described, but an upward vertical extension 12·5 or 15 cm long at the outer end of the oblique incision is essential.

The superficial fat, veins, glands and deep fascia are dissected as far as the saphenofemoral junction and the internal saphenous vein ligated and divided at this point. The bloc of tissue thus mobilized is still attached by some strands of tissue containing lymphatics which connect via the femoral canal with the external iliac glands. The inguinal ligament has now to be divided. As a preliminary to its division, the upper skin flap is retracted upwards and the inguinal canal opened by incision of the external oblique aponeurosis outwards and slightly upwards from the subcutaneous ring, as in an inguinal hernia operation but prolonged 10 or 12·5 cm farther. The spermatic cord or round ligament of the uterus is identified and held in tissue forceps, whilst the internal oblique and transversus muscle fibres are severed in an outward and upward direction for 10 or 12·5 cm lateral to the internal inguinal ring. The transversalis fascia is cut or broken through and the deep circumflex iliac and inferior epigastric branches of the external iliac artery are exposed and divided. The peritoneum can now be brushed upwards off the iliac fossa exposing the iliacus and psoas muscles and the external and common iliac artery. A slight Trendelenburg tilt helps at this stage. The lower flap of the external oblique aponeurosis and the inguinal ligament can now be divided, most conveniently just lateral to the external iliac artery, and the inner part dissected up off the vessels and femoral canal to allow the strand of tissue still tethering the mobilized subinguinal tissues to be lifted out of the canal. Whilst the peritoneum is retracted medially and forwards the dissection proceeds upwards along the external iliac vessels at least as far as the bifurcation of the common iliac, and as much farther as can conveniently be managed. At the same time any glands or fatty connective tissues on the medial side of the obturator internus muscle are removed as far posteriorly as possible. If the truth be told, the amount of additional glandular tissue obtained by the extension of the operation above the inguinal ligament is usually disappointly small, and, in the ten extended dissections of this kind that I have done, evidence of growth above the ligament was discovered in only one.

The reconstruction of the musculoaponeurotic structures of the inguinal region, which is more safely accomplished by a series of fine catgut sutures rather than by any form of non-absorbable suture material, can usually be effected in a fairly adequate manner, and incisional hernia has not occurred in any of my cases. As regards closure of the skin wound, reference should be made to the notorious tendency of these wounds after inguinal node dissection (superficial or deep) to develop necrosis of the skin with resulting separation and slow healing by granulation. This development is partly attributable to the poor blood supply to the skin in this region, but an additional factor is the accumulation of serum in the wound lifting the flaps off the underlying structures. Suction drainage (e.g. Zimmer or Redivac) is, therefore, particularly valuable in these cases. But, even with it, necrosis and separation may occur, and one effect may be to leave the femoral vessels exposed in an open granulating wound. To guard against this contingency it is a good plan, before suturing the skin, to mobilize the upper part of the sartorious muscle so that it may be drawn over the femoral artery and vein, as originally recommended by Baronofsky (1948) and also practised by Milton et al. (1968) and Gupta (1969). The best way to do so is to divide the muscle at its upper end and then to rotate the superior portion of the muscle belly, so that its former lateral edge becomes the medial edge and overlies the femoral vessels. Using fine chromic catgut sutures the new medial margin and the cut upper border of the muscle are attached in turn to the adductor longus, pectineus and inguinal ligament. Incidentally, in female patients it is always wise to insert an indwelling urethral catheter to avoid soiling of the inguinal wound postoperatively.

LATE RESULTS

The over-all results of treatment of squamous cell carcinoma of the anus have usually been poorer than those of adenocarcinoma of the rectum. Thus Sweet (1947) found that of a series of 77 cases presenting with squamous cell epitheliomas of the anus or anal canal at the Palmer Memorial Hospital, Boston, and treated by surgery, irradiation or a mixture of the two, only 13 (17·3%) were alive and well five years later, which contrasts with an absolute five-year survival rate of approximately 30% for adenocarcinomas of the rectum (see p. 642). The best results in Sweet's series were obtained in the 48 cases subjected to abdominoperineal excision: 12 of these or nearly 30% achieved five-year survivals, as compared with only one five-year survivor out of 19 patients treated solely by irradiation. A more encouraging report of the outcome of treatment for squamous cell cancer of the anal region is that provided by Grinnell (1954). He found that of 49 patients treated for this lesion at the Presbyterian Hospital, New York, between 1916 and 1952, 21 (42·9%) were alive five years later; in the group of 30 cases having some form of surgical excision the five-year survival rate was 63%. As Grinnell emphasizes, however, the series of cases seen at his hospital seem to have been of a less advanced kind that those usually encountered. Richards et al. (1962) in a survey of 109 patients with squamous cell carcinoma of the anus or anal canal seen at the Mayo Clinic, 73 of which had been treated five or more years previously, reported an over-all five-year survival rate of 53·4%. If only cases submitted to abdominoperineal excision were considered, there was a 62% five-year survival rate. Dillard et al. (1963) had a 39% absolute or over-all five-year survival rate in 79 cases of squamous cell cancer of the anal margin and canal dealt with at the Ellis Fischel Cancer Hospital and the Barnes Hospital, St Louis, from 1940 to 1957. There were 58% of five-year survivors in 46 patients treated by abdominoperineal excision, but only 28% in 14 patients having a purely local excision. Specially interesting in this connection is the progressive improvement in more recent years in the achievements of treatment for this condition reported from the Memorial Hospital, New York, by Stearns and Quan (1970). Before 1944, 125 patients were treated at this hospital with a five-year survival rate over-all of 29%, or in surgically treated cases of 41%, but between 1944 and 1963 109 patients presented, with a five-year survival rate over-all of 53%, or in surgically treated cases of 57%.

The results reported from St Mark's Hospital, London, by Gabriel (1960, 1963) are particularly valuable because of their comprehensiveness and detail. Of 28 cases *with growths of the anal margin and perianal region* 27 were treated by local excision with 16 five-year survivors (59%). One patient had a combined excision of the rectum and also survived five years. Of 87 cases *with lesions of the anal canal* 70 were considered operable and were treated by combined excision, a resectability rate of 80%. Of 56 operation survivors 29 (51%) were alive five or more years later. (This figure is to be compared with the crude five-year survival rate of 55·8% after synchronous combined excision and 55·5% after perineoabdominal excision for adenocarcinoma of the rectum at that hospital recorded by Bussey et al. (1960); see also p. 644.) Stearns and Quan (1970) have recorded a similar difference in the five-year survival rate, depending on whether the growth was located at the anal margin and was treated by local excision or lay in the anal canal and was managed by abdominoperineal excision—66% for 30 cases in the former group, and 58% for 59 cases in the latter.

Effect of Involvement of Inguinal Lymph Nodes on Ultimate Prognosis. Some of the experiences reported in the past in the treatment of inguinal node metastases in this disease have been most discouraging. For example, Judd and De Tar (1955) found that there were no five-year survivors among the patients with involvement of the groin glands in association with squamous cell carcinoma of the anus or anal canal at the Mayo Clinic, even when inguinal block dissection was performed. Grinnell (1954) had equally depressing results. But in recent years more favourable results have been recorded, and an important prognostic point that has emerged is whether the metastases are clinically apparent when the patient first presents or only became evident on follow-up some time after the primary lesion has been treated. Thus, Dillard et al. (1963) found that 11 of their 78 patients, when first examined, had palpably involved inguinal nodes. Six of the 11 were treated by colostomy only, because of other metastases. The remaining five patients were subjected to groin dissection, as well as surgical excision of the primary lesion, and two have survived free of cancer for seven and eight years respectively. Seven patients, whose inguinal glands were originally considered on clinical examination to be normal, subsequently developed groin metastases after treatment of their primary tumours—in all instances within six months of their original reference to hospital. The primary lesion had been controlled in three of the seven cases and these three patients have survived without evident recurrence after groin dissection. Wolfe and Bussey (1968) report that of 170 cases 49 had obvious inguinal node metastases when first seen, but only 19 were deemed suitable for block dissection; five of these were alive and well five years later. But, of 17 patients developing clinically evident groin metastases subsequently, nine proceeded to block dissection with five five-year survivors. Stearns and Quan (1970) state that in their series of 109 cases 14 had clinically obvious inguinal metastases when they first presented; all 14 underwent block dissections,

but only two survived for five years. On the other hand, 21 patients developed inguinal metastases subsequently; 20 were deemed suitable for block dissection and, of these, 15 achieved five-year survival.

MANAGEMENT OF INOPERABLE CASES

Unfortunately many cases arrive at a late stage of the illness when the condition has advanced beyond the scope of surgical excision. For these cases reliance has to be placed mainly on radiotherapy. If this is unavailing or unsuitable, and pain is a distressing feature as it often is with anal carcinoma, sedatives should be used freely and intrathecal injection of phenol or chordotomy may be required.

Squamous Cell Carcinoma of the Rectum

As pointed out by Richards et al. (1962), an epidermoid carcinoma occasionally arises in the rectum quite remote from the anal canal (and not as an extension of an advanced carcinoma of the cervix uteri). It is difficult to explain the development of such a tumour in this situation and one can only surmise that it has occurred as a malignant change in an area of squamous metaplasia. The growth is clinically indistinguishable as a rule from a scirrhous type of adenocarcinoma. Biopsy may give the diagnosis—or may not, because these are usually highly anaplastic growths and it may be difficult for the pathologist to decide on the tissue of origin. The final recognition of the precise nature of the lesion may thus depend on careful histopathological examination of the whole specimen. As may be deduced from these remarks on the pathological features, the prognosis is very poor. Of six cases of squamous cell carcinoma of the rectum seen at St Mark's Hospital, London, only one achieved a five-year cure (Gabriel, 1963).

Bowen's Disease of the Anus and Perianal Region

A form of slowly-growing intraepidermal squamous cell carcinoma, which masquerades as a chronic dermatosis, was described by Bowen (1912) and may occur in the anal and perianal region, where it is apt to be mistaken for conditions such as pruritus ani, senile keratosis or psoriasis. According to Strauss and Fazio (1979) only 112 cases have been reported in the world literature. If this lesion is suspected, the affected area of skin should be extensively biopsied and the specimens examined by frozen section. If intraepidermal cancer is demonstrated, all the involved skin is excised and this may well entail the removal of the entire circumference of the anal and perianal region, so that subsequent immediate split-thickness skin-grafting may be required. The prognosis is apparently very good. If recurrence should take place, it is usually amenable to further local excision.

BASAL CELL CARCINOMA

The anal skin is rarely the site of a basal cell carcinoma or rodent ulcer. The incidence of this type of growth has been given as twice in 3000 anorectal neoplasms during 13 years at the Mayo Clinic (Buie and Brust 1933); four times in approximately 1000 anorectal carcinomas at the Leeds General Infirmary from 1938 to 1954; 10 times in over 4000 malignant growths of the rectum and anal region at St Mark's Hospital, London, from 1928 to 1956 (Morson 1960a); four times in 237 rodent ulcers reviewed by Wakeley and Childs (1949); and twice in 706 rodent ulcers reviewed by Sutherland (1953). From their survey of the literature Armitage and Smith (1954) were able to collect 23 examples of basal cell carcinoma of the anal region, including their own four personally recorded cases, to which should now be added Morson's (1960a) ten cases.

CLINICAL FEATURES

The patient usually complains of 'piles' or of an ulcer or sore spot in the anal region. On examination an ulcer is found usually at or touching the anal margin, with an irregular outline and hard or slightly raised edges, and usually measuring about 1 × 2 cm. A lesion much larger than this is unlikely to be a rodent ulcer. In many of the recorded cases new growth was *not* suspected till reported by the pathologist and this emphasizes again the value of taking biopsies from any doubtful lesion in the anal region. The inguinal lymph glands are not implicated, though there may rarely be some inflammatory swelling due to septic absorption from the ulcerated area of the primary lesion.

TREATMENT AND PROGNOSIS

Just as for rodent ulcer in other situations, there is probably little to choose in effectiveness between radiotherapy and simple local excision. Unlike facial rodents, however, these anal lesions raise no cosmetic problems in regard to unsightly scars, and my own preference would therefore be for surgical excision in their treatment. Few good follow-up reports are available in the literature; what there are suggest that the prognosis is good.

MALIGNANT MELANOMA

Malignant melanoma is a rare tumour and Raven (1948), who has made a most comprehensive survey of the subject, was able to discover only about 100 cases recorded in the world literature. Morson (1960b) states that there have been only ten of these growths in over 4000 cases of malignant tumour of the anorectum at St Mark's Hospital, London, from 1928 to 1956. Though in some of these published cases the growth appeared to originate in the rectum proper, almost invariably the lower pole of the lesion connected with the epidermoid lining of the anal canal. Chalier and Bonnet (1912), Raven (1948) and most other writers are of the opinion that these growths are in fact ectodermal in origin. They have a very high metastasizing potential so that, even when the primary growth is small, wide dissemination may already have taken place via the lymphatic system and blood stream to the lungs, liver, brain, bony skeleton, lymph glands and skin.

CLINICAL FEATURES AND DIAGNOSIS

The lesion may present as a small polypoid tumour projecting into the lumen of the anal canal or at the anal orifice, and resembling a thrombosed haemorrhoid because of its bluish-black colour. Alternatively it may have a more papillomatous appearance, or may be frankly ulcerating and indurated, suggesting its neoplastic nature. In advanced cases a massive tumour may be present in the anal region with enlarged, hard inguinal glands. With smaller early lesions there may be few symptoms apart from the complaint of a swelling or 'piles'. With larger lesions pain, bleeding, discharge of pus and slime and alteration of bowel habit may all occur.

The diagnosis may be suggested by the dark coloration of the lesion as seen at the anal orifice or on proctoscopy, but confirmation by biopsy is required and in the majority of cases the diagnosis has depended entirely on pathological examination. Not infrequently the true nature of the lesion has only been revealed after histological section of the specimen removed in the course of a 'haemorrhoidectomy'.

TREATMENT AND PROGNOSIS

As Raven (1948) has shown, malignant melanoma is not sensitive to radiotherapy and the only prospect of cure seems to lie with surgical removal, best carried out as a radical abdominoperineal excision with high ligation of the inferior mesenteric vessels, followed later by bilateral block dissection of the inguinal glands. Gabriel (1963) has emphasized the necessity for avoiding delay in proceeding to excision, and in cases suspected clinically to have melanoma has urged that the shortest possible interval should be allowed to elapse between the confirmatory biopsy and the performance of rectal excision. In this connection a frozen section may be of special value. It must be admitted, however, that even with wide abdominoperineal excision the prognosis is very poor, and Braastad et al. (1949) were able to discover in the world literature reports of only three cases observed long enough after operation to be regarded as lasting clinical cures. Of the nine cases seen at St Mark's Hospital, London, two were inoperable, and seven had a 'radical' excision of the rectum, but one succumbed from the operation, three died within a year, two within two years and one lived just over three years (Morson 1960b). Of four cases reported by Sinclair et al. (1970), all rapidly recurred following treatment. Of the 14 patients with anorectal malignant melanoma diagnosed in Finland between 1953 and 1967, 13 died of the disease despite treatment, but one is still alive 13 years after operation (Husa and Höckerstedt 1974).

PRIMARY COLLOID OR ADENOCARCINOMA OF THE ANAL CANAL AND PERIANAL REGION (CLOACOGENIC CARCINOMA)

PATHOLOGY

Very rarely adenocarcinomas may arise primarily in the anal canal region or perianal tissues (Zimberg and Kay 1957; Dukes and Galvin 1956; Cabrera et al. 1966; Harrison et al. 1966; Sink et al. 1978), instead of reaching these parts by direct extension from a primary rectal carcinoma, or as an implantation metastasis from a colorectal cancer on to a raw area (e.g. a haemorrhoidectomy wound) in the anal canal (see p. 399). The exact histogenesis of these primary anal adenocarcinomas is controversial and probably varies from case to case. A well recognized association is some cases is with a long-standing anal fistula (see p. 177), which seems to predispose to the development of a malignant tumour in relation to the fistulous track. Though the growth arising in connection with a fistula is sometimes a squamous carcinoma, more commonly it is a colloid carcinoma, which does not involve the lining of the anal canal or rectum. The site of origin of primary adenocarcinoma of the anal region is debatable. Dukes and Galvin (1956) postulate that it commences in *unusual reduplications of the anorectal mucosa*, but Zimberg and Kay (1957) think that the *anal intermuscular glands* (see p. 9) are the most likely source. Indeed these latter authors consider these glands the most likely starting point for the majority of primary adenocarcinomas of the anal and perianal region. Another site of origin may be the *transitional epithelium lining the suprapectinate part of the anal canal*, from which mucoepidermoid carcinoma, consisting of a combination of squamous and mucus-producing carcinoma, may arise (Morson and Volkstädt 1963; Morson and Pang 1968). Yet another possible source of anal adenocarcinoma is the *apocrine glands of the perianal skin* (Grodsky 1960; Nelson 1960).

CLINICAL FEATURES AND DIAGNOSIS

A notable feature of some primary adenocarcinomas of the anal canal and perianal region is that they do not manifest themselves on the inside of the canal—the so-called extramucosal adenocarcinomas—but spread in an annular extraluminal fashion around the bowel, infiltrating widely in the perianal tissues and involving regional nodes extensively. They may also erupt through the perianal skin or occasionally give rise to a peculiar, scaling, erythematous eczema of the perianal region, comparable to Paget's disease of the nipple. (However, such perianal Paget's disease may also occur with certain primary rectal adenocarcinomas spreading extensively downwards to the anal region, as Morson (1960b) has emphasized.)

Because a lesion of the anal lining itself is often absent, it is very easy to confuse some of these adenocarcinomas of the anal region with an inflammatory condition. Perianal Paget's disease may readily be mistaken for ordinary pruritus ani or Crohn's disease. The important diagnostic measure is a deep biopsy from representative tissues.

TREATMENT

The treatment of these primary adenocarcinomas follows closely that of squamous cell carcinoma of the anal canal (see p. 669). Where possible, an abdominoperineal excision of the rectum with wide removal of the perianal tissues is performed, and, in addition, a block dissection of the inguinal nodes is employed as required. But many cases are inoperable and have to be managed by radiotherapy or symptomatic treatment. In general the prognosis appears poor.

REFERENCES

ARMITAGE, G. and SMITH, I. B. (1954) Rodent ulcer of the anus. *Br. J. Surg.*, *42*, 395.

BACON, H. E. (1949) *The Anus, Rectum and Sigmoid Colon*, 3rd ed. Philadelphia: Lippincott.

BARONOFSKY, I. D. (1948) Technique of inguinal node dissection. *Surgery, St Louis*, *24*, 555.

BINKLEY, G. E. (1950) Epidermoid carcinoma of the anus and rectum. *Am. J. Surg.*, *79*, 90.

BOWEN, J. T. (1912) Precancerous dermatoses: a study of two cases of atypical epithelial proliferation. *J. cutan. Dis.*, *30*, 241.

BRAASTAD, F. W., DOCKERTY, M. B. and DIXON, C. F. (1949) Melano-epithelioma of the anus and rectum. *Surgery, St Louis*, *25*, 82.

BRODERS, A. C. (1925) the grading of carcinoma. *Minn. Med.*, *8*, 726.

BUIE, L. A. and BRUST, J. C. M. (1933) Malignant anal lesions of epithelial origin. *Journal-Lancet*, *53*, 565.

BUSSEY, H. J. R., DUKES, C. E. and LOCKHART-MUMMERY, H. E. (1960) Results of the surgical treatment of rectal cancer. In *Cancer of the Rectum*, ed. C. E. Dukes. Edinburgh: Livingstone.

CABRERA, A., TSUKADA, Y. and PICKREN, J. W. (1966) Adenocarcinomas of the anal canal and perianal region. *Ann. Surg.*, *164*, 152.

CATTELL, R. B. and WILLIAMS, A. C. (1943) Epidermoid carcinoma of the anus and rectum. *Archs Surg., Chicago*, *46*, 336.

CHALIER, A. and BONNET, P. (1912) Les tumeurs mélaniques primitives du rectum. *Rev. Chir., Paris*, *46*, 336.

DILLARD, B. M., SPRATT, J. S., Jr., ACKERMAN, L. V. and BUTCHER, H. R., Jr. (1963) Epidermoid cancer of the anal margin and canal. *Archs Surg., Chicago*, *86*, 772.

DUKES, C. E. and GALVIN, C. (1956) Colloid carcinoma arising within fistulae in the anorectal region *Ann. R. Coll. Surg. Engl.*, *18*, 246.

FRANKLYN, A. and PARKS, A. G. (1979) Anal cancer treated by fast-reaction irradiation. *Br. J. Surg.*, in the press.

GABRIEL, W. B. (1932) The results of perineal excision and of radium in the treatment of cancer of the rectum. *Br. J. Surg.*, *20*, 234.

—— (1941) Squamous-cell carcinoma of the anus and anal canal. *Proc. R. Soc. Med.*, *34*, 139.

—— (1960) Discussion on squamous cell carcinoma of the anus and anal canal. *Proc. R. Soc. Med.*, *53*, 403.

—— (1963) *Principles and Practice of Rectal Surgery*, 5th ed. London: H. K. Lewis.

GILCHRIST, R. K. and DAVID, V. C. (1938) Lymphatic spread of carcinoma of the rectum. *Ann. Surg.*, *108*, 621.

GORDON-WATSON, C. (1930) Treatment of carcinoma of the rectum with radium. *Br. J. Surg.*, *17*, 643.

GRINNELL, R. S. (1954) An analysis of forty-nine cases of squamous cell carcinoma of the anus. *Surgery Gynec. Obstet.*, *98*, 29.

GRINVALSKY, H. T. and HELWIG, E. B. (1956) Carcinoma of the anorectal junction. *Cancer*, *9*, 480.

GRODSKY, L. (1960) Extramammary Paget's disease of the perianal region. *Dis. Colon Rect.*, *3*, 502.

—— (1969) Current concepts on cloacogenic transitional cell anorectal cancers. *J. Am. med. Ass.*, *207*, 2057.

GUPTA, T. K. (1969) Radical groin dissection. *Surgery Gynec. Obstet.*, *129*, 1275.

HARRISON, E. G., BEAHRS, O. H. and HILL, J. R. (1966) Anal and perianal malignant neoplasms: pathology and treatment. *Dis. Colon Rect.*, *9*, 255.

HARVEY, H. D. (1946) Epithelioma of the anus. *Ann. Surg.*, *124*, 245.

HUSA, A. and HÖCKERSTEDT, K. (1974) Anorectal malignant melanoma. *Acta chir. scand.*, *140*, 68.

JUDD, E. S. Jr. and DE TAR, B. E., Jr. (1955) Squamous cell carcinoma of the anus: results of treatment. *Surgery, St Louis*, *37*, 220.

KHEIR, S., HICKEY, R. C., MARTIN, R. G., MACKAY, B. and GALLAGHER, H. S. (1972) Cloacogenic carcinoma of anal canal. *Archs Surg., Chicago*, *104*, 407.

McQUARRIE, H. B. and BUIE, L. A. (1950) Epithelioma of anus. *Postgrad. Med.*, *7*, 402.

MILTON, G. W., WILLIAMS, A. E. J. and BRYANT, D. H. (1968) Radical dissection of the inguinal and iliac lymph nodes for malignant melanoma of the leg. *Br. J. Surg.*, *55*, 42.

MORSON, B. C. (1959) The pathology and results of treatment of cancer of the anal region. *Proc. R. Soc. Med.*, Suppl. *52*, 117.

—— (1960a) Discussion on squamous cell carcinoma of the anus and anal canal. *Proc. R. Soc. Med.*, *53*, 416.

—— (1960b) Rare malignant tumours of the rectum and anal canal. In *Cancer of the Rectum*, ed. C. Dukes. Edinburgh and London: Livingstone.

—— and PANG, L. S. C. (1968) Pathology of anal cancer. *Proc. R. Soc. Med.*, *61*, 623.

—— and VOLKSTÄDT, H. (1963) Muco-epidermoid tumours of the anal canal. *J. clin. Path*, *16*, 200.

NELSON, T. F. (1960) Perianal Paget's disease. *Dis. Colon Rect.*, *3*, 135.

RAVEN, R. W. (1941) Squamous-cell carcinoma of the anus and anal canal. *Proc. R. Soc. Med.*, *34*, 157.

—— (1948) Anorectal malignant melanoma. *Proc. R. Soc. Med.*, *41*, 469.

RICHARDS, J. C., BEAHRS, O. H. and WOOLNER, L. B. (1962) Squamous cell carcinoma of the anus, anal canal and rectum in 109 patients. *Surgery Gynec. Obstet.*, *114*, 475.

ROSSER, C. (1931) The etiology of anal cancer. *Am. J. Surg.*, *11*, 328.

ROUX-BERGER, J. L. and ENNUYER, N. (1948) Carcinoma of the anal canal. *Am. J. Roentgen.*, *60*, 807.

SAUER, I. and BACON, H. E. (1952) A new approach for excision of carcinoma of the lower portion of the rectum and anal canal. *Surgery Gynec. Obstet.*, *95*, 229.

SINCLAIR, D. M., HANNAH, G., McLAUGHLIN, I. S., PATRICK, R. S., SLAVIN, G. and NEVILLE, A. M. (1970). Malignant melanoma of the anal canal. *Br. J. Surg.*, *57*, 808.

SINK, J. D., KRAMER, S. A., COPELAND, D. D. and SEIGER, H. F. (1978) Cloacogenic carcinoma. *Ann. Surg.*, *188*, 53.

STEARNS, M. W., Jr. (1955) Epidermoid carcinoma of the anal region. Inguinal metastases. *Am. J. Surg.*, *90*, 727.

—— and QUAN, S. H. Q. (1970) Epidermoid carcinoma of the anorectum. *Surgery Gynec. Obstet.*, *131*, 953.

STRAUSS, R. J. and FAZIO, V. W. (1979) Bowen's disease of the anal and perianal area. A report and analysis of twelve cases. *Am. J. Surg.*, *137*, 231.

SUTHERLAND, T. W. (1953) Quoted by Armitage and Smith (1954).

SWEET, R. H. (1947) Results of treatment of epidermoid carcinoma of the anus and rectum. *Surgery Gynec. Obstet.*, *84*, 967.

WAKELEY, SIR C. and CHILDS, P. (1949) Basal-cell carcinoma (rodent ulcer), with special reference to lesions on neck, trunk and limbs. *Br. med. J.*, *1*, 737.

WILLIAMS, I. G. (1962) Carcinoma of the anus and anal canal. *Clin. Radiol.*, *13*, 30.

WOLFE, H. R. I. and BUSSEY, H. J. R. (1968) Squamous cell carcinoma of the anus. *Br. J. Surg.*, *55*, 295.

ZIMBERG, Y. H. and KAY, S. (1957) Anorectal carcinomas of extramucosal origin. *Ann. Surg.*, *145*, 344.

20

Rarer Tumours of the Colon, Rectum and Anus

BENIGN TUMOURS

LYMPHOMA

A simple lymphoma of the rectum, consisting of an aggregation of lymphoid tissue with a covering of normal mucous membrane, is the commonest benign non-epithelial tumour of the large intestine, and is confined virtually entirely to the rectum and rectosigmoid. Granet et al. (1950), Hayes and Burr (1952) and Cornes et al. (1961) have given good reviews of the subject. At proctoscopy or sigmoidoscopy a lymphoma is usually seen as a single (occasionally multiple), reddish, purple or grey, rounded polyp varying in diameter from a few millimetres to 3 cm. Rarely is it larger or pedunculated. Symptoms may be absent, the tumour being discovered incidentally, or there may be bleeding or discharge. The treatment is removal by diathermy snare or simple local excision, usually on an erroneous diagnosis of a benign adenoma.

Histologically the appearances may be not unlike those of a lymphosarcoma, and roughly half of a series of 70 cases of benign lymphoma reported by Helwig and Hansen (1951) were thus misdiagnosed in the first instance. As Stout (1959) has emphasized, there is no evidence that benign lymphomas tend to become lymphosarcomatous, so that, even if histological examination shows that the polyp has not been completely removed, there is no urgent necessity to attempt further excision of the remnant. A follow-up study by Cornes et al. (1961) confirms the soundness of this advice, for, of 75 patients traced, many for more than five years, after simple (often incomplete) local excision of lymphomas, none developed malignant changes.

LIPOMA

This is the next least uncommon simple connective tissue tumour of the large intestine. As has been shown by Mayo et al. (1963) in a series of 119 cases with intestinal lipomas seen at the Mayo Clinic from 1935 to 1961, these growths are most frequently found in the caecum and right colon in females (a favourite site being the ileocaecal valve itself), and in the left colon in males, and are less commonly encountered in the rectum or rectosigmoid in either sex. The usual pathological appearance of a lipoma of the bowel is of a submucous growth projecting in polypoid fashion into the lumen, but rarely it may occupy a subserous position. The size of the lesion varies from a few millimetres to 6 cm or more, and the larger forms may completely encircle the bowel, especially in the caecal region. Usually lipomas occur singly, but in 20% of the series of Mayo et al. (1963) two or more growths were present. Erosion of the overlying mucosa may take place with resultant ulceration. The lipoma may form the apex of an intussusception, or may undergo infection or gangrene or be the seat of a haemorrhage.

The clinical manifestations vary greatly. There may be no symptoms at all and the lipoma may be discovered in the course of a laparotomy for some other condition or be found in an operative specimen removed for some other lesion, as happened in many of the cases in Mayo et al.'s (1963) series. The rare rectal lipoma is also usually detected in an asymptomatic state on routine sigmoidoscopy. At the other end of the scale, the condition may present as an acute abdominal emergency due to the occurrence of a complicating intussusception. Between these extremes many patients have less severe symptoms, often of a rather vague kind, such as abdominal pain, alteration of bowel habit, bleeding and anaemia, or a palpable abdominal mass. Mayo et al. (1963) have made the observation that the larger the lipoma the more likely it is to be associated with some complaint. Radiological examination to investigate symptoms or clinical signs will often show a polypoid lesion and its benign nature may sometimes be surmised, but in other instances the appearances are quite equivocal or more closely resemble those of carcinoma, especially in the right colon, as in many of the Mayo Clinic cases (Mayo et al. 1963).

If the condition has been discovered as a polyp on sigmoidoscopy, a biopsy will be taken at the same time (or the entire lesion removed) and histological examination will show its exact nature. No further treatment is required. If, as is much more usual, the tumour lies in the colon and is disclosed by barium study or at laparotomy, the necessity to exclude a malignant lesion with certainty will demand operative intervention. Depending on the degree of suspicion of carcinoma, this may take the form of a partial colectomy or a colotomy and enucleation. Mayo et al. (1963) point out that in the earlier cases in their series radical resections were frequently used, but in the later ones there was a trend towards more conservative excisions.

Leiomyoma

The classical paper on the pathological aspects of intestinal leiomyomas (and leiomyosarcomas) is that of Golden and Stout (1941) of Columbia University, New York, and another excellent general review has been provided by Morton et al. (1956) of Rochester, New York. These tumours arise in the muscle coat of the bowel wall and may remain in an intramural position or may project into the lumen or into the peritoneal cavity. They usually occur singly, but instances of multiple leiomyomas are on record. The smaller tumours are rubbery, firm rounded nodules which have a whorled, grey or pink appearance on section; the larger ones tend to become lobulated. Histologically the lesion is composed essentially of spindle-shaped cells arranged in interlacing bundles, but there is frequently a considerable admixture of fibrous tissue, so that they might logically be termed 'fibromyomas'. Usually leiomyomas of the colon are not encapsulated, but according to Anderson et al. (1950) those in the rectum often

have a capsule. The crucial histopathological consideration in regard to these tumours is their differentiation from leiomyosarcomas, which may be far from easy. As Golden and Stout (1941) emphasize, the absence of encapsulation does not necessarily indicate malignancy. The smooth muscle cells in leiomyosarcomas may be as well differentiated as in a leiomyoma, and the tumour can only be distinguished from a benign one by the presence of mitoses. A leiomyoma may undergo malignant change, but it seems to be impossible to predict with certainty whether this will occur or not.

Leiomyoma of the large intestine may be found at any age and in either sex. In Stout's (1959) series they affected the colon rather more often than the rectum, but at the Mayo Clinic this was reversed, for Anderson et al. (1950) found 10 rectal leiomyomas in the records there between 1911 and 1946 (during which time over 2000 rectal tumours were treated), but during a similar period at that institution Mackenzie et al. (1954) could discover only eight leiomyomas of the colon. It would appear that these tumours usually grow to a size of 1–2 cm and never increase any further. Only rarely does one become large enough to cause symptoms. Ulceration of the overlying mucosa with resulting haemorrhage may occur as in a case described by Ghabrial (1955), but this is most unusual. Generally the condition is discovered during routine rectal examination.

The management of a suspected leiomyoma of the rectum must be governed largely by the biopsy findings, but, as Sanger and Leckie (1959) point out, the clinical findings are also important. If the biopsy strongly suggests that the lesion is benign and it is small or pedunculated and easily circumscribed, it should be removed by local excision, as was done in all the 10 cases reported by Anderson et al. (1950) without recurrence, and in Ghabrial's (1955) case. If there is some doubt about the histological interpretation of the biopsy material and the tumour seems clinically capable of being enucleated, it would be justifiable to attempt local removal and to be guided by the pathologist's report on the whole tumour as to whether more radical surgery should be undertaken later. If the biopsy shows unequivocal evidence of leiomyosarcoma or if the tumour is large a radical excision of the rectum should be carried out (see also Leiomyosarcoma, p. 684).

A leiomyoma of the colon large enough to cause symptoms drawing attention to it would probably be diagnosed preoperatively as a probable carcinoma. At laparotomy it would be wise to treat it as such by a radical colectomy.

HAEMANGIOMA

This is another very rare tumour of the large intestine, of which Hunt was able to collect only 21 examples from the literature in 1941; a further seven or eight cases were published up to 1955, when Hellström et al. reported another two examples of rectal haemangioma. More recently Allred and Spencer (1974) have reported 40 cases from the Mayo Clinic. In most cases the rectum or distal colon has been the part affected, but it may occur anywhere in the colon. The tumour varies greatly in size and may be small, consisting of a few reddish purple nodules in the submucosa, or may form a complete cuff round a segment of colon or rectum, and may even implicate surrounding structures. Though Brown (1924) has described the occurrence of intestinal obstruction due to massive submucous haemangiomas, in most cases the condition reveals itself by producing haemorrhage, and this is a cause that should be borne in mind in investigating cases of rectal bleeding of obscure aetiology.

If the angioma is in the rectum or distal sigmoid, it will be revealed by sigmoidoscopy. The exact diagnosis may be suggested by the finding of dilated veins in the submucosa, but in other cases, as in those described by Aylett (1954), with smaller lesions the appearances may not be typical and it is not till the biopsy is examined that the nature of the growth is established. Rarely, as Bensaude and Bensaude (1932) have pointed out, a haemangioma of the lower rectum may extend to the anal margin or into the perianal region. Another sign that may be of diagnostic value is the detection on plain X-ray examination of the pelvis of multiple small phleboliths in the part of the rectal wall affected by the haemangioma. Such phleboliths were present in one case of diffuse cavernous haemangioma of the rectum described by Jacques (1952) and in two cases reported by Hellström et al. (1955). Further radiological confirmation of the diagnosis in cases of suspected rectal haemangioma can be obtained by selective inferior mesenteric angiography. In a case of haemangioma of the colon, where the lesion is small, its recognition may be difficult even at laparotomy due to the fact that the tumour is often confined to the mucosa and submucosa and produces no abnormality on the serosal aspect. Rutter (1956) has described a case of this kind. The patient had had two previous negative laparotomies to discover a cause for rectal haemorrhage. Only at a third laparotomy, undertaken whilst bleeding was in progress, was the condition detected. Nowadays

mesenteric arteriography performed whilst haemorrhage was occurring would offer a good chance of making a preoperative diagnosis in such a case (Baum et al. 1969). A similar condition which may give rise to mysterious severe haemorrhage is solitary or multiple angiodysplasias of the intestinal wall. These minute lesions are usually quite undetectable by ordinary barium enema study or even at laparotomy. Their diagnosis rests mainly on mesenteric arteriography preferably whilst bleeding is taking place. Colonoscopy might be helpful. Whitehouse (1973) gives a good review.

TREATMENT

If the haemangioma is *in the rectum* and small, it may be possible to destroy it with diathermy through the sigmoidoscope, as in Aylett's (1954) two cases and in many of the Mayo Clinic cases (Allred and Spencer 1974), or to remove it by a local excision if low down, as in one of Gabriel's (1948) patients. But if the tumour is of diffuse type involving a considerable segment of bowel, no simple treatment of this kind is feasible, and the prognosis is much more serious, several of the recorded cases ending fatally. The haemorrhage may be checked temporarily by rectal packing but its ultimate arrest demands urgent surgical treatment. For a haemangioma extending down to the anal canal the choice of operation in the past usually lay with abdominoperineal excision, though this could be a technically difficult and daunting procedure because of excessive bleeding. Very successful results with it were recorded by Flaschka (1924), Hunt (1941), Jacques (1952), Hellström et al. (1955) and Scott and Brand (1957). Gabriel (1948), in dealing with a patient with a very large pulsating rectal haemangioma, instead established a proximal colostomy and tied the superior haemorrhoidal artery, with a good permanent result, the colostomy eventually being closed. However, this manoeuvre would seem to be unreliable, as shown by the fact that, following its use in another case by Bancroft (1930), the bleeding recurred and rectal excision was ultimately necessary. The most interesting development in recent years has been the adoption by Jeffrey et al. (1976) of a sphincter-saving technique of resection for this condition, with excision of the upper two-thirds of the rectum, dissecting out of the mucosa of the anorectal remnant from the pectinate line upwards and a colo-anal sleeve anastomosis, as in the Soave (1964) procedure for Hirschsprung's disease and in the treatment of some villous papillomas (see p. 353). They

intact or only s
usually movab
tinal wall like
polyp, but it i
have a yellowis
not usually r
tumour becom
so that it cl
grosser type o
stases in lymph
stream as well.
difference in th
the colon and
colon carcinoi
to have metast
only two had t
tumours and l
son's (1956) fin
carcinoid tum
London, were
were of the sr
showed the m
cinoid of rect
whilst only on
ulcerated prim
of a malignant
the superior ha
But Peskin and
incidence of m
less than 10 o
invasive forms
beyond the m
lymphatic or l
the ten maligna
than 2 cm.

Clinically cai
simple polyps
tinguishable fi
rectal examin
tumours of thi
Treatment of th
noid of the co
by radical col
sphincter-savir
smaller polyp-
sigmoid a loca
plete removal
normal mucos
the underlying
operative spec
examination t
has been left b
these cases tu
metastasizing l

report five patients so treated with very good functional results.

Haemangioma *of the colon* discovered during exploratory laparotomy calls for a segmental resection.

MISCELLANEOUS OTHER BENIGN TUMOURS

Stout (1959) mentions several other benign connective tissue tumours which are excessively rarely met with in the colon or rectum—*lymphangioma, mesothelioma, granular cell myeloblastoma, fibroma, neurofibroma, ganglioneuroma and teratoma*. These will not be further discussed here.

Hypertrophied anal papillae are in a sense fibromas. Their appearances and management are described on p. 131.

ENDOMETRIOSIS

For an account of the aetiology and pathology of endometriosis in general reference should be made to standard gynaecological texts, to the excellent articles by Masson (1935) or MacLeod (1946), or to Goodall's (1943) monograph on the subject. Here only those aspects of endometriosis that have a bearing on the surgery of the rectum or colon will be considered.

Endometriosis may affect the rectum, sigmoid or rarely the caecum of female patients, usually in association with endometriosis of the ovaries and uterus. The condition is naturally restricted to the reproductive years, but most cases apparently occur between 30 and the menopause. As a rule the lesion in the bowel wall is confined to the serosal aspect or to the muscularis or submucosa, the mucosa remaining intact. It may consist of a small discrete nodule or may extend circumferentially round the bowel producing a stenosis, which at laparotomy may appear indistinguishable from a constricting carcinoma. According to Cattell (1937), Mayo and Miller (1940) and Jenkinson and Brown (1943), some degree of obstruction was present in nearly 50% of the cases of endometriosis of the sigmoid or rectum coming under their care.

SYMPTOMS

Only about half the patients with endometriosis of the rectum or colon have any symptoms referable to the lesion in the bowel. One of the most frequent complaints is of a *more or less constant rectal or pelvic pain* of a dull aching character, aggravated by defaecation and *especially by menstruation*. Very rarely slight rectal bleeding may occur at the menstrual periods. There may be gradually increasing constipation or slight diarrhoea. Additional symptoms frequently present are dysmenorrhoea and pain in the lower abdomen and back. An important feature is that the symptoms are usually of long duration and go back many months or even years.

EXAMINATION

Digital palpation of the rectum may be negative as the lesion of endometriosis is *usually situated in the upper part of the rectum or distal sigmoid*. However, sometimes the finger detects a mass high up in the rectosigmoid region. Sigmoidoscopy will confirm the presence of a swelling projecting into or constricting the lumen, but shows that the mucosa covering the lesion, though possibly puckered, is intact. Jenkinson and Brown (1943) have claimed that the appearances or endometriosis of the rectum and sigmoid on barium enema examination are characteristic, with a long filling defect with sharp regular borders, intact mucosa and marked local tenderness and fixation on palpation during screening; but Cattell (1937) and Mayo and Miller (1940) could observe no special distinguishing features on radiological examination.

DIAGNOSIS

The relationship of the symptoms to menstruation, and the length of the history together with the patient's good general condition may possibly suggest the diagnosis of endometriosis. More often the bowel lesion is discovered during routine examination in a patient with vague lower abdominal, gynaecological or rectal symptoms. Sigmoidoscopy is apt to be equivocal unless a good biopsy is obtained, when the diagnosis may be immediately established. Barium enema examination is usually unhelpful and, as Kelly and Schlademan (1949) emphasize, the great majority of cases come to operation on an uncertain diagnosis or the condition is discovered for the first time at laparotomy. Even then it may be thought to be a carcinoma.

TREATMENT

Many cases of endometriosis of the colon or rectum have been treated by resection of the bowel on a mistaken diagnosis of carcinoma, and only after the pathological examination of the specimen was the

correct
the slig
the cor
be per
nosis
sigmoi
laparor
in one
the pe
frozen
ment a

Rem
a retrc
This is
in you
severe
resulti
interfe
bearin
ever, i
apprec
regarc
oophc
extent
ovarie

Rese
metho
sible.
rectos
the fo
perma

IMPLA

Duke
descri
to tra
by a
tomy
epithe
accur
Clinic
a ben
treate
repor
inade
years
coinc

extremely difficult. Sarcomas of the colon will produce the same radiological appearances as a carcinoma on barium enema examination and will likewise be indistinguishable at laparotomy.

The prognosis with sarcomas of the large intestine is very bad, but not quite hopeless. Thus Stout (1959) reported that there was only one long-term survivor in 37 cases of lymphosarcoma, of which the specimens were examined in his laboratory. Dawson et al. (1961) had rather more favourable results, with three of 24 cases surviving for 15 years or longer; they concluded that the prospects with giant follicular lymphosarcoma were better than with reticulum cell sarcoma. Surprisingly, they, like Marshall and Meissner (1950), found that the prognosis was unrelated to the occurrence of regional lymph node involvement. Dawson et al. (1961) also emphasized that nodes observed to be grossly enlarged at laparotomy were frequently found on histological examination not to contain growth. The best prospects of cure appear to lie with surgical excision, if technically feasible, and this was the method used in the successful cases of Stout (1959) and Dawson et al. (1961). Though lymphosarcomas in general are radiosensitive, radiotherapy for these tumours in the large bowel has not been successful in providing any lasting cures, though it has often afforded good temporary palliation, with relief of symptoms, improvement in general health, and even reduction in the size of abdominal masses (Stout 1959; Dawson et al. 1961). Possibly, with the more powerful forms of irradiation now available, the results in the future might be better.

LEIOMYOSARCOMA

Leiomyosarcoma of the large gut has roughly the same over-all incidence as benign leiomyoma and occurs rather more frequently in the rectum than in the colon. In the records of the Mayo Clinic there were ten cases each of leiomyosarcoma and leiomyoma of the rectum (Anderson et al. 1950), and five cases of leiomyosarcoma and eight of leiomyoma of the colon. Malignant myomas may occur in either sex, most patients being over the age of 50. The tumours originate in the muscle coat and tend to project either into the lumen or on the external aspect of the bowel. They are usually larger than simple leiomyomas and may be as big as a grapefruit or larger. Some of them are rubbery firm in consistency and coarsely lobulated, others are

softer. The mucosa overlying the tumour may be intact, but in roughly half the cases it is ulcerated, usually in a punched-out or umbilicated fashion, and haemorrhage may then occur. Occasionally the tumour may obstruct the lumen by its bulk or by causing constriction.

Histologically these growths may vary widely from well differentiated lesions, composed of sheets of spindle-shaped cells, not very different from a benign leiomyoma, to tumours consisting of immature, shorter, plumper cells of varying size and shape with more oval, deeply staining nuclei. Giant cells may be present and many normal and pathological mitoses may be evident. There may be great difficulty in distinguishing between leiomyoma and leiomyosarcoma (see Leiomyoma, p. 679). The most important evidence of malignancy is the presence of mitoses. The finding of bizarre cells without mitoses is insufficient for a diagnosis of leiomyosarcoma, and conversely a well differentiated smooth muscle tumour must be considered malignant if mitoses are evident (Stout 1959).

Leiomyosarcomas spread chiefly by direct continuity or by the blood stream. A feature of local spread is that sometimes there are apparently isolated nodules of growth in the submucosa, perirectal or ischiorectal fat, or mesocolon. However, microscopical examination shows that there is intervening tumour connecting such outlying deposits to the parent tumour. Blood spread may result in metastases in liver, lungs or other tissues and this is the usual cause of death (Morson 1960). It is generally considered that involvement of the lymph nodes does not occur with this tumour of the large bowel (Anderson et al. 1950; MacKenzie et al. 1954; Morson 1960), but Thorlakson and Ross (1961) report a case of rectal leiomyosarcoma with deposits in a perirectal lymph node.

The symptoms of these growths are not at all distinctive. Some of the more common complaints with rectal leiomyosarcomas have been pain or a feeling of fullness in the rectum, rectal bleeding, passage of mucus, change of bowel habit to constipation or diarrhoea and loss of weight and energy (Anderson et al. 1950). Severe haemorrhage has occurred on occasion and required emergency abdominoperineal excision for its arrest (Sanger and Leckie 1959). The clinical manifestations of leiomyosarcomas of the colon are similar except that the pain is located in the abdomen; it may be a constant dull ache or more of a colic, and sometimes there is acute intestinal obstruction from the occurrence of an intussusception or even of perforation at the site of the growth (MacKenzie et al. 1954). Rarely the finding of an abdominal mass may be the presenting symptom.

In a case of leiomyosarcoma of the colon there may be no abdominal physical signs in the abdomen, or a palpable mass or area of tenderness and guarding may be present, and exceptionally there will be the signs of an intestinal perforation or obstruction. Usually barium enema examination shows a projecting or constricting lesion not readily distinguishable from a carcinoma. This will lead to laparotomy, at which the diagnosis will probably still be in doubt, and a radical resection will be performed if the lesion is removable. This was feasible in nine of ten cases treated at the Mayo Clinic (MacKenzie et al. 1954); two of the patients were alive and well four and a half and nine years after the operation.

Leiomyosarcomas of the rectum are invariably detected on rectal examination, usually with the finger because they are nearly always situated in the lower rectum. If the mucosa is intact, this may arouse suspicion that the lesion is not an ordinary rectal carcinoma, but usually the initial clinical diagnosis is carcinoma and it is not till the biopsy report is available that this error is corrected. As explained above and under Leiomyoma (see p. 679), the pathologist may have the greatest difficulty in deciding whether he is dealing with a benign or malignant smooth muscle tumour, and the clinical findings may be equally important in helping to make this distinction, which is essential in planning correct treatment. Unless the tumour is small (not more than 2 or 3 cm) or the biopsy report by an experienced pathologist unequivocally diagnoses the tumour as benign, it would be wise to regard it as a leiomyosarcoma and to treat it accordingly.

Local excision of leiomyosarcomas of the rectum has sometimes been practised in the past, occasionally on a doubtful diagnosis of simple muscle tumour, but the result has almost invariably been recurrence of the lesion. Thus six of the ten cases reported by Anderson et al. (1950) were treated by local excision; one could not be traced, but the other five all recurred, three of them developing further recurrences after repeated local excisions. Four of 14 cases at St Mark's Hospital were similarly treated, but all recurred (Morson 1960). The results of radiotherapy alone or in conjunction with local removal have been equally bad in the experience of Hunt (1921), Golden and Stout (1941), Oppenheim and O'Brien (1950) and Anderson et al. (1950), which is not perhaps surprising as the tumours are often very well differentiated. Possibly modern radiotherapy might have more to offer. The most satisfactory treatment for rectal leiomyosarcomas would seem to be radical removal by abdominoperineal excision, with the emphasis on wide ablation of the rectum itself rather than on extensive removal of lymphatics which are seldom involved in this condition. In reporting 12 cases of rectal leiomyosarcoma treated by radical removal of the rectum at St Mark's Hospital, London, Morson (1960) mentions that three patients lived for five or more years, but died eventually of recurrence. He believes that despite the good five-year survival rate the ultimate prognosis is poor.

MISCELLANEOUS OTHER MALIGNANT TUMOURS

Other tumours which have been recorded as occurring very rarely in the anorectum or colon are *rhabdomyosarcoma, haemangiopericytoma* and *plasmacytoma* (Stout 1959; Pack et al. 1963), and *endothelioma* (Morgan 1932; Norbury 1932).

MALIGNANT MELANOMA

Malignant melanomas occur rarely in the lower rectum or anal canal, but they derive from melanoblasts in the squamous epithelium of the anal canal. They have, therefore, been dealt with in this book in connection with carcinoma of the anal canal (p. 675).

EXTRARECTAL TUMOURS

During a digital examination of the rectum an abnormal extrarectal mass is not infrequently encountered. Indeed the palpation of such masses is one of the most important diagnostic signs in surgery. It may be useful to recapitulate some of the more common 'tumours' felt in this way.

ANTERIORLY

1. Pelvic abscesses.
2. Secondary deposits in the rectovesical or rectovaginal pouch.
3. Carcinoma of the sigmoid.
4. Ovarian cyst or carcinoma.

5. The normal cervix uteri, fibroids, carcinoma of the utrerus or a normal pregnancy.
6. Carcinoma of the bladder.
7. Carcinoma or benign enlargement of the prostate (see also p. 914).

POSTERIORLY

1. Chronic abscess in the retrorectal space secondary to injection treatment for rectal prolapse or haemorrhoids, or to escape of barium through a tear in the rectal wall during a barium enema examination.
2. Ordinary soft tissue tumours such as lipoma, liposarcoma, fibroma, fibrosarcoma, haemangioma, neurofibroma or neurolemmoma of the retrorectal space.
3. Bony tumours of the sacrum and coccyx—osteoma, osteosarcoma, chondroma, chondrosarcoma, giant cell tumours, bone cysts and bony metastases from visceral carcinomas.
4. Meningocele.
5. Teratoma.
6. Dermoid cyst.
7. Chordoma.

Most of the masses liable to be felt anteriorly are commonplaces of clinical practice and do not require further consideration in this work. However, a few comments may be appropriate in regard to retrorectal swellings. Useful surveys of large series of cases with posterior extrarectal swellings are given by Jackman et al. (1951), Mayo et al. (1958), Swinton and Lehman (1958) and Freier et al. (1971). Such tumours in infants and young children often assume a formidable size and present as large external swellings of the sacrococcygeal region rather than strictly retrorectal lesions. Good accounts of them from the paediatric aspect are provided by Gross et al. (1951), McCarty et al. (1952) Mahour et al. (1974) and Izant and Filston (1975), and Miles and Stewart (1975) consider the condition in adults. Unquestionably the commonest retrorectal tumours are the congenital conditions—the teratomas, the dermoid cysts and the chordomas—and my remarks will be confined to these conditions.

TERATOMA

Teratomas are initially encapsulated cystic or solid tumours containing a mixture of tissues. Though largely confined to infants, a few have been recor-

ded in adults, 12% of them being malignant (Killen and Jackson 1963). Superadded infection is a common occurrence and may mask the underlying condition. Also the tumour may burst into the rectum. X-ray examination may be helpful in diagnosis by showing bone formation or teeth. Because of their tendency to become infected and to rupture, teratomas should be excised, if possible. Usually this can be done through a sacral approach, the patient being in a kneeling or crouching position and the coccyx and terminal part of the sacrum being excised, but occasionally an abdominal or abdominoperineal approach is required. If the lesion is benign and is removed intact, the prognosis is excellent. Incomplete removal results in recurrence. The outlook for malignant teratomas is poor.

DERMOID CYST

Dermoid cysts are presumably due to faulty inclusion of ectoderm when the embryo coalesces. Usually they do not appear till adult life and are much more common in women than men. They may be unilocular or multilocular and vary in size from an average diameter of 2–5 cm up to 10 cm. They are very prone to be complicated by infection and may thus be confused with ordinary anorectal abscesses and fistulas. The prognosis as to life is excellent, but recurrence after operation is not infrequent, because of incomplete removal due to the size of the lesion or its adherence to surrounding parts. Excision can often be effected from below after disarticulating the coccyx, but, with bigger cysts situated higher up, an abdominal or abdominoperineal approach is necessary (Swinton and Lehman 1958; Jackman et al. 1951).

CHORDOMA

Sacral chordomas arise from remnants of the fetal notochord in the sacral region. They may occur in either sex at any age, but are most often seen in men past middle life. They slowly enlarge over the years causing sacral or sciatic pain and later interfering with the sphincters or sexual function. In 10% of cases distant metastases are found. On rectal palpation the tumour is felt as an elastic, sometimes lobulated, swelling. X-ray examination reveals circular or oval areas of translucency in the sacrum corresponding to the lesion; there may also be trabeculation or calcification. Biopsy shows characteristic vacuolated mucus-containing cells. Chordomas have usually been treated by excision through a sacral approach, but the operation required is often very extensive and difficult and a combined abdominal and sacral approach is often best. According to McCarty et al. (1952) the distal two or even three pieces of sacrum can be removed without impairment of bladder function provided that the third sacral nerve on at least one side is preserved, and Localio et al. (1967) claim to have removed all but the first sacral segment—and including S2 bilaterally—without detriment. Both these groups of authors given an encouraging account of what can be accomplished by bold surgery in these cases. Excellent palliation is often achieved for a time, but it is only rarely that a lasting cure is achieved, and in addition many tumours are found to be beyond the scope of even this very radical type of surgery. As a consequence most patients eventually die of the condition (McCarty et al. 1952; Freier et al. 1971). Chordomas are generally considered to be radio-insensitive but Windeyer (1959) has reported excellent results with supervoltage therapy for this condition—of eight patients treated six were without symptoms or signs of the disease five years later. Rosenqvist and Saltzman (1959) also urge the advantages of megavoltage radiotherapy; apart from cure, it may afford considerable relief of pain. My own experience of four patients submitted to this treatment has been disappointing, and their severe discomfort persisted till they had intrathecal injections of phenol (see p. 655).

REFERENCES

ALLRED, H. W., Jr. and SPENCER, R. J. (1974) Hemangiomas of the colon, rectum and anus. *Mayo Clin. Proc.*, *49*, 739.

ANDERSON, P. A., DOCKERTY, M. B. and BUIE, L. A. (1950) Myomatous tumours of the rectum (leiomyomas and myosarcomas). *Surgery, St Louis, 28*, 642.

AYLETT, S. O. (1954) *Surgery of the Caecum and Colon.* Edinburgh: Livingstone.

BANCROFT, F. W. (1930) Haemangioma of the sigmoid and colon. *Ann. Surg., 94*, 828.

BAUM, S., STEIN, G. N., NUSBAUM, M. and CHAIT, A. (1969) Selective arteriography in the diagnosis of hemorrhage in the gastrointestinal tract. *Radiol. Clins N. Am., 7*, 131.

BENSAUDE, R. and BENSAUDE, A. (1932) Sur une forme particulière d'angiome caverneux du rectum, l'angiome cutanéo-muquex ou génito-périnéo-rectal. *Presse méd., 40*, 1739.

BIÖRCK, G., AXEN, O. and THORSON, A. (1952) Unusual cyanosis in a boy with congenital pulmonary stenosis and tricuspid insufficiency. Fatal outcome after angiocardiography. *Am. Heart J., 44*, 143.

BROWN, A. J. (1924) Vascular tumours of the intestine. *Surgery Gynec. Obstet., 39*, 191.

CATTELL, R. B. (1937) Endometriosis of the colon and rectum with intestinal obstruction. *New Engl. J. Med., 217*, 715.

CORNES, J. S. (1961) Multiple lymphomatous polyposis of the gastrointestinal tract. *Cancer, 14*, 249.

—— WALLACE, M. H. and MORSON, B. C. (1961) A summary of the clinical features of 100 cases of benign lymphoma of the rectum and anal canal. *Proc. R. Soc. Med., 54*, 729.

DAWSON, I. M. P., CORNES, J. S. and MORSON, B. C. (1961) Primary malignant lymphoid tumours of the intestinal tract. Report of 37 cases with study of factors influencing prognosis. *Br. J. Surg., 49*, 80.

DUKES, C. E. (1929) Submucous implantation cysts of the rectum. *Proc. R. Soc. Med., 22*, 715.

—— and BUSSEY, H. J. R. (1947) Sarcoma and melanoma of the rectum. *Br. J. Cancer, 1*, 30.

FLASCHKA, A. (1924) Über einen Fall von diffusem kavernösem Haemangiom des Rektum und Sigma. *Wien. klin. Wschr., 64,*, 993.

FREIER, D. T., STANLEY, J. C. and THOMPSON, N. W. (1971) Retrorectal tumours in adults. *Surgery Gynec. Obstet., 132*, 681.

GABRIEL, W. B. (1948) *Principles and Practice of Rectal Surgery*, 4th ed. London: H. K. Lewis.

—— and MORSON, B. C. (1956) Carcinoid of rectum with lymphatic and liver metastases. *Proc. R. Soc. Med., 49*, 472.

GHABRIAL, F. (1955) Leiomyoma of the rectum. *Lancet, 2*, 325.

GOLDEN, T. and STOUT, A. P. (1941) Smooth muscle tumours of the gastrointestinal tract and retroperitoneal tissues. *Surgery Gynec. Obstet., 73*, 784.

GOODALL, J. R. (1943) *A Study of Endosalpingiosis, Endocervicosis and Peritoneo-ovarian Sclerosis.* Philadelphia: Lippincott.

GRANET, E., KAGAN, M. B. and SOLOMON, C. (1950) Lymphomas of the anorectum. *Am. J. Surg., 80*, 311.

GROSS, R. E. CLATWORTHY, H. W., Jr and MELKER, I. A., Jr. (1951) Sacrococcygeal teratomas in infants and children. *Surgery Gynec. Obstet., 92*, 341.

HAYES, W. T. and BURR, H. B. (1952) Benign lymphomas of the rectum. *Am. J. Surg., 84*, 545.

HELLSTRÖM, J., HULTBORN, K. A. and ENGSTEDT, L. (1955) Diffuse cavernous haemangioma of the rectum. *Acta chir. scand., 109*, 277.

HELWIG, E. B. and HANSEN, M. C. (1951) Lymphoid polyps (benign lymphoma) and malignant lymphoma of the rectum and anus. *Surgery Gynec. Obstet., 92*, 233.

HUNT, V. C. (1921) Myoma of the rectum: report of four cases. *Ann. Surg., 74*, 236.

—— (1941) Haemangioma of the large bowel. *Surgery, St Louis, 10*, 651.

IZANT, R. T., Jr. and FILSTON, H. C. (1975) Sacro-coccygeal teratomas: analysis of forty-three cases. *Am. J. Surg., 130*, 617.

JACKMAN, R. J., CLARK, P. L. and SMITH, N. D. (1951) Retrorectal tumours. *J. Am. med. Ass., 145*, 956.

JACQUES, A. A. (1952) Cavernous haemangioma of the rectum and rectosigmoid colon. *Am. J. Surg., 84*, 507.

JEFFERY, P. J., HAWLEY, P. R. and PARKS, A. G. (1976) Colo-anal sleeve anastomosis in the treatment of diffuse cavernous haemangioma involving the rectum. *Br. J. Surg., 63*, 678.

JENKINSON, E. L. and BROWN, W. H. (1943) Endometriosis. *J. Am. med. Ass., 122*, 349.

KELLY, F. J. and SCHLADEMAN, K. R. (1949) Endometriosis—its surgical significance. *Surgery Gynec. Obstet., 88*, 231.

KILLEN, D. A. and JACKSON, L. M. (1963) Sacrococcygeal teratoma in adult. *Archs Surg., Chicago, 88*, 425.

LOCALIO, S. A., FRANCES, K. C. and ROSSANO, P. G. (1967) Abdomino-sacral resection of sacrococcygeal chordoma. *Ann. Surg., 166*, 394.

MCCARTY, C. S., WAUGH, J. M., MAYO, C. W. and COVENTRY, M. B. (1952) Surgical treatment of presacral tumours: a combined problem. *Proc. Staff Meet. Mayo Clin., 27*, 73.

MACKENZIE, D. A., MCDONALD, J. R. and WAUGH, J. M. (1954) Leiomyoma and leiomyosarcoma of the colon. *Ann. Surg., 139*, 67.

MACLEOD, D. H. (1946) Endometriosis: a surgical problem. *Br. J. Surg., 34*, 109.

MAHOUR, G. H., WOOLLEY, M. M., TRIVEDI, S. N. and LANDING, B. H. (1974) Teratomas in infancy and childhood: experience with 81 cases. *Surgery, St Louis, 76*, 309.

MARSHALL, S. F. and MEISSNER, W. A. (1950) Sarcoma of stomach. *Ann. Surg., 131*, 824.

MASSON, J. C. (1935) Surgical significance of endometriosis. *Ann. Surg., 102*, 821.

MASSON, P. (1928) Carcinoids and nerve hyperplasia of appendicular mucosa. *Am. J. Path., 4*, 131.

MAYO, C. W., BAKER, G. S. and SMITH, L. R. (1958) Presacral tumours: differential diagnosis and report of a case. *Proc. Staff. Meet. Mayo Clin. 28*, 616.

—— and MILLER, J. M. (1940) Endometriosis of the sigmoid, rectosigmoid and rectum. *Surgery Gynec. Obstet., 70*, 136.

—— PAGTALUNAN, R. J. G. and BROWN, D. J. (1963) Lipoma of the alimentary tract. *Surgery, St Louis, 53*, 598.

MILES, R. M. and STEWART, G. S. (1973) Sacro-coccygeal teratomas in adults. *Am. Surg., 179*, 676.

MORGAN, J. G., MARKS, C. and HEARN, D. (1973) Carcinoid tumours of the gastrointestinal tract. *Ann. Surg., 180*, 720.

MORGAN, C. N. (1932) Endothelioma of the rectum. *Proc. R. Soc. Med., 25*, 1020.

MORSON, B. C. (1960) In *Cancer of the Rectum*, ed. C. E. Dukes, p. 92. Edinburgh and London: Livingstone.

MORTON, J. H., STABINS, S. J. and MORTON, J. J., Jr. (1956) Smooth muscle tumours of the alimentary tract. *Ann. Surg., 144*, 487.

MORTON, W. A. and JOHNSTONE, F. R. C. (1965) Rectal carcinoids. *Br. J. Surg., 52*, 391.

NIGAM, R. (1947) A case of dermoid arising from the rectal wall. *Br. J. Surg., 35*, 218.

NORBURY, L. E. C. (1932) Specimen of endothelioma of rectum. *Proc. R. Soc. Med., 25*, 1021.

OPPENHEIM, A. and O'BRIEN, J. P. (1950) Unusual anal, rectal, and perirectal tumours palpable by rectal examination. *Am. J. Surg., 79*, 302.

ORLOFF, M. J. (1971) Carcinoid tumours of the rectum. *Cancer, 28*, 175.

PACK, G. T., MILLER, T. R. and TRINIDAD, S. S. (1963) Pararectal rhabdomyosarcoma: report of two cases. *Dis. Colon Rect., 6*, 1.

PESKIN, G. W. and ORLOFF, M. J. (1959) A clinical study of 25 patients with carcinoid tumours of the rectum. *Surgery Gynec. Obstet., 109*, 673.

ROSENQVIST, H. and SALTZMAN, G.-F. (1959) Sacrococcygeal and vertebral chordomas and their treatment. *Acta radiol., 52*, 177.

RUTTER, A. G. (1956) Submucous telangiectasis of the colon. *Lancet, 2*, 1077.

SANGER, B. J. and LECKIE, B. D. (1959) Plain muscle tumours of the rectum. *Br. J. Surg., 47*, 196.

SCOTT, W. McC and BRAND, N. E. (1957) Giant haemangioma of the rectum. *Br. J. Surg., 45*, 294.

SOAVE, F. (1964) Hirschprung's disease: a new surgical technique. *Archs Dis. Childh., 39*, 116.

STOUT, A. P. (1942) Carcinoid tumours of the rectum derived from Erspamer's pre-enterochrome. *Am. J. Path., 18*, 993.

—— (1955) Tumours of the colon and rectum (excluding carcinoma and adenoma). *Surg. Clins N. Am.*, 1283.

—— (1959) Tumours of the colon and rectum (excluding carcinoma and adenoma). In *Diseases of the Colon and Anorectum*, ed. R. Turell, vol. 1, p. 295. Philadelphia and London: W. B. Saunders.

SWINTON, N. W. and LEHMAN, G. (1958) Presacral tumours. *Surg. Clins N. Am., 38*, 849.

THORLAKSON, R. T. and ROSS, H. M. (1961) Leiomyosarcoma of the rectum. *Ann. Surg., 154*, 979.

WHITEHOUSE, G. H. (1973) Solitary angiodysplastic lesions in the ileocaecal region diagnosed by angiography. *Gut, 14*, 977.

WILSON, E. (1964) Rectal cyst. *Aust. N. Z. J. Surg., 34*, 32.

WINDEYER, B. W. (1959) Chordoma. *Proc. R. Soc. Med., 52*, 1088.

21

Ulcerative Colitis

As generally understood the term ulcerative colitis denotes a form of colitis of unknown aetiology, characterized by ulceration of the mucosa, and originally described by Wilks and Moxon (1875). Actually the emphasis on macroscopic ulceration is a little misleading for it has generally been taken to imply the existence of discrete ulcers, but in some of the patients ordinarily classed as suffering from the disease no such gross ulceration is present, the mucosa instead showing to the naked eye just a diffuse thickening and granularity—though it is microscopically ulcerated. Also the failure to designate the rectum in the title is unfortunate in view of the fact that it is involved in the great majority of cases, sometimes being the part of the large bowel mainly or solely affected. Undoubtedly the expression 'non-specific or idiopathic proctocolitis' would be more accurate, but the name 'ulcerative colitis' is so firmly entrenched in medical parlance and literature that it is hard to believe it will ever be displaced in the interests of more precise terminology.

EPIDEMIOLOGY

AGE AND SEX INCIDENCE

It is a matter of common clinical experience that ulcerative colitis is a disease predominantly of young adults, particularly women. This impression has been confirmed by the epidemiological studies of Cullinan and MacDougall (1957), Edwards and Truelove (1963) and Watts et al. (1966c, d). The data provided by the last group were derived from an analysis of my own cases (Table 52); they show that roughly half the patients were between 20 and 39 years of age at the commencement of their colitis, and that at all ages females preponderated over males in the ratio of about 4 : 3. It is interesting to note, however, that in the series of

TABLE 52. *Age and Sex Incidence of Patients under Care of Author at the General Infirmary, Leeds, 1955–63*

Age at onset (years)	Male	Female	Total
0–19	30	40	70
20–39	93	138	231
40–59	50	72	122
60–79	17	24	41
All ages	190	274	464

After Watts et al. (1966*d*).

cases of colitis commencing in childhood reported by Canby and Mehlhop (1964), Michener et al. (1964) and Ross (1964) there was a reversal of the sex ratio.

GEOGRAPHICAL INCIDENCE

Because ulcerative colitis remains generally an unreportable disease it is usually impossible to obtain statistics as to its prevalence in entire populations. But Melrose (1955, 1956) has

TABLE 53. *Incidence of Ulcerative Colitis in Different European Countries*

Country	Incidence (per 10 000 hospital admissions)
Switzerland	5·8
Scotland	6·9
Finland	7·0
Denmark	7·8
Belgium	10·8
England	14·8

After Melrose (1956).

studied the incidence of colitis in different parts of Britain and the continent of Europe, deriving his information from grouped hospital statistics supplied by collaborators in each of the centres included in his survey. Some of his findings are recorded in Table 53, from which it will be noted that colitis appeared to be twice as common in England as in Scotland or certain other European countries. Similar studies by Carleson et al. (1962) and Chojecki (1963) estimate the frequency of colitis in Sweden and Poland as 3·5 and 6·6 respectively per 10 000 hospital admissions.

National figures of prevalence are, however, available for two countries with excellent vital statistics—Norway and New Zealand. The incidence or rate of recognition of ulcerative colitis in Norway rose from 8·6 per million during 1951–6 to 20·6 per million between 1956 and 1960 (Gjone and Myren 1964). The corresponding annual rate of incidence of the disease in New Zealand during 1954–8 is given as 50 to 60 per million of population as deduced from study of state medical service hospital records by Wigley and Maclaurin (1962).

CONSTITUTIONAL AND OTHER FACTORS

Race. In New Zealand Wigley and Maclaurin (1962) found that colitis was much more prevalent among the population of European stock than among the Maoris. The disease also appears to be rarer among Negroes than white people in America (Monk et al. 1967), and may also be rarer in American Indians (Bebchuk et al. 1961). There is now strong statistical evidence that colitis is two or three times as frequent amongst Jews as among non-Jews (Weiner and Lewis 1960; Acheson and Nefzger 1963). It is interesting to note, however, that amongst Jews in Israel considerable differences in the prevalence of colitis occur according to their ethnic origin (Birnbaum et al. 1960).

Social Status and Intellect. In Acheson and Nefzger's (1963) study of United States Army personnel it was found that colitis was commoner among officers than among enlisted men, and among former salesmen than among former agricultural workers. The greater frequency of colitis in urban than country dwellers is also pointed out by Wigley and Maclaurin (1962) in New Zealand. One factor contributing to this difference is the much higher proportion of Jews in city populations than in rural areas. The influence of superior intellect in predisposing to the occurrence of the disease is debatable, as contradictory findings were obtained in two controlled studies (Acheson and Nefzger 1963; Fullerton et al. 1962).

Blood Groups. In two recent studies by Boyd et al. (1961) and Maur et al. (1964) it has been confirmed that there is no correlation between the incidence of colitis and the ABO and MN blood groups or secretor status, but a positive correlation was found with Rhesus type CC (Boyd et al. 1961; Thayer and Bove 1965).

Familial Occurrence. The familial incidence of ulcerative colitis has been stressed by Sloan et al. (1950b), Barker (1962) and Kirsner and Spencer (1963) among others, and our observations in Leeds (Goligher et al. 1968) provide support for this concept. We have reckoned that the series of 465 patients with ulcerative colitis analysed by us had around 5500 first- and second-degree relatives at risk. According to the natural regional incidence of the disease it would be reasonable to expect four or five of these relatives to develop colitis. But no less than 40 did, and in eight instances there were two relatives affected (in addition to our

patient). No less than 23 of the 40 relatives were first-degree relatives. On the basis of these findings, therefore, it seems justifiable to assert that there is a genuine familial predisposition to colitis. It is important to remember, however, that at least 90% of the patients have no familial history of the disease.

AETIOLOGY

Though a number of theories as to the aetiology of ulcerative colitis have been advanced from time to time, none of them has proved generally applicable and, if the truth be told, we are still almost totally ignorant of the cause of this disease. In this section only a bare outline of the subject will be attempted, and for fuller information reference should be made to the surveys of Warren and Berk (1957), Taylor and Truelove (1962), Almy and Lewis (1963), Mackay and Wood (1964), Almy and Plaut (1965), Goligher et al. (1968), de Dombal et al. (1969) and Burch et al. (1969). Aetiological factors that have been considered, and to a greater or lesser extent discarded, are the following:

Infection

Bargen's (1924) claim that ulcerative colitis was due to a specific diplococcus has never been substantiated and no other specific organism has ever been isolated. Of course, infection with suppuration and destruction of tissue probably plays a part in producing some of the pathological changes found in ulcerative colitis, but so far as we know this is due entirely to organisms ordinarily resident in the colon and filling the role of secondary invaders. Several workers, notably Hurst and Knott (1936), Felsen (1945), Stewart (1950) and Brooke (1954), have suggested that damage to the colon by a preceding attack of dysentery, bacillary or amoebic, may often be the factor that initiates ulcerative colitis. But, even if it is allowed that there is such a thing as a post-dysenteric form of non-specific ulcerative colitis, the vast majority of cases of colitis met in practice have clearly had no antecedent attack of dysentery.

Lysozyme and Mucinases

Lysozyme occurs in high concentration in the stools of patients suffering from ulcerative colitis, and Meyer et al. (1948) postulated that it might be the primary aetiological factor by dissolving the layer of mucus protecting the colonic mucosa and exposing it to digestion and secondary infection. Sammons (1951), however, has disposed of this theory by showing that the occurrence of lysozyme in the faeces of colitis is due simply to its presence in pus cells and that it is thus dependent on secondary infection and not an initiating agent. Other mucinases, which occur independently of the amount of pus in the faeces, have been isolated by Sammons (1951) in cases of colitis, but their role in the aetiology has not been clearly elucidated.

Psychological Influences

It is generally stated that patients with ulcerative colitis are often highly strung and introspective and their attacks frequently coincide with periods of increased stress (Murray 1930; Wittkower 1938; Paulley 1956; Groen and van der Valk 1956). The interesting studies by Grace et al. (1951) show, moreover, that emotional influences can produce changes in the colon mucosa up to frank ulceration. Though Paulley (1956, 1971) has claimed dramatic, almost invariable, clinical improvement in patients with ulcerative colitis by means of psychotherapy, most clinicians find the results of psychological treatment less consistent, and usually only a partial success.

Our experience in Leeds (Goligher et al. 1968) is that less than 5% of our colitis patients had ever attended a psychiatrist. Another 9% admitted on questioning that they considered their relapses of colitis to be related to emotional trauma (usually adding that they had frequently been told that their colitis was due to 'nerves'). The remaining 86% of our patients denied a relationship between the onset of their colitis and any emotional stress, and most of them seemed to be normal, well-adjusted individuals whose attitude to life and emotional make-up did not obviously differ from that of the population at large. Our rather crude assessment corresponds closely with a more sophisticated psychiatric evaluation of colitis patients by Feldman et al. (1967). It is also noteworthy that, after surgical treatment, even the colitis patients exhibiting some psychopathic stigmata preoperatively soon lose them, suggesting that they are probably an effect rather than a cause of the disease.

Immunological Factors

The most popular theory at the moment is that ulcerative colitis represents an immunological response to antigens, which may be *alimentary* (foods, chemicals or drugs), *bacterial* or *autogenous*.

ALIMENTARY ANTIGENS

The American physician Andresen first focused attention on this possibility in 1925 by describing a case of ulcerative colitis which he considered was due to food allergy. He continued his studies of colitis from this point of view and by 1942 was able to report that in 50 patients with this disease no less than 33 were instances of allergy to food, the responsible allergen in the majority being milk, but rarely other foods, such as wheat, tomatoes, oranges, potatoes and eggs, being incriminated. He recommended the use of elimination diets to identify the causal food and subsequently as a form of therapy.

On the experimental side Gray et al. (1940) showed in animals and man that the colon and small bowel could be sensitized to certain foods, and Kirsner and Elchlepp (1957) managed to produce a sort of colitis in rabbits by making them hypersensitive to egg albumin. Unfortunately the lesions created in the colon in these experiments have not been identical with those of ordinary ulcerative colitis. A useful survey of this work is provided by Kirsner and Goldgraber (1960).

In recent years there has been a considerable revival of clinical interest in the concept of colitis being caused by allergy to certain foods. Thus Rider et al. (1960) studied the reaction of the rectal mucosa to injections of extracts of various food substances in patients suffering from colitis and in normal individuals. They found that negative responses were usually elicited in the control subjects, but the colitic patient frequently gave a positive response to one or more of the test foods. Furthermore, withdrawal of the foods to which they reacted seemed to be followed by a clinical improvement in these patients' illness, though no properly controlled trial was organized to evaluate this impression. Truelove and his colleagues in Oxford have conducted a number of studies to examine the hypothesis of milk allergy. Truelove (1961) reported that in a small series of patients with ulcerative colitis removal of milk and milk-products from the diet was followed by a clinical remission, whilst their reintroduction into the diet seemed to lead to an aggravation of symptoms in the course of the next few days or weeks. Taylor and Truelove (1961) estimated the serological reaction to purified cow's milk protein in patients with colitis and in normal subjects and found that the colitics were more liable to have a high titre than were the normals. Acheson and Truelove (1961) also pointed out that patients suffering from colitis were twice as likely to have been weaned from the breast within one month of birth as were a control group of the same age and sex distribution.

Despite this suggestive evidence, the theory that ulcerative colitis represents an immunological reaction to certain foods has still to be proved, for it has yet to be shown that withholding of certain food substances can cure *all* patients of their disease.

AUTOGENOUS ANTIGENS

It is possible that ulcerative colitis may be an autoimmune disease (like Hashimoto's thyroiditis, certain forms of haemolytic anaemia and thrombocytopenic purpura, and systemic lupus erythematosus). Broberger and Perlmann (1959) were able to demonstrate circulating antibodies to human fetal colon (and liver and kidney) in the sera of children with ulcerative colitis; these antibodies were not present in the sera of normal healthy subjects. Similar observations have been reported by Polcak and Vokurka (1960) and Calabresi et al. (1961) using different techniques, but it is possible that these positive findings represent serological reactions to bacterial antigens. 'Colitis' has been produced experimentally in animals by immunological means (Callahan et al. 1963; Kraft et al. 1963; Ford and Kirsner 1964), but the resulting lesions do not closely resemble the disease as seen in the human subject, and in one study (Shean et al. 1964) the antigen used appears to have been grossly contaminated by bacterial products. Broberger (1964) himself subsequently sounded a note of caution in regard to the acceptance of an autoimmune process as the main aetiological factor in ulcerative colitis.

Indirect evidence in favour of autoimmunity as a basis for the development of ulcerative colitis has been provided by Burch et al. (1969). They point out that the age and sex distributions in several published series of cases of colitis in different parts of the world are remarkably similar, and argue that, where the age patterns of initiation of a disease are virtually independent of the geographical areas from which they are recorded, there must be a close correlation between this unvarying pattern and the underlying pathogenesis. If the surrounding environment does not significantly affect the kinetics of initiation of a disease, either the primary factor initiating it is constant throughout the world or the primary cause is largely independent of extrinsic factors.

Ulcerative Colitis as a Generalized Disease

Although colitis is by definition a disease of the large intestine, in a fair proportion of the cases other tissues remote from the colon are affected, with the production of arthritis, ankylosing spondylitis, erythema nodosum, pyoderma gangrenosum, iritis and episcleritis and hepatitis (see pp. 727–30). It is notable that often several of these associated lesions occur together and that sometimes they appear to precede the onset of the bowel condition itself. These considerations have raised the question as to whether these 'complications' are secondary to the diseased colon, or whether colitis is to be regarded as a generalized disease, the main target organ being the large intestine but other organs and tissues also being primarily susceptible. Edwards and Truelove (1964) discuss this suggestion critically. At first sight the fact that spondylitis or liver disease may sometimes antedate the occurrence of bowel symptoms may seem unassailable evidence in favour of the theory of a generalized disease, but it must be remembered that it may be extremely difficult to determine the exact starting point of a colitis. Known colitic patients who are in complete symptomatic remission are often found to show sigmoidoscopic evidence of the disease, such as contact bleeding and the discharge of mucopus. It could well be, therefore, that in patients whose spondylitis etc. has preceded the development of classical bowel symptoms mild inflammatory changes have been present in the colon all the time. Another point supporting the conception of colitis as a generalized disease is that, unlike the local complications, the severity of the so-called systemic complications often bears little relationship to the severity of the colitis itself, and patients with very severe pyoderma or joint disease may have negligible bowel symptoms.

The strongest argument against this theory and in favour of regarding the remote 'complications' of colitis as being secondary to the disease in the colon is the markedly beneficial effect on them usually observed after removal of the entire large intestine by ileostomy and protocolectomy. Though there have been exceptions to this finding, particularly in regard to spondylitis (Fernandez-Herlihy 1959) and to pyoderma gangrenosum (Margoles and Wenger 1961), my own experience is that proctocolectomy has practically always provided a complete cure for remote complications (see pp. 727–30).

Carrageenan Ingestion in Experimental Animals

Watt and Marcus (1971) have produced a state of ulceration in the large intestine of guinea-pigs, closely resembling ulcerative colitis in human subjects, by feeding them with a 5% aqueous solution of degraded carrageenan derived from the red seaweed *Eucheuma spinosum*. It is not suggested that this has any bearing on the causation of the human disease, but it provides an experimental model that might be useful for the study of various aspects of the pathology and therapy of ulcerative colitis.

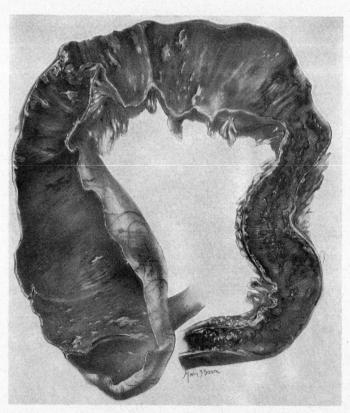

Fig. 512. Specimen of colon obtained by emergency colectomy from a case of chronic relapsing colitis during a severe exacerbation of the illness. The changes are most marked in the left colon where extensive ulceration is present and the circular muscular coat is bared in the floor of the ulcers. Discrete ulcers are evident also in the right colon.

SURGICAL PATHOLOGY

One of the consequences of the increased use of radical surgery in the treatment of patients with ulcerative colitis is that it has made available large numbers of operative specimens, study of which has greatly furthered our knowledge of the pathology of this disease. Good accounts of the morbid anatomical changes have been given by Warren and Sommers (1949, 1954), Brooke (1954), Dukes (1954), Counsell (1956), Lockhart-Mummery (1956) and Dukes and Lockhart-Mummery (1957). They may be considered as follows:

Mucosal Appearances

Most cases show ulceration of the mucosa in some part of the affected bowel. This may take the form of discrete ulcers, the mucosal lining being mainly intact though thickened; or the ulcers may have coalesced over a considerable area to produce a 'sea of ulceration', dotted with small islets of surviving mucosa (Figs 512 and 513). More extensive ulcers tend to be elongated in the long axis of the colon, and sometimes lie along the line of the taeniae. In the floor of the larger areas of ulceration the circular muscle coat is often laid quite bare so that the transversely running muscle bundles can be clearly perceived. The intervening mucosa is oedematous and swollen, and in cases with extensive ulceration, and usually a long history of recurrent and severe attacks of colitis, the mucosal remnants often become grossly protuberant, forming a series of polyps. These are not adenomatous in structure but are composed essentially of granulation or fibrous tissue with an epithelial covering, and to distinguish them from adenomas they are referred to as *pseudopolyps*, which is terminologically inaccurate (see p. 321) and is better replaced by the expression *inflammatory polyps*. In their gross appearance also they differ from ordinary adenomatous polyps in being less regularly formed. Sometimes, if the original destruction of mucosa was particularly widespread, the inflammatory polyps consist of widely scattered stunted stalks (Fig. 514A). In other cases the polyps are more closely packed and have an almost grape-like appearance (Fig. 514B). whilst in yet others they resemble stalactites or stalagmites and often have an attachment to the opposite colonic wall or to neighbouring polyps (Fig. 515). Sometimes this process of fusion produces an extensive branching network—the so-called 'sea wrack appearance'. The intervening areas of bowel in cases with inflammatory polyposis may show active ulceration, but more usually in

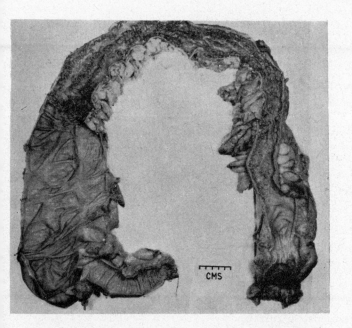

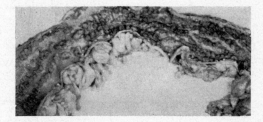

Fig. 513. Proctocolectomy specimen showing extensive ulceration in which small 'islands' of mucosa remain, mostly arranged in linear position in the long axis of the bowel. *Right*, Close-up of part of colon mainly affected.

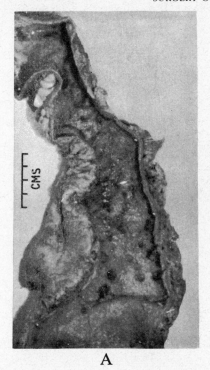

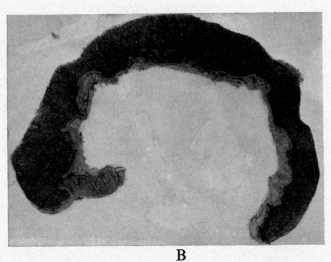

A   B

Fig. 514. Operative specimens showing different forms of inflammatory polyps encountered in ulcerative colitis. (A) Stunted polypoid tags in the sigmoid in a woman of 51 with colitis of many years' standing. (B) Abundant grape-like polyps, which were present throughout the greater part of the colon in a man of 24 with an 18 months' history of colitis.

operative specimens they have become partly healed and recovered by a mucosal lining of sorts. Though inflammatory polyps may occur throughout the entire colon, extending up to the ileocaecal valve and even into the terminal ileum in certain cases with ileal involvement, they very seldom occur in the rectum, even though it is nearly always implicated by the disease. This is a distinction, of considerable practical importance, from the true adenomatous polyps of familial polyposis, which are found in abundance in the rectal ampulla.

In some cases of colitis, however, macroscopic ulceration is completely absent; instead the mucosa merely shows a diffuse thickening and granularity and is immobile on the underlying muscle coat (Fig. 516). Indeed in perhaps the majority of cases with frank ulceration, there are considerable areas of bowel mucosa—usually in the proximal part of the affected segment and in the rectum—that reveal only such granularity and immobility. Examination of this granular mucosa with a powerful hand lens often reveals the presence of minute ulcers imperceptible to the unaided eye and, as will be mentioned later, microscopical examination shows that there is a considerable loss of surface epithelium throughout the granular areas (p. 695).

CHANGES IN THE COLON WALL

The characteristic changes in the colon wall are that it loses its haustration and becomes thickened and rigid (Figs 516 and 517). However, the extent to which these alterations occur varies greatly, usually in conformity with the severity of the mucosal changes, and in areas where the mucosa shows only slight granularity the colon wall may be of normal thickness and haustration may be well preserved—an important consideration in the interpretation of radiological findings. In some cases indeed of a more acute nature the wall of the colon is thinned out by massive gaseous distension (Fig. 518)—the *toxic megacolon* of Lumb et al. (1955). Even when the bowel wall is typically thickened and indurated and the lumen is somewhat reduced, neither the thickening nor the narrowing as a rule

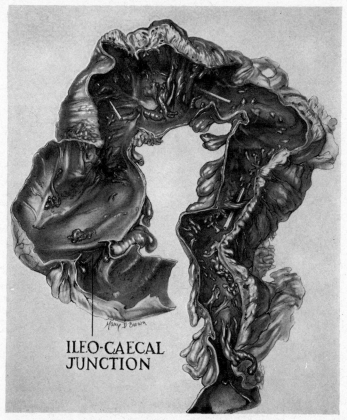

ILEO-CAECAL
JUNCTION

Fig. 515. Drawing of the colon showing ulcerative colitis with gross inflammatory polyposis, many of the polyps forming bridges across the lumen of the bowel, especially in the transverse colon. In this patient the rectum was uninvolved, so that the condition was one of so-called segmental ulcerative colitis and may thus have been really a case of Crohn's disease. He remains in excellent health with a normal rectum 15 years after colectomy and ileorectal anastomosis.

reach anything like that in Crohn's disease of the small intestine. Localized narrowings—the so-called 'fibrous strictures'—may also occur, but as Counsell and Dukes (1952) have clearly shown, such strictures should be regarded with considerable suspicion for histological examination sometimes reveals the presence of an atypical form of carcinoma in the thickened area of bowel wall (see Fig. 537).

The appearances of the colon from the serosal aspect in this disease are seen to best advantage when the intact bowel is viewed at laparotomy before there has been any interference with its blood supply and normal coloration. In the affected segments the peritoneal coat shows a characteristic pallor with numerous fine tortuous vessels ramifying in or underneath it (Plate IV). In some of the more acute cases there may actually be a thin fibrinous covering on certain parts of the colon. Normal haustration is diminished or completely abolished. The bowel wall feels oedematous on palpation and is *extremely friable*.

HISTOLOGICAL FINDINGS

Microscopically the changes are confined chiefly to the mucosa and submucosa. *At the site of frank ulceration* the mucosa may have disappeared completely, but in what remains of it, and more particularly in the submucosa, there is a heavy infiltration with round cells, plasma cells, eosinophils and macrophages. Occasionally the infiltration extends into the muscle coat as well and there may even be small interstitial abscesses in this part of the bowel wall.

In areas showing only granularity of the mucosal lining there is the same infiltration of the mucosa and submucosa with mononuclear cells, and with it usually some loss of the surface epithelium and of

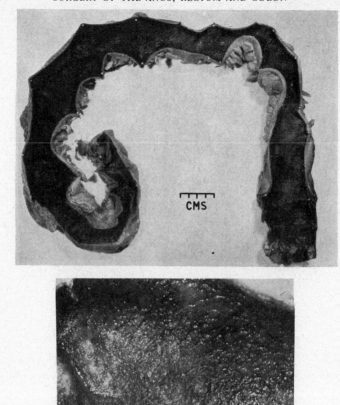

Fig. 516. (A) Proctocolectomy specimen from a girl of 12 years with colitis of three years' duration. Macroscopically the mucosa of the large intestine shows a diffuse fine granularity and immobility, but histological section reveals widespread superficial ulceration. (B) Close-up view of the granular mucosa.

the superficial parts of the mucosal glands. A feature that has been particularly commented on by Warren and Sommers (1949) is the occurrence of crypt abscesses in the deeper extremities of the gland tubules. Eventually several of these abscesses may coalesce to form a larger lacunar abscess, which undermines the mucosa and ultimately causes it to separate, producing a macroscopic ulcer. This is probably the way in which gross ulceration often commences in colitis.

THE PROCESS OF REPAIR

The colonic mucosa has a remarkable capacity for repair and such reparative processes probably begin as soon as there is any remission of the disease. When the mucosal loss has been superficial, rapid epithelial repair is achieved by cells growing from the depths of the surviving glands. When there has been complete destruction of the mucosa to its full depth, epithelial repair takes place from the periphery, from the epithelial cells in the islands of surviving mucosa. The epithelium is at first very thin and elongated, but individual cells later become cubical and columnar and even mucus-secreting. A condensation of tissue forms a new subepithelial layer, but there are no new mucous glands, and the normal depth of submucosa and mucosa is never regained.

DISPLACEMENT OF EPITHELIAL CELLS IN THE COLON WALL

Occasionally groups of epithelial cells are found in the submucosa of the colon in cases of ulcerative colitis, as pointed out by Dukes (1954). These are

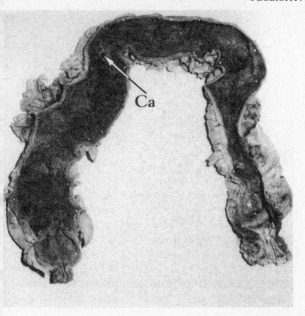

Ca

Fig. 517. Proctocolectomy specimen removed from a patient who had had colitis for nine years. Note the gross thickening of the colon wall and the coarse granularity of the muscosal surface. An early carcinoma was present close to the hepatic flexure. The patient was alive and well eight years after operation.

not malignant cells but have the appearance of normal glandular epithelium which has become displaced. They are only seen in cases in which there has at some time been deep ulceration and subsequent repair.

CHANGES IN THE MUSCLE COATS

As Lockhart-Mummery (1956) has emphasized, microscopical examination shows that the thickening of the bowel wall in chronic cases, which has in the past usually been attributed to fibrosis, is in fact due to thickening of the muscle coat. Moreover the areas of narrowing, often referred to as 'fibrous strictures', are often due to localized muscular thickening and not fibrosis. This is a most significant observation because it means that some of the changes, formerly regarded as indicative of fibrosis and therefore irreversible, are caused by muscle hypertrophy, which in most instances is probably reversible.

APPEARANCES ON ELECTRON MICROSCOPY

Studies of the histological changes in ulcerative colitis have been conducted by Donnellan (1966), Gonzalez-Licea (1966), Gonzalez-Licea and Yardley (1966) and Jenkinson and Dawson

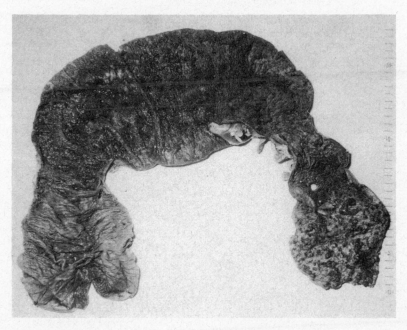

Fig. 518. Colectomy specimen from a patient who was operated on during a severe acute phase of colitis in which she developed 'acute toxic megacolon'. Note that the dilatation is maximal in the transverse colon.

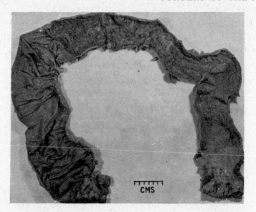

Fig. 519. Proctocolectomy specimen from a case of ulcerative colitis, in which the pathological changes extended only as far proximally as the hepatic flexure.

(1971), whose papers should be consulted by readers interested in the subject.

ANATOMICAL DISTRIBUTION OF THE LESION IN THE LARGE BOWEL

The classical conception of ulcerative colitis is of a disease extending from the anal canal to the caecum, stopping sharply at the ileocaecal junction (Figs 512 and 514B). A study of operative specimens, however, shows that the distribution of the lesion in the bowel does not always conform to this pattern.

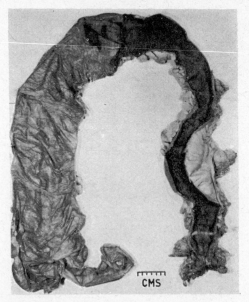

Fig. 520. Proctocolectomy specimen showing ulcerative colitis confined to the bowel distal to the middle of the transverse colon.

Whilst the distal limit is situated with remarkable constancy at the mucocutaneous junction in the anal canal, its proximal limit is very variable. In a small proportion of cases it extends beyond the ileocaecal valve into the terminal ileum for a few centimetres as a retrograde or 'backwash' ileitis. More frequently it falls short of the caecum, in some cases only reaching as far as the hepatic flexure or midtransverse colon, in others stopping at the splenic flexure or in the descending or sigmoid colon (Figs 519–21). Even in the cases where the whole large bowel is affected, the pathological changes are generally noted to be most marked in the distal part of the left colon. It is difficult to resist the conclusion that in most instances ulcerative colitis is primarily a left-sided condition, which shows a tendency to extend proximally. That this is the manner in which cases of universal colitis usually evolve is further substantiated by the clinical experiences of Sloan et al. (1950a), Bochus et al. (1956), Lennard-Jones et al. (1962) and ourselves (Watts et al. 1966a, b), that many mild, relatively symptomless lesions, originally localized by sigmoidoscopy and barium enema examination to the rectum or rectum and distal sigmoid, have in the course of months or years gradually spread proximally to involve the entire colon and produce severe symptoms requiring radical surgical treatment (see also p. 704).

The distribution of ulcerative colitis revealed in a survey of colectomy specimens obviously differs from that encountered in actual clinical practice, because extremely distal lesions only rarely come to operation, as when associated with very severe constitutional disturbance in elderly subjects or with a rectovaginal fistula or other troublesome local complications. It is of more value to study the frequency of involvement of the different segments of large bowel as determined clinically—that is by a combination of sigmoidoscopy, radiology, operative findings, and pathological examination of operative material—even though such localization is less precise than one based entirely on morbid anatomical studies. The distribution will clearly vary according to the type of practice from which the cases are derived. Our figures in Leeds (Table 54) may be taken as representative of the experience of a large general hospital with a well-known interest in ulcerative colitis. It will be seen that the rectum and sigmoid colon were the parts most constantly affected, but that in a very small proportion of cases (3·4%) the rectum was known to be spared by the disease; these were examples of so-called 'right-sided' or segmental colitis.

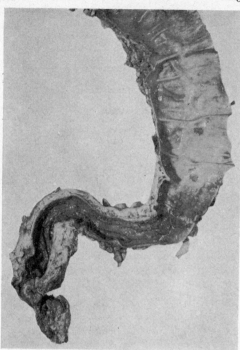

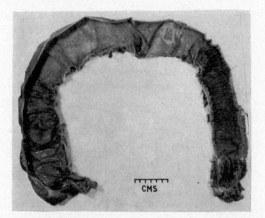

Fig. 521. More distal forms of ulcerative proctocolitis which were nonetheless severe enough to demand radical surgical treatment.

RIGHT-SIDED OR SEGMENTAL COLITIS

The term 'right-sided colitis' was apparently introduced by Crohn and his colleagues at the Mount Sinai Hospital, New York (see particularly Crohn and Berg 1938; Crohn et al. 1947) to designate cases of colitis where the disease originated in the right colon. In many such cases, as Crohn and Berg (1938) were able to show by serial radiographic studies, the process gradually spread proximally into the caecum and, as a 'backwash' phenomenon, into the lower ileum, or distally into the transverse and left colon but not usually reaching as far as the rectum till a very late stage. Actually in the group of 77 cases with right-sided colitis reported by Crohn et al. (1947), which represented about 10% of all the cases of colitis seen by them, the disease was confined to the right

TABLE 54. *The Maximal Extent of Involvement of the Bowel in 465 Clinical Cases of Ulcerative Colitis seen at the General Infirmary, Leeds (1955–63 inclusive)*

Part of bowel affected	Percentage of cases
Rectum only	18·1
Rectum + sigmoid	13·8
Rectum + sigmoid + descending colon	15·0
Rectum + sigmoid + descending + transverse colon	15·0
Rectum + all colon	30·1
Segmental (i.e. sparing the rectum)	3·4
Ileal involvement	6·9
Maximal extent undetermined	4·6

colon in only 22; in 33 the lower ileum was also implicated and in 55 parts of the left colon were involved. In some of the latter the lesion had occurred as a localized segment of colitis in the left or transverse colon and had never at any stage been present in the right colon. Clearly the application of the term 'right-sided colitis' to a varied collection of cases of this kind is somewhat misleading.

The alternative expression, 'regional or segmental colitis' used by Bargen and Weber (1930), is likewise not entirely satisfactory, for it suggests a lesion restricted to a very short segment of the colon, and has apparently been used in this case by Wells (1952) and Kellock (1957). As employed by Barbosa et al. (1945), however, the term has been taken in effect to include all forms of colitis, involving long, short or multiple segments of the bowel, *but sparing the rectum*, at any rate in the first instance. In their survey of 201 cases of segmental colitis at the Mayo Clinic, Neuman et al. (1954) found that in two-thirds the lesions involved segments of both right and left halves of the colon in continuity. In the remaining third the disease was confined to one or other half of the colon or involved both halves discontinuously. The lower ileum was affected in about a quarter of the cases.

As regards the actual pathology of right-sided or segmental colitis, Crohn and Berg (1938) were at considerable pains to emphasize that the pathological features were essentially similar to those of the more common, primarily left-sided, forms of ulcerative colitis. Originally I was very sceptical of this claim and believed that most cases described in the literature as segmental colitis were really examples of Crohn's granulomatous enteritis occurring as an extension into the proximal colon from a lesion in the terminal ileum, as first described by Colp (1934), Mixter (1935), Crohn and Rosenak (1936) and Clark and Dixon (1939), or arising quite independently in the large bowel. Then we encountered several cases ourselves (Watkinson et al. 1960), which were suffering from a brand of ulcerative colitis macroscopically and microscopically indistinguishable from ordinary ulcerative colitis except that it did not implicate the rectum in the first instance and appeared particularly suitable for treatment by colectomy and ileorectal anastomosis (Fig. 522). We did, however, emphasize that the ultimate outcome after operation would be of particular interest in these patients, because of the uncertainty about the pathological nature of the lesion. If it were really a form of diffuse ulcerative colitis, it might be expected that it would carry the excellent prognosis of the latter condition after radical surgery in that it virtually never recurs in the small bowel (see pp. 779 and 794). If, on the other hand, it were more akin to Crohn's, fairly frequent reassertion of the condition in the ileum or jejunum might be anticipated from the analogy of the results of surgical treatment for Crohn's disease occurring primarily in the small bowel. In the event, as I have already reported (Goligher 1961a, 1965), two of nine cases of segmental ulcerative colitis previously published by us (Watkinson et al. 1960) subsequently developed typical Crohn's lesions in the terminal ileum proximal to the ileorectal anastomosis but the others have remained well, several of them for 12 and 15 years since colectomy. (It could be that these two patients who later produced Crohn's lesions in the ileum did originally have an ulcerative colitis type of lesion in the larger bowel, but, though a dual pathology of this kind has been postulated by Cave (1945) and Colcock et al. (1961), I should prefer to explain this occurrence on the basis of a single pathological process.) As a consequence I am now always dubious about the diagnosis of a rectum-sparing form of ulcerative colitis, however emphatic the pathologist may be in his report, and have difficulty in shaking off a suspicion that it will turn out to be a manifestation of Crohn's disease (see also p. 830). Moreover I strongly suspect that many of the cases of right-sided or segmental colitis reported by Crohn et al. (1947), Neuman et al. (1954) and Manning et al. (1955) were really suffering from granulomatous enteritis; the fact that some of Neuman et al.'s (1954) patients had 'skip' lesions is very suggestive of the latter condition.

Another recently recognized cause of a segmental form of colitis in older patients is acute or chronic insufficiency of the arterial supply to the colon (see Ischaemic colitis, p. 858).

ILEOCOLITIS

It may be convenient to summarize the forms of ileocolitis that may be found in patients presenting with apparent ulcerative colitis:

Ulcerative colitis with 'backwash ileitis'—the so-called coloileitis. This is by far the commonest variety. The incidence of retrograde ileitis in ulcerative colitis has been variously estimated, but Counsell (1956), in a careful pathological study of a large series of colectomy specimens from cases with ulcerative colitis,* found evidence of retrograde ileitis, involving the terminal 1–35 cm of ileum, in 17%. The incidence in my own patients coming to operation for ulcerative colitis is very similar, 18·3% (Watts et al 1966a). The changes in the affected part of the

* It is possible that a few of these specimens of ulcerative colitis might now be diagnosed pathologically as Crohn's disease of the colon.

ileum are essentially the same as those in the diseased colon with granularity and ulceration of the mucosa, even with polyposis.

Crohn's disease of the terminal ileum with a direct extension to the right colon or a 'skip' lesion elsewhere in the colon. See Chapter 22.

Crohn's disease of the terminal ileum in association with typical ulcerative colitis. In some of the recorded cases of ileocolitis the ileal lesion has been clearly a hyperplastic enteritis of Crohn's type, whilst the colonic lesion has equally definitely been described as an ordinary ulcerative colitis. Thus Crohn (1949) found that 22 of a series of 306 cases of regional ileitis had a concomitant ulcerative colitis, and Pemberton and Brown (1937) and Pugh (1945) found a similar incidence of associated colitis in their smaller series of cases of ileitis. Conversely Cave (1945) reported seven cases with inflammatory lesions of the small bowel resembling Crohn's regional enteritis in his series of 80 patients with ulcerative colitis. Colcock et al. (1961) have also described the association of regional enteritis and ulcerative colitis in the large series of patients suffering from these conditions at the Lahey Clinic. Lockhart-Mummery and Morson (1964), however, state that they have never seen this combination and, as already explained (p. 522), I would always suspect that such cases may have been entirely Crohn's disease involving both large and small gut.

A form of ileocolitis or enterocolitis described by Brooke and Cooke (1951). These authors reported a form of ileocolitis characterized by the occurrence of 'flea-bite' ulcers in the small bowel mucosa and typical changes of ulcerative colitis in the large bowel. Though they based their conception of the condition on 17 clinical cases, in only two of them did they have pathological material, but they stressed that the histological appearances were unlike those of Crohn's disease. Other workers such as Counsell (1956), Bochus et al. (1956), Dukes and Lockhart-Mummery (1957) and Watkinson et al. (1959, 1960) in clinical and pathological analyses of large series of cases of ulcerative colitis were unable to find any clear and unequivocal examples of this variety of enterocolitis. In 1965, Brooke admitted that further follow-up study of their cases has shown most of them in fact to be suffering from Crohn's disease.

Ileitis following ileostomy with or without colectomy for ulcerative colitis. This somewhat different but related topic is discussed on pp. 765–79.

Associated Mucosal Changes in the Stomach and Small Intestine

It has generally been considered that, apart from the changes sometimes observed in the terminal ileum due to 'reflux ileitis' in association with extensive ulcerative colitis, the rest of the gastro-intestinal tract in this disease shows no abnormality. However, observations by Salem et al. (1964) have cast some doubt on this popular belief. They studied the state of the mucosa of the stomach and small intestine in 25 patients with colitis, using peroral gastric and small intestinal biopsy, faecal fat estimations and a test of vitamin B12 absorption. During an actual attack of colitis they found varying degrees of histological abnormality in the mucosa of the small gut in roughly half the patients, but when the patients were symptom-free the small bowel mucosa was usually normal. Faecal fat excretion was likewise increased in about half the patients during an attack of colitis, usually in cases showing histological mucosal abnormalities. Vitamin B12 absorption was usually within normal limits, but a few patients showed some impairment of this function. Gastric biopsy revealed that superficial gastritis was common during an attack of colitis, but that the mucosa appeared normal when patients were symptom-free.

The cause and significance of these changes is a matter for speculation. Possibly they arise from reflux or mechanical disturbance of the upper gastrointestinal tract secondary to the disease of the large bowel. Another explanation invokes the hypothesis that ulcerative colitis may be a generalized disease, the brunt of which usually falls on the colon though other tissues, such as the liver, the eyes, joints and possibly the small intestine and stomach, may be affected. A third possibility is that the small intestinal mucosa may become abnormal whenever a patient is seriously ill, regardless of the nature of his disease, for the epithelium of the mucosa has a very rapid rate of turnover, which may make it specially susceptible to damage by the metabolic effects of any severe illness. Possibly the wasting associated with severe exacerbations of colitis may be partly attributable to the mucosal changes in the small bowel.

CLINICAL FEATURES

Symptoms

DIARRHOEA WITH PASSAGE OF BLOOD AND MUCUS

This is the main complaint in most cases of ulcerative colitis, and broadly speaking its severity varies with the extent and severity of the changes in the bowel wall. In cases with only a mild proctitis or distal proctocolitis, diarrhoea may be minimal and amount to nothing more than a slight looseness of the motions, which the patient may not think worthy of mention, or there may actually be constipation. But even in these latter cases there is usually a little bleeding and, on careful inter-rogation, a history of passing some slime. Indeed the patient may complain that, though he passes faeces infrequently and only with the aid of pur-gatives, he has to go to the lavatory several times a day to evacuate small quantities of blood and slime.

With extensive lesions the diarrhoea is much more troublesome and during a phase of exacer-bation the patient may have 10, 12 or 20 motions in the 24 hours and, due to exhaustion, weakness and indifference, may be virtually incontinent. The motions may consist of a mixture of liquid faeces, blood and mucopus, or may be composed almost entirely of blood-stained mucopurulent material. During a phase of remission of symptoms the diarrhoea may disappear completely, but more usually a slight frequency persists with three or four soft or liquid motions per day and some blood and slime continues to be passed. Mallet et al. (1978) have emphasized that in addition to the increased frequency of stools in colitis there is usually great urgency of defaecation with a tendency to precipit-ate incontinence, which may prove a very in-capacitating aspect of the illness.

ABDOMINAL PAIN

A fair amount of abdominal pain of colicky nature is usually experienced in the more extensive and severe cases. Severe pain of an intermittent or continuous kind may also occur in major acute exacerbations of the disease, due possibly to some degree of peritoneal irritation, and should always be regarded with considerable suspicion as possibly heralding the development of a perforation of the bowel.

LOSS OF ENERGY AND WEIGHT, ANAEMIA

Even with milder, distal forms of colitis there is often a definite, if slight, impairment of general health and of the capacity for sustained work during active phases of the disease. In severe cases the constitutional effects are profound and during exacerbations the patient rapidly becomes bed-ridden and grossly debilitated and emaciated. A loss of 20–30 kg in weight over a period of several weeks is not uncommon. During remission the general condition improves and weight is regained, but usually the improvement falls considerably short of the patient's normal health, so that he is usually left in a thin, semi-invalid state. With each phase of recurrence and remission the residual debility becomes more pronounced. Mallet et al. (1978) have stressed that lassitude is quite a disabling feature in many patients with colitis.

PYREXIA

Phases of exacerbation in all but the most distal forms of colitis and proctitis are associated with some elevation of the temperature, but a pyrexia of more than 38°C (101–102° F) is unusual except in the very rare fulminating type of colitis, or in cases with septic complications such as perianal abscesses or pyoderma gangrenosum.

Examination

GENERAL APPEARANCE

Patients with milder distal forms of the disease often look perfectly well, but more typical cases are emaciated, often profoundly so, anaemic and unmistakably ill.

ABDOMINAL EXAMINATION

Usually examination of the abdomen is unhelpful apart from confirming that the patient may have lost a good deal of weight, but in some cases there is tenderness over the iliac colon or other parts of the large intestine. This is particularly so in patients suffering from acute exacerbations, when a combination of extreme local tenderness and some degree of abdominal distension should alert the clinician to the possibility of acute dilatation or imminent perforation of the colon.

RECTAL EXAMINATION INCLUDING SIGMOIDOSCOPY AND FIBRE-OPTIC COLONOSCOPY

This is the most important item of examination in the majority of cases. Before passing a finger or any instrument it is essential to carry out a *careful inspection of the anal region* to exclude the presence of local anal complications such as a perianal abscess, a fistula or fissure or a marked degree of anal spasm and stenosis, all of which might render instrumentation painful and difficult and thus contraindicate further examination without a general anaesthetic.

On digital palpation it is often possible to feel the granularity and thickening of the rectal mucosa and sometimes appreciate the rigidity of the rectal wall, or the presence of an actual stricture. More usually, however, no abnormality can be detected, though blood or blood-stained mucopus may be observed on the fingertip after withdrawal.

Proctoscopy and sigmoidoscopy may reveal a variety of appearances. In severe cases the rectum contains abundant free blood and mucus or mucopus, making inspection of the mucosa at first difficult or impossible. However, after the fluid has been swabbed or sucked away, the mucosa is seen to be thickened and granular and to be bleeding freely (Plate IIID and E). In less severe cases there may be little or no free fluid in the rectal lumen, but the mucosa may have a partial covering of mucopurulent or fibrinous exudate, removal of which discloses a granular surface which usually bleeds vigorously, at first as numerous punctate haemorrhages, later as a diffuse ooze (Plate IIIc). In mild cases, and in patients who are in a phase of remission following a severe attack, the mucosa may at first appear normal. Careful scrutiny, however, will usually show that it lacks the moist glistening appearance of a normal mucosa, being matt and perhaps slightly granular (Plate IIIB). The vascular pattern is absent or patchy and interspersed with areas of pallor due to fibrosis, particularly in patients who have had previous attacks. The most important sign of active proctocolitis is the occurrence of '*contact bleeding*' on rubbing the mucosa gently. Absence of this sign indicates that whatever may have been the condition of the mucosa in the past, any inflammatory process is now completely quiescent.

Discrete ulceration is but rarely seen on sigmoidoscopy even in the severest examples of ulcerative colitis. Quite often what apears to be an ulcer is only a patch of mucopurulent or fibrinous exudate, and gentle swabbing of the mucosa removes the 'ulcer'. Genuine localized ulceration always suggests that the condition is really one of Crohn's colitis (see p. 834).

As mentioned previously, inflammatory polyps seldom occur in the rectal ampulla, and if in a case of colitis polyps are present, they are not usually encountered on sigmoidoscopy till the end of the instrument has entered the upper rectum. They then appear quite suddenly in a cluster which crowds into the lumen of the sigmoidoscope and which make further passage difficult, especially as there is often some narrowing of the bowel at the lower limit of the polypoid area (Plate IIIF). These polyps are usually quite easily distinguished from the more perfectly formed adenomatous polyps of familial polyposis, the inflamed state of the rectal mucosa also serving to dispel any doubt as to their true nature.

The Reliability of Various Sigmoidoscopic Signs in the Recognition of Colitis

The consistency with which the various sigmoidoscopic appearances of colitis are recorded by different observers examining the same areas of mucosa has been the subject of two carefully controlled studies (Baron et al. 1964; Watts et al. 1966e). They showed that there was a considerable variation in the frequency with which signs such as 'oedema', 'congestion', 'excess mucus', or even the time-honoured 'granularity' were recorded, but that there was pretty close agreement in the use of the terms 'absence of vessel pattern' or 'presence of contact bleeding' as well as in the over-all assessment of the normality or otherwise of the mucosa.

Sigmoidoscopic Biopsy

There has been some difference of opinion as to the value of biopsy of the rectal mucosa in the detection of colitis. Matts (1961) contended that examination of a biopsy specimen may sometimes reveal microscopical changes of colitis when the mucosa has been considered macroscopically to be normal, so that biopsy may be helpful occasionally in making the diagnosis of colitis in the face of a negative sigmoidoscopy, or in showing in a known case of colitis, thought to be completely quiescent, that the disease process is still present. Truelove and Richards (1956) share these views and have devised a special suction tube for taking the biopsies. Morson and Dawson (1972) also rate the value of rectal biopsy highly in colitis and Crohn's disease; they consider it specially useful in conducting serial studies of these conditions and in recognizing premalignant changes in colitis (see pp. 723 and 740). A controlled study by us (Watts et al. 1966e) showed biopsy to be less helpful because biopsy specimens from our normal control subjects often showed mild 'inflammatory changes'. I used to consider that rectal biopsy added little to the diagnostic accuracy of a careful sigmoidoscopic examination, but recognized that it was often very useful in distinguishing between ordinary ulcerative colitis and a granulomatous colitis, but I have to admit that sometimes biopsy can disclose a quiescent colitis when the sigmoidoscopic appearances are perfectly normal.

Cytological Study of the Mucosal Surface

Anthonisen and Riis (1961) have described a method of studying the cells present in the mucus lying on the rectal mucosa. A circular cover slip, 10 mm in diameter, covered with albumen and held firmly on a special carrier, is passed down the lumen of the sigmoidoscope and held lightly in contact with the mucosa for a few seconds. Subsequently it is dried, fixed and stained. Depending on whether inflammatory cells are demonstrated in the mucosal exudate or not, the cytological appearances are graded as 'active' or 'inactive'. Our experience of this cytological technique led us to conclude that it was probably at least as reliable as close macroscopic inspection at sigmoidoscopy or the detection of microscopical mucosal abnormalities, but much less convenient to carry out (Watts et al. 1966e).

Fibre-optic Colonoscopy

Recently the fibre-optic colonoscope has been increasingly used in cases of inflammatory disease of the colon to supplement radiological examination (Williams and Muto 1972). Apart from inspection, it permits multiple mucosal biopsies of doubtful areas. Unlike sigmoidoscopy, it should *follow, not precede*, barium enema study.

BARIUM ENEMA EXAMINATION

In cases with very localized, distal forms of proctocolitis and proctitis the lesion may be entirely within the reach of the sigmoidoscope. More commonly the upper limit of the disease lies farther proximally and a barium enema examination is necessary to give a complete picture of the con-

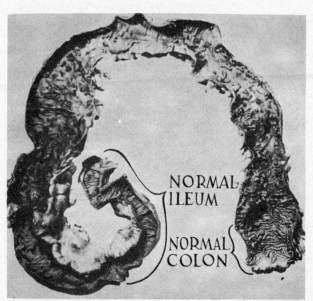

Fig. 522. Colectomy specimen showing right-sided colitis which extends from 17·5 cm proximal to the ileocaecal valve to the upper sigmoid colon. The histological section was typical of ulcerative colitis. Colectomy with ileorectal anastomosis was performed 19 years ago and the patient has continued in excellent health to the present.

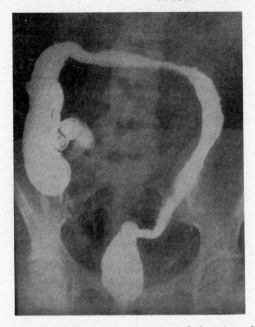

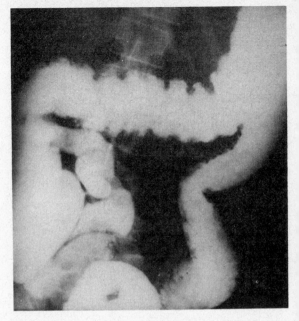

Fig. 523. Barium enema plate in a case of ulcerative colitis with marked contraction of the colon, loss of haustration and irregularity of outline.

Fig. 524. Barium enema plate of a case of severe ulcerative colitis, showing deep ulceration with undermining of the mucosa, especially in the sigmoid and descending colon.

dition. The radiological appearances of colitis are well known, and it is only necessary to emphasize and illustrate a few points (see Geffen et al. 1968).

Loss of haustration and considerable reduction in the calibre of the colon are the most constant findings (Fig. 523). Rarely a form of 'pseudohaustration' is present, which may mimic true haustration but lacks the smoothness and regularity of the latter. When gross ulceration and polyposis are present, the edge of the bowel, instead of being straight, is fluffy or shaggy and in cases with deep ulcers extensively undermining the mucosa, the bowel outline may be very irregular indeed with lacunae of barium seen lying actually outside the lumen (Figs 524, 525). Polyps are best demonstrated by means of a double contrast enema but often show well on ordinary barium enema films (Fig. 526). Single or multiple strictures of the colon may be revealed (Fig. 527); however smooth the edges of these may be it is always wise to assume that they may be due to the development of a colitis carcinoma. Occasionally a more typically carcinomatous filling defect may occur in cases with malignant change (Figs 528 and 536B).

The distribution of the changes revealed in the barium enema examination is very variable, as would be expected from what has previously been said about the pathology of the disease. Often the sigmoid or sigmoid and descending colon alone

show any abnormality (Fig. 529); in other cases the changes extend much farther proximally to involve the greater part or all of the colon. Reflux of barium through the ileocaecal valve into the small bowel is very common on barium enema examination and in cases with extensive colitis it may sometimes be possible to demonstrate changes in the lower ileum (Fig. 530). The reliability of the radiological assessment of the extent of the disease in the colon has often been questioned. Our experience, like that of others, shows that it is possible for the radiologist to miss mild changes in the mucosa unassociated with any loss of haustration or irregularity of the bowel outline on X-ray examination, and as these slighter changes are most liable to be found at the upper end of the lesion, the radiological error usually lies in a faulty judgement of the upper limit of the disease. But by and large there has been very close correlation between the radiological and pathological findings, except in the right colon, where the tendency has been towards underestimation of the extent of the disease by the radiologist.

Changes in the Radiological Extent of the Colitis during the Course of the Disease

The alterations in the extent of the disease revealed by repeat barium enema studies have been carefully investigated in 46 patients by Ricketts et al.

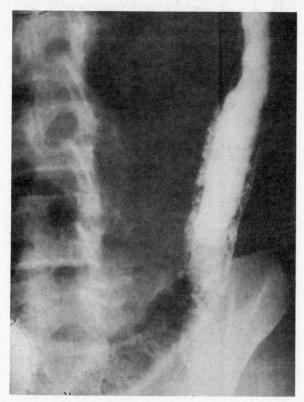

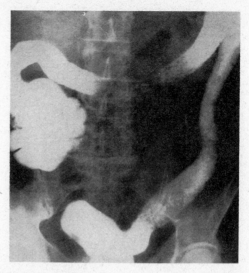

Fig. 526. Barium enema film from a case of ulcerative colitis showing numerous inflammatory polyps in the sigmoid and transverse colon.

Fig. 525. Radiograph of colon filled partly with barium and partly with air, depicting deep ulceration in colitis—the 'double contour' appearance.

(1948). They found that the disease remained static in 65%, was progressive in 24% and regressive in 11%, and thus concluded that the extent of the bowel involved usually remained relatively constant. Sloan et al. (1950a, b), reviewing 2000 cases of ulcerative colitis, drew similar conclusions. They noted progression of the disease in 184 (9·2%) and regression in 47 (2·3%), but it is not stated what proportion of their large series of patients were followed up by means of repeated barium studies. Edling and Eklöf (1960, 1961) analysed by repeat barium enema examinations 154 patients with ulcerative colitis and found that the extent of the disease increased in 18 and diminished in three. Our own studies (Watts et al. 1966a) with serial investigations comprised 128 patients with ulcerative colitis and disclosed the following findings: (a) In 50 patients the disease was confined to the rectum at the time of their initial clinical examination; at their most recent assessment, the disease was still restricted to the rectum in 36, had spread to involve substantial areas of the colon in

11 and had become total in seven. (b) In 51 patients the disease initially involved a substantial part of the colon; at the time of their subsequent barium study, the disease was confined to the rectum in two, showed no great change in 44 and had spread to involve the entire bowel in five. (c) In 27 patients with total involvement at their first examination, the subsequent barium study showed that the colon was still totally involved in 26, there was no instance of regression to 'substantial' involvement, but in one patient, only the rectum was affected. (It is important to emphasize that in this study it was the *extent* of involvement rather than the severity of the changes that was being considered. Thus, a case categorized as showing no alteration in the extent of disease at subsequent examination might none the less reveal a considerable qualitative improvement in the radiological appearances of disease, and the term regression was applied only if some of the more proximally affected part of bowel had become completely normal.)

To summarize our conclusions, then, it would appear that both progression and regression of ulcerative colitis frequently take place. However, progression of disease initially confined to the rectum occurred in 36% of our cases, compared with regression, which was noted in only 3% of patients with initial substantial or total involvement. This theme is examined in greater detail by de Dombal et al. (1968). It is only fair to add that Powell-Tuck et al. (1977a) found idiopathic proctitis

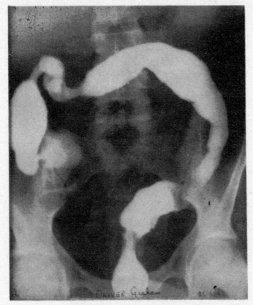

Fig. 527. Radiological appearances of two strictures just proximal and distal to the hepatic flexure and one in the upper rectum in a long-standing case of colitis; pathological examination of the colon after colectomy showed no evidence of carcinoma.

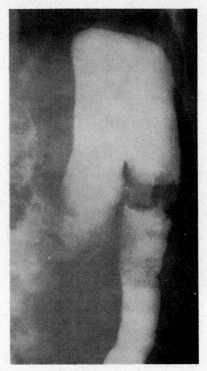

Fig. 528. Barium enema plate showing 'colitis carcinoma' just below the splenic flexure.

to be a much more static condition, so far as change in the extent of disease is concerned, than we did. They reckoned that the cumulative probability of the disease extending to involve the descending colon is about 5% at five years and 12% at ten years, the corresponding figures for extension to the hepatic flexure being 4% at five years and 6% at ten years.

Widening of the Retrorectal Soft Tissue Space as a Sign of Colitis

Edling and Eklöf (1963) have drawn attention to the widening of this space as shown on a lateral X-ray exposure as a fairly constant feature in patients with chronic ulcerative colitis (see Fig. 531). Of 197 cases with long-standing colitis 103 were found to have a space over 1 cm in width, the actual width corresponding roughly to the severity of the disease. Chrispin and Fry (1963) have placed the upper limit of normal size for this space at 1.5–2 cm. The widening in patients with colitis is presumably due to perirectal inflammation, oedema and fat. Obese patients may normally have a wider space, and widening also occurs in cases of carcinoma of the prostate or rectum according to Chrispin and Fry (1963). It should be added that Kinsey et al. (1964) have strongly disputed the reliability of widening of the presacral space as a sign of colitis.

PLAIN X-RAY EXAMINATION OF THE ABDOMEN

The plain X-ray plate of the abdomen can also give useful information in ulcerative colitis. The shadow cast by the gas-filled colon may reveal the characteristic features of the colitic large bowel with absence of haustration and possibly irregularity due to ulceration and polyposis (Fig. 532). The plain X-ray examination is *particularly valuable in acute phases of colitis* in revealing the occurrence of toxic dilatation (Fig. 533 and see p. 714).

SELECTIVE MESENTERIC ARTERIOGRAPHY

Selective mesenteric arteriography, using the Seldinger technique of introducing the catheter into the inferior or superior mesenteric arteries via the femoral artery, has been employed in recent years to study the vascular changes in the wall of the large bowel in cases of ulcerative colitis and Crohn's disease (Busson and Hernandez 1965; Boijsen and Reuter 1966; Lunderqvist 1967; Knutsson et al. 1968; Brahme 1971; Erikson et al. 1971). It was hoped initially that such arteriographic studies might define more accurately the extent of the disease in the bowel than does

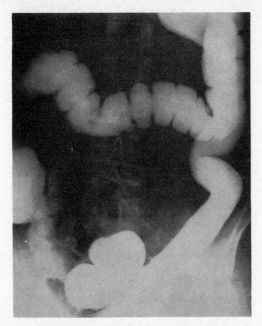

Fig. 529. Distal proctocolitis shown by barium enema examination; the disease extends as far proximally as the splenic flexure, the transverse and right colons being normal.

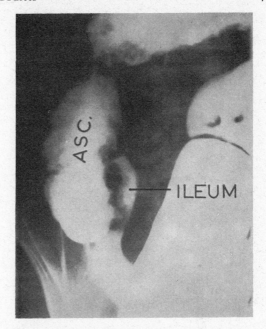

Fig. 530. Retrograde or 'backwash' ileitis in a case of ulcerative colitis shown in the barium enema film.

ordinary barium enema examination, and further that they might help in the differentiation between ulcerative colitis and Crohn's disease, which is sometimes extremely difficult on conventional radiological, and even pathological, examination. But these early hopes do not appear to have been realized, for it seems from the work of Brahme (1971), Fagerberg (1971) and Erikson et al. (1971) that in both diseases rather similar hypervascularization is usually evident with an increased frequency of shunts, but sometimes there is relatively sparse vascularization. It is thus difficult to distinguish between the two conditions on arteriographic examination. As for the extent of the disease in the intestine, arteriography is sometimes more accurate, sometimes less so, than barium enema study. Altogether, it cannot be claimed that arteriographic investigation has much to contribute to the assessment of these cases.

Diagnosis

Usually the diagnosis of ulcerative colitis or proctocolitis is very simple. The symptoms are highly suggestive and confirmation is readily obtained by sigmoidoscopy and barium enema examination. The importance of sigmoidoscopy cannot be overemphasized and no case of suspected colitis can be considered to have been fully investigated till this examination has been done. The conditions which may temporarily obtrude themselves in the differential diagnosis, such as dysentery and other forms of specific proctitis and colitis, benign and

malignant neoplasms of the rectum and colon, and irradiation proctitis, are easily excluded as a rule by a careful sifting of the history and physical findings, supplemented if necessary by appropriate bacteriological tests. Four special problems, however, require to be mentioned:

Haemorrhoids

Milder cases of proctocolitis often reach the surgeon misdiagnosed as haemorrhoids, because their presenting symptom is bleeding and, as there may be no disturbance of bowel habits, the family doctor refers them to a rectal clinic with a tentative diagnosis of piles. If the surgeon is not careful, he too may fall into the same error, for many of these patients resolutely deny having diarrhoea and at the time of attendance at hospital they may be in a phase of relative remission. The changes in the mucosa may then be very slight and easily overlooked unless a vigilant routine of mucosal assessment with particular reference to 'contact bleeding' is enforced in all rectal cases. If injections are given as for haemorrhoids in these cases of proctitis, they usually produce no benefit whatsoever, which in itself should arouse suspicion of a wrong diagnosis, for even with the grossest internal piles injection therapy is usually successful in checking the bleeding for a time. I frequently see patients who a short

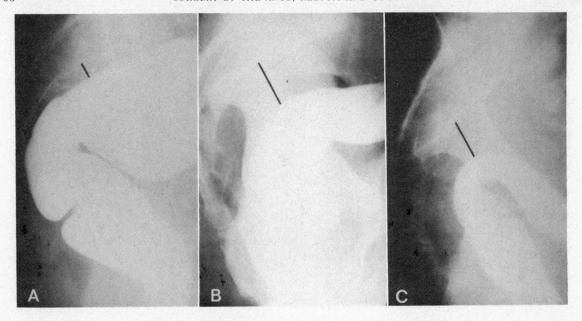

Fig. 531. Lateral radiographs of the rectum and sigmoid filled with barium. (A) In a normal individual. (B, C) In patients with chronic ulcerative colitis, showing the much wider space between the sacrum and the rectum in the latter two.

time previously have had unsuccessful injection treatment for 'haemorrhoids' elsewhere and are found at my clinic to be suffering from proctitis or proctocolitis.

Crohn's Disease

The increasing frequency with which Crohn's disease is now being encountered in the large intestine makes it important to bear this condition in mind in dealing with patients who are ostensibly suffering from ulcerative colitis. Sometimes the clinical and radiological features are such as to make the diagnosis of Crohn's enteritis only too obvious, as for example when 'skip lesions' are present or there appears to be extensive involvement of the small bowel as shown by progress barium meal or the demonstration of malabsorption by fat balance study. Another very suggestive finding is extensive ulceration in the anal region. Though broad anal fissures and abscesses may occur in ulcerative colitis, ulceration extending widely into the perianal skin is almost pathognomonic of Crohn's disease. When the rectum is spared by the disease the condition may be an example of the very rare segmental variety of ulcerative colitis, but, as emphasized on p. 699, it is very likely to turn out to be Crohn's lesion.

In other cases it may be much more difficult or impossible to distinguish on clinical grounds between ulcerative colitis and Crohn's disease of the large intestine. Points that would raise the suspicion of the latter condition are: a less severe form of diarrhoea despite extensive disease, bleeding slight or absent, considerable narrowing or deformity of the colon on radiological examination and the presence of asymmetrical changes or of a spiky 'rose thorn' edge to the barium shadows of the bowel, a 'cobblestone' appearance of the rectal mucosa on sigmoidoscopy or patchy changes there with intervening areas of normal mucosa. Sometimes a biopsy of the rectal lesion or of an anal ulcer may clarify the diagnosis by displaying the characteristic histological features of Crohn's disease, although a lot depends on the expertise of the pathologist.

Ischaemic Colitis

As pointed out on p. 859, though ischaemic colitis may closely resemble clinically a very severe attack of ordinary ulcerative colitis, there are certain points of difference, which generally enable a distinction to be made from this condition. Ischaemic colitis is apt to occur in elderly subjects, who may well give a history of previous cardio-

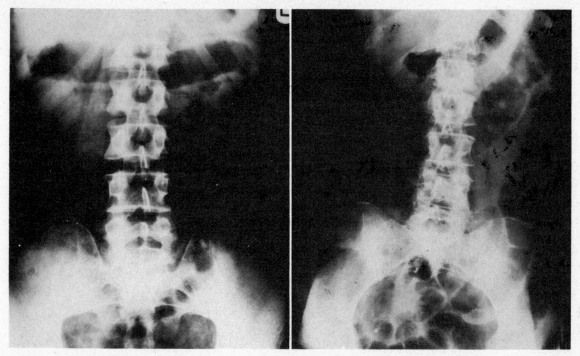

Fig. 532. Plain radiographs of abdomen in two cases of ulcerative colitis showing gas shadows of colon, particularly the transverse, devoid of normal haustrations.

vascular disease; the onset is particularly abrupt; sigmoidoscopy usually shows a normal rectum, for the lesion is generally confined to the upper left colon; and the radiological appearances may be distinctive.

Functional Diarrhoea, Irritable Colon, Cathartic Colon

These conditions are separately considered on pp. 932 and 933. It is only necessary here to make the point that a distal form of proctocolitis confined to the rectum will often escape detection on barium enema study, and that sigmoidoscopy is essential for its reliable diagnosis. If sigmoidoscopy has not been performed, it is easy to miss this form of colitis and to resort to other more or less unsatisfactory diagnoses, as, for example, functional diarrhoea or irritable colon. Clearly such diagnoses should never be considered till distal proctocolitis has been confidently excluded by sigmoidoscopic examination. It is also important to remember that the appearance of a rectal mucosa on sigmoidoscopy in cases of colitis may return to normal during phases of remission of the disease (perhaps rectal biopsy may be more reliable in disclosing evidence of past inflammation, as claimed by Morson and Dawson (1972), but see p. 703). Therefore, before excluding

this condition, it is well to repeat the examination when symptoms are actually present.

Clinical Course

It is customary to recognize several clinical types of ulcerative colitis depending on the course pursued by the disease (see Bochus et al. 1956):

Chronic Relapsing Colitis

This is easily the most common variety and I would say that it comprises at least 95% of all cases of ulcerative colitis. After a period of a few weeks, perhaps longer, the initial attack of the disease undergoes a spontaneous remission. During the interval that follows the patient may be completely symptom-free and may return to normal health, but more usually he continues to have mild symptoms and to show some impairment of general health. Sigmoidoscopically, too, the rectal mucosa may sometimes be restored to complete normality during the phase of remission, with a normal vessel pattern and no vestige of contact bleeding, but it is rather more common for some of the stigmata of mild proctocolitis to persist. Similarly the radiological abnormalities of colitis, even when gross and apparently irreversible, may sometimes disappear completely, as Ricketts et al. (1948) and Bargen (1956) have convincingly shown, but in other cases some changes remain. The period of remission may last for weeks, months or years, but eventually another exacerbation occurs. This may be of similar severity and duration to the previous one or may be milder or worse. In due course it undergoes remission and the same cycle of events may be repeated many times. It is always possible that one of the exacerbations may prove fatal or one of the remissions may herald a permanent arrest of the disease. Alternatively the course of the colitis may be interrupted by successful treatment. If, however, the recurrences continue the patient's condition steadily declines, and after two or three years of this sort of existence he is reduced to a state of partial or complete invalidism.

In cases of distal proctocolitis and proctitis the same periodic exacerbations and remissions of symptoms also occur, but the severity of the attacks is very much less and the patients often continue with this alternation of phases for many years without serious impairment of general health. There are, however, important exceptions to this generalization, for sometimes these mild distal cases end by becoming more extensive and producing grave constitutional disturbances.

Chronic Continuous Colitis

In this form of colitis the symptoms are usually only of moderate severity, but they show no tendency to abate. After they have continued relentlessly for five or six months, the term chronic continuous colitis may reasonably be applied to the condition (Bochus et al. 1956), but it will be obvious that in many cases with symptoms that continue beyond two or three months the natural course of events is liable to be terminated by a resort to surgical treatment. It is then impossible to say whether the condition was really one of chronic continuous colitis or merely a very prolonged initial attack of the chronic relapsing form of the disease. It is for this reason that chronic continuous ulcerative colitis has been excessively rare in my experience.

Acute Fulminating Colitis

This very acute form of colitis, which is associated with particularly severe symptoms, including a pyrexia to 39°C (102–103°F) or higher, produces a profound and rapid deterioration in the patient's condition often culminating in a fatal termination within a few weeks of the onset of symptoms. However the term 'fulminating colitis' is also used rather loosely by many writers to describe any very severe exacerbation of chronic relapsing colitis and is not reserved for particularly florid initial attacks.

Prognosis

Almost on a par with its baffling aetiology has hitherto been the unpredictability of ulcerative colitis as regards both the outcome of the particular episode from which the patient was suffering at the moment and the possibility of later recurrence. One patient with a very severe attack might recover spontaneously when almost all hope had been abandoned and might have no further trouble with colitis for years, whilst another patient with negligible initial symptoms due to a proctitis might end up with an attack of severe total colitis, for which urgent operation was required. However, our understanding of the prognosis in ulcerative colitis has been clarified by very detailed and comprehensive studies of the natural history of the disease undertaken by Edwards and Truelove (1963) in Oxford, by our own group in Leeds (Watts et al. 1966a, b), by Jalan et al. (1970a, b) in Edinburgh and by Ritchie et al. (1978) at St Mark's Hospital, London. From these surveys it has been possible to secure much more accurate information regarding the outcome in patients suffering from the disease under modern conditions of treatment, and to formulate some guidelines for prognosis. It should be explained that in all four series the patients had been treated primarily along medical lines with resort to surgical treatment only when conservative measures had failed, either urgently at the height of an acute attack that had failed to remit, or in the long run on account of chronic ill-health or other considerations. There are some slight differences in the findings of the four enquiries but a substantial measure of agreement. For full details readers should consult the original articles. It will perhaps suffice here to summarize the conclusions reached by us on the basis of our observations in Leeds:

OUTCOME OF INITIAL ATTACK

The outcome of the first attack is adversely affected by several factors: the rapidity of onset of the symptoms, the severity of the attack, the extent of involvement of the large bowel and the age of the patient. Of these the last is the most decisive and no less than five of the eight deaths in the initial attack in our series occurred in the group of 29 patients aged 60 years or over. Furthermore, if these 29 patients are excluded, the mortality of the remaining 175 patients under the age of 60 is only 1·7% instead of 3·4% for the whole series.

SUBSEQUENT COURSE AND ULTIMATE OUTCOME

If the patient survives the initial attack on medical treatment, he has a very considerable chance of having subsequent attacks. Thus after three years of follow-up 75% of our patients had experienced one or more additional attacks. These subsequent attacks were just as common in patients whose initial disease was confined to the rectum as in those who had had extensive or total colitis at that stage. But the age of the patient in each subsequent year exercised an influence on the likelihood of further attacks, the frequency diminished with increasing age.

As for the severity and mortality of subsequent attacks, these were found to be affected chiefly by the *extent of the colitis at the time of that particular attack* (and it is important to emphasize, as has been done by Sloan et al. (1950a, b), Kirsner et al. (1951), Bochus et al. (1956), Banks et al. (1957), Texter (1957), Lennard-Jones et al. (1962), Watts et al. (1966a) and Ritchie et al. (1978), that the extent of involvement of the bowel in colitis is not static but may alter at different stages of the disease; see also p. 704) and by the *age of the patient also at that time*. Patients with total or near-total colitis were more liable to have very severe, potentially fatal attacks than those with distal disease. In regard to age the more severe attacks occurred in patients over 60 or under 20. This was reflected also in a higher mortality in the older patients thus affected but not in the younger ones.

It must be admitted that Jalan et al. (1970b) reached contradictory conclusions in regard to the effect of the age of the patient on the subsequent mortality in colitic patients. They found that elderly patients with colitis, who survived the first referred attack without operation, suffered no greater mortality than did elderly subjects without colitis, but younger patients fared considerably worse.

ADDITIONAL FACTORS INFLUENCING OR GUIDING PROGNOSIS

VARIATIONS IN SERUM PROTEIN LEVELS

Some work by de Dombal (1968, 1969) shows that the prognosis in colitis can be gauged with considerable accuracy from variations in the levels of the serum protein fractions. Thus in *severe attacks* remission on conservative treatment is less likely if the gammaglobulin level is low or falling, whilst *during a period of quiescence of the colitis* the finding of a raised alpha-2 globulin fraction indicates that a further attack is imminent. Earlier studies by de Dombal (1967) on the electrophoretic pattern of the blood in the inferior mesenteric artery and vein in patients with colitis had suggested that there is a local production or release of alpha-2 globulins and a fixation or destruction of gamma-globulins by the diseased colon.

MALIGNANT CHANGE

An important prognostic consideration in certain cases of long-standing ulcerative colitis is the development of carcinoma in the affected large bowel. This serious complication and its bearing on prognosis are considered on p. 719.

CHILDHOOD

In the examination of the factors affecting the prognosis in our cases of colitis in Leeds (pp. 710–11), the age of the patient was seen to be specially significant (Watts et al. 1966a, b). Though the outlook was poorest in elderly patients, it was also worse in younger persons than in those of middle years. There are several reports in the literature emphasizing the poor prognosis in children and the frequent need to resort to operative treatment at this age (Helmholz 1923; Davidson 1939; Jackman et al. 1940; Benson and Bargen 1943; King et al. 1959; Michener et al. 1961, 1964; Ehrenpreis and Ericsson 1964; Wolfman et al. 1965; Ein et al. 1970; Patterson et al. 1971). Two additional problems arise with colitis in childhood to render the prognosis with medical treatment management less satisfactory and strengthen the indication for surgical treatment. One is the *impairment of growth and normal development* that may result from continued severe colitis in young children or adolescents. The other is the increased *risk of malignant change* in colitis commencing in early childhood, which has been specially stressed by Swedish workers (Rosenqvist et al. 1959; Edling and Eklöf 1961), and will be discussed further on p. 721.

SEX

In general no significant difference was noted in the prognosis in male and female patients respectively in our series of colitis patients (Watts et al. 1966a, b), and this has been the experience also of Cullinan and MacDougall (1957), Bochus et al. (1956) and Edwards and Truelove (1963). However, in women the effect of pregnancy on colitis requires to be considered.

PREGNANCY

Ever since 1909 when Gossage and Price presented to the Royal Society of Medicine four patients who developed ulcerative colitis during or just after a pregnancy, there has been much speculation and comment on the association of these two occurrences (Yeomans 1921; Barnes and Hayes 1931; Bargen et al. 1938; Felsen and Wolarsky 1948; Tumen and Cohn 1950; Sloan et al. 1950a, b; Abramson et al. 1951; Kleckner et al. 1951; Patterson and Eytinge 1952; Kallett 1952; Machella 1952; MacDougall 1956; Crohn et al. 1956; Banks et al. 1957; de Dombal et al. 1965b). Of course, pregnancy and colitis are both conditions encountered not infrequently in any large group of women of child-bearing age. It is hardly surprising, therefore, that they should sometimes coincide in the same individual. Indeed, there is general agreement amongst those who have studied the matter that at least two-fifths of women who develop ulcerative colitis before the age of 45 subsequently become pregnant, although the percentage varies slightly from one series to another (MacDougall 1956, 49%; Banks et al. 1957, 41%; de Dombal et al. 1965b, 31%). Naturally all these estimates under-rate the percentage of women with ulcerative colitis who will eventually become pregnant, because many of the patients still have a significant portion of their reproductive span before them. Two questions arise:

1. *What is the effect of ulcerative colitis on the pregnancy?* Our investigations (de Dombal et al. 1965b) confirm the findings of MacDougall (1956) and Crohn et al. (1956) that pregnancy is largely unaffected by ulcerative colitis. The vast majority of pregnancies in our patients culminated in the delivery at full term of a normal healthy baby, and the spontaneous abortion rate (6·5%) was below previous estimates of the national average (10%, Baird 1950). Moreover, activity of a patient's colitis in the first two trimesters did not seem to predispose to abortion.

2. *What is the effect of pregnancy on the colitis?* This is variable, for in some patients the bowel condition seems to improve or remain unchanged whilst in others it undergoes an exacerbation during the pregnancy or puerperium. However in any large series of cases it is found that a considerable proportion experience a deterioration of their colitis (Machella 1952, 50%; MacDougall 1956, 33%; Crohn et al. 1956, 75%; de Dombal et al. 1965b, 33%). Combining these estimates it seems fair to say that about 46% of women of child-bearing years with colitis who become pregnant will have a relapse of their colitis symptoms during the succeeding 12 months. But a question left uncon-sidered by most writers on the subject is the chance of a relapse of colitis occurring during a 12-month period of follow-up in a control group of female patients aged between 15 and 45 years, who are *not* pregnant. Our data have enabled us to answer this query (de Dombal et al. 1965b), and we find that the relapse rate in a control group of this kind is approximately the same, namely 47·5%. It appears, therefore, that a young female patient with colitis has about an even chance of experiencing an attack of colitis during any year *whether she is pregnant or not*, and that contrary to popular belief pregnancy has no *over-all* adverse effect on the course of the colitis.

The total relapse rate in the 12 months covering pregnancy and the puerperium is thus shown to be the same as in other years of follow-up. However, our figures also confirm the earlier findings of Crohn et al. (1956) that *such attacks of colitis as do take place more commonly occur around the third month of pregnancy and in the first three months of the puerperium.* Various theories have been advanced to explain this pattern of incidence. It has been suggested that the first trimester and the puerperium are the times of maximum psychological stress or of the greatest normal response of the gastrointestinal tract to the disturbance of pregnancy (Maddix 1962). The low incidence of relapses in the second and third trimesters has also been attributed to a rise at these times of the levels in the plasma of certain hormones, particularly of oestrogen and progesterone (Crohn et al. 1956) or of cortisol (de Dombal et al. 1965b).

Therapeutic Implications of Pregnancy

When colitis and pregnancy occur together they constitute a perplexing therapeutic problem, which has evoked a variety of opinions.

The aspect of treatment that has aroused the greatest contro-versy has been the question of therapeutic abortion and sterilization (Abramson et al. 1951; Crohn et al. 1956; Felsen and Wolarsky 1948; Krawitt 1959; Maddix 1962). Our experience inclines us to find little place for this measure. In only three of our patients was therapeutic abortion undertaken during an attack of colitis in the first three months of pregnancy, and two of these three patients failed to improve after therapeutic abortion. On the other hand, a total of 23 attacks of colitis were treated during pregnancy by medical measures alone, without resort to radical surgery or termination of the pregnancy. Only one of these 22 attacks was complicated by spontaneous abortion, and only three of them failed to respond to medical treatment. In the remaining 19 attacks medical treatment led to prompt remission of symptoms.

As for sterilization, Maddix (1962) aptly comments that this is unlikely to control the basic disease process of ulcerative colitis and that surgery should be directed at the gastrointestinal tract, not at the reproductive system.

Our numbers of patients are small and no definite comparison is possible between various forms of medical treatment, but it is our clinical impression that sulphasalazine is the drug of choice for pregnant colitic patients. After all, the plasma level of cortisol rises during pregnancy to around two and a half times the normal level and, if this fails to control the disease, it is unlikely that the intermittent external administration of similar substances will do so. However, steroids may be of value during the first few weeks of the puerperium, and the prophylactic administration of gradually decreasing doses of hydrocortisone during this period may well be worth a therapeutic trial.

Fortunately, none of our patients have required radical surgery for colitis during the period of pregnancy, and reports of such operations during pregnancy are rare in the literature. Clearly the operative risks of such a situation are likely to be considerable, whatever procedure is employed; but, despite the greater technical difficulties, it would seem logical from what has been written on p. 733 to aim at removal of the cause of the illness by ileostomy and subtotal colectomy (Abramson et al. 1951), rather than to be content with the easier but less effective measure of ileostomy alone (Maddix 1962). Flatmark et al. (1971) recorded a case of acute fulminating colitis in the terminal stages of pregnancy where Caesarean section and ileostomy with sub-total colectomy were combined in the one stage with a successful outcome for mother and child.

COMPLICATIONS OF ULCERATIVE COLITIS

Local Complications

PERFORATION

This is the most immediately serious local com-plication of ulcerative colitis. It was recognized as a hazard of the disease by Wilks and Moxon (1875) in their original description, and since then over 300 cases of perforation have been reported in the literature (de Dombal et al. 1965a).

INCIDENCE

The incidence of this complication has varied greatly from author to author, depending largely on the number of gravely ill patients included in their series of cases. Thus Sloan et al. (1950a, b) had a perforation rate of 2% in an unselected group of 2000 colitis patients at the Mayo Clinic, but van Prohaska and Siderius (1962) found the incidence of perforation in a surgically treated group of 88 patients to be as high as 14%. In the follow-up survey of 624 patients with colitis treated at the Radcliffe Infirmary, Oxford, from 1938 to 1962, Edwards and Truelove (1963) reported perforations in 3·2%. In our own series of 465 patients treated at the General Infirmary, Leeds, between 1955 and 1963, 13 cases had perforated, an overall incidence of 2·8%, the total number of perforations being 20. But perforation is most common *during the first attack of colitis*, and many of our patients were first seen during subsequent attacks. Of the 204 patients who presented to us during their first attack, 11 (5·4%) suffered a perforation of the colon in this or subsequent attacks, which is probably a more accurate reflection of the true incidence of this complication in colitis.

The incidence of perforation is very much influenced by the *severity of the initial attack* and the *extent of the disease in the bowel*, which are partly interdependent. Thus the chance of a colonic perforation occurring in all patients during their first attack was 3·9%, but in patients with a severe attack it was 9·7%. In patients who had total involvement at the time of their first attack the incidence of perforation was 14·6% and, if this initial attack was also a severe one, 19·2% of the patients developed a perforation during it.

Some previous series have placed the *site of perforation* as fairly evenly distributed throughout the colon, being perhaps slightly more common in the transverse colon than elsewhere (Sloan et al. 1950a, b; Brown et al. 1951; Bruce and Cole 1962). However, both our series (de Dombal et al. 1965a) and that of Edwards and Truelove (1964) suggest that the commonest location of perforation is the sigmoid colon, 11 of our 13 patients having at least one perforation in this segment.

Colonic dilatation (toxic megacolon) has been said to predispose to perforation and it is true that gross distension was present in five of our 13 patients in whom perforation occurred. However, a further 20 patients came to emergency operation without suffering a perforation, and nine of these patients were also found at operation to have dilatation of the diseased colon (de Dombal et al. 1965a). Thus the incidence of colonic dilatation in patients coming to emergency surgery was roughly the same whether perforation had occurred or not (but see Toxic megacolon, p. 714).

The suspicion that *steroid therapy might induce perforation* in colitic patients has evoked considerable controversy. Bargen drew attention to this danger in 1955, and Brooke (1956b) reported examples of colonic disintegration, which were claimed only to occur in steroid-treated patients. In the last few years several other reports have emphasized this hazard of steroid therapy in colitis (Rosenak et al. 1958; Kiefer 1960; Bruce and Cole 1962), but another group of authors have affirmed with equal conviction that steroids do not increase the risk of perforation (Goldgraber et al. 1957; Truelove and Witts 1959; Smith et al. 1962; Spencer et al. 1962; Korelitz and Lindner 1964; Edwards and Truelove 1964). Contrary to my previous opinion on this issue (Goligher 1961b), our subsequent more detailed observations overwhelmingly support the belief that steroid or ACTH therapy does not predispose to perforation of the colon, for we find that there is an almost identical incidence of perforation in severe attacks treated by steroids or ACTH (4·3%) and in those managed without these agents (4·1%). It seems more reasonable, therefore, to account for perforation of the colon as a consequence of the colitis itself—usually a severe initial attack—rather than to attribute it to steroid therapy.

DIAGNOSIS

It might seem that the occurrence of this complication would constitute a clear and definite indication for operation. But the difficulty of diagnosing with confidence on clinical grounds a perforation of the colon in connection with ulcerative colitis needs emphasis. This springs from the fact that abdominal physical signs often seem to be unreliable in patients suffering from severe acute manifestations of this disease (Graham et al. 1971). Certainly the development of any abdominal pain or tenderness suggestive of peritoneal irritation should arouse suspicion of perforation and lead to plain X-ray examination of the abdomen. But occasionally a patient who exhibits the classical symptoms and signs of a perforated intestine with an exquisitely guarded abdomen is found at laparotomy to have no such complication.

Our own detailed experience from 1955 to 1963 (de Dombal et al. 1965a) reflects this difficulty in diagnosis. During this period 30 of our patients came to emergency operation because of a rapid deterioration in their general condition. No less than 11 of them (37%) were found to have one or more perforations of the colon; and, although in six of the 11 perforation was suspected pre-operatively, in the remaining five there were no clear abdominal signs of perforation. Further-more, in another three patients who came to emergency operation with a confident preoperative diag-nosis of colonic perforation, no evidence of perforation was found, though two of them had peritonitis. We, therefore, believe that rapid deterioration in the general condition of any patient despite intensive medical treatment for his severe attack of colitis demands emergency opera-tion, for in such a patient the risk of perforation is considerable.

TREATMENT

From what has been said about the difficulties in clinical recognition of perforation in colitis, it is understandable that some patients with this compli-cation may inadvertently have been treated along conservative lines and have survived. We only know of the failures of such treatment when they come to necropsy. However, the vast majority of surgeons and physicians will unquestionably prefer surgical treatment, which involves immediate exploratory laparotomy.

The conditions encountered at laparotomy in these cases may vary. The perforation may have taken place anywhere in the caecum, colon or intra-peritoneal part of the rectum, but in the 21 patients with this complication dealt with by me (Goligher et al. 1970) the commonest site was the sigmoid. Perforations were not infrequently multiple, so that there was a total of 31 perforations in these 21 cases. The colon wall was often so thin and friable that it resembled wet blotting paper and was liable to give way even on gentle handling. 21 of my 31 perfora-tions had become sealed off by adhesion to the parietal peritoneum or to another viscus, but 10 were still open perforations into the peritoneal cavity. Occasionally, indeed, the colon was in a semi-pultaceous state over a considerable part of its length. In one of my patients the peritoneal cavity was found at laparotomy to be tightly distended with air from a tiny perforation of the sigmoid, which had probably been present for 24 hours according to the history and physical signs, but there was no gross evidence of peritonitis, nor did infection develop postoperatively.

Operative Procedure

Though occasional recoveries have followed ileostomy and suture of the perforation (Rice-Oxley and Truelove 1950; Brooke 1956a), the procedure usually employed has been ileostomy and colec-tomy or proctocolectomy. Ripstein (1953a, b), Peskin and Davis (1960), Bruce and Cole (1962) and van Prohaska and Siderius (1962) have reported a total of 32 patients with perforation treated by this operation, 23 of whom survived. My own results (Goligher et al. 1970) are equally encouraging: 21 patients came to emergency proctocolectomy (or colectomy) and 15 recovered. In cases with sealed perforations it may be advantageous to avoid colec-tomy which unseals the perforation and leads to faecal contamination, and instead to use a simple ileostomy combined with a decompressing trans-verse colostomy, as practised by Turnbull et al. (1970) with encouraging results (but see p. 743 for full discussion).

ACUTE DILATATION OF THE COLON OR 'TOXIC MEGACOLON'

Extreme dilatation of the colon occurring during an acute phase of ulcerative colitis—the so-called 'toxic megacolon'—is a complication that has received a good deal of attention in recent years (Madison and Bargen 1951; Lumb et al. 1955; McConnell et al. 1958; Roth et al. 1959; Marshak et al. 1960; Peskin and Davis 1960; Klein et al. 1960; Sampson and Walker 1961; Smith et al. 1962; McInerney et al. 1962). The information from these papers is to some extent conflicting, but certain generalizations seem justified.

INCIDENCE

Peskin and Davis (1960) found that marked dilata-tion of the colon combined with severe toxaemia was present in nine (6%) of 154 patients admitted to the hospital of the University of Pennsylvania from 1953 to 1958, whilst Sampson and Walker (1961) noted it in 14 (9%) of 168 cases of ulcerative colitis undergoing operation in the Department of Surgery of the University of Birmingham, England. McIner-ney et al. (1962) surveyed 1230 patients admitted to the Mayo Clinic for ulcerative colitis from 1954 to 1959. Of these, 379 were ill enough to require blood transfusion, or had a temperature of 39°C (102°F) or more during their stay in hospital; 36 of this group presented the clinical and radiological appearances of toxic megacolon. Of these 36 cases 16 were having their first episode of ulcerative colitis, 16 were suffering from the relapsing remit-tent type of the disease and had experienced severe attacks before, and four were patients with chronic continuous colitis.

CLINICAL FEATURES

Associated with the dilatation are often pronounced abdominal distension, local or diffuse tenderness of the abdomen, feeble or absent peristaltic sounds, cramping abdominal pains, mental confusion, diminution in the number of stools, and fever. McInerney et al. (1962), however, emphasize that frequently many of these classical signs were absent in cases in which gross dilatation of the colon was evident radiologically. It is thus probable that instances of megacolon may be overlooked unless it is a routine practice to have plain radiographs of the abdomen in all cases of colitis admitted in an acute phase of the disease.

RADIOLOGICAL FEATURES

In 35 of McInerney et al.'s (1962) cases the maximum dilatation was in the transverse colon, the greatest recorded diameter being 17 cm, with an average of 9–10 cm. Jones and Chapman (1969) reckon that the radiological upper limit of normal for the diameter of the transverse colon on the midline of the abdomen is 5·5 cm on a plain radiograph and 6·5 cm on a double-contrast enema film). Gas was present in several loops of small intestine in 34 patients, and distension of the small intestine was severe enough in five cases to suggest a mechanical obstruction. In Fig. 533 the plain film is illustrated in a case of mine with gross dilatation of the transverse colon occurring in the course of an acute exacerbation of ulcerative colitis.

AETIOLOGY

Several factors have been incriminated by different authors, but there is no general agreement.

Steroid therapy. All but one of Sampson and Walker's (1961) patients had had steroids previously, but no less than 24 of McInerney et al.'s (1962) 36 patients had never received any form of corticoid therapy.

Barium enema examination. Smith et al. (1962) and McInerney et al. (1962) both express the view that barium enema examination has sometimes seemed to precipitate the onset of colonic dilatation.

Use of anticholinergic drugs. Smith et al. (1962) are impressed by the possible causal effect of anticholinergic drugs.

Potassium deficiency. Hypokalaemia has been invoked by some writers to explain dilatation, but Sampson and Walker (1961) found that plasma potassium levels were normal in all but one of their 14 patients.

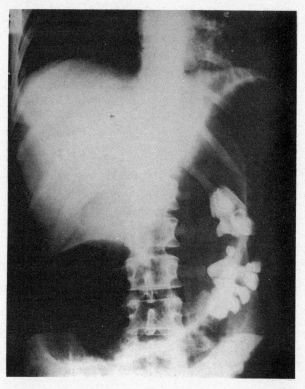

Fig. 533. Plain X-ray plate of the abdomen of a patient with a severe acute attack of colitis, showing 'toxic megacolon' affecting the transverse colon. Large stag-horn calculi present in left kidney. The colectomy specimen removed in this case is illustrated in Fig. 518.

Involvement of the myenteric nerve plexus or smooth muscle-fibres. Bochus et al. (1958) have suggested that it is destruction of the myenteric plexus that is responsible. Sampson and Walker (1961), however, found the ganglion cells of this plexus to be normal in appearance in four of their cases in which the colon specimen was specially examined from this point of view. They believe that it is more probably damage to the smooth-muscle cells of the bowel wall that causes the dilatation.

PROGNOSIS

The condition is noteworthy especially for the grave prognosis it carries. There seems to be considerable danger of perforation, as shown by the occurrence of this complication in 10 of McInerney et al.'s (1962) 36 cases, seven of Peskin and Davis' (1960) nine cases, and four of Sampson and Walker's (1961) 14 cases. Partly on this account the overall mortality of toxic megacolon is very high: McConnell et al.'s (1958), 23%; Sampson and

Walker (1961), 28%; and McInerney et al. (1962), 28%.

(Some writers seem to use the term 'toxic megacolon' as synonymous with 'acute fulminating colitis'. This is quite wrong, for this extreme dilatation of the colon with toxaemia may occur in patients who are having not their initial attack but one of many periodic exacerbations of a long-standing relapsing colitis. Further, some patients with a very severe attack of colitis necessitating emergency operation may have no particular dilatation of the colon at all, and may be found to have a perforation without preceding dilatation.)

TREATMENT

Opinion amongst various authorities is divided as to the merits of medical and surgical treatment for this condition. Roth et al. (1959) and McInernery et al. (1962) have argued in favour of continued medical treatment and the avoidance of operation if possible. In support of their conservative attitude McInerney et al. (1962) quote their experience of 28 patients with toxic megacolon treated medically with five deaths, whilst of their eight patients subjected to operation five died. Other writers give a relatively more favourable picture of the results of emergency colectomy or proctocolectomy for this condition. Thus, of 28 cases reported by McConnell et al. (1958), 13 were treated medically with five deaths and 11 surgically with one death; Peskin and Davis (1960) operated on all their nine cases with one death, as did Sampson and Walker (1961) on all their 14 cases with four deaths; and van Prohaska et al. (1964) report five deaths in their group of 16 surgically treated patients. My personal experience comprises 48 patients with acute colonic dilatation, all but one of whom were operated on, 21 being found to have an associated perforation, usually sealed, at laparotomy. The 47 surgically treated cases all had proctocolectomy or colectomy with eight deaths, a mortality of 17%.

My own feeling is that the finding of toxic megacolon in a patient suffering from a severe attack of ulcerative colitis is best regarded as an indication for emergency operation. Whether at laparotomy the condition should always be dealt with by colectomy or proctocolectomy is more debatable, because Turnbull et al.'s (1970) reported experience with the operation of diverting ileostomy combined with a decompressing colostomy in the treatment of cases of severe acute colitis with toxic megacolon has been most impressive. The method seems specially suited to patients who are found on exploration to have sealed perforations, for its application does not involve unsealing these perforations and contaminating the peritoneal cavity. (But see p. 743 for further discussion.)

MASSIVE HAEMORRHAGE

Bleeding from the bowel is a fairly prominent symptom in many cases of colitis, particularly those suffering from severe attacks, and blood transfusion is frequently required. Sometimes, when the blood loss is brisk, transfusion may be required very urgently and have to be continued rapidly for some time. Just when the definition 'massive haemorrhage' should be applied will depend on the clinician's use of this term. According to some, such as Edwards and Truelove (1964), a really big haemorrhage necessitating forceful and determined transfusion before the situation is eventually controlled is not unnaturally designated by this term. Using this definition they reported that there were 21 cases of massive haemorrhage in the 624 cases of colitis analysed by them in Oxford. Others, such as ourselves, have reserved the expression 'massive haemorrhage' essentially for cases in which the bleeding continues despite transfusion and is an urgent indication for operation. Such patients are very rare, for in our Leeds series of 465 colitis cases seen between 1955 and 1963 there was only one patient for whom the paramount indication for urgent operation was massive haemorrhage (Watts et al. 1966a), though there were two other cases where major bleeding was an important additional consideration.

SURGICAL TREATMENT

If, exceptionally, surgical intervention should be required for continued severe bleeding, ileostomy alone is obviously an uncertain, probably ineffective measure, and even ileostomy and subtotal colectomy may prove disappointing, for major bleeding may persist from the sigmoidorectal remnant. What is required is a complete proctocolectomy.

BENIGN STRICTURE

The *incidence* of non-malignant strictures of the rectum or colon in ulcerative colitis has been given as 11% by Sloan et al. (1950a), 9.5% by Jackman (1954), and 6.3% by Edwards and Truelove (1964).

TABLE 55. *Incidence of Stricture at Varying Sites in the Colon and Rectum*

Site	No. of patients with involvement by colitis	No. of strictures
Rectum	428	34 (7·9%)
Sigmoid	344	8 (2·3%)
Descending colon	280	7 (2·5%)
Transverse colon	210	11 (5·2%)
Ascending colon	140	7 (5·0%)

After de Dombal et al. (1966a).

Our own estimate (de Dombal et al. 1966a) is similar, for of 465 patients 52 had strictures (11·2%). In a number of these patients more than one stricture was present, the total number of strictures being 67, 50 of which were diagnosed by rectal examination or barium enema study and 17 were detected for the first time on examining the operative specimen.

The *site* of the strictures in our cases is shown in Table 55, which also indicates the frequency with which each segment of the large bowel was involved by colitis. The rectum is seen to be the commonest site for stricture formation, but this was largely due to the fact that this part of the bowel was more often implicated by colitis than any other area of the colon. Of the 428 patients with involvement of the rectum 7·9% developed a rectal stricture; although the ascending colon was only affected by colitis in 140 patients, 5% developed stricture at this site.

Stricture of the colon is generally held to be a manifestation of chronic forms of colitis. However, one-quarter of our patients who came to operation during their first attack of the disease were found to have a stricture at that time, and in two of these six patients the stricture was unsuspected clinically. It thus appears that stricture formation may not infrequently begin during a severe initial attack of colitis, although such a stricture may not become clinically apparent until some years later.

PATHOLOGICAL FEATURES

In 55 instances the stricture was localized and the narrowing of the lumen was confined to 2 or 3 cm in length. The remaining 11 strictures were more diffuse, the bowel being narrowed for a distance of up to 30 cm. Precise histological details were available on 28 strictures. The predominating feature in the majority of these lesions was marked submucosal fibrosis, which was found in 20 cases. Mucosal hyperplasia was seen in five strictures and muscular hypertrophy in the remaining three.

CLINICAL SIGNIFICANCE

There are two important differential diagnoses for the clinician to bear in mind when faced with a stricture in a case of ulcerative colitis: colitis carcinoma and a stricture due to Crohn's disease. Sometimes the distinction from a carcinoma may be difficult or impossible, but at other times a confident diagnosis of benign stricture may be made. For example, rectal strictures in colitis often have a characteristic delicacy and give way readily as the finger is forced through them, though they may be firm, hard, more suspicious narrowings. Biopsies of such rectal lesions should always be possible and may be very helpful. Strictures above the reach of the finger or sigmoidoscope will have to be demonstrated by barium enema studies (see Fig. 527); at best the differentiation from carcinoma may be uncertain—for example, in a series of 23 patients with colitis carcinomas demonstrated on barium enema study, Fennessy et al. (1968) reported that only 12 cases (40%) were confidently diagnosed by the radiologist as having carcinoma. Indeed Edwards and Truelove (1964) considered stricture formation an indication for laparotomy in order to excise the colon and secure histological examination, but fibre-optic colonoscopy now permits biopsy and accurate tissue diagnosis in many cases. Certainly, if there is the slightest doubt about the benign nature of the condition, operation is advisable. The other possibility to remember is that the underlying condition in the colon is really Crohn's disease and that the stricture is a complication of this process, for stricture formation is undoubtedly commoner in Crohn's colitis than in ordinary ulcerative colitis (see p. 829). In fact, Morson (1968) maintains that stricture formation is excessively rare in ulcerative colitis and its presence nearly always means that one is dealing with Crohn's disease. Though this may be an extreme view, there is an element of truth in his contention.

INFLAMMATORY POLYPOSIS

It is convenient to include under this heading all three types of inflammatory polyp described by Dukes (1954) in ulcerative colitis: (a) polypoid oedematous mucosal tags; (b) polyps composed of granulation tissue covered by mucous membrane; and (c) polyps composed of connective tissue covered by a layer of glandular epithelium. So defined, inflammatory or non-adenomatous polyps occurred in 58 of our 465 patients with ulcerative colitis, an incidence of 12·5% (de Dombal et al.

1966a), which is similar to that recorded by Sloan et al. (1950a), Brown et al. (1951), Edwards and Truelove (1964) and Jalan et al. (1969a).

EFFECT OF EXTENT, SEVERITY AND DURATION OF COLITIS ON THE OCCURRENCE OF POLYPOSIS

No patients whose disease was restricted to the rectum developed polyposis, but nearly 20% of patients with total or substantial involvement of the colon were found to have polyps. It is generally held that polyposis is a manifestation of severe disease. It may arise in the *first* attack of colitis; thus, of 204 patients seen by us during their initial attack, 18 (8·8%) were found to have polyposis at that time, whilst of 41 patients first seen during a *severe* initial attack of colitis, 12 (29·3%) were discovered at that stage to have polyposis.

DISTRIBUTION OF POLYPS

It has been claimed that polyposis occurs most commonly in the rectum (Sloan et al. 1950a), and in the left side of the colon (Edwards and Truelove 1964). Our findings on clinical examination, including assessment by sigmoidoscopy and barium enema studies (see Fig. 526), supported this opinion except that we have always been impressed by the fact that inflammatory polyps—unlike adenomatous polyps—practically never seem to affect the rectal ampulla but only the upper rectum (see Plate IIIF). However, in 25 cases direct inspection of the excised colon and rectum was possible after proctocolectomy. The extent of the polyposis in these patients was much greater than we had previously supposed after clinical and radiological examination. In the majority of these patients involvement began proximally in the ascending colon and extended distally as far as the rectosigmoid junction. In the few with rectal polyposis this complication was rare within 10 cm of the anal verge.

THE FATE OF INFLAMMATORY POLYPS AND THEIR RELATIONSHIP TO THE DEVELOPMENT OF CARCINOMA

Once polyposis has developed my experience is that the condition usually persists indefinitely with little change, though the associated colitis may become completely quiescent. However, Edwards and Truelove (1964) claim that complete regression can occasionally occur. Shands et al. (1952) and Bacon et al. (1956) allege that inflammatory polyposis is a precancerous condition, and the latter group mention

that they have had 48 cases of colitis with polyposis, nine of which developed carcinoma. In addition Dawson and Pryse-Davies (1959) claim to show examples of a transitional stage between inflammatory and adenomatous polyps. We have found in our colitis patients that the incidence of carcinoma of the colon and rectum is slightly higher in those with inflammatory polyposis than in those without, but we believe that this increased incidence is due to the extent and severity of the disease in the colon rather than to any specific pre-malignant change in the polyps. Counsell and Dukes' (1952) findings and opinion were similar; moreover, they were unable to discover any clear causal relationship between the polyps and the carcinomas in their pathological material. The suggestion that polyposis in colitis predisposes to the development of carcinoma is also emphatically rejected by the careful data of Edling and Eklöf (1961). 41 of their colitis cases had polyps demonstrated radiologically; in only two of these cases did carcinoma subsequently occur. By contrast 163 of their cases were radiologically free of polyps; 20 of them eventually developed malignant growths.

MANAGEMENT

The presence of polyposis does not affect the plan of treatment, which depends essentially on the characteristics of the colitis which gave rise to the polyposis. Most patients with polyposis have total involvement of the large bowel (Jalan et al. 1969a) or are seen in a severe attack, so that radical surgery is often needed irrespective of the presence or absence of polyps. (Interestingly, Jalan et al. (1969a) have shown that the prognosis in severe attacks seems to be somewhat better in the patients with polyposis than in those without this complication.) But occasionally patients are encountered with polyposis in association with a distal colitis; in these cases the management would in the ordinary way probably be conservative, and there is no indication to contemplate colectomy solely for the purpose of eradicating the patient's polyposis.

ANORECTAL COMPLICATIONS (ANAL FISSURE, ANORECTAL ABSCESS AND FISTULA, AND RECTOVAGINAL FISTULA)

In our series of 465 cases of colitis 82 (17·6%) had anorectal complications (de Dombal et al. 1966b). This is a higher incidence than that found by many other workers (Sloan et al. 1950a; Jackman 1954;

TABLE 56. *The Incidence of Anorectal Complications among 465 Patients with Ulcerative Colitis*

Complications	No. of patients
Perianal or ischiorectal abscess	28 (6·0%)
Fistula-in-ano	25 (5·4%)
Rectovaginal fistula	10 (2·2%)
Fissure-in-ano	57 (12·3%)
One or more complications	82 (17·6%)

After de Dombal et al. (1966*b*).

Hightower et al. 1958; Edwards and Truelove 1964; Waugh et al. 1964), probably attributable to the fact that during our survey practically all the patients were submitted to rectal examination and some who had not been attending the clinic regularly were found to have previously unrecorded anorectal complications. The incidence of the different types of anorectal complications in our patients is indicated in Table 56, from which it will be seen that often more than one complication was present and that the commonest was anal fissure which occurred in 12·3% of the patients.

RELATIONSHIP BETWEEN THE ONSET OF ANORECTAL COMPLICATIONS AND THE COURSE OF THE COLITIS

Investigation of both the severity and the extent of colitis at the commencement of the anorectal complications was possible because these complications usually produced uncomfortable symptoms, which drew the attention of the patient to them as soon as they developed. Anorectal complications differ in this respect from other local complications such as stricture, which may remain symptomless for a considerable time before clinical detection.

The relationship between the course of colitis and the development of anorectal complications has been investigated by several writers, with discordant results. Hurst (1935) alleged that anorectal complications might arise at any time during the course of colitis, whilst Bochus et al. (1956) claimed that these were always associated with other manifestations of colitis, and Gallart-Monés (1956) and Hightower et al. (1958) regarded anorectal abscess as a complication of severe disease. But Edwards and Truelove (1964) found that abscess and fistula may occur at any stage of the disease, though the development of these complications does imply active disease in the bowel.

Our study (de Dombal et al. 1966*b*) indicates an over-all association between severe attacks of colitis and the development of anorectal complications. All complications occurred most frequently during the year of the first attack; after this year the duration of colitic symptoms had little effect on the incidence of anorectal complication. The incidence of fissure-in-ano was significantly raised when extensive colitis was present, but that of abscess and fistula varied little with the extent of the colitis.

CLINICAL FEATURES AND DIAGNOSIS

As already pointed out, anorectal complications may be associated with relatively distal forms of proctocolitis causing few constitutional symptoms. They may also often appear during the early stages of the disease. They may thus to some extent dominate the clinical picture and, if the patient's local pain makes endoscopy difficult without an anaesthetic, it is very easy to miss the diagnosis of the underlying bowel condition, as I have seen happen not infrequently. This is a serious oversight which could lead to faulty management of an anal fistula (see p. 140). An error in the diagnosis of an anal fissure is also possible, though the anal fissures occurring in ulcerative colitis are unlike ordinary idiopathic fissures in that they are usually much broader, are not always situated in the posterior or anterior midline, are often double, and frequently are associated with a fair amount of suppuration. Sigmoidoscopy is urgently required, under a short general anaesthetic if necessary, to show the state of the rectal mucosa before embarking on any active surgical treatment.

TREATMENT

See p. 714.

CARCINOMA OF THE COLON AND RECTUM

INCIDENCE

It was Bargen (1928) who first seriously drew attention to the increased risk of malignant change in the colon and rectum in patients suffering from chronic ulcerative colitis. Since then many workers have investigated the relationship between these two conditions (Bargen et al. 1938, 1954; Sauer and Bargen 1944, 1949; Cattell and Boehme 1947; Svartz and Ernberg 1949; Gleckler and Brown 1950; Sloan et al. 1950*a*; Lyons and Garlock 1951; Brown et al. 1951; Counsell and Dukes 1952; Dennis and Karlson 1952; Weckesser and Chinn 1953; Bacon et al. 1956; Goldgraber et al. 1958a, b; Rosenqvist et al. 1959; Dawson and Pryse-Davies 1959; Slaney and Brooke 1959; Lindner et al. 1960; Bargen and Gage 1960; Edling and Eklöf 1961; Bruce and Cole 1962; Nefzger and Acheson 1963; Edwards and Truelove 1964; MacDougall 1964; de Dombal et al. 1966a). As a result of these and other surveys it is now widely accepted that there is an undoubted predisposition to the development of carcinoma of the large bowel in ulcerative colitis. However, controversy still exists as to the magnitude of this danger, for the incidence of carcinoma in reported series of cases of ulcerative colitis has varied considerably—for example Sloan et al. (1950a) put it at 5% in 2000 cases; Counsell and Dukes (1952) at 11·1% in 63 cases; Wheelock and Warren (1955) at 8·8% in 319 cases; Svartz (1954) at 3·9% in 403 cases; Dawson and Pryse-Davies (1959) at 2·9% in 663 cases; Slaney and Brooke (1959) at 6·7% in 222 cases; Edwards and Truelove (1963) at 3·5% in 624 cases; de Dombal et al. (1966a) at 1·7% in 465 cases; and Lennard-Jones et al. (1977) as 3% in nearly 170 cases. But most of these variations in estimate of the risk can probably be explained by differences in the types of cases making up the parent series, for it is known that the incidence is much affected in this way. Factors that have been discussed in this connection are the following:

The Duration of the Colitis. This is the predisposing factor about which there is most agreement, for it has been generally found that the incidence of carcinoma has risen progressively with the increasing length of history of colitis. Thus Cattell (1948) reported that a complicating carcinoma of the colon or rectum had been discovered in 7% of all the cases of colitis on which he had operated, but that the incidence of carcinoma rose to over 30% in those patients who had had symptoms for nine years or longer. Dawson and Pryse-Davies (1959) found that their over-all incidence of carcinoma in 663 mixed medical and surgical cases of colitis was 2·9%, but that in 127 patients with a history of colitis of more than 15 years it was 10·2%. Slaney and Brooke (1959) observed a complicating carcinoma in 6·7% of 222 cases of colitis treated surgically by them, the frequency increasing to 17% in those patients who had had their colitis for more than 10 years. Edwards and Truelove (1964) have calculated the steadily increasing incidence of carcinoma according to the duration of ulcerative colitis in their large, carefully followed-up series of cases,

and show that the annual risk of developing cancer is almost 20 times as high in those who have had colitis for more than 20 years as it is in those who have had colitis for under five years.

The Extent of Involvement of the Bowel by Colitis. It has often been surmised that more localized distal forms of colitis probably predispose less to the development of carcinoma than do extensive or total forms of the disease, but it is only in recent years that this point has received proper emphasis. Edling and Eklöf (1961) surveyed the outcome in 204 cases of colitis treated in the medical department of the Karolinska Sykhuset, Stockholm, between 1940 and 1946 inclusive. They found that of 86 patients in whom the entire colon and rectum were involved no less than 18 (21%) developed carcinomas, but of the remaining 118 patients with various forms of partial, mainly distal, colitis only four produced growths (3·4%). Edwards and Truelove (1964) divided their cases into two groups according to the maximum extent of involvement by colitis at any stage of their disease: 236 with total involvement and 388 who at no stage were more than partially involved; 17 of the former group developed carcinoma, an incidence of 7·2%, but only five of the latter, an incidence of 1·3%. MacDougall (1964) in his follow-up of colitis cases treated at the Gordon Hospital, London, between 1947 and 1963 has classified the patients into three groups according to the extent of their colitis at the latest attendance—total, distal colon, and rectum only. Of 196 cases with total involvement, nine (4·6%) developed carcinoma; of 291 with colitis confined to the distal colon only, one (0·34%) was complicated by the occurrence of carcinoma; and of 132 with rectal involvement only, none developed a carcinoma.

Our experience in the follow-up of 465 cases of colitis attending our clinic in Leeds between 1954 and 1963, which was summarized by de Dombal et al. (1966a), was very similar to that of MacDougall. Of the eight patients who developed carcinoma of the colon or rectum all had suffered from total or substantial colitis, and in none of the 218 patients with disease confined to the rectum or left side of the colon did a growth develop. As the danger of malignant change in colitis seems to apply almost exclusively to patients with total or subtotal involvement we thought it would be interesting to examine the effect of the duration of colitic symptoms on the incidence of carcinoma in this specially predisposed group. Fig. 534 shows the steady increase in the *yearly* incidence of growth, which reached the figure of 5·8% per annum after 20 years of colitic symptoms. In Fig. 535 is plotted the *cumulative* expected incidence of carcinoma in these patients, and it will be seen that it amounted to no less than 13% after 15 years, and no less than 41·8% after 25 years. It will also be noted from Fig. 534 that any patient with total involvement of the rectum and colon, first seen 20 years or more after the onset of colitis, had a risk of developing carcinoma of at least 5% each year for the rest of his life. In a study of 234 cases of extensive colitis in Göteborg, Kewenter et al. (1978) found that the cumulative incidence of carcinoma 25 years after the onset of disease was 34% and for those with an onset of colitis before 25 years of age it was 48%.

incidence of 22·7%; whilst of 160 patients whose colitis began after this age only 12 produced growths, an incidence of 7%. The reason that immediately suggests itself for this difference is that the cases starting with colitis in childhood are likely to have the disease for a longer time than those beginning in adult life. However, Edling and Eklöf (1961) point out that this cannot be the correct explanation, for the mean duration of the colitis originating before and after the age of 15 years was approximately the same, namely 17·6 and 17·2 years respectively. They believe that the difference

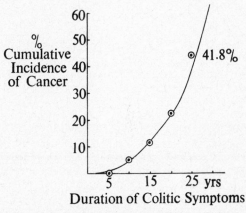

Fig. 535. The cumulative incidence of large bowel cancer in a series of patients with *total* colitis according to the duration of colitic symptoms. (*From de Dombal et al. 1966a*)

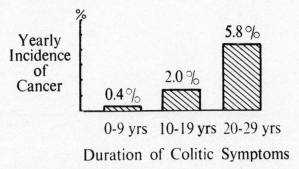

Fig. 534. The yearly incidence of colitis carcinoma increases in patients with *total* colitis according to the duration of the colitis. (*From de Dombal et al. 1966a*)

But in a recent very important article on this subject Lennard-Jones et al. (1977) paint a much less alarming picture of the cancer risk in long-standing colitis. They calculated the annual risks in terms of patient-years of follow-up in 169 patients with total or extensive colitis. In 578 patient-years of follow-up during the first decade after the onset of the colitis no carcinomas were discovered. In 200 patient-years of follow-up during the second decade one carcinoma was found. In 60 patient-years of follow-up during the third decade one further carcinoma was detected.

The Age of the Patient at the Onset of the Colitis. It has been strongly suggested by Jackman et al. (1940), Rosenqvist et al. (1959) and Edling and Eklöf (1961) that carcinoma is much more likely to develop in patients whose colitis starts in childhood than in those who are first afflicted in adult life. Thus in Edling and Eklöf's (1961) series there were 44 patients with colitis starting before the age of 15 years and 10 of these developed carcinomas, an

in malignant potential of the two groups of cases is accounted for by the fact that patients with an early onset of colitis more often had an extensive or total colitis of considerable severity than did cases developing colitis in adult life. Thus in their series the ratio of total colitis to less extensive colitis was 34 : 10 in patients with an onset of the disease under 15 years, but 52 : 108 in patients whose onset was after that age.

Edwards and Truelove (1964) have analysed their cases in terms of age at onset of ulcerative colitis and find that one in eight of those patients in whom colitis began before the age of 10 subsequently developed carcinoma, compared with one in 25 of those in whom the onset of colitis occurred in the next two decades. The percentage affected with carcinoma fell steadily over the next three decades, and none of the 56 patients aged 60 or more at the start of colitis developed cancer.

The Presence of Inflammatory Polyposis in the Bowel. As already pointed out on p. 712, there is some differ-

TABLE 57. *Sites of Colitis Carcinomas*

Site of growth	No. of growths				
	Counsell and Dukes (1952)	Slaney and Brooke (1959)	Edwards and Truelove (1963)	Author's series	Collective series
Caecum	—	—	2	1	3
Ascending colon	—	2	2	5	9
Hepatic flexure	—	2	—	3	5
Transverse colon	3	1	8	4	16
Splenic flexure	—	2	—	2	4
Descending colon	1	1	2	1	5
Sigmoid colon	1	5	7	5	18
Rectosigmoid	—	3	—	6	9
Rectum	7	5	6	7	25
Not determined	1	1	—	—	2
All sites	13	22	27	34	96
No. of cases with multiple growths	1	3	5	7	16

ence of opinion as to whether inflammatory polyps *per se* are to be regarded as pre-malignant. The majority view is that, whilst cases of colitis showing polyposis may be slightly more likely to develop carcinoma than cases without such polyps, this is to be attributed to the fact that both polyposis and carcinoma occur more frequently in long-standing severe cases of colitis.

Age Incidence of Colitis Carcinoma

Carcinoma arising as a complication of ulcerative colitis occurs as a rule at an earlier age than does ordinary large bowel cancer. Thus in Slaney and Brooke's (1959) series of cases of colitis carcinoma collected from the world literature, the average age incidence was 42·5 years, compared with 63·2 years in 710 cases of ordinary carcinoma of the colon and rectum treated at hospitals in the Birmingham area during 1954. Edwards and Truelove (1964) state that the age distribution of their 22 patients with colitis carcinoma at the time of diagnosis of the tumour ranged from 20 to 72 years, the average being 41.

PATHOLOGICAL FEATURES

Site. Edling and Eklöf (1961) have commented on the distribution of the colitis carcinomas in their cases being different from that of ordinary carcinomas of the large bowel. Of their 23 growths one-quarter were in the rectum or sigmoid and three-quarters lay more proximally (with ordinary carcinomas of the large intestine approximately three-quarters are concentrated in the rectum and sigmoid). But this has not been the experience of most other writers, who have found that the siting of colitis carcinomas does not differ materially from that of ordinary large bowel carcinomas, as is shown in Table 57, which records the distribution in four series of cases of colitis carcinomas in this country, making a total of 96 growths.

Multiplicity. A notable feature of colitis carcinomas (also shown in Table 57) is the high incidence of multiple primary growths (one in seven) which is about four times greater than that found with carcinoma of the colon in general (one in 30).

Gross Appearances. The individual growth may exhibit the gross features of an ordinary malignant ulcer of bowel (Fig. 536c), but, as pointed out by Counsell and Dukes (1952), they may be quite atypical in their appearances and may present rather as relatively inconspicuous thickenings of the colon wall, which merge gradually into the adjoining colon or rectum and are no more ulcerated than the rest of the bowel (Figs 537–8). The resemblance of these areas to so-called 'fibrous' strictures is thus very close, and it seems possible indeed that in the past some of these growths may have been wrongly diagnosed at autopsy as simple strictures and their neoplastic nature not appreciated. Usually colitis carcinomas have spread extensively by the time they come to the surgeon or pathologist.

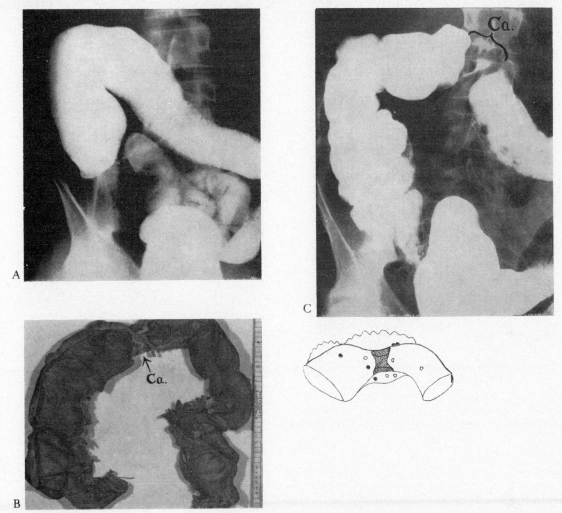

Fig. 536. (A) Barium enema plate in 1956 of a man of 25 who had had severe chronic relapsing colitis for seven years; note typical changes of colitis. (B) Barium enema plate of the same case in 1959 showing tight stricture in the right transverse colon. (C) Procto-colectomy specimen removed from this case, displaying the appearances of diffuse ulcerative colitis with in addition an annular carcinoma of the transverse colon. *Inset:* Gland dissection chart of the growth showing several involved glands (shaded black).

Histological Structure. On microscopic section these growths have usually been found to be highly active, often anaplastic carcinomas, but occasionally better differentiated lesions are encountered (Counsell and Dukes 1952; Dawson and Pryse-Davies 1959; Lennard-Jones et al. 1977).

Morson and Pang (1967) have found that in all colectomy specimens removed for ulcerative colitis and containing a colitis carcinoma there are extensive histological changes in the mucosa, not only near the carcinoma but elsewhere, which they regard as pre-malignant. These alterations consist of dysplasia of the epithelial tubules, which are irregular in shape and lined by epithelium showing stratification of the nuclei (Fig. 539). The latter are hyperchromatic and vary in size and shape. Such changes correspond to what many pathologists would designate as 'carcinoma-in-situ' and have been termed by Morson and Pang (1967) in this context as 'precancer'. These authors state that similar precancerous appearances are also present in some colitis patients who have no invasive cancer

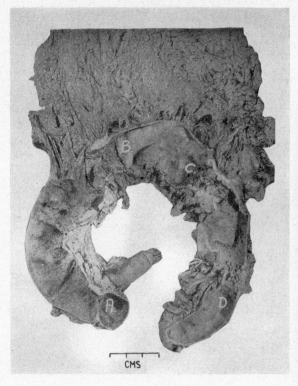

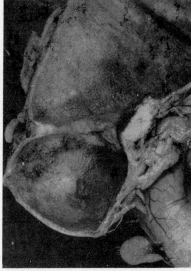

Fig. 537. Specimen of colon and rectum removed by proctocolectomy from a patient with ulerative colitis. Four separate primary carcinomas are present (A, B, C, and D). *Inset:* Close-up of growth A showing that it has the appearance of a localized thickening of the colon wall rather than that of a typical malignant ulcer (Sir Clifford Naunton Morgan's case).

but give a long history of total colitis. In such cases they are usually patchy in distribution and confined mainly to the distal colon and rectum, but may rarely be found diffusely throughout the entire large intestine. Morson and Pang (1967) consider that detection of 'precancer' on rectal biopsy in cases of colitis might be helpful in indicating which patients have developed or are specially likely to develop carcinoma, but this needs to be substantiated by careful follow-up studies on conservatively treated patients. It is already apparent that epithelial dysplasia may be patchy in distribution and thus missed on biopsy, hence the need for multiple biopsies through the sigmoidoscope and by means of the colonoscope (Cook and Goligher 1975). Also the histopathological diagnosis of epithelial dysplasia and its differentiation from reactive hyperplasia, which is not uncommon in colitis, may be quite difficult for the average pathologist (Cook and Goligher 1975).

A significant contribution to the assessment of the value of recognition of epithelial dysplasia on rectal and colonoscopic biopsies has been provided by Lennard-Jones et al. (1977). In a survey of 229 patients with extensive or total colitis, whom they have been following up and from whom regular biopsies have been taken, their findings regarding the incidence of epithelial dysplasia and of carcinoma were as follows:

1. In 196 patients no epithelial dysplasia was found on biopsy and no carcinomas were observed. (This group of patients comprised 501 patient-years of follow-up in the first decade after the onset of colitis symptoms, 301 in the second decade and 139 in the third.)

2. In 20 patients moderate dysplasia was noted and one carcinoma was found.

3. In 13 patients severe dysplasia was observed. Seven of these came to operation, carcinoma being found in four, severe dysplasia only in two and no dysplasia in one. Six patients continue to be managed conservatively; in five of these subsequent biopsies failed to show dysplasia and in one a decision about operation is pending.

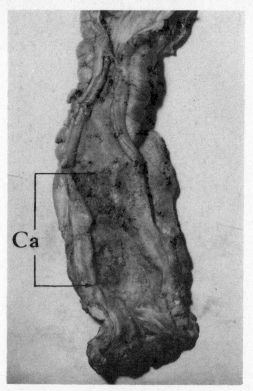

Fig. 538. The rectal part of a proctocolectomy specimen removed from a patient who had had colitis for 24 years, showing a carcinoma of rather diffuse imperceptible kind.

CLINICAL FEATURES AND DIAGNOSIS

The difficulties in the way of early diagnosis of carcinoma arising as a complication of ulcerative colitis will be readily appreciated. Because of the pre-existing colitis the patient has already had the sort of symptoms that would normally draw attention to the occurrence of an intestinal growth, and it is natural therefore to attribute any aggravated complaint of this kind to an exacerbation of his colitis. If the carcinoma lies in the rectum and the symptomatic 'relapse' leads to routine rectal examination, the lesion may possibly be detected right away by the finger or the sigmoidoscope. But, as pointed out on p. 722, these growths may be very unusual in their appearances and may not be easily recognized. An important point is always to submit to biopsy any areas about which even the slightest doubt is felt, particularly in patients who have had their colitis for a number of years. Alternatively the carcinoma may be shown by barium enema study, if

this is undertaken. But in a certain number of patients in most reported series—either because repeat radiological examination has not been carried out or has been considered to be negative—the diagnosis of colitis carcinoma is first made at laparotomy or even on examination of the operative specimen. As will be gathered from the previous paragraph the finding of severe epithelial dysplasia on rectal or colonoscopic biopsy should alert the clinician to the possible presence of a small early carcinoma, and, if dysplasia is confirmed on repeat biopsies, it could be an indication *per se* for proctocolectomy.

Svartz and Ernberg (1949), Svartz (1954), Rosenqvist et al. (1959), Dawson and Pryse-Davies (1959) and Slaney and Brooke (1959) warn that carcinoma may sometimes develop in patients who have been symptom-free for from one to several years. Other writers, such as Nefzger and Acheson (1963) and ourselves (de Dombal et al. 1966a), have noted that the symptoms of colitis in patients who produce a carcinoma may be relatively mild.

PROGNOSIS

Because of the active nature of these growths and the delay that often attends their diagnosis, many of them have reached an advanced inoperable or incurable stage by the time they present for surgical treatment, but occasional cases are more favourable. Slaney and Brooke (1959) have calculated from a series of 358 patients with colitis carcinoma collected from the literature that the average five-year survival rate was no higher than 18·6%. Brooke (1969) has reported somewhat more encouraging results in his own personal series of cases, and Lennard-Jones et al. (1977) state that all five carcinomas detected by them in their series of colitis patients being very carefully followed-up had very early favourable growths—four Dukes A and one Dukes B—which ought to give a good prognosis with surgical treatment. In the treatment of established colitis carcinomas, if the growth is operable, the ideal is an excision of the entire large intestine, for more limited resections are very liable to be followed by the development of further carcinomas in the remaining colon or rectum (Hultén et al. 1971).

BEARING ON TREATMENT OF ULCERATIVE COLITIS

It is clear from these experiences that the chances of cure of colitis carcinoma once it has arisen may be

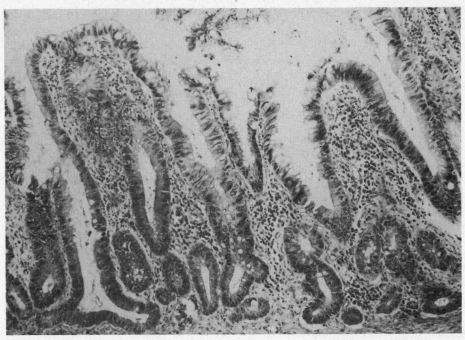

Fig. 539. Photomicrograph of rectal mucosa from a proctocolectomy specimen. The patient, female, aged 46 years, had an eight-year history of ulcerative colitis and was found to have a stage A carcinoma of the rectum. An irregular almost villous configuration of the mucosa is associated with changes in the epithelial cells. These comprise a variation in size, shape and hyperchromicity of the nuclei, occasional mitoses, and a loss of polarity in the nuclear arrangement. These are the features of epithelial dysplasia in the rectum. H & E × 120. (*Slide kindly prepared by Dr Martin Cook*)

rather poor, and this raises the question of preventing the development of this complication in long-standing cases of colitis by prophylactic proctocolectomy. Opinion on the advisability of this step has been very divided. Texter (1957) stated that the frequency of malignant degeneration was insufficient to warrant total colectomy for this reason alone. By contrast Dennis and Karlson (1961) advocated removal of any colon which still shows radiological abnormality four years after the onset of the colitis. Though Michener et al. (1961), like Rosenqvist et al. (1959), emphasized the special predisposition of children with colitis towards the development of cancer, they made no definite recommendation about preventive proctocolectomy. Nefzger and Acheson (1963) discussed the question at some length. They found preventive colectomy difficult to justify from their own figures, but clearly they had been handicapped in this respect by a high surgical mortality in their collective series of colitis patients. Carleson et al. (1962) were also unable to share the view that the risk of cancer justifies an increased use of colectomy. Edwards and Truelove (1964) considered that in general the risk of carcinoma is out-weighed by the other dangers of colitis, but concluded that the

mortality of elective proctocolectomy is probably substantially less than that of carcinoma developing in certain 'high risk' groups, whilst MacDougall (1964) recommended prophylactic proctocolectomy to all patients with total involvement of the colon and rectum after 10 years of colitic symptoms.

At one stage I certainly did advocate offering prophylactic operation routinely to all patients with total or extensive colitis of ten or more years duration (de Dombal et al. 1966a). Furthermore, it seemed to me that for the purposes of cancer prophylaxis the operation *must include the establishment of an ileostomy and complete excision of the affected large bowel*. Operations which left part or all of the diseased intestine, even if it was 'defunctioned', did not in my view provide adequate protection, for in the 304 cases of carcinoma complicating colitis collected by Slaney and Brooke (1959) there were 34 which had been treated solely by ileostomy, caecostomy or appendicostomy. In addition, 11 cases in which an ileostomy and subtotal colectomy had been performed developed a carcinoma in the retained unused rectal stump, and three cases in which colectomy and ileorectal anastomosis had been carried out were also complicated later by the occurrence of carcinoma in the rectum. Further reports of the subsequent development of carcinoma in the rectal remnant after colectomy and ileorectal anastomosis for colitis have come from Griffen et al. (1963; two growths in 50 cases so treated), MacDougall (1964; five growths in 237 cases), Aylett (1971; seven growths in some 300 cases) and Baker et al. (1978; 22 growths in 374 cases, there being a steady increase in the incidence the longer the follow-up).

But the whole question of prophylactic proctocolectomy has now to be looked at afresh in the light of Lennard-Jones et al.'s (1977) instructive experience in the follow-up of patients with extensive colitis using regular rectal and colonoscopic biopsies for evidence of epithelial dysplasia to monitor the risk at any time of carcinogenosis. As explained on p. 724, they were able to select from their series of 196 cases 20 with moderate epithelial dysplasia and 13 with severe dysplasia and to reserve consideration of a preventive operation for this small group of 33 patients. In the event operation was performed on only eight of them, five being found to have early favourable carcinomas (and no other carcinomas having, so far as Lennard-Jones et al. (1977) are aware, developed in their series). Operation was withheld in the other 25 cases with dysplasia for several reasons, mainly because of the mildness of the changes or the inability to find clear evidence of dysplasia on repeat biopsy, or because of the reluctance of the patients to accept surgical treatment.

From this experience it would seem that, if good collaboration can be obtained from one's pathologist, as Lennard-Jones has from Morson, an initially conservative attitude to the malignant potential of ulcerative colitis is fully justified, the patients specially at risk with total or subtotal colitis being observed annually, sigmoidoscoped and submitted each time to several rectal biopsies (after the disease has been present for 10 years colonoscopic biopsies being added). If the biopsies prove negative for epithelial dysplasia, it is assumed that the patient can safely be left to conservative management for another 12 months. If, however, the biopsies turn out to be positive and show undoubted dysplasia, it is probably wise to arrange for a repeat set of biopsies in three or four months, and if these are also positive to urge operation on the patient.

LYMPHOSARCOMA

Another form of malignant tumour that may occur in association with ulcerative colitis is intestinal lymphosarcoma. Six instances of this combination have been collected from the literature by Cornes et al. (1961) and more recently another case has been described by Walker and Weaver (1964). Malignant lymphoid tumours of the bowel are rare, which suggests that the concomitant occurrence with colitis might not be mere coincidence. Since the degenerative and inflammatory changes that take place in the colon wall in ulcerative colitis involve also structures of mesenchymal origin, it would seem possible that the development of a lymphosarcoma might be provoked by long-standing colitis.

The diagnosis of lymphosarcoma in this connection has usually not been made till laparotomy or necropsy. The condition is probably best treated by colectomy if possible, but alternative or supplementary measures are chemotherapy or irradiation. However the prognosis is very poor.

Systemic (Remote or Metastatic) Complications

ARTHRITIS

It has long been recognized that the course of ulcerative colitis may be punctuated by bouts of arthritis, but estimates of the frequency of this complication have varied widely from 4·5% (Bargen 1929) to 22% (Bochus et al. 1956) and even 45% (Wright and Watkinson 1965a). It used to be believed that the arthritis was usually of rheumatoid type, but by applying the Rose-Waaler differential agglutination test, which is held to be specific for rheumatoid arthritis, Bywaters and Ansell (1958) and Wright and Watkinson (1959) have distinguished a separate form of arthritis peculiar to ulcerative colitis. Though this latter concept of a specific *colitic arthritis* has been challenged by some workers, such as Rotstein et al. (1963), others have provided supporting evidence (Ford and Vallis 1959; McEwen et al. 1962). Recently attention has also been focused on the possible special relationship of *ankylosing spondylitis* to ulcerative colitis (Steinberg and Storey 1957; Fernandez-Herlihy 1959; Acheson 1960; McEwen et al. 1962; McBride et al. 1963; Wright et al. 1965; Wright and Watkinson 1965b).

Wright and Watkinson (1965a) have described the results of a forward-planned review of 269 unselected patients with ulcerative colitis at our Colitis Clinic in Leeds, the cases being assessed simultaneously and independently by a gastroenterologist and a rheumatologist. The incidence of the various types of arthritis elicited by them is indicated in Table 58, from which it will be seen that colitic arthritis occurred in 11·5% of their cases, and ankylosing spondylitis and sacroiliitis in 6·4%.

TABLE 58. *Frequency of Different Forms of Rheumatic Disorder Present in 269 Patients with Ulcerative Colitis*

Disorder	No. of cases
Osteo-arthritis	33
Lumbar disc lesion	16
History of rheumatic fever	5
Rheumatoid arthritis	4
Psoriatic arthritis	1
Specific *colitic arthritis*	31
Ankylosing spondylitis and *sacroiliitis*	19

After Wright and Watkinson (1965a).

COLITIC ARTHRITIS

The clinical characteristics of this complication have been defined by Wright and Watkinson (1965a). The arthritis usually commences between the ages of 25 and 44 years (rheumatoid arthritis 35–65 years). It begins as an acute synovitis in a large single joint of the lower limb as a rule, most commonly the knee, secondly in order of frequency the ankle. Thereafter other joints may be affected, again predominantly in the legs, and involvement is usually asymmetrical. The arthritis generally subsides within six weeks with little or no residual deformity. Subsequent attacks follow a similar pattern. Subcutaneous nodules and tendon sheath effusions never occur and muscle wasting is rare. Small bony erosions have been reported as residue of colitic arthritis by Bywaters and Ansell (1958), but no such changes were observed radiologically by Wright and Watkinson (1965a) in any of their patients.

Relation of the Arthritis to the Colitis and Other Colitic Complications. Wright and Watkinson (1965a) found that patients with long-standing colitis were more prone to develop recurrent arthritis, but arthritis began before symptoms of colitis had been present for six months as often as it did later. Colitic arthritis was more frequent in patients with a chronic intermittent or continuous course than in those with acute fulminating disease. In women the frequency of the arthritis varied with the extent of the colitis, being more common when the entire colon was involved. This association was not seen among men. Colitic arthritis usually manifested itself at a time when bowel symptoms were worse and the bowel and joint symptoms tended to remit simultaneously.

There was a striking association between both local and systemic complications of ulcerative colitis and colitic arthritis. The arthritis was significantly more common in patients with perianal disease and inflammatory polyposis. Similarly it was significantly more common in colitics with recurrent ulceration of the buccal mucosa, and eye and skin lesions.

Prognosis and Response to Treatment. Arthritis has often been regarded in the past as an urgent indication for colectomy (Brooke 1954), but Wright and Watkinson (1965a) record that in many of their patients complete subsidence of the arthritis followed remission of the colitis and persisted for many years, as long as the colitis remained quiescent. Edwards and Truelove (1964) have had similar experiences. On the other hand, Wright and Watkinson (1965a) are able to confirm that when required colectomy is capable of affording a certain cure of arthritic symptoms. My own experience of 24 patients with colitic arthritis treated by proctocolectomy is that they have all been completely relieved of their joint trouble.

ANKYLOSING SPONDYLITIS AND SACROILIITIS IN ASSOCIATION WITH ULCERATIVE COLITIS

As Jayson and Bouchier (1968) point out, in several published series of cases of ankylosing spondylitis the incidence of ulcerative colitis has ranged from 1·5 to 3·9% (which is probably much higher than the frequency of colitis in ordinary hospital admissions—see p. 690), but these estimates underrate the incidence because sigmoidoscopy and barium enema examination was not performed on all patients. In Jayson and Bouchier's (1968) series of 77 patients with ankylosing spondylitis, on whom these investigations were performed routinely, the frequency of colitis was found to be 18%. Conversely, among patients with colitis many authors have in recent years discovered a certain number suffering from ankylosing spondylitis, two of the highest incidences being 5% and 6·4% reported by Fernandez-Herlihy (1959) and Wright and Watkinson (1965a) respectively (see Table 58). But these estimates all underrate the frequency of spondylitis in colitic patients because in none of these series was any attempt made to carry out routine radiographs, particularly of the sacro-iliac region and lumbar spine. To secure a more accurate assessment Wright and Watkinson (1965b) have re-examined from this point of view 234 of the patients previously surveyed (Wright and Watkinson 1965a; Table 58), and in addition have surveyed a control population. They report that the incidence of severe sacroiliitis was 12 times greater in patients with colitis than in the controls (5·1% to 0·4%) and moderate sacroiliitis was three times as common (12·8% to 4·3%). These differences are highly significant.

Relation of Sacroiliitis to the Colitis and to Other Colitic Complications. Sacroiliitis was slightly more common and more severe the more extensive the colitis, and the incidence of sacroiliitis was also marginally greater in long-standing cases of colitis. But there was none of the close parallelism that exists between the activity of colitic arthritis and the state of the bowel lesion. It is also interesting to note that the onset of bowel symptoms was sometimes preceded by the occurrence of sacroiliitis, on occasions by many years. (By contrast colitis was never antedated by the development of colitic arthritis.) Further, there was no association of sacroiliitis with local complications of ulcerative colitis, such as perianal disease or polyposis, nor with systemic complications, such as buccal mucosal ulceration or uveitis. But there was a very definite correlation in female colitis patients between sacroiliitis and colitic arthritis; over three times as many women with colitic arthritis had sacroiliitis compared with women without colitic arthritis.

Response to Surgical Treatment of the Colitis. Fernandez-Herlihy (1959) reports that of 15 colitic patients with spondylitis treated by colectomy and ileostomy at the Lahey Clinic 12 had progressive symptoms postoperatively referable to the spinal condition. I have performed proctocolectomy on only three colitic patients with clinically diagnosable ankylosing spondylitis: two have cleared up completely since operation; the third has persisted, but may be a case of Reiter's syndrome.

SKIN LESIONS

ERYTHEMA NODOSUM

This well recognized complication of ulcerative colitis was noted in eight (1·7%) of our series of 465 cases and in a roughly similar percentage of the series of cases reported by Edwards and Truelove (1964) and Johnson and Wilson (1969). It is almost confined to female patients, as it is when it occurs apart from ulcerative colitis. It is frequently found in association with arthritis. Usually the appearance of the erythema coincides with an attack of colitis, either an initial one or a relapse. Edwards and Truelove (1964) also describe the occasional occurrence of erythema before the onset of the colitis, but this is contrary to our experience. There is no close correlation between the extent of the colitis and the development of this complication, for it can occur in patients with total involvement or with limited disease.

PYODERMA GANGRENOSUM

This rare skin lesion is seldom encountered in practice except in association with ulcerative colitis, and even then is usually held

PLATE III.

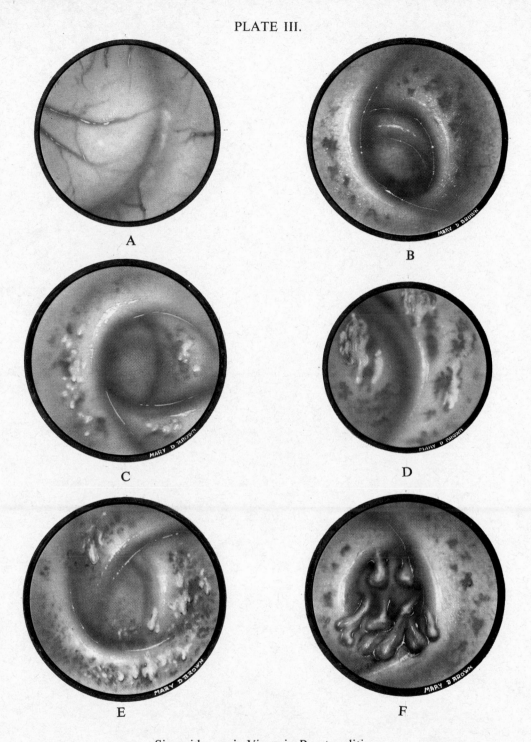

Sigmoidoscopic Views in Proctocolitis

A,   Normal rectal mucosa. Note obvious vessel pattern

B,   Mild granular proctitis with 'contact' bleeding and absent vessel pattern

C,   More severe proctitis with flecks of purulent discharge

D, E, Grosser forms of protocolitis with more haemorrhage and suppuration

F,   Colitis with numerous inflammatory polyps appearing at rectosigmoid junction

to be very uncommon. Thus Edwards and Truelove (1964) had only four instances of it in their 624 cases of colitis. Actually of our 465 patients 13 (2·8%) were complicated by the occurrence of pyoderma. Suppuration and scabbing are perhaps the salient features of the lesion, which occurs usually on the lower limb, though gangrene may also be evident. There may be considerable associated constitutional disturbance; whilst this may emanate partly from the colitis, frequently the associated bowel lesion is relatively mild. Butler (1948) and Corbett (1952) have stressed the dramatic efficacy of excision of the affected bowel in clearing up the skin lesion, and this has been my experience also.

OTHER SKIN ERUPTIONS

Edwards and Truelove (1964) describe various other skin lesions in 15·9% of their cases. These consisted of areas of dermatitis; macular, papular, pustular or urticarial rashes; boils and superficial abscesses; ulceration; and abnormalities of the skin and hair. It is difficult to know how many of these were related to the colitis and how many were due to drugs or quite independent. The only one of these lesions specially noted in our series was leg ulceration, which occurred in eight cases, an incidence of 1·7%

RESPONSE OF SKIN COMPLICATIONS TO TREATMENT OF COLITIS

Of our 29 patients with erythema nodosum, pyoderma or leg ulcers, one with pyoderma died in the immediate postoperative period after proctocolectomy, leaving 28 for analysis of the response of the skin lesion to medical or surgical management of the bowel condition. 15 patients were treated along medical lines; in seven the skin lesion cleared. 13 patients had proctocolectomy, following which there was a complete subsidence of the cutaneous complication in 11.

EYE LESIONS

The frequency of eye complications has been estimated by Edwards and Truelove (1964) as 7·5% and by Billson et al. (1967) in our Leeds series of 465 cases as 3·6%; the incidence being slightly greater in women than men in both studies. All but two of our 17 cases with these complications were young adults, the mean age when the eye condition developed being 35 years. The most common ophthalmic lesions were iritis and episcleritis. The eye lesions developed and flared up in association with severe attacks of colitis. The extent of colitic involvement of the bowel had little effect on the incidence of eye complications. The presence of eye lesions was always associated with the existence of at least one other systemic manifestation of colitis, and *all* patients with iritis also suffered from joint symptoms. It is interesting to note that in three patients with eye lesions the latter *commenced before the onset of bowel symptoms.*

In nine of our colitic patients with eye lesions the colitis was treated medically, with complete clearance of the eye complications in two. In eight patients radical surgery was undertaken for the bowel condition, with cure of the eye lesions in all of them.

LIVER AND BILIARY TRACT DISEASE

LIVER DISEASE

Earlier reports by Comfort et al. (1938) and Tumen et al. (1947) of *sporadic cases* suggested that cirrhosis of the liver might be

specially common in patients with ulcerative colitis. But *routine necropsy studies* by Warren and Sommers (1949), Jones et al. (1951) and Parker and Kendall (1954) failed to show that cirrhosis was significantly more frequent in patients dying of colitis, though they did reveal fatty changes in the liver in between 25 and 50% of the cases. However, a further study by Palmer et al. (1964) implied that cirrhosis might be as much as 12 times commoner in patients dying of colitis than in a control group.

The incidence of frank cirrhosis elicited in a *retrospective survey of a large clinical series of cases* of ulcerative colitis by Edwards and Truelove (1964) was a 2·5%, and in the Leeds clinical series we reckon it to be roughly similar—namely 1·6%. These estimates are probably slightly higher than the incidence of cirrhosis for hospital patients in general, but are fairly reassuring. *More detailed clinical studies of the state of the liver*, however, by Pollard and Block (1948), Ross and Swarts (1948), Kleckner et al. (1952), Boden et al. (1959), Brooke et al. (1961), Mistilis et al. (1965), de Dombal et al. (1966c), Dordal et al. (1967) and Eade (1970), utilizing liver function tests and liver biopsies by needle or at laparotomy, have been less encouraging, for they have revealed that a high proportion of patients have hepatic dysfunction and histopathological changes in the liver. Particularly impressive are the findings on biopsy, with histopathological abnormalities being observed in the great majority of cases. Though there have been considerable variations in the abnormal appearances observed in different biopsy studies and in their interpretation, the commonest findings include: (*a*) fatty change in about half the cases, (*b*) portal tract infiltration by inflammatory cells in 10–50% of cases; and (*c*) cirrhosis in less than 5% of cases.

It was the impression in Leeds (de Dombal et al. 1966c) and Birmingham (Brooke et al. 1961; Eade 1970), from the operative biopsies done in both centres on patients coming to colectomy or proctocolectomy, that the severity of the liver changes, particularly the fatty infiltration, was related to the severity of the colitis at the time of operation, being much more marked in patients operated on in severe unremitting attacks than in those undergoing elective operation. But Boden et al. (1959) claimed that mild chronic ulcerative colitis could be associated with pericholangitis, and Eade (1970) found that portal fibrosis occurred irrespective of the extent of the colitis, but was commoner in patients over 50 years of age who had had their bowel trouble for more than 10 years. Both in Birmingham and Leeds it was noted that there was a higher operative mortality in the patients whose biopsies at laparotomy showed severe liver damage.

As regards the mechanisms of production of the liver changes in ulcerative colitis, it has been suggested by Brooke et al. (1961) that 'toxic substances', normally contained within the lumen of the bowel, escape into the portal venous system and are thereby conveyed to the liver. In support of this hypothesis is the infiltration of the portal tracts in the liver with inflammatory cells (giving rise to what has been badly termed pericholangitis), and the finding by Brooke and Slaney (1958) of bacteria in the lumen of the portal vein in one-quarter of a group of patients undergoing operation for ulcerative colitis. It is not clear, however, what significance should be attached to such positive portal blood cultures in the pathogenesis of the hepatic histological changes, in view of the extreme rarity of frank liver abscess in colitis patients.

Of great interest is the bearing of these liver changes in colitis on the ultimate well-being of the patients and the possible indication for radical surgical treatment. Specially valuable in this connection has been the follow-up study by Eade et al. (1970) of the 138 patients from whom biopsy specimens had been taken at operation in Birmingham, three to seven years after colectomy: 21 patients died, 13 in the postoperative period and eight in subsequent years. Of five patients shown by biopsy to have cirrhosis at colectomy, only one died (four years after operation), and this was the only death attributable to liver disease. Needle biopsy was performed on 33 of the patients on follow-up—these were all cases showing biochemical evidence of disordered liver function. Fatty infiltration was still present in 45% of the cases, but it was less noticeable than at the time of operation. Infiltration of the portal tracts with inflammatory cells was reduced in frequency from 42% to 15% of cases, and fibrosis and bile duct proliferation were also less in the follow-up specimens. But in 11 of the 33 patients having follow-up biopsies, who had been left with a rectal stump the seat of persisting disease, no reduction in hepatic histological changes was observed, which suggests that the course of liver disease can be to some extent halted or reversed by complete proctocolectomy. On the other hand, it must be admitted that Mistilis et al. (1965) and Dordal et al. (1967) noted, on serial liver biopsies, regression of inflammatory liver changes in colitis on successful medical treatment, though Mistilis et al. (1965) also found that of 14 patients with pericholangitis present for periods of over 10 years under conservative management, three eventually developed cirrhosis. It will be seen, therefore, that it is difficult to take a strong line on the advisability in patients with colitis and liver disorder of proceeding to proctocolectomy to prevent progression of the liver condition and ultimate development of cirrhosis, particularly when the rather higher recorded immediate mortality of this operation in patients with hepatic changes is borne in mind.

The Incidence of Colitis in Patients with Established Liver Disease. Another way of looking at the relationship of hepatic changes to ulcerative colitis is to study the frequency of colitis in patients known to be suffering from liver disease, as has been done by Holdsworth et al. (1965). They found that colitis was present in 5% of their cases with disease of the liver. In the group with colitis, four types of liver disorder were observed: (*a*) intrahepatic cholestasis in three cases; (*b*) post-necrotic cirrhosis in seven cases; (*c*) 'juvenile' cirrhosis in eight cases; and (*d*) unclassifiable chronic liver disease unassociated with jaundice in four cases.

SCLEROSING CHOLANGITIS

Thorpe et al. (1967) have described four instances of primary sclerosing cholangitis occurring in patients suffering from ulcerative colitis. There was no relationship between the severity and duration of the colitis and the episodes of jaundice. It was not possible to distinguish this sclerosing cholangitis of the extra- and intrahepatic ducts from intrahepatic biliary disease except at laparatomy.

CANCER OF THE BILE DUCT

Cases of ulcerative colitis with carcinoma of the bile ducts have been recorded by Parker and Kendall (1954), Nefzger and Acheson (1963), Palmer et al. (1964), Edwards and Truelove (1964), Rankin et al. (1966), Dordal et al. (1967) and Babb et al. (1970). Cancer of the bile duct is such a rare condition that its occasional association with ulcerative colitis may well be more than just fortuitous.

STOMATITIS

Stomatitis is a relatively common systemic complication of ulcerative colitis which occurred in 10% of Edwards and Truelove's (1964) cases and in 16·5% of our series. Though in most instances the stomatitis is an aphthous condition, it is important, as Edwards and Truelove (1964) have emphasized, to be on the alert for candidal infections, which sometimes occur and can be dangerous by becoming generalized. For this reason, oral candidiasis should be promptly treated with nystatin tablets to suck, which are usually effective. Generalized candidiasis can also be treated by nystatin, locally or systemically, and if this is not soon successful amphotericin B should be exhibited parenterally.

In Edwards and Truelove's (1964) experience and ours stomatitis occurred more often in severe attacks of colitis than in moderate or mild ones. Of our 37 colitic patients with stomatitis who had medical treatment for their bowel condition only eight were cured, but 38 patients who underwent proctocolectomy were all completely cleared of their stomatitis.

OESOPHAGITIS

Rosendorff and Grieve (1967) have reported a case in which ulcerative oesophagitis occurred in association with ulcerative colitis, and they refer to several similar cases recorded in the literature.

OTHER SYSTEMIC COMPLICATIONS

Other complications that occurred in our series of 465 patients were: venous thrombosis of the legs, 4·7%; severe mental derangement, 1·3%; physical retardation, 0·6%; and nephrotic syndome, 0·2%.

MEDICAL TREATMENT OF ULCERATIVE COLITIS

It is generally agreed that the management of many cases of colitis ought to be along medical or expectant lines in the first instance. Whilst certainly no comprehensive account of medical treatment is called for in a surgical work of this kind, a few general and practical comments may be appropriate:

1. No specific medical therapy exists for this disease, and the aim of the physician is to encourage a spontaneous remission of symptoms by various non-specific measures such as bedrest, nourishing diet, blood transfusions, psychotherapy, antispasmodics, sedatives, intestinal antiseptics, corticosteroids (and, recently, immunosuppressive drugs).

2. The precise evaluation of any therapeutic measure in the treatment of colitis is rendered particularly difficult by the uneven course of the disease, with its naturally occurring exacerbations and remissions. This accounts for the widely divergent views of physicians on the importance of different items of medical management.

3. *Corticosteroid therapy.* Nowhere has the conflict of medical opinion been more evident than in regard to the value of cortisone and ACTH (corticotrophin). Fortunately much of the earlier acrimonious controversy on the advantages and disadvantages of these agents has been settled by the conduct of carefully controlled therapeutic trials. The value of *systemic corticosteroid therapy* has been subjected to a comprehensive controlled enquiry in this country by Truelove and Witts (1955, 1959) with the collaboration of a number of other physicians in Oxford, Leeds, Edinburgh, London and Birmingham. Their investi-

gation seems to have established beyond doubt that cortisone materially enhances the prospect of securing a remission of symptoms in patients who are having their first attack of colitis. Its value in obtaining remission in patients who have had previous attacks is considerably less. A disappointing feature was the high relapse rate subsequently, for by the end of nine months after completion of the course of cortisone only 41% of the patients had not had further symptoms as compared with 35% of the patients who had been treated by a dummy preparation. Attempts to reduce the incidence of relapse by continuing the cortisone therapy indefinitely in a later trial (Truelove and Witts 1959) were only very slightly successful. Spencer et al. (1962) have claimed that using much larger maintenance doses of steroid (e.g. 15–20 mg of prednisone daily) 38% of their patients could be kept in remission and another 28% remained improved. But to do so they had to accept a formidable array of side effects from the steroid therapy, and furthermore their assessment of results was not conducted as part of a properly controlled trial. But more recently such a double-blind trial of higher doses of prednisone in maintenance therapy has been reported by Lennard-Jones et al. (1965); they were unable to demonstrate that the steroid was any more effective than the dummy preparation in avoiding relapses. A comparison of the results of oral cortisone and ACTH showed that the latter was rather more effective in securing remissions, but the improvement was not so well maintained as with cortisone and there was a higher incidence of complications referable to corticosteroid therapy with it than with cortisone (Truelove and Witts 1959). The charge that corticosteroids predisposed to perforation of the colon in colitis was not substantiated in the Truelove and Witts' (1955) trial for they found that there were no perforations in their series of 109 cases having cortisone as compared with two perforations in the 101 cases treated by a dummy preparation. More recently controlled comparisons of intravenous hydrocortisone and ACTH showed them to be equally effective in the management of acute attacks of colitis (Kaplan et al. 1975; Powell-Tuck et al. 1977b).

Topical corticosteroid therapy. Prompted by the favourable results obtained by the use of topical hydrocortisone in affections of the skin, eyes and joints, Truelove (1956) first advocated its local use in ulcerative colitis in the form of hydrocortisone retention enemas. This type of therapy seemed specially suitable for milder distal forms of colitis, particularly as the patients could be taught to give themselves the enemas nightly at home and thus avoid having to come into hospital. Alternative preparations to hydrocortisone hemisuccinate sodium to use for this purpose are prednisolone 21-phosphate or betamethasone, and instead of the vehicle of an enema a suppository (of prednisolone) may be employed. One of the advantages claimed for topical steroid therapy is that the compound is not absorbed and side effects are not observed; this is true except in regard to betamethasone, which is 50 times more potent than hydrocortisone and does tend to be absorbed unless the dosage is reduced to relatively ineffective levels (Watkinson 1962). Controlled trials of topical therapy have confirmed its value when used alone (Truelove 1958; Watkinson 1958; Matts 1960) or in combination with oral prednisone (Truelove 1960). Popular proprietary preparations for topical therapy are Predsol enema (containing prednisone), Cortenema (containing hydrocortisone), Retenema (containing betamethasone) and Colifoam (containing hydrocortisone acetate). The enemas should be administered last thing at night before retiring, in the hope that the steroid may be retained all night. Their use should be continued for at least two or three weeks, and often much longer.

4. *Sulphasalazine.* Though various intestinal antiseptics of sulphonamide or antibiotic nature have been tried in ulcerative colitis, the one that has undoubtedly secured the greatest sup-

port in recent years is sulphasalazine (Salazopyrin). It was introduced by Svartz of Stockholm in 1942 and strongly recommended by her (Svartz 1948) and Bargen (1956) for the treatment of ulcerative colitis. According to some reports (Svartz 1954, 1960; Moertel and Bargen 1959) as many as three-quarters of the patients treated by it showed improvement. From a clinical trial Lennard-Jones et al. (1960) concluded that sulphasalazine was probably as effective in securing remissions as prednisone, but slower in its action. Truelove et al. (1962) compared combined oral and topical corticosteroid therapy with sulphasalazine over a 14-day period and found the former to be significantly more effective. Baron et al. (1962) and Dick et al. (1964) conducted double-blind trials contrasting sulphasalazine with a placebo in the management of mild or moderate cases of ulcerative colitis and proctitis. Both groups were able to show a statistically significant advantage for sulphasalazine over the inert control tablet on a three-week course, though there was a high incidence of unpleasant side effects (nausea, vomiting, anorexia, diarrhoea, dizziness and skin rashes) which in a few cases required termination of the treatment. Toxic haemolytic anaemia with the presence of Heinz bodies and agranulocytosis are two more serious complications which have also been reported (Spriggs et al. 1958; Thirkettle et al. 1963). Despite these drawbacks sulphasalazine has become popular, usually in combination with topical corticosteroids. The prophylactic value of maintenance therapy with sulphasalazine 2 g daily in lessening the incidence of relapses is emphasized by Misiewicz et al. (1965) and Dissanayake and Truelove (1973), who recommend that this medication should be continued indefinitely. Riis et al. (1973) were less impressed with the prophylactic value of sulphasalazine, as am I.

5. *Immunosuppressive drugs.* A treatment that has generated a great deal of controversy is the use of immunosuppressive agents such as 6-mercaptopurine, azathioprine and nitrogen mustard (Bean 1962, 1966; Bowen et al. 1965; Winkelman and Brown 1965) on the basis that this disease may be a manifestation of an autoimmune response (see p. 691). However, initial enthusiasm for this form of therapy was somewhat tempered by the report of a severe marrow depression as a complication of it (Jones et al. 1966) and by the attention drawn by Penn and Starzl (1970) to the possible development of neoplasms in patients on long-term immunosuppression. Furthermore, there is a lack of good objective data on the effects of such treatment on the course of the bowel condition, though Jewell and Truelove (1974), on the basis of a controlled trial of azathioprine in the management of ulcerative colitis, came to the conclusion that it was of some value and as a consequence they have now incorporated this drug in their overall plan of therapy for this disease (Truelove et al. 1978). Most clinicians, however, continue to adopt a distinctly cautious attitude towards treatment with these drugs.

6. Two drugs which have recently been tried in the treatment of colitis are disodium cromoglycate and metronidazole. Disodium cromoglycate (DSCG) is of proven clinical value in the management of allergic bronchial asthma, where it is thought to reduce the degranulation of mast cells in the bronchial mucosa. In colitis mast cell degranulation is a frequent feature in rectal biopsies. It seemed pertinent, therefore, to Heatley et al. (1975) to try the effect on this disease of DSCG given topically (200 mg in an enema twice daily) or orally (200 mg thrice daily). On the basis of a controlled trial they reached a cautiously favourable verdict on the value of the drug, as also did Mani et al. (1976). However, further trials by Dronfield and Langman (1978), Bucknell et al. (1978) and Willoughby et al. (1978) have shown DSCG to be useless.

As for metronidazole, now so fashionable as an intestinal antiseptic specially effective against anaerobic organisms, the rationale for its use in colitis is not clear, for there is no definite evidence that bacterial invasion is a primary causal factor in this condition, though it may play a secondary role. Anyway, in a controlled trial Davies et al. (1977) were unable to produce any evidence that metronidazole had been of benefit in cases of proctitis.

7. In view of the great advances made in the administration of parenteral alimentation in recent years, it may be wondered what this regimen has to offer patients with severe episodes of ulcerative colitis. The theoretical advantages of intravenous feeding are that it permits complete rest of the intestinal tract so far as feeding is concerned and at the same time provides an adequate supply of calories and other essentials to combat the malnutrition which is such a pronounced feature in these cases. A combination of total parenteral feeding and intensive steroid therapy would thus seem eminently logical (Reilly et al. 1976). Truelove et al. (1978) report enthusiastically on the use of intravenous feeding in patients undergoing intensive medical treatment for acute attacks of colitis. But for a proper assessment a controlled trial is essential, and this takes some time to organize and to produce results. Actually such a trial involving 40 patients with severe acute episodes of colitis has now been completed in Leeds (Dickinson et al. 1979). Unfortunately it has failed to show that intravenous feeding and total bowel rest made a significant difference to the prospects of securing a remission. It could, of course, be argued that it may have been of benefit by enhancing the patients' ability to withstand the hazards of the urgent operations which then became necessary, but this is difficult to establish.

8. The use of an elemental diet in severe attacks of colitis has also been suggested (Voitk et al. 1973; Rocchio et al. 1974; Axelsson and Jarnum 1977). It has some of the advantages of total parenteral feeding but avoids the risk of intravenous feeding. On the evidence available, which is based mainly on uncontrolled observations, I am not convinced that this diet has been clearly established on an objective basis to be of value in acute episodes of this disease, but it may well be of assistance in long-term nutritional support (Goode et al. 1976).

9. Though it now seems to be established beyond question that both corticosteroids and sulphasalazine are agents of definite value in the treatment of colitis and they are now at present widely used in medical practice, their very considerable limitations and drawbacks should not be forgotten. Even with their aid many patients with acute exacerbations of colitis cannot be induced to enter a phase of remission, as the surveys of Edwards and Truelove (1963) and of my own group (Watts et al. 1966b) have clearly demonstrated. It has been thought by some observers, such as Brooke (1956b) and myself (Goligher 1961b), that prolonged administration of corticoids in acute attacks of colitis, which have failed to remit, may allow the patient's local condition to deteriorate considerably under a mask of general improvement and predispose to the occurrence of colonic perforation. The evidence on this point is equivocal (see p. 713), but many surgeons retain a lingering suspicion, and it is probably wise in treating acute attacks of colitis not to continue corticosteroid therapy beyond 10 days if there is no obvious symptomatic and objective improvement in that time. Previous treatment with corticosteroids certainly introduces special problems into the conduct of surgical treatment (see pp. 746–8). But unquestionably the greatest weakness of corticosteroids or sulphasalazine is their inability, when continued as maintenance therapy, to prevent the occurrence of further attacks of colitis, and it is disappointing in the extreme to find that patients who have remitted during one attack—with or without steroids or sulphasalazine—eventually relapse and come to operation during a subsequent attack or as a result of recurrent ill-health. This failure of these drugs seriously to alter the long-term course of the disease has been well demonstrated by our survey (Watts et al. 1966d), for many of our patients who relapsed were on maintenance therapy.

MEDICAL MANAGEMENT OF AN ATTACK OF COLITIS

Because of confusion in initial diagnosis or the surgeon's special interest in this field, patients with acute episodes of colitis sometimes come immediately under his care. It may be helpful, therefore, to outline briefly the practical medical management of this emergency state (Watkinson 1962; Truelove 1964; Truelove and Jewell 1974).

A SEVERE ATTACK

General Measures. Dehydration, electrolyte depletion, hypoproteinaemia and anaemia require to be corrected by suitable infusion of fluid, electrolytes, plasma and blood. A high-calorie diet with plenty of first-class protein is desirable, but its ingestion may be rendered difficult by nausea and vomiting. Vitamin supplements are also advisable and may have to be administered parenterally. Barbiturate sedatives are useful to allay the patient's apprehensions and help him to get a reasonable amount of sleep, but opiates should be avoided because they are liable to blur the clinical picture.

Corticosteroids. Corticosteroids may be given *systemically*, either 10–15 mg of prednisone six-hourly by mouth or, if vomiting is a symptom in a severe fulminating attack, 100 mg of hydrocortisone intramuscularly every six hours or intravenously as a continuous infusion, 400 mg in 24 hours. Alternatively 40–60 units of ACTH (corticotrophin) gel may be given by intramuscular injection twice daily. If the patient can tolerate them, which he seldom can, *topical* corticosteroids are administered twice daily in the form of Predsol enemas, Retenemas, Cortenemas or Colifoam enemas.

Sulphasalazine. In a very severe attack sulphasalazine may be given in doses of up to 2 g six-hourly, as well as systemic and topical steroid therapy, or, if the attack is not so severe, the sulphasalazine may be used as a substitute for systemic steroids but in combination with topical steroids. Unfortunately some patients are unable to tolerate sulphasalazine in full doses because of frequent side effects—anorexia, nausea, vomiting, headaches, dizziness, skin rashes or anaemia.

Antibiotics. Antibiotics should be used with caution in colitis for they may aggravate the diarrhoea, if given orally, by causing irritation of the intestinal tract or predisposing to candidal or resistant staphylococcal infection. If there is a high temperature which may be due to secondary infection of the colon, a short course of broad-spectum antibiotic *given parenterally* may be beneficial (e.g. tetracycline 100 mg six-hourly or by intravenous drip for three or four days).

A MILD OR MODERATE ATTACK

Many patients with mild attacks, particularly in association with distal forms of proctocolitis or proctitis, can be managed with topical steroid therapy supplemented usually by oral sulphasalazine 1–2 g six-hourly and occasionally by prednisone 5 mg four times daily. This treatment can often be satisfactorily carried out in the home. When the patient becomes symptom-free, the enemas may be reduced in frequency from nightly to every other night for another two or three weeks, but the sulphasalazine should be continued at somewhat reduced dosage for several months—and perhaps indefinitely at a small dose of 0·5 g twice daily, as a sort of prophylactic against the development of further attacks.

SURGICAL TREATMENT OF ULCERATIVE COLITIS

Evolution of Surgical Methods

Perhaps the most remarkable thing about the surgical treatment of ulcerative colitis is the way in which it has evolved from the relatively minor operations of appendicostomy and simple ileostomy to its present extremely radical form, usually comprising excision of the entire large intestine. It is interesting to see how these changes have occurred (Goligher 1978).

APPENDICOSTOMY

This operation was first suggested by Keetley (1895) of the West London Hospital, and first performed by Weir (1902) of the Roosevelt Hospital, New York. It had the great virtue of extreme simplicity—a most attractive feature in any operation intended for very ill colitis patients—the appendix being brought out through a small gridiron incision which was then closed around it. Either at the conclusion of the operation or a week later amputation of the appendix was carried out 1 cm or so beyond

the level of the adbominal skin, and a fine rubber catheter inserted through the appendicular stump into the caecum and fixed in position by a silk ligature. An immediate irrigation was performed with 1–1·5 litres of a warm solution of sodium bicarbonate, a stout rubber tube being inserted into the anus beforehand to prevent accumulation of the fluid in the rectum and colon. The irrigations were repeated twice daily, the appendicostomy catheter being worn constantly to prevent stenosis of the opening. In some cases the appendicostomy was maintained indefinitely, in others it was allowed to close after several months or a year or so.

J. P. Lockhart-Mummery (1934) was one of the chief exponents of appendicostomy and stated that he had performed it on 79 cases of ulcerative colitis with 12 deaths but very satisfactory results in the remaining patients. In retrospect, however, it seems that many of the alleged cures with this operation were in fact examples of spontaneous remission of symptoms, which is such a characteristic feature of this disease. The 'last stand' of the appendicostomists in this country was made at a meeting of the Royal Society of Medicine in 1940 when Lockhart-Mummery, Gabriel and Norbury spoke in favour of appendicostomy, and Hurst, Ogilvie and Corbett strongly advocated ileostomy, which by then had taken firm root in America. Shortly afterwards appendicostomy dropped out of surgical practice in Britain.

ILEOSTOMY WITH SUBSEQUENT EXCISION OF THE LARGE INTESTINE

The logical step of performing ileostomy to secure a total faecal diversion away from the diseased colon was first suggested by Brown (1913) of St Louis (who at the same time incidentally established a caecostomy to allow irrigation of the large bowel). This operation only gradually found favour, but by the middle 1930s and early 1940s it had been adopted by several influential American surgeons such as Strauss (Strauss et al. 1924); Rankin (Bargen et al. 1932); McKittrick and Miller (1935); Cattell (1935); Cave (1939); Lahey (1941). Its acceptance in Britain took longer and was due to the advocacy chiefly of Hurst (1940), Ogilvie (1940), Corbett (1940, 1945) and Maingot (1942). At first it was hoped that by resting the colon in that way it might be enabled to recover completely, so that eventually the ileostomy might be closed, and patients were indeed sometimes induced to have the operation on this understanding. However, experiences such as those of Cattell (1948) showed that this was seldom possible without recrudescence of the disease, and it came reluctantly to be realized that the ileostomy had practically invariable to be permanent—hence the dictum 'once an ileostomy, always an ileostomy'.

Further, it was soon found that not only had the ileostomy to be maintained indefinitely, but in many instances some or all of the large bowel had to be removed as well, for a variety of reasons. Sometimes it was necessary because the patients did not make a full recovery of general health after ileostomy alone, or because metastatic complications such as arthritis or skin lesions persisted till all the diseased bowel had been removed. In other cases the continuance of a troublesome discharge per anum from the rectum and colon was the indication for colectomy and rectal excision. Finally the realization that there was an undoubted predisposition to carcinomatous change in the chronically inflamed intestine, as Bargen (1928), Cattell (1948), Counsell and Dukes (1952) and MacDougall (1954) among others so clearly showed, convinced most surgeons that the diseased bowel was safer removed as a routine than merely defunctioned by permanent ileostomy and the regular operative plan adopted by Cattell

(1948, 1953), Gabriel (1952) and many others, was a three-stage procedure consisting of ileostomy, subtotal colectomy with exteriorization of the sigmoid stump as a suprapubic colostomy and abdominoperineal excision, at intervals of approximately three months.

Ileostomy with Immediate Colectomy or Proctocolectomy

The next major advance in the surgical treatment of colitis was made by Miller et al. (1949) of Montreal, and Crile and Thomas (1951) of Cleveland, who suggested that combining colectomy with ileostomy as the primary procedure might have advantages. In severe colitis there is presumably a considerable amount of toxic absorption from the septic colon. In addition the diffusely ulcerated surface of the bowel with its constant discharge of exudate represents an important source of protein loss. Gardner and Miller (1951) claimed that up to 100–200 g of protein per day might be lost in this way. Our own estimates (Smiddy et al. 1960) are distinctly lower than this—not more than 30 g daily—but continued losses even of this order might produce considerable depletion in an ill patient. It seemed reasonable, therefore, to suppose that ileostomy with immediate colectomy, though inflicting a much more major operation on the patients in the first instance, might be followed by a more rapid and certain recovery than simple ileostomy. These advantages might be expected to be most evident in the more severely toxic cases, operated on during an acute exacerbation of the disease that had not responded to medical treatment, and for which experience in the past had shown ileostomy alone to be too frequently unavailing. The results claimed by Gardner and Miller (1951) certainly appeared to substantiate their contentions, for they were able to report 69 patients subjected to ileostomy and immediate colectomy with a mortality of only 4·4%. In their treatment of these cases the distal end of the colon was usually brought out as a suprapubic colostomy, and the colorectal remnant removed by abdominoperineal excision at a second operation, but in two cases the principle of primary excision of diseased bowel was pursued to its logical conclusion by removing the rectum as well at the initial intervention, so that the operation performed was an ileostomy with primary proctocolectomy.

Ileostomy with primary excision of the large bowel soon became widely accepted in the treatment of colitis in America and this country, and several large series of cases treated along these lines have been reported by Goligher (1954, 1961b, 1965), Scarborough (1955), Brooke (1956a), Cooper et al. (1956), Bruce and Cole (1962), van Prohaska and Siderius (1962), Waugh et al. (1964), Rhodes and Kirsner (1965) and Watts et al. (1966b). The opinion of surgeons, however, is divided as to the choice of technique for accomplishing this operation:

Ileostomy with Complete Proctocolectomy. In a sense this method, which is the one I prefer, is the more logical procedure of removing a disease that usually involves the greater part or all of the large intestine, including the rectum. If the surgeon is accustomed to the technique of synchronous combined abdominoperineal excision of the rectum for carcinoma, as is now commonly used in Britain, it is a simple matter to extend this operation upwards into the abdomen to provide also for complete removal of the colon and the creation of a terminal ileostomy. For surgeons not familiar with the synchronous technique of rectal excision there are several other ways of performing com-

plete proctocolectomy in one stage (see p. 753), or they may be wiser to do an ileostomy with subtotal colectomy in the first instance.

Ileostomy with Subtotal Colectomy. This method is preferred by many surgeons, the initial operation being confined to formation of an ileostomy and removal of the greater part or all of the colon, the top of the sigmoidorectal or rectal stump being brought out as an inactive suprapubic colostomy or closed by suture and dropped back into the pelvis. An undoubted advantage of this technique is that, if the surgeon does not normally do many rectal excisions, he will be glad not to have to combine excision of the rectum with complete colectomy in the same operation on a patient who may be pretty ill with colitis. Another argument often advanced in its favour is that it gives the disease in the rectum a chance to settle down, so that subsequent restoration of continuity may be possible (see p. 736). It could also be argued for ileostomy and subtotal colectomy that it protects the pelvic autonomic nerves from injury, which might result in sexual dysfunction, an important consideration in a young man, but this protection is afforded only as long as the rectum is left in situ. Temporary retention of the rectum to exclude with absolute certainty derangement of sexual function might have something to commend it under certain circumstances (but see p. 772 for further discussion). The chief drawback to ileostomy with subtotal colectomy is the persistence of a troublesome discharge of mucus and blood from the retained rectal stump that occurs in many cases and the occasional development of septic complications or very rarely of carcinoma. In addition the patient has to face all the physical and psychical trauma of yet another major abdominal operation if the rectal remnant has subsequently to be removed, which becomes necessary in over 10% of the cases according to Moss and Keddie (1965) and Binder et al. (1976). For these reasons ileostomy with subtotal colectomy was confined in my practice in the past mainly to those few patients who were deemed too ill to stand the additional strain of proctocolectomy in one stage, or could not make up their minds to accept a permanent ileostomy right away, but more recently I have made greater use of it mainly to keep open for the patient the option of a secondary ileorectal anastomosis (see p. 736) or even an ileo-anal pull-through operation combined with an ileal reservoir (see p. 738). The disadvantage of retaining the rectum is that it is somewhat unsettling psychologically for the patient, who continues to ask about the possibility of it being put into use subsequently and the ileostomy dispensed with. A full acceptance of ileostomy is more readily achieved when it is combined with a complete proctocolectomy.

Development of Technique of Ileostomy and Design of Ieostomy Appliances

INCONTINENT ILEOSTOMY

Pari passu with the introduction of the plan of treatment of ulcerative colitis by means of a terminal ileostomy and subsequent or immediate colectomy and rectal excision, there were significant changes in the technique of construction of the ileostomy itself and its after-care. Originally the method employed was to leave the terminal 5 cm or so of ileum projecting beyond the abdominal wall with a Paul's glass tube or a stout rubber catheter tied into it. After five to seven days the tube would separate, and by then a thick coating of granulation tissue had usually formed on the exposed serosal surface of the intestinal spout. Moreover the wall of the projecting portion of intestine would be quite oedematous and its lumen was often somewhat obstructed by the thickened wall. Over the next two weeks or so the granulation tissue became converted into fibrous tissue and contracted, the ileal mucosa being gradually everted and drawn down to the abdominal skin. Unfortunately this fibrous ring was very liable to undergo narrowing producing a troublesome stenosis at skin level (Fig. 540). The weakness of this method was the not infrequent occurrence of partial obstruction giving rise to the so-called ileostomy dysfunction (Warren and McKittrick 1951; Counsell and Goligher 1952), due to the initial intestinal oedema or subsequent fibrosis and stenosis (see p. 765).

Dragstedt et al. (1941) introduced the method of covering the peritoneal surface of the projecting ileum by Thiersch grafts to produce a *penile* type of ileostomy. These generally took well, and Black and Sholl (1954), who used this technique in 80 cases, reported favourably on it. Waugh (1952), however, found that in the long run, presumably due to the digestive action of the ileostomy fluid bathing the projecting spout of bowel as it dipped into the ileostomy bag, the grafted skin tended to undergo contraction, often leading to stenosis, and I myself had the same experience in a few cases treated by this method. A further report by Waugh et al. (1964) indicated that the skin-grafted ileostomy was the least satisfactory of several methods essayed by them. Monroe and Olwin (1949) and Wells (1952) used a method in which the projecting ileum was covered with a pedicle of abdominal skin, but this never became popular.

In 1951 Patey and in 1952 Butler advocated immediate suture of the cut end of the bowel and the skin in the construction of colostomies. In 1952 Brooke and in 1953 Turnbull adopted this principle of *immediate mucocutaneous suture* in constructing ileostomies, only they made the bowel project more, so that its terminal part had to be turned back to reach the skin. In the technique described by Brooke (1952) the whole thickness of the last centimetre or two or so of the ileal wall was everted and its cut edge stitched to the edges of the separate skin incision used for making the ileostomy. Turnbull's method (Turnbull 1953; Crile and Turnbull 1954) involved a preliminary excision of the serosal and muscular coats from the terminal portion of the ileum, so that the part turned back was merely the mucosa. It is difficult to discern any clear advantage in Turnbull's technique over the much simpler one of everting the whole thickness of the ileal wall. Admittedly, as the everted portion of bowel in the Turnbull method is denuded of its peritoneal covering, it is possibly more likely to adhere to the inner tube, so that recession or prolapse of the ileostomy but, which sometimes develop in ileostomies made by full-thickness eversion and primary suture, may be less likely to occur, but this is speculative. My own experience

of the Turnbull technique in a few cases impressed me with the tediousness of dissecting off the other layers from the mucosal flap and the risk of 'button-holing' the latter. More recently Turnbull (1975*b*) has introduced what might be regarded as a modification of this technique, in which, as an alternative to complete excision of the serosal and muscle coat from the terminal 5 cm or so of the ileal stump, these coats are simply snicked with scissors down to the submucosa with a series of criss-cross cuts before the end of the bowel is turned back for suture to the skin. Frankly, the theoretical advantages of this myotomy manoeuvre are not clear to me and I doubt if it will ever be widely used. Meanwhile the Brooke technique of full-thickness eversion and primary suture (see p. 757 for details) has become the conventional method of making ileostomies in most centres.

ILEOSTOMY APPLIANCES

All the ileostomies described in the preceding paragraphs are incontinent stomas, and an integral part of their management is the constant wearing of an appliance to catch the escaping faeces. In the early days of ileostomy surgery the appliances used were simple bags or boxes, which had an opening on their posterior aspect, which was pressed firmly against the abdominal wall immediately around the stoma. This arrangement was sometimes reasonably satisfactory during the day, when the patient was up and around, for, if the ileostomy projected beyond the abdominal skin, the discharge dropped immediately into the bottom of the bag. But at night, when the patient was recumbent, the ileal fluid in the bag tended to gravitate into the upper part of the appliance in contact with the ileostomy and skin, and leakage was common, making anything like a fastidious existence with an ileostomy impossible.

The great innovation that revolutionized ileostomy care and made ileostomy a really acceptable surgical procedure was the development of the *adherent ileostomy bag* by Koenig, a patient of Strauss (Strauss and Strauss 1944) of Chicago, who collaborated with Rutzen to produce the Koenig–Rutzen appliance on a commercial basis. The mental tranquility and feeling of confidence that this water-tight, leak-proof arrangement for collecting faeces engendered in the minds of ileostomy patients can readily be imagined, as can the enormous increase in the range of their activities and enjoyment of life. Needless to say, consequent upon the acceptance of the principle of the adherent ileostomy bag, many different patterns of appliance incorporating this idea have been marketed, and a full account of the types of bags now available is given on p. 767.

To stick the bags to the skin, reliance was at first placed on the use of proprietary cements, issued by the firms manufacturing the appliances, or of double-sided adhesive plasters. These forms of adhesion were found to be satisfactory in the great majority of cases, but when, as occasionally happened due to leakage of faeces, the skin around the stoma became red, sore and digested, these agents ceased to be effective and allowed still further leakage to occur, with progressive aggravation of the situation. One of the great advances in ileostomy care, designed to deal with this particular predicament, was the introduction some 12–15 years ago by Turnbull (1975*a*) of *karaya gum powder* (Sterculia gum or Indian tragacanth, derived from the tree or bush *Sterculia urens*, which is related to the cocoa tree), which, when mixed with a little water to produce a paste or with glycerine to form a *washer*, possesses the dual properties of being very soothing to an inflamed skin and of acting as an extremely efficient adhesive on such a raw surface. No recital of the salient steps in the evolution of colitis surgery would be complete without mention of this very practical aid. A full account of the methods of using various

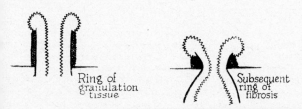

Fig. 540. How stenosis develops at skin level in ileostomies (and colostomies) fashioned by the now obsolete, simple projection, non-suture method. (*From Goligher 1954*)

adhesives to affix ileostomy appliances is given on p. 767. Another adhesive agent particularly effective on sore skin and soothing to such skin is the recently introduced proprietary preparation *Stomahesive* which is a compressed wafer of gelatin, pectin, sodium carboxymethylcellulose and polyisobutylene.

Finally, it should be pointed out that these developments in 'ileostomy' care have had their repercussion on colostomy care in which adherent appliances are being increasingly employed, at any rate in Britain (see p. 625).

CONTINENT OR RESERVOIR TYPE OF ILEOSTOMY

Unquestionably the most challenging development in regard to ileostomy in recent years has been the introduction by Kock (1969, 1971*a*, *b*, 1973, 1976*a*, *b*) of Göteborg, Sweden, of the so-called reservoir ileostomy. The principle of this operation is that instead of the patient wearing an external bag on the ileostomy to collect the faeces escaping incontinently from it, the surgeon constructs an internal bag out of the 45–50 cm of ileum immediately above the stoma and the faeces accumulate in it till they are evacuated by periodic passage of a tube. Ideally, in between intubations the ileostomy should be continent and no external appliance should be required, just a covering of gauze. Certainly when the operation works according to plan, the result is gratifying in the extreme, but the plain fact is that in practice the results have quite frequently proved disappointing because of failure to achieve continence or the occurrence of complications. Accordingly there is still considerable controversy as to the precise value of the reservoir operation and the best technique for performing it. The whole subject is dealt with in detail on p. 796, after consideration of the various aspects of the more conventional and established methods of surgical treatment for ulcerative colitis.

ILIAC OR TRANSVERSE COLOSTOMY WITH RECTAL EXCISION OR DISTAL PROCTOCOLECTOMY

Naturally in patients with colitis severe enough to require surgical treatment the disease has usually involved most, if not all, of the large bowel. But occasionally relatively distal procto-colitis or proctitis may reach sufficient severity to require operation. The question arises as to whether in such cases it may suffice to remove only the distal diseased portion of rectum and colon. If the disease is so localized that it can be circumscribed by an abdominoperineal excision of the rectum and distal sigmoid, leaving the patient with an iliac colostomy, this may possibly be preferable to having an ileostomy. But such cases are very rare, and the surgeon is always worried lest the disease should extend further proximally than he thinks at operation. In fact I have only five times felt sufficiently confident in operating for colitis to restrict my efforts to abdominoperineal excision, and two of these patients subsequently had to have the remaining colon excised because of reassertion of the disease in this part of the large bowel.

As for cases of more extensive colitis which, however, appears to spare the right and transverse colon, the treatment by distal proctocolectomy finishing off with a terminal transverse colostomy would seem to offer no advantages over a straight-forward complete proctocolectomy with ileostomy. A transverse colostomy is probably less manageable and less attractive to the patient than an ileostomy. There is a real risk of overlooking the

existence of disease in the right colon or of finding that it starts up later in this part. I have never employed this method in treating colitis, but I have seen two patients who had had distal proctocolectomy with transverse colostomy performed by other surgeons and in whom further colitis had developed in the right colon by the time they came to me some two or three years later. In one patient it seemed likely from the history that there had been disease in the proximal colon at the time of the original operation. Stahlgren and Ferguson (1959*b*), in a helpful paper on this subject, recorded 18 cases in which the proximal colon was retained at the initial operation for colitis. In 11 of these patients excision of this part was subsequently required because it became the seat of further colitis, but many of them went for several years before this became necessary.

COLECTOMY WITH ILEOSIGMOID OR ILEORECTAL ANASTOMOSIS

WITH ILEOSIGMOID ANASTOMOSIS

Lilienthal (1903), Reinhoff (1925) and Arn (1931) were the first to attempt the treatment of ulcerative colitis by ileosigmoidostomy with or without later excision of the intervening bowel. But it was Devine (1943; Devine and Devine 1948) of Melbourne who principally focused attention on the possibilities of anastomotic operations with retention of the functioning rectum and anal sphincter apparatus in this disease. He devised a method of conducting ileosigmoidostomy by an extraperitoneal technique, which seemed likely to be safer than a sutured anastomosis between the ileum and the diseased friable sigmoid colon. At the same time the other ends of the divided ileum and sigmoid were exteriorized, and at a later stage, after the external opening at the ileosigmoidostomy had been closed and the patient's general health considerably restored, the entire excluded bowel was excised. Though Devine (1943; Devine and Devine 1948) claimed generally satisfactory results with this operation, he gave no precise details as to immediate mortality, functional results or the subsequent progress of the inflamed rectal mucosa. Gabriel (1952) reported that in four or five patients, on whom he had performed Devine's operation with ileosigmoidostomy, severe symptoms referable to the residual proctitis compelled him to separate the anastomosis and establish an ileostomy. Corbett (1953) treated 12 patients with colitis by ileosigmoidostomy, there was one operative death, one case was too recent for assessment, two patients were failures, but eight were very well from six months to four years after operation.

WITH ILEORECTAL ANASTOMOSIS

More recently the chief advocate of an anastomotic type of operation has been Aylett (1953, 1957, 1960, 1963, 1966, 1970). His method of performing this operation has varied. Latterly he had preferred to use a simple end-to-end anastomosis between the end of the ileum and the top of the rectum, but the loop of the ileum immediately proximal to the junction is brought to the surface as a double-barrelled ileostomy to protect the suture line in the bowel for three weeks or so. A point on which Aylett (1960) lays great stress is that the superior haemorrhoidal vessels should be divided in preparing the rectal stump, for he believes that this step somehow assists in the resolution of inflammation in the rectum. He has apparently used colectomy and ileorectal anastomosis almost as his routine procedure in the surgical treatment of colitis. In 1963 he gave a detailed account of the results in 213 cases so treated by him and his colleagues at the

Gordon Hospital, London. There were 11 immediate post-operative deaths, (5·1%) and seven unrelated subsequent deaths. A fairly common late complication was acute intestinal obstruction due to adhesions. 13 patients have had to be converted to ileostomy for a variety of reasons, but 183 patients are rated as successful cases (10 with minor social limitations), and it is implied that most of them have not more than six motions in the 24 hours. This represents between 88 and 94% of highly satisfied patients. No full report is given in any of Aylett's (1953, 1957, 1960, 1963) papers of the sigmoidoscopic findings after ileorectal anastomosis. Further information on the outcome in Aylett's patients has been provided by certain of his colleagues. Price (1968) and Bell and Lewis (1968) comment on the high incidence of anastomotic dehiscence in these cases, which the former author finds unrelated to whether the patients had had steroid therapy or not, and which the latter authors claim is due to the use by the anaesthetist of neostigmine to reverse the action of relaxant drugs given during the operation (but see p. 437 for discussion). Jagelman et al. (1969) report on the findings of a postal enquiry conducted on 200 patients chosen randomly from Aylett's group of some 400 cases treated by colectomy and ileorectal anastomosis for ulcerative colitis. 174 replied to the questionnaire. Though roughly 25% still had six or more stools per day, over 90% of the patients considered that the operation had been an enormous success.

In this connection, however, it must be borne in mind that the term ulcerative colitis, as already pointed out (p. 698), is a misnomer: the condition is really a proctocolitis, for the rectum is nearly always involved. Consequently, if it is treated by colectomy and ileorectal anastomosis (or ileosigmoidostomy), this means keeping and using a diseased distal segment of large bowel, which might reasonably be expected to give rise to further trouble in a fair proportion of the patients. But what matters in medicine is not what should but what actually does happen, and the results obtained by Aylett with this operation have been so impressive that they have induced a number of surgeons in different parts of the world—almost against their better judgement in some instances—to give the operation a trial. It must be admitted right away that no-one has succeeded in reproducing Aylett's remarkable achievements with ileorectal anastomosis, and most of the results have fallen far short of those reported by Aylett and his colleagues. Thus when I tried the operation some 25 years ago (Goligher 1954, 1961b), I found, as have several others since, such as Muir (1959), Ault (1960), the surgeons of St Mark's Hospital, London (Anderson 1960; Baker 1970), Wangensteen (Griffen et al. 1963), Adson et al. (1972) and Grüner et al. (1975) that at least half the cases were failures and many eventually came to ileostomy. A feature stressed by Grüner et al. (1975) is dyspareunia in half their female patients so treated, with anal incontinence often triggered off by sexual intercourse. More favourable reports have been those of Fallis and Barron (1960), Barker and Ozeran (1963), Turnbull (1975a), Brown et al. (1962), Hughes (Watts and Hughes 1977) and Jones et al. (1977), but even Turnbull and Hughes have had failure rates of 25% and 21% respectively and have reservations about the results in a number of other cases. Turnbull (1966) thought that the eventual failure rate in his hands might well be about 50%.

Admittedly it is not easy to define what constitutes failure after colectomy and ileorectal anastomosis, for much depends on the attitude of the surgeon and patient towards the alternative of ileostomy. If the latter is regarded with abhorence, then the less than perfect results of ileorectal anastomosis will tend to be accepted as reasonably satisfactory, whilst, if it is recognized that an ileostomy is compatible with a full and active life, the results of ileorectal anastomosis are looked at more critically and considered in many cases to represent a less satisfactory

functional state than that of an ileostomy. Another difficulty is that most patients improve remarkably in their general health after colectomy and ileorectal anastomosis. Consequently, even if they continue to have rather severe changes in the rectal stump and to experience quite severe diarrhoea with up to 8–10 motions a day, they may none the less be so pleased with their overall condition that they are prepared to put up with this state of affairs indefinitely rather than have an ileostomy, against which they may have been warned rather vehemently before operation. I have now had to convert a number of patients to ileostomies following unsuccessful colectomies and ileorectal anastomoses for colitis, mostly done elsewhere. Without exception they have found the ileostomy a blessed relief from their incessant diarrhoea and have bitterly regretted not having proceeded to it sooner.

Some surgeons have proposed that most patients with colitis requiring operation should first be given a chance with colectomy and ileorectal anastomosis, on the grounds that, even if it fails in 20–50%, the failures can always be converted subsequently to ileostomy. There are three disadvantages to this plan. Firstly such a conversion operation may be technically difficult and is frequently associated with contamination and an unpleasant amount of sepsis. Secondly, there is the problem, already mentioned, of inducing patients with poor results to accept a further operation involving an ileostomy. And thirdly, if the disease persists in the rectal mucosa—which it did on routine sigmoidoscopy in over two-thirds of Watts and Hughes' (1977) 69 cases, including many with a reasonably satisfactory functional result—the patient is exposed to the undoubted risk of developing a carcinoma in the rectal stump. Griffen et al. (1963) have encountered this complication in two of 52 cases treated by colectomy and ileorectal anastomosis and MacDougall (1964) reported finding five carcinomas in the rectum and a series of 240 patients treated by this operation. Originally Aylett (1960) belittled this danger but in a recent publication (Aylett 1971) he admits that, of 350 patients surviving colectomy and ileorectal anastomosis under his care, seven have now developed rectal carcinomas. Most of these growths occurred in patients who had been followed-up for at least 10 or 15 years after operation. It seems probable that, when his entire series has been followed for a similar period since operation, more carcinomas will be encountered. Adson et al. (1972) reported the development of two rectal carcinomas, both fatal, in 34 patients followed-up for 6 to 21 years after colectomy and ileorectal anastomosis for ulcerative colitis, Grüner et al. (1975) had two carcinomas developing in 44 cases and Baker et al. (1978) noted the occurrence of 22 rectal carcinomas in 374 patients followed for 1–23 years. I feel strongly that the surgeon has a bounden duty in operating on patients with colitis to protect them from the risk of producing a colitis carcinoma, and that one of the weaknesses of colectomy and ileorectal anastomosis has been that it has hitherto failed to provide this protection. (But this may now be compensated for to a considerable extent by the possibility of being able to anticipate malignant change by rectal biopsy—see below—though these need to be carried out regularly and with good pathological cooperation to be of real value.)

The particularly frustrating thing about colectomy and ileorectal anastomosis is that it seems impossible to forecast with certainty which cases will do well and which badly with it (Baker 1970). Presumably those patients with relatively mild changes in the rectum should offer the best prospects for this method, though I know from my own experience that even they may fare badly and others surprisingly do well. Nonetheless it should be mentioned that there has recently been a definite revival of interest in this operation (Parks 1975; Hawley 1975; Jones et al. 1977; Khubchandani et al. 1978). My own practice at the present time is to reserve ileorectal anastomosis for such patients with lesser degrees of rectal involvement who are specially anxious to avoid a permanent ileostomy. The operation is performed preferably as a second stage procedure after a preliminary subtotal colectomy and ileostomy with retention of a sigmoido-rectal stump, but if done as a primary procedure it is *covered by a temporary loop ileostomy* (see p. 759) to lessen the risks of anastomotic dehiscence. It is highly desirable that after the operation the patient should be carefully followed-up and sub-jected to periodic sigmoidoscopy and rectal biopsy to detect the onset of changes of epithelial dysplasia which might signify a special predisposition to the development of carcinoma in the rectal stump (see p. 723) and indicate the need to proceed to rectal excision—if the patient can be induced to accept this proposal.

COLECTOMY AND PARTIAL RECTAL EXCISION WITH ILEO-ANAL 'PULL-THROUGH' ANASTOMOSIS

To remove the entire diseased large intestine in ulcerative colitis (or familial polyposis coli) Ravitch (1948) devised an operation consisting of complete colectomy, excision of the upper part of the rectum, and coring out the mucosa from the lower part down to the mucocutaneous junction in the anal canal. The terminal ileum was then drawn down through the bared tube of rectal muscle coat and anal canal and stitched to the anal skin (Fig. 541A). Ravitch hoped that sensory endings in the retained muscle layer of the rectum would be responsive to distention of the terminal ileum and that rectal sensation, so essential for anal continence, would thereby be preserved. He claimed very satisfactory functional results in actual practice (Ravitch and Handelsman 1951), as did Devine and Webb (1951), and Schneider (1955), though often only after a prolonged and complicated convalescence. Wangensteen and Toon (1948), Best (1948), and myself (Goligher 1951) on the other hand have found our patients after this operation to be severely handicapped by great frequency of defaecation and a good deal of incontinence.

Moreover, because of the presence of considerable fibrosis in the submucosa in cases of colitis, dissecting out the rectal mucosa could be technically extremely difficult in such patients. A few further cases treated by this type of anal ileostomy were reported by Drobni (1964) and MacDermott (1964) with generally satis-factory results, but most surgeons remained unconvinced and for the most part the operation has not been accepted in surgical practice. However, more recently Martin et al. (1977) have aroused interest in it again by their account of 17 young patients with ulcerative colitis submitted to this procedure. Fifteen patients achieved perfect continence, though several took 6–12 months to reach this very satisfactory functional state and still have very frequent motions, up to seven or eight per day. Martin et al. (1977) stress the importance of establishing a covering loop ileostomy until the ileo-anal anastomosis is well healed. However, Ravitch (1977) still remains somewhat disillusioned about the value of this operation for colitis, though he is more enthusiastic about it for familial polyposis, where the removal of the rectal mucosa, preferably from above, as in the Soave procedure for Hirschprung's disease (see p. 290), is much easier than in colitis. In some ways a more promising proposition would seem to be a *combination of an ileal reservoir or pouch (without nipple-valve) with an ileo-anal pull-through anastomosis* and covering loop ileostomy (Fig. 541B). Ferrari and Fonkalsrud (1978) have employed such an operation successfully and Parks and Nicholls (1978) have recently reported five patients with colitis treated along these lines with encouraging results (see pp. 814, 940).

OPERATIONS ON THE NERVOUS SYSTEM

Vagotomy was at one stage advocated by Dennis et al. (1948), and Eddy (1951) for the treatment of ulcerative colitis. It is, however, difficult to discern any convincing rationale for an operation on the nerve supply to the right colon for a disease that is usually maximal in the left colon and may indeed be confined to that side of the large intestine. It is well known that vagotomy for duodenal ulcer is often followed by quite troublesome diarrhoea, so that this operation might even be expected to exaggerate the symptoms of ulcerative colitis on occasions.

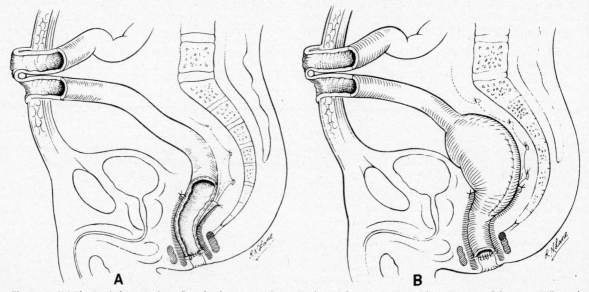

Fig. 541. (A) The Ravitch operation of total colectomy and proximal partial proctectomy, with coring out of the mucosa from the distal half of the rectum and pull-through ileo-anal anastomosis. (B) A combination of the Ravitch operation with an ileal reservoir.

The attempts made by Schlitt et al. (1951) to affect the course of ulcerative colitis by *operative division of the pelvic autonomic nerves* are mentioned only to be condemned, as likely to imperil bladder and sexual function in pursuit of a very dubious hypothesis.

Levy et al. (1956) subjected a group of five patients suffering from ulcerative colitis and associated psychiatric disease to *prefrontal lobotomy*, and reported that two went into remission of their colitis. More recently Bucaille (1962) has employed the less damaging technique of electrocautery to divide selectively part of the association fibres between the frontal cortex and the thalamic-hypothalamic system, thus avoiding the profound psychological disturbances of prefrontal lobotomy. Again a proportion of the patients thus treated improved, but without a large-scale trial with proper controls it is impossible to distinguish between spontaneous remission and that possibly resulting from the treatment.

Indications for Conventional Surgery

FOR ELECTIVE OPERATION

INTRACTABILITY AND CHRONIC INVALIDISM

This is the commonest reason for resorting to elective operation. In some cases the indication on these grounds is only too obvious, as when a patient with a history of severe colitis for several years presents in a state of extreme emaciation of Belsen type, with gross extensive changes in the large bowel on sigmoidoscopic and radiological examination, and often with local or systemic complications. Even the most conservatively minded of physicians would nowadays admit that the only chance of restoring such an individual to a reasonable state of health and a useful existence lies with surgery.

In certain other cases surgical treatment is just as clearly *contra*indicated. These are patients with mild distal forms of the disease confined to the rectum and possibly the distal sigmoid who, remarkably enough, often present first not to the physician but to the surgeon at his rectal clinic, because constitutional symptoms are often negligible, diarrhoea may be absent (indeed there may be constipation) and the main complaint is of bleeding as if from haemorrhoids. But the condition is quickly recognized for what it is on proctoscopy and sigmoidoscopy, and frequently the upper limit of the disease can be demonstrated at the latter examination. Generally speaking, no question of surgery arises in such cases as long as the disease is thus restricted, although occasionally severe distal proctocolitis or proctitis in elderly subjects or proctitis complicated by extensive abscess formation and fistulation may necessitate radical surgical treatment. However, it is important to appreciate that the idea advocated by Brooke (1954), that distal proctocolitis is a different disease

from ordinary ulcerative colitis and remains localized throughout its life history, is erroneous. There seems to be no essential difference in the pathological changes in the bowel wall in these two conditions, only a variation of the extent of involvement, and we know from our follow-up studies (Watts et al. 1966a, b) this is by no means fixed. Thus in no less than 36% of 50 patients who came to us in their first attack with proctitis alone, the disease eventually progressed proximally to produce total or substantial colitis, for which radical surgical treatment was sometimes required. If, therefore, one is not to slip up in one's management of patients with proctocolitis, it is important to be constantly alert to the possibility of proximal extension of the disease in this way.

Between these extremes of severe total colitis on the one hand and mild proctitis or distal proctocolitis on the other, there is a wide spectrum of patients with disease of varying degrees of severity and extent of involvement of the bowel, associated with more or less diarrhoea and constitutional disturbance, for whom the verdict for or against surgery has often in the past been a very fine one indeed. One of the difficulties hitherto in reaching a decision in these cases has been the lack of really reliable information regarding the outcome of continued conservative measures. However, this defect in our knowledge has been largely remedied recently by the careful follow-up studies of Edwards, and Truelove (1963, 1964) in Oxford, and of our own group (Watts et al. 1966c, d) in Leeds (see also p. 711), which show that, after an initial attack of colitis and often despite maintenance therapy with steroids or sulphasalazine, patients usually have further attacks. Indeed, if the follow-up is carried on long enough—say eight to ten years—virtually all patients have had one or more such additional attacks. These may be mild, moderate or severe (about a sixth of them turn out to be severe), and, contrary to the finding of Edwards and Truelove (1963), there is no close correlation between the severity of the first attack and that of subsequent ones. Our data have demonstrated that the patients most likely to develop severe attacks which medical management often fails to arrest, resulting in resort to emergency surgery with all the risks that this entails, are those *with total or near-total involvement* of the large bowel and those *over 60 years of age*. It is in these two groups of cases—particularly those with extensive or total colitis—that the need for elective surgery is most likely to arise. To patients with total or near-total colonic involvement I usually mention that operative treatment may eventually be required, but it is not till they have had one or more further major attacks that they are usually prepared to consider seriously accepting this recommendation. Furthermore, the follow-up studies of Lennard-Jones et al. (1977) show that many such patients may continue for a long time or indefinitely without coming to urgent or elective surgical treatment. With regard to patients over 60 years even with more limited disease, radical surgery may well be advisable, but the possible operative risks need to be carefully gauged. Frankly, I have been disturbed by the high operative mortality in older patients with a too liberal policy of surgical intervention and now tend to withhold operation unless strongly indicated on symptomatic grounds.

The seriousness of the decision for the patient for or against an ileostomy should certainly not be underrated. She is often young, in her teens or early twenties, and, quite apart from any other fears she may have about an ileostomy, not unreasonably (but usually wrongly—see p. 722) she may feel that it puts an end to all romantic aspirations. Without doubt the best way to allay her misgivings is to ask another patient—of the same age and social background—who has had an ileostomy established some time previously, to come and talk to her. Almost invariably, such a practical demonstration of the results of surgical treatment is successful in persuading her to accept operation. Indeed, such a meeting is an excellent preparation for any patient who is about to undergo ileostomy and colectomy, for it gives her an encouraging picture of what she may look forward to after operation, to sustain her through a convalescence that may sometimes be marred by troublesome and prolonged complications.

THE RISK (OR ACTUAL DEVELOPMENT) OF MALIGNANT CHANGE

Another reason that used to be advanced for not allowing patients with extensive colitis to drag on indefinitely on medical treatment was the risk of carcinomatous change. As pointed out on p. 719, this danger applied particularly to patients with total or subtotal colitis of 10 or more years duration, especially perhaps if the disease commenced in childhood, and, as the resulting tumours were apt to carry a poor prognosis, a case could be argued for advising a prophylactic proctocolectomy to this selected group of high risk patients (see p. 726). However, more recently the experience of Lennard-Jones et al. (1977) suggests that a reliable way of monitoring these patients on conservative lines is to carry out yearly sigmoidoscopic or colonoscopic biopsies and to reserve surgical treatment for those showing good evidence of epithelial dysplasia, which can be regarded as a pre-cancerous change indicative of a significant risk of carcinoma developing somewhere in the affected large bowel (see p. 724). I would now accept this policy for managing the potential risk of malignant change in colitis.

The occurrence of *signs that prove or strongly suggest the actual development of a carcinoma* may be the indication for operation in a patient who has previously rejected operative treatment. Sometimes there is no doubt about the diagnosis, as when a rectal stricture is present and has been shown by biopsy to be malignant. Then the only circumstance that might contraindicate operation is if the lesion were found to be grossly inoperable on clinical grounds. On other occasions, as for example when a localized narrowing of the colon is revealed on barium enema examination (see Figs 527, 528, 536B), the diagnosis may be more or less equivocal depending on the detailed radiological appearances. In the past under these circumstances abdominal exploration was undertaken in several of my patients and proctocolectomy performed, the subsequent pathological examination demonstrating that the strictures were in fact benign. But in more recent years colonoscopy has provided a histological diagnosis in such cases and avoided laparotomy. As pointed out on p. 718, the occurrence of multiple inflammatory polyps in colitis is not considered to carry any intrinsic risk of carcinogenesis.

POSSIBLE RETARDATION OF GROWTH AND DEVELOPMENT

In children or adolescents the possibility of physical retardation due to continued colitis must also be seriously considered and may be an additional reason for advising operation. Fig. 542 is a photograph of a girl who appears to be about 15 years of age, just reaching puberty. She is in fact a women of 24 who failed to grow or develop properly because of severe chronic relapsing colitis since she was 11 years of age. I only saw her a year before this picture was taken and removed a grossly diseased colon and terminal ileum, but as her epiphyses had already united there was no chance of further growth at that stage. This case certainly serves to emphasize the dangers of neglecting colitis in childhood. While it is particularly regrettable to have to advise an ileostomy to a young person, it seems to me that to allow a child to develop into a half-girl, halfwoman like this is far worse than inflicting an ileostomy on her. Actually, my experience, like that of many other authors (see p. 711), of colitis in young children and infants is that surgery is often required and that ileostomy is well accepted and seems to cause no particular psychological upset.

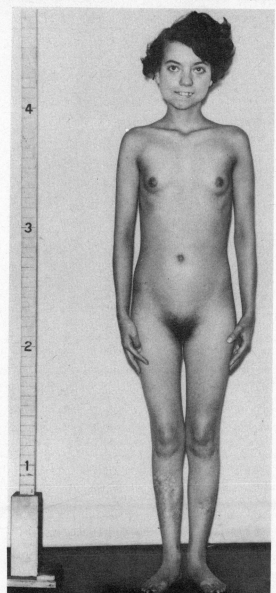

Fig. 542. This patient, who has the appearance of a girl of about 15 or 16 years of age, is in fact a woman of 24! She had colitis since she was 11 years old. Shortly after this photograph was taken she underwent proctocolectomy for it. Menstruation occurred for the first time after operation. Within 18 months she was engaged and has since married, giving birth to a child recently. Due to her continued small physique a Caesarean section was necessary for the delivery. (*From Goligher 1959*)

LOCAL ANORECTAL COMPLICATIONS—
FISSURES, ABSCESSES AND FISTULAS

These local complications often show a remarkable degree of spontaneous improvement as the colitis itself undergoes remission. Fissures and fistulas may heal or enter a quiescent phase causing the patient little trouble, though still producing a little puru-

lent discharge periodically. This gives the keynote in immediate management of these complications, which in most cases should be conservative (de Dombal et al. 1966*b*). Admittedly, abscesses may need simple incision for drainage, but often have already ruptured by the time they are recognized and may only require baths and dressings. For fistulas Jackman (1954) and Edwards and Truelove (1964) recommend local surgery, but my limited experience of such operations is that they are usually followed by very slow healing of the wound, which seems to depend largely on subsidence of the colitis. I would now always counsel expectant management in the first instance, whilst observing the course of the underlying bowel condition, and would postpone operation till the colitis showed signs of undergoing remission. Similarly I would advise conservative treatment for anal fissures as a rule.

In the long run these conditions are apt to recur coincident with relapses of the colitis, and eventually radical surgical treatment by ileostomy and proctocolectomy may be required. But this is usually determined largely by the state of the bowel lesion and only to a much lesser extent by the anorectal complications. However, in a few patients with these complications in a severe form—as for example with a rectovaginal fistula present—the colitis may yet be confined to the rectum and distal colon and there may be little constitutional disturbance. In such patients the anorectal infective complications may be the major consideration in deciding on radical surgery, and, because the general condition is so good, there may be great reluctance to accept this treatment. Bruce and Cole (1962) emphasize the dangers of perineal sepsis, if proctocolectomy is carried out in one stage in the presence of extensive perianal and perirectal infection. They recommended in these circumstances ileostomy and colectomy in the first instance, with later rectal excision. We have not had serious troubles of this kind with ileostomy and proctocolectomy.

REMOTE OR SYSTEMIC COMPLICATIONS

Remote complications such as arthritis (p. 727), skin lesions (p. 728) like pyoderma gangrenosum or erythema nodosum, and eye lesions (p. 729) may also subside as the colitis improves, but they may persist or recur till radical surgical treatment is undertaken. As indicated on pp. 728–9 thorough excisional surgery affords an excellent prospect of eliminating these manifestations of colitis. It is important to emphasize, however, that ileostomy alone, or even ileostomy and colectomy, sparing the rectum, may fail to bring about a resolution of the skin, joint or eye lesions. I have known such complications to persist as long as a diseased rectal stump was allowed to remain and to clear up dramatically after its removal.

FOR URGENT OR EMERGENCY OPERATION

Despite the introduction of steroid therapy and sulphasalazine for the treatment of ulcerative colitis, a fair proportion of patients suffering from acute episodes of this disease—either initial attacks or subsequent relapses—fail to achieve a remission of symptoms on conservative management, as is well shown by the reports of Truelove and Witts (1955), Edwards and Truelove (1963), and Watts et al. (1966c), Truelove et al. (1978). Under these circumstances the physician looks to the surgeon to undertake urgent operation. As pointed out on p. 710, the factors which seem to predispose to failure of medical treatment during an acute episode and to the likelihood of having to resort to urgent operation are: great severity and rapidity of onset of the attack, total involvement of the large bowel, and the age of the patient over 60 or less than 20 years.

TIMING OF URGENT OPERATION

There has been much controversy in the past as to when medical treatment should be abandoned in favour of urgent surgical intervention. One group of gastroenterologists—Gallagher et al. (1962) of Sydney—have, indeed, recommended that, in dealing with patients in severe attacks of colitis, medical treatment should be confined to a brief, three- or four-day period of resuscitation essentially designed to prepare the patient for urgent operation. But the great majority of physicians have preferred to make a determined effort to secure remission of the attack with the aid of steroid therapy and possibly sulphasalazine, together with other supportive measures, as outlined on p. 732. This has also been the policy pursued by us, in conjunction with our physician colleagues at the Leeds General Infirmary, in the treatment of most such cases. However, we have considered it important to recognize the limitations of this treatment and to be prepared to abandon it, after a set period, if there have been no clear signs of improvement in that time (Goligher 1961b). For a number of years we accepted 10–14 days as the limit, for it had been our experience that, if remission were going to

TABLE 59. *Outcome of Severe Attacks of Colitis*

Outcome	1955–63 (124 attacks)	1964–69 (134 attacks)
Remission	65 (52·4%)*	62 (46·3%)
Resort to surgery	40 (32·3%)	72 (53·0%)
Deaths		
Under medical treatment	6 (4·8%)	1 (0·7%)**
Operative	8 (20%)	5 (7·0%)
Total	14 (11·3%)	6 (4·5%)

After Goligher et al. (1970).
* Excludes a further 13 patients (10·5%) who were not brought to surgery but continued for over 12 months with chronic bowel symptoms.
** Death was due to status asthmaticus and was unrelated to the colitis.

occur, it usually took place by then. But a review of our experience in the management of these cases in the latter part of 1963 showed that we still had a disturbingly high mortality, and we resolved to make it our practice to intervene surgically at an earlier stage in severe attacks—say after three or four days if no unequivocal signs of remission were evident—in the hope of avoiding some of these deaths. During these few days the patient was given intensive steroid therapy as before. A comparison of our experience in the treatment of severe attacks of ulcerative colitis up to the end of 1963 and since then (Goligher et al. 1970) has shown a decided lowering of the mortality in the second period (Table 59). This applied to the operative mortality, which was reduced from 20 to 7%, and to the overall mortality, which dropped from 11·3 to 4·5%. A striking feature was that, despite the shorter period of preliminary medical treatment on average since 1964, roughly the same proportion of patients underwent spontaneous remission of their attacks as in the years before 1964. It would be tempting to attribute the improvement in the results to the change in the policy of treatment, but we have to admit that this may not be so and that instead the lowering of mortality may be largely or entirely fortuitous and due to a change in the character of the cases presenting with severe colitis to our service since 1964. However, the results at present being obtained by us with a fairly ready resort to urgent surgical intervention seem to us to be quite gratifying and we would feel disposed to continue with this plan of management. Flatmark et al. (1969, 1975) also report very encouraging results with early colectomy in severe ulcerative colitis as do Truelove et al. (1978).

RESORT TO EMERGENCY OPERATION

Apart from the need to resort to *urgent* operation at the end of a set period of intensive medical therapy, if remission has not by then occurred, an *emergency* intervention may be called for at any stage in response to sudden deterioration in the patient's general condition or the development of local abdominal signs suggesting that perforation of the colon has taken place, to the occurrence of acute colonic dilatation (which may be regarded as liable to lead rapidly to perforation), or to the onset of really severe haemorrhage from the bowel difficult to make good by blood transfusion. Clearly, these very ill patients require close clinical supervision during this probationary period of medical treatment, and there is much to be said for taking the surgeon into consultation from the very beginning. A very important precaution to detect toxic megacolon at the earliest stage is a plain X-ray examination of the abdomen on admission and again each day subsequently, even if there is no clinically obvious abdominal distension.

CHOICE OF OPERATIVE METHOD IN URGENT OR EMERGENCY OPERATIONS

When *ileostomy alone* was the elective procedure of choice for ulcerative colitis, it was naturally also the surgical measure to which the surgeon turned when called upon to operate urgently for an attack which had not remitted. Unfortunately, the results were often bitterly disappointing, for all too frequently it failed to halt the progress of the disease, and in many instances perforation of the colon took place even after the establishment of an ileostomy (Crile and Thomas 1951). The operative mortality of ileostomy done as an emergency procedure was thus very high, an average of 50% being found by Crile and Thomas (1951) in a survey of published statistics. It must be admitted, however, that some of the deaths were almost certainly due to ileostomy complications that would now be avoided or better treated, so that this operation might conceivably be attended by a somewhat lower mortality at the present time.

The introduction of the operation of *ileostomy and primary colectomy or proctocolectomy* appeared to offer hope of considerable improvement in the results of surgery in these more acute cases. It is easy to see the theoretical advantages of immediate removal of the diseased large intestine, if it could be accomplished without too much operative risk. This latter point is, of course, the crux of the matter, for some of these patients are extremely ill, indeed almost moribund, when they come to operation, and to advise an operation of this magnitude might seem to court a prohibitively high mortality for them. The earlier published reports of Gardner and Miller (1951), Crile and Thomas (1951) and Ripstein (1953) suggested that primary colectomy or proctocolectomy was in fact a safer and more reliable operation than ileostomy alone in these more acute forms of colitis. However, a great deal depends on exactly what sort of cases are included under the terms 'acute toxic' or 'fulminating' colitis, for the significance attached to these expressions seems to vary considerably from one author to another. Certainly some of the subsequent, more extensive, statistics relating to the results of primary colectomy or proctocolectomy for severe acute attacks of colitis have been much less impressive and have underlined that these operations carry grave risks. Thus Lennard-Jones and Vivian (1960) reported a mortality of 30·8% in 32 colectomies for fulminating colitis at St Mark's Hospital, London (elective mortality 4·4%); Brooke and Sampson (1964) had a mortality of 16·1% in 62 urgent colectomies at the Queen Elizabeth Hospital (elective mortality 6%). My own experience is similar (see Table 59), for I had an immediate mortality of 13·6% in 184 urgent or emergency colectomies or proctocolectomies for colitis (as against an elective mortality of 2·8). In extenuation of these results, it should be emphasized that all 184 patients were seriously ill, many of them being *in extremis*, and no less than 24 of them having one or more perforations of the colon. Under the circumstances it might be considered that the mortality figure was not too discreditable.

Most surgeons in carrying out urgent radical operations for colitis have preferred ileostomy and subtotal colectomy rather than proctocolectomy because it spares an ill patient the additional strain of a rectal excision. Having had many septic complications in connection with a retained colorectal remnant after subtotal colectomy—as well as a perforation of this part and severe haemorrhage from it—I have been strongly in favour of complete proctocolectomy in one stage (which is the method I have employed in 97 of my 112 cases). An additional advantage of this operation is that in certain patients coming to emergency operation the colitis may be confined to the distal half or less of the colon; if these cases are treated by subtotal colectomy, a considerable part of the diseased segment of the large intestine responsible for the patient's acute illness may be retained. Analysis of the causes of death in our 97 cases treated by urgent or emergency procto-colectomy does not suggest that the fatal outcome was due particularly to the use of this more major operation, except possibly in one instance, where postoperative collapse, attributed to adrenal in-sufficiency, was the lethal factor. It is obviously impossible to be sure, but apart from this single case it does not seem that the results would have been any better if ileostomy and subtotal colectomy had been employed instead of proctocolectomy. Provided one has a good organization for proc-tocolectomy, such as described on p. 748, and can perform excision of the rectum in a quick and relatively bloodless fashion, complete excision of the large intestine is, in my experience, remarkably well borne even by these very ill patients. But if the surgeon lacks good facilities and experience in rectal excision, he would probably be wise to avoid the more major operation and use ileostomy and subtotal colectomy instead in emergency cases. This latter operation will also occasionally be advisable even for the specially experienced surgeon when dealing with some particularly ill patients or if he accepts the policy of conserving the rectum as far as possible in the first instance in order to keep open for the patient the chance of a subsequent res-toration of continuity by ileo-rectal or ileo-anal anastomosis (see pp. 736–8).

As has been mentioned (p. 712), perforation of the colon is a not infrequent finding when operat-ing during severe attacks of colitis. This may be a frank opening from the bowel into the general peritoneal cavity leading to a diffuse faecal periton-itis, or alternatively it may be found that the part of the colon penetrated is firmly adherent to the anterior or lateral abdominal wall or to an adjacent viscus, so that the hole in the bowel is in effect sealed off and there is no general peritoneal contamination. With regard to *open* perforations, it is obvious that, whatever is done surgically at operation, postoperative peritonitis will be one of the major hazards and will require management as outlined on p. 441, including peritoneal irrigation at the conclusion of the laparotomy with, say, noxythiolin, and massive systemic antibiotic therapy during and after operation. Probably the best operative plan in these patients with open perforations is to press on with ileostomy and colectomy, making an effort to control further leakage of faecal material into the peritoneal cavity by the judicious use of the sucker inserted into the bowel in an upward and downward direction in the earlier stages of the operation, and by tying a sheet of some waterproof material round the colon at the site of the perforation as soon as it has been sufficiently mobilized to make this possible.

In dealing with patients with *sealed* perforations, however, obviously if a colectomy is performed, this will result in unsealing the perforation with conse-quent faecal contamination of the periton-eum—that is, unless a disc of the parietal periton-eum and the deeper layers of the musculo-aponeurotic tissues of the abdominal parietes adherent to the bowel at the site of the perforation can be excised en bloc with the colon. (This latter manoeuvre sounds easy, but in my experience leakage nearly always occurs before the disc can be completely freed.) An alternative plan in cases with sealed perforations would be to avoid colectomy and instead to return to minimal procedures such as ileostomy alone or caecostomy as suggested by Klein et al. (1960). It must be admitted that till recently the reported cases treated by these lesser operations in the last decade or two were too few in number to enable any firm conclusion to be reached as to their value, but, so far as they went, the results had not been particularly impressive. Thus, Brooke (1956a), who normally favoured primary colectomy, recorded six cases of emergency ileostomy with two deaths. Truelove et al. (1965) employed a double-barrelled ileostomy combined with instillation of steroid solutions into the colon in 14 emergency operations for colitis and had four failures (as indicated by operative death or by the need for a subsequent emergency colectomy). But in the last year or two Turnbull of Cleveland (Turn-bull et al. 1970) has lent the weight of his great authority to the use of this lesser type of operation in cases of sealed perforation and toxic megacolon. He has favoured a *loop ileostomy* combined with a *decompressing transverse (and possibly sigmoid)* colostomy (Fig. 543). The construction of the loop ileostomy to provide a stoma that is readily manageable by ilestomy appliances is described on p. 759. As regards the making of the decompressing transversostomy, this is done through a 5 cm long transverse incision dividing the upper part of the right rectus muscle and other tissues of the ab-dominal wall overlying the dilated proximal trans-verse colon. This incision is made whilst the abdomen is open. After closing the left paramedian exploratory wound, the distended transverse colon can be seen pressing up against the under surface of the right transrectus incision. The cut edges of the anterior rectus sheath in this wound are then sutured circumferentially to the seromuscular layers of the colon by means of a continuous very fine chromic catgut suture. A second suture of similar

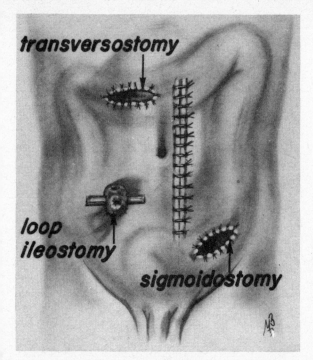

Fig. 543. Loop ileostomy and decompressing transversostomy and sigmoidostomy as advocated by Turnbull et al. (1970). This manoeuvre is specially suitable for patients with toxic megacolon and a sealed colonic perforation.

material now approximates the subcutaneous fat to the serosa of the colon within the ambit of the previous stitch. Next, the exposed transverse colon is aspirated with a stout needle and syringe and then incised transversely in the line of the skin incision, the cut edges of bowel being sutured to the cut edges of skin. If it is elected to make a decompressing sigmoidostomy, a similar technique is used for its construction.

Turnbull et al. (1970) described their encouraging results in 26 patients treated by diverting ileostomy and decompressing colostomy for severe attacks of colitis. There was only one operative death. Of the 25 survivors, four continued in a very ill state after the operation and between the twelfth and eighteenth postoperative days came to emergency colectomy without mishap. Another eight patients had to be readmitted during the next six months to undergo urgent colectomy because of re-activation of their colitis. Another 12 patients proceeded to elective colectomy after six months and one patient awaits this operation. Turnbull et al. (1970) emphasize that abscess formation at the site of former sealed perforations is common after

such subsequent colectomies and recommend the use of rubber drains to these sites, for periods up to 21 days after operation. In a more recent report Turnbull et al. (1977) state that 49 patients have now been treated by ileostomy–colostomy with only one death.

The Proportion of Patients Requiring Surgical Treatment

The proportion of patients receiving surgical treatment for colitis varies from clinic to clinic depending not only on how the balance is held between surgeon and physician in that particular centre, but also on the type of clinical material presenting, particularly as regards the number of milder cases of distal proctocolitis and proctitis being seen and the number with more severe colitis being referred from other hospitals specifically for surgical treatment. Thus operation was required in 26% of the series of 630 patients with colitis reported by Cattell (1948) from the Lahey Clinic, in 19% of Bacon and Trimpi's (1950) series of 249 cases at the Temple University, Philadelphia, in 48% of Wheelock and Warren's (1955) group of 483 cases at the Massachusetts General Hospital, in 21% of 400 cases at the University of Chicago (van Prohaska and Siderius 1962) and in 16·7% of 1230 cases at the Mayo Clinc (Waugh et al. 1964). In my own series of just over 1000 patients suffering from colitis of varying degrees of severity, ranging from proctitis to total proctocolitis, approximately 45% have come eventually to radical surgery, but many of these cases were referred to me specifically for surgical treatment after prolonged but unsuccessful courses of medical treatment elsewhere. Ritchie et al. (1978), on the basis of their survey at St Mark's Hospital, provide the interesting generalization that one patient in 50 with proctitis, one in 20 with moderately extensive colitis and one in three with really extensive colitis will require surgical treatment within five years of the onset of the disease.

Preoperative Treatment

This follows the general lines of preparation for any major intestinal operation, with special reference to the following points:

Correction of Anaemia and Depletion of Plasma Proteins by Blood Transfusion and Administration of Plasma. Most patients requiring surgical treatment for colitis are moderately or severely anaemic. For nearly all of them preoperative blood transfusion is necessary to bring their haemoglobin up to 11·0–12·0 g/litre, and unquestionably this is the most important single factor in making these patients fit for operation. Depleted plasma proteins may also provide an indication for plasma infusions.

Restoration of Electrolyte Balance. Estimation of the plasma electrolyte levels and correction of any imbalance by oral or intravenous administrations is essential, as patients with severe colitis may suffer serious depletions of potassium or sodium. It is in cases undergoing emergency operations during acute phases of the disease that the most difficult problems are encountered, for on admission to hospital many of these patients are grossly dehydrated and deficient in electrolytes, the plasma potassium level sometimes being below 2 mmol/litre. Less well known is the fact that they may also be depleted in calcium and magnesium (see pp. 763–4).

Intravenous Feeding. Patients with ulcerative colitis, who are so frequently suffering from gross malnutrition, would seem to be very appropriate subjects for intensive parenteral alimentation, and with the increased safety of intravenous feeding in recent years, this method of treatment has been more widely used in such patients. As pointed out on p. 732, there is no objective evidence available as yet to show that a regimen of total parenteral nutrition providing 'complete bowel rest', when combined with the other elements of conventional medical treatment for *acute episodes* of colitis, significantly enhances the prospects of securing a spontaneous remission. But if remission is not secured, surgery will be required and it could reasonably be argued that the patient might be better able to withstand the risks of operation if his nutrition has been assisted by intravenous feeding during the preliminary period of medical treatment (Hill et al. 1977). By the same token it could be claimed that in undernourished patients coming to *elective* surgery for colitis, a similar course of preoperative nutritional support by intravenous feeding or oral administration of an elemental diet would be rational and might prove beneficial. But to have a chance to be effective it would probably need to be prolonged and other factors such as the cost and economic inconvenience to the patient have to be taken into consideration. The routine use of these measures at any rate in elective colitis surgery will continue to be *sub judice* till harder data

on their cost-effectiveness are produced (see Allardyce and Groves 1974; Reilly et al. 1976).

Bowel Preparation. Obviously no attempt at mechanical cleansing of the colon by aperients or enemas is required, but bacteriological preparation by intestinal antiseptics, as in cases of carcinoma of the rectum or colon (see p. 449) is most important, because, however carefully the operation is done, the friable bowel is occasionally torn and the peritoneal cavity contaminated. Fortunately, sulphasalazine is a moderately efficient intestinal antiseptic and most of these colitis patients have been taking this drug as part of their medical treatment for some weeks before they come to operation.

Respiratory and General Exercises. Some of these patients are clearly too ill to be made ambulant before operation, as when urgent or semi-urgent colectomy is being undertaken. But whenever practicable it is a good plan to interrupt the phase of complete bed rest that has often prevailed in the medical ward by getting the patient up for a short period each day. This may help to restore the circulation in his lower limbs and reduce the tendency to postoperative pulmonary embolism. In addition general and respiratory exercises are initiated at this stage under the tutelage of the physiotherapist.

Finding the Best Site for the Ileostomy Bag. A very important preoperative measure is to affix the ileostomy bag to the abdominal skin at the site that would usually be chosen for the ileostomy (see Fig. 544), and to note how securely and comfortably it remains stuck in that position during a trial period of 12–24 hours. Whilst the bag is being worn in this way—preferably containing 100 ml or so of water—the patient should be as active as possible in order to give the fixation of the appliance a thorough testing during walking, standing and sitting as well as lying. As a result of this experience it may be found that a slightly different position may be preferable for the ileostomy. When the best site has been found the skin is marked to indicate this point as a guide to the surgeon at operation.

The Special Problem of Patients Who Have Had Previous Corticosteroid Therapy

Corticosteroids are now so widely used in the medical treatment of ulcerative colitis that it is extremely difficult for a patient suffering from this disease to reach the surgeon at the present time without having had corticosteroid therapy. Unfortunately this prior administration of adrenocortical hormones may expose him to certain additional hazards during the course of surgical treatment:

The Risk of Suppression of Normal Pituitary–Adrenal Responses leading to Postoperative Adrenal Insufficiency. Acute stress such as surgical operation in some way stimulates the secretion of corticotrophin by the pituitary gland and this in turn leads to an increased secretion of adrenocortical hormones. The therapeutic administration of these latter hormones, however, inhibits the normal mechanism, so that, after such treatment has been discontinued, pituitary and adrenocortical functions usually remain impaired for a time. During this period, though the adrenals may be capable of secreting enough corticosteroids to satisfy ordinary daily requirements, the response to stress is subnormal and severe stress may cause acute circulatory collapse or death from acute adrenocortical insufficiency. That this is a genuine hazard in practice is shown by the numerous reports of fatal or near-fatal cases with this complication (Fraser et al. 1952; Salassa et al. 1953; Lundy 1953; Harnagel and Kramer 1955; Downs and Cooper 1955; Hayes and Kushlan 1956; Allanby 1957; Slaney and Brooke 1957; Treadwell et al. 1963). As Salassa et al. (1953) and Graber et al. (1956) have pointed out, the period of impairment of the pituitary–adrenal response to stress after steroid therapy may persist for several months or even as long as two years. It seems a sound policy therefore that *any patient coming to operation who has had such therapy in the preceding two years should have full corticosteroid cover during the operative and postoperative period.* It is no less important to emphasize too that *the same corticosteroid cover is required if the patient should develop serious complications, such as intestinal obstruction, some time after the initial operation,* for there is a natural tendency to overlook this requirement, particularly if the second operation is undertaken in a different hospital.

Defective Healing and Impaired Resistance to Infection. The experimental work of Ragan et al. (1949) and Baxter et al. (1951) emphasized that intensive corticosteroid therapy exerted a deleterious effect on the healing of wounds and the resistance to infections in animals, but there is considerable difference of opinion as to whether these ill-effects apply in clinical practice or not (Thorn 1954;

Popert and Davis 1958; Slaney and Brooke 1958; van Prohaska et al. 1962; Kellner et al. 1963; Watts et al. 1966a, b; Jalan et al. 1970c). The evidence is equivocal and would certainly not justify withholding the intensive continued corticosteroid therapy necessary to obviate the risk of postoperative adrenal insufficiency.

SCHEDULE OF DOSAGE RECOMMENDED FOR CORTICOSTEROIDS DURING THE OPERATIVE PERIOD

The patient will probably be having some form of oral corticosteroid preparation up to five hours or so before operation. This is changed to parenteral administration of hydrocortisone hemisuccinate to cover the actual operation and the first few postoperative days till feeding by mouth is well reestablished. The plan followed by me is to give 100 mg of hydrocortisone intramuscularly six-hourly, commencing the morning of the day of operation or the evening before. In addition 100 mg of hydrocortisone is administered with the anaesthetic premedication, and if desired another 100 mg may be given in the intravenous drip infusion during the operation itself.

When oral corticosteroids are recommenced after operation, say about the fourth or fifth day in the average uncomplicated case, a dosage of prednisone 15 mg is given six-hourly (or its equivalent in other preparations) for five or six days. The dose is then reduced to 15 mg twice daily for four or five days, and thereafter tailed off over a period of two weeks or so, provided that the convalescence is entirely uneventful. The occurrence of any significant complication which might increase the demands on the adrenals calls for a temporary increase in steroid medication.

MANAGEMENT OF ACUTE ADRENOCORTICAL INSUFFICIENCY

Acute adrenocortical failure may arise postoperatively in patients who have had prolonged steroid therapy and not been protected by adequate cover during and after operation. It is readily recognized by the development of severe hypotension unassociated with other causes—such as gross dehydration, uncorrected haemorrhage, or infection—and unresponsive to the normal measures of blood volume replacement. It is often accompanied by acute gastric dilatation, lassitude and drowsiness. The only condition likely to be confused with it is an acute staphylococcal enterocolitis which may produce a similar state of collapse. If an eosinophil count is done, it is found to be high (100–200/ml³) in acute adrenal failure, by contrast with the normal state of affairs after operation, when the count is below 50/ml³. The condition calls for energetic treatment by intravenous hydrocortisone, 400 mg being given in 500 ml of normal saline, plasma or dextran. If adrenocortical failure is the cause of the shock, the response is usually rapid, and the blood pressure is restored to a normal level within 15–20 minutes. The subsequent management consists in the institution of adequate corticosteroid cover for the rest of the postoperative period as outlined above. Rarely the response to hydrocortisone is much less dramatic and dosages of up to 600 mg to 1 g may have to be employed and supplemented by a noradrenaline drip infusion.

Conventional Operative Technique

ILEOSTOMY WITH PROCTOCOLECTOMY OR SUBTOTAL COLECTOMY

POSITION OF THE PATIENT

If the surgeon is familiar with the synchronous combined technique for abdominoperineal excision of the rectum, as described on p. 525, it is a simple matter to adapt it to the needs of a total proctocolectomy. This greatly facilitates the performance of this extensive operation which can then

usually be completed without haste in 2–2¼ hours. The patient is placed in exactly the same position as for a purely rectal excision by the synchronous method with the thighs strongly abducted on Lloyd-Davies leg rests, the sacrum resting on a special sacral support, and the shoulders held in place by shoulder rests, permitting the assumption of a moderate Trendelenburg tilt. In addition, however, to facilitate the exposure and mobilization of the right and left halves of the colon, and particularly the colic flexures, during the colectomy, it is an advantage, if not absolutely essential, to have the patient tilted in turn to one side and then the other. A table capable of a 25–30° lateral tilt is thus desirable. To prevent the patient slipping sideways off the table during these manoeuvres it is necessary to fit side supports to hold the trunk firmly in position. The general arrangement of the instrument tables, sterile towelling, assistants and lighting is as for synchronous combined rectal excision, but during the respective halves of the colectomy it is essential to have a light stationed behind the surgeon and shining into that section of the abdominal cavity in which the dissection is then taking place.

If the synchronous technique is not being used, the legs will be placed flat on the table, with the knees correctly positioned and shoulder rests fitted, so that a Trendelenburg tilt can be assumed during the abdominal dissection for removal of the rectum, as in the Miles operation. The arrangements for lateral tilting of the patient and for side lighting are as already described. During the perineal phase of the rectal excision the patient has to be moved on to

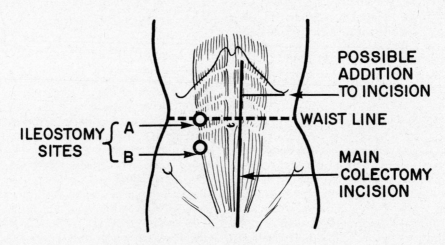

Fig. 544. The main incision used for primary colectomy or proctocolectomy and the sites favoured for the ileostomy.

his side or placed in an exaggerated lithotomy position.

INCISION

A long left paramedian rectus-displacing incision extending from the pubis almost to the costal margin gives excellent access as a rule to all parts of the colon and the rectum, particularly if side tilting is used as required (Fig. 544); but a median incision skirting the umbilicus on the left side is also satisfactory. It is often said that in severe ulcerative colitis requiring operation the shrinkage of the colon draws the colic flexures down from underneath the lower ribs and renders them more accessible to the surgeon (see Fig. 523), but in my experience this is only occasionally true. Usually the flexures lie in their normal position and require the same steps to facilitate their safe exposure as are employed in operations for carcinoma coli. However, only very rarely is it necessary to supplement this long vertical incision by a transverse cut across the left rectus muscle to facilitate the access to a particularly high and difficult splenic flexure.

ASSESSMENT OF THE EXTENT OF THE DISEASE

A word of warning is necessary regarding the interpretation of the operative findings in ulcerative colitis, for they may be most misleading. In the majority of cases the diseased bowel, as seen from the serosal aspect, has a highly characteristic appearance compounded of a dead white pallor of the overlying coat and the presence of numerous leashes of fine tortuous vessels ramifying in this coat (Plate IV). After the bowel has been handled a few times these appearances may give way to a diffuse blush with many minute ecchymoses (Plate IV). In addition the affected colon usually feels thickened and firmer than normal on palpation, though very gross thickenings should suggest rather Crohn's type of enteritis. Another feature that may be noted is the presence of enlarged soft glands in the lower ileal mesentery and ileocaecal region when proximal colon is affected. But in other cases, bowel which the radiological examination has shown to be extensively diseased may, on first opening the abdomen, appear and feel quite normal. This discrepancy may apply to the greater part of the large gut, but is more often noted in the right colon, which may make it difficult to determine the proximal limit of the disease process with accuracy. As mentioned on p. 704, the radiological findings in colitis are not always absolutely reliable, but I would say that in general they are distinctly more trustworthy than the evidence provided by laparotomy. My advice therefore would always be to proceed on the basis of the radiological and clinical assessment and not to be misled into rejecting ileostomy and colectomy and adopting any more limited operation. This temptation may arise particularly when all but the sigmoid, or sigmoid and lower descending colon, appears normal, and it might seem that the condition could be adequately treated by transverse colostomy with or without excision of the rectum and distal colon. Experience shows, however, that, when this has been done, the colostomy, which was thought to be entirely above the colitis, is often placed in diseased bowel and even when it is clear of the disease the colitis may make its appearance later in the proximal colon. Altogether, then, the surgeon would be most unwise to depart from the preconceived plan of ileostomy and proctocolectomy or subtotal colectomy with which the laparotomy was commenced.

Nowhere perhaps is the difficulty in detecting evidence of the disease on examination at laparotomy greater than in the terminal ileum. Though a retrograde ileitis occurs in about a sixth of all cases of diffuse ulcerative colitis, this involvement is only occasionally revealed by visible changes on the serosal aspect or by an alteration in the texture of the ileal wall on palpation. However, it is a simple matter to inspect the mucosa of that part of the terminal ileum attached to the excised colon immediately after removal, and if it is diseased up to the proximal limit of the operative specimen another 5 or 7.5 cm of ileum may be resected and similarly examined, the process being repeated as required. I am not convinced that the alternative scheme, favoured by Dennis and Karlson (1952), of preparing a frozen section of the ileum for histological examination gives any more reliable information than simple macroscopic inspection. Indeed for many years I did not bother particularly to ensure that the ileostomy had been accurately sited proximal to the upper limit of any retrograde ileitis, for I had noted that in two cases in which it was inadvertently placed in diseased ileum, no harm seemed to result, the patients doing well, and the ileitis rapidly clearing up. Brooke (1956a) has had a similar experience (but see also p. 779). More recently, however, because of the greater frequency of Crohn's disease and difficulty often experienced in distinguishing between it and ulcerative colitis till the specimen is examined postoperatively, I have been careful to avoid leaving any macroscopically abnormal ileum, in case it should be the seat of a Crohn's enteritis.

THE GENERAL CONDUCT OF THE COLECTOMY

The technique for removal of the colon is merely a combination of right and left hemicolectomy for carcinoma as described on pp. 453, 456, the only essential difference being that, as the lymphatics need not be removed widely, it suffices to divide the colic vessels and the medial leaves of the peritoneum and the mesocolon quite close to the bowel. Similarly most of the greater omentum may be left attached to the stomach. Each half of the colectomy is completed in turn before altering the patient's position for the second side, though, of course, the transverse colon is not at any stage divided. It is unnecessary to attempt reperitonealization of the areas of the posterior abdominal wall denuded of peritoneum by the removal of the colon. It is a great assistance in the conduct of the colectomy if, as a preliminary, *the small gut is turned out of the abdominal cavity and enclosed in a plastic Lahey bag*, as described on p. 532. Then, as the surgeon is working in different parts of the abdomen in turn, the small intestine is readily displaced to the opposite side.

COMPLETION OF THE OPERATION AS A SUBTOTAL COLECTOMY

If after the colon has been completely mobilized down to the lower sigmoid, the patient's condition is such as to suggest that removal of the rectum at this stage would carry considerable risk, or if for any reason it is desired to retain the rectum in the first instance, the operation will be finished as a subtotal colectomy. The simplest way of doing so is to divide the sigmoid between Cope's clamps about its middle or a little lower, allowing the proximal part to be removed along with the rest of the colon, whilst the distal end is brought out at the lower extremity of the main paramedian wound as a suprapubic colostomy (Fig. 545). This method is quick and easy, avoids all pelvic dissection and leaves no suture line in the abdomen which might leak. Unfortunately, a certain amount of sepsis in the abdominal wall in the vicinity of the colon stump is not an uncommon occurrence in my experience. The colorectal remnant may be removed by abdominoperineal excision three or four months later, or alternatively may be left indefinitely to see if the disease subsides in this segment.

An alternative method, which I have used occasionally when the disease in the rectum and lower sigmoid has been relatively slight, consists in dividing the bowel at, or slightly above the rectosigmoid junction, so that there is an intraperitoneal stump which is closed and invaginated by suture in the same way as a duodenal stump in a Polya gastrectomy (see Figs 483–5). The superior haemorrhoidal vessels may be divided as in preparing the

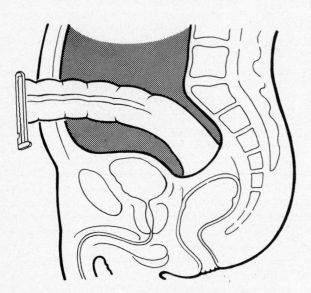

Fig. 545. The method of completion of colectomy by exteriorization of the terminal sigmoid still attached to the rectum as a suprapubic colostomy.

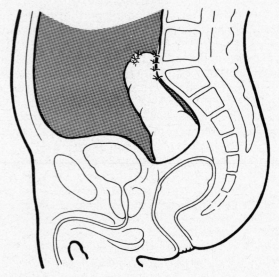

Fig. 546. Termination of subtotal colectomy by division of bowel at or just above the sigmoidorectal junction, with closure of the stump by suture and its fixation by further sutures to the tissues of the posterior abdominal wall to facilitate subsequent ileorectal anastomosis, if this should be considered desirable.

rectal stump for a high anterior resection (see p. 573), or kept intact as in preparing the rectum for an ileorectal anastomosis for familial polyposis (see p. 366). I have usually left a suprapubic drain down to the closed upper end of the rectum for a few days. Subsequent rectal excision necessitates an abdominoperineal approach. Because of the possibility of a secondary ileorectal anastomosis being performed instead, it is perhaps well to suture the top of the sigmoidorectal stump to the posterior or anterior abdominal wall with a few silk sutures to prevent it receding into the pelvis and keeping it more readily available for such an anastomosis (Figs 546, 547).

COMPLETION OF THE OPERATION AS A TOTAL PROCTOCOLECTOMY

If, on the other hand, it is decided to proceed with removal of the entire rectum along with the colon, this may be accomplished in several ways:

*As a Straightforward Synchronous Combined Abdominoperineal Excision.** If the patient has been positioned to allow simultaneous abdominal and perineal operating, the operation is rapidly completed by a

---

* In recent years, when performing elective complete proctocolectomy on patients whose fitness for the whole operation has never been in doubt, it has been my practice to make rectal excision the first step and to proceed therefrom proximally, finishing with the fashioning of the ileostomy.

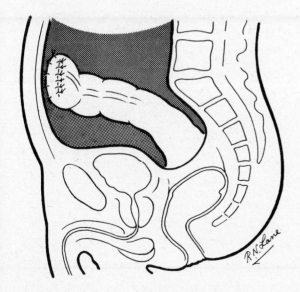

Fig. 547. Fixation of the closed sigmoidorectal stump to the anterior abdominal wall by suture.

synchronous combined rectal excision more or less as described on p. 525. It is specially important, however, in young male patients to *make every effort to avoid injury to the autonomic nerves, which might result in sexual dysfunction.* Thus, during the isolation and ligation of the superior vascular pedicle, which is usually carried out just below the level of the aortic bifurcation, the vessels should be carefully separated from the underlying presacral nerve. Subsequently, after division of the pedicle and whilst the rectum is being lifted forward off the point of the sacrum, it is important to brush the two terminal branches of the nerve off the back and sides of the bowel to avoid the risk of them being torn when the hand is inserted into the sacral cavity during the posterior dissection. It is, unfortunately, not possible to be so certain about excluding injury to the parasympathetic nerves, but the separation of the rectum from the sacrum and coccyx is better carried out entirely by the abdominal operator, who usually strikes a plane closer to the bowel—and, therefore, less likely to damage the sacral autonomic nerves—than does the perineal operator. Similarly the lateral ligaments are divided by the abdominal operator as close as possible to the rectum to lessen the chance of injuring the parasympathetic fibres on the pelvic side wall.

The perineal phase of the dissection is also best conducted essentially as in the operation for carcinoma, though there is no necessity to take a particularly wide sweep of tissue. The coccyx may be removed or left as desired; the posterior vaginal wall should be preserved if possible in younger patients unless rectovaginal fistulation makes this impossible. The pelvic phase is then completed by suture of the pelvic peritoneum by the abdominal operator and by partial or complete suture of the perineal wound, with open or closed drainage or a pelvic pack, depending on the adequacy of the haemostasis and the occurrence of faecal or purulent contamination during the operation (see also p. 556).

A more conservative type of section may also be considered. Many years ago I experimented with a perineal technique for colitis cases which left the levator muscles and anal sphincters intact. Through a circumcision close to the anus the lining of the anal canal was dissected off the underlying internal sphincter to the upper end of the canal. The rectal muscle coat was then divided all round to enter the plane of the pelvic dissection reached from above. Unfortunately drainage from the pelvis through the intact sphincters was often impeded and convalescence thereby prolonged. Also tearing of the anal canal during the dissection was a not uncommon occurrence, with resulting contamination and sepsis. As a consequence I abandoned this technique. But recently Fonkalsrud and Ament (1978) have employed an extension of this technique, preserving not only the sphincters but also the rectal muscle coat up to the level of the anterior peritoneal reflection, the mucosal tube being dissected out mainly from above. They claim encouraging results in five cases.

Recently Lytle and Parks (1977) have similarly advocated a more conservative perineal phase, the

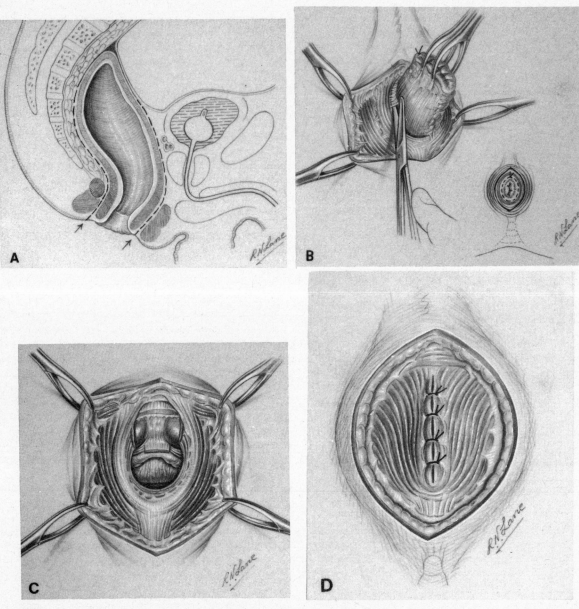

Fig. 548. Intersphincteric dissection for perineal phase of rectal excision for inflammatory bowel disease. (A) The plane of dissection. (B) The purse-string suture of the anus followed by a close oval incision and subsequent dissection up between the sphincters. (C) The resulting wound after the rectal excision has been completed, showing the intact external sphincter and levator musculature. (D) Suture of sphincter muscles, preparatory to complete closure of the skin wound. Two sump drains are inserted into the pelvic cavity from the suprapubic region.

plane of dissection from below being taken, not between the anal lining and the internal sphincter, but between the internal and external sphincters. The steps of this *intersphincteric technique* of perineal dissection are depicted in Fig. 548. The perineal wound is finally closed completely by suture, suction drainage of the pelvic cavity being secured by two sump suction drains inserted suprapubically or through the perineum lateral to the wound. This technique is not as easy to perform as might be inferred from Fig. 548. One of the difficulties is that the access to the pelvis from below for purposes of haemostatis is much more limited than when the plane of dissection is outside the sphincters. Contamination from tearing of the rectal wall during the operation is also not uncommon, predisposing to subsequent sepsis. Lytle and Parks (1977) claim for this intersphincteric technique of perineal dissection that it is less liable to be followed by neurogenic impairment of sexual function but their data are far from convincing to me on this point. It would seem likely that if there is any reduction in the incidence of sexual dysfunction in their cases it is due rather to keeping the pelvic dissection from above specially close to the rectum, for disorders of sexual function after rectal excision can occur after low anterior dissection, when there is no perineal dissection at all.

As a Miles Operation. When the synchronous technique is not being used it is probably best to carry out rectal excision by the classical Miles method as described on p. 561. With the patient in the Trendelenburg position, the colon is divided between Cope's clamps in the lower sigmoid, the proximal portion being removed with the rest of the mobilized colon. The inferior mesenteric vessels are then ligated and divided and the sigmoidorectal remnant is dissected free on all aspects as far as the anorectal junction, turned down into the presacral space, and covered over by suture of the pelvic peritoneum. Finally, after bringing out the ileal stump, the abdomen is closed and the patient turned on her side for the perineal dissection. The completion of the ileostomy is postponed till after this dissection or can be done earlier if desired, with a change of instruments before doing the perineal phase.

As an Extended Hartmann's Operation with Immediate or Later Removal of the Anal Canal. A third possibility is to remove the rectum as far as possible from the abdomen by an extended Hartmann's operation, with which it is sometimes possible by vigorous traction on the bowel to reach almost to the anal orifice. The peritoneum is then reconstituted over the pelvic cavity, drainage being provided through the remnant of the anal canal. Alternatively, at the conclusion of the laparotomy the mucocutaneous lining may be cored out of the tiny anal stump from below, as recommended by Fallis and Baron (1953). My criticism of these techniques is that it is almost impossible to avoid contamination in the pelvis when the bowel is divided and, further, that they are liable to be followed by poor drainage from the pelvic cavity through the anal canal, unless the intact sphincters are divided.

CONSTRUCTION OF THE ILEOSTOMY

The importance of meticulous care in making the ileostomy cannot be overestimated for successful ileostomy management commences in the theatre with proper fashioning of the ileostomy itself, and no amount of attention lavished on the subsequent fitting of ileostomy appliances can atone for serious errors of operative technique at this stage. The following are the points demanding closest consideration:

The Site of the Ileostomy

It is essential to place the ileostomy so that there is an area of flat smooth skin all round it to which the ileostomy bag may be securely stuck. This means that it should not be made in the line of the main wound, the scar of which above and below might make the subsequent attachment of the ileostomy bag more difficult, but a separate stab wound, an adequate distance away from the main incision and from the umbilicus and anterior superior iliac space. As already explained on p. 746, the *exact site for the ileostomy will have been chosen preoperatively* with these considerations in mind and thoroughly tested for its suitability as regards fixation of the appliance before the patient comes to operation. I think that for really secure fixation of the bag the best place to put the ileostomy is in the waist line, lateral to the umbilicus and opposite the outer third of the right rectus muscle (Fig. 544A), for in this situation the appliance can be very firmly supported by a belt or corset as a reinforcement or substitute for adhesives. However, most patients object to this site because it interferes with the use of the waist for suspending clothing, and—a very important consideration for women anxious to wear tight-fitting dresses—it spoils the waist-line of their figure. An alternative site, frequently chosen therefore, is one a little lower down (Fig. 544B), but it suffers the disadvantage that tightening of the supporting belt tends to pull the bag upwards out of place. Also this situation may be distinctly concave in many emaciated colitis patients when they have their operation, so that the fixation of the ileostomy bag here may at first be very troublesome till they put on some weight. It is important, too, to make sure that the ileostomy is not so low that when the right hip is flexed to less than a right-angle, as in sitting on a low chair, the lower edge of the flange of the appliance is not pushed up by the front of the thigh against the ileostomy bud, with resulting damage (see p. 776).

Making the Ileostomy Wound

The best type of wound for the ileostomy is a circular or 'trephine'-shaped wound with removal of a disc of skin and subcutaneous fat and cruciate division—or even disc-removal if preferred—of the musculoaponeurotic structures and peritoneum of the abdominal wall. It is important to bear in mind that, in the presence of a vertical abdominal wound, the oblique and transverse abdominal muscles undergo considerable lateral retraction and to correct this tendency by catching with forceps the layers of the abdominal wall revealed in the right edge of the paramedian wound opposite to the proposed site of the ileostomy, drawing them well to the left before making the actual ileostomy wound. Another way of avoiding distortions of this kind is to make the ileostomy wound as the first step of the operation, before the abdomen is opened. But I have not usually done this because I find it a convenience to have the abdominal wall pushed well forwards by the fingers of the left hand or the end of a proctoscope inside the abdomen at the site of the trephine wound; this facilitates the division of the layers and helps in the control of bleeding.

Some surgeons such as Rapaport (1956) use a metal tube with a sharp edge at one end like a corkborer to make the wound, but I find it quite easy to create a satisfactory opening with scalpel and dissecting forceps. First of all, a cone of skin and subcutaneous fat is lifted up with the forceps and amputated so as to leave a skin wound approxi-

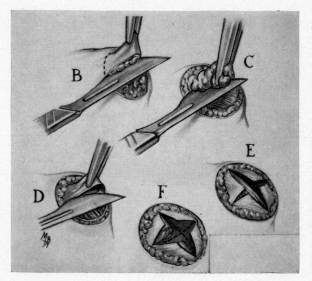

Fig. 549. Making the ileostomy wound. The cut right edge of the main paramedian wound is held taut with artery or tissue forceps. The surgeon is standing on the left side of the patient. (A) A disc of skin is excised at the approved site lateral to and just below the level of the umbilicus. (B) The subcutaneous fat is similarly removed baring the external oblique aponeurosis (C). If desired a disc of the anterior rectus sheath may now be excised (D), followed in due course by similar removals from the rectus muscle and posterior rectus sheath to produce a 'trephine wound' through the abdominal wound. Alternatively the musculoaponeurotic layers may be simply incised in cruciate fashion, which is simpler (E and F). (A, *from Goligher 1958*)

mately 2·5 cm in diameter (Fig. 549A, B). The remaining fat is then treated in the same way, (Fig. 549C) and, possibly with a little additional dissection, the aponeurosis is completely bared of subcutaneous tissue in the floor of the wound. If all fat is not removed in this way, the view of the musculo-aponeurotic layers during their subsequent division is obscured and haemostasis impeded. A disc of tissue may be excised from each of these layers in turn (Fig. 549D), but my own preference is to incise the anterior rectus sheath, the rectus muscle and the posterior sheath and parietal peritoneum in cruciate fashion (Fig. 549E, F), the incisions being kept deliberately too short in the first instance, to provide an opening that will accommodate two fingers snugly. If necessary, the cuts can be subsequently extended somewhat to afford an aperture of requisite size.

Closure or Elimination of the Paraileostomy Gutter

If the ileum is now drawn through this wound in the anterior abdominal wall, it will be found that a large peritoneal foramen exists on its outer side, and it is clear from the reports of Hardy et al. (1949), Bliss (1963) and Hughes et al. (1963) that there is a real danger of a loop of small gut becoming strangulated in this space if it is left unclosed. It should therefore be obliterated at the time of operation, and one way of doing so is to employ a technique similar to that used by me for closing the comparable lateral space in colostomy cases (see p. 542). In this method the paraileostomy gutter is approached through the main laparotomy wound and this is done before the ileum is taken forwards to the anterior parietes. Access is obtained by elevating the right half of the abdominal wall either by two retractors or by the simple device of inserting a pair of 27·5 cm scissors or long artery forceps into the peritoneal cavity through the ileostomy wound and lifting up their blades. A purse-string suture of non-absorbable material such as linen thread is then inserted, starting with a bite in the musculature of the abdominal wall revealed in the ileostomy wound and continuing along the anterior parietal peritoneum, the fat of the posterior abdominal wall where the caecum or ascending colon was, and the cut edge of the ileal mesentery up to a point 7·5 cm from the clamp on the end of the bowel (Fig. 550). When this stitch is tied it effectively closes the lateral space. Then—and only then—is the ileum threaded through the abdominal wall.

An alternative method, which I have used almost exclusively in recent years to obviate troubles with the lateral space, is to avoid entirely the formation of a lateral space by bringing the ileum forward, not through the peritoneal cavity, but *in the extra-peritoneal tissues* round its lateral edge (see Goligher 1958). In this technique the surgeon abstains from making the ileostomy wound in the first instance and instead turns his attention to the making of an extraperitoneal tunnel from inside the abdomen. Whilst the right edge of the main abdominal wound is held strongly forwards by the assistant, he catches with long artery forceps the cut margin of peritoneum at the outer border of the raw area on the back wall of the abdomen, where the caecum and ascending colon have been (Fig. 551A). As this is lifted up, he dissects in the extraperitoneal tissues, first with scissors then with the finger round the lateral wall of the peritoneum, to enter the plane between the anterior parietal peritoneum and the internal oblique muscle. The separation is pursued till a point is reached directly opposite the site selected for the ileostomy. The assistant now places his hand in the extraperitoneal space with the tip of his middle finger, bearing a metal thimble, pressed forwards against the anterior abdominal wall at this point, whilst the surgeon, now working from the front, makes a circular wound as described previously (see Fig. 549). When this is deepened through the internal oblique, it enters the extraperitoneal space lateral to the separated anterior peritoneum, and the surgeon can pass his fingers from behind and in front to meet in the resulting tunnel (Fig. 551B). The ileal stump with its controlling Cope's clamp is then threaded through this tunnel to emerge on the anterior abdominal wall (Fig. 552A). Next, using a continuous fine catgut suture on a small curved atraumatic needle, the cut edge of the lateral parietal peritoneum is sutured, from above downwards in turn, to the medial leaf of peritoneum or connective tissue in front of the second part of the duodenum, to the cut edge of the ileal mesentery and finally to the anterior surface of the mesentery as far as the ileum itself (Fig. 552B). Actually experience shows that for this reperitonealization to be easily carried out it is necessary not merely to create an extraperitoneal tunnel for the ileum but to mobilize the lateral parietal peritoneum widely so that it drapes itself freely over the ileum and its mesentery. Finally, if the last coil of ileum in the peritoneal cavity is lifted forwards it is found that there is a small raw area (Fig. 553), which is closed by a continuous fine catgut stitch between the medial edge of peritoneum and the peritoneal covering of the mesentery (Fig. 553). The utmost delicacy is required in the

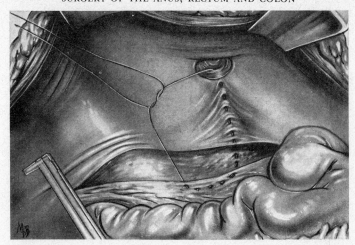

Fig. 550. Closure of the paraileostomy gutter by purse-string suture. View obtained by the surgeon of the right half of the inside of the abdomen as he stands on the left side of the patient, the assistant meanwhile retracting strongly on the right edge of the paramedian wound with retractors (or, better, with a long pair of scissors threaded into the peritoneal cavity through the ileostomy wound). A purse-string suture of linen thread is then inserted along the anterior parietal peritoneum, the fat of the posterior abdominal wall where the caecum was, and the cut edge of the ileal mesentery to within 7·5 cm of the Cope's clamp. When tied this stitch effectively closes the lateral space. *Only then is the ileum brought through the abdominal wall.*

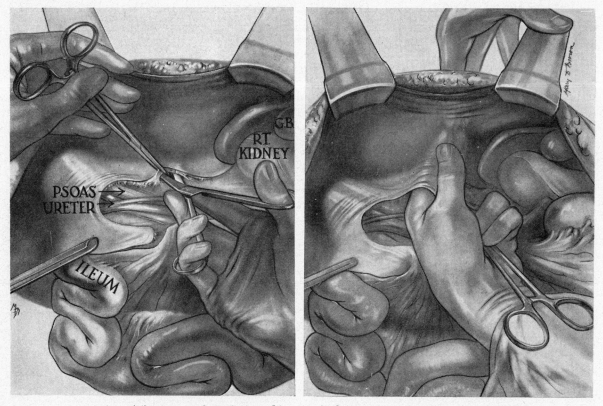

Fig. 551. Extraperitoneal ileostomy. *Left*, Beginning of inner end of extraperitoneal tunnel. View obtained by the surgeon, standing on the left side of the abdomen, of the right half of the abdominal cavity at the completion of the colectomy. Peritoneal leaf at the outer edge of the raw area corresponding to the ascending colon being elevated and extraperitoneal space opened up. *Right*, Completion of extraperitoneal tunnel. Fingers of left hand being passed along tunnel from its inner end to meet those of right hand inserted through the outer end. (*From Goligher 1958*)

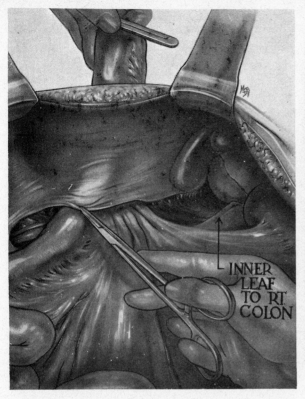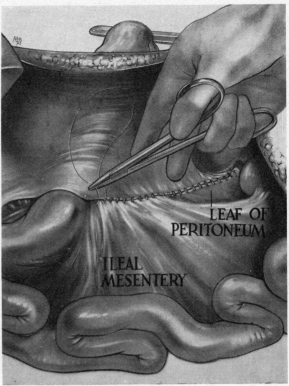

Fig. 552. Extraperitoneal ileostomy. *Left*, Drawing the ileal stump and mesentery through the extraperitoneal space to emerge at the separate ileostomy wound. *Right*, Suture of the outer leaf of peritoneum in turn to inner leaf of peritoneum to right colon, to front of ileal mesentery as far as the ileum. (*From Goligher 1958*)

insertion of this suture to avoid pricking one of the mesenteric vessels.

It is, in fact, preferable to fix the ileal stump to the musculoaponeurotic layers of the abdominal parietes in the ileostomy wound, as described below, before carrying out the reperitonealization just outlined.)

Completion of the Ileostomy
The ileostomy is fashioned by the method of *eversion and primary mucocutaneous suture*. The first step in the application of this technique is to draw the ileal stump sufficiently far through the ileostomy wound, so that, when it is turned back on itself and the cut edge of the bowel is sutured to the skin, there will still be an adequate spout of mucosal-covered ileum projecting beyond the abdominal skin. The crucial question is what constitutes an adequate projection of the finished ileostomy, and the answer would vary somewhat from surgeon to surgeon. All would agree that a stoma showing no protrusion and lying completely flush with the skin surface is most unsatisfactory, for it almost invariably leads to leakage despite the most meticulous application of an adherent bag. Similarly most surgeons would feel that a projection of 5 cm or more is too great, for this may tend to push off the ileostomy bag and may be objectionable to the patients also by causing a slight bulge, which shows through the clothes. Something in between these two extremes is what is required. I personally have usually aimed at a final projection of 2·5–4 cm, but many surgeons of my acquaintanceship regard a 1–2 cm spout as ideal. One of the difficulties, however, is to gauge accurately how much uneverted ileum should project beyond the abdominal skin in order to produce a final protrusion of the desired length. Theoretically, an initial projection of uneverted ileum of 6–7·5 cm should be halved when the bowel is everted, leaving a final ileostomy bud of 3–4 cm. But, certainly in obese subjects, the initial ileal projection is often reduced by a good deal more than half by eversion, owing to the fact that the

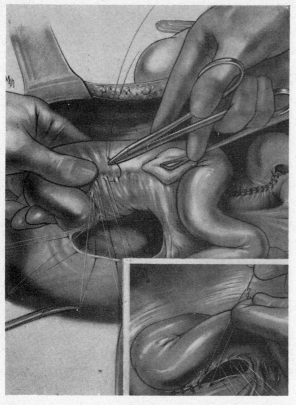

Fig. 553. Extraperitoneal ileostomy. Suture of deep aspect of ileal mesentery (or of ileum itself) to the inner leaf of peritoneum. Care must be taken to catch only the peritoneal covering of the mesentery and not the underlying vessels. *Inset:* Sutures tied. (*From Goligher 1958*)

of the ileum and mesentery from the musculo-aponeurotic layers and drawing the bowel farther out of the abdominal cavity (see p. 782).

Having decided on the amount of ileum to withdraw from the abdomen through the ileostomy wound, the *next step* is to fix this inner tube of bowel and its related mesentery to the musculature of the abdominal wall in this small wound. Most surgeons probably achieve this fixation by means of sutures inserted from inside the abdomen between the anterior parietal peritoneum and posterior rectus sheath and the ileal mesentery (Fig. 554). But when using the extraperitoneal technique for making the ileostomy this manoeuvre is not practicable. Instead, it is necessary to secure fixation by sutures passed through the anterior part of the ileostomy wound as shown in Fig. 554. At one stage I used to eschew direct suture of the ileum itself to the musculoaponeurotic layers, for fear of producing necrosis of the ileal wall with subsequent formation of a subcutaneous faecal fistula. Reliance was placed on sutures of very fine silk or chromic catgut passed between the medial leaf of the ileal mesentery and the inner cut edge of the anterior rectus sheath as seen on looking into the ileostomy wound from the front. But during the past 10 or 12 years I have also been inserting similarly fine sutures between the ileal wall itself and the anterior rectus sheath in the rest of the circumference of the ileostomy wound. Fig. 555 shows the suture arrangement now used. I must emphasize that the bites of bowel wall are very superficial and do not penetrate deeper than the muscle coat, so that, if necrosis should take place subsequently, it would presumably not open the lumen. So far, no troubles from fistulas have been encountered in over 400 cases done by this technique, including some emergency operations.

The *third step* in the construction of the ileostomy is the turning back of the projecting ileum and the suture of its cut end to the edges of the circular skin wound (Fig. 556A). The stitches may be of fine serum-proof silk or chromic catgut and are passed between the end of the bowel and the skin, but do not take a bite of the inner tube of bowel. (In other words the projection of the everted bowel will be maintained solely by the fixing sutures that were passed at an earlier stage between the anterior rectus sheath and the bowel and mesentery.) To start with, two stay sutures are inserted; these divide the mucocutaneous junction into halves, in each of which further stitches are placed as required, usually up to a total of 8 to 12. The full extent of the projection of the everted ileum is often not appreci-

inner tube of bowel seems to sag back into the thick layer of subcutaneous fat. It is a wise precaution, therefore, in such cases to allow for an initial projection of uneverted ileum of 8·5–10 cm. It is also well to bear in mind that, if the finished ileostomy turns out to project rather too much, it is a relatively simple operative manoeuvre, either at the conclusion of the initial operation or on a subsequent occasion, to separate the cut end of the ileum from the skin, to unevert it, to amputate some more bowel and to resuture the severed ileal end to the skin—all of which can be done without disturbing the fixation of the inner tube of bowel to the musculoaponeurotic layers or opening the abdomen again (see p. 776). But, if the completed ileostomy protrudes inadequately, any refashioning operation—certainly at a second intervention—is rather more difficult, because it involves separation

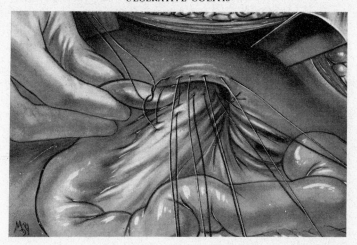

Fig. 554. Suture of the leaf of ileal mesentery to the anterior parietal peritoneum as viewed from inside the abdomen, the surgeon standing on the left side of the patient and the right edge of the main wound being strongly retracted forwards.

ated till the suturing has been completed and pressure is made with the finger tips on the surrounding skin; the bud then expands and lengthens in a most impressive manner, often doubling or trebling its length (Fig. 556B).

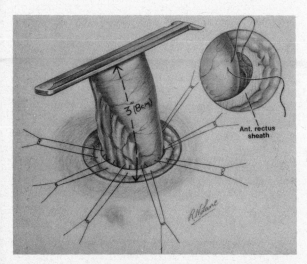

Fig. 555. Fixation of the ileal stump to the musculo-aponeurotic layers of the abdominal wall by a circumferential series of 3/0 silk sutures between the anterior rectus sheath and the ileal wall and leaf of the ileal mesentery. View of the ileostomy wound with the surgeon standing on the right side of the patient. *Inset:* The bites of the suture in the wall of the ileum are very superficial.

Immediate Application of the Ileostomy Bag in the Theatre

With the ileostomy sited in a separate wound with normal skin around, and using the technique of immediate mucocutaneous suture, there is no reason why an adherent ileostomy bag should not be applied immediately at the conclusion of the operation. I have done this for many years and it has greatly simplified the immediate postoperative care of these cases.

ILEOSTOMY ALONE

Though simple ileostomy without simultaneous colectomy or proctocolectomy had at one stage almost completely disappeared from surgical practice, there has more recently been some revival of its use as a *loop ileostomy*, particularly in very ill patients undergoing operation for toxic megacolon (see p. 744) or as a safety measure proximal to an ileorectal anastomosis (see p. 738) or reservoir ileostomy (see p. 808). It has often been stated that a loop ileostomy is an unsatisfactory one for the patient to manage subsequently because of the difficulty in fitting an appliance to it. But this need not be so if the technique suggested by Turnbull (1975a) of providing a protruding active opening and a receding inactive one is employed, as shown in Figs 577–60. It will be noted that a glass rod not longer than 5–7 cm is used to support the loop, which allows a Hollister bag with a 8 cm flange to be fitted

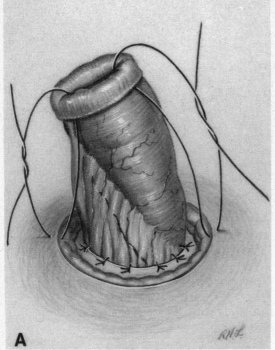

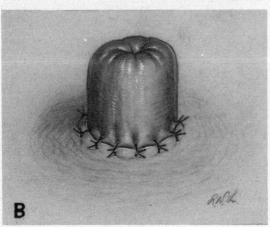

Fig. 556. The end of the ileum is sutured to the skin by interrupted stitches of fine silk or chromic catgut as shown in (A), the final result being a bud or spout of about 4 cm, as depicted in (B).

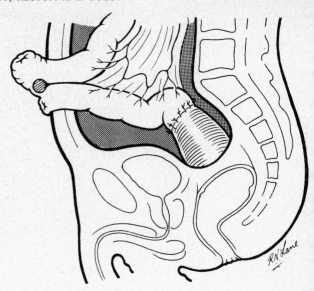

Fig. 557. Proximal loop ileostomy with protruding active opening in conjunction with end-to-end ileorectal anastomosis.

fashion a loop ileostomy in such patients whose ileal mesentery is laden with fat, making preparation of a sufficiently long ileal stump for an end-ileostomy quite difficult. In these patients, in whom the large bowel has been removed, the end of the ileum is closed by suture and tucked against the other limb of the ileal loop with a few stitches. It should be mentioned further that, as with terminal ileostomies, Turnbull (1975b) often carries out a myotomy on the 7–8 cm piece of bowel to be used for making a loop ileostomy. This is accomplished by means of a series of longitudinal and transverse scissor cuts down to the submucosa. I have no experience of this additional manoeuvre in connection with loop ileostomies and would be apprehensive about its use in the very ill acute patients who might need loop ileostomy. I find that the protruding opening of the loop ileostomy maintains its projection quite well without incorporating a myotomy in the technique of manufacture.

A *terminal* ileostomy alone is an exceptionally rare operation in the hands of most surgeons, but Truelove et al. (1965) have advocated its use in certain cases of inflammatory bowel disease, in the hope that the inflammation in the colon and rectum will eventually resolve with defunctioning, possibly aided by systemic steroid therapy or steroids introduced into the large bowel through an inactive ileostomy opening. The operation is best per-

securely to the surrounding skin at the end of the operation. The rod is removed after 14 days and then a smaller bag may be employed.

Turnbull (1975a) has also favoured a loop technique in more obese patients undergoing even elective ileostomy with proctocolectomy or subtotal colectomy, because he believes that it is easier to

PLATE IV

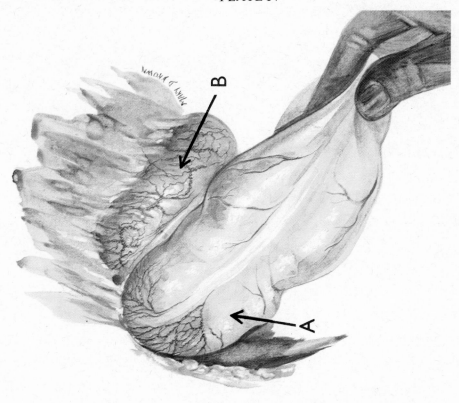
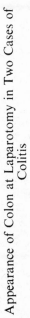

Appearance of Colon at Laparotomy in Two Cases of
Colitis

A, Normal large bowel
B, Colon affected by colitis. In one case this is indicated by
pallor of the wall and fine tortuous vessels; in the other
(after handling) by marked congestion with a fine network of
vessels

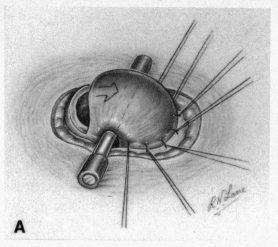

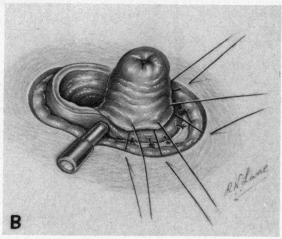

A

B

Fig. 558. Construction of a loop ileostomy with protruding afferent limb and receding efferent limb. Patient viewed from the right side with the afferent limb uppermost. (A) A 6 cm glass rod through the mesentery supports the loop whilst a semicircular row of 3/0 silk sutures is inserted between the anterior rectus sheath and the wall of the afferent limb. An incision with diathermy is made in the efferent limb of bowel. (B) The cut bowel of the efferent limb is now turned back on the efferent limb and sutured to the skin to produce a protruding stoma.

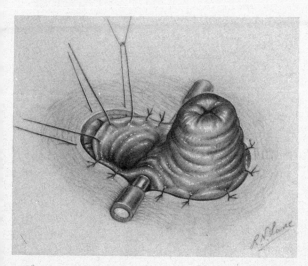

Fig. 559. Loop ileostomy. The other edge of the cut efferent limb of bowel is next sutured to the skin of the rest of the ileostomy wound.

formed through a left paramedian or median laparotomy wound. When the decision is made to proceed with a simple ileostomy, there are two variants of technique available with regard to the disposal of the distal ileal end. In one, favoured by Rankin (in Bargen et al. 1932), the ileum is divided close to the caecum, leaving a 2·5 cm ileal stump, which is closed by suture and invaginated almost flush with the caecal wall. The active other end of ileum is brought out as a terminal ileostomy at a separate trephine wound in the right abdomen, employing the same technique essentially as in making an ileostomy in connection with a procto-colectomy (see p. 753), but with a little more difficulty in closing the lateral paraileostomy space (Hardy et al. 1949). Though this method is open to the theoretical objection that in these debilitated colitis patients the blind ileal stump might rupture, Counsell and Goligher (1952) found that this complication had not occurred in any of a large series of cases of simple ileostomy conducted along these lines at St Mark's Hospital. The alternative scheme, which was favoured by Cattell (1944), is to divide the ileum between Cope's clamps 15 cm or so from the ileocaecal junction, or as far from it as is necessary to get above any extension of the disease into the small bowel. The two ends of bowel are then brought to the surface—the active end at a separate trephine ileostomy wound and fashioned into a proper ileostomy after removal of the clamp, as described above, the other through the lower part of the main laparotomy wound or through a further small separate stab wound between the main wound and the ileostomy and sufficiently far away from the latter so as not to interfere with the

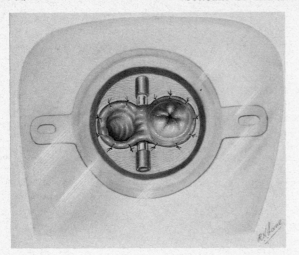

Fig. 560. Loop ileostomy. Finally a Hollister drainage bag with 7 cm flange is fitted to the skin around the ileostomy, the karaya ring lying just outside the ends of the 6 cm glass rod.

fitting of the ileostomy bag. This inactive end of bowel can be left with the Cope's clamp on and supported by gauze till it separates by sloughing of the clamped tissue in five to six days. Cattell (1944) made a special point of suturing the cut edge of the divided ileal mesentery between the two ends of bowel to the anterior parietal peritoneum to obviate the gap there through which a loop of small bowel might slip and be strangulated, but this is not always easy to do.

PARTIAL AND SUBTOTAL COLECTOMY WITH ANASTOMOSIS

Partial colectomy is occasionally indicated for localized segmental forms of colitis; it follows recognized lines and is completed by end-to-end anastomosis between ileum or normal colon proximally and normal colon distally. More extensive lesions of this kind may involve a subtotal or total colectomy with ileosigmoid or ileorectal anastomosis. In uniting ileum and distal sigmoid or rectum I use a straightforward end-to-end or side-to-side anastomosis, as employed in the treatment of polyposis coli (see p. 366 and Figs 273–275), but in addition I usually establish a temporary loop ileostomy 20–25 cm proximal to the anastomosis (Fig. 557) to help to lessen the risk of anastomotic

dehiscence. For a good functional result with ileorectal anastomosis it is desirable to *retain as much of the rectum as possible and preferably to make the anastomosis at the rectosigmoid junction.* This has the additional advantage that it provides a peritoneal-covered cuff of rectum for the actual anastomosis, which should increase the security of the suture. Whether the superior haemorrhoidal vessels are divided, as recommended by Aylett (1960), or left intact (see p. 736–8) seems immaterial. A suction or corrugated rubber drain is left down to the anastomosis for at least four or five days.

RESERVOIR ILEOSTOMY

The evolution and some of the outstanding problems of this type of ileostomy will be discussed on pp. 796–814. Its operative technique, postoperative care and complications, and the indications for its use are dealt with in that section.

Postoperative Care and Early Complications of Conventional Ileostomy Surgery

Much of the immediate postoperative care follows the general lines of treatment after any major abdominal operation, and the usual complications are liable to be met (see p. 463). If, as is so frequently the practice now, the ileostomy is but part of a complete proctocolectomy, the perineal wound will, of course, require the same attentions and pursue much the same course as after abdominoperineal excision of the rectum for cancer; however, slow healing is a noticeable feature in many colitis patients and convalescence may be greatly prolonged on that account, especially in very ill cases submitted to urgent or emergency operations (see p. 789). If on the other hand a subtotal colectomy with exteriorization of the sigmoid stump has been performed, the Cope's clamp on the projecting end of bowel usually separates in five or six days. Thereafter the resulting protuberant colostomy gradually shrinks as oedema subsides and eventually, after three or four weeks, the opening may be almost flush with the skin. In some cases indeed it tends to recede within the abdomen, leaving an area of granulation tissue on the surface at the lower end of the wound. Sometimes the skin grows over it, and when this happens a superficial abscess occasionally forms in the suprapubic region, eventually bursting to the surface.

In ileostomy cases, however, two considerations dominate this background of ordinary postoperative care: the maintenance of fluid and electrolyte balance and the management of the ileostomy opening itself.

MAINTENANCE OF FLUID AND ELECTROLYTE BALANCE

LOSSES OF FLUID, ELECTROLYTES AND NITROGEN FROM THE ILEOSTOMY

Clearly accurate replacement therapy must depend on precise information as to fluid and electrolyte losses in any particular case. The average surgeon may be to some extent guided by general rules formulated on the basis of special studies on ileostomy patients conducted by Coghill et al. (1956), Crawford and Brooke (1957), Smiddy et al. (1960) and Nuguid et al. (1963), the findings of which—with particular reference to our own investigations—may be summarized as follows:

Volume of Fluid. In the average case, though there may be some ileostomy actions on the first postoperative day, it is usually not until 24–48 hours after operation that the ileostomy starts to act properly. At first the discharge is very liquid and voluminous, and the quantities passed daily may amount to anything from 0·5 litre to 1·5 litres; losses in excess of this are exceptional in cases uncomplicated by ileostomy dysfunction. After about a week as a rule the faecal losses gradually diminish and at the same time become much firmer. By the end of seven to ten days the quantity of faeces has reduced to that of a long-established ileostomy, namely about 400–500 ml per day, the consistency being rather similar to that of stiff porridge.

Sodium. Our investigations show that, contrary to the observations of Crawford and Brooke (1957), the concentration of sodium in the ileostomy fluid remains remarkably constant at about 120 mmol/litre, despite wide fluctuations in the quantity of fluid being passed. Only when the volume becomes really excessive, say over 1·5 litres, does the sodium concentration depart from this level and then it drops only slightly—in one of our cases to 110 mmol/litre. With an average daily excretion of about 1000 ml of ileostomy fluid during the first week after operation the total loss of sodium from the stoma will be of the order of 144 mmol per day, which is many times greater than the faecal loss of this electrolyte in a normal individual (2–10 mmol per day) but about the same as that lost per anum in the average patient with severe colitis before ileostomy and colectomy (9–170 mmol per day).

Potassium. We found that the concentration of potassium in the ileostomy fluid was very variable even in the same individual and

ranged from 6 to 18 mmol/litre at different times in the postoperative period. However, even at peak periods the concentration is relatively low, and the total daily faecal loss, which varied from 1 to 11 mmol, never exceeded that of a normal person (6–12 mmol per day). This compares strikingly with the state of affairs in patients with severe colitis before operation, in whom the faecal losses of potassium may be considerable—up to 90–167 mmol per day.

Calcium. Nuguid et al. (1963) report that the average concentration of calcium in the fluid output from recent ileostomies is 35 mmol/litre and the average daily loss about 18 mmol, whilst the average concentration in the faeces from established ileostomies is 25 mmol/litre and the approximate daily loss 15 mmol.

Magnesium. Nuguid et al. (1963) give as an average figure for the concentration of magnesium in the discharge from a recent ileostomy 15 mmol/litre and the average daily loss 7 mmol, and for the concentration and average daily loss in the faeces from an established ileostomy 15 mmol/litre and 15 mmol respectively.

Nitrogen. Nitrogen excretion from ileostomies is usually quite small during the first two postoperative weeks, and amounts to between 0·4 and 1·8 g per day, the loss being least in the first few days, when the patient is not eating, and increasing as a solid diet is resumed. Even in the case with a long-established ileostomy the nitrogen loss does not exceed 1·5 g per day. This can usefully be compared with the faecal nitrogen losses in normal persons and in preoperative patients with severe ulcerative colitis. In a normal individual having 100 g of protein in the diet per day (= approx. 16 g of nitrogen) the nitrogen excretion in the faeces is 10% of this amount or 1·6 g. In colitis patients before operation the nitrogen loss in the faeces is approximately 20–30% of that ingested, which, with an intake of 16 g daily, amounts to 3·2–5 g per day.

Effect of Corticosteroids. The excretion of fluid and electrolytes from the ileostomy is affected by the systemic administration of corticoids, which is so often necessary postoperatively at the present time, as pointed out on p. 746, because of its previous use by the physician. The influence of corticosteroids during the immediate postoperative period is to depress the output of fluid and sodium, so that there is no initial 'peak' of excretion for these substances. The volume of ileostomy discharge varies little throughout and gradually reduces to that of a long-established ileostomy. The concentration of sodium in the ileostomy fluid is constant, but slightly less than that found in non-cortisone treated cases, namely about 80 mmol/litre. As in ileostomy patients not receiving corticosteroids, the excretion of potassium through the stoma is variable but tends to be raised.

Effect of Intraperitoneal Sepsis. We have noted in several cases that the occurrence of peritonitis or intraperitoneal abscesses is invariably associated with the development of a profuse outpouring of fluid from the ileostomy, with volumes up to 3 and 4 litres being passed daily. This cause of ileostomy diarrhoea should be borne in mind by the clinician.

ADMINISTRATION OF FLUID AND ELECTROLYTES

From the foregoing remarks it will be evident that potassium losses per ileostomy are so small that they may be largely disregarded in considering treatment. Attention may therefore be concentrated on the fluid and saline requirements. The excretion of sodium in the ileostomy fluid at a more or less constant concentration of 120 mmol/litre makes this fluid roughly isotonic with normal saline (= 130 mmol of sodium per litre). A good working rule, therefore, is to replace the amount of fluid lost from the ileostomy by the same volume of normal saline intravenously or, if the patient is taking oral fluids as well, by the same amount of water by mouth together with sodium chloride capsules up to 9 g for each litre of ileostomy fluid passed. Any vomitus or aspirate on gastric or intestinal suction should, of course, also be replaced by an equivalent amount of normal saline by the intravenous route.

If the patient has had a colectomy or proctocolectomy in addition to the ileostomy, an intravenous drip will already have been instituted to cover the course of the operation and allow of the administration of blood as necessary. This infusion should be continued during the next 36–48 hours, or till the ileostomy is acting freely, and during that time it will be wise to give most of the fluids intravenously, though oral feeding is started cautiously right away. If the ileostomy discharge rapidly becomes profuse and the patient is still unable to manage mouth fluids freely, it may be necessary to continue or recommence the intravenous administration for a little longer in order to maintain the fluid and saline intake at a sufficient level to combat the severe losses that are being sustained. Also if obstructive symptoms should occur, with vomiting, fluids may have to be given intravenously for a considerable time and supplemented by gastric aspirations and possibly further blood transfusion as required. It is a good plan to have periodic estimations of the plasma electrolyte levels on any patients undergoing prolonged intravenous administrations as an additional guide to correct replacement therapy.

LONG-TERM EFFECT OF ILEOSTOMY ON TOTAL BODY WATER AND BODY SODIUM

Clarke et al. (1968) have drawn attention to a state of latent chronic dehydration and sodium depletion in patients with established ileostomies. Total body water and total exchangeable sodium were measured in a group of ileostomy patients who were otherwise well. Compared with a control group the ileostomy patients showed on the average an 11% reduction in total body water and a 7% deficit in total exchangeable sodium. The urinary excretion of water and sodium in the ileostomy patients was also significantly reduced. However, the patients exhibited no symptoms attributable to dehydration or sodium depletion. Singer et al. (1973) have also noted that apparently healthy individuals with an ileostomy show a reduced volume of urine with a lowered sodium content compared with normal subjects, or even with patients after colectomy and ileorectal anastomosis.

MAGNESIUM DEFICIENCY

A few words may perhaps be helpful on magnesium depletion and its management, for the importance of this electrolyte has only recently been recognized and is still imperfectly understood. Using atomic absorption spectrophotometry (Dawson and Heaton 1961) to determine the serum magnesium concentration, Heaton (1964) found that the normal range of values lay between 1·72 and 2·28 mg/100 ml. In 59 of my patients suffering from ulcerative colitis, Duthie et al. (1964) demonstrated low serum magnesium levels in five; in 50 of these patients, who had only mild colitis, there was only one with hypomagnesaemia, but in nine with severe colitis there were four with gross magnesium depletion. As Heaton et al. (1967) point out, the clinical features of this condition are ill-defined and their elucidation is complicated by the almost invariable concomitance of other electrolyte imbalances. Muscular weakness with incoordination, twitching, tremor and abdominal cramps may occur. Cardiovascular symptoms have been described with hypertension and tachycardia and the ECG may show low voltage potentials. Psychic disturbances and depression are probably the most frequent manifestations of severe deficiency and agitation or delirium with hallucinations have been observed. Sudden fits of anger, as observed in one of our patients, may require very heavy sedation. Tetany occurred in three of our patients when hypocalcaemia was associated with magnesium deficiency.

Hypomagnesaemia produces severe clinical symptoms in only a few cases. In these patients treatment is clearly essential and is generally followed by a dramatic improvement. In the majority of cases, however, symptoms may be ill-defined and correction of the deficiency is less spectacular, though improvement in the general condition of the patient is the rule. Apart from its direct effects, correction of magnesium depletion may greatly assist in the correction of other electrolyte disorders. The administration of magnesium salts alone has been shown to raise the serum calcium concentration in patients with hypomagnesaemia and hypocalcaemia after intestinal resection (Heaton and Fourman 1965).

The treatment of magnesium deficiency is usually not difficult. In cases with severe depletion 20 mmol of magnesium chloride or sulphate should be given intravenously or intramuscularly and repeated on alternate days as necessary. This must be combined with the oral administration of magnesium salts continued daily for several weeks. In less severe cases oral supplements alone are adequate and magnesium hydroxide suspension has proved in our experience to be more acceptable than soluble magnesium salts. Magnesium hydroxide, 20 ml daily in divided doses, is generally adequate, although this dose has been doubled on some occasions. Large amounts of magnesium salts have a cathartic effect, but diarrhoea has only occasionally been found with the regimen outlined above.

EARLY MANAGEMENT OF THE ILEOSTOMY OPENING

Most of the troubles that used to occur in ileostomy patients from digestion of the skin by the ileal discharge have been eliminated by the present method of applying the adherent bag in the operating theatre. In the majority of cases now the ileostomy appliance remains firmly attached for five to seven days after the initial attachment. Thereafter, whilst the ileostomy discharge is very liquid it may need to be re-applied rather more frequently as leakage occurs, say every two or three days, but as the motion becomes firmer this tendency to leakage lessens, and finally it will be found that the adherent flange can be retained for a week or so. In most cases, indeed, this is so throughout and no trouble with leakage is experienced at any stage.

ILEOSTOMY COMPLICATIONS DURING THE IMMEDIATE POSTOPERATIVE PERIOD

SKIN IRRITATION

In some patients unfortunately leakage occurs frequently and the skin around the ileostomy becomes digested, red and raw. With each leakage the skin becomes more excoriated and less well able to retain an adherent flange, so that a vicious circle is rapidly established. It is not always possible in such cases to be sure what has initiated the leakage, but the excessively liquid character of the motions at this stage is often apparently the main factor, whilst in some very emaciated cases the concavity of that part of the anterior abdominal wall in which the ileostomy is situated may be partly responsible. Occasionally an unusual sensitivity to the material of the appliance or to the adhesive is responsible for the trouble (see p. 781).

In the management of this complication two measures are specially valuable:

The Use of Stomahesive Squares. The very special virtues of Stomahesive as a washer between the skin and the flange of the appliance in patients with a sore peristomal skin are emphasized on pp. 736, 781.

Administration of Drugs to Render the Motions less Liquid. A valuable auxiliary measure is the prescription of codeine phosphate, Lomotil or loperamide, (see p. 780), which are usually successful in reducing the fluidity and volume of the faeces. If the patient is not already receiving systemic corticosteroid therapy to cover the operation and postoperative period, the possibility of giving steroids, in the hope that they may help to control the loss of fluid and electrolytes, as mentioned on p. 763, may also be considered.

ILEOSTOMY DYSFUNCTION

This expression was coined by Warren and McKittrick (1951) of Boston to denote a condition of partial obstruction at the ileostomy opening resulting in irregular ileostomy action. It is a complication that used to be extremely common as is shown by the fact that it occurred in 130 of Warren and McKittrick's (1951) series of 210 patients treated by ileostomy, and in nearly half of 60 patients with ileostomy reported by Counsell and myself from St Mark's Hospital in 1952. The symptoms usually began about a week after operation, the patient complaining of abdominal pains, distension and vomiting, and the ileostomy either ceasing to act or producing an excessive amount of very liquid motion often reaching 2–3 litres in 24 hours. The symptoms and signs suggested a mechanical obstruction rather than a paralytic ileus, but, if treated conservatively with gastric suction and administration of intravenous fluids, the patients usually recovered satisfactorily, though such a regimen might have had to be continued for more than two weeks. When patients were submitted to laparotomy for this complication, as sometimes happened when the surgeon suspected that a true mechanical obstruction was present, no obstructive lesion of the small gut was found as a rule, but it was noted that the ileum was dilated right down to the ileostomy opening in the abdominal wall. These experiences showed that in the management of these obstructive episodes it was best to persist with conservative measures. An important part of these latter was the insertion of a soft rubber catheter for a distance of 15–30 cm into the terminal ileum. This was often followed by the escape of 200–300 ml of ileal contents apparently under pressure. It was repeated two or three times a day and sometimes the catheter was left *in situ*, especially during the night.

As shown by Warren and McKittrick (1951) and by Counsell (1956), cases with a severe degree of ileostomy dysfunction might develop an ileitis proximal to the partially obstructed stoma. Doubtless the profuse watery motions that occurred with dysfunction were due, at any rate in part, to this ileitis. A more serious manifestation of severe and prolonged dysfunction was the development of a perforation of one of the numerous small stercoral ulcers found in severe ileitis of this kind. (Such a perforation requires to be distinguished from certain other forms of perforation that may occur in the terminal ileum after ileostomy; see Ileitis, Ileal perforation or Oedema, p. 779).

more severe form, as a tightly constricting fibrous ring developed. Warren and McKittrick (1951) advised that, in cases that did not respond satisfactorily to conservative measures, the ring of granulation and young fibrous tissue should be divided to release the constriction. Actually, at the present time, most surgeons faced with this situation would probably prefer to refashion the ileostomy completely, using the technique of im-

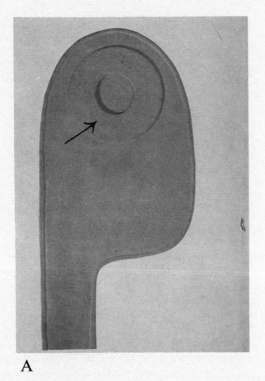

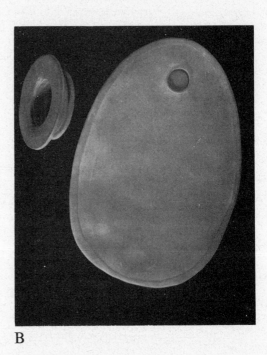

A   B

Fig. 561. Rubber ileostomy appliances—museum pieces! (A) The one-piece adherent bag manufactured by Salt & Son of Birmingham. Back view of appliance showing the opening into which the ileostomy fits, surrounded by the rubber flange indicated by an arrow. The spout at the lower end is for emptying the bag; it is normally kept closed by being folded and turned back on itself and kept in that state with a rubber band. (B) The two-piece adherent bag made by Down Bros. of London. Back view of appliance showing more rigid flange separated from bag. When the flange has been stuck to the abdominal wall the bag is fixed to the flange by stretching the opening shown on the upper part of its back wall and fitting the rim into the groove near the front edge of the side wall of the flange. The bag is emptied by an opening on the lower part of the front wall, normally closed by a screw cap.

Our understanding of the precise pathology of ileostomy dysfunction was greatly clarified by the work of Warren and McKittrick (1951), Turnbull (1953) and Crile and Turnbull (1954), who showed that the obstruction at the stoma is due to the 'serositis', oedema, granulation tissue formation, and early fibrosis associated with the old-fashioned method of making ileostomies. As the oedema subsided the dysfunction might diminish or recur in

mediate mucocutaneous suture. The employment of this method of ileostomy constructed at the original operation is the important measure of prophylaxis against this complication, for since I have been using this technique—which is followed by primary union in all but some 3% of the cases, in which partial separation of the circumferential mucocutaneous suture line takes place—serious ileostomy dysfunction has virtually ceased to occur in my patients. However, the report that the motions, in a patient convalescing after an ileostomy operation, have again become more liquid and profuse should always lead to a careful digital examination of the stoma to make sure that a stenosis has not developed. If no local cause is found in the ileostomy itself, the possibility of intraperitoneal sepsis being present should be seriously considered, as pointed out on p. 763.

OTHER FORMS OF ILEITIS

See p. 779.

The Ultimate Management of the Patient with a Conventional Ileostomy

ILEOSTOMY APPLIANCES

As explained on p. 735, the original type of appliance used by ileostomy patients, when the operation was first taken up by surgeons, was a relatively simple bag or box, held firmly by a belt against the abdominal wall at the site of the stoma. But this comparatively inefficient pattern of appliance has been completely supplanted by adherent bags, many models of which in rubber or plastic have been produced in America, Britain and Scandinavia, following their initiation by Koenig-Rutzen (Strauss and Strauss 1944). A good impartial appraisal of the numerous American bags was provided a few years ago by Lenneberg and Sohn (1972). In this book attention will not unnaturally be devoted to those appliances marketed in Britain. For descriptive purposes it will be convenient first of all to consider very briefly the longer-established rubber appliances, which are still used by a steadily dwindling group of patients, and then to discuss in greater detail the newer plastic bags, which have become increasingly popular in recent years.

RUBBER APPLIANCES

These are of two main types, depending on whether the appliance is made all in one piece or whether the portion that is stuck to the skin can be separated from the bag proper.

One-Piece Appliances

A good example of this type of bag is that manufactured by Salt and Son of Birmingham, England, which is closely modelled on the original Koenig–Rutzen bag (Fig. 561A). It consists of a bag, which bears near the upper border of its posterior surface an opening, into which the ileostomy bud normally projects.

Surrounding this hole is a flat disc of firm rubber, with a central perforation corresponding to the aperature on the bag. This disc, which is known as the *flange*, is the part actually stuck to the skin. As an additional precaution a special belt is also worn to hold the appliance to the body. The bag is emptied through an opening at its lower end, which is normally kept clipped off with a rubber band. The usual procedure is to empty the bag every four hours or so as required, usually every time the patient goes to the lavatory to micturate. Removal of the appliance for washing and replacement by a clean bag need only be carried out at intervals of a week or so, if the bag is made of black rubber, which is more odour-resistant than ordinary rubber. The bags are available in two sizes, normal and extra-large, the latter being specially suited to persons whose ileostomy discharge is unduly profuse. Various sizes of flange opening are also available, ranging from 2·5 to 5 cm in diameter, the size most commonly used being about 3 cm.

Two-Piece Appliances

Two of the most commonly used British appliances of this type are those manufactured by Down Bros. and by Franklin (Fig. 561B), both of London. These consist of: (1) an upper portion known as the *flange*, made of more rigid rubber or firm plastic material, which is stuck to the skin of the abdomen (and usually held in place also by a belt or special corset); and (2) the *bag proper* made of finer, preferably black, rubber with an opening on the back near the upper end to fit on to the flange, and another with a screw cap on the front near the lower end for emptying the bag. As with the one-piece appliance, various sizes of flange are available and two sizes of bag are made.

The main advantage of the two-piece appliance is that it is easier to site the flange accurately around the stoma when there is no bag attached to it and the ileostomy spout can be seen to emerge through the ring of the flange. The disadvantage of this type of appliance is that the bag may tend to slip off the groove on the flange. This is most apt to occur at night when the bag has become filled with flatus; as the patient turns round in bed the distended bag may be caught by the bedclothes and torn off. This mishap is more often encountered when the rubber of the appliance has perished somewhat and for that reason obtains a less secure grip on the top of the flange.

Adhesives Available for Sticking Rubber Appliances

Four main types of adhesive are available at the present time for sticking ileostomy appliances to the skin:

1. *Proprietary Cements*. A good example is that issued by Salt & Son with their bags.

2. *Double-sided Adhesive Squares or Circles*. Probably the most commonly used of these in Britain are the Chiron (made by Down Bros. of London) and Meredith made by Eschmann Bros. and Walsh Ltd.). Another pattern is the Stomaseal made by the 3M Company; in my experience it is kinder to the skin than the other two, but, perhaps as a consequence, it does not provide quite such secure fixation.

3. *Karaya Gum Washers*. Though originally used as a powder, which when a little water was added to it produced a glue, karaya gum is at present generally employed in the form of washers, prepared commercially (e.g. by C. S. Bullen of Liverpool) by mixing the karaya with glycerine. Several plastic appliances now incorporate a karaya washer (see below), but separate washers are

available for sticking on rubber appliances. These come in disc form and should be kept within the plastic waterproof covering, in which they are supplied, until they are about to be used, otherwise they become dry and hard. The central opening in the disc is cut to a size that will fit snugly round the stoma, covering all the skin up to the mucocutaneous junction. The flange of the appliance is then applied to the washer and held firmly in position for a few minutes. Finally strips of non-irritating adhesive strapping, such as Micropore, are placed along the edge of the flange, partly on the flange and partly on the skin, to seal off the exposed edge of washer. Karaya does not usually provide as prolonged adhesion as does ordinary adhesive plaster—three to four days being a common maximum for the former as against seven to ten days for the latter, though there are exceptions. The great virtue of karaya is that it is an effective adhesive even on a raw oozing skin, which would be quite unable to take ordinary adhesive plasters.

4. *Stomahesive Squares*. Yet another fairly recently introduced adhesive is Stomahesive, made by E. & R. Squibb, which provides very secure adhesion even on sore skin, but it is quite expensive (approximately £0·70 for each square in June 1979) and for that reason is usually better reserved for patients who are suffering from soreness of the peristomal skin.

PLASTIC APPLIANCES

The present trend in life in general towards replacement of older materials, such as rubber, by plastic

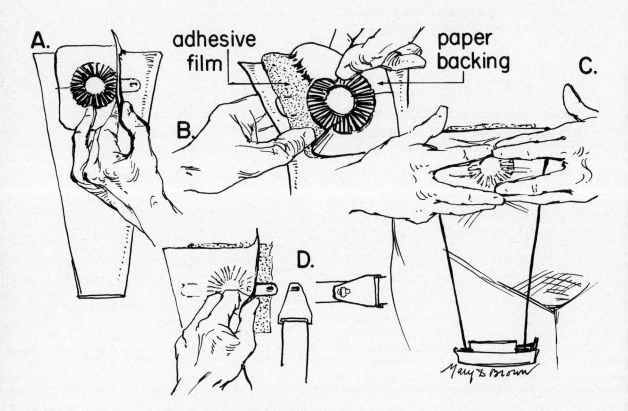

Fig. 562. Hollister plastic ileostomy bag. (A) Back view of the appliance showing opening into which ileostomy protrudes. Incorporated in the bag immediately surrounding this opening is a thin ring of plastic material with two side-arms. Covering the ring is a thick karaya gum washer, and more peripherally there is an adhesive square, which is protected by covering paper till the appliance is about to be used. In this illustration the adhesive square and paper are folded over at one side to display the side-arm to the plastic ring. (B) Protective covering being removed from the adhesive square. (C) Front view of appliance after it has been placed on the abdominal wall, the karaya gum washer and adhesive square being firmly pressed against the skin around the stoma. Note that the open lower end of the bag has been closed by a special clip, which is released when it is desired to empty the bag. (D) Again a front view of the appliance, the edge of which near the top has been turned over to display the rigid plastic side-arm to which the belt is attached. Because of the tendency for the peripheral adhesive square in the original version of the Hollister drainage appliance to irritate the skin, it was usually advisable to place a Stomahesive square between it and the skin. In the current version the peripheral square has been replaced by a square of Micropore adhesive tape, which is non-irritating.

substances is nowhere more evident than in regard to ileostomy appliances. During the past few years a number of plastic ileostomy bags have been designed as substitutes for rubber bags and now dominate the market. They have the advantage that they are disposable, which saves the time and effort that is required for washing rubber bags.

As with rubber ileostomy bags, it is convenient to consider plastic bags under the general headings of one-piece and two-piece appliances.

One-Piece Appliances

By contrast with colostomy bags (pp. 625–8), one-piece ileostomy appliances need to have a drainage opening to allow them to be emptied at least three or four times a day, whilst the appliance itself is usually left adherent to the skin for several days on end. The sticking of the bag to the skin may be by ordinary adhesive, as in the Simpla-Sassco appliance, but most bags now incorporate a karaya gum washer. In the very popular Hollister appliance (Fig. 562) fixation is achieved by a combination of a karaya washer, immediately surrounding the hole on the back of the bag for the ileostomy spout, and a square of adhesive material more peripherally. In the original pattern of appliance the peripheral adhesive was apt to prove very irritating to the skin and to avoid this complication it was often necessary for the patient to wear a square of Stomahesive between the plastic and the skin. In a more recent pattern the peripheral adhesive is of microporous tape and much less likely to irritate. Another disadvantage of the Hollister appliance relates to its translucency, for many patients find the overt display of its faecal contents objectionable. But this objection can be

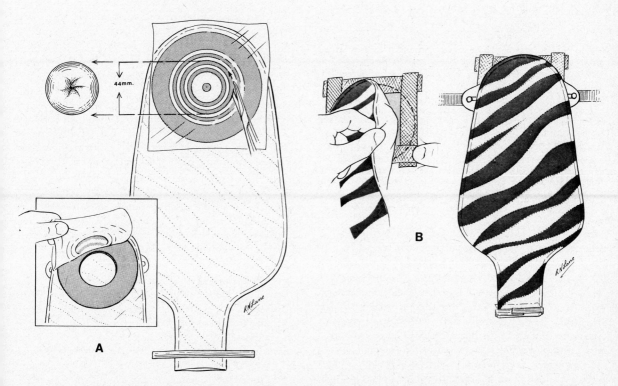

Fig. 563. Coloplast K-flex one-piece drainage appliance. (A) Back view of the appliance showing the circular flange which surrounds the opening near upper end into which the ileal spout will be fitted. The flange has a karaya washer on it, which is covered by a square sheet of thin plastic material with concentric markings to facilitate cutting the central hole to an appropriate size for the stoma. (It should be made slightly larger than the stoma, rather than the exact same size as shown here, to avoid injurious pressure by the cut edge of the flange on the ileal spout.) *Inset:* After the central hole has been suitably enlarged, the plastic sheet is peeled off, preparatory to fitting the bag. (B) Front view of fitted appliance, with flange adherent to the abdominal wall around the stoma and the belt in place. Note the gaily patterned material of which the front wall of the bag is constructed to conceal the faeces. The metal strip at the lower end has been folded on itself to close the exit conduit. *Inset:* The way in which the fixation of the flange to the abdominal skin is re-inforced by four strips of bland adhesive along the edge.

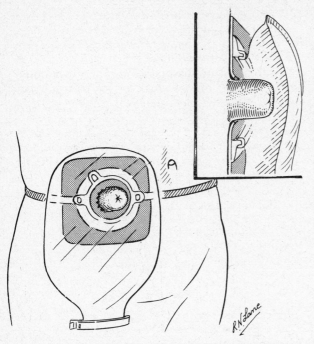

Fig. 564. Surgicare System 2 two-piece drainable appliance. (For more details of the structure of the appliance see Fig. 496 which describes the non-drainable version.) Central hole in Stomahesive square of flange piece has been cut to an appropriate size for the stoma and the edges of the opening snicked with a series of radiating short scissor cuts. The flange has then been applied to the abdominal wall around the stoma and the bag and belt fitted. In the early postoperative period a transparent bag is used, as here, to allow easy inspection of the state of the stoma. Subsequently an opaque grey bag is preferred, for it does not show the faecal content. *Inset:* Sectional view to illustrate how the Stomahesive fits snugly round the ileostomy spout, the snicked edge actually resting against the bowel mucosa.

plastic bag is fitted. A good example is the Translet appliance (see Fig. 495), the plastic bag of which has to be removed from the flange and discarded each time emptying is required. Down Bros. also make a two-piece appliance along similar lines, except that the plastic bag has an open spout at its lower end which is controlled by a clip. Another two-piece appliance that has recently come on the market is the Surgicare System 2, similar to that shown in Fig. 496 for use in connection with colostomies but with a drainage bag instead of a blind pouch (Fig. 564). The employment of Stomahesive as the fixing agent in this appliance should make it specially useful in ileostomy cases, particularly if there are any problems with skin soreness.

Detailed Routine for Changing Appliances

The changing of the appliance and fixing of a clean bag are best carried out in a combined toilet and bathroom, but, if this is not available, it is preferable to use the bathroom and to dispose of dirty materials subsequently partly in the toilet and partly elsewhere (see discussion on disposal of plastic colostomy appliances on p. 627). Some patients, indeed, have had a small washbasin installed in their toilet to enable them to carry out the whole procedure there. It is as well for them to have a small cupboard set aside in the bathroom or lavatory for keeping all the things needed for the care of the ileostomy and if they should have to do any travelling, it is a good plan to purchase a wide sponge-bag with zip fastener to carry the ileostomy equipment.

The used appliance is removed by peeling the flange off the skin, using the non-inflammable fat-solvent carbon tetrachloride to help dissolve any ordinary adhesive plaster holding the flange if it does not separate easily. If, on the other hand, fixation has been entirely by karaya or Stomahesive, no fat-solvent is needed. When the separation has been completed, the skin around the ileostomy should be thoroughly cleansed of all remnants of ordinary adhesive material, using a swab of cellulose tissue or Kleenex tissues soaked in carbon tetrachloride for this purpose. The ileostomy and skin should then be gently washed with soap and water and dried, and, finally, if the appliance being used is to be stuck even partly with ordinary adhesives, the skin (but not the stoma itself) is swabbed once again with carbon tetrachloride and allowed to dry for a minute or two. Some patients follow this with the application of Tr. Benz. Co., which on drying makes the skin quite sticky. But if the appliance is to be stuck entirely with karaya or

overcome by fitting a cloth or paper bag over the plastic one to conceal the faeces (and also in some cases to avoid irritation of the skin by the plastic material). The Coloplast bag (Fig. 563) obviates this problem by being made of an attractive patterned opaque plastic material; the flange of this appliance is stuck to the skin entirely with a karaya gum washer, but it is usual to place strips of non-irritating adhesive plaster, such as Dermaplast or Micropore, along the edges of the flange. Other very satisfactory one-piece drainage bags held in place partly or entirely by karaya gum washers or other relatively non-irritating adhesives are made by firms such as Salt and Eschmann.

Two-Piece Appliances

These appliances have a flange of more rigid plastic material (or rubber), on which the flimsy

Stomahesive, the use of carbon tetrachloride or Tr. Benz. Co. in this way is unnecessary and probably better avoided.

Attention is now turned to the fresh appliance that is going to be used. It will have been selected to be of an appropriate size of flange if, for example, it is a Hollister type, or if it is one with a karaya or Stomahesive washer that needs to have its central aperture enlarged as necessary by cutting with scissors, as in the Coloplast or Surgicare System 2 appliances, this is now done, the opening being made large enough to provide a fairly snug fit round the ileal spout without exposing it to the pressure and friction of an edge of the appliance. Finally any plastic or paper coverings are removed from the adhesive surface of the flange and it alone or with the bag attached (depending on whether a two- or one-piece appliance is being used) is apposed to the peristomal skin, care being taken to have the stoma sited exactly in the centre. Firm pressure is maintained on the flange for one or two minutes to obtain a secure adhesion to the skin. If a karaya or Stomahesive washer reaches to the periphery of the flange, it is a good plan to seal off the edge of the washer by applying four strips of non-irritating 2 cm strapping along the outer margin of the flange, partly on the flange and partly on the skin. Lastly the belt is applied and adjusted.

If a Stomahesive square is being used in conjunction with a Hollister appliance to avoid soreness of the skin from the adhesive peripheral to the karaya washer, a hole is cut in the central part of the square large enough to transmit the projecting ileal spout and a few radial snicks are made in the margin of the opening to avoid any injurious constriction. The paper covering is then peeled off and the square is applied to the peristomal skin with firm pressure for a few moments. Next the flange of the appliance is placed accurately over the square and held firmly in position for a couple of minutes or so. Finally peripheral strips of Micropore are applied and the belt fitted.

Supply of Appliances
In Britain ileostomy appliances can be obtained free on the National Health scheme. This is fortunate because the expense can be quite considerable, particularly to a patient who has recently had a major illness and operation and whose earning capacity is temporarily reduced or completely abolished for a while. Current prices (June 1979) for several of the appliances mentioned are as follows: Coloplast K-Flex drainage bag £0·80, Hollister drainage bag £0·80 to £1·00, Surgicare

System 2 flange £0·78, drainage bag £0·35, Stomahesive squares, ordinary size £0·74.

Disposal of Plastic Bags
The disposal of plastic ileostomy bags involves some problems, which are discussed in connection with plastic colostomy bags (see p. 627).

DEODORANTS

Though not by any means as malodorous as faeces escaping from a colostomy, the discharge from an ileostomy carries a peculiar aroma, which is somewhat offensive. Usually the odour is completely contained within the appliance and no smell is detectable by other people in the ordinary way. But occasionally the aroma seems to escape from within the appliance, either because it is more pungent or because the material of the bag is less odour-resistant, as, for example, when a rubber bag is starting to perish. If malodour is a persistent problem deodorants may be used in the bag, as described on p. 632. Sparberg (1974) in a controlled trial recently found oral bismuth subgallate 400 mg in capsules before each meal to be effective in controlling ileostomy odour.

DIET

There is no need for the ileostomy patient to follow a special diet though he may find it advisable to make a few minor dietetic adjustments. Much fruit or vegetables, especially in an uncooked condition, may produce very liquid motions which are more liable to leak from the appliance. If there is a tendency to leakage therefore it may be necessary among other precautions to restrict somewhat the amounts of these articles in the diet. Beer, stout and spirits are apt to have a similar effect and may have to be curtailed for the same reason. But these minor restrictions should not prevent the patient having a full and varied diet including moderate amounts of green vegetables and fruit.

BATHS

Many ileostomy patients imagine that because of the ileostomy appliance they can only have baths infrequently, in fact only at the times of changing the flange. This is incorrect. Certainly if *a double-sided adhesive square or a cement is being used* to fix the appliance, there is no reason why the patient should not have baths with the bag in position. Provided the water is not too hot, the appliance will remain securely attached, but it is a good plan to change the narrow strips of adhesive plaster on the front of the flange after the bath. If, on the other hand, *karaya gum or Stomahesive is being employed as the main fixing agent*, baths may have a deleterious effect, leading to some erosion of the adhesive, so that some caution is required. However, usually the bag remains securely in position despite baths.

CAPACITY FOR WORK AND RECREATION

The patient can be assured that there are countless persons in all walks of life who are enjoying perfect health and living full normal lives despite the fact that they possess an ileostomy, and that in due course when he regains his normal strength and has learned to look after his ileostomy, he will be able to do likewise. The actual time required before this state of affairs is reached will obviously depend on the occurrence and course of any complications. In certain cases, however, it may be advisable for the patient not to return to his former occupation (see p. 787).

Reassurance may also be given to the patient that his ileostomy will not debar him from mixing with other people and taking part in social life. Many men and women with ileostomies take part in athletics or games such as cricket, tennis or golf. Soccer and rugby, which involve rough bodily contacts, may well displace the ileostomy bag and are better avoided. Surprisingly enough, swimming occasions no difficulty whatsoever, for the ileostomy bag remains firmly adherent despite submersion in water, and it need not show through a thick double-fronted bathing costume. There are special rubber belts available to wear instead of the ordinary belt when swimming, but most people find that the appliance is held sufficiently securely in position with the adhesive alone aided by the support of the swim-suit. However, the outer strips of adhesive strapping are better changed after the swim.

SEXUAL FUNCTION

IN THE FEMALE

Unmarried women can be reassured that ileostomy does not prove an insuperable, or even major, obstacle to matrimony, for very many of my younger female patients seem to have experienced little difficulty about becoming engaged and getting married since ileostomy and proctocolectomy. As to the relative chances of such women becoming pregnant and the relative hazards of pregnancy after this operation, possibly the prospects of pregnancy are somewhat diminished, as after any other major lower abdominal operation, because of adhesion formation in the vicinity of the uterine tubes, and conceivably the risks of the actual pregnancy and confinement might be marginally increased. But to elicit such slight differences would necessitate massive statistics, which we do not have. Certainly a large number of my patients have gone through pregnancy and parturition *per vias naturales* without incident; indeed the absence of the anorectum facilitated the performance of episiotomy in a few instances! Roy et al. (1969), Ritchie (1971*b*) and Hudson (1972) record equally reassuring limited experiences. Accordingly, I feel that, if a patient with an ileostomy is anxious to have a child, she should be encouraged to do so.

As to whether the act of sexual intercourse is altered after operation, information is scanty and somewhat superficial. Watts et al. (1966*b*) interviewed from this point of view 67 of my female patients after ileostomy and proctocolectomy: five stated that they had had considerable mechanical difficulties with intercourse (because of a perineal sinus, vaginal stenosis, pain, urinary incontinence and fear of dislodging the ileostomy flange, respectively). Most of the remaining 62 patients claimed that their sexual relationships had been enhanced since operation, this usually being attributed to improvement in general health: Burham et al.'s (1977) report on a larger postal survey of 175 married female ileostomists is similar but somewhat less reassuring. About 50% of the patients considered the ileostomy to be something of an embarrassment and felt that it rendered them sexually less attractive, but this view was shared by only 6% of their spouses. Between 10 and 14% found that sexual intercourse was more difficult because of the ileostomy, mainly on account of a fear, usually unrealized, that the bag might come off during the act. Nearly 30% of female patients complained that they had some new perineal or vaginal discomfort at intercourse, but the proportion of women experiencing orgasm increased slightly following proctocolectomy.

IN THE MALE

Disturbance of sexual function in the male from damage to the pelvic autonomic nerves is a well recognized complication, which, as pointed out on p. 621 occurs in some two-thirds of the patients having rectal excision *for carcinoma*. Fortunately, the advanced age of many of these patients lessens the disability resulting from this complication. Much more serious significance attaches to this consequence of rectal excision when it occurs as a result of treatment *for ulcerative colitis*, for patients suffering from this disease are usually younger and deprivation of this function may have grave psychological and social repercussions. It has generally been held that the risk of neurogenic disturbance of sexual function by rectal excision in male colitics is slight because of the more restricted dissection in these cases (Dennis and Karlson 1952; Brooke 1956a; Stahlgren and Ferguson 1959a; Donovan and O'Hara 1960; Bacon et al. 1960; Barker 1961; van Prohaska and Siderius 1962). For example, Stahlgren and Ferguson (1959a) interrogated 25 male patients, who had had abdominoperineal excision as part of the surgical treatment of their colitis during the previous 10 years, and found that 18 had normal sexual function, two claimed enhanced prowess and five reported some dysfunction (partial impotence in five, failure of ejaculation in two).

A similar survey of some of my male colitis patients after ileostomy and proctocolectomy (Watts et al. 1966b) has been slightly less reassuring: 41 patients over the age of puberty at the time of operation were followed up for a mean period of four years. 30 reported normal sexual function and 11 some impairment of function (failure of ejaculation in two; temporary impotence, which eventually recovered, in two; and permanent impotence in seven). It seemed that the *age of the patient at the time of the operation was an important factor* in determining the risks of sexual dysfunction, for none of eight patients aged less than 30 years noticed any alteration of sexual function, five of 25 patients aged between 30 and 50 years suffered some form of sexual dysfunction—fortunately permanent impotence in only one—and six of eight older patients (mean age 59 years) became completely impotent. It is difficult to offer an adequate explanation on technical grounds for the difference in the results according to the age of the patients (which was also observed by Stahlgren and Ferguson, 1959a), for the same sort of pelvic dissection, with reasonable care to avoid damage to the autonomic nerves, was employed in all of them. It may well be that in the older patients the abolition of potence was merely a reflection of the psychological effect of a major operation, culminating in the creation of an artificial anus, on an individual whose sexual function was already on the wane.

An investigation by May (1966) at St Mark's Hospital reached similar conclusions. 46 male patients, who were under 40 at the time of operation and had rectal excision as part of the surgical treatment of their colitis, were interviewed. 35 claimed to have normal sexual function, three complained of transient disturbances of this function postoperatively and eight had permanent impairment (including complete impotence in three and partial impotence in three). The disorders of sexual function were more frequent in the older age groups. In Burnham et al.'s (1977) recent postal survey of 128 male ileostomists 5% were found to be completely impotent, and 10% partially so, whilst 7·6% noted failure of ejaculation. The age of the patient seemed to be an important factor in regard to the incidence of these complaints, for five of the instances of complete impotence occurred in the 35 patients over the age of 45 and none in the 61 patients under the age of 35.

What makes these reports on disturbances of sexual function so disappointing is that the dysfunction has arisen often despite particular efforts on the part of the surgeon to keep very close to the rectum during his pelvic and perineal dissection. It is difficult to see what more can be done to obviate these complications of rectal excision for inflammatory bowel disease, though Lytle and Parks (1976) claim that an intersphincteric plane of dissection in the perineal part of the operation may lessen the risks of damage to the autonomic nerves (see p. 735).

SEXUAL FUNCTION AFTER ILEORECTAL ANASTOMOSIS

There have been no really thorough surveys of sexual function after colectomy and ileorectal anastomosis, but Grüner et al. (1975) noted that dyspareunia was complained of by over half their female patients treated by this operation and in a number anal incontinence seemed to be triggered off by intercourse. Several of the women given ileorectal anastomoses by me had similar complaints which only emerged on determined questioning.

BOOKLET OF ADVICE ON ILEOSTOMY MANAGEMENT

To supplement the practical instruction given to the patient on the care of her ileostomy before her discharge from hospital, I have found it useful to provide her with a small blooklet of advice incorporating most of the information comprised in pp. 765–72 above. This is written in clear and simple language readily understood by lay people and has apparently been much appreciated by my patients. It is also incidentally very helpful in instructing medical students and nurses in the essentials of ileostomy care. Of course, similar booklets are provided by some firms manufacturing stomal appliances, but one is always apprehensive that they may reflect commercial bias. Comprehensive texts on all aspects of stomal care are those of Walker (1975) and Todd (1978), but these are designed more for professional readers than for ileostomists.

ILEOSTOMY ASSOCIATIONS

During the past couple of decades ileostomy clubs have been established in a number of centres in America and this country for persons with ileostomies. The first such club took the title of QT because the majority of its members had had their operations done in the Q and T wards of the Mount Sinai Hospital, New York (Lyons 1952). Many other ileostomy clubs, which were formed subsequently in the United States, have also adopted this non-committal name, and there has recently been an amalgamation of most of these groups.

The Ileostomy Association of Great Britain was founded in 1956 and has a national committee and many local divisions in different parts of the country. The organization functions by distributing a quarterly magazine and by holding periodic divisional meetings, at which new ileostomy appliances are displayed and subjects of interest to 'ileostomists' are discussed. Further information about QT in America can be obtained from United Ostomy Association Inc., Secretary: Bernice T. Kaufman, 373 Avenue S, Brooklyn, New York, and about the British Ileostomy Association from the National Secretary, Mr C. J. W. Penny, 1st floor, 23 Winchester Road, Basingstoke, Hants RG21 1VE.

Late Complications of Conventional Ileostomy

Ileostomy has had an evil reputation in the past for the frequency of complications and sequelae, often necessitating further operations. For example, Bargen (1956) in a follow-up of 124 patients submitted

to ileostomy at the Mayo Clinic between 1940 and 1949 reported that no less than 86% had complications referable to their stomas during the first postoperative year and 43% of those surviving that year had further complications. The result was that very many patients had one, two or more revision operations on the ileostomies. Rhodes and Kirsner (1965) have given an equally depressing account of the frequency of complications after ileostomy. These numerous complications may have been representative of the outcome after ileostomy made by the methods prevalent in the 1940s, but they are certainly not typical of the results obtainable by the modern technique of terminal ileal eversion and immediate mucocutaneous suture (see p. 753). This is the method which I have used exclusively since 1952 and a follow-up by Watts et al. (1966b) of 115 of my ileostomy patients operated on between 1955 and 1963 gives a reliable impression of the complication rate of ileostomy at the present time (Table 60).

STENOSIS

Stenosis has already been referred to (p. 765) as a complication of ileostomy made by the old-fashioned technique without mucocutaneous suture, due in the early stages to oedema of the stoma, and later to fibrous stenosis at the junction of the mucosa and skin, which may eventually reduce its lumen at this level to less than the width of a lead pencil. In an endeavour to prevent the development of such stenosis it has often been

TABLE 60. *Late Ileostomy Complications in 115 Patients Operated on between 1955 and 1963*

Ileostomy complications	No. of patients
Stenosis	2
Prolapse	
sliding	2
fixed	1
Recession	
sliding	13
fixed	9
Ulceration and fistula formation	1
Hernia	3
Abscess	2
Stitch sinus	2
Ileitis or oedema	2
Granulomatous polyps	1
Profuse watery stools	4
Intermittent skin irritation	30

After Watts et al. (1966b).

recommended that the patient should pass a finger into the stoma every time the bag is changed. I think the value of this practice is in the highest degree dubious; it may be, indeed, that it merely serves to promote stenosis by tearing the tissues slightly each time the finger is inserted, with resulting increased fibrosis.

The only reliable way to prevent this complication of ileostomy is to abandon the technique that produced it and to employ a method embodying immediate mucocutaneous suture. The incidence of stenosis in ileostomies made by the old-fashioned method was estimated by Counsell and Lockhart-Mummery (1954) to be 30% and by Brooke (1956a) some 25%. By comparison, the chances of stenosis occurring with the modern technique of eversion and primary suture are very slight; thus, Brooke (1956a) found that narrowing had developed in only one of 74 patients whose ileostomies were made in this way, and I observed only two stenoses in 115 ileostomies similarly constructed (see Table 60). Ritchie (1967, 1971a) records incidences of ileostomy stenosis of only 1 and 2·5% respectively in series of 200 and 405 cases followed-up by her, the operative technique employed having apparently been that of primary mucocutaneous suture.

Considerable stenosis may be present without causing any symptoms. The sort of complaint eventually produced by a severe degree of narrowing is cramping abdominal pain, difficulty with the ileostomy actions, and frequently very liquid voluminous motions. Rarely perforation of the terminal ileum has occurred through a stercoral ulcer with resulting peritonitis and a fatal outcome unless surgical treatment has been promptly carried out (see p. 779).

The treatment of an established ileostomy stenosis involves excision of the strictured stoma together with a surrounding disc of skin and subcutaneous fat (see p. 783).

PROLAPSE

This used to be a common complication of simple ileostomy (made by the non-suture technique), the bowel often projecting as much as 12–15 cm (Fig. 565). Thus, in a group of 60 cases treated by ileostomy alone, Counsell and I (1952) found severe prolapse in nine. But in the series of 115 cases treated by ileostomy and proctocolectomy by me and referred to in Table 60, there were only three instances of ileostomy prolapse. Ritchie (1967, 1971a) had a similarly low incidence of prolapse in the large series of cases followed-up by her after ileostomy and proctocolectomy. It is difficult to understand the greater rarity of this complication with the method of eversion and immediate suture (combined with proctocolectomy), because this technique might perhaps on theoretical grounds have been expected to predispose to prolapse, and it is interesting to find that, in actual practice it did not do so. Perhaps more attention has been lavished on the fixation of the inner tube of bowel to the musculo-aponeurotic layers of the abdominal wall in association with this latter technique than was customary in the making of ileostomies 25 or 30 years ago.

Two types of prolapse may be recognized: (a) A *sliding prolapse* in which the ileostomy bud projects excessively at some times—usually when the patient is upright or straining, but occasionally in a more capricious way—and at other times is of normal length or less. Presumably the condition has arisen because fixation of the inner tube of ileum to the opening in the abdominal wall was either initially inadequate or subsequently gave way. (b) A *fixed excessive projection*, where the ileostomy bud per-

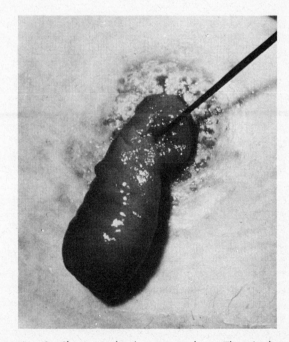

Fig. 565. Ileostomy showing gross prolapse. There is also a fistula (indicated by probe) through the ileostomy bud near to the level of the abdominal skin due to the friction of the ileostomy appliance, a stenosis is present, and the stoma has been placed too low—altogether a good example of how *not* to make and manage an ileostomy!

manently protrudes too much. This is really due to faulty judgement at operation as to the amount of ileum to be retained beyond the site of fixation of the inner tube of bowel.

A mild degree of excessive fixed projection or sliding prolapse may occasion little inconvenience and be compatible with normal ileostomy management, though a fastidious female ileostomist may object to the bulky protuberant stoma. But a major degree of over-projection or prolapse is a serious handicap, because it tends to push the appliance off and cause leakage with resultant digestion of the skin. The prolapse may even become stuck in the flange of the appliance, as happened in one case in my experience! For these grosser forms of prolapse operative treatment is indicated and may take one of three forms:

Amputation of the Projecting Bowel (comparable to rectosigmoidectomy for prolapse of the rectum) has sometimes been recommended. But, for a *sliding prolapse*, this method is entirely unsatisfactory, because it does absolutely nothing to prevent recurrence of the prolapse and thus merely sacrifices valuable small bowel to no useful end. For a *fixed over-protruberant stoma*, however, this operation can be successfully employed. It is best to make the initial circumcision through the outer tube of ileum at the mucocutaneous junction and to un-evert the bowel to its full length. An appropriate portion can then be amputated from the end of the extended segment, so that, when the ileum is everted once more and sutured to the skin, a suitable-sized ileostomy projection is produced.

Re-fixation of the Ileum and Mesentery to the Abdominal Wall by an Operation confined to the Ileostomy Itself. A circumcision is made round the base of the 'bud' accurately at the mucocutaneous junction (Fig. 569). This is deepened to expose the inner tube of ileum and its related mesentery (Figs 570, 571), which in these cases will usually be found to be quite unattached to the parietes. The next step is to re-fix the leaf of the ileal mesentery and the ileum to the anterior rectus sheath by a close series of fine serum-proof silk sutures as shown in Fig. 556. If the aperture in the parietes is a trifle too wide, it may be partly closed by one or two silk sutures, but *any gross widening of this kind or weakness of the surrounding muscles calls for the use of an entirely different technique* (see below). Finally, the distal cut edge of the ileum is resutured to the skin margin (Fig. 557).

Re-siting of Ileostomy. If before or during operation it is found that the aperture in the parietes through which the ileum passes is unduly wide and the musculature surrounding it is thin and stretched, it will probably be better not to attempt fixation of the bowel in this site, but to re-site the ileostomy (see p. 782), choosing a place where the musculature is good and taking care to make the opening of such a size that it fits the ileum snugly, as, for example, on the opposite side of the abdomen.

ULCERATION AND FISTULA FORMATION

It will be seen from Table 60 that there was only one instance of ulceration of the ileostomy in our group of 115 ileostomists surveyed. This complication may arise in two main ways. If the bud is longer than normal, and particularly if a definite prolapse has developed, friction of the bag against the end of the protruded bowel may result in superficial ulceration. Alternatively, if the flange of the ileostomy bag grips the ileostomy too tightly, this may result in ulceration developing at the neck of the bud, especially on the under aspect, probably because the flange is pushed up against the stoma when the thigh is flexed in sitting. If this state of affairs is allowed to continue, the ulcerative process may continue till the ileostomy is eroded through to the lumen of the bowel, thus producing a fistula just superficial to the level of the skin (Fig. 565). This is a troublesome state of affairs, for the escape of ileal contents in this situation tends to unstick the flange and produce leakage. In fact, satisfactory ileostomy management is usually impossible till the stoma has been completely re-fashioned (see p. 783). In this little operation all bowel distal to the fistula is amputated and the ileum is drawn farther out of the abdomen and fixed by sutures of silk to the anterior rectus sheath as in Fig. 556A, to allow of an adequate protrusion after eversion and resuture of the skin.

In the avoidance of mucosal ulceration and fistulation of the ileostomy it is clearly important that the aperture in the plastic (or rubber) part of the appliance should be sufficiently wide to allow a gap between it and the stomal spout. But there is no objection to the edge of a karaya washer or Stomahesive square being in contact with the bowel, for they are soft and non-injurious.

HERNIATION

In my experience herniation has been very unusual with terminal ileostomies made at a separate wound by the technique described on p. 754, and occurred in only three of 115 patients (Table 60). Ritchie (1971a) had an even lower incidence. This is indeed remarkable when the frequent, almost invariable, association of herniation with colostomies fashion-

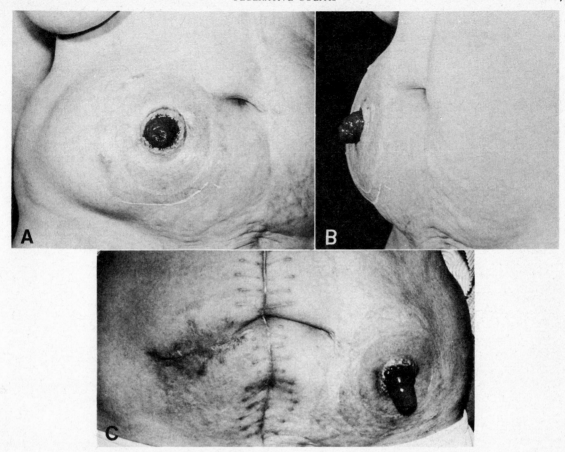

Fig. 566. Large peri-ileostomy hernia seen *en face* (A) and in profile (B). This was treated by transplantation of the stoma to the left half of the abdomen, as shown in (C).

ed by a very similar technique is recalled. I can offer no explanation for this difference. Para-ileostomy hernias have been commoner in cases where the stoma was established in the line of the main incision and some degree of separation of the wound took place subsequently, or where the ileostomy was of loop variety and had been made at a fairly large gridiron incision in the right iliac region. Fortunately, such errors of initial operative procedure are now rare.

Herniation around an ileostomy is a serious handicap, as a rule, for it interferes with the firm retention of the ileostomy appliance (Fig. 566A, B). The only satisfactory management for this state of affairs is to re-site the ileostomy, usually on the other side of the abdomen (Fig. 566C).

FIXED INADEQUATE PROTRUSION OR SLIDING
RECESSION

The ideal ileostomy projects 2·5–4 cm (Fig. 567) and the amount of protrusion should vary only slightly

with alterations in the posture of the patient. In certain cases, however, due to faulty judgement at operation an inadequate ileostomy bud has been provided (Fig. 572). In others, though the pro-trusion is adequate when the patient is standing or straining, or pressure is exerted by the examiner's fingers on the surrounding abdominal wall (Fig. 568A), the ileostomy recedes into the abdomen in recumbency and may even disappear completely below the level of the skin (Fig. 568B).

The practical significance of these abnormalities is that they predispose to leakage despite a well fitted adherent ileostomy bag, and a severe degree of recession on recumbency almost invariably leads to nocturnal soiling. For this reason it is important in the initial fashioning of the ileostomy to secure an adequate protrusion and to fix the inner tube of bowel by suture to the musculo-aponeurotic layers of the abdominal wall to avoid recession. I used not to stitch the ileum directly to the parietes, for fear of producing necrosis of bowel and faecal fistulation, but instead relied on suturing of the ileal mesentery. However, using this technique in 115 cases, it will be seen from Table 60 that I have had no less than 13 instances of sliding ileostomy recession. At reoperation on several of these patients it seemed that, though the mesenteric fixation was still secure, the inner tube of bowel itself had failed to adhere and was able to swing round about this *point d'appui* into and out of the abdominal cavity. As a result of this experience I have more recently been suturing the ileum itself at the initial operation, as pointed out on p. 758, and the incidence of recession seems now to be lessened. It will also be noted in Table 60 that I have had nine cases in which the ileostomy was considered on review to show a fixed inadequate projection. Some of these were undoubtedly due to errors of judgement at operation; others were due to the fact that

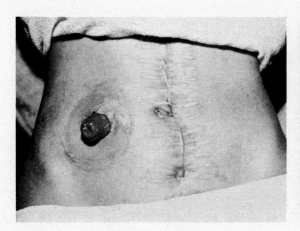
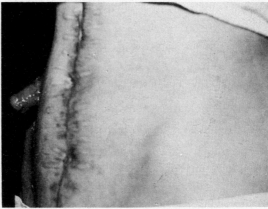

Fig. 567. *En face* and profile views of a well-formed ileostomy, which projects 3 cm beyond the abdominal skin, does not recede materially when the patient is recumbent, and is supple and free from any suggestion of stenosis at the mucocutaneous junction.

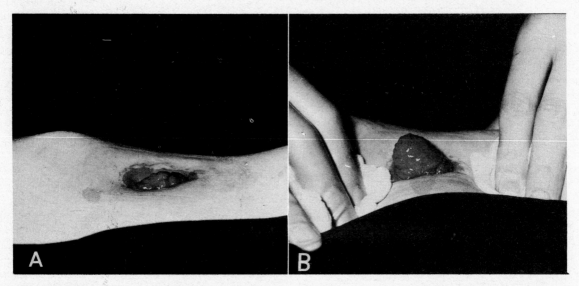

Fig. 568. Ileostomy recession. (A) Tangential view of abdomen with patient recumbent, showing that ileum does not project beyond the abdominal skin. (B) Similar view with pressure exerted on the surrounding skin causing the stoma to protrude nearly 2·5 cm. (*From Goligher 1963*).

the patient had put on a great deal of weight subsequently, making a previously adequate ileal protrusion insufficient.

Mild degrees of inadequate protrusion or sliding recession may cause little or no trouble, but, if the condition is at all marked, the patient will amost certainly find it more difficult to avoid leakage and irritation of the skin. However, by paying particular attention to the details of application of the ileostomy bag, this difficulty may be largely overcome, and this is the treatment one would always recommend in the first instance. A grossly deficient projection or recession of the stoma will almost invariably be found to result in frequent leakage and excoriation, despite the most meticulous efforts devoted to ileostomy care, and operative treatment should be seriously considered. In essence this consists of detaching the ileostomy and terminal ileum from the abdominal wall and re-fixing the bowel in such a way that it projects adequately and is held in this position so that it cannot slide in or out. This may often be accomplished by a simple circumcision around the base of the ileostomy bud, deepened on the inner tube of bowel and carried along it into the peritoneal cavity to free the ileum and mesentery (Figs 569–571). The ileum is then re-attached by suture and the ileostomy remade (Figs 555, 556). If, however, the gap in the musculo-aponeurotic layers is wide, it is better to do a formal laparotomy and re-site the ileostomy in order to secure a more snugly-fitting hole in the abdominal wall, which will help fixation of the ileum to the parietes.

ABSCESS

Two of my patients developed abscesses on the lateral side of their ileostomies many months after their operations. There was no connection with the bowel lumen and it was difficult to understand why they should have arisen in otherwise healthy individuals. Both abscesses were opened by a small incision through the abdominal wall well lateral to the stoma, so as not to damage the skin immediately around the ileostomy, to which the flange of the adherent bag is applied. It seemed that the pus had possibly accumulated in the extraperitoneal space created by the extraperitoneal technique (see p. 755) used for the formation of most of my ileostomies. No unabsorbed suture material was found to account for the infection. In both cases the abscess cleared up very rapidly after drainage and there has been no trouble since.

STITCH SINUS

Considering that non-absorbable silk sutures are usually employed to fix the ileal mesentery (and possibly the ileum itself) to the abdominal wall, and that some degree of contamination of the wound is probably inevitable during the completion of the ileostomy, it is surprising that persistent sepsis around stitches is not more common. I have had this trouble in only two of my cases. They both developed a smouldering infection, which did not clear up till several silk sutures were extruded—in one case the process being assisted by plucking some of the stitches out with a crochet-hook.

ILEITIS, ILEAL PERFORATION OR OEDEMA

In the 1940s the development of ileitis in the terminal ileum immediately proximal to the ileostomy was much discussed as a serious and fairly common complication of this operation. Sometimes even perforation of the diseased small bowel occurred, often in the early postoperative period, as in the cases recorded by Crandon et al. (1944) and Madell and Golden (1955). It was believed by Crandon et al. (1944), McCready et al. (1949), Lyons and Garlock (1954) and Colcock and Mathiesen (1956) that this state of affairs usually resulted from making the ileostomy in bowel already the seat of 'backwash' or retrograde ileitis at the time of the original operation. But, following the exposition by Warren and McKittrick (1951) of the significant role of ileostomy dysfunction (see p. 734) in the aetiology of terminal ileitis and ileal perforation, it became widely accepted that this was probably the main cause of these complications (Counsell 1956). With the introduction of the technique of ileal eversion and primary mucocutaneous suture in the construction of ileostomies, stenosis at the stoma due to early oedema or later fibrosis has become exceedingly rare (see pp. 765 and 774) in my experience and in that of most surgeons of my acquaintance. Similarly ileitis seems to have largely disappeared as a postoperative complication or sequel so far as patients originally suffering from ulcerative colitis are concerned. (It is quite different in patients having ileostomy for Crohn's disease, see p. 874). In fact I have met with only one instance of such ileitis in some 240 patients whose ileostomies were made by the modern technique. In that case—which is not included in the series analysed in the compilation of Table 60—there was no ileostomy stenosis or dysfunction to account for it, and the original proctocolectomy specimen showed typical gross and histopathological features of ordinary ulcerative colitis and no evidence of Crohn's enteritis. The segment of diseased ileum, which was removed at a subsequent operation two years later, was thought by our pathologist to be the seat of Crohn's disease.

I have had two patients who developed a peculiar *transient oedema of the ileostomy and the terminal ileum.* This occurred one and two years respectively after the operation and presented by causing a swelling and stiffness of the ileostomy spout with partial intestinal obstruction. A sigmoidoscope passed through the stoma into the lower ileum showed only oedema of the mucosa. This oedematous state of the terminal ileum was confirmed at laparotomy in one of the cases on which active surgical treatment was carried out. The condition subsided spontaneously in both patients in five to seven days and the ileostomy and intestinal function returned to normal. In one case there was a mild recurrence of the condition some 12 months later, again with spontaneous subsidence. I am quite unable to explain this occurrence and have been unable to discover any similar cases recorded in the literature.

More recently there have been four reports of an ileitis not histopathologically typical of Crohn's disease developing in the terminal ileum following ileostomy and colectomy for ulcerative colitis. Tolstedt and Bell (1961) observed 10 examples of this phenomenon in 33 patients so treated; Kellner et al. (1963) in five of 66 patients; Turnbull et al. (1964) in 35 of 250 patients; and Knill-Jones et al. (1970) in five cases, the size of the parent series not being stated. No less than 18 of this collective group of 55 patients with ileitis presented acutely, and of these 12 had ileal perforations. The great majority of these cases proceeded to further operation, at which the diseased lower ileum was resected, often with very gratifying results. I find it extremely difficult to reconcile the findings of these authors regarding the incidence of terminal ileitis after ileostomy with my own very different experience. Though it is stated that the primary condition for which the colectomy was performed in these cases was ordinary ulcerative colitis, I cannot help wondering if in some of them it was not Crohn's disease of the large bowel and the resuting ileitis was not a further manifestation of this condition (see p. 847). I am particularly prompted to make this comment in regard to Turnbull et al.'s (1964) patients, because in a personal communication two years later he explained that a more recent assessment of the pathological features of his colitis material, using different histological criteria, had shown a high proportion of the patients to be suffering from Crohn's enteritis of the large bowel.

FORMATION OF POLYPOID GRANULOMAS ON THE EXPOSED ILEOSTOMY MUCOSA

I have now encountered multiple nodules about the size of split peas on the external surface of the ileostomy bud in five other patients in addition to the one listed in Table 60. Examination of the lower ileum with the sigmoidoscope revealed no similar lesions in the lining mucosa, and a barium progress meal and fat balance study on two of the cases demonstrated no definite abnormality. Biopsy of the nodules indicated that they are composed of granulation tissue without any special diagnostic features. I am unable to explain their formation.

No active treatment seems to be required, for they are compatible with normal functioning and management of the ileostomy.

PROFUSE ILEOSTOMY DISCHARGE

Most patients with an ileostomy done for ulcerative colitis find that within two or three weeks of their operation the ileostomy discharge has reduced itself to 400–500 ml per day and has acquired a firmer consistency. (When this operation has been done for Crohn's colitis often a good deal of terminal ileum has to be excised along with the large bowel so that a persistently profuse ileostomy discharge is a not infrequent sequel, see p. 849.) With certain colitics this state of affairs is never reached; instead the ileostomy continues to pour out 1200 or 1500 ml or more of very liquid faeces each 24 hours (Hill et al. 1975a). Though some degree of ileostomy stenosis, with resulting dysfunction, may account for a few of these examples of ileostomy diarrhoea—and the treatment is then obvious (see p. 774)—more usually no such local cause is evident. In these latter cases passage of a sigmoidoscope into the ileostomy shows no abnormality of the mucosa of the terminal ileum. Barium progress studies usually reveal rapid transit of the barium through the small bowel but no other abnormality. (It is of course very important to be on the alert for 'recurrent' Crohn's disease even if the pathological report on the proctocolectomy specimen diagnosed it as ordinary ulcerative colitis.) The condition is compatible with excellent general health; the difficulty arises in connection with ileostomy management, for these very liquid motions predispose to leakage. Salt depletion may also occur. Efforts may be made to secure firmer motions by avoidance of certain items of diet by prescribing large dose of codeine phosphate (60–120 mg four times daily), Lomotil (two tablets four times daily) or—perhaps best of all according to a recent report by Tytgat and Huibregtse (1975)—loperamide (4 mg twice or thrice a day), though I have known all these drugs to fail. The systemic administration of steroids may also be tried for their anti-diarrhoeal effect. To help to avoid leakage the use of Stomahesive squares to fix the appliance is usually advisable. Correction of any electrolyte depletion by suitable intravenous or oral supplements may be necessary. Where exceptionally severe diarrhoea makes it impossible for the patient to keep her appliance on without leakage, consideration may have to be given to the desirability of a re-operation to reverse a short segment—say

10 cm—of lower ileum to act as an antiperistaltic brake, as suggested by Ellis and Coll (1968), Javett and Brooke (1971) and Cohen et al. (1975). Sometimes this works well, but in some cases it is relatively ineffective. An alternative is to convert to a reservoir type of ileostomy, but this sort of case puts the continence of the reservoir to a very severe test (see p. 796).

SKIN IRRITATION

This is easily the most frequent complication of ileostomy and at some stage occurred in 26% of my patients (see Table 60), but fortunately in most of them it was very transient and responded to appropriate management, so that these patients no longer have this complaint, though they know that they are liable to it if they are not careful. From the patient's point of view irritation is troublesome because it interferes with the firm fixation of the appliance and may thus lead to considerable bodily discomfort. Also it is the mode of presentation of several of the other complications of ileostomy, because the most common cause of skin irritation is leakage and any condition which predisposes to leakage may manifest itself first by producing digestion and excoriation of the skin. Very rarely the prime cause of the irritation is a sensitization of the skin to the material of the ileostomy appliance or to one of the ingredients in the fixing cement or adhesive plaster. But even then the leakage that ensues, when the appliance cannot be securely stuck on, rapidly aggravates the skin condition.

In the management of this disturbing complication, therefore, the first consideration is to look for a primary cause of leakage. The *stoma* itself is viewed critically with reference to the presence of fistulation, the amount of protrusion, and any tendency to recession; depending on the findings, it may be necessary to advise re-siting or refashioning of the ileostomy, though naturally these steps would only be recommended for gross structural defects when simpler measures have failed. It is also important to enquire about the *consistency of the motions*, for very liquid motions may cause frequent leakages, even if the ileostomy itself has been satisfactorily constructed. Advice regarding diet and possibly the prescription of medicaments such as codeine phosphate, Lomotil or loperamide (see above) may be required to secure firmer motions. Finally, if it is suspected that *skin sensitization* may be a factor, this may be investigated by sticking the appliance on some other part and noting whether any reaction results. If the skin becomes irritated in the new site, patch tests may then be carried out to determine whether it is the material of the bag or the adhesive that is responsible. (As mentioned on p. 769, a common cause of skin soreness when using the Hollister drainage bag is sensitivity to the adhesive on the plastic square peripheral to the karaya washer, which can be avoided or corrected by using a square of Stomahesive between the appliance and the skin or changing to the pattern of Hollister bag with a microporous adherent flange.)

It must be admitted that in many instances no obvious initiating cause for the skin irritation can be discovered. In such cases it may be that the condition arose out of a transient leak, which led to some digestion of the skin making adhesion of the bag difficult, so that further leakage occurred. To break this vicious circle—and this will be required also in cases where a primary cause has been found and removed—the use of Stomahesive as a washer, as described on p. 769, is invaluable. After the skin has been soundly healed with this regimen, a return is made to the use of ordinary adhesives again or Stomahesive may be continued indefinitely.

GASTROENTERITIS WITH DEPLETION OF FLUID AND SALT

Patients with ileostomies may have occasional bouts of vomiting and diarrhoea, just as do ordinary individuals, due presumably to a mild transient non-specific gastroenteritis or dietetic indiscretion. The special significance of these attacks in ileostomy patients is that, due to a combination of vomiting and profuse ileostomy actions, depletion of fluid and electrolytes, particularly sodium, may take place with astonishing rapidity. I have seen several patients re-admitted in a very ill condition with gross dehydration and sodium deficiency after such an attack lasting 24–36 hours. The moral is that all ileostomists and their doctors should be warned of the dangers of gastrointestinal upsets and strongly advised that, if these do not rapidly subside, the patients should seek re-admission to hospital, where accurate fluid and electrolyte control may be established.

INJURY TO ILEOSTOMY

Because of the way in which it projects, an ileostomy would seem to be specially exposed to the risk of injury, and it is for this reason that the ileostomist is advised against indulging in so-called 'body contact' sports. No doubt occasional injuries of this kind have occurred but I am not aware of any having been published. However, I do know of one instance of injury to an ileostomy by a seat belt during a motor car accident (Wilkinson and Humphreys 1978). The effect was to produce a 4 cm tear at the mucocutaneous junction which caused severe bleeding requiring suture. I also know of one patient who tried unsuccessfully to cut off her rather unduly projecting ileostomy spout because of an obsession about its unsightliness and phallic qualities! She did not quite succeed and some months later I converted her to a reservoir ileostomy with a very satisfactory result from all points of view.

Conventional Ileostomy Reconstruction

Though there have been significant advances in the technique of ileostomy construction and in its after-care, this operation is still occasionally followed by troublesome leakage and soreness of the skin, as pointed out on p. 781. This is most frequently due to faulty ileostomy management and can be corrected by a change of appliance or alteration of the routine for its fixation to the abdominal wall. But sometimes the trouble persists despite the most assiduous attention to the details of ileostomy care, and in the majority of these patients the explanation lies in the fact that the ileostomy has been badly sited or made.

As explained on p. 753, there are differences of opinion even among experienced colon surgeons as to the best site for an ileostomy. But there is fairly general agreement that *certain sites are thoroughly bad*. Thus, placing the stoma too close to the umbilicus or to the anterior superior iliac spine, so that the flange of the appliance overlies these structures, is very liable to result in leakage. Similarly, if the opening is made too high, so that the bag impinges on the rib margin, it is apt to be uncomfortable and to leak; whilst if it is sited too low, pressure on the inferior margin of the flange by the front of the thigh during flexion of the hip may press it upwards against the ileostomy spout and lead to ulceration or fistulation and leakage. It is certainly better to have the stoma emerging not in the line of a main wound scar, which renders fixation of the appliance more difficult, but through a separate snugly-fitting wound, so that it is surrounded by smooth flat skin.

In the actual reconstruction of the ileostomy, the modern technique now favoured has been described on p. 753. It must be admitted, however, that, even with considerable familiarity with this technique, it is not too difficult to err at operation in one's judgement as to the site, amount of projection, or degree of fixation of an ileostomy. In addition the structure of the stoma, which may be satisfactory in the first instance, may subsequently deteriorate due to factors more or less beyond the surgeon's control. I have to confess that of the 504 cases treated by me by ileostomy and procto-colectomy (or colectomy) for ulcerative colitis, 25 (5%) have subsequently had to undergo a re-fashioning or re-siting of their stomas for various reasons—the re-fashioning having to be repeated in nine of these patients. (In addition, I have had occasion to re-make ileostomies in another 71 patients, whose original operations had been performed by other surgeons.) The frequency of reconstruction or re-siting of the ileostomy recorded by other authors in their own cases in recent times has been similar—Daly and Brooke (1967) 6%, Roy et al. (1969) 9·7% and Ritchie (1971a) 10·8%. I should add that in more recent years I have also converted quite a number of conventional ileostomies to reservoir ileostomies, sometimes after reconstruction as a conventional stoma has failed to give satisfaction (see p. 796).

INDICATIONS

Of my 96 ileostomy re-operations, 46 have been re-fashionings at the same site and 50 have involved re-siting of the stoma. The indications are listed in Table 61.

OPERATIVE TECHNIQUE

RECONSTRUCTION AT THE SAME SITE

There are three ways of reconstructing the ileostomy in its original location.

TABLE 61. *Indications for Re-fashioning or Re-siting 96 Ileostomies*

Indication	No. of cases
Inadequate protrusion or recession	31
Faulty siting	40
Prolapse	7
Stomal ulceration or fistulation	9
Depressed scar at the side of the ileostomy	14
Ileostomy hernia	3
Recurrent abscesses and sinuses	2
Stenosis	2

Note: In some patients there was more than one indication for re-operation, so that there are more indications listed in this table than there were operations.

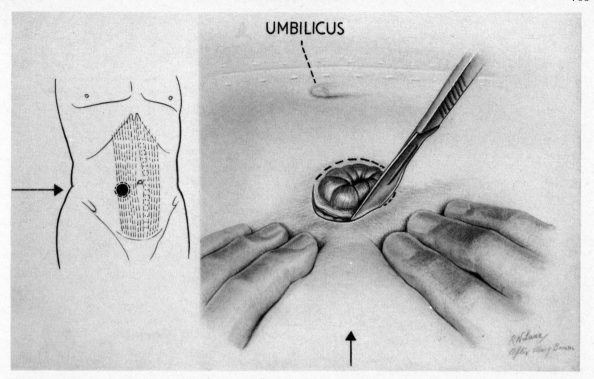

UMBILICUS

Fig. 569. Ileostomy re-fashioning at the same site. *Left*, The abdominal wall showing outline of circumcision around the ileostomy. *Right*, The view as seen by a surgeon standing on right side of patient as incision is made through tautened peri-ileostomy skin. (*From Goligher 1963*)

Through a Simple Circumcision at the Base of the Ileostomy Spout

In my experience adequate access for reconstruction of an ileostomy at the same site can usually be obtained through this approach. The incision is made at or just wide of the mucocutaneous junction (Fig. 569). The cut edge of the end of the ileum is caught with four artery or tissue forceps, and firm upward traction is exerted on them whilst the incision is deepened to expose the junction of the ileum and the ileal mesentery with the anterior rectus sheath (Fig. 570). The plane of dissection is cautiously continued to separate the bowel and its mesentery from the entire thickness of the anterior abdominal wall, so that they can be freely drawn out of the abdomen—either out of a general peritoneal cavity, if the ileostomy had originally been made directly through the anterior parietal peritoneum (see p. 755), or out of the extra-peritoneal space, if an extraperitoneal technique of ileostomy formation had been used (see p. 755).

The next step is to re-make the ileostomy. The terminal fringe of skin and fat at the end of the ileum is trimmed off with scissors (Fig. 571). The position of the bowel is then adjusted, so that its cut distal end projects approximately 7·5 cm beyond the anterior abdominal skin, and a series of interrupted sutures of fine chromic catgut or Dexon, No. 3/0 on atraumatic needles, is passed between the anterior rectus sheath and the ileum and its mesentery (Fig. 556). (Because these ileostomy re-fashioning wounds inevitably become to some extent contaminated, I consider it better not to use non-absorbable material for this purpose.) Usually four or five stitches are placed in one leaf of the mesentery, and another four or five in the ileum round to its mesenteric border on the opposite side, but not extending on to the other surface of the mesentery. The utmost care must be exercised in inserting the sutures in the ileal wall to take only very superficial bites not entering the lumen. These stitches are conveniently left untied till all have been placed. They are then tied, and the end of the ileum is sutured back to the edges of the circular skin wound, giving a mucosal-covered bud, which normally projects 3–4 cm beyond the skin surface (Fig. 557).

When the aperture in the musculoaponeurotic layers seems at operation to be slightly enlarged, I have sometimes narrowed it a fraction by two or three catgut (or Prolene) sutures; but, if there is a gross widening of the gap in the abdominal wall, appreciable clinically before operation, I have preferred to re-site the ileostomy entirely, in order to obtain a really snug opening for transmission of the bowel.

A good example of what can be achieved by this technique in the correction of an inadequately projecting ileostomy is shown in Fig. 572.

By Means of a Formal Laparotomy

This alternative is technically easier for the surgeon, but subjects the patient to more discomfort and possibly to more risk, for it involves opening the abdomen widely. The incision is best taken through the scar of the left paramedian proctocolectomy wound. Working from the left side of the patient the surgeon then has a good view of the inside of the right half of the abdomen. The ileum and mesentery going to the site of the ileostomy are clearly defined. The further procedure will depend on the reason for the reconstruction. If it is for a sliding prolapse or recession, the ileum will be drawn into, or pushed out of, the abdomen sufficiently to make the ileostomy project about 3–4 cm. It is then fixed in this position by a close circumferential series of fine silk sutures

passed between the anterior parietal peritoneum around the opening in the parietes and the ileal wall and leaf of the mesentery. Additional stitches may be inserted between the anterior abdominal wall and the last 7·5 cm of intra-abdominal ileum to provide increased anchorage against prolapse. If, on the other hand, the re-fashioning is being performed for a fixed deformity of the ileostomy or for a fistula, it is necessary to free the bowel and its mesentery from the anterior abdominal wall by a circumcision and appropriate dissection. Finally, after the terminal fringe of ileum has been trimmed off (or, in the case of a fistula, all bowel distal to the fistula excised), the ileostomy is re-made at the same site in the usual way—or elsewhere if this seems indicated because of the size of the aperture in the musculoaponeurotic layers or for any other reason—particular attention being devoted to the fixing sutures.

Simple Suturing of the Inner and Outer Tubes of Ileum in the Projecting Ileostomy Spout

In cases of sliding recession where the mesenteric attachment is still sound, Brooke and Walker (1962) have proposed that the operative treatment shall be confined to forcing the ileostomy into maximum projection by pressure on the surrounding abdominal wall and then suturing together the inner and outer

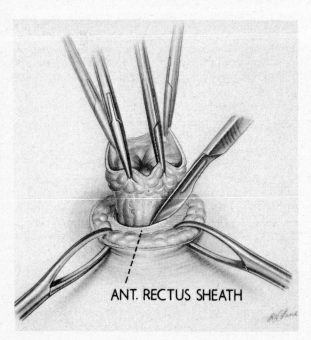

Fig. 570. The incision has been deepened down to the anterior rectus sheath, and the ileum and its mesentery are being dissected free from the musculoaponeurotic layers. (*From Goligher 1963*)

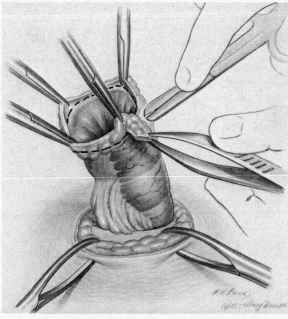

Fig. 571. Free ileum and mesentery have been drawn out of the abdomen, and the terminal fringe of skin and fat is being excised. (*From Goligher 1963*)

tubes of bowel in the ileostomy spout. To afford access to the space between these two layers for the purpose of inserting these sutures a longitudinal incision is made through the outer tube along the antimesenteric border of the ileostomy spout. This is converted into a T-shaped incision by a half-circumferential cross cut near the base of the spout. Two flaps of outer tube of ileum are then elevated exposing the inner tube of bowel. A continuous longitudinal suture of fine catgut is now inserted on either side between the flap of outer tube 12 mm or so from its cut edge and the inner tube. Finally, the flaps of outer tube are sutured back in place.

I have not myself used this method for ileostomy reconstruction, but several years ago occasionally adopted a somewhat similar device for attempting to secure adhesions between the two tubes of ileum in the ileostomy spout in freshly made ileostomies, where the stoma tends to recede into the subcutaneous tissues, as in obese patients. The spout was first of all forced into maximum projection by firm pressure on the adjacent abdominal wall. Then the extreme end of the spout was caught with two pairs of fine tissue forceps at the mesenteric and antimesenteric borders respectively. Whilst traction was exerted on these forceps the surgeon inserted his left index finger into the spout as far as the abdominal wall, with the palmar aspect directed towards the antimesenteric border. With the other hand he then passed a row of fine interrupted chromic catgut sutures on an atraumatic needle along the antimesenteric border, each stitch penetrating the outer tube of bowel, taking up a bite of the inner tube (but not entering the lumen, the left index finger serving as a guide to the depth of the stitches), and then emerging through the outer tube again. When all these had been placed they were tied. Sometimes an additional row of stitches was inserted on either lateral wall of the spout as well.

I used this technique in about 10 cases. Usually the sutures came away about 10–14 days afterwards. No fistulation or other

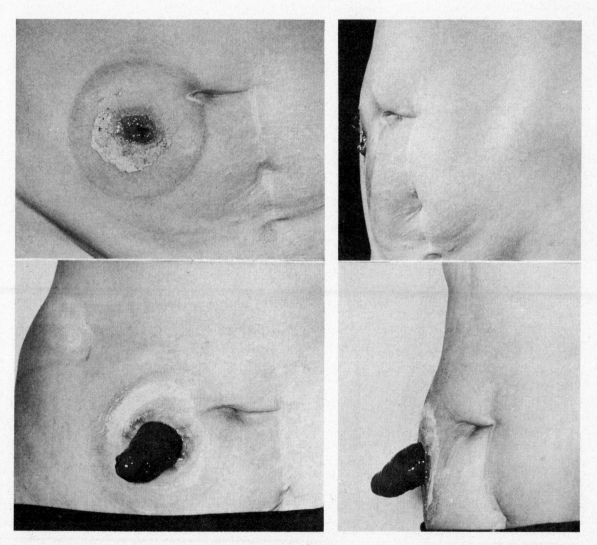

Fig. 572. Fixed inadequate ileostomy protrusion. *Above, En face* and tangential views of abdomen *before* re-fashioning. *Below, En face* and tangential views *after* reconstruction at the same site. (*From Goligher 1963*)

ill-effect resulted in any case, and it was my impression that the suturing sometimes helped to give the ileostomy greater prominence but frankly I have not employed the method more recently.

RE-SITING OF THE ILEOSTOMY

Sometimes it is possible to find a suitable area of skin for a new site in the same half of the abdomen; but in other cases there is insufficient space between the rib margin and the scar that would result from the suture of the old ileostomy site to accommodate a new ileostomy on the same side. Under these circumstances it is necessary to seek a new site in the opposite half of the abdominal wall, as I have now done in 50 patients.

In performing a re-siting it is sometimes possible, especially in thin patients, to achieve the re-location by separating the old ileostomy from the abdominal wall as shown in Figs 569–71, then passing a finger inside the peritoneal cavity to impinge from within on the anterior abdominal wall at the new site, where a fresh wound is created and the ileal stump is brought to the surface (Taylor et al. 1978). More usually it is necessary to carry out a formal laparotomy, and, in doing so, it is important to place the wound for this exploration where it will not encroach on the proposed site for the new stoma. Thus, if the re-siting is to take place in the right half of the abdomen, a left paramedian rectus-sliding incision, preferably in the line of the original proctocolectomy incision (or a median incision), is very satisfactory (Fig. 573). If on the other hand it is intended to bring the new ileostomy out of the left abdomen, a right paramedian incision will be more convenient (Fig. 574), and a median incision would also do. During the laparotomy the old ileostomy is freed by a close circumcision of the skin, deepened through the abdominal wall. The new ileostomy wound is made at the site selected by removal of a disc of skin and subcutaneous fat and by cruciate incision of the muscles and aponeuroses of the abdominal wall through to the peritoneal cavity, the opening being of such a size that it just fails to allow the passage of two fingers through it. The ileal stump is then drawn down to the surface, fixed in position by sutures inserted through the front of the wound (see Fig. 555) and the end turned back and stitched to the skin (see Fig. 556). With left-sided ileostomies it is not possible to close the lateral space by suture, because the peritoneal cavity at this level is divided into two more or less equal spaces by the ileum and its mesentery extending forwards from the right side of the lumbar spine to a left-sided ileostomy. Perhaps a greater danger exists of

obstruction occurring with this form of ileostomy than with the orthodox arrangement of an ileostomy in the right abdomen, with closure or avoidance of a paraileostomy gutter, but the special troubles that call for re-siting in the left abdomen in these cases justify the acceptance of such extra risks. So far, no complications or sequelae from obstruction have been encountered in my 50 cases treated in this way.

Two patients whose ileostomies required to be re-sited on the same side and the opposite side of the abdomen, respectively are illustrated in Figs 575 and 576.

RESULTS

Immediate Postoperative Course

There have been no deaths or serious complications in the 96 cases treated by ileostomy reconstruction. 14 patients developed signs of *cellulitis in the subcutaneous tissues* surrounding the

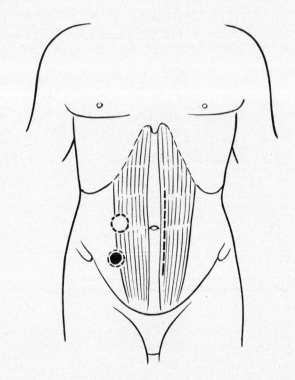

Fig. 573. Incisions used for re-siting the ileostomy at a higher level on the right side of the abdomen. A left paramedian incision is employed for the laparotomy, the old ileostomy is detached from the abdominal wall by a close circumcision, and a disc wound is made at the site selected for the new ileostomy on the same side. (*From Goligher 1963*)

stoma; in 10 the condition subsided without suppuration under antibiotic therapy, but pus formed in the other four. In two of the latter the resulting abscess discharged satisfactorily through the crevice between the ileum and the skin, and the inflammation subsequently resolved completely. In the other two, spontaneous drainage was inadequate and an incision had to be made in the skin wide of the area in contact with the flange of the ileostomy appliance, in order to secure proper evacuation of the pus. This small drainage wound had subsequently to be re-explored in one case to remove several of the silk sutures fixing the ileal mesentery to the anterior rectus sheath, before the discharge ceased. In the remaining 82 cases healing occurred without incident, which is very gratifying considering that a certain amount of contamination of the wound is inevitable in re-fashioning operations. To deal with such contamination a preoperative course of intestinal antiseptics (kanamycin or neomycin with or without metronidazole) was prescribed in all cases, and systemic antibiotic

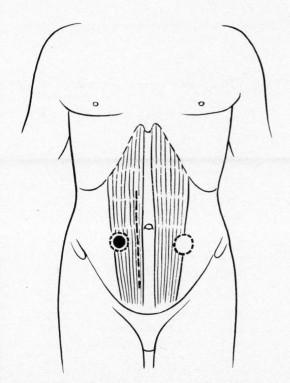

Fig. 574. Incision employed for re-siting the ileostomy on the left side of the abdomen. A right paramedian incision is used for the laparotomy, the old ileostomy is separated by a circumcision, and the new ileostomy is established in a disc wound at a suitable site on the left side. (*From Goligher 1963*)

therapy with various antibiotics was given postoperatively as a routine. In order to obviate the risk of stitch sinuses developing in the event of wound infection, chromic catgut or Dexon sutures have more recently been substituted for the silk sutures previously used to fix the ileal mesentery and ileum to the anterior rectus sheath in reconstruction operations.

Functional State and Ultimate Results

The amount of projection and the siting achieved by the reconstruction were deemed to be satisfactory in 87 of the cases, and this was quickly reflected in an improved functional state with complete avoidance of leakage, or a very considerable reduction in its incidence in these patients. In nine cases, however, the immediate results of re-fashioning were disappointing, because of failure to correct the original deformity completely, with resulting continuation of some of the symptoms.

Of great interest and importance is the durability of the reconstructions, for it would be reasonable to suppose that a tendency to recession or prolapse might re-assert itself and in the long run produce a recurrence of the original defect. Of the 87 immediately successful cases seven are known to have developed further recession or prolapse but most of the others on a fairly complete follow-up seem to be satisfactory.

Rehabilitation After Conventional Ileostomy

The inconvenience occasioned by an ileostomy varies greatly depending on several circumstances: the mechanical success achieved with the ileostomy appliance, the psychological reaction of the patient to ileostomy life and the nature of the occupation to which he or she ultimately aspires to return. Though minor transient difficulties, mostly with skin irritation, may not infrequently occur, especially at first, and a few patients may require to have their ileostomies re-made because of structural deficiencies impeding efficient ileostomy care, it is our experience that with perseverance practically all ileostomists can eventually be provided with a *modus vivendi* acceptable to the average well-adjusted individual. However, there are a few patients, who, because of their innate hostility to an artificial anus, cannot bring themselves to accept the fact that the arrangement which they have been given is compatible with a full and active existence. Five of a group of 119 of my patients with an ileostomy who

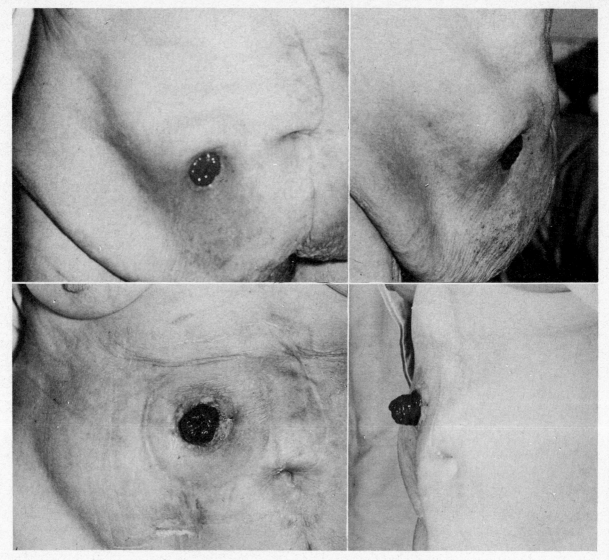

Fig. 575. Re-siting of a receded ileostomy at a higher level on the right side. *Above, En face* and tangential views of ileostomy *before* re-fashioning with the patient in the erect position. Her ileostomy projected adequately when she was recumbent, but she was very obese and, when she stood, the anterior abdominal skin and subcutaneous fat descended some 5–7 cm like an apron, so that the ileal stump became too short and the stoma was drawn in. *Below,* The ileostomy was re-sited quite high up in the epigastric region on the same side of the abdomen, and the resulting stoma *after* operation was very satisfactory, as is shown in the photographs, both taken with the patient erect. (*From Goligher 1963*)

were surveyed by Watts et al. (1966*b*), fell into this latter category. Clearly, we would have liked to have avoided submitting these individuals to an operation involving the creation of an ileostomy, but it was not possible to select them with confidence in advance. Moreover, the prognosis without operation seemed to be very poor, and our results with colectomy and ileorectal anastomosis would not have encouraged us to offer it as an alternative to proctocolectomy and ileostomy.

As regards fitness for work, the vast majority of patients reported that since their operation they have enjoyed a far higher standard of general health and physique than they had known for years. Indeed one of the commonest complaints was that they were putting on too much weight! There was always the excuse that the sort of diet that would help them to lose weight might upset their ileostomy. Though usually capable of strenuous physical effort, ileostomists were debarred from

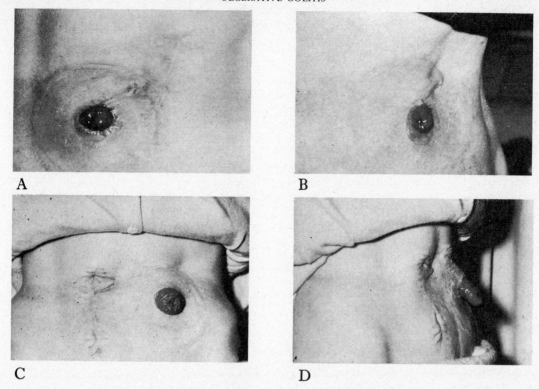

Fig. 576. Re-siting of an inadequately projecting and badly sited ileostomy on the left side of the abdomen. The ileostomy *before* re-fashioning is shown in (A) and (B), from which it will be noted that it was so close to the umbilicus that the flange of the appliance overlay the latter, and also that it scarcely projected beyond the abdominal skin. There was an insufficient area of smooth unscarred skin between the costal margin, the anterior superior iliac spine and the umbilicus for the ileostomy to be re-sited on the left side. Consequently re-siting was performed on the left side as shown in (C) and (D).

certain occupations which might displace the appliance or injure the stoma, such as mining (at the coal face) and manual labour involving the resing of heavy objects against the abdominal wall. Similar objections applied to 'body-contact' sports, such as rugby football or wrestling. But a wide range of employment and vigorous recreations was still open to these patients including cricket, tennis, golf and swimming. At the time of review 105 of our 119 ileostomists had returned to their full preoperative (or pre-colitis) work, and 112 of them claimed that their social activities were not restricted in any way. Our findings, therefore, are in full agreement with those of Brooke (1956a), Hughes et al. (1963), Wilson (1964), Daly (1968), Roy et al. (1969) and Ritchie (1971b) in showing that all but a small minority of ileostomists can be completely rehabilitated in society. Lenneberg and Rowbotham (1970) reach the same conclusion, but state that in their experience about 9% of ileostomists encountered discrimination against them in seeking

work, and some 8% found it necessary to change their employment because of the ileostomy.

Ultimate Healing of the Perineal Wound

There is a fairly general impression amongst surgeons that delay in the healing of the perineal wound is much more common after rectal excision for colitis than after this operation for cancer (Dennis 1945; Bacon and Nuguid 1962; van Prohaska and Siderius 1962; Hughes 1965; Waugh et al. 1964; Roy et al. 1969; Jalan et al. 1969b; Grüner et al. 1977). We have adopted an arbitrary definition of 'perineal sinus' as a perineal wound unhealed for more than six months after operation, a state of affairs which occurred in 24.7% of our 93 patients who underwent rectal excision (Watts et at. 1966b). Analysis of this group of patients has enabled us to implicate several factors that may play some part in determining the rapidity of perineal healing.

The complication was more common in females than in males—which suggests that lack of anterior support in the perineum may have a deleterious effect on healing (although it was rarely necessary to include any part of the vaginal wall in the excision). A prolonged history or the presence of severe rectal or pararectal disease (abscess, fistula, fissure) appeared to increase the incidence of perineal sinus. Patients developing a perineal sinus also had a much higher incidence of severe postoperative perineal wound sepsis. It is a matter for speculation whether this sepsis occurred because of tissue changes consequent on prolonged severe local disease or whether it was instrumental in prolonging the time of wound healing. We favour the former view, as sepsis alone in other wounds (as for example in the perineal wound after rectal excision for cancer) produces only a moderate delay in the rate of healing.

We have shown elsewhere that increased severity of disease at the time of operation delays healing in both abdominal and perineal wounds (Watts et al. 1966a); but, contrary to the finding of Bacon et al. (1960), this factor was found to exert no influence on the occurrence of perineal sinus. It has also been stated by Bacon et al. (1960) and Hughes (1965) that the incidence of perineal sinus is greater if a conservative type of rectal excision has been performed avoiding wide excision of perineal skin. All our patients, however, had a wide cutaneous excision, not very different from that used in a cancer operation, and perineal drainage was provided, yet the incidence of perineal sinus was 25%.

We have also investigated the effect of steroid therapy prior to operation and subsequently on the occurrence of perineal sinus. The over-all incidence in patients receiving these drugs was only marginally higher than in those who had not been so treated within a year prior to operation. However, further analysis of the steroid-treated group showed that the frequency of perineal sinus was increased four-fold if administration of the steroids had continued for more than six months prior to surgery. This relationship between *prolonged* steroid administration and delayed healing of the perineal wound is interesting but its significance is uncertain. It could be that the indication for the long-continued use of these agents was the presence of extensive and severe colonic and rectal disease, and that it was these local conditions which affected the rapidity of perineal wound healing rather than prolonged steroid administration.

Treatment of Perineal Sinus
If the perineal wound continues discharging after several months, the surgeon may feel compelled to try to assist healing by further operation. This may take the form of a simple curettage of the sinus or of a backward incision from the sinus to recreate the perineal wound as a tent-shaped cavity with its apex superiorly and its base on the perineum. By either of these manoeuvres and by subsequent meticulous attention to dressing of the perineal wound, complete healing may sometimes be obtained. But quite frequently the sinus re-establishes itself. Some of my patients have had three or four such re-operations, and a very vew of them still have persistent sinuses. Ritchie (1971a) records that, of 263 survivors of operations for ulcerative colitis who left hospital with a perineal wound, in 101 this wound was still unhealed after six months and 33 required re-admission for further operation on the perineum, a total of 46 re-operations being performed.

Some surgeons have favoured more elaborate manoeuvres in the treatment of perineal sinuses than the laying open and curetting described above. Thus, Silen and Glotzer (1974) have employed a method that involves excision of the coccyx and possibly the terminal two pieces of sacrum and turning in a flap of skin to provide a lining for part of the saucerized wound. They claim very good results in hitherto intractable cases. Anderson and Turnbull (1976) advocate the application of split-skin grafts two or three days after the sinus had been saucerized, the patient being maintained on ACTH at a dose of 40 units a day throughout the period in hospital. They report some encouraging experiences with this method. Another possibility is to use a pedicled graft of gracilis muscle, prepared as mentioned on p. 318, to fill the perineal wound cavity (Block 1978).

Prevention of Persistent Sinus Formation
I have no magic formula to suggest for the prevention of persistent perineal sepsis after rectal excision in these cases. In my own patients the perineal wound has been variously managed according to individual circumstances and one's inclination at that particular period—by partial suture with open drainage or packing, or by complete suture with supraputic or perineal suction drainage. Perineal sinuses have formed in a proportion of the patients managed by these different methods.

Intestinal Obstruction

Quite apart from an early oedematous or later fibrous stenosis at the ileostomy (see pp. 765, 774), causing difficulty in the passage of faeces, a true mechanical intestinal obstruction may develop either in the early postoperative period or subsequently. Indeed, of all abdominal operations ileostomy and proctocolectomy is perhaps the one most likely to be followed by this complication. A variety of mechanisms of obstruction is possible. The small bowel may become adherent to the laparotomy wound, to the line of suture of the pelvic peritoneal floor, to the posterior abdominal wall, or to the vicinity of the ileostomy. A factor considered by Hughes (1965) to predispose to the development of a mechanical obstruction is the retention of a diseased rectal stump (after either colectomy and ileostomy or colectomy and ileorectal anastomosis), contamination around which he believes provokes the formation of adhesions. Certainly intestinal obstruction seems to be quite common after colectomy and ileorectal anastomosis, for Aylett (1963) and Anderson (1960) both report an incidence of some 10% in their series treated by this operation, and no less than three of my 24 cases with diffuse colitis submitted to this procedure were similarly complicated. Another well recognized mechanism of obstruction is strangulation of a loop of small gut in the paraileostomy gutter (Fig. 577), the danger of which was originally pointed out by Hardy et al. (1949), and has recently been re-emphasized by Hughes (1965). But it can be obviated by closure or avoidance of this space in the construction of the ileostomy at the initial operation, as described on p. 755.

Two types of obstruction may be recognized: *complete* or unrelenting, which requires operation for its relief, and *incomplete* or transient, which resolves on conservative management, usually within 24 to 36 hours. The latter type has also often been referred to as a *bolus obstruction*, but it is only very rarely that anything like an obstructing bolus is passed when the obstruction relieves itself and the ileostomy starts to act again. It also happens not uncommonly that patients who have recovered spontaneously from a so-called bolus obstruction are re-admitted on a subsequent occasion with a complete obstruction that necessitates operation, at which a kink or twist of the bowel due to adhesions is revealed. It seems probable, therefore, that an incomplete version of the latter mechanism is the factor responsible for most transient obstructions.

Several authors have reported the frequency of complete intestinal obstruction in large series of patients followed-up for 1 to 10 or more years after ileostomy and colectomy or proctocolectomy: Wheelock and Warren (1955) 11·2% in 233 cases; Barker (1961) 13% in 107 cases; van Prohaska and Siderius (1962) 12·5% in 79 cases; Hughes (1965) 6·2% in 162 cases; Watts et al. (1966b) 8·4% in 119

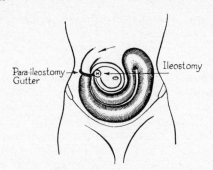

Fig. 577. Strangulation of a loop of small bowel in the para-ileostomy gutter. (*From Goligher 1954*)

cases; Daly and Brooke (1967) 9% in 100 cases; and Ritchie (1971a) 9·3% in 453 cases (which included 35 cases of Crohn's colitis). Ritchie (1971a) gives some interesting particulars regarding the 42 patients who developed complete obstruction in the collective series of 453 cases reviewed by her. Actually two patients required two operations on separate occasions (my experience is that repeated obstructions are even commoner than that), making 44 operations in all. The cause of the obstruction was found at laparotomy to be adhesions in 27 cases, volvulus of the small gut in five cases, kinking in relation to a rectal stump in two cases, snaring in the paraileostomy space in six cases and miscellaneous other causes in four cases. Fifteen of the obstructions arose in the immediate postoperative period, with four deaths, whilst 29 developed after discharge from hospital, with only one death. In this same review of 453 cases Ritchie (1971a) noted that 22 patients had developed incomplete or transient obstructions (with a total of 26 admissions). These were all treated successfully along conservative lines, but four of the patients required laparotomy for complete obstruction at a subsequent re-admission. Wheelock and Warren (1955) and Watts et al. (1966b) have emphasized that the danger of developing obstruction is greatest in the early years after colectomy, but, from analogy with other postoperative adhesive obstructions and from my personal experience of many obstructions in ileostomy patients, I would have little doubt that the risk of this complication continues indefinitely.

The over-all mortality resulting from intestinal obstructive episodes is not always clearly reported but is estimated by Cattell (1953) as approximately 3%, by Wheelock and Warren (1955) as 1·7%, by Watts et al. (1966b) as 0·7% and by Ritchie (1971a) as 1·1%.

The diagnosis of intestinal obstructions after ileostomy and colectomy or proctocolectomy is not usually difficult, except when it occurs during the immediate postoperative period before the ileostomy action has become thoroughly established. At this stage confusion with a paralytic ileus may arise (see p. 609) and ileostomy dysfunction (see p. 765)—though excessively rare with modern techniques of ileostomy construction—must also be borne in mind. The latter can be excluded by passing a finger into the stoma and finding that it enters easily, and by inserting a catheter into the terminal ileum and failing to withdraw any fluid. When obstruction arises in a patient who has left hospital and is leading an ordinary existence, it is very characteristic. There is a sudden onset of severe colicky abdominal pain, followed by nausea and vomiting and cessation of ileostomy actions. By the time the patient comes to hospital, perhaps 8–10 hours later, the ileostomy bag remains empty, the abdomen may be slightly or not at all distended, there is usually no abdominal tenderness, though a little tenseness may be appreciated, and auscultation detects vigorous peristalic sounds. Digital examination of the stoma reveals no stenosis and no fluid escapes on withdrawal. A plain X-ray examination of the abdomen usually shows gaseous distension of loops of small bowel with fluid levels.

The problem in such a case is not to diagnose the obstruction but to decide whether it is a mechanical obstruction due to adhesions, which requires urgent laparotomy, or a 'bolus obstruction', which may relieve itself spontaneously in time or be overcome by a wash-out given into the ileostomy. It is difficult to give firm guidance on this issue. If the symptoms have been present for 24 hours or longer and there has been no discharge from the ileostomy in all that time, I should proceed to laparotomy as soon as the patient can be quickly re-hydrated by intravenous fluids. In reopening the abdomen of such a case it is best to go through the old left paramedian laparotomy incision. On the other hand, if the symptoms began only a few hours before and if the general condition is good and there is no area of abdominal tenderness to raise the suspicion of a strangulation obstruction, I should prefer to temporize for 8–12 hours. During that time intravenous fluids should be given and the effect of a wash-out tried. The state of intestinal distension should be assessed radiologically at the beginning and end of the probationary period. If the ileostomy has not acted by 24 hours from the commencement of the pain the abdomen should be explored.

Urinary Lithiasis

It has been claimed by Deren et al. (1962) in North America, Maratka and Nedbal (1964) in Czechoslovakia, Bennett and Jepson (1966) in South Australia and Bennett and Hughes (1972) in Victoria, Australia, that urolithiasis is specially liable to occur as a complication of colitis, especially when treated by ileostomy. Maratka and Nedbal (1964) reported one case of urinary lithiasis in 438 colitic patients treated medically, and nine cases (12%) in 74 colitics who had had surgical treatment. Bennett and Jepson (1966) found urolithiasis in six or 8·3% of 72 ileostomists, the stones in a high proportion of the cases being composed of uric acid. Bennett and Hughes (1972) elicited an incidence of urinary calculi of 4% in 125 medically treated colitics and of 8·4% in 352 surgically treated colitics, again the stones not infrequently being of radiotranslucent uric acid type; it was reckoned that the average incidence of urolithiasis in ordinary hospital admissions in the state of Victoria was 0·7%.

Analysis of our own cases of colitis in Leeds has failed to provide any confirmation of this contention. Of 465 patients with colitis seen between 1952 and 1963 and all carefully followed up since their initial attendance or admission, six developed urinary calculi, three in the group of 297 cases treated along purely medical lines and three in the group of 168 cases treated surgically. Two of the latter three occurred some years after ileostomy and proctocolectomy but one of them was possibly present before operation. There is no significant difference in these incidences of calculus formation in medically and surgically treated patients. Moreover the overall incidence of urolithiasis in this series of 465 colitic patients (1·3%) is very similar to that calculated for the general population in the Leeds area by Williams (1965)—normally 1%.

A follow-up study of 300 ileostomy patients in Birmingham by Alexander (1970) has uncovered only two cases of urolithiasis, an incidence of 0·7%. But in a similar survey of 371 ileostomists in London by Ritchie (1971b), it was found that 16 patients (4·3%) had developed urinary calculi since operation. The majority of the stones were composed partly of calcium and were radiopaque.

Altogether, despite these discrepancies in the reported incidences of urinary stones in colitic patients and those having ileostomies, it seems possible that ulcerative colitis or the possession of an ileostomy may predispose patients to the occurrence of urolithiasis, perhaps because of the persistent loss of fluid and electrolytes in the diarrhoea or ileostomy discharge in these cases. Factors such as diet, geography and climate may also be involved, as they apparently are in the genesis of primary urinary calculi, and the varying extent to which they are operative in different groups of patients with colitis or after ileostomy may account for the recorded variations in frequency of stone in such people.

Cholelithiasis

In ileostomy patients who have had some ileal resection, bile salt deficiencies might be expected to occur (see p. 43), with consequent increase in the incidence of cholelithiasis (Hill et al. 1975*b*), but this combination of ileostomy and ileal resection is a feature rather of the treatment of Crohn's colitis than of ordinary ulcerative colitis (see p. 845).

Gastric Hypersecretion and Peptic Ulceration

It is known from the work of Landor and Baker (1964) and Frederick et al. (1965) that gastric hypersecretion follows massive small bowel resection in dogs and apparently in humans, with a possible predisposition to resulting peptic ulceration (see Buxton 1974 for a good review). Landor et al. (1966) demonstrated a similar hypersecretion in dogs following colectomy and ileorectal anastomosis. However, some unpublished studies of basal and maximal gastric acid secretion before and after ileostomy and proctocolectomy in 23 patients in my department by M. Corman and M. C. Mason failed to show any consistent increase after operation.

Mortality of Conventional Surgical Treatment

IMMEDIATE DEATHS

There is general agreement amongst surgeons with experience in the treatment of ulcerative colitis that the immediate mortality of operations for this condition has declined significantly since the early days of colitis surgery. It is equally evident that the postoperative course of these patients is now much smoother than formerly, though it still provides quite a few complications and anxieties, particularly in the cases undergoing operation as an urgent or emergency procedure. A number of factors would seem to be responsible for these improvements in the results of surgical treatment: firstly, the increased safety of surgery in general in recent years; secondly, the better understanding of the problems of ileostomy technique and management, and thirdly, perhaps, the introduction of primary colectomy and proctocolectomy as the operation of election in colitis.

A good demonstration of the effect of these first two factors alone, the form of operative procedure adopted remaining the same, is provided by the figures published from the Lahey Clinic (Cattell 1953; Cattell and Colcock 1955). Between 1928 and 1946 the patient mortality for the three-stage operation used at that clinic (ileostomy, colectomy, and excision of the rectum) was 22·2% in 147 cases. During the years 1947–52, the patient mortality for the same three-stage operative programme used in the treatment of 208 cases was only 5%. Most of the deaths recorded in both periods under review occurred in connection with the initial ileostomy.

The immediate results with primary colectomy and proctocolectomy in some of the earlier reported series treated by this method have been particularly encouraging. Thus Ripstein et al. (1952) had an operative mortality of only 4·1% in 72 cases treated by these operations. In 1954 I myself published a collective series of 74 cases treated by primary colectomy or proctocolectomy at St Mark's Hospital during 1951–4 with an immediate mortality of only 2·7%. This contrasts very strikingly with the immediate mortality of surgery for colitis at that hospital during 1942 to 1950 when ileostomy alone was the 'sheet anchor' of treatment—which was 21·6% (Counsell and Goligher 1952). However, it would certainly not be correct to attribute the improvement solely to the change of operative procedure to primary excision, for undoubtedly the standard of postoperative care and ileostomy management since 1950 was much higher than that available in the 1940s and particularly during the war years, and these considerations alone might have been sufficient to account for the difference in the results.

The results recorded more recently for primary colectomy or proctocolectomy have been less striking with rather higher mortality rates: van Prohaska and Siderius (1962) 7% in 85 cases; Waugh et al. (1964) 8·8% in 205 cases; Hughes (1965) 8·5% in 188 cases; Rhodes and Kirsner (1965) 10·6% in 170 cases; Watts et al. (1966*a*) 11·9% in 151 cases; Daly (1968) 10·4% in 442 cases; and Ritchie (1972*b*) 8·1% in 246 cases. But comparison of achievements in different centres, where the criteria for acceptance of cases for operation may vary significantly, is open to fallacy. Certainly a most important factor in determining the immediate outcome of surgical treatment is the type of case presenting for operation. Unquestionably the risks are greatly increased if operation has to be undertaken during a severe exacerbation which has failed to remit and the patient's condition is steadily deteriorating. This is well shown in my own personal series of 504 cases treated by primary proctocolectomy (or colectomy). There were 34 operative deaths, an over-all operative mortality of 6·7%, but included in the series were 184 gravely ill patients (24 with perforation of the colon), on whom operation was being performed in the course of a severe attack of

TABLE 62. *Operative Mortality of Primary Proctocolectomy and Colectomy for Ulcerative Colitis*

Type of operation	No. of cases	Operative mortality
Elective	320	9 (2·8%)
Urgent	141	15 (10·7%)
Emergency	43	10 (23·3%)
Total	504	34 (6·7%)

TABLE 63. *Causes of 34 Immediate Postoperative Deaths in 504 Primary Proctocolectomies and Colectomies for Ulcerative Colitis*

Principal cause	No. of fatal cases
Intra-abdominal sepsis	9
Pulmonary embolism	6
Septicaemia	5
Primary haemorrhage	2
Bronchopneumonia	4
Necrotizing enteritis	1
Lung abscess	1
Small bowel obstruction	1
Adrenal failure	1
Electrolyte imbalance	1
Diabetic imbalance	1
Cerebral haemorrhage	2

the disease. In Table 62 the cases are grouped according to the urgency of the intervention. The term *elective* operation is self-explanatory but the expressions urgent and emergency operation, which are very similar, call for definition. An *urgent* operation was one required to terminate an acute attack that had not responded to medical treatment, but the patient's general conditions was fairly well maintained and the intervention could if necessary have been postponed for a day or so. An *emergency* operation was one that had to be undertaken immediately, absolutely without delay, because of a sharp deterioration in the patient's general state or the development of some complication such as perforation. It will be seen that most of the deaths occurred after urgent or emergency operations. This contrasts with the mortality rate of just under 3% for elective operations. Ritchie (1972b) records a very similar difference in operative mortality depending on the urgency of intervention in 246 patients with colitis at St Mark's Hospital. The prospects of lessening the mortality of severe attacks by a readier resort to surgical intervention at an earlier stage are discussed on p. 742. The causes of operative death are listed in Table 63, from which it is apparent that the two main lethal factors were infection and pulmonary embolism. To lessen the latter danger the possible routine use of antithrombosis measures such as mini-dose heparin might be considered, but, certainly until recently, I have had misgivings about anticoagulant therapy of this kind in patients with the large raw areas left after a protocolectomy.

LATE DEATHS AND COMPLICATIONS

The deaths and complications occurring during the immediate postoperative period do not unfortunately represent the sum total of the mortality and morbidity referable to the surgical treatment of colitis. As already stressed a number of late complications are liable to be encountered in patients who have undergone radical surgical treatment for ulcerative colitis—in connection with the ileostomy (p. 774) and with the perineal wound (p. 789) and in the form of acute intestinal obstruction (p. 790). These complications not infrequently demand further operative treatment and though these further interventions may often be relatively slight, such as the curettage of an unhealed perineal wound, they do constitute a considerable inconvenience to the patient. Also they may on occasions be more major (e.g. laparotomy for intestinal obstruction) and carry a risk to life.

The *late mortality* after radical surgery for colitis is derived from three sources—from the late morbidity just referred to, from the original disease (especially when a carcinoma has been present at the time of the original operation) and from intercurrent disease or accidental trauma. This is well shown by the follow-up by Watts et al. (1966b) on 131 of my patients, operated on between 1955 and 1963, the causes of the six late deaths among which are listed in Table 64 (to which I may add that in another 335 cases, treated before and since that series but followed up less thoroughly, there were ten known late deaths due to: intestinal obstruction one, suicide one, non-intestinal carcinoma three, recurrent colitis carcinoma three, cardiovascular accident two). The over-all late mortality rate was thus 4·6% but, if deaths caused by unrelated conditions are excluded, the mortality attributable to the primary operative treatment was 2·3%. Watts et al. (1966b) calculated that the *annual* risk to life referable to the original operation was about 0·7%, or more correctly about 1% for each of the

TABLE 64. *Analysis of Late Mortality after Radical Surgery in 131 Patients Treated between 1955 and 1963*

Cause	Age at death	Time after operation (months)
Attributable to operation		
Perforation of ileum	38	4
Pulmonary embolus etc.	54	10
Intestinal obstruction	65	14
Unrelated to operation		
Recurrence of rectal cancer present at time of palliative proctocolectomy	29	12
Fractured femur	85	16
Road accident	41	4

After Watts et al. (1966*b*).

first two years and thereafter considerably less. It is interesting to note that this risk is much less than that which applied to our specially analysed series of 465 colitis patients under primarily medical treatment, for in this latter group the annual mortality was 1·1%, or 2·7% in the group with total involvement, which is more comparable to a surgically treated series (Watts et al. 1966*d*).

The over-all late mortality after radical surgery reported by Cattell (1953) was 3·2% and by Brooke 1956*a*) 3%. It would seem that most of the late deaths in these series were due to intestinal obstruction. But in four series (Rhodes and Kirsner 1965; Parks 1965; Daly 1968; Ritchie 1972*a*) recurrence of carcinoma present in the original operative specimen has been stressed as a major cause of subsequent deaths. Ritchie's (1972*a*) study was undertaken at the instigation of the Ileostomy Association of Great Britian, and consisted of a survey of the causes of death among its 4000-odd members during the period 1960–70. Unfortunately there is doubt as to the exact size and composition of the parent series from which these deaths were derived, for ileostomists belonging to the Association include not only colitis patients but also some suffering from large-bowel Crohn's disease, from polyposis and from bladder cancer, and a few colostomists manage to slip in as well! There were 213 deaths, the causes of which are listed in Table 65.

Daly's (1968) data were derived from a follow-up survey of a collective series of 427 patients treated by radical operation for ulcerative colitis in Birmingham in the years 1947–65. There were 85 subsequent deaths, 46 in the early postoperative period and 39 later. The causes of these 39 late deaths are shown in Table 66.

TABLE 65. *Causes of Death Among Ileostomy Association Members 1960–70*

Cause of death	No. of cases
Certainly or possibly attributable to the disease, its complications or surgery	
Metastases from carcinoma in colitis	42
Small bowel obstruction	14
Cirrhosis of the liver	6
Postoperative deaths after re-operations	15
Crohn's disease	11
Suicide	4
Miscellaneous	9
Total	101
Unrelated to the disease or operation	
Malignant tumours in sites other than the colon or rectum	32
Coronary thrombosis	17
Heart failure	12
Cerebrovascular accident	14
Pulmonary disease	14
Renal failure	7
Accidental death	6
Miscellaneous	10
Total	112

After Ritchie (1972*a*).

After excluding all deaths occurring within one year of operation and all deaths due to recurrent colitis carcinoma, Daly and Brooke (1967) compared the number of observed deaths occurring in this series of ileostomists with the number of deaths that might be expected in a group of the general population of similar age and sex composition. They found that there was no significant difference and concluded that once the early postoperative hazards have been surmounted the expectation of life after radical surgical treatment for ulcerative colitis (not complicated by the development of an intestinal cancer) is not materially impaired.

TABLE 66. *Cause of Late Death After Radical Operation for Ulcerative Colitis, Birmingham, 1947–65*

Cause of death	No. of cases
Recurrent carcinoma of large bowel	15
Primary carcinoma elsewhere	4
Liver failure	7
Small bowel obstruction	2
Cerebrovascular accidents	3
Coronary disease	2
Miscellaneous causes	6
Total	39

After Daly (1968).

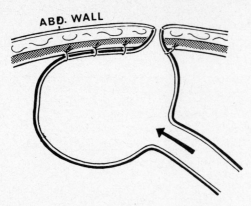

Fig. 578. Mark I pattern of reservoir ileostomy.

2. In this modification the reservoir was connected to the surface by means of a short conduit of *antiperistaltically placed ileum* (Fig. 579).

3. This technique utilized an *orthoperistaltically placed* outflow segment of ileum (Fig. 580).

4. In this technique the connection of the reservoir to the surface was also achieved by means of an *orthoperistaltically placed* ileal conduit (Fig. 581). But the lack of antiperistalsis in the ileal conduit was compensated for by the construction of a nipple-valve at its base.

A survey by Kock in 1973 of 90 patients given reservoir ileostomies using these various techniques led him to conclude that the one affording the best prospect of complete continence was Mark 4 (Fig. 581). As a consequence, this method became that of first choice for him and for most other surgeons who have adopted the reservoir operation for some of their patients (Cameron 1973; Beahrs et al. 1974; Beahrs 1975; Goligher and Lintott 1975; Halvorsen and Heimann 1975; Madigan 1976; Gelernt et al. 1977; Halvorsen et al. 1978; Kock et al. 1979;

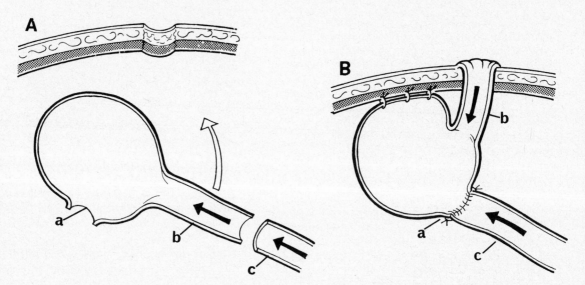

Fig. 579. Mark II pattern of reservoir ileostomy, the *anti*peristaltic exit conduit being obtained by rotating the reservoir.

The Reservoir or Continent Ileostomy

When Kock (1969, 1971a) introduced the concept of the reservoir ileostomy, it was his original idea—now known to be erroneous—that, if a loop of terminal ileum were folded on itself, opened and anastomosed to form a sac in a certain way (see Figs 584–7, 595), the motor activities of the various parts of its wall might counteract one another to produce a reservoir that would be relatively aperistaltic and unable to empty itself except when intubated. He experimented with four techniques for connecting such a reservoir to the surface:

1. In this plan one corner of the reservoir was left open (Fig. 578) and was drawn through a small 'trephine' wound in the right iliac region of the anterior abdominal wall for direct suture to the skin. The weakness of this method was that the bowel tended to retract into the abdomen, with resulting infection, granulation and stenosis.

Palmu and Silvula 1978; Beart et al. 1979; Kock and Myrvold 1979).

But as Kock (1976a, b) and Kock and Myrvold (1979) have also discovered, there is a considerable tendency for the nipple-valve (Fig. 582), which is the significant feature of this method in regard to continence, to become extruded from the reservoir, an occurrence that is very convincingly demonstrated by radiological examination after injection of an opaque medium into the reservoir, such as we have employed (Goligher and Lintott 1975; Goligher 1978) and as done also by Standerskjöld-Nordenstam et al. (1979). Examples of these 'pantaloonograms' demonstrating nipple-valves in or out of place are given in Fig. 583.

It is possible to re-operate to replace the extruded valve (Fig. 600) or more usually to create a new valve (Fig. 601) or to make a new reservoir. Surgeons who have much experience with patients with reservoir ileostomies know that re-operation—sometimes for a second or even a third or fourth time—is not infrequently required to deal with displaced valves (Kock 1973, 1976;

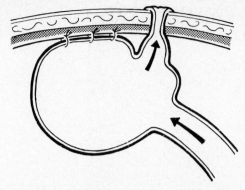

Fig. 580. Mark III pattern of reservoir ileostomy with short *ortho*peristaltic exit conduit.

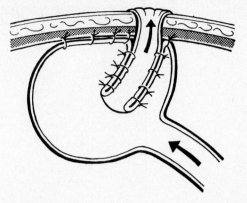

Fig. 581. Mark IV pattern of reservoir ileostomy with long exit conduit invaginated into the reservoir to make a 'nipple-valve'.

Madigan 1976; Goligher and Lintott 1975; Halvorsen et al. 1978; Palmu and Silvula 1978; Beart et al. 1979; Kock and Myrvold 1979). In addition in the early postoperative period, re-intervention is sometimes needed to cope with septic complications or other urgent surgical mishaps. In my own series of 62 reservoir ileostomy operations, there has been a re-operation rate of nearly 50% and, though it is not always easy to cull this sort of information from published reports, I have formed the impression from personal contacts and visits to other centres that a similarly high re-operation rate is quite usual amongst other surgeons undertaking fair numbers of these cases. If the patient is firm in her resolve to seek a continent ileostomy and is prepared to submit to repeat operations as necessary the chances of a successful outcome in the long run are really quite good, but not unnaturally some patients—or surgeons!—lose their determination after several setbacks and settle for a conventional ileostomy.

More fundamental considerations are (*a*) why the nipple-valve becomes displaced despite the great care exercised at operation to maintain it in position by suturing together the entering and leaving layers of the bowel in the valve and by fixing the reservoir to the anterior abdominal wall around the base of the exit conduit, and (*b*) what better precautions can be taken to safe-guard the integrity of this structure so crucially important for the attainment of continence? Kock (1976*a*, *b*) now believes that the weak point in the construction of the nipple-valve has hitherto been on the mesenteric side, where sutures between the entering and leaving parts of the bowel have been strenuously avoided in order not to imperil the blood supply to the valve. The consequence is that a considerable unsutured gap exists corres-ponding to the mesentery and Kock (1976*a*, *b*; Kock et al. 1978) contends that it is through it that the extrusion of the valve

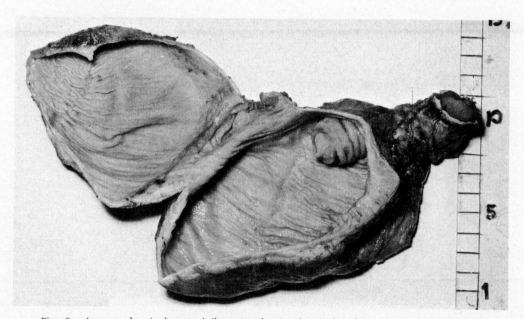

Fig. 582. An opened excised reservoir ileostomy showing the nipple-valve projecting into the lumen.

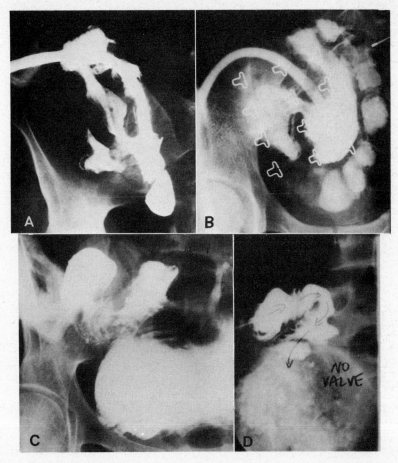

Fig. 583. Pantaloonograms made by radiographing ileal reservoirs after injecting a barium mixture. (A, B) Well-formed nipple-valves hugging the tube; both patients were continent. (C, D) Displaced valves; both patients were incontinent and unable to pass the tube into the reservoir.

probably takes place as a rule (Fig. 589c). He has developed a new technique for making the valve, in which the mesentery is split into two portions which are separated from one another in the valve, so that there are two small gaps rather than one big one (Figs 590–4). He claims that since adopting this technique the incidence of valve extrusion in his patients has dropped from 54 to 26% (Kock and Myrvold 1979). I must record, however, that in 20 patients given reservoir ileostomies more recently by me employing this new technique valve extrusion took place in seven, and in two patients necrosis of the valve occurred. Consequently I remain to be convinced that this particular variation of technique is the complete solution to the valvular problem.

CONSTRUCTION OF RESERVOIR

The construction of a reservoir ileostomy by Kock's Mark 4 technique (see Fig. 581) incorporating a nipple-valve is illustrated in Figs 584–598, which with the accompanying captions give a clear account of this operation, only requiring to be supplemented by a few additional comments to emphasize certain points. Figs 587–9 show the original method favoured for making the valve, fixation being achieved by two or three longitudinal rows of silk sutures passing through all layers of tissue in the wall of the nipple, but avoiding the mesenteric area. Note the wide mesenteric gap left (Fig. 589c). If this method of valve construction is to be employed, it is important to supplement the endocavitary suturing with one or two circumferential rows of Lembert sutures of silk at the base of the valve, taking the sutures right up to the mesenteric leaf on either side. It might even be wise to carry out preliminary excision of a triangular portion of the peritoneum covering either side of the mesentery together with some of the mesenteric fat (Figs 590,

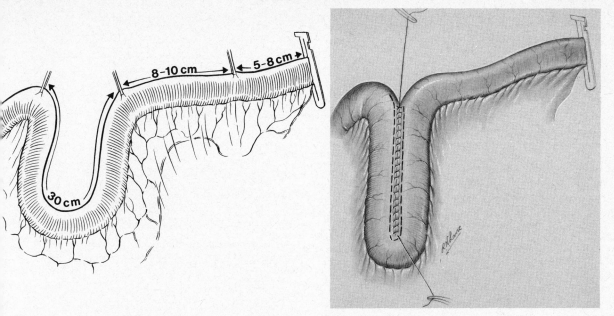

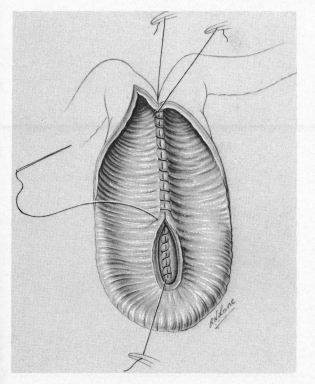

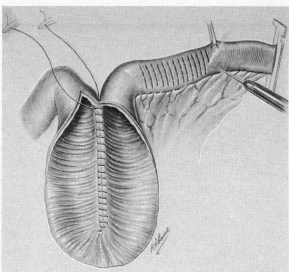

Fig. 584. Construction of Mark IV reservoir ileostomy. Lengths of bowel needed for making reservoir, nipple-valve and conduit through anterior abdominal wall.

Fig. 585. Construction of Mark IV reservoir ileostomy. Insertion of posterior Lembert suture.

Fig. 586. Construction of Mark IV reservoir ileostomy. Opening the loop of bowel and insertion of posterior through-and-through suture.

Fig. 587. Construction of Mark IV reservoir ileostomy. Diathermizing the serosal and muscle coats of the segment of bowel that will be used to make the nipple-valve.

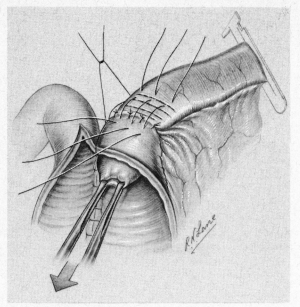

Fig. 588. Construction of Mark IV reservoir ileostomy. Drawing the exit conduit into the reservoir as nipple-valve and insertion of Lembert sutures of silk.

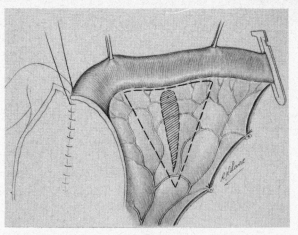

Fig. 590. Construction of Mark IV reservoir ileostomy, alternative technique for making nipple-valve, Outline of the amount of peritoneal leaves of mesentery to be excised and of the site of mesenteric division.

591) with the object of narrowing the mesentery to make it less bulky as it is eventually drawn into the valve and possibly to promote adhesions within the valve.

Figs 590–4 show the method of preparing the nipple-valve by splitting the mesentery, and also, for what it is worth, excising a triangle of mesenteric peritoneum on either side. The removal of the peritoneum in the way depicted in Figs 590 and 591 is quite straightforward, though a little finicky and tedious, in cases having a reservoir ileostomy made at the time of the procto-

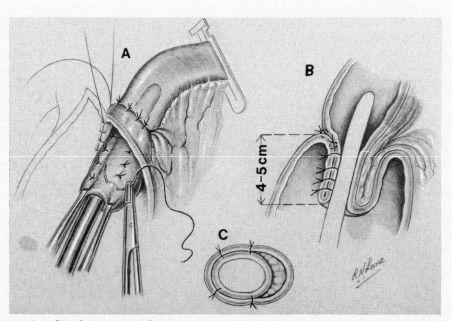

Fig. 589. Construction of Mark IV reservoir ileostomy. (A) Nipple-valve fully invaginated, through-and-through sutures of silk being inserted through all layers to try to maintain invagination; Hegar's dilator in lumen of valve to prevent sutures picking up opposite side by mistake. (B) Diagrammatic longitudinal section of valve and sutures. (C) Diagrammatic transverse section to show the large mesenteric gap.

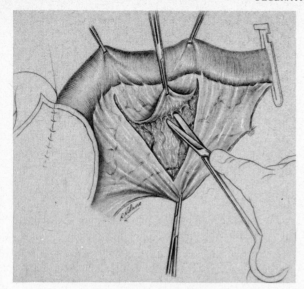

Fig. 591. Construction of Mark IV reservoir ileostomy, alternative technique for making nipple-valve. Dissecting up one of the leaves of peritoneum.

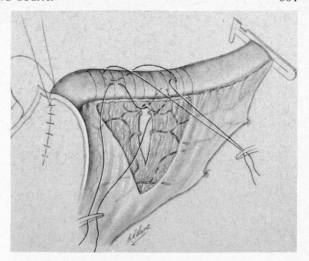

Fig. 592. Construction of Mark IV reservoir ileostomy, alternative technique for making nipple-valve. Seromuscular coats of bowel have been diathermized and relating sutures have been inserted.

colectomy, but in patients who are having a conventional ileostomy converted to a reservoir type, the dissection necessary to free the ileum from the abdominal wall and make a satisfactory stump of bowel and mesentery for the new ileostomy usually leaves a very patchy mesenteric peritoneal covering and formal excision of triangular leaves of peritoneum, as shown in Fig. 591, is often im-

possible or very difficult. But the fact that the peritoneal leaves already are incomplete renders the more formal manoeuvre unnecessary. The rotation sutures shown in Figs 592 and 593 may be found difficult to understand at first viewing or until practised on the cadaver or at operation. The finished nipple-valve is illustrated in Fig. 594A, but the diagram in Fig. 594B is not quite accurate in so

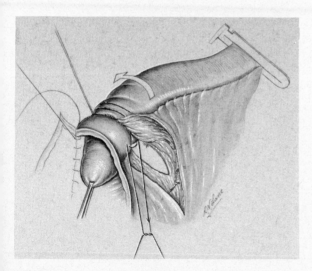

Fig. 593. Construction of Mark IV reservoir ileostomy, alternative technique for making nipple-valve. Exit conduit being drawn into reservoir whilst rotating sutures are tied.

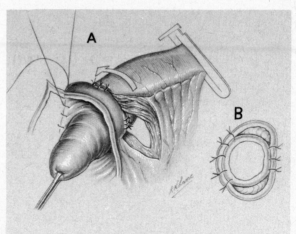

Fig. 594. Construction of Mark IV reservoir ileostomy, alternative technique for making nipple-valve. (A) Nipple-valve completed, its maintenance in position depending on several layers of Lembert sutures of silk, the splitting of the mesentery into two halves making their insertion easier. (B) Diagrammatic transverse section to show the placing of the Lembert sutures between the two segments of the mesentery (but the mesenteric gaps are usually rather smaller than shown in this illustration).

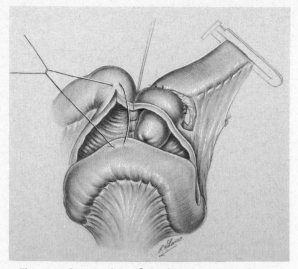

Fig. 595. Construction of Mark IV reservoir ileostomy. Closing the reservoir by folding the plate of bowel.

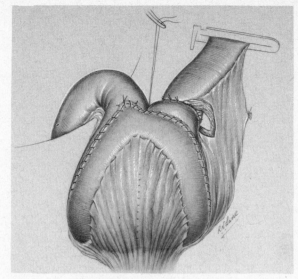

Fig. 596. Construction of Mark IV reservoir ileostomy. Suture of reservoir completed by a continuous Lembert suture of 3/0 chromic catgut or Dexon.

far as the mesenteric gaps in the suturing shown on either side of the valve are not usually as wide as here portrayed. It should also be emphasized that when the reservoir has been closed (Figs 595 and 596), it is possible and advisable to insert further Lembert sutures of silk at the base of the nipple-

valve to invaginate it still further, care being taken not to narrow the two spaces left in the circumferential rows of sutures for transmission of the two portions of the mesentery. It will be noted that this technique of preparing the nipple-valve entirely

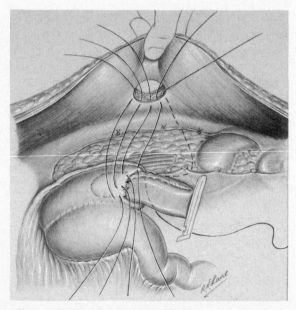

Fig. 597. Fixing the reservoir to the anterior abdominal wall. The posterior row of fine silk sutures being inserted between the posterior half of the circumference of the circular ileostomy wound in the abdominal wall and the reservoir just behind the base of the exit conduit before exit conduit is taken through abdominal wall. Suture are also placed to close the lateral space.

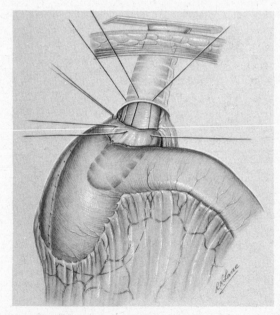

Fig. 598. Fixing the reservoir to the anterior abdominal wall. The anterior row of fine silk sutures being inserted after exit conduit has been drawn through the ileostomy wound in the abdominal wall.

eschews endocavitary suturing through all coats of the valve, because occasionally such sutures have been followed by the development of a fistula through the substance of the valve with resultant loss of continence (Kock 1976*b*; Palmu and Sivula 1978).

After completion of the reservoir and reinforcement of the inturning of the nipple-valve by further silk sutures at its base, the competence of the valvular mechanism should be tested by clipping the afferent limb of ileum with an intestinal spring clamp 10–12 cm proximal to the reservoir, passing a tube into the reservoir through the exit conduit and valve and inflating with a bladder syringe full of air. The reservoir and afferent limb distal to the spring clamp become obviously distended, but no air escapes. The tube is then quickly withdrawn and if the valve is competent the distension persists. However, when the tube with its proximal end, not attached to the bladder syringe but open, is passed again, the air escapes with an audible puff and the reservoir and distal afferent ileal limb immediately collapse. The tube is then withdrawn and the end of the exit conduit left open or re-clipped with a Cope's clamp.

The next step is the passage of the exit conduit through the trephine wound made specially for it in the abdominal wall and the secure fixation of the reservoir to the parietes around this wound. It is best to proceed in the manner shown in Figs 597 and 598. Whilst the right half of the anterior abdominal wall is elevated the posterior sutures between the reservoir and the posterior margin of the ileostomy wound are inserted loosely and then tied *before the exit conduit is taken through*. The exit conduit is then drawn through the trephine wound and the anterior row of fixing silk sutures is inserted and tied. Attention is next turned to the extremity of the exit conduit. The Cope's clamp is removed from it and sufficient bowel amputated to leave a cut edge which scarcely projects beyond the skin level. The bowel wall and the edge of the circular skin wound are sutured with interrupted stitches of fine silk or chromic catgut. Finally a plastic ileostomy tube is passed through the stoma into the reservoir, the surgeon's hand within the abdomen guiding it if necessary and certainly ensuring that the tip of the tube projects beyond the end of the valve and impinges lightly on the opposite wall of the reservoir. With the tip so sited a strong silk ligature is tied round the tube where it emerges out of the stoma, as a marker to help in the post-operative management. The tube is also fixed by a suture to the skin or to the rubber flange of a two-piece ileostomy appliance which has been stuck to the skin around the stoma, but without the bag itself being fitted.

USE OF STAPLING DEVICES FOR CONSTRUCTION OF RESERVOIR ILEOSTOMY

Recently Steichen (1978) has worked out an interesting and ingenious technique for making the nipple-valve and most of the reservoir with the USS Corporation's GIA and TA staplers. The steps of the method are clearly shown in Fig. 599. It should be pointed out that the GIA stapler, used for approximating the posterior wall of the reservoir and for fixing the nipple-valve, has an SCMA loading unit, which contains a specially prepared push-bar assembly without a knife blade. This makes it possible to place four parallel rows of staples without division of tissue. It will be noted that the basal half of the two sides of the front of the reservoir are opposed *serosa-to-serosa* with a TA stapler, but the difficult half of the front suture line adjacent to the base of the exit conduit is left for a hand-placed suture.

At the time of writing I personally have only used the stapling technique a few times and my appraisal of it can thus only be tentative and incomplete. Its great attraction is that it would speed up considerably the process of making a reservoir ileostomy, not perhaps that that is a very important consideration. It would still leave what most surgeons would regard as the most difficult and dangerous part of the preparation of a reservoir ileostomy to hand suture. As for the construction of the valve, the double or treble application of a GIA stapler with SCMA loading unit—preferably on either side of the mesentery and on the antimesenteric wall—is a neater and quicker method than the insertion of through-and-through silk sutures shown in Fig. 589A, B. But it seems to me that there might still be a considerable risk of valve extrusion unless the stapling is supplemented by quite a lot of hand suturing from outside at the base of the valve close to the mesentery. (See Appendix C, p. 940, for information regarding a fascial sling method of retaining the mesentery of the nipple-valve in place.)

POSTOPERATIVE MANAGEMENT

The postoperative management after reservoir ileostomy follows basically the pattern of care given after major abdominal surgery in general.

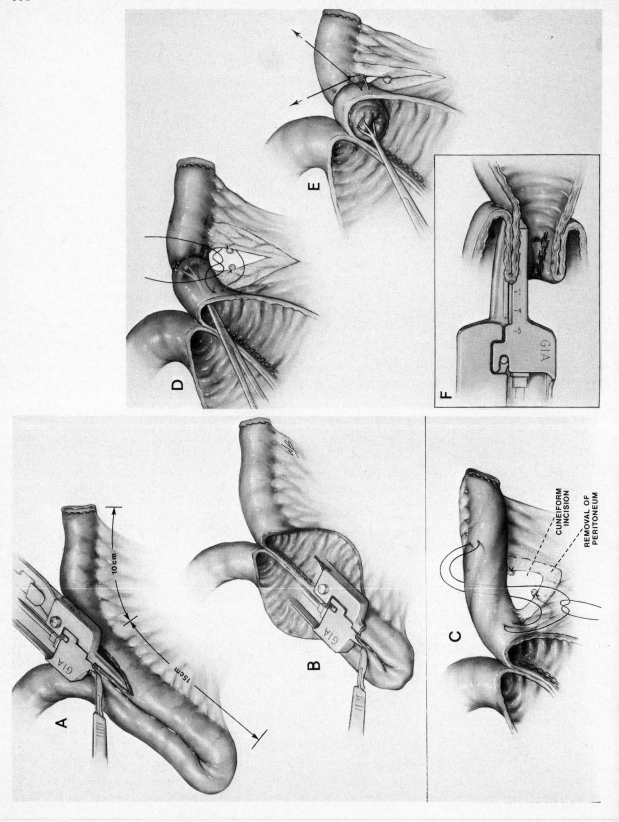

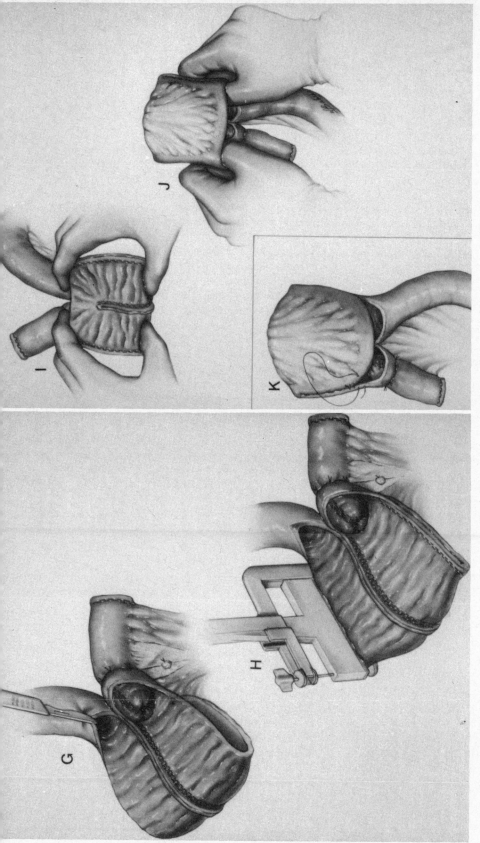

Fig. 599. (A) Kissing stab wounds are made in the apposed lateral borders of the bowel segments 15 cm from the distal end of the ileal loop. The arms of the GIA instrument, loaded with special staple cartridges, are introduced into the bowel lumina, the pusher bars are advanced and the four posterior staple lines are created. Prior to removal of the instrument, the anterior bowel walls, corresponding to the 4–5 cm suture line obtained with each GIA application, are incised on to the GIA forks used as a cutting guide. (B) The GIA is applied a total of four more times to complete the posterior wall of the pouch. Each time the small bowel is incised anteriorly on to the forks of the instrument. (C) The peritoneal leaves of the part of the ileal mesentery that will be involved in the creation of the nipple-valve are excised and the mesentery is split and a rotating suture is placed as on Figs 590–4. (D, E) The nipple is created by grasping the anterior wall of the exit conduit with Babcock or Allis forceps 5 cm from the lumen of the future pouch. The bowel is intussuscepted into the pouch and simultaneously rotated by tying the suture. (The serosa of the bowel to be intus-suscepted should have been stroked with diathermy before invagination.) (F) The shape of the nipple is maintained by two lateral applications of the GIA instrument loaded with special stapling units. (G) The anterior wall of the entrance conduit is then snicked for 1–2 cm. The flat bowel plate representing the future pouch is then turned upon itself along a trans axis and the serosal surfaces are apposed. (H) The lateral walls of the pouch are enclosed with two applications of the TA 90 stapler and excess tissue is encised using the edge of the stapler as a guide. (I, J) The TA 90 staple lines are converted into inverting suture lines by turning the pouch right side out, thus giving the pouch its permanent shape. (K) The anterior bowel edges extrud-ing between the nipple and the afferent bowel are closed with a running suture of catgut reinforced with interrupted silk sutures. The nipple is also further inserted with interrupted silk Lembert sutures at its base. (*From Steichen 1978*)

Intravenous fluids are administered for a few days or longer depending on the occurrence of paralytic ileus or temporary mechanical hold-up. The intravenous infusion is monitored by regular plasma electrolyte estimations. By mouth only ice or small hourly feeds of 30–60 ml of water are allowed until there is a free discharge of faeces from the ileostomy. A close watch is kept on the patient's general and abdominal condition for any evidence of peritonitis or leakage.

MANAGEMENT OF THE ILEOSTOMY

The patient returns from the operating room with a plastic catheter tied in the ileostomy and connected to a urinary bag for continuous drainage, and one of the most important aspects of after-care is close supervision of this arrangement. To start with, the ileal mucosa exposed at the stoma needs to be examined periodically for the first 24–36 hours or longer to see that it is a good pink colour, particularly if at the completion of the operation any doubts were entertained regarding the viability of the exit conduit. As for the tube, sometimes it drains easily and automatically and occasions no anxiety, but in many cases it is otherwise and the surgeon is plagued by worry as to whether the failure of the tube to drain properly is due to faulty siting. For the first two or perhaps three days as a rule all that comes out of the reservoir is blood-stained serous fluid, perhaps 50–100 ml daily. Then, in a straightforward case, the fluid assumes a faecal character and thenceforth drainage may continue to be entirely satisfactory. In other cases true faecal material fails to appear for several days and in addition there may be some abdominal distention or fair amounts of fluid may be aspirated from the nasogastric tube. The question that arises is whether the failure of faeces to emerge is due to some degree of paralytic ileus, to a mechanical obstruction of the small bowel proximal to the reservoir or to retention in the reservoir due to faulty siting of the tube, as, for example, from it having slipped out a little from oedema and enlargement of the valve, whereby the tip of the catheter no longer projects beyond the end of the valve. Obviously it is very important to try to make a distinction between these possible causes, for their proper management differs drastically.

First of all, a check is made to see that the tube has not slipped out slightly, as indicated by the strong silk ligature on the tube being no longer flush with the stoma but having become separated from it by say 1–2 cm. If this is the state of affairs, its correction by inserting the tube slightly further may be immediately effective with the sudden escape of faecal matter. But sometimes the response to this move is less impressive and uncertainty will remain as to whether the tip of the catheter is clear of the end of the valve. It might be thought that, if the tube is simply pushed into the reservoir as far as it will go, that should solve the problem, but it must be remembered that in its early days the reservoir is of relatively small size and the valve stretches right across it to reach almost to the opposite wall. If the tube impinges firmly on this wall it may become kinked and obstructed if pressed further and, if the pressure is maintained, necrosis of the wall of the reservoir could occur. (It seems possible that this may have been the causal mechanism of leakage in two of my patients whose reservoirs leaked seven to ten days after operation with resulting peritonitis.)

There are two ways of trying to determine whether the tip of the catheter is clear of the end of the valve. One is to inject 15–20 ml of saline from a bladder-type syringe via the tube and into the reservoir, and immediately afterwards to attempt to aspirate it back with the syringe. If the tip of the catheter is in the lumen of the reservoir, the fluid should be largely recoverable in this way; if the tip is still in the valve, aspiration should be unavailing (Kock 1976b). I have had rather equivocal results with this test, and, if the first aspiration proves unrewarding, there is a natural tendency to try injecting a little more fluid and repeating the test, which could be dangerous to the integrity of the reservoir.

Another way to check on the siting of the tip of the tube, and the one that I have found more reliable, is by radiological examination. The tube itself shows faintly but sufficiently on plain X-ray plates. A very small injection of a water-soluble radiopaque medium (e.g. Gastrografin) will give an outline of the reservoir and show the position of the valve (Fig. 583). In a few cases recently I have at the time of making the valve and reservoir placed one Liga-clip (Ethicon) on the extreme end of the valve and another on the wall of the reservoir immediately opposite the valve, as markers to indicate the relative positions of these structures and of the tip of the catheter on plain X-ray examination in the postoperative period. This measure seems promisingly helpful but more experience with it is needed. Of course, if the reservoir—or at least the nipple-valve—was constructed with staples, these will show on a plain X-ray examination.

If the siting of the catheter appears to be satisfactory and there are no overwhelmingly strong indications on clinical (and radiological) grounds of a mechanical intestinal obstruction proximal to the reservoir to account for the failure of faeces to escape from the tube, an expectant attitude is indicated, with continued intravenous infusion and nasogastric aspiration. Often after a further day or two on this regimen the reservoir begins to discharge faecal matter, but, if inactivity of the ileostomy is prolonged beyond five or six days from the time of operation, the need for reoperation to resolve the problem at laparotomy will arise.

Once a free faecal flow from the reservoir has commenced, a major hurdle of the postoperative period has been surmounted. Oral fluids may now be given freely and a light mainly fluid diet started, but during the first two or three weeks it is wise to stick to low-residue items of diet, otherwise the faeces may become bulky and firm in consistency and tend to block the tube, with resulting cessation of drainage and abdominal pain. This blockage can be dealt with by irrigating the tube and reservoir with saline injected from a bladder type syringe, but to do this irrigation effectively often requires a good deal of force, which one is reluctant to use on a recently made ileostomy. It is thus better to avoid this problem by dietetic restraint during this early delicate period in the reservoir's existence.

It is quite customary, and certainly my practice, to keep the tube in position for at least three and preferably four weeks. During the first three weeks it is allowed to drain continuously. At the end of this period it is useful, but not essential, to have a 'pantaloonogram' made after a small gently given injection of Gastrografin into the reservoir (Fig. 583) to show that it is intact and has a good valve. The tube is then allowed still to drain continuously at night but during the day it is clipped off and released only for 10 minutes or so every three hours, and this routine is maintained for another four to seven days. After four weeks the indwelling tube is withdrawn and intermittent intubation is practised, at first every three hours during the day and perhaps once at night, but gradually over the next week or 10 days the nightly intubation is omitted and the daily intubations are made rather less frequent. At first the tube is passed by a member of the surgical staff, but gradually the patient herself is taught the process and usually rapidly masters the intricacies of her particular exit conduit.

Periodic Intubation

A convenient tube for this purpose is a translucent plastic one, size 28 Charrière, made by A. B. Medena of Kungsbacka, Sweden; the agent in this country is Henleys Medical Supplies Ltd, Clarendon Road, Hornsey, London N8 ODL. Messrs Franklin of High Wycombe, Buckinghamshire, England, make a similar tube. Whilst the patient stands or sits, the rounded end of the well-lubricated tube is introduced into the stoma, being directed backwards, inwards and slightly downwards, or in whatever direction experience has shown to be appropriate for that individual. When the reservoir is entered, usually at a depth of about 7–10 cm, there is a gush of intestinal contents along the tube, the external end of which is held over a jug, dish or lavatory bowl to catch the discharge. Emptying is assisted by to-and-fro movement of the tube combined with a little pressure by the other hand on the lower abdomen.

If the contents are unduly thick, as may happen if the patient has been eating a lot of vegetables, they may obstruct the tube. This will necessitate its removal for washing clean and then reintroduction, or else irrigation through the tube in position with water from a large plastic bladder syringe to break up and liquify the faeces in the reservoir. The length of time required for complete evacuation of the reservoir varies from three or four to 10–15 minutes, depending on the consistency of the faeces and other factors.

Between intubations, if perfect continence has been achieved, the stoma is simply covered with a piece of dry gauze and strapping, but, if there is occasional leakage of faeces, it may be necessary to wear an ordinary ileostomy bag continuously or for some part of the 24 hours.

In my experience dieting is quite often necessary, at any rate in the early stages, in patients with reservoir ileostomies, to reduce the amount of roughage, which may make the faeces too stiff for evacuation through the tube.

IMMEDIATE COMPLICATIONS

LEAKAGE FROM THE SUTURE LINE IN THE
RESERVOIR WITH RESULTING DIFFUSE
PERITONITIS OR LOCALIZED ABSCESS
FORMATION

In my series of 62 reservoir operations, leakage from the reservoir occurred in seven cases, with the development of fulminating diffuse peritonitis in three and of a localized abscess in four (pelvic in two, subphrenic in one, and in the right iliac region in one). The three patients with *diffuse peritonitis* all came to emergency re-laparotomy, at which holes were discovered in the suture lines of the reservoirs (in the fundus in two and at the base of the valve in one), and excision of the reservoir with establishment of a conventional ileostomy was performed; they all made good recoveries. The four patients with *localized abscesses* were treated more conservatively in the first instance, the abscess simply being drained (or bursting spontaneously), with subsequent formation of a faecal fistula from the reservoir. In one case early excision of the reservoir and formation of a conventional ileostomy was undertaken. In the other three an attempt was made to get the fistulae to heal with prolonged total parenteral feeding, but after two to three months of this regimen the fistulous track persisted in all three patients. One elected then to have the reservoir removed and be converted to an ordinary ileostomy; the other two proceeded to a further laparotomy at which the hole in the reservoir was found to be in the fundus and was closed by suture, the operation being completed by establishment of a proximal loop ileostomy (see Figs 557–60). In both cases the fistula was thereby cured and eventually the loop ileostomy was closed, putting the reservoir back into use.

It should be added that in another two of my cases treated by reservoir ileostomy signs highly suggestive of the development of peritonitis appeared and led to re-laparotomy, at which no definite peritonitis was found. However, a proximal loop ileostomy was made on the left side of the abdomen 35 cm proximal to the reservoir. Both patients did well and the loop ileostomy was closed in due course.

So far as I can gather these septic complications of the operation appear to be rather less common in the hands of several other surgeons doing reservoir ileostomies than in mine, but the published reports are not always very forthcoming on this matter. Thus Kock (1973) does not state exactly how many of his patients had non-fatal peritonitis, abscesses or fistulas, though he admits to 15% of his 275 patients requiring re-operation in the immediate postoperative period for non-lethal complications. In Cameron's (1973) series of six patients, two developed abscesses which had a fistulous connection with the exit conduit, but the fistulas closed spontaneously. Halvorsen et al. (1978) reported that seven of their 36 patients produced fistulas from the reservoir to the surface; four closed spontaneously. Beahrs (1975) records no septic complications in 37 reservoir cases.

Madigan (1975) had three leaks from the reservoir in 19 patients; two apparently healed spontaneously and one required operative closure. In Failes's (1976) group of seven patients given reservoir ileostomies, one developed a faecal fistula which healed on conservative treatment. Gelernt et al. (1977) had two fistulas from the reservoir in 54 patients; both healed spontaneously, one only after a temporary proximal loop ileostomy. Palmu and Sivula (1978) report two ruptures of the reservoir with diffuse peritonitis (one fatal) and four faecal fistulas which all healed with conservative treatment.

In the light of all these experiences, including my own, I would say that if the patient develops an acute diffuse peritonitis due to leakage from a reservoir ileostomy, the correct plan is to remove the reservoir, but if a more localized peritonitis occurs with abscess formation, an initially conservative surgical approach is reasonable. The abscess should be drained, and either total parenteral nutrition provided, or a loop ileostomy established proximal to the reservoir. The fistula may then close spontaneously or after two months or so a further operation can be performed, either to close it if it is suitably situated (e.g. with the opening in the fundus of the reservoir rather than at the base of the exit conduit), or to remove the reservoir if the patient is anxious for a quick certain solution.

NECROSIS OF THE EXIT CONDUIT

In many cases during the preparation of the nipple-valve at operation the intussuscepted piece of ileum becomes decidedly blue and the surgeon experiences some apprehension regarding its ultimate viability. Similarly the exit conduit may look quite cyanosed when it is fixed in place in the abdominal wall. Fortunately, despite these alarming developments at operation, the nipple valve and exit conduit almost invariably seem to survive satisfactorily. But in two of my patients, on both of whom the 'split mesentery' technique (Figs 590, 594) of making the nipple valve was practised, necrosis did occur. In one the nipple valve and conduit eventually sloughed completely, but by the time the necrotic tissue separated the reservoir had become firmly adherent to the anterior abdominal wall and no peritonitis or abscess ensued. The granulating track without epithelial lining leading from the reservoir through the abdominal wall to the skin surface naturally showed a great tendency to contract despite attempted regular stretching with

Hegar's dilators, and in the absence of a nipple-valve the reservoir was incontinent. Eventually this patient came to re-operation, at which the reservoir was rotated and a new valve constructed as shown in Fig. 601 with an excellent result. In the other instance of necrosis the exit conduit remained viable, but the entire nipple-valve sloughed and was discharged through the stoma after 12 days. The loss of the valve deprived this patient also of her continence but she has since undergone a re-operation to make a new valve as in Fig. 601, so far with an excellent result.

Most other publications on reservoir ileostomy do not mention these vascular complications, but from conversation with other surgeons doing these operations I know that necrosis of the valve or exit conduit has occasionally been encountered.

INCONTINENCE

Incontinence can occur in the early postoperative period when intermittent intubation is commenced, and was in my experience almost universal in those patients given reservoirs without nipple-valves (Goligher and Lintott 1975). But it has been not infrequent also after some of the currently popular operative techniques providing a nipple-valve, though in these cases it occurs more often as a late complication and will be considered together with other later complications (see below).

IMMEDIATE MORTALITY

In my series of 62 cases given reservoir ileostomies (roughly half done as a secondary operation, half as a primary procedure together with an elective proctocolectomy or subtotal colectomy) there were no operative deaths, though, as will be deduced from the foregoing account of the complications that occurred, several patients were exceedingly ill for a while and may perhaps be considered fortunate to have survived.

Kock and Myrvold (1979), in a series of 275 patients given reservoir ileostomies (roughly half as primary operations and half as secondary procedures), had seven deaths clearly related to complications of the reservoir. Cameron (1973) had no hospital deaths in six cases; Madigan (1976) one in 19 cases; Failes (1976) none in seven cases; Gelernt et al. (1977) none in 54 cases; Palmu and Sivula (1978) one in 51 cases; Halvorsen et al. (1978) three in 36 cases; and Beart et al. (1979) none in 250 cases.

LATER COMPLICATIONS

INCONTINENCE

As mentioned on p. 797 almost above everything else, it is its failure to afford lasting continence to all the patients submitted to it that has bedevilled and to some extent discredited the reservoir operation. Estimates of the frequency of this complication have varied. When methods of making the reservoir *without a nipple-valve* were used, some degree of incontinence was the rule in my experience (Goligher and Lintott 1975), and, though Kock (1973) gave a substantially more favourable report in this respect on these techniques, most surgeons now consider that it is not worth the effort to make a reservoir without a valve mechanism. But, *even with a nipple-valve*, there has been a fairly high incidence of subsequent incontinence as reported by different authors though the precise frequency is not always easily deduced from the relevant publications. The figures for incontinence for different authors seems to be roughly as follows: Cameron (1973) 25% in four cases; Bearhs (1975) 30% in 22 cases; Madigan (1976) 27% in 18 cases; Kock (1976a) 33% in 113 cases; Gelernt et al. (1977) 9% in 54 cases; Goligher (1978) 38% in 54 cases; Palmu and Sivula (1978) 39% in 51 cases; Halvorsen et al. (1978) 35% in 36 cases; and Beart et al. (1979) 41% in 125 cases.

It is now believed that incontinence arising in patients who were given nipple-valves in their reservoirs is due to deterioration in the efficacy of the valve, either because of its partial or complete extrusion (Goligher and Lintott 1975; Madigan 1976; Kock 1976a, b; Pamu and Sivula 1978), or rarely because of the development of a perforation and fistula through the valve near its base at the site of one of the through-and-through silk fixing sutures (Kock 1976a, b; Palmu and Sivula 1978). Certainly valve extrusions can be well demonstrated by pantaloonograms, i.e. radiological films made after injection of barium into the reservoir (Fig. 583B, C, D). Kock (1976b) claims that if the valve remains in position for three months from the time of operation, it is then most unlikely to become displaced. I consider this a good general rule, though both Palmu and Sivula (1978) and I can recall patients who developed incontinence and valve extrusion up to six to twelve months after operation.

When incontinence does occur, it may vary in severity from a slight leakage of flatus and faeces to a considerable faeculent discharge. In cases with lesser degrees of the condition it is usually possible for the tube still to be passed periodically into the reservoir, but in cases with gross incontinence intubation is often impossible because of the angulated course of the exit conduit due to the extruded valve (Fig. 583D). In these latter instances the patient has to wear a bag and manage the ileostomy as if it were a conventional one. For minor degrees of incontinence it may suffice for the patient to change the piece of gauze covering the stoma rather more frequently, but sometimes she prefers to wear a bag for at least part of the 24 hours, say at night. In the long term, too, the patient may elect to continue with these conser-

vative measures, however great the incontinence, and to accept that the operation has failed to provide a continent ileostomy, or she may be keen to try further operative treatment. Certainly it is possible to offer the chance of correcting this state of affairs by another operation, which, however, is better postponed for at least three months from the time of the previous operation to allow adhesions to absorb and facilitate the dissection. Several surgical methods are available depending on the precise findings at re-laparotomy:

Reconstruction of the Original Nipple-Valve. Occasionally it is possible, after the abdomen has

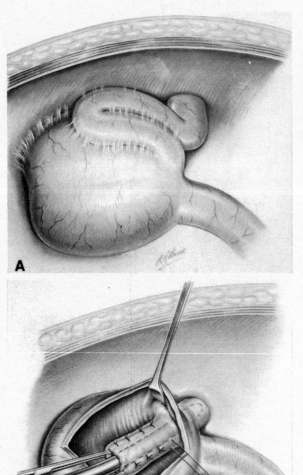

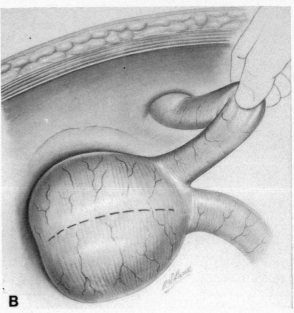

Fig. 600. Reconstruction of extruded nipple-valve. (A) The extruded knuckle of bowel is seen wrapped in adhesions. (B) The adhesions have been divided and the exit conduit converted into a free loop. (C) The reservoir has been opened and the exit conduit largely drawn into it to make a new nipple-valve, which is being sutured in place.

been opened and residual adhesions have been divided exposing the reservoir, to define and free outside the reservoir the piece of intestine that represents the extruded valve (Fig. 600A, B). Then the reservoir is opened (Fig. 600C) and the redundant portion of the exit conduit is drawn into the lumen to reform the valve, which is then fixed either by silk sutures inserted inside the reservoir or by two or three rows of silk Lembert sutures at the base of the valve, particularly in the region of the mesenteric gap, the reservoir is subsequently closed. Depending on the build and obesity of the patient it may or may not be possible to do all this with the end of the exit conduit still attached to the stoma, but more usually it is necessary to free the intestine entirely from the abdominal wall to get proper access. Also it is possibly wiser to split the mesentery and rotate the bowel as it is intussuscep-

ted to form the valve (Figs 590–4) or to use a metal stapling technique (Fig 599).

Construction of a New Nipple-Valve. More usually it is necessary to adopt this procedure, which is generally performed as shown in Fig. 601. The principle of the operation is that, after freeing the reservoir and the exit conduit from the abdominal wall, the entire extruded nipple-valve and exit conduit are excised, leaving a hole on the reservoir. The entrance conduit is then divided 15–20 cm from the reservoir and a new nipple-valve is fashioned out of the portion still attached to the reservoir. Finally the lower end of the main part of the small gut is sutured to the hole in the reservoir and the latter is rotated to enable the proximal end of the portion of the entrance conduit that was used to make the new nipple-valve to be used as a new

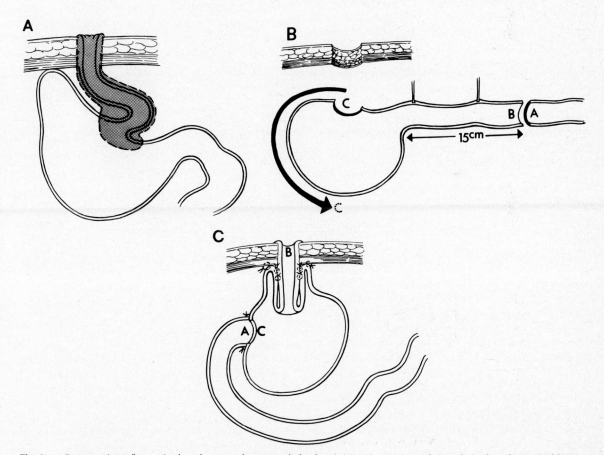

Fig. 601. Construction of new nipple-valve to replace extruded valve. (A) Previous exit conduit and nipple-valve excised leaving a hole in the wall of the reservoir. (B) Entrance conduit divided 15 cm or more from the reservoir, the part attached to the reservoir is then made into a nipple-valve. (C) Finally the reservoir is rotated, so that the former entrance conduit becomes the exit conduit and is taken through the anterior abdominal wall, whilst the remainder of the small intestine is anastomosed to the hole in the reservoir.

exit conduit and to form a new stoma. This same technique of excising the old valve and exit conduit and making a new valve and new exit conduit is used when the old valve has a fistula through its basal part (Kock 1976a), though alternatively an attempt might be made just to close the fistula by suture.

An alternative procedure is to excise the extruded nipple-valve and exit conduit and then to provide a new exit conduit and new valve by isolating a 15–20 cm segment of small bowel with its mesentery intact (from a point 7–10 cm or so above the reservoir) and inserting it between the reservoir and the abdominal wall. The continuity of the rest of the small intestine is restored by end-to-end anastomosis. The reservoir is *not* rotated in this operation.

Excision of Reservoir and Construction of Entirely New Reservoir with New Nipple-Valve. In three cases in which the entrance conduit of ileum was caught up inextricably in adhesions around the extruded valve and was inadvertently opened in two or three places during attempts to isolate it, I elected to sacrifice the entire existing reservoir and make a new one out of the terminal 50 cm or so of remaining small bowel. Kock (1976b) advises against this step because of apprehension about the quality of continence to be expected of a reservoir dealing with the somewhat looser faeces at this higher level in the bowel, but my three patients so treated all had good immediate and two satisfactory late results.

LEAKAGE OF MUCOID MATERIAL

A condition which does not seem to have attracted the attention of other authors, but which has proved a considerable nuisance to several of my patients, has been leakage from the stoma of mucoid material unassociated with faeces or flatus. In view of the continence of the reservoir *per se*, the discharge presumably comes from the exit conduit, but, when the interior of the conduit and the reservoir was inspected by passing a narrow bore sigmoidoscope, no discharging abscess or local ileitis was observed to account for the complaint. I have not been able to advise any effective treatment and the patients have simply carried on with rather more frequent changes of the pads covering the stoma. One of them found Hollister colostomy caps useful.

RETENTION

Five of my patients developed this complication as an acute crisis six to seven weeks after their operation. They found one day that they could not pass the tube into the reservoir, and, as nothing leaked out of the reservoir, within 12 hours they were becoming extremely uncomfortable. In one case I was able to pass a finger down the exit conduit to the tip of the valve and then to repeat the performance in conjunction with a tube, guiding the latter into the reservoir. In the other four cases a general anaesthetic was necessary to enable this to be done. The tube was then left in place for a few days. On removal, intermittent intubation was at first quite easy and satisfactory, but eventually after two or three weeks the trouble recurred. In two patients the difficulty gradually lessened so that they were able to manoeuvre the tube into place themselves during these episodes, and now have no problems with intubation two and two-and-a-half years later. In the other three patients, however, the trouble persisted and they all came to re-operation to re-align the valve by further suturing from within and without the reservoir, but unfortunately the benefit was short-lived. All three declined further operation to make an entirely new valve and elected to have their reservoirs removed and to be converted to a conventional ileostomy.

Most other writers do not seem to have encountered this complication. Kock (1976b) suggests that it represents the earliest stage of extrusion of the nipple-valve, but my conservatively treated patient has not developed a frank valvular extrusion in two years.

STOMAL STENOSIS

One of my patients developed stenosis following sloughing of the exit conduit and nipple-valve. After re-operation to provide a new exit conduit and valve there was slight separation of the bowel from the skin edge with resulting further slight fibrous stenosis, which requires periodic dilatation.

ILEITIS IN THE RESERVOIR

Kock (1976b) described 14 instances of a non-specific ileitis occurring in the reservoir. The condition proclaimed itself by the development of diarrhoea with liquid profuse faeces, sometimes containing a little blood. Some of the patients became dehydrated and depleted in sodium. Endoscopy showed the mucous membrane of the reservoir to be inflamed and to manifest contact bleeding, sometimes discrete ulcers. The treatment recommended by Kock (1976a) is continuous drainage of the reservoir by an indwelling tube through the stoma and the administration of sulphasalazine. He has seen complete resolution take place in a few weeks or months. Halvorsen et al. (1978) noted ileitis of the reservoir in five of their 36 patients. In two of these patients the reservoir had eventually to be removed.

VOLVULUS OF THE RESERVOIR

This remarkable complication occurred in one of my earlier cases and caused acute intestinal obstruction. At laparotomy the reservoir was found to have rotated several times round the attachment of the exit conduit to the anterior abdominal wall. As some necrosis had already taken place the reservoir was excised.

BIOLOGICAL CONSEQUENCES

In a sense the reservoir ileostomy is a blind intestinal loop and it would be reasonable to expect that the stasis in it might predispose to bacterial proliferation with resulting mucosal irritation and possibly impairment of absorption.

Bacteriological studies show that after a conventional ileostomy there is an increased number of micro-organisms in the lower ileal contents compared with normal and a preponderance of colonic anaerobes (Gorbach et al. 1967; Finegold et al. 1970). After a reservoir ileostomy these changes are even more marked and the bacterial flora of the reservoir has a character midway between that of the normal lower ileum and the rectum (Brandberg et al. 1972; Philipson et al. 1975). Though fluctuations in the numbers and proportions of different bacteria can be demonstrated by cultures at different times, the bacterial population is fairly stable and there appears to be no consistent tendency to progressive deterioration.

Morphological studies of the mucosa of the reservoir by means of serial biopsies have also revealed changes in the form of reduced height of the villi and increased depth of the crypts (Philipson et al. 1975). There was also an increased mitotic index. These alterations were evident within one month of the operation, but subsequent studies do not show significant further changes on either light microscopy or dissection microscopy. These appearances are considered to indicate that there is an accelerated epithelial turn-over in the reservoir.

As regards *absorption*, information is available from Jagenburg et al. (1971) that there is no difference in the absorption of L-phenylalanine, D-xylose and fat in reservoir ileostomy patients as compared with those with a conventional ileostomy, but absorption of vitamin B_{12} seemed to be decreased in the reservoir cases. Further investigation by Jagenburg et al. (1975), however, involving estimations of serum levels and repeated Schilling tests, was re-assuring in showing that malabsorption of this vitamin was infrequent. Philipson et al. (1975) were also able to demonstrate good absorption of vitamin B_{12} after its direct instillation into the reservoir. But Halvorsen et al. (1978) found malabsorption of vitamin B_{12} in four of seven patients tested from this point of view. In view of the recognized failure of patients with conventional ileostomy to absorb the normal amount of sodium from the intestine, so that in the long run they suffer chronic depletion of this electrolyte (Clarke et al. 1968), it would be interesting to know how reservoir ileostomy patients behave in this respect. Unfortunately no such information is yet available. Altogether these investigations are re-assuring for though there are mucosal changes as a result of creating the ileal reservoir, absorptive function seems pretty well maintained. Certainly the general health of my patients with reservoir ileostomies, some of them now done six and seven years ago, seems fully on a par with that of conventional ileostomy patients.

CURRENT INDICATIONS FOR RESERVOIR ILEOSTOMY

Regarding the place of the reservoir ileostomy in the overall strategy of contemporary surgical treatment for ulcerative colitis, caution must still be exercised in making pronouncements. Obviously this type of operation carries intrinsic risks of leakage and infection that apply scarcely at all to a conventional ileostomy. As these hazards are likely to be increased during acute phases of the disease, consideration of this procedure should be reserved exclusively for patients whose colitis is in complete remission and who are in reasonably good general condition. At one stage Kock (1971b) advised against the use of a reservoir operation in anyone who had been having intensive and prolonged steroid therapy in the recent past, but so many colitis patients have inevitably had treatment with steroids, this is scarcely a practicable contraindication. Even apparently fit patients should be left in no doubt that the choice of a reservoir ileostomy somewhat increases the risks of operation. It is also important to stress to the patient that it is impossible to guarantee that complete continence will be obtained without possible further surgical intervention. Accordingly a strong sense of dedication on the part of the patient to the idea of having a continent ileostomy is highly desirable to enable her to surmount the various set-backs that may beset the course to this objective. Unquestionably the most satisfactory type of patient in many ways to be considered for a reservoir ileostomy is one who has already had a proctocolectomy or subtotal colectomy with conventional ileostomy, and who, because of persistent physical or phychological problems in relation to the stoma, is anxious to try a reservoir operation. In this connection I ought to mention that the factor inducing most of the patients coming to me for a primary or secondary reservoir ileostomy to seek this type of operation has been their hope—not always realized unfortunately—of improving their sex life by avoiding the necessity for wearing an external appliance. On the credit side, it must be emphasized that the results of reservoir ileostomies seem to be improving in recent years and, whatever the difficulties associated with this operation, when it works well the outcome is so pleasing as to make both the patient and the surgeon feel that it was thoroughly worth the trouble.

FUTURE DEVELOPMENTS IN REGARD TO THE RESERVOIR ILEOSTOMY

COMBINING A MAGNETIC CLOSING DEVICE WITH A RESERVOIR

As continence is not always perfect with a reservoir ileostomy even when provided with a nipple-valve, an obvious development would be to combine one of the new magnetic colostomy devices (see p. 633) with a reservoir ileostomy. This could be done at the time of the original reservoir operation, the nipple-valve being dispensed with and a magnetic ring being inserted into the abdominal wall around the emerging exit conduit instead. As stressed in connection with the making of magnetic colostomies, there would have to be no protrusion of the stoma beyond the level of the skin and no indrawing of the latter; in other words the junction of the bowel wall and abdominal skin should be an exact right angle. Alternatively the magnetic ring could be implanted secondarily in patients the continence of whose reservoir, made with a nipple-valve, has been found to be somewhat imperfect. Admittedly there would be a greater chance of infection following secondary implantations of this kind. Though many surgeons, including myself, have often discussed the possibility of incorporating a magnetic device in a reservoir ileostomy in either of these ways, I am aware of only five or six cases where this has been done with encouraging results and also of two or three other cases where a magnetic device was used in connection with a conventional ileostomy *without* reservoir with indifferent results. Clearly this idea warrants further exploration. Another even more ambitious plan would be to place the stoma of the valveless ileal reservoir in the perineum after proctocolectomy and to combine with it a magnetic closing device, but it is rather doubtful whether a sufficiently flat skin surface would be obtained in that situation to permit of the secure fitment of a magnetic cap. Also the presence of the rather heavy magnetic device in the perineum might prove uncomfortable to the patient.

BRINGING THE EXIT CONDUIT OF A RESERVOIR ILEOSTOMY TO THE ANUS THROUGH A DENUDED RETAINED LOWER RECTUM AND ANAL CANAL

Another possibility is to revert to the original Ravitch (1948) conception of an ileo-anal pull-through anastomosis after denuding the anorectal remnant of its lining, but creating an ileal reservoir without a nipple-valve immediately above the anastomosis to reduce the pressure under which faeces will reach the sphincter mechanism. The denuding of the anorectal remnant is achieved as described in connection with abdomino-transanal resection (see p. 577), though it is desirable to excise all the mucosa down to the pectinate line in order to remove all the disease, and, if a long rectal segment is being preserved, it might be necessary to effect some of the mucosal excision from above. When I employed the original Ravitch technique many years ago, the excision of the inflamed adherent and friable mucosa from the muscle coat of the anorectal remnant proved far from easy and I was not at all impressed by the functional results. But our methods of dissecting out mucosa from such a rectal remnant have improved through practice in connection with the method of abdominotransanal excision of the rectum for carcinoma or villous papilloma (see pp. 350, 577), and the presence of an ileal reservoir above the anal canal might greatly improve the prospects of achieving continence. The tendency of ileal reservoirs and pull-through anastomoses to give rise to septic complications would make many surgeons reluctant to adopt such a daring operative plan, but a covering proximal loop ileostomy might substantially lessen the risks. Ferrari and Fonkalsrud (1978) have used this technique successfully in dogs.

Actually since the above comment was written Parks and Nicholls (1978) have described five patients treated by a combination of an ileal reservoir without nipple-valve and an ileo-anal anastomosis with covering loop ileostomy along these lines with encouraging results. There were no deaths, two cases developed temporary pelvic abscesses and some degree of anastomotic dehiscence or stenosis occurred in two cases. The functional results are rated as excellent in four cases, evacuation being achieved by passing a tube three or four times a day, complete continence being afforded by the sphincters between intubations. Spontaneous defaecation did not occur. The fifth patient was a failure in so far as he found the anal intubations disturbing, and he was eventually given a conventional abdominal ileostomy. Certainly Parks and Nicholls' (1978) achievements with this ingenious technique are challenging and should encourage other surgeons to consider such an operation for carefully selected patients. (See Appendix C, p. 940, for more practical details.)

REFERENCES

ABRAMSON, D., JANKELSON, I. R. and MILNER, L. R. (1951) Pregnancy in idiopathic ulcerative colitis. *Am. J. Obstet. Gynec.*, *61*, 121.

ACHESON, E. D. (1960) An association between ulcerative colitis, regional enteritis, and ankylosing spondylitis. *Q. Jl Med.*, *29*, 489.

—— and NEFZGER, M. D. (1963) Ulcerative colitis in the United States Army in 1944. Epidemiology: Comparisons between patients and controls. *Gastroenterology*, *44*, 7.

—— and TRUELOVE, S. C. (1961) Early weaning in the aetiology of ulcerative colitis: A study of feeding in infancy in cases and controls. *Br. med. J.*, *2*, 929.

ADSON, M. A., COOPERMAN, A. M. and FARROW, G. M. (1972) Ileorectostomy for ulcerative disease of the colon. *Archs Surg., Chicago*, *104*, 424.

ALEXANDER, F. G. (1970) Quoted by Ritchie (1971*b*).

ALLANBY, K. D. (1957) Deaths associated with steroid-hormone therapy: an analysis of 18 cases. *Lancet*, *i*, 1104.

ALLARDYCE, D. B. and GROVES, A. C. (1974) A comparison of nutritional gains resulting from intravenous and external feeding. *Surgery Gynec. Obstet.*, *139*, 179.

ALMY, T. P. and LEWIS, C. M. (1963) Ulcerative colitis: a report of progress, based upon the recent literature. *Gastroenterology*, *45*, 515.

ALMY, T. P. and PLAUT, A. G. (1965) Ulcerative colitis: a report of progress, based upon the recent literature. *Gastroenterology, 49,* 295.

ANDERSON, A. F. (1960) Colectomy and ileorectal anastomosis in surgical treatment of ulcerative colitis. *Aust. N.Z. J. Surg., 30,* 107.

ANDERSON, R. and TURNBULL, R. B., Jr. (1976) Grafting the unhealed peroneal wound after coloproctectomy for Crohn's disease. *Archs Surg., Chicago, 111,* 335.

ANDRESEN, A. F. R. (1942) Ulcerative colitis—allergic phenomenon. *Am. J. dig. Dis., 9,* 91.

ANTHONISEN, P. and RIIS, P. (1961) A new diagnostic approach to mucosal inflammation in proctocolitis. *Lancet, 2,* 81.

ARN, E. R. (1931) Chronic ulcerative colitis; surgical treatment of refractory cases. *Ohio St. med. J., 27,* 121.

AULT, G. W. (1960) Selective surgery for ulcerative colitis. *Proc. R. Soc. Med., 52,* 11.

AXELSSON, C. and JARNUM, S. (1977) Assessment of the therapeutic value of an elemental diet in chronic inflammatory bowel disease. *Scand. J. Gastroent., 12,* 89.

AYLETT, S. O. (1953) Discussion on the surgery of ulcerative colitis. *Proc. R. Soc. Med., 46,* 1032.

—— (1957) Total colectomy and ileo-rectal anastomosis in diffuse ulcerative colitis. *Br. med. J., 1,* 489.

—— (1960) Diffuse ulcerative colitis and its treatment by ileorectal anastomosis. *Ann. R. Coll. Surg., Engl., 27,* 260.

—— (1963) Ulcerative colitis treated by total colectomy and ileorectal anastomosis: a ten-year review. *Proc. R. Soc. Med., 56,* 183.

—— (1966) Three hundred cases of diffuse ulcerative colitis treated by total colectomy and ileorectal anastomosis. *Br. med. J., 1,* 1001.

—— (1970) Delayed ileorectal anastomosis in the surgery of ulcerative colitis. *Br. J. Surg., 57,* 812.

—— (1971) Cancer and ulcerative colitis. *Br. med. J., 1,* 203.

BABB, R. R., LEE, R. H. and PECK, O. C. (1970) Cancer of the bile duct and chronic ulcerative colitis. *Am. J. Surg., 119,* 337.

BACON, H. E., BRALOW, S. P. and BERKLEY, J. L. (1960) Rehabilitation and long-term survival after colectomy for ulcerative colitis. *J. Am. med. Ass., 172,* 324.

—— and NUGUID, T. P. (1962) The management of large bowel obstruction. *Minn. Med., 45,* 402.

—— and TRIMPI, H. D. (1950) The selection of an operative procedure for patients with medically intractable ulcerative colitis. *Surgery Gynec. Obstet., 91,* 409.

—— YANG, L., CARROLL, P. T., CATES, B. A., VILLALBA, G. and McGREGOR, R. A. (1956) Non-specific ulcerative colitis, with reference to mortality, morbidity, complications and long-term survivals following colectomy. *Am. J. Surg., 92,* 688.

BAIRD, D. (1950) *Combined Textbook of Obstetrics and Gynaecology for Students and Practitioners.* Edinburgh: Livingstone.

BAKER, W. N. W. (1970) The results of ileorectal anastomosis at St Mark's Hospital from 1953 to 1968. *Gut, 11,* 235.

—— GLASS, R. E., RITCHIE, J. K. and AYLETT, S. O. (1978) Cancer of the rectum following colectomy and colorectal anastomosis for ulcerative colitis. *Br. J. Surg., 65,* 862.

BANKS, B. M., KORELITZ, B. I. and ZETZEL, L. (1957) The course of non-specific ulcerative colitis: review of 20 years' experience and late results. *Gastroenterology, 32,* 983.

BARBOSA, J. DE C., BARGEN, J. A. and DIXON, C. F. (1945) Regional segmental colitis. *Surg. Clins N. Am., 25,* 939.

BARGEN, J. A. (1924) Experimental studies on the etiology of chronic ulcerative colitis. *J. Am. med. Ass., 83,* 332.

—— (1928) Chronic ulcerative colitis associated with malignant disease. *Archs Surg., Chicago, 17,* 561.

—— (1929) Complications and sequelae of chronic ulcerative colitis. *Ann. intern. Med., 3,* 335.

—— (1943) Ileostomy for chronic ulcerative colitis (end results and complications in 185 cases). *Ann. intern. Med., 18,* 43.

—— (1955) Present status of hormonal and drug therapy of ulcerative colitis. *Sth. med. J., Nashville, 48,* 2.

—— (1956) Complications and problems associated with the management of ulcerative colitis. *Gastroenterologia, 86,* 674.

—— BROWN, P. W. and RANKIN, F. W. (1932) Indications for and technique of ileostomy in chronic ulcerative colitis. *Surgery Gynec. Obstet., 55,* 196.

—— and GAGE, R. P. (1960) Carcinoma and ulcerative colitis: prognosis. *Gastroenterology, 39,* 385.

—— JACKMAN, R. J. and KERR, J. G. (1938) Studies on the life histories of patients with chronic ulcerative colitis (thrombo-ulcerative colitis), with some suggestions for treatment. *Ann. intern. Med., 12,* 339.

—— SAUER, W. G., SLOAN, W. P. and GAGE, R. P. (1954) The development of cancer in chronic ulcerative colitis. *Gastroenterology, 26,* 32.

—— and WEBER, H. M. (1930) Regional migratory chronic ulcerative colitis. *Surgery Gynec. Obstet., 50,* 964.

BARKER, W. F. (1961) Surgical treatment of ulcerative colitis. *Am. J. Surg., 102,* 176.

—— (1962) Familial history of patients with ulcerative colitis. *Am. J. Surg., 103,* 25.

—— and OZERAN, R. S. (1963) Ileorectal anastomosis for ulcerative colitis. *Am. J. Surg., 106,* 348.

BARNES, C. S. and HAYES, H. M. (1931) Ulcerative colitis complicating pregnancy and the puerperium. *Am. J. Obstet. Gynec., 22,* 907.

BARON, J. H., CONNELL, A. M. and LENNARD-JONES, J. E. (1964) Variation between observers in describing mucosal appearances in proctocolitis. *Br. med. J., 1,* 89.

—— —— —— and JONES, F. AVERY. (1962) Sulphasalazine and salicylazosulphadimidine in ulcerative colitis. *Lancet, 1,* 1094.

BAXTER, H., SCHILLER, C., WHITESIDE, J. H. and SRAITH, R. E. (1951) Influence of cortisone on skin and wound healing in experimental animals. *Plast. reconstr. Surg., 7,* 24.

BEAHRS, O. H. (1975) Use of ileal reservoir following proctocolectomy. *Surgery Gynec. Obstet., 141,* 363.

—— KELLY, K. A., ADSON, M. A. and CHONG, G. C. (1974) Ileostomy with ileal reservoir rather than ileostomy alone. *Ann. Surg., 179,* 634.

BEAN, R. H. D. (1962) The treatment of chronic ulcerative colitis with 6-mercaptopurine. *Med. J. Aust., 49,* 592.

—— (1966) Treatment of ulcerative colitis with antimetabolites. *Br. med. J., 1,* 1081.

BEART, R. W., KELLY, K. and BEAHRS, O. H. (1979) Personal communication.

BEBCHUK, W., ROGERS, A. C. and DOWNEY, J. L. (1961) Chronic ulcerative colitis in a North American Indian. *Gastroenterology, 40,* 138.

BELL, C. M. A. and LEWIS, C. B. (1968) Effect of neostigmine on integrity of ileorectal anastomoses. *Br. med. J., 3,* 587.

BENNETT, R. C. and HUGHES, E. S. R. (1972) Urinary calculi and ulcerative colitis—a Victorian survey. *Br. med. J., 2,* 494.

—— and JEPSON, R. P. (1966) Uric acid stone formation following ileostomy. *Aust. N.Z. J. Surg., 36,* 153.

BENSON, R. E. and BARGEN, J. A. (1943) Chronic ulcerative colitis as a cause of retarded sexual and somatic development. *Gastroenterology*, *1*, 147.

BEST, R. R. (1948) Anastomosis of the ileum to the lower part of the rectum and anus. A report on experiences with ileorectostomy and ileoproctostomy, with special reference to polyposis. *Archs Surg., Chicago*, *57*, 276.

BILLSON, F. A., DE DOMBAL, F. T., WATKINSON, G. and GOLIGHER, J. C. (1967) Ocular complications of ulcerative colitis. *Gut*, *8*, 102.

BINDER, S. C., MILLER, H. H. and DETERLING, R. A., Jr. (1976) Fate of the retained rectum after subtotal colectomy for inflammatory disease of the colon. *Am. J. Surg., 131*, 201.

BIRNBAUM, D., GROEN, J. J. and KALLNER, G. (1960) Ulcerative colitis among the ethnic groups in Israel. *Archs intern. Med., 105*, 843.

BLACK, B. M. and SHOLL, P. R. (1954) Surgical treatment of chronic ulcerative colitis: the skin-grafted ileac stoma. *Archs Surg., Chicago, 68*, 454.

BLISS, B. P. (1963) Dehiscence of lateral space following its closure in colostomy and ileostomy. *Br. J. Surg., 50*, 730.

BLOCK, G. (1978) Personal communication.

BOCHUS, H. L. (1943–6) *Gastroenterology*, Vol. 2. Philadelphia and London: Saunders.

—— ROTH, J. L. A., BUCHMAN, E. and KALSER, M. (1958) In *Modern Trends in Gastroenterology*, 2nd series, ed. Jones, F. Avery, p. 296. London: Butterworth.

—— —— —— STAUB, W. R., FINKELSTEIN, L. and VALDES-DAPENA, A. (1956) Life history of non-specific ulcerative colitis: relation of prognosis to anatomical and clinical varieties. *Gastroenterologia, 86*, 549.

BODEN, R. W., RANKIN, J. G., GOULSTON, S. J. M. and MORROW, W. (1959) The liver in ulcerative colitis: the significance of raised serum alkaline phosphatase levels. *Lancet, 2*, 245.

BOIJSEN, E. and REUTER, S. (1966) Mesenteric angiography in the evaluation of inflammatory and neoplastic disease of the intestine. *Radiology, 87*, 1028.

BOWEN, G. E., IRONS, G. V., RHODES, J. B. and KIRSNER, J. B. (1965) Precautionary early experiences with immunosuppressive medication (azathioprine) in ulcerative colitis. *Gastroenterology, 48*, 807.

BOYD, W. C., HEISLER, M. and OROWAN, E. (1961) Correlation between ulcerative colitis and Rh. blood groups. *Nature, Lond., 190*, 1123.

BRAHME, F. (1971) Roentgenology. In *Regional Enteritis (Crohn's Disease)*, ed. A. Engel and T. Larsson. Stockholm: Nordiska Bokhandelns Förlag.

BRANDENBURG, Å., KOCK, N. G. and PHILIPSON, B. (1972) Bacterial flora in intra-abdominal ileostomy reservoir. *Gastroenterology, 63*, 413.

BROBERGER, O. (1964) Immunologic studies in ulcerative colitis. *Gastroenterology, 47*, 229.

—— and PERLMANN, P. (1959) Autoantibodies in human ulcerative colitis. *J. exp. Med., 110*, 657.

BROOKE, B. N. (1952) The management of ileostomy. *Lancet, 2*, 102.

—— (1954) *Ulcerative Colitis and Its Surgical Treatment*. Edinburgh: Livingstone.

—— (1956a) The outcome of surgery for ulcerative colitis. *Lancet, 2*, 532.

—— (1956b) Cortisone and ulcerative colitis: an adverse effect. *Lancet, 2*, 1175.

—— (1965) Discussion on regional enterocolitis. *Dis. Colon Rect.. 8*. 3.

—— (1969) Ulcerative colitis and carcinoma of the colon. *J. R. Coll. Surg. Edinb., 14*, 274.

—— and COOKE, W. T. (1951) Ulcerative colitis. *Lancet, 2*, 463.

—— DYKES, P. W. and WALKER, F. C. (1961) A study of liver disorder in ulcerative colitis. *Postgrad. med. J., 37*, 245.

—— and SAMPSON, P. A. (1964) An indication for surgery in acute ulcerative colitis. *Lancet, 2*, 1272.

—— and SLANEY, G. (1958) Portal bacteraemia in ulcerative colitis. *Lancet, 1*, 1206.

—— and WALKER, F. C. (1962) A method of external reversion of an ileostomy. *Br. J. Surg., 49*, 401.

BROWN, C. H., TURNBULL, R. B., Jr. and DIAZ, R. (1962) Ileorectal anastomosis in ulcerative colitis. *Am. J. dig. Dis., 7*, 585.

BROWN, J. Y. (1913) Value of complete physiological rest of large bowel in ulcerative and obstructive lesions. *Surgery Gynec. Obstet., 16*, 610.

BROWN, M. L., KASICH, A. M. and WEINGARTEN, B. (1951) Complications of chronic ulcerative colitis. *Am. J. dig. Dis., 18*, 52.

BRUCE, D. and COLE, W. H. (1962) Complications of ulcerative colitis. *Ann. Surg., 155*, 768.

BUCAILLE, M. (1962) Selective frontal lobe operation for the treatment of some diseases of the digestive tract with special reference to ulcerative colitis. *Surgery, St Louis, 52*, 690.

BUCKNELL, N. A., GOULD, S. R. and DAY, D. W. (1978) Controlled trial of disodium cromoglycate in chronic persistent ulcerative colitis. *Gut, 19*, 1140.

BURCH, P. R. J., DE DOMBAL, F. T. and WATKINSON, G. (1969) Aetiology of ulcerative colitis. II. A new hypothesis. *Gut, 10*, 277.

BURNHAM, W. R., LENNARD-JONES, J. E. and BROOKE, B. N. (1977) Sexual problems amongst married ileostomists. *Gut, 18*, 673.

BUSSON, A. and HERNANDEZ, C. (1965) L'artériographie sélective mésentérique dans la rectocolite hémorrhagique et la colite ulcéreuse d'emblée. *Arch. Mal. Appar. dig., 54*, 441.

BUTLER, E. C. (1948) Spreading ulceration of the skin associated with idiopathic ulcerative colitis. *Proc. R. Soc. Med., 41*, 474.

—— (1952) Some observations on the treatment of carcinoma of the rectum. *Proc. R. Soc. Med., 45*, 41.

BUXTON, B. (1974) Progress report: small bowel resection and gastric acid secretion. *Gut, 15*, 229.

BYWATERS, E. G. L. and ANSELL, B. M. (1958) Arthritis associated with ulcerative colitis: a clinical and pathological study. *Ann. rheum. Dis., 17*, 169.

CALABRESI, P., THAYER, W. R., Jr. and SPIRO, H. M. (1961) Demonstration of circulating anti-nuclear globulins in ulcerative colitis. *J. clin. Invest., 40*, 2126.

CALLAHAN, W. S., GOLDMAN, R. G. and VIAL, A. B. (1963) The Auer phenomenon in colon-sensitized mice. Histopathology of colonic lesions. *J. surg. Res., 3*, 395.

CAMERON, A. (1973) The continent ileostomy. *Br. J. Surg., 60*, 785.

CANBY, J. P. and MEHLHOP, F. H. (1964) Ulcerative colitis in children. *Am. J. Gastroent., 42*, 66.

CARLESON, R., FRISTEDT, B. and PHILIPSON, J. (1962) Ulcerative colitis: a follow-up investigation of a 20-year primary material. *Acta med. scand., 172*, 647.

CATTELL, R. B. (1935) Surgical treatment of ulcerative colitis. *J. Am. med. Ass.,* *104,* 104.

—— (1944) Technic of total colectomy for ulcerative colitis. *Surg. Clins N. Am.,* *24,* 661.

—— (1948) The surgical treatment of ulcerative colitis. *Gastroenterology,* *10,* 63.

—— (1953) Discussion on the surgery of ulcerative colitis. *Proc. R. Soc. Med.,* *46,* 1022.

—— and BOEHME, E. J. (1947) The importance of malignant degeneration as a complication of ulcerative colitis. *Gastroenterology,* *8,* 695.

—— and COLCOCK, B. P. (1955) Surgical treatment of ulcerative colitis. *Postgrad. Med.,* *17,* 114.

CAVE, H. W. (1939) The surgical management of chronic intractable ulcerative colitis. *Am. J. Surg.,* *46,* 79.

—— (1945) Surgical experiences with ulcerative colitis. *Surg. Clins N. Am.,* *25,* 301.

CHOJECKI, Z. (1963) Epidemiology of ulcerative colitis. *Polskie Archwm Med. wewn.,* *33,* 1239.

CHRISPIN, A. R. and FRY, I. K. (1963) The presacral space shown by barium enema. *Br. J. Radiol.,* *36,* 319.

CLARK, R. L. and DIXON, C. F. (1939) Regional enteritis. *Surgery, St Louis,* *5,* 277.

CLARKE, A. M., CHURNSIDE, A., HILL, G. L. and POPE, G. (1968) Chronic dehydration and sodium depletion in patients with established ileostomies. *Lancet,* *2,* 740.

COGHILL, N. F., LUBRAN, M., MCALLEN, P. M., EDWARDS, F. and RICHENBERG, C. S. (1956) Sodium and potassium absorption and excretion in patients with ulcerative colitis before and after colectomy. *Gastroenterologia,* *86,* 724.

COHEN, S. E., MATOLO, N. M., MICHAS, C. A. and WOLFMAN, E. F., Jr. (1975) Antiperistaltic ileal segment in the prevention of ileostomy diarrhoea. *Archs Surg., Chicago,* *110,* 829.

COLCOCK, B. P. and MATHIESON, W. L. (1956) Complications of surgical treatment of chronic ulcerative colitis. *Archs Surg., Chicago,* *72,* 399.

—— VANSANT, J. H. and CONTRERAS, O. (1961) Surgical treatment of coexisting regional enteritis and ulcerative colitis. *Surgery Gynec. Obstet.,* *112,* 96.

COLP, R. (1934) A case of non-specific granuloma of the terminal ileum and cecum. *Surg. Clins N. Am.,* *14,* 443.

COMFORT, M. W., BARGEN, J. A. and MORLOCK, C. G. (1938) The association of chronic ulcerative colitis (colitis gravis) with hepatic insufficiency: report of 4 cases. *Med. Clins N. Am.,* *22,* 1089.

COOK, M. and GOLIGHER, J. C. (1975) Carcinoma and epithelial dysplasia complicating ulcerative colitis. *Gastroenterology,* *68,* 1127.

COOPER, D. R., STAHLGREN, L. H. and FERGUSON, L. H. (1956) Postoperative care following surgical treatment of chronic ulcerative colitis. *Ann. Surg.,* *144,* 19.

CORBETT, R. S. (1940) Discussion on the surgical treatment of idiopathic ulcerative colitis and its sequelae. *Proc. R. Soc. Med.,* *33,* 647.

—— (1945) A review of the surgical treatment of chronic ulcerative colitis. *Proc. R. Soc. Med.,* *38,* 277.

—— (1952) Recent advances in the surgical treatment of chronic ulcerative colitis. *Ann. R. Coll. Surg., Engl.,* *10,* 21.

—— (1953) Discussion on the surgery of ulcerative colitis. *Proc. R. Soc. Med.,* *46,* 1028.

CORNES, J. S., SMITH, J. C. and SOUTHWOOD, W. F. W. (1961) Lymphosarcoma in chronic ulcerative colitis with a report of 2 cases. *Br. J. Surg.,* *49,* 50.

COUNSELL, P. B. (1956) Lesions of the ileum associated with ulcerative colitis. *Br. J. Surg.,* *44,* 276.

—— and DUKES, C. E. (1952) The association of chronic ulcerative colitis and carcinoma of the rectum and colon. *Br. J. Surg.,* *39,* 485.

—— and GOLIGHER, J. C. (1952) The surgical treatment of ulcerative colitis. *Lancet,* *2,* 1045.

—— and LOCKHART-MUMMERY, H. E. (1954) Ileostomy: Assessment of disability: management. *Lancet,* *1,* 113.

CRANDON, J. H., KINNEY, T. D. and WALKER, I. J. (1944) Perforation of the ileum following late ileostomy for ulcerative colitis. *New Engl. J. Med.,* *230,* 419.

CRAWFORD, N. and BROOKE, B. N. (1957) Ileostomy chemistry. *Lancet,* *1,* 864.

CRILE, G., Jr. and THOMAS, C. Y., Jr. (1951) Treatment of acute toxic ulcerative colitis by ileostomy and simultaneous colectomy. *Gastroenterology,* *19,* 58.

—— and TURNBULL, R. B., Jr. (1954) The mechanism and prevention of ileostomy dysfunction. *Ann. Surg.,* *140,* 459.

CROHN, B. B. (1949) *Regional Ileitis.* London: Staples Press.

—— and BERG, A. A. (1938) Right-sided (regional) colitis. *J. Am. med. Ass.,* *110,* 32.

—— GARLOCK, J. H. and YARNIS, H. (1947) Right-sided (regional) colitis. *J. Am. med. Ass.,* *134,* 334.

—— and ROSENAK, B. D. (1936) A combined form of ileitis and colitis. *J. Am. med. Ass.,* *106,* 1.

—— YARNIS, H., CROHN, E. B., WALTER, R. I. and GABRILOVE, L. J. (1956) Ulcerative colitis and pregnancy. *Gastroenterology,* *30,* 391.

CULLINAN, E. R. and MacDOUGALL, I. P. (1957) The natural history of ulcerative colitis. *Lancet,* *1,* 487.

DALY, D. W. (1968) Outcome of surgery for ulcerative colitis. *Ann. R. Coll. Surg. Engl.,* *42,* 38.

—— and BROOKE, B. N. (1967) Ileostomy and excision of the large intestine for ulcerative colitis. *Lancet,* *2,* 62.

DAVIDSON, S. (1939) Infantilism in ulcerative colitis. *Archs intern. Med.,* *64,* 1187.

DAVIES, P. S., RHODES, J., HEATLEY, R. V. and OWEN, E. (1977) Metronidazole in the treatment of chronic proctitis: a controlled trial. *Gut,* *18,* 680.

DAWSON, I. M. P. and PRYSE-DAVIES, J. (1959) The development of carcinoma of the large intestine in ulcerative colitis. *Br. J. Surg.,* *47,* 113.

DAWSON, J. B. and HEATON, F. W. (1961) The determination of Mg in biological materials by atomic absorption spectrophotometry. *Biochem. J.,* *80,* 99.

DE DOMBAL, F. T. (1967) Serum proteins in ulcerative colitis: electrophoretic patterns in the inferior mesenteric artery and vein. *Gut,* *8,* 482.

—— (1968) Prognostic value of the serum proteins during severe attacks of ulcerative colitis. *Gut,* *9,* 144.

—— (1969) Prognostic value of estimating serum proteins in cases of ulcerative colitis in remission. *Gut,* *10,* 491.

—— BURCH, P. R. J. and WATKINSON, G. (1969) Aetiology of ulcerative colitis. I. Review of past and present hypotheses. *Gut,* *10,* 270.

—— GEFFEN, N., DARNBOROUGH, A., WATKINSON, G. and GOLIGHER, J. C. (1968) The radiological appearances of ulcerative colitis: an evaluation of their clinical significance. *Gut,* *9,* 157.

DE DOMBAL, F. T., GOLDIE, W., WATTS, J. McK. and GOLIGHER, J. C. (1966c) Hepatic histological changes in ulcerative colitis. *Scand. J. Gastroent., 1*, 120.

—— WATTS, J. M., WATKINSON, G. and GOLIGHER, J. C. (1965a) Intraperitoneal perforation of the colon in ulcerative colitis. *Proc. R. Soc. Med., 58*, 713.

—— —— —— —— (1965b) Ulcerative colitis and pregnancy. *Lancet, 2*, 599.

—— —— —— —— (1966a) Local complications of ulcerative colitis: stricture, pseudopolyposis and carcinoma of the colon and rectum. *Br. med. J., 1*, 1442.

—— —— —— —— (1966b) The incidence and management of anorectal abscess, fistula and fissure, occurring in patients with ulcerative colitis. *Dis. Colon Rect., 9*, 201.

DENNIS, C. (1945) Ileostomy and colectomy in chronic ulcerative colitis. *Surgery, St Louis, 18*, 435.

—— and KARLSON, K. E. (1952) Surgical measures as supplements to the management of idiopathic colitis; cancer, cirrhosis, and arthritis as frequent complications. *Surgery, St Louis, 32*, 892.

—— —— (1961) Cancer risk in ulcerative colitis: formidability per patient-year of late disease. *Surgery, St Louis, 50*, 568.

—— EDDY, F. D., FRYMAN, H. M., McCARTHY, A. M. and WESTOVER, D. (1948) The response to vagotomy in idiopathic ulcerative colitis and regional enteritis. *Ann. Surg., 128*, 479.

DEREN, J. J., PORUSH, J. G., LEWITT, M. F. and KHILNANI, M. T. (1962) Nephrolithiasis as a complication of ulcerative colitis and regional enteritis. *Ann. intern. Med., 56*, 843.

DEVINE, H. (1943) Method of colectomy for desperate cases of ulcerative colitis. *Surgery Gynec. Obstet., 76*, 136.

—— and DEVINE, J. (1948) *Surgery of the Colon and Rectum*. Bristol: Wright.

DEVINE, J. and WEBB, R. (1951) Resection of the rectal mucosa, colectomy and anal ileostomy with normal continence. *Surgery Gynec. Obstet., 92*, 437.

DICK, A. P., GRAYSON, M. J., CARPENTER, R. G. and PETRIE, A. (1964) Controlled trial of sulphasalazine in the treatment of ulcerative colitis. *Gut, 5*, 437.

DICKINSON, R. J., ASHTON, M. G. and AXON, A. R. (1979) Failure of intravenous hyperalimentation and bowel rest as primary therapy in acute colitis: results of a randomized controlled trial. *Gut*, in the press.

DISSANAYAKE, A. S. and TRUELOVE, S. C. (1973) A controlled therapeutic trial of long-term maintenance treatment of ulcerative colitis with sulphasalazine (Salazopyrin). *Gut, 14*, 923.

DONNELLAN, W. L. (1966) Early histological changes in ulcerative colitis. A light and electron microscope study. *Gastroenterology, 50*, 519.

DONOVAN, M. J. and O'HARA, E. T. (1960) Sexual function following surgery for ulcerative colitis. *New Engl. J. Med., 262*, 719.

DORDAL, E., GLASGOV, S. and KIRSNER, J. B. (1967) Hepatic lesions in chronic inflammatory bowel disease. I. Clinical correlations with liver biopsy diagnoses in 103 patients. *Gastroenterology, 52*, 239.

DOWNS, J. W. and COOPER, W. G. J. (1955) Surgical complications resulting from ACTH and cortisone medication. *Am. Surg., 21*, 141.

DRAGSTEDT, L. R., DACK, G. M. and KIRSNER, J. B. (1941) Chronic ulcerative colitis. A summary of evidence implicating bacterium necrophorum as an etiologic agent. *Ann. Surg., 114*, 653.

DROBNI, A. (1964) One-stage proctocolectomy with anal ileostomy. *Dis. Colon Rect., 7*, 416.

DRONFIELD, M. W. and LANGMAN, M. J. S. (1978) Comparative trial of sulphasalazine and oral sodium cromoglycate in the maintenance of remission in ulcerative colitis. *Gut, 19*, 1136.

DUKES, C. E. (1954) The surgical pathology of ulcerative colitis. *Ann. R. Coll. Surg. Engl., 14*, 389.

—— and LOCKHART-MUMMERY, H. E. (1957) Practical points in the pathology and surgical treatment of ulcerative colitis: a critical review. *Br. J. Surg., 45*, 25.

DUTHIE, H. L., WATTS, J. M., DE DOMBAL, F. T. and GOLIGHER, J. C. (1964) Serum electrolytes and colonic transfer of water and electrolytes in chronic ulcerative colitis. *Gastroenterology, 47*, 525.

EADE, M. N. (1970) Liver disease in ulcerative colitis. I. Analysis of operative liver biopsy in 138 consecutive patients having colectomy. *Ann. intern. Med., 72*, 475.

—— COOKE, W. T. and BROOKE, B. N. (1970) Liver disease in ulcerative colitis. II. The long-term effect of colectomy. *Ann. intern. Med., 70*, 489.

EDDY, F. D. (1951) Late results of vagotomy in the treatment of idiopathic ulcerative colitis and regional enteritis. *Surgery, St Louis, 29*, 11.

EDLING, N. P. G. and EKLÖF, O. (1960) A roentgenologic study of the course of ulcerative colitis. *Acta radiol., 54*, 397.

—— —— (1961) Radiological findings and prognosis in ulcerative colitis. *Acta chir. scand., 121*, 299.

—— —— (1963) The retrorectal soft-tissue space in ulcerative colitis. *Radiology, 80*, 949.

EDWARDS, F. C. and TRUELOVE, S. C. (1963) The course and prognosis of ulcerative colitis. Part I. Short-term prognosis. Part II. Long-term prognosis. *Gut, 4*, 299.

—— —— (1964) The course and prognosis of ulcerative colitis. Part III. Complications. Part IV. Carcinoma of the colon. *Gut, 5*, 1.

EHRENPREIS, T. and ERICSSON, N. O. (1964) Surgical treatment of ulcerative colitis in childhood. *Surg. Clins N. Am., 44*, 1521.

EIN, S. H., LYNCH, M. J. and STEPHENS, C. A. (1970) Ulcerative colitis in children under one year: a twenty-year review. *J. pediat. Surg., 6*, 264.

ELLIS, H. and COLL, I. (1968) Antiperistaltic segment for profuse ileostomy diarrhoea. *Br. med. J., 1*, 290.

ERIKSON, U., FAGERBERG, S., KRAUSE, U. and OLDING, L. (1971) Angiographic studies in Crohn's disease and ulcerative colitis. *Am. J. Roentg., 110*, 385.

FAGERBERG, S. (1971) In discussion of paper by Brahme (1971).

FAILES, D. (1976) Kock continent ileostomy: a preliminary report. *Aust. N.Z. J. Surg., 46*, 25.

FALLIS, L. S. and BARRON, J. (1953) Modified technique for total colectomy in ulcerative colitis. *Archs Surg., Chicago, 67*, 363.

—— —— (1960) Ileorectal anastomosis in ulcerative colitis. *Archs Surg., Chicago, 81*, 444.

FELDMAN, F., CANTOR, D., SOLL, S. and BACHRACH, W. (1967) Psychiatric study of a consecutive series of 34 patients with ulcerative colitis. *Br. med. J., 3*, 14.

FELSEN, J. (1945) *Bacillary Dysentery, Colitis and Enteritis*. Philadelphia and London: Saunders.

—— and WOLARSKY, W. (1948) Chronic ulcerative colitis and pregnancy. *Am. J. Obstet. Gynec., 56,* 751.

FENNESSY, J. J., SPARBERG, M. B. and KIRSNER, J. B. (1968) Radiological findings in carcinoma of the colon complicating chronic ulcerative colitis. *Gut, 9,* 388.

FERNANDEZ-HERLIHY, L. (1959) The articular manifestations of chronic ulcerative colitis. An analysis of 555 cases. *New Engl. J. Med., 261,* 259.

FERRARI, B. T. and FONKALSRUD, E. W. (1978) Endorectal ileal pull-through operation with ileal reservoir after total colectomy. *Ann. Surg., 136,* 113.

FINEGOLD, S. M., GUTTER, U. L., BOYLE, J. D. and SHIMADA, K. (1970) The normal flora of ileostomy and colostomy effluents. *J. infect. Dis., 122,* 376.

FLATMARK, A. L., FRETHEIM, B. and GJONE, E. (1969) Early colectomy in severe ulcerative colitis. *Scand. J. Gastroent., 4,* 505.

—— —— —— (1975) Early colectomy in severe ulcerative colitis. *Scand. J. Gastroent., 10,* 427.

—— NORDÖY, A. and GJONE, E. (1971) Radical surgery for ulcerative colitis during pregnancy. *Scand. J. Gastroent., 6,* 45.

FONKALSRUD, E. W. and AMENT, M. E. (1978) Endorectal mucosal resection without proctectomy as an adjunct to abdominoperineal resection for nonmalignant conditions: clinical experience with five patients. *Ann. Surg., 188,* 245.

FORD, D. K. and VALLIS, D. G. (1959) The clinical course of arthritis associated with ulcerative colitis and regional ileitis. *Arthritis Rheum., 2,* 526.

FORD, H. and KIRSNER, J. B. (1964) 'Auer colitis' in rabbits induced by intrarectal antigen. *Proc. Soc. exp. Biol. Med., 116,* 745.

FRASER, C. G., PREUSS, F. S. and BIGFORD, W. D. (1952) Adrenal atrophy and irreversible shock associated with cortisone therapy. *J. Am. med. Ass., 149,* 1542.

FREDERICK, P. L., SIZER, J. S. and OSBORNE, M. P. (1965) Relation of massive bowel resection to gastric secretion. *New Engl. J. Med., 272,* 509.

FULLERTON, D. T., KOLLAR, E. J. and CALDWELL, A. B. (1962) A clinical study of ulcerative colitis. *J. Am. med. Ass., 181,* 463.

GABRIEL, W. B. (1940) Discussion on the surgical treatment of idiopathic ulcerative colitis and its sequelae. *Proc. R. Soc. Med., 33,* 643.

—— (1952) The surgical treatment of chronic ulcerative colitis. *Br. med. J., 1,* 881.

GALLAGHER, N. D., GOULSTON, S. J. M., WYNDHAM, N. and MORROW, W. (1962) The management of fulminant ulcerative colitis. *Gut, 3,* 306.

GALLART-MONÉS, X. (1956) Anatomia pathologica de la colitis ulcerativa grave. *Gastroenterologia, 86,* 632.

GARDNER, C. and MILLER, G. G. (1951) Total colectomy for ulcerative colitis. *Archs Surg., Chicago, 63,* 370.

GEFFEN, N., DARNBOROUGH, A., DE DOMBAL, F. T., WATKINSON, G. and GOLIGHER, J. C. (1968) The radiological signs of ulcerative colitis: an assessment of their reliability by means of observer variation studies. *Gut, 9,* 150.

GELERNT, I. M., BAUER, J. J. and KREEL, I. (1977) The reservoir ileostomy: early experience with 54 patients. *Ann. Surg., 185,* 179.

GJONE, E. and MYREN, J. (1964) Ulcerative colitis in Norway. *Nord. Med., 71,* 143.

GLECKLER, W. J. and BROWN, C. H. (1950) Carcinoma of the colon complicating chronic ulcerative colitis. *Gastroenterology, 14,* 455.

GOLDGRABER, M. B., HUMPHREYS, E. M., KIRSNER, J. B. and PALMER, W. L. (1958a) Carcinoma and ulcerative colitis; a clinical-pathologic study. I. Cancer deaths. *Gastoenterology, 34,* 809.

—— —— —— —— (1958b) Carcinoma and ulcerative colitis, a clinical-pathologic study. II. Statistical analysis. *Gastroenterology, 34,* 840.

—— KIRSNER, J. B. and PALMER, W. L. (1957) The role of ACTH and adrenal steroids in perforation of the colon in ulcerative colitis. *Gastroenterology, 33,* 434.

GOLIGHER, J. C. (1951) The functional results after sphincter-saving resections of the rectum. *Ann. R. Coll. Surg., Engl., 8,* 421.

—— (1954) Primary excisional surgery in the treatment of ulcerative colitis. *Ann. R. Coll. Surg. Engl., 15,* 316.

—— (1958) Extraperitoneal colostomy or ileostomy. *Br. J. Surg., 46,* 98.

—— (1959) The surgery of ulcerative colitis. *Scot. med. J., 4,* 1.

—— (1961a) Non-malignant ulcerative diseases of the large intestine. *Trans. med. Soc. Lond., 78,* 17.

—— (1961b) Surgical treatment of ulcerative colitis. *Br. med. J., 1,* 151.

—— (1963) Ileostomy reconstruction. *Br. J. Surg., 50,* 259.

—— (1965) Treatment of chronic ulcerative colitis. *Current Problems in Surgery*, August. Chicago: Year Book Medical Publishers.

—— (1978) The surgery of colitis—past, present and future. *Ann. R. Coll. Surg. Engl., 60,* 258.

—— DE DOMBAL, F. T., WATTS, J. McK. and WATKINSON, G. (1968) *Ulcerative Colitis*. London: Baillière, Tindall & Cassell.

—— HOFFMAN, D. C. and DE DOMBAL, F. T. (1970) Surgical treatment of severe attacks of ulcerative colitis, with special reference to the advantages of early operation. *Br. med. J., 4,* 703.

—— and LINTOTT, D. J. (1975) Experience with 26 reservoir ileostomies. *Br. J. Surg., 62,* 893.

GONZALEZ-LICEA, A. (1966) Ulcerative colitis: electron microscopic observations on rectal biopsy. *Dis. Colon Rect., 9,* 417.

—— and YARDLEY, J. H. (1966) Nature of the tissue reactions in ulcerative colitis. Light and electron microscopic findings. *Gastroenterology, 51,* 825.

GOODE, A., FEGGETTER, J. G. W., HAWKINS, T. and JOHNSON, I. D. A. (1976) Use of an elemental diet for long-term nutritional support in Crohn's disease. *Lancet, 1,* 122.

GORBACH, S. L., NAHAS, L. and WEINSTEIN, L. (1967) Studies of intestinal microflora, IV. The microflora of ileostomy effluent: a unique microbial ecology. *Gastroenterology, 53,* 874.

GOSSAGE, A. M. and PRICE, F. W. (1909) Statistics of ulcerative colitis from the London hospitals. *Proc. R. Soc. Med., 2,* 151.

GRABER, A. L., NEY, R. L., NICHOLSON, W. E., ISLAND, D. P. and LIDDLE, G. W. (1956) Natural history of pituitary-adrenal recovery following long-term suppression with corticosteroids. *J. clin. Endocr., 25,* 11.

GRACE, W. J., WOLF, S. and WOLFF, H. G. (1951) *The Human Colon*. London: Heinemann.

GRAHAM, N. G., DE DOMBAL, F. T. and GOLIGHER, J. C. (1971) Reliability of physical signs in patients with severe attacks of ulcerative colitis. *Br. med. J., 2,* 746.

Gray, I., Harten, M. and Walzer, M. (1940) Studies in mucous membrane hypersensitiveness. IV. The allergic reaction in the passively sensitized mucous membranes of the ileum and colon in humans. *Ann. intern. Med., 13*, 2050.

Griffen, W. O., Lillehei, R. C. and Wangensteen, O. H. (1963) Ileoproctostomy in ulcerative colitis: long-term follow-up extending in early cases to more than 20 years. *Surgery, St Louis, 53*, 705.

Groen, J. and van der Valk, J. M. (1956) Psychosomatic aspects of ulcerative colitis. *Gastroenterologia, 86*, 591.

Grüner, O. P. N., Flatmark, A., Naas, R., Fretheim, B. and Gjone, E. (1975) Ileorectal anastomosis in ulcerative colitis. *Scand. J. Gastroent., 10*, 641.

—— Naas, R., Flatmark, A., Fretheim, B. and Gjone, E. (1977) Proctectomy in ulcerative colitis. *Scand. J. Gastroent., 12*, 65.

Halvorsen, J. F. and Heimann, P. (1975) The continent ileostomy of Kock (ileal intra-abdominal reservoir). *Br. J. Surg., 62*, 52.

—— —— Hoel, R. and Nygaard, K. (1978) The continent reservoir ileostomy: review of a collective series of 36 patients from three surgical departments. *Surgery, St Louis, 83*, 252.

Hardy, T. L., Brooke, B. N. and Hawkins, C. F. (1949) Ileostomy and ulcerative colitis. *Lancet, 2*, 5.

Harnagel, E. E. and Kramer, W. G. (1955) Severe adreno-cortical insufficiency following joint manipulation; report of patient receiving cortisone orally. *J. Am. med. Ass., 158*, 1518.

Hawley, P. R. (1975) Personal communication.

Hayes, M. A. and Kushlan, S. D. (1956) Influence of hormonal therapy for ulcerative colitis upon course of surgical treatment. *Gastroenterology, 30*, 75.

Heatley, R. V., Calcraft, B. J., Rhodes, J., Owen, E. and Evans, B. K. (1975) Disodium cromoglycate in the treatment of chronic proctitis. *Gut, 16*, 559.

Heaton, F. W. (1964) Magnesium metabolism in surgical patient. *Clinica chim. Acta, 9*, 327.

—— Clark, C. G. and Goligher, J. C. (1967) Magnesium deficiency complicating intestinal surgery. *Br. J. Surg., 54*, 41.

—— and Fourman, P. (1965) Magnesium deficiency and hypocalcaemia in intestinal malabsorption. *Lancet, 2*, 50.

Helmholz, H. F. (1923) Chronic ulcerative colitis in childhood. *Am. J. Dis. Child., 26*, 418.

Hightower, N. C., Jr., Broders, A. C., Jr., Haines, R. D., McKerney, J. F. and Sommer, A. W. (1958) Chronic ulcerative colitis: 11 complications. *Am. J. dig. Dis., 3*, 861.

Hill, G. L., Blackett, R. K., Pickford, I. R. and Bradley, J. A. (1977) A survey of protein nutrition in patients with inflammatory bowel disease—a rational basis for nutritional therapy. *Br. J. Surg., 64*, 894.

—— Mair, W. S. J. and Goligher, J. C. (1975a) Cause and management of high volume output salt-depleting ileostomy. *Br. J. Surg., 62*, 720.

—— —— —— (1975b) Gallstones after ileostomy and ileal resection. *Gut, 16*, 932.

Holdsworth, C. D., Hall, E. W., Dawson, A. M. and Sherlock, S. (1965) Ulcerative colitis in chronic liver disease. *Q. Jl Med., 34*, 211.

Hudson, C. N. (1972) Ileostomy in pregnancy. *Proc. R. Soc. Med., 65*, 281.

Hughes, E. S. R. (1965) The treatment of ulcerative colitis. *Ann. R. Coll. Surg., Engl., 37*, 191.

—— Russell, I. S., Cuthbertson, A. M. and Carden, A. B. (1963) Ileostomy for ulcerative colitis. *Aust. N.Z.J. Surg., 32*, 215.

Hultén, L., Kewenter, J. and Kock, N. G. (1971) the long-term results of partial resection of the large bowel for intestinal carcinomas complicating ulcerative colitis. *Scand. J. Gastroent., 6*, 601.

Hurst, A. F. (1935) Prognosis of ulcerative colitis. *Lancet, 11*, 1194.

—— (1940) Discussion on the surgical treatment of idiopathic ulcerative colitis and its sequelae. *Proc. R. Soc. Med., 33*, 645.

—— and Knott, F. A. (1936) British dysenteric infections. *Lancet, 2*, 1197.

Jackman, R. A. (1954) Management of anorectal complications due to chronic ulcerative colitis. *Archs intern. Med., 94*, 420.

Jackman, R. J., Bargen, J. A. and Helmholz, H. F. (1940) Life histories of 95 children with chronic ulcerative colitis. *Am. J. Dis. Child., 59*, 459.

Jagelman, D. G., Lewis, C. B. and Rowe-Jones, D. C. (1969) Ileorectal anastomosis: appreciation by patients. *Br. med. J., 1*, 756.

Jagenburg, R., Dotevall, G., Kewenter, J., Kock, N. G. and Philipson, B. (1971) Absorption studies in patients with intra-abdominal ileostomy reservoirs and in patients with conventional ileostomies. *Gut, 12*, 437.

—— Kock, N. G. and Philipson, B. (1975) Vitamin B12 absorption in patients with continent ileostomy. *Scand. J. Gastroent., 10*, 141.

Jalan, K. N., Prescott, R. J., Sircus, W., Card, W. I., McManus, J. P. A., Falconer, C. W. A., Small, W. P., Smith, A. N. and Bruce, J. (1970a) An experience of ulcerative colitis. II. Short-term outcome. *Gastroenterology, 59*, 589.

—— —— —— —— —— —— —— —— —— (1970b) An experience of ulcerative colitis. III. Long-term outcome. *Gastroenterology, 59*, 598.

—— Smith, A. N., Sircus, W., McManus, J. P. A., Small, W. P. and Falconer, C. W. A. (1970c) The influence of corticosteroids on the results of surgical treatment for ulcerative colitis. *New Engl. J. Med., 282*, 588.

—— Sircus, W., Walker, R. J., McManus, J. P. A., Prescott, R. J. and Card, W. I. (1969a) Pseudopolyposis in ulcerative colitis. *Lancet, 3*, 555.

—— Smith, A. N., Ruckley, C. V., Falconer, C. W. A., Small, W. P. and Prescott, R. J. (1969b) Perineal wound healing in ulcerative colitis. *Br. J. Surg., 56*, 749.

Javett, S. L. and Brooke, B. N. (1971) Reversed ileal segment for ileostomy diarrhoea. *Lancet, 1*, 291.

Jayson, M. I. V. and Boucher, I. A. D. (1968) Ulcerative colitis in patients with ankylosing spondylitis. *Proc. R. Soc. Med., 61*, 340.

Jenkinson, J. A. and Dawson, I. M. P. (1971) The value of electron microscope studies in diagnosing malignant change in ulcerative colitis. *Gut, 12*, 110.

Jewell, D. P. and Truelove, S. C. (1974) Azathioprine in ulcerative colitis: report on a controlled trial. *Lancet, 4*, 627.

Johnson, M. L. and Wilson, H. T. H. (1969) Skin lesions in ulcerative colitis. *Gut, 10*, 255.

Jones, F. A., Lennard-Jones, J. E., Hinton, J. M. and Reeves, W. G. (1966) Dangers of immuno-suppressive drugs in ulcerative colitis. *Br. med. J., 1*, 1418.

Jones, G. W., Baggenstoss, A. M. and Bargen, J. A. (1951) Hepatic lesions and dysfunction associated with chronic ulcerative colitis. *Am. J. med. Sci., 221,* 279.

Jones, J. H. and Chapman, M. (1969) Definition of megacolon in colitis. *Gut, 10,* 562.

Jones, P. F., Munro, A. and Ewen, W. B. (1977) Colectomy and ileorectal anastomosis for colitis: report on a personal series, with a critical review. *Br. J. Surg., 64,* 615.

Kallett, H. I. (1952) Influence of pregnancy on chronic ulcerative colitis. *Am. J. Surg., 84,* 574.

Kaplan, H. P., Portnoy, B., Binder, H. J., Amatruda, T. and Spiro, H. (1975) A controlled evaluation of intravenous adrenocorticotrophic hormone and hydrocortisone in the treatment of acute colitis. *Gastroenterology, 69,* 91.

Keetley, C. B. (1895) Quoted by Corbett, R. S. (1945).

Kellner, H., Hersch, R. A. and Barker, W. (1963) Effect of adrenocortical steroids on the postoperative course of patients with ulcerative colitis, with discussion of spontaneous rupture of the small bowel. *Gastroenterology, 45,* 27.

Kellock, T. D. (1957) Acute segmental ulcerative colitis. *Lancet, 2,* 660.

Kewenter, J., Ahlman, H. and Hultén, L. (1978) Cancer risk in extensive ulcerative colitis. *Ann. Surg., 188,* 824.

Khubchandani, I. T., Trimpi, H. D., Sheets, J. A., Stasik, J. J. and Kleckner, F. S. (1978) Ileorectal anastomosis for ulcerative colitis and Crohn's disease. *Am. J. Surg., 135,* 751.

Kiefer, E. D. (1960) ACTH and the corticosteroid hormones in the management of chronic ulcerative colitis. *Med. Clins N. Am., 44,* 567.

King, R. C., Linder, A. E. and Pollard, H. M. (1959) Chronic ulcerative colitis in childhood. *Archs Dis. Child., 34,* 257.

Kinsey, I., Hornes, N., Anthonisen, P. and Riis, P. (1964) he radiological diagnosis of non-specific haemorrhagic proctocolitis (haemorrhagic proctitis and ulcerative colitis). *Acta med. scand., 176,* 181.

Kirsner, J. B. and Elchlepp, J. (1957) The production of an experimental ulcerative colitis in rabbits. *Trans. Ass. Am. Physns, 70,* 102.

—— and Goldgraber, M. B. (1960) Hypersensitivity, autoimmunity and the digestive tract. *Gastroenterology, 38,* 536.

—— Palmer, W. L. and Klotz, A. P. (1951) Reversibility in ulcerative colitis—clinical and roentgenologic observations. *Radiology, 57,* 1.

—— and Spencer, J. A. (1963) Family occurrence of ulcerative colitis, regional enteritis and ileocolitis. *Ann. intern. Med., 59,* 133.

Kleckner, M. S., Jr., Bargen, J. A. and Banner, E. A. (1951) Chronic ulcerative colitis and pregnancy. *Am. J. Obstet. Gynec., 62,* 1234.

—— Stauffer, M. H., Bargen, J. A. and Dockerty, M. B. (1952) Hepatic lesions in a living patient demonstrated by needle biopsy. *Gastroenterology, 22,* 13.

Klein, S. H., Edelman, S., Kirschner, P. A., Lyons, A. S. and Baronofsky, I. D. (1960) Emergency caecostomy in ulcerative colitis with acute toxic dilatation. *Surgery, St Louis, 47,* 399.

Knill-Jones, R. P., Morson, B. C. and Williams, R. (1970) Prestomal ileitis: clinical and pathological findings in five cases. *Q. Jl Med., 154,* 287.

Knutsson, H. and Lunderqvist, A. (1968) Vascular changes in Crohn's disease. *Am. J. Roentgen., 103,* 380.

Kock, N. G. (1969) Intra-abdominal reservoir in patients with permanent ileostomy. *Archs Surg., Chicago, 99,* 223.

—— (1971a) Ileostomy without external appliances: a survey of 25 patients provided with intra-abdominal intestinal reservoir. *Ann. Surg., 173,* 545.

—— (1971b) Personal communication.

—— (1973) Continent ileostomy. In *Progress in Surgery*, Vol. 12, ed. Allgöwer, M., Bergentz, S. E., and Calne, R. Y. p. 180. Basle: Karger.

—— (1976a) Present status of the continent ileostomy: surgical revision of the malfunctioning ileostomy. *Dis. Colon Rectum, 19,* 200.

—— (1976b) Personal communication.

—— Darle, N., Hultén, L., Kewenter, J., Myrvold, H. E. and Philipson, B. (1979) Ileostomy. *Current Prob. Surg., 14,* 8.

—— and Myrvold, H. E. (1979) Progress report on the continent ileostomy. *Wld J. Surg.,* in the press.

Korelitz, B. I. and Lindner, A. E. (1964) The influence of corticotrophin and adrenal steroids on the course of ulcerative colitis: a comparison with the presteroid era. *Gastroenterology, 46,* 671.

Kraft, S. C., Bregman, E. and Kirsner, J. B. (1962) Criteria for evaluating autoimmune phenomena in ulcerative colitis. *Gastroenterology, 43,* 330.

—— Fitch, F. W. and Kirsner, J. B. (1963) Histologic and immunohistochemical features of the Auer 'colitis' in rabbits. *Am. J. Path., 43,* 913.

Krawitt, E. L. (1959) Ulcerative colitis and pregnancy. *Obstet. Gynec., N.Y., 14,* 354.

Lahey, F. H. (1941) Ulcerative colitis. *N.Y. St J. Med., 41,* 475.

Landor, J. H., Azcancia, E. Y. and Fulkerson, C. C. (1966) Effect of colectomy on gastric secretion in dogs. *Am. J. Surg., 113,* 32.

—— and Baker, W. K. (1964) Gastric hypersecretion produced by massive small bowel resection in dogs. *J. Surg., Res., 4,* 518.

Lennard-Jones, J. E., Cooper, G. W., Newell, A. C., Wilson, C. W. E. and Jones, F. Avery (1962) Observations on idiopathic proctitis. *Gut, 3,* 201.

—— Longmore, A. J., Newell, A. C., Wilson, C. W. E. and Jones, F. Avery (1960) An assessment of prednisone, salazopyrin and topical hydrocortisone hemisuccinate used as out-patient treatment for ulcerative colitis. *Gut, 1,* 217.

—— Misiewicz, J. J., Connell, A. M., Baron, J. H. and Jones, F. Avery (1965) Prednisone as maintenance treatment for ulcerative colitis in remission. *Lancet, 1,* 188.

—— Morson, B. C., Ritchie, J. K., Shove, D. C. and Williams, C. B. (1977) Cancer in colitis: assessment of the individual risks by clinical and histological criteria. *Gastroenterology, 73,* 1280.

—— and Vivian, A. B. (1960) Fulminating ulcerative colitis: recent experience in management. *Br. med. J., 2,* 96.

Lenneberg, E. and Rowbotham, J. L. (1970) *The Ileostomy Patient. A Descriptive Study of 1425 Persons.* Springfield, Ill.: Charles C. Thomas.

—— and Sohn, N. (1972) Modern concepts in management of patients with intestinal and urinary stomas. *Clin. Obstet. Gynec., 15,* 542.

LEVY, R. W., WILKINS, H., HERRMANN, J. D., LISLE, A. C., Jr. and RIX, A. (1956) Experiences with prefrontal lobotomy for intractable ulcerative colitis. *J. Am. med. Ass., 160,* 1277.

LILIENTHAL, H. (1903) Extirpation of the entire colon, the upper portion of the sigmoid flexure and four inches of the ileum for hyperplastic colitis. *Ann. Surg., 37,* 616.

LINDNER, A. E., KING, R. C. and BOLT, R. J. (1960) Chronic ulcerative colitis. A clinical appraisal and follow-up study. *Gastroenterology, 39,* 153.

LOCKHART-MUMMERY, H. E. (1956) Surgical Pathology of Ulcerative Colitis. M.D. thesis, University of Cambridge.

—— and MORSON, B. C. (1964) Crohn's disease of large intestine. *Gut, 5,* 493.

LOCKHART-MUMMERY, J. P. (1934) *Diseases of the Rectum and Colon,* 2nd ed. London: Baillière, Tindall and Cox.

LUMB, G., PROTHERO, R. H. B. and RAMSAY, G. S. (1955) Ulcerative colitis with dilatation of the colon. *Br. J. Surg., 43,* 182.

LUNDERQVIST, A. (1967) Arteriography in ulcerative colitis. *Am. J. Roentgen., 99,* 18.

LUNDY, J. S. (1953) Cortisone problems involving anaesthesia. *Anesthesiology, 14,* 376.

LYONS, A. S. (1952) Ileostomy Club. *J. Am. med. Ass., 150,* 812.

—— and GARLOCK, J. H. (1951) The relationship of chronic ulcerative colitis to carcinoma. *Gastroenterology, 18,* 170.

—— —— (1954) The complications of ileostomy. *Surgery, St Louis, 36,* 784.

LYTLE, J. A. and PARKS, A. G. (1977) Intersphincteric excision of the rectum. *Br. J. Surg., 64,* 413.

MCBRIDE, J. A., KING, M. J., BAIKIE, A. G., CREAN, G. P. and SIRCUS, W. (1963) Ankylosing spondylitis and chronic inflammatory diseases of the intestines. *Br. med. J., 2,* 483.

MCCONNELL, F. C., HANELIN, J. and ROBBINS, L. L. (1958) Plain film diagnosis of fulminating ulcerative colitis. *Radiology, 71,* 674.

MCCREADY, F. J., BARGEN, J. A., DOCKERTY, M. B. and WAUGH, J. M. (1949) Involvement of the ileum in chronic ulcerative colitis. *New Engl. J. Med., 240,* 119.

MACDERMOTT, E. N. (1964) Anal ileostomy with sphincter preservation. *Dis. Colon Rect., 7,* 386.

MACDOUGALL, I. P. M. (1954) Ulcerative colitis and carcinoma of the large intestine. *Br. med. J., 1,* 852.

—— (1956) Ulcerative colitis and pregnancy. *Lancet, 2,* 641.

—— (1964) The cancer risk in ulcerative colitis. *Lancet, 2,* 655.

MCEWEN, C., LINGG, C. and KIRSNER, J. B. (1962) Arthritis accompanying ulcerative colitis. *Am. J. Med., 33,* 923.

MACHELLA, T. A. (1952) Problems in ulcerative colitis. *Am. J. Med., 13,* 760.

MCINERNEY, G. T., SAUER, W. G., BAGGENSTOSS, A. H. and HODGSON, J. R. (1962) Fulminating ulcerative colitis with marked colonic dilatation: a clinicopathologic study. *Gastroenterology, 42,* 244.

MACKAY, I. R. and WOOD, I. J. (1964) Auto-immunity as a cause of disease. *Med. Ann., 24.*

MCKITTRICK, L. S. and MILLER, R. H. (1935) Idiopathic ulcerative colitis; review of 149 cases with particular reference to the value of and indications for surgical treatment. *Ann. Surg., 102,* 656.

MADDIX, B. L. (1962) Ulcerative colitis and pregnancy. *Minn. Med., 45,* 1097.

MADELL, S. H. and GOLDEN, R. (1955) The ileum following colectomy. *Radiology, 65,* 539.

MADIGAN, M. R. (1976) The continent ileostomy and isolated ileal bladder. *Ann. R. Coll. Surg. Engl., 58,* 62.

MADISON, M. S. and BARGEN, J. A. (1951) Fulminating chronic ulcerative colitis with unusual segmental dilatation of the colon: report of a case. *Proc. Staff Meet. Mayo Clin., 26,* 21.

MAINGOT, R. (1942) Terminal ileostomy in ulcerative colitis. *Lancet, 2,* 121.

MANI, V., GREEN, F. H. Y., LLOYD, G., FOX, H. and TURNBERG, L. A. (1976) Treatment of ulcerative colitis with oral disodium cromoglycate: a double-blind controlled study. *Lancet, 1,* 439.

MALLET, S. J., LENNARD-JONES, J. E., BINGLEY, J. and GILON, E. (1978) Colitis. *Lancet, 3,* 619.

MANNING, J. H., WARREN, R. and ADI, A. S. (1955) Segmental colitis; results of surgery. *New Engl. J. Med., 252,* 850.

MARATKA, Z. and NEDBAL, J. (1964) Urolithiasis as a complication of the surgical treatment of ulcerative colitis. *Gut, 5,* 214.

MARGOLES, J. S. and WENGER, J. (1961) Stomal ulceration associated with pyoderma gangrenosum and chronic ulcerative colitis: report of two cases. *Gastroenterology, 41,* 594.

MARSHAK, R. H., KORELITZ, B. I., KLEIN, S. H., WOLF, B. D. and JANOWITZ, H. D. (1960) Toxic dilatation of the colon in the course of ulcerative colitis. *Gastroenterology, 38,* 165.

MARTIN, L. W., LECOULTRE, C. and SCHUBERT, W. K. (1977) Total colectomy and mucosal proctectomy with preservation of continence in ulcerative colitis. *Ann. Surg., 186,* 477.

MATTS, S. G. F. (1960) Local treatment of ulcerative colitis with prednisolone-21-phosphate enemata. *Lancet, 1,* 517.

—— (1961) The value of rectal biopsy in the diagnosis of ulcerative colitis. *Q. Jl Med., 30,* 393.

MAUR, M., TORANZO, J. C. and FRAISE, A. M. (1964) Sistemas sanguineos ABO, Rh en proctologia colonica. *Semana méd.,B. Aires, 124,* 634.

MAY, R. E. (1966) Sexual function following rectal excision for ulcerative colitis. *Br. J. Surg., 53,* 29.

MELROSE, A. G. (1955) The geographical incidence of chronic ulcerative colitis in Britain. *Gastroenterology, 29,* 1055.

—— (1956) Observations on the European incidence of chronic ulcerative colitis. *Gastroenterologia, 86,* 626.

MEYER, K., GELLHORN, A., PRUDDEN, J. F., LEHMAN, W. L. and STEINBERG, A. (1948) Lysozyme activity in ulcerative alimentary disease. II. Lysozyme activity in chronic ulcerative colitis. *Am. J. Med., 5,* 496.

MICHENER, W. M., BROWN, C. H. and TURNBULL, R. B., Jr. (1964) Ulcerative colitis in children. *Am. J. Dis. Child., 108,* 230.

—— GAGE, R. P., SAUER, W. G. and STICKLER, G. B. (1961) The prognosis of chronic ulcerative colitis in children. *New Engl. J. Med., 265,* 1075.

MILLER, C. G., GARDNER, C. McG. and RIPSTEIN, C. B. (1949) Primary resection of the colon in ulcerative colitis. *J. Can. med. Ass., 60,* 584.

MISIEWICZ, J. J., LENNARD-JONES, J. E., CONNELL, A. M., BARON, J. H. and JONES, F. AVERY. (1965) Controlled trial of sulphasalazine in maintenance therapy for ulcerative colitis. *Lancet, 1,* 185.

MISTILIS,, S. P., SKYRING, A. P. and GOULSTON, S. J. M. (1965) Effect of long-term tetracycline therapy, steroid therapy and colectomy on pericholangitis associated with ulcerative colitis. *Ann. intern. Med., 63*, 17.

MIXTER, C. G. (1935) Regional ileitis. *Ann. Surg., 102*, 674.

MOERTEL, C. G. and BARGEN, J. A. (1959) A critical analysis of the use of salicylazosulfapyridine in chronic ulcerative colitis. *Ann. intern. Med., 51*, 879.

MONK, M., MENDELOLI, A. T., SIEGEL, C. R. and LILIENFIELD, A. (1967) An epidemiologic study of ulcerative colitis and regional enteritis amongst adults in Baltimore. I. *Gastroenterology, 53*, 198.

MONROE, C. W. and OLWIN, J. H. (1949) Use of an abdominal flap graft in construction of a permanent ileostomy. *Archs Surg., Chicago, 59*, 565.

MORSON, B. C. (1968) In *Ulcerative Colitis*, by J. C. Goligher, F. T. de Dombal, J. McK. Watts, and G. Watkinson. London: Baillière, Tindall and Cassell.

—— and DAWSON, I. M. P. (1972) *Gastro-intestinal Pathology*. Oxford: Blackwell Scientific.

—— and PANG, L. S. C. (1967) Rectal biopsy as an aid to cancer control in ulcerative colitis. *Gut, 8*, 423.

MOSS, G. S. and KEDDIE, N. (1965) Fate of rectal stump in ulcerative colitis. *Archs Surg., Chicago, 91*, 967.

MUIR, E. G. (1959) The results of ileo-rectal anastomosis. Anglo-American Conference on Proctology. *Proc. R. Soc. Med.*, Suppl. 25.

MURRAY, C. D. (1930) Psychogenic factors in the etiology of ulcerative colitis. *Am. J. med. Sci., 180*, 239.

NEFZGER, M. D. and ACHESON, E. D. (1963) Ulcerative colitis in the United States Army in 1944. Follow-up with particular reference to mortality in cases and controls. *Gut, 4*, 183.

NEUMAN, H. W., BARGEN, J. A. and JUDD, E. S., Jr. (1954) Clinical study of 201 cases of regional (segmental) colitis. *Surgery Gynec. Obstet., 99*, 563.

NUGUID, T. P., BACON, H. E. and BOUTWELL, J. (1963) The ileostomy: its physical characteristics and clinical behaviour. *Dis. Colon Rect., 6*, 293.

OGILVIE, W. H. (1940) Discussion on the surgical treatment of idiopathic ulcerative colitis and its sequelae. *Proc. R. Soc. Med., 33*, 640.

PALMER, W. L., KIRSNER, J. B., GOLDGRABER, M. B. and FUENTES, S. S. (1964) Disease of the liver in chronic ulcerative colitis. *Am. J. Med., 36*, 856.

PALMU, A. and SIVULA, A. (1978) Kock's continent ileostomy—results of 51 operations and experiences with correction of nipple-valve insufficiency. *Br. J. Surg., 65*, 645.

PARKER, R. G. F. and KENDALL, E. J. C. (1954) The liver in ulcerative colitis. *Brit. med. J., 2*, 1030.

PARKS, A. G. (1965) Prognosis of patients with an ileostomy. *Proc. R. Soc. Med., 58*, 793.

—— (1975) Personal communication.

—— and NICHOLLS, R. J. (1978) Proctocolectomy for ulcerative colitis without ileostomy. *Br. med. J., 2*, 85.

PATEY, D. H. (1951) Primary epithelial apposition in colostomy. *Proc. R. Soc. Med., 44*, 423.

PATTERSON, M. and EYTINGE, E. J. (1952) Chronic ulcerative colitis and pregnancy. *New Engl. J. Med., 246*, 691.

—— CASTIGLIONI, L. and SAMPSON, L. (1971) Chronic ulcerative colitis beginning in children and teenagers: a review of 43 patients. *Am. J. dig. Dis., 16*, 289.

PAULLEY, J. W. (1956) The emotional factors in ulcerative colitis. *Gastroenterologia, 86*, 709.

—— (1971) Medical management of ulcerative colitis. *Proc. R. Soc. Med., 64*, 97.

PEMBERTON, J. DE J. and BROWN, P. W. (1937) Regional ileitis. *Ann. Surg., 105*, 855.

PENN, I. and STARZL, T. E. (1970) Incidence of malignant disease in patients on azathioprine for transplants. *Int. J. clin. Pharmac., 3*, 49.

PESKIN, G. W. and DAVIS, A. V. O. (1960) Acute fulminating ulcerative colitis with colonic distension. *Surgery Gynec. Obstet., 110*, 269.

PHILIPSON, B., BRANDBERG, Å. and JAGENBURG, R. (1975) Mucosal morphology, bacteriology and absorption in intra-abdominal ileostomy reservoir. *Scand. J. Gastroent., 10*, 145.

POLCAK, J. and VOKURKA, V. (1960) Auto-immune reactions in the course of ulcerative colitis. *Am. J. dig. Dis., 5*, 395.

POLLARD, H. M. and BLOCK, M. (1948) Association of hepatic insufficiency with chronic ulcerative colitis. *Archs intern. Med., 82*, 159.

POPERT, A. J. and DAVIS, P. S. (1958) Surgery during long-term treatment with adrenocortical hormones. *Lancet, 1*, 21.

POWELL-TUCK, J., BUSKELL, N. A. and LENNARD-JONES, J. E. (1977b) A controlled comparison of corticotrophin and hydrocortisone in the treatment of severe proctocolitis. *Scand. J. Gastroent., 12*, 971.

—— RITCHIE, JEAN K. and LENNARD-JONES, J. E. (1977a) The prognosis of idiopathic proctitis. *Scand. J. Gastroent., 12*, 727.

PRICE, L. A. (1968) The effect of systemic steroids on ileorectal anastomosis in ulcerative colitis. *Br. J. Surg., 55*, 839.

PUGH, H. L. (1945) Regional enteritis. *Ann. Surg., 122*, 845.

RAGAN, C., HOWES, E. L., PLOTZ, C. M., MEYER, K. and BLUNT, J. G. (1949) Effect of cortisone on production of granulation tissue in the rabbit. *Proc. Soc. exp. Biol., N.Y., 72*, 718.

RANKIN, J. G., SKYRING, A. P. and GOULSTON, S. J. M. (1966) Liver in ulcerative colitis: obstructive jaundice due to bile duct carcinoma. *Gut, 7*, 433.

RAPAPORT, L. M. (1956) The technique of ileostomy with description of a new stomal cutter. *Surgery, St Louis, 39*, 794.

RAVITCH, M. M. (1948) Anal ileostomy with sphincter preservation in patients requiring total colectomy for benign conditions. *Surgery, St Louis, 24*, 170.

—— (1977) In discussion of Martin et al. (1977).

—— and HANDELSMAN, J. C. (1951) One-stage resection of entire colon for ulcerative colitis and polypoid adenomatosis. *Bull. Johns Hopkins Hosp., 88*, 59.

REILLY, J., RYAN, J. A., STROLE, W. and FISCHER, J. E. (1976) Hyperalimentation in inflammatory bowel disease. *Am. J. Surg., 131*, 192.

REINHOFF, W. F. (1925) The surgical treatment of chronic ulcerative colitis by ileo-sigmoidostomy. *Ann. clin. Med., 4*, 430.

RHODES, J. B. and KIRSNER, J. B. (1965) The early and late course of patients with ulcerative colitis after ileostomy and colectomy. *Surgery Gynec. Obstet., 121*, 1303.

RICE-OXLEY, J. M. and TRUELOVE, S. (1950) Complications of ulcerative colitis. *Lancet, 1*, 607.

RICKETTS, W. E., KIRSNER, J. B. and PALMER, W. L. (1948) Chronic non-specific ulcerative colitis: a roentgenologic study of its course. *Gastroenterology, 10, 1.*

RIDER, J. A., MOELLER, H. C., DEVERAUX, R. G. and WRIGHT, R. R. (1960) The use of an intramucosal test to demonstrate food hypersensitivity in ulcerative colitis. *Acta allerg., 15, Suppl. 7, 486.*

RIIS, P., ANTHONISEN, P., WULFFE, H. R., FOLKENBORG, O., BONNEVIE, O. and BINDER, V. (1973) The prophylactic effect of salazo-sulphapyridine in ulcerative colitis during long-term treatment. *Scand. J. Gastroent., 8, 71.*

RIPSTEIN, C. B. (1953a) Primary resection of the colon in acute ulcerative colitis. *J. Am. med. Ass., 152, 1093.*

—— (1953b) Primary resection of colon in fulminating ulcerative colitis. *Surg. Forum, 117.*

—— MILLER, G. G. and GARDNER, C. McG. (1952) Results of the surgical treatment of ulcerative colitis. *Ann. Surg., 135, 14.*

RITCHIE, J. K. (1967) Ileostomy: the sequelae of 216 operations. *Proc. R. Soc. Med., 60; 35.*

—— (1971a) Ileostomy and excisional surgery for chronic inflammatory disease of the colon: A survey of one hospital region. Part I. Results and complications of surgery. *Gut, 12, 528.*

—— (1971b) Ileostomy and excisional surgery for chronic inflammatory disease of the colon: A survey of one hospital region. Part II. The health of the ileostomists. *Gut, 12, 536.*

—— (1972a) The causes of late mortality in ileostomists. *Proc. R. Soc. Med., 65, 73.*

—— (1972b) Ulcerative colitis treated by ileostomy and excisional surgery. Fifteen years' experience at St Mark's Hospital. *Br. J. Surg., 59, 345.*

—— POWELL-TUCK, J. and LENNARD-JONES, J. E. (1978) Clinical outcome of the first ten years of ulcerative colitis and proctitis. *Lancet, 2, 1140.*

ROCCHIO, M. A., CHA, C.-J. M., HAAS, K. F. and RANDALL, H. T. (1974) Use of chemically defined diets in the management of patients with acute inflammatory bowel disease. *Am. J. Surg., 127, 467.*

ROSENAK, B. D., PICKETT, R. D., van VACTOR, H. D., HAMMOND, J. B., HEALEY, R. J. and MOSER, R. H. (1958) The present status of the treatment of chronic ulcerative colitis with steroid hormones. *Gastroenterology, 34, 879.*

ROSENDORFF, C. and GRIEVE, N. W. (1967) A cases of ulcerative oesophagitis in association with ulcerative colitis. *Gut, 8, 344.*

ROSENQVIST, H., ÖHRLING, H., LAGERCRANTZ, R. and EDLING, N. (1959) Ulcerative colitis and carcinoma coli. *Lancet, 1, 906.*

ROSS, J. R. and SWARTS, J. M. (1948) Hepatic dysfunction and cirrhosis in chronic ulcerative colitis. *Gastroenterology, 10, 81.*

ROSS, S. T. (1964) Surgical treatment of ulcerative colitis. *Surgery, St Louis, 55, 782.*

ROTH, J. L., VALDES-DAPENA, A., STEIN, G. N. and BOCHUS, H. L. (1959) Toxic megacolon in ulcerative colitis. *Gastroenterology, 37, 239.*

ROTSTEIN, J., ENTEL, I. and ZEVINER, B. (1963) Arthritis associated with ulcerative colitis. *Ann. rheum. Dis., 22, 194.*

ROY, P. H., SAUER, W. G., BEAHRS, O. H. and FARROW, G. M. (1969) Experience with ileostomies. Evaluation of longterm rehabilitation in 497 patients. *Am. J. Surg., 119, 77.*

SALASSA, R. M., BENNETT, W. A., KEATING, F. R., Jr. and SPRAGUE, R. G. (1953) Postoperative adrenal cortical insufficiency; occurrence in patients previously treated with cortisone. *J. Am. med. Ass., 152, 1509.*

SALEM, S. N., TRUELOVE, S. C. and RICHARDS, W. C. D. (1964) Small-intestinal and gastric changes in ulcerative colitis: a biopsy study. *Br. med. J., 1, 394.*

SAMMONS, H. G. (1951) Mucinases in ulcerative colitis. *Lancet, 2, 239.*

SAMPSON, P. A. and WALKER, F. C. (1961) Dilatation of the colon in ulcerative colitis. *Br. med. J., 2, 1119.*

SAUER, W. G. and BARGEN, J. A. (1944) Chronic ulcerative colitis followed by carcinoma: report of 26 cases. *Proc. Staff Meet. Mayo Clin., 19, 311.*

—— —— (1949) Chronic ulcerative colitis and carcinoma. *J. Am. med. Ass., 141, 982.*

SCARBOROUGH, R. (1955) Surgical treatment of chronic ulcerative colitis. *Am. J. Surg., 89, 1224.*

SCHLITT, R. J., McNALLY, J. J. and SHAFIROFF, B. G. (1951) Pelvic autonomic neurectomy for ulcerative colitis. *Gastroenterology, 19, 812.*

SCHNEIDER, S. (1955) Anal ileostomy: experiences with a new three-stage procedure. *Archs Surg., Chicago, 70, 539.*

SHANDS, W. C., DOCKERTY, M. B. and BARGEN, J. A. (1952) Adenocarcinoma of the large intestine associated with chronic ulcerative colitis. *Surgery Gynec. Obstet., 94, 302.*

SHEAN, F. C., BARKER, W. F. and FONKALSRUD, E. W. (1964) Studies on active and passive antibody-induced colitis in the dog. *Am. J. Surg., 107, 337.*

SILEN, W. and GLOTZER, D. (1974) The prevention and treatment of the perineal sinus. *Surgery, St Louis, 75, 535.*

SINGER, A. M., BENNETT, R. C., CARTER, N. G. and HUGHES, E. S. R. (1973) Blood and urinary changes in patients with ileostomies and ileorectal anastomoses. *Br. med. J., 3, 141.*

SLANEY, G. and BROOKE, B. N. (1957) Postoperative collapse due to adrenal insufficiency following cortisone therapy. *Lancet, 1, 1167.*

—— —— (1958) Septicaemia in modern therapy. *Lancet, 1, 505.*

—— —— (1959) Cancer in ulcerative colitis. *Lancet, 2, 694.*

SLOAN, W. P., BARGEN, J. A. and BAGGENSTOSS, A. H. (1950a) Local complications of chronic ulcerative colitis based on the study of 2,000 cases. *Proc. Staff Meet. Mayo Clin., 25, 240.*

—— —— and GAGE, R. P. (1950b) Life histories of patients with chronic ulcerative colitis: a review of 2,000 cases. *Gastroenterology, 16, 25.*

SMIDDY, F. G., GREGORY, S. D., SMITH, I. B. and GOLIGHER, J. C. (1960) Faecal losses of fluid and electrolytes before and after ileostomy for colitis. *Lancet, 1, 14.*

SMITH, F. W., LAW, D. H., NICKEL, W. F., Jr. and SLEISENGER, M. H. (1962) Fulminant ulcerative colitis with toxic dilation of the colon: medical and surgical management of eleven cases with observations regarding etiology. *Gastroenterology, 42, 233.*

SPARBERG, M. (1974) Bismuth subgallate as an effective means for the control of ileostomy odor: a double blind study. *Gastroenterology, 66, 476.*

SPENCER, J. A., KIRSNER, J. B., MILYNARYK, P., REED, P. I. and PALMER, W. L. (1962) Immediate and prolonged therapeutic effects of corticotrophin and adrenal steroids in ulcerative colitis: observations in 340 cases for period up to 10 years. *Gastroenterology, 42, 113.*

SPRIGGS, A. I., SMITH, R. S., GRIFFITH, H. and TRUELOVE, S. C. (1958) Heinz-body anaemia due to salicylazosulphapyridine. *Lancet, 1,* 1039.

STAHLGREN, L. H. and FERGUSON, L. K. (1959*a*) Effects of abdominoperineal resection on sexual function in 60 patients with ulcerative colitis. *Archs Surg., Chicago, 78,* 604.

—— —— (1959*b*) Is ileostomy always necessary in surgical treatment of segmental ulcerative colitis? *Surgery, St Louis, 46,* 847.

STANDERTSKJÖLD-NORDENSTAM, C.-G., PALMU, A. and SIVULA, A. (1979) Radiological assessment of nipple-valve insufficiency in Koch's continent reservoir ileostomy. *Br. J. Surg., 66,* 269.

STEICHEN, F. M. (1978) The creation of autologous substitute organs with stapling instruments. *Am. J. Surg., 134,* 659.

STEINBERG, V. L. and STOREY, G. (1957) Ankylosing spondylitis and chronic inflammatory lesions of the intestines. *Br. med. J., 2,* 1157.

STEWART, G. T. (1950) Post-dysenteric colitis. *Br. med. J., 1,* 405.

STRAUSS, A. A., FRIEDMAN, J. and BLOCH, L. (1924) Colectomy for ulcerative colitis. *Surg. Clins N. Am., 4,* 667.

—— and STRAUSS, S. F. (1944) Surgical treatment of ulcerative colitis. *Surg. Clins. N. Am., 24,* 211.

SVARTZ, N. (1942) Salazopyrin, a new sulfanilamide preparation. *Acta med. scand., 110,* 577.

—— (1948) Treatment of 124 cases of ulcerative colitis with salazopyrine and attempts at desensibilization in cases of hypersensitiveness to sulfa. *Acta med. scand., 130,* 465.

—— (1954) The treatment of ulcerative colitis. *Gastroenterology, 26,* 26.

—— (1960) Colitis ulcerosa. Proc. int. Congr. Gastroenterology, Leyden. Amsterdam, *Excerpta med. int. Congr. Ser., 31,* 383.

—— and ERNBERG, T. (1949) Cancer coli in cases of colitis ulcerosa. *Acta med. scand., 135,* 444.

TAYLOR, K. B. and TRUELOVE, S. C. (1961) Circulating antibodies to milk proteins in ulcerative colitis. *Br. med. J., 2,* 924.

—— —— (1962) Immunological reactions in gastrointestinal disease: a review. *Gut, 3,* 277.

TAYLOR, R. L., ROMBEAU, J. L. and TURNBULL, R. B. (1978) Transperitoneal relocation of the ileal stoma without formal laparotomy. *Surgery Gynec. Obstet., 146,* 955.

TEXTER, E. C. (1957) The natural history of ulcerative colitis. *J. chron. Dis., 5,* 347.

THAYER, W. R. and BOVE, J. R. (1965) Blood groups and ulcerative colitis. *Gastroenterology, 48,* 326.

THIRKETTLE, J. L., GROUGH, K. R. and READ, A. E. (1963) Agranulocytosis associated with sulphasalazine (Salazopyrin) therapy. *Lancet, 1,* 1395.

THORN, G. W. (1954) In *Medical Uses of Cortisone*, ed. F. D. W. Lukens, chap. 2. New York: Blakiston.

THORPE, M. E. C., SCHEUER, P. J. and SHERLOCK, S. (1967) Primary sclerosing cholangitis, the biliary tree and ulcerative colitis. *Gut, 8,* 435.

TODD, I. P. (1978) *Intestinal Stomas.* London: Heinemann Medical.

TOLSTEDT, G. E. and BELL, J. W. (1961) Intestinal obstruction following total colectomy for ulcerative colitis. *Ann. Surg., 153,* 241.

TREADWELL, B. L. C., SAVAGE, O., SEVER, E. D. and COPEMAN, W. S. (1963) Pituitary adrenal function during corticosteroid therapy. *Lancet, 1,* 355.

TRUELOVE, S. C. (1956) Treatment of ulcerative colitis with local hydrocortisone. *Br. med. J., 2,* 1267.

—— (1958) Treatment of ulcerative colitis with local hydrocortisone hemisuccinate sodium; a report on a controlled therapeutic trial. *Br. med. J., 2,* 1072.

—— (1960) Systemic and local corticosteroid therapy in ulcerative colitis. *Br. med. J., 1,* 464.

—— (1961) Ulcerative colitis provoked by milk. *Br. med. J., 1,* 154.

—— (1964) The treatment of ulcerative colitis. *Prescriber's J., 4,* 24.

—— ELLIS, H. and WEBSTER, C. U. (1965) Place of a double-barrelled ileostomy in ulcerative colitis and Crohn's disease of the colon: a preliminary report. *Br. med. J., 1,* 150.

—— and JEWELL, D. P. (1974) Intensive intravenous regimen for severe attacks of ulcerative colitis. *Lancet, 1,* 1067.

—— and RICHARDS, W. C. D. (1956) Biopsy studies in ulcerative colitis. *Br. med. J., 1,* 1315.

—— WATKINSON, G. and DRAPER, G. (1962) Comparison of corticosteroid and sulphasalazine therapy in ulcerative colitis. *Br. med. J., 2,* 1708.

—— WILLOUGHBY, C. P., LEE, E. G. and KETTLEWELL, M. G. W. (1978) Further experience in the treatment of severe attacks of ulcerative colitis. *Lancet, 4,* 1086.

—— and WITTS, L. J. (1955) Cortisone in ulcerative colitis; final report on a therapeutic trial. *Br. med. J., 2,* 1041.

—— —— (1959) Cortisone and corticotrophin in ulcerative colitis. *Br. med. J., 1,* 387.

TUMEN, H. J. and COHN, E. N. (1950) Pregnancy and ulcerative colitis. *Gastroenterology, 16,* 1.

—— MONAGHAN, J. F. and JOBB, E. (1947) Hepatic cirrhosis as a complication of chronic ulcerative colitis. *Ann. intern Med., 26,* 542.

TURNBULL, R. B. (1953) Management of an ileostomy. *Am. J. Surg., 86,* 617.

—— (1966) Personal communication.

—— (1975*a*) The surgical approach to the treatment of inflammatory bowel disease (IBD): a personal view of techniques and prognosis. In *Inflammatory Bowel Disease*, ed. J. B. Kirsner and R. G. Shorter, p. 338. Philadelphia: Lea and Febiger.

—— (1975*b*) Advances in the technique of ulcerative colitis surgery: endoanal proctectomy and two-directional myotomy ileostomy. *Surg. Ann., 7,* 315.

—— and GILL, N. (1960) Accurate application of the ileostomy pouch. The use of a paper training sleeve. *Ileostomy Quarterly,* Spring.

—— WEAKLEY, F. L. and FARMER, R. G. (1964) Ileitis after colectomy and ileostomy for nonspecific ulcerative colitis: report of 35 cases. *Dis. Colon Rect., 7,* 427.

—— —— and HAWK, W. A. (1977) Choice of operation for the toxic megacolon phase of non-specific ulcerative colitis. In *Colitis Ulcerosa*, ed. K. Kremer and H. Kivelitz, p. 96. Stuttgard: Georg Thieme.

—— —— —— and SCHOFIELD, P. (1970) Choice of operation for the toxic megacolon phase of non-specific ulcerative colitis. *Surg. Clins N. Am., 50,* 1151.

TYTGAT, G. N. and HUIBREGTSE, K. (1975) Loperamide and ileostomy output: placebo-controlled double-blind crossover study. *Br. med. J.*, *2*, 667.

VAN PROHASKA, J., DRAGSTEDT, L. R., III and THOMPSON, R. G. (1962) Surgical problems in corticosteroid treated patients. *Ann. Surg.*, *159*, 408.

—— GREER, D., Jr. and RYAN, J. F. (1964) Acute dilatation of the colon in ulcerative colitis. *Archs Surg., Chicago, 89*, 24.

—— and SIDERIUS, N. H. (1962) The surgical rehabilitation of patients with chronic ulcerative colitis. *Am. J. Surg., 103*, 42.

VIOTK, A. J., ECHAVE, V., FELLER, J. H., BROWN, R. A. and GURD, F. N. (1973) Experience with elemental diet in the treatment of inflammatory bowel disease. *Archs Surg., Chicago, 107*, 329.

WALKER, F. C. (1975) *Stomal Care.* London: MacMillan.

—— and WEAVER, J. P. A. (1964) Lymphosarcoma in ulcerative colitis. *Br. J. Surg., 51*, 475.

WANGENSTEEN, O. H. and TOON, R. W. (1948) Primary resection of the colon and rectum with particular reference to cancer and ulcerative colitis. *Am. J. Surg., 75*, 384.

WARREN, I. A. and BERK, J. E. (1957) The etiology of chronic non-specific ulcerative colitis. A critical review. *Gastroenterology, 33*, 395.

WARREN, R. and McKITTRICK, L. S. (1951) Ileostomy for ulcerative colitis; technique, complications and management. *Surgery Gynec. Obstet., 93*, 555.

WARREN, S. and SOMMERS, C. S. (1949) Pathogenesis of ulcerative colitis. *Am. J. Path., 25*, 657.

—— —— (1954) Pathology of regional ileitis and ulcerative colitis. *J. Am. med. Ass., 154*, 189.

WATKINSON, G. (1958) Treatment of ulcerative colitis with topical hydrocortisone hemisuccinate sodium: a controlled trial employing restricted segmental analysis. *Br. med. J., 2*, 1077.

—— (1962) The medical treatment of ulcerative colitis. *Postgrad. med. J., 38*, 688.

—— THOMPSON, H. and GOLIGHER, J. C. (1959) Segmental colitis. *Gastroenterologia, 92*, 157.

—— —— —— (1960) Right-sided or segmental ulcerative colitis. *Br. J. Surg., 47*, 22.

WATT, J. and MARCUS, R. (1971) Carrageenan-induced ulceration of the large intestine in the guinea-pig. *Gut, 12*, 164.

WATTS, J. McK., de DOMBAL, F. T. and GOLIGHER, J. C. (1966a) The early results of surgery for ulcerative colitis. *Br. J. Surg., 53*, 1005.

—— —— —— (1966b) Long-term complications and prognosis following major surgery for ulcerative colitis. *Br. J. Surg., 53*, 1014.

—— —— WATKINSON, G. and GOLIGHER, J. C. (1966c) The early course of ulcerative colitis. *Gut, 7*, 16.

—— —— —— —— (1966d) The long term prognosis of ulcerative colitis. *Br. med. J., 1*, 1447.

—— and HUGHES, E. S. R. (1977) Ulcerative colitis and Crohn's disease: results after colectomy and ileorectal anastomosis. *Br. J. Surg., 64*, 77.

—— THOMPSON, H. and GOLIGHER, J. C. (1966e) Sigmoidoscopy and cytology in the detection of microscopic disease of the rectal mucosa in ulcerative colitis. *Gut, 7*, 288.

WAUGH, J. M. (1952) Personal communication.

—— PECK, D. A., BEAHRS, O. H. and SAUER, W. G. (1964) Surgical management of chronic ulcerative colitis. *Archs Surgs., Chicago, 88*, 556.

WECKESSER, E. C. and CHINN, A. B. (1953) Carcinoma of the colon complicating chronic ulcerative colitis. *J. Am. med. Ass., 152*, 905.

WEINER, H. A. and LEWIS, C. M. (1960) Some notes on the epidemiology of nonspecific ulcerative colitis. An apparent increase in incidence in Jews. *Am. J. dig. Dis., 5*, 406.

WEIR, R. F. (1902) Quoted by Corbett (1945).

WELLS, C. A. (1952) A skin-covered spout ileostomy. *Br. J. Surg., 39*, 309.

WHEELOCK, F. C., Jr. and WARREN, R. (1955) Ulcerative colitis: follow-up studies. *New Engl. J. Med., 252*, 421.

WIGLEY, R. D. and MACLAURIN, B. P. (1962) A study of ulcerative colitis in New Zealand, showing a low incidence in Maoris. *Br. med. J., 2*, 228.

WILKINSON, A. J. and HUMPHREYS, W. G. (1978) Seatbelt injury to ileostomy. *Br. med. J., 3*, 1249.

WILKS, S. and MOXON, W. (1875) *Lectures on Pathological Anatomy*, 2nd ed. London: Churchill.

WILLIAMS (1965) Personal communication.

WILLIAMS, C. and MUTO, T. (1972) Examination of the whole colon with the fibreoptic colonoscope. *Br. med. J., 3*, 278.

WILSON, E. (1964) The rehabilitation of patients with an ileostomy established for ulcerative colitis. *Med. J. Aust., 1*, 842.

WINKELMAN, E. L. and BROWN, C. H. (1965) Nitrogen mustard in the treatment of chronic ulcerative colitis and regional enteritis: a preliminary report. *Cleveland clin. Q., 32*, 165.

WITTKOWER, E. (1938) Ulcerative colitis: personality studies. *Br. med. J., 2*, 1356.

WOLFMAN, E. F., SCHWARTZ, S. and TREVINO, G. (1965) Management of chronic idiopathic ulcerative colitis in children. *Archs Surg., Chicago, 91*, 321.

WRIGHT, R., LUMSDEN, K., LUNTZ, M. H., SEUEL, D. and TRUELOVE, S. C. (1965) Abnormalities of the sacro-iliac joints and uveitis in ulcerative colitis. *Q. Jl Med., 34*, 229.

WRIGHT, V. and WATKINSON, G. (1959) The arthritis of ulcerative colitis. *Medicine, Balt., 38*, 243.

—— —— (1965a) The arthritis of ulcerative colitis. *Br. med. J., 2*, 670.

—— —— (1965b) Sacro-iliitis and ulcerative colitis. *Br. med. J., 2*, 675.

YEOMANS, F. C. (1921) Chronic ulcerative colitis. *J. Am. med. Ass., 77*, 2043.

22

Crohn's Disease
(Granulomatous Enteritis)

Though this form of non-specific enteritis had previously been described by others, such as Moynihan (1907) and Mayo-Robson (1908) of Leeds and Dalziel (1913) of Glasgow, it is to Burrill Crohn of New York that we are indebted for establishing it as a clinical and pathological entity. It is for this reason that most clinicians and pathologists in Britian persist in calling the condition Crohn's disease, but in America it is generally referred to as regional or granulomatous enteritis. In their original paper Crohn et al. (1932) described the disease as occurring in the terminal ileum, but it was soon realized that it could occur anywhere in the intestinal tract—or, indeed, in the duodenum or stomach (Fielding et al. 1970; Burgess et al. 1971), oesophagus (Madden et al. 1969), pharynx or mouth (Croft and Wilkinson 1972), or even in situations remote from the alimentary system such as the skin of the submammary region (Mountain 1970) or the scrotum and prepuce (Atherton et al. 1978). This wide distribution of the condition in areas other than the intestine renders an eponymous designation additionally desirable in that it obviates the use of the occasionally inept word 'enteritis'.

That the large bowel could be affected by Crohn's disease in conjunction with an ileal lesion, either as a direct extension of the latter into the caecum and right colon, or as a discrete lesion in the colon separated from the disease in the ileum by a 'skip' segment of normal large intestine, was shown by Colp (1934), Mixter (1935), Crohn and Rosenak (1936), Clark and Dixon (1939), Pugh (1945), Wells (1952), Watkinson et al. (1960), Morson and Lockhart-Mummery (1959a) and Brooke (1959). That an entirely isolated colonic lesion of this disease could occur without any concomitant involvement of the small bowel was demonstrated by Pugh (1945), Lockhart-Mummery and Morson (1960, 1964), Cornes and Stecher (1961), and Lewin and Swales (1966), the writings of Lockhart-Mummery and Morson being particularly influential in this connection.

The acceptance of Crohn's disease of the large intestine was at first strangely resisted by Crohn (1965) and many of his fellow countrymen. It is probable, however, that some of the cases labelled by Crohn et al. (1947), Neuman et al. (1954) and Manning et al. (1955) as segmental ulcerative colitis were in fact examples of Crohn's disease in the large gut. But the existence of a granulomatous colitis has been acknowledged by some American authors (Marshak et al. 1959; Wolf and Marshak 1962; Lindner et al. 1963; Bochus 1965; Ross 1965; Hawk et al. 1967; Korelitz 1967; Glotzer et al. 1970; Zetzel 1970). In Britian and Scandinavia Crohn's disease of the large bowel is now widely accepted, and a common experience on the part of surgeons who do a good deal of colonic surgery in these countries is that this condition is at present being encountered far more frequently than it was a few years ago (Goligher et al. 1971a, b; Krause 1971). The apparent rise in incidence may be partly due to a readier recognition by pathologists of this disease process in specimens that would previously have been diagnosed as showing ordinary ulcerative colitis, for there is now a greater awareness in pathological circles of Crohn's disease as a lesion of the large intestine. But many of the cases now presenting are fairly obviously diagnosable as Crohn's disease—and presumably always would have been—even by the crudest clinical and pathological criteria, so that one is driven to the conclusion that this condition has become genuinely commoner in the large bowel. Krause (1971) has emphasized, too, that, in the area of Sweden studied by him, the increase in frequency of Crohn's disease had not been accompanied by any corresponding fall in the incidence of ordinary ulcerative colitis. In my experience at the present time, when a patient is referred ostensibly with ulcerative colitis, there is at least an even chance that the condition, on more careful scrutiny, will be found to be Crohn's disease of the large bowel and not colitis. It is thus important for the clinician—and the radiologist and pathologist—to be on the alert for the special characteristics of this lesion.

EPIDEMIOLOGY

RELATIVE INCIDENCE OF CROHN'S DISEASE IN DIFFERENT PARTS OF THE ALIMENTARY TRACT

No doubt the relative frequency of the disease in the small and large intestine respectively in any group of cases will be influenced by the special interests of the clinicians concerned. Thus in my personal series of 517 patients with Crohn's disease treated between 1958 and 1977 there may have been a bias towards locations in the large intestine because of my abundant colitis clientele. In 102 cases the pathological changes were confined entirely to the small intestine (with associated 'skip' lesions in the duodenum or stomach in five patients), in 221 they occurred only in the large intestine, and in 194 they affected both small and large bowel but with the main emphasis on the small bowel in 63 and on the large bowel in 131. There were thus 165 patients with disease *mainly or entirely in the small intestine* and 353 with disease *chiefly or solely in the large intestine*. In 29% of 517 cases 'skip' lesions occurred in small or large intestine. In the 353 cases with essentially large bowel disease the rectum was implicated in 78%, it and a variable amount of the sigmoid being the only parts affected in 22·1%.

GEOGRAPHICAL AND SECULAR TRENDS OF INCIDENCE

Though few precise data exist relating to the frequency of Crohn's disease in different countries (Evans 1972), it would appear, mainly from conversation with colleagues in other parts of the world, that, as with ulcerative colitis (see p. 689), there are considerable variations in the incidence of the condition from one country to another. Chronic Crohn's disease seems to be commonest in Britain, several western European countries such as Scandinavia, USA and Canada, is much less common in Mediterranean countries, and is very rare in most parts of Africa and Asia. In the countries in which the disease has occurred with some frequency, there appears to be an increase in both the overall incidence and the incidence of large bowel lesions. As already mentioned (p. 827) this is certainly true of Britain, at least in the practice of surgeons such as myself with a special interest in colorectal surgery and, I think, more generally as well.

TABLE 67. *Age and Sex Distribution of 517 Patients with Crohn's Disease*

Age (years)	Males	Females	Total
10–19	21	33	54
20–9	59	79	138
30–9	44	61	105
40–9	53	71	124
50–9	12	41	53
60–9	10	23	33
70–9	4	5	9
80–9	1	–	1
All ages	204	313	517

AGE AND SEX INCIDENCE

Though Crohn's disease is generally held to occur with roughly equal frequency in the two sexes (Evans 1972), analysis of my cases shows that there is a 2 : 3 male/female ratio of incidence (Table 67) and this slight female preponderance held for both patients with mainly small bowel disease and for those with mainly large bowel lesions. As regards age-specific incidence rates, as Table 67 shows, the disease is encountered at any age from early childhood up to advanced old age, but over 70% of the patients are between 20 and 49 years with maximal incidence in the 20–9 and 40–9 periods. A similar age distribution applies equally to patients with chiefly small bowel disease and to those with disease affecting mainly the large bowel.

FAMILIAL INCIDENCE

A number of authors have reported the frequency with which their patients with Crohn's disease have had similarly affected relatives. Thus Crohn and Yarnis (1958) noted this occurrence in 12 of 542 cases, Cornes and Stecher (1961) in one of 45 cases with large bowel Crohn's disease, Kirsner and Spencer (1963) in 12 of 185 cases, and Lennard-Jones (1968) in nine of 145 cases. Several instances of Crohn's disease in identical twins have also been recorded (Almy and Sherlock 1966; McConnell 1971). Analysis some years ago of 332 cases of Crohn's disease in Leeds showed nine patients with probable Crohn's disease in 'first-degree' relatives—that is in a father, mother, sibling, son or daughter—and a further eight patients with probable ulcerative colitis in a 'first-degree' relative.

But Kirsner (1970) has reported that cases of ulcerative colitis and Crohn's disease occur in approximately 25% of the members of families with inflammatory bowel disease. The significance of this observation would depend in part on the reliability of the criteria employed to differentiate between ulcerative colitis and Crohn's disease of the large intestine.

EFFECT OF RACIAL AND SOCIAL FACTORS ON INCIDENCE

The apparent differences in geographical incidence may be attributable partly to environmental and partly to racial factors, but it is difficult to evaluate these elments. However, there seem to be clear differences in the incidence in three racial groups resident in the United States—namely the Negroes, the Jews and the Caucasians. Acheson (1960a) demonstrated a four-fold greater risk of developing Crohn's disease amongst service veterans professing the Jewish faith than amongst other white veterans. Monk et al. (1967) reached a similar conclusion for Jewish and non-Jewish white male residents of Baltimore. Acheson (1960a) was also able to show that Crohn's disease was about 2½ times more common in non-Jewish whites than in Negroes.

Kyle (1971a) suggested that the proportion of unskilled workers amongst sufferers from Crohn's disease is higher than in the general population, whilst Monk et al. (1969) concluded that the incidence of the disease was slightly greater in better educated persons. In Leeds, however, we have not discerned any differences in social class distribution as between patients with Crohn's disease and the general population (de Dombal 1971).

AETIOLOGY

Until a few years ago it could truthfully be said that so far as the cause of Crohn's disease (as of ulcerative colitis) was concerned, ignorance reigned supreme, and this state of affairs was well demonstrated by the Skandia Symposium (Engel and Larsson 1971). More recently there have been some interesting and initially very exciting developments in our understanding of the aetiology of the disease; but unfortunately they have not maintained their original momentum and seem to have bogged down in disagreements and contradictions.

A Possible Aetiological Agent Transmissible from Crohn's Disease Tissue. Work on this idea began with Mitchell and Rees (1970) who prepared homogenates from fresh tissue (bowel wall or related lymph nodes) taken from an operative specimen of histologically proven Crohn's disease of the terminal ileum. As controls, homogenates were also prepared from para-aortic or inguinal lymph nodes obtained during operations for arterial grafting or varicose veins. Samples of the homogenates were injected into the hind footpads of six normal and six immunologically deficient female CBA strains of mice 12 weeks old. Samples of the homogenates were also injected into guinea-pigs and cultured on Löwenstein–Jensen medium to detect the presence of mycobacteria. No mycobacteria were isolated on culture or in guinea-pigs from any of the Crohn's tissue homogenates. But in eight of 48 footpads from 24 mice given Crohn's tissue homogenates lesions developed, which on histological examination 169–500 days after the injections were found to contain epithelioid and giant cell granulomas typical of Crohn's disease. None of the 95 footpads given non-Crohn's lymph node homogenates showed these characteristics when examined at the same time intervals. These experiments seemed to provide good evidence for the existence of a transmissible aetiological agent.

Cave et al. (1975) then took this concept a step further by injecting homogenates prepared from the fresh ileum or colon of patients with histologically proven Crohn's disease into the intestinal wall of New Zealand white rabbits. Of 22 animals so injected nine developed granulomatous changes considered to be very similar to those of human Crohn's disease, whilst no such changes appeared in any of the 22 control inoculated rabbits.

Regrettably, two other groups of workers, who have repeated the experiments of Mitchell and Rees (1970) and of Cave et al. (1975), have been unable to confirm their findings. Heatley et al. (1975) also prepared homogenates of Crohn's tissue and injected them into the ileum of rats, mice and rabbits and also into the footpads of rats. Altogether bowel homogenates from 17 patients with Crohn's disease were given to 91 experimental animals, without being able to produce any macroscopic or microscopic changes indicative of Crohn's disease. Simonowitz et al. (1977) also performed experiments involving injection of Crohn's tissue homogenates and control normal tissue homogenates into the wall of the ileum of rabbits. They were able consistently to produce changes in the ileum in those animals receiving the Crohn's homogenates, but not in those animals given control homogenates. However Simonowitz et al. (1977) did not consider that the abnormalities thus created were at all characteristic of Crohn's disease.

On the conflicting evidence available one must conclude that the existence of a transmissible causal agent in Crohn's disease has not been established.

Immunological Factors. The other subject that has been much discussed for several years is the possible role of immunosuppression in the aetiology and pathogenesis of Crohn's disease. A welter of conflicting information is available in the literature, which I am certainly not competent to evaluate, but the reader may find helpful a recent paper by MacPherson et al. (1976), which concludes that immunity is qualitatively normal in Crohn's disease.

Other Factors. More detailed consideration of the factors mentioned above, and discussion of other possible aetiological agents will be found in Martini and Malchow (1979).

PATHOLOGY OF CROHN'S DISEASE OF LARGE BOWEL

GROSS APPEARANCES

These may closely resemble the appearances of Crohn's disease of the small gut, with marked thickening of the bowel wall and encroachment on the lumen, and with fissuring of the mucosa to produce a 'cobblestone' effect on the mucosal surface. Also the lesion may be confined to a relatively limited segment of the colon or rectum or may take the form of a short stricture. Similarly 'skipping' may occur with two or more lesions separated by normal bowel (Fig. 602). But one of the most frequent patterns of distribution of Crohn's disease of the large bowel is that shown in Fig. 603 in which the right colon, transverse colon and descending colon are affected together with the terminal ileum, but the sigmoid and rectum are largely spared. When such typical appearances are present there is usually no difficulty in recognizing the condition as one of Crohn's disease.

But in other cases the changes may be much less characteristic and indeed scarcely distinguishable from those of ordinary diffuse ulcerative colitis. The wall of the bowel may be quite thin and there may be no narrowing or stricture formation. The mucosa is extensively ulcerated with or without polyposis, and the greater part or all of the large intestine may be implicated.

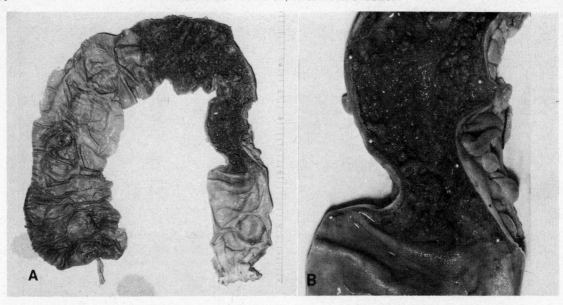

Fig. 602. (A) Proctocolectomy specimen showing a segment of Crohn's disease of the left colon. (B) Close-up view of affected part to demonstate the 'cobblestone' appearance of the mucosa.

MICROSCOPIC ANATOMY

The most reliable diagnostic feature of Crohn's disease on histological examination is the *sarcoid reaction*, as pointed out by Hadfield (1939). Unfortunately this is not always present, even in macroscopically typical lesions of the small bowel, which do not admit of any other diagnosis. Lockhart-Mummery and Morson (1964) were able to demonstrate sarcoid foci in some 87% of a series of 70 cases of Crohn's disease of the large bowel, but they emphasize that the foci were often very scanty, so that many histological sections were sometimes required to detect them.

But there are other histopathological features of Crohn's disease that help to distinguish it from ulcerative colitis. Thus, as pointed out by Warren and Sommers (1954) and confirmed by Lockhart-Mummery and Morson (1964) and Williams (1964), there is a difference in *the depth to which the bowel wall is involved* in these two diseases. In colitis the changes are maximal in the submucosa and mucosa, usually with considerable mucosal ulceration, and seldom go any deeper. In Crohn's disease on the other hand there is generally involvement of all coats, often through to the serosa, with cellular infiltrate composed of lymphocytes arranged generally in follicular fashion. The *presence of 'fissures' or microscopic sinuses*, passing from the mucosal surface deep into the bowel wall and sometimes into the peri-

intestinal tissues has been commented on particularly by Lockhart-Mummery and Morson (1964) as a helpful diagnostic feature of Crohn's disease. Such 'fissures' were found in 25% of their large bowel cases of Crohn's disease.

In specimens with Crohn's disease of the large bowel, sarcoid foci may also sometimes be demonstrated in the regional lymph nodes—in 25% of the cases according to Lockhart-Mummery and Morson (1964). But it is important to note that not infrequently nodes that are macroscopically enlarged may on histological section show only nonspecific reactive changes (Cook 1972).

DISTRIBUTION OF LESIONS IN BOWEL

As already pointed out, the lesions of Crohn's disease of the large intestine may occur as short segments or be a more diffuse process involving a major part or all of the large bowel; may be single or multiple, and may or may not be associated with a lesion of the small intestine. In some 25% of the patients with Crohn's disease mainly or entirely of the large bowel, the rectum and a variable amount of the distal colon are uninvolved; in another 12·8% the lesion is confined entirely to the rectum or rectum and sigmoid—the so-called anorectal Crohn's disease (Fig. 603), which tends to occur in older patients, is associated with a high incidence of

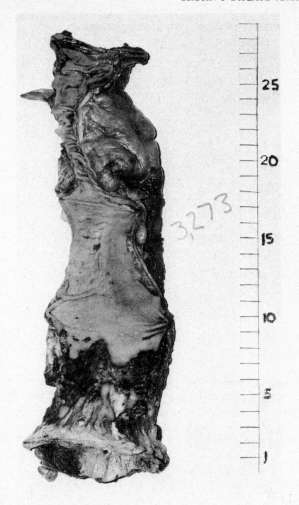

Fig. 603. Abdominoperineal excision specimen showing localized Crohn's disease of the rectum, ressembling somewhat a rectal carcinoma.

anal complications, and generally carries a specially good prognosis with conservative or operative treatment (Ritchie and Lennard-Jones 1976; Ritchie and Lockhart-Mummery 1973).

PATHOLOGICAL DIAGNOSIS

Warren and Sommers (1954) and Lockhart-Mummery and Morson (1964) claim that it is nearly always possible on pathological examination of the operative specimen to decide with confidence between a Crohn's lesion and ulcerative colitis. But my pathologists occasionally find it very difficult to reach a firm diagnosis between these two conditions, as do Lewin and Swales (1966). Sometimes

the gross appearances are not at all typical of Crohn's disease, and yet the histological examination may show characteristic giant cell follicles. In other cases the histological features may also be unhelpful, but the distribution of the disease in the bowel wall, with for example non-involvement of the rectum, may strongly suggest Crohn's disease rather than ulcerative colitis. A useful discussion of these difficulties is provided by Cook and Dixon (1973).

RELATIONSHIP OF ULCERATIVE COLITIS TO
CROHN'S DISEASE OF THE SMALL BOWEL

Another point on which there is great difference of opinion is the relationship of ulcerative colitis in the large intestine to regional enteritis of the small intestine. Warren and Sommers (1954) maintain that these two diseases seldom coexist and Lockhart-Mummery and Morson (1964) go further and claim that these lesions never occur in the same patient either at the same time or subsequently. Yet other authors have reported series of cases in which these conditions were found together or consecutively (Colcock et al. 1961; Valdes-Dapena and Vilardell 1962; Truelove and Reynell 1963), whilst Kirsner and Spencer (1963) have drawn attention to the frequent occurrence of regional enteritis and ulcerative colitis in the same family. The crucial consideration would seem to be the interpretation of the original pathological changes in the large intestine in these cases which, as has just been emphasized, can be difficult and open to dispute. My own experience is that very occasionally patients, who have had radical operation for what was reported by the pathologist to be ulcerative colitis or an indeterminate brand of colitis, return with an obvious Crohn's lesion of the terminal small bowel immediately proximal to the ileostomy or to an ileocolic anastomosis (Goligher 1972). The pathologist then usually finds no difficulty, on re-examining the histological sections of the colon specimen, in coming to the conclusion that the original condition was really a Crohn's colitis! This practice certainly helps to support the philosophy that ulcerative colitis and Crohn's disease do not coexist in the same patient.

THE RISK OF MALIGNANT CHANGE IN
CROHN'S DISEASE

An important question related to the pathology of Crohn's disease is whether the now well-documented predisposition of ulcerative colitis to form intestinal cancers also applies to Crohn's

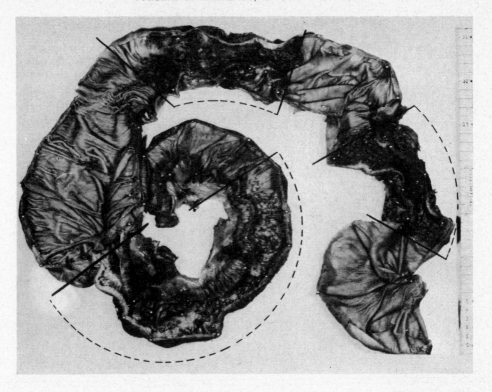

Fig. 604. Colectomy specimen from a man aged 27 with Crohn's disease of the terminal ileum and two separate 'skip' lesions of the transverse and descending colon respectively. Histological examination showed typical appearances of Crohn's disease in both the ileal and colonic lesions. The patient was alive and well 11 years after operation.

disease, particularly of the large bowel. At least 15 or 16 well-authenticated cases of carcinoma arising in large or small bowel, the seat of Crohn's disease, have now been reported (Shiel et al. 1968; Parrish et al. 1968; Morowitz et al. 1968; Perrett et al. 1968; Jones 1969; Wyatt 1969; Rha et al. 1971), and it seems unwise at the present stage to rule out the possibility that long-standing granulomatous enteritis, particularly of the small bowel, may potentiate the development of intestinal cancer. From a survey of the recorded cases of carcinoma of the bowel in cases of Crohn's disease, Darke et al. (1973) conclude that there is a small but significant increase in the risk of cancer developing, both in the small and the large intestine, in Crohn's disease. The most recent report of carcinoma arising in cases of Crohn's disease is that of Greenstein et al. (1978) from the Mount Sinai Hospital, New York City. They describe seven instances of carcinoma developing in excluded bowel after diversionary surgery for Crohn's enteritis mostly of the lower ileum; six of the tumours were located in bowel actually the seat of the disease.

CLINICAL FEATURES AND COMPLICATIONS WITH SPECIAL REFERENCE TO CROHN'S DISEASE OF LARGE BOWEL

SYMPTOMS

Though Crohn's disease of the large bowel may present with similar symptoms to those of ulcerative colitis, with diarrhoea, passage of blood and slime and failure of general health, there are frequently slight differences which may be suggestive. The *diarrhoea* is often *less severe* than in colitis and is frequently associated with *abdominal pain*. *Bleeding* is apt to be a *less frequent* or severe symptom in Crohn's disease than in colitis. There may be considerable loss of weight and the patients often look just as ill with Crohn's disease of the colon as they do with long-standing severe colitis. Occasionally patients may present in an *acutely ill condition* indistinguishable clinically from severe ulcerative colitis, sometimes with toxic megacolon, colonic perforation or

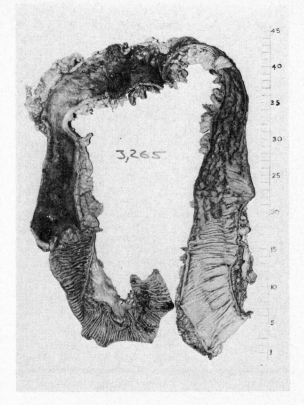

Fig. 605. Subtotal colectomy specimen from a patient aged 38, showing what is perhaps the most common distribution of Crohn's disease affecting mainly the large bowel—namely terminal ileum, right and transverse colon, descending colon and upper sigmoid.

severe haemorrhage, and only after the operative specimen is examined pathologically following emergency colectomy is it recognized that the lesion is Crohn's disease and not ordinary colitis (Hawk and Turnbull 1966; Javett and Brooke 1970; Goligher et al. 1970).

ABDOMINAL PHYSICAL SIGNS

There may be some tenderness on palpation over the affected parts of the colon, as in ulcerative colitis, but occasionally a *distinct mass* is palpable either in the colon or in the coincidentally involved ileum and this never occurs in colitis. Rarely an external abdominal fistula may be present (see p. 834).

ANAL EXAMINATION

Unquestionably one of the most distinctive features of Crohn's disease of the small or large intestine is the *occurrence of anal lesions*, the frequency of which in recorded series of cases has been variously estimated—14% by Crohn and Yarnis (1958), 18% by Edwards (1964), 50% by Morson and Lockhart-Mummery (1959b), 76% by Fielding (1972), and 45% in my own series of 517 cases of Crohn's disease. These variations in incidence are partly explained by the relative proportions of patients with small and large bowel lesions of the disease in the series concerned; for anal complications are commoner in association with lesions of the large than of the small bowel. Thus, in Morson and Lockhart-Mummery's (1959b) series 68% of patients with Crohn's disease of the colon or rectum had anal lesions, but only 27% of those with small bowel disease. Fielding (1972) observed a similar difference. In my series of cases anal complications were noted in 20% of the patients whose intestinal lesions were confined to the small bowel, in 44% of patients with mixed small and large bowel lesions, and in 55% of those with only large bowel disease; of patients whose rectum was involved 68% had anal lesions. Lockhart-Mummery (1972) reckons that anal lesions of some kind occur in 75% of patients with Crohn's disease of the large bowel, and when the rectum itself is involved the incidence of such lesions is nearly 100%. However I can recall patients with rectal involvement who had no obvious anal lesions.

The commonest anal lesion is an *anal fissure*, which like the fissures encountered in colitis differs from idiopathic anal fissures in being really a broad ulcer rather than a crack, in occurring anteriorly and laterally as often as posteriorly, and in often being multiple. Associated with such fissures are often oedematous *skin tags. Anal abscesses* and *fistulas* are also common. But such fissures, abscesses and fistulas are also well-recognized complications of ulcerative colitis (see p. 718) which reduces their diagnostic significance in Crohn's disease. Unquestionably the most characteristic of the anal lesions of Crohn's disease is *gross anal* and *perianal ulceration* (Plate V, A, B, C and D), the features of which have been so clearly demonstrated by Lockhart-Mummery and Morson (1964). These ulcers are indolent and undermined and often exude a little thin pus. They extend from the anal margin both outwards into the perianal region and inwards up the anal canal. Their size is very variable; some are 2–3 cm in diameter, others are very extensive and reach forwards on to the vulva and laterally as far as the ischial tuberosity, whilst deeply they may invade the ischiorectal fat and sphincter muscles, sometimes producing great destruction of tissue. An important point about these anal ulcers is that they never occur in ordinary ulcerative colitis, and, when found in cases of Crohn's disease, are invariably associated with involvement of the rectum itself.

Not infrequently the anal complications are the presenting manifestation of Crohn's disease, and, as emphasized on p. 176, every apparently idiopathic anal abscess or fistula should be regarded as possibly indicating the existence of an underlying Crohn's lesion of the intestinal tract. Histological examination of the granulation tissue in the wall of the abscess or fistula may reveal the typical appearances of Crohn's disease, and further investigation by radiological study may disclose an associated lesion in the small or large bowel. As Morson and Lockhart-Mummery (1959*b*) and Gray et al. (1965) have pointed out, sometimes an intestinal lesion cannot be demonstrated at the time, but becomes evident after an interval of months or years.

RECTAL EXAMINATION AND SIGMOIDOSCOPY

Digital palpation may detect rigidity of the rectal wall, a 'cobbled' mucosa or a stricture of the rectum, but is just as frequently quite negative. Sigmoidoscopy may also fail to reveal any abnormality for, as already pointed out, the rectum itself is spared by Crohn's disease of the large intestine in about half the cases. But even in these cases some pus or blood may be observed through the sigmoidoscope descending from above and, if the examination can be pressed to reach the sigmoid, the lower end of the diseased area may possibly be glimpsed. In patients with involvement of the rectum I agree entirely with Lockhart-Mummery and Morson (1964) that the *sigmoidoscopic findings are often quite distinctive* and usually differ strikingly from those seen in ulcerative colitis. In some cases the mucosa has the typical 'cobblestone' appearance, in others there are patchy changes with discrete ulcers separated by normal or nearly normal rather oedematous mucosa—highly suggestive findings of Crohn's disease, which may be confirmed on rectal biopsy.

OTHER COMPLICATIONS

ABDOMINAL FISTULAS

A characteristic of Crohn's disease is the tendency to produce abdominal abscesses, which subsequently discharge to the exterior or into a related viscus, such as another loop of bowel, the urinary bladder, the vagina or the ureter and thus form either an external or an internal fistula—or a combination of both. In an analysis of some years ago of 332 of my cases of Crohn's disease, 81 were found to have developed abdominal fistulas, and, as some patients had multiple fistulas, the total number of fisulas was 94. Forty-five were external and 49 internal (to other parts of the intestinal tract in 33 and to the genitourinary tract in 16). The incidence of abdominal fistulation varied according to the site of the primary intestinal lesion, being 23% with purely small bowel lesions, and 21% with mixed small and large bowel lesions, but only 9% with disease confined to the large bowel. As regards fistulae connecting with the urinary tract, the tendency for Crohn's disease of the ileum to fistulate into the bladder is well known and as Williams (1954) pointed out this is perhaps the second commonest cause of an intestinovesical fistula.

In 75 cases of large-bowel Crohn's disease, Lockhart-Mummery and Morson (1964) noted the existence of abdominal fistulas in 10; two were coloenteric, one each to the duodenum and small bowel, two were colocutaneous and four were rectovaginal. Such abdominal fistulas do not occur with ulcerative colitis, except for rectovaginal fistulas, which were present in 3·6% of a series of 275 female colitic patients under my care (de Dombal et al. 1966)—and this may be a helpful additional point of differentiation between these two forms of colitis.

CUTANEOUS ULCERATION

As emphasized on p. 833, ulceration may occur in the perianal skin in cases of Crohn's disease of the large bowel and may extend widely in the perineum and sometimes into the external genitalia, with the production of an extensive raw area. In addition, however, cutaneous ulceration may appear in the abdominal wall alongside a colostomy or ileostomy, which is itself the seat of Crohn's disease—comparable to the spreading ulceration that may arise in relation to a colostomy in a case of amoebic dysentery (see p. 866)—or an isolated area of ulceration may occur, say, in the submammary fold of skin in a patient suffering from intestinal Crohn's disease (Mountain 1970). In any of these forms of cutaneous ulceration it is usually possible to demonstrate a typical sarcoid reaction on biopsy of the ulcer.

ULCERATION OF THE MOUTH, PHARYNX AND LARYNX

In a few recent cases of Crohn's disease of the intestine, lesions have been described in the lips, mouth, pharynx and larynx, which have presented clinical and histological features suggesting that they are also affected by this condition (Croft and Wilkinson 1972; Bishop et al. 1972).

PSOAS ABSCESS

A rare complication of Crohn's disease of the small or large intestine is the occurrence of a psoas abscess, the features of which in this connection have been reviewed by Kyle (1971b) and Ramus and Shorey (1975). I have encountered psoas or lumbar abscesses on three occasions in association with Crohn's disease of the large bowel.

SEPTIC ARTHRITIS OF HIP

London and Fitton (1970) describe two cases of septic arthritis arising in the hip joint as a direct extension from contiguous intestinal lesions of Crohn's disease.

NON-SUPPURATIVE ARTHRITIS, SKIN COMPLICATIONS, EYE COMPLICATIONS

Quite apart from the septic arthritis and cutaneous ulceration described above, patients with Crohn's disease can develop as systemic complications non-suppurative arthritis and certain skin and ocular manifestations in exactly the same way as do patients with ulcerative colitis, as Hammer et al. (1968) and Thayer (1970) have emphasized. These extraintestinal complications may arise simultaneously with the lesion in the bowel or may apparently precede or follow its appearance.

Arthritis. This seems to be of two types. One is a subacute, migratory asymmetrical polyarthritis, usually involving the knees and ankles, although almost any joint may be involved. Tests for rheumatoid arthritis are negative and the condition usually undergoes complete resolution without limitation of movement. Hammer et al. (1968) noted this type of arthritis in 22% of their cases of Crohn's disease.

The second type of arthritis is ankylosing spondylitis, which may be either asymptomatic (diagnosed only radiologically) or severely crippling (Acheson 1960b; Ansell and Wigley 1964). There is no close correlation between the severity of the arthritis and that of the bowel lesion, and the joint condition does not always improve on removal of the intestinal condition.

Both types of arthritis were found in 9% of our patients with Crohn's disease in Leeds.

Skin Manifestations. These have been reviewed by McCallum and Kinmont (1968) and include erythema nodosum, pyoderma gangrenosum and psoriasis; 6% of our patients with Crohn's disease in Leeds had such skin complications.

Ocular Manifestations. Uveitis, keratitis, episcleritis and conjunctivitis have all been described in Crohn's disease (Korelitz 1967). Collectively these ocular complications occurred in 5% of our series of 332 cases of Crohn's disease.

Finger Clubbing. This complication was noted by Fielding and Cooke (1971a) in 58% of 181 patients with Crohn's disease. It was related to the activity but not the site of the enteritis, and usually disappeared within two or three months of the latter becoming quiescent.

Diffuse Periostitis. Symmetrical periostitis has been recorded in Crohn's disease by Neale et al. (1968).

HEPATOBILIARY DISEASE

There is good evidence of an increased incidence of hepatic and biliary tract disease in Crohn's enteritis, comparable to that which occurs in ulcerative colitis (see p. 729).

Hepatic Disease. One of the best studies is that of Eade et al. (1970). In 100 consecutive patients with Crohn's disease, liver function tests were performed, and in 49 of them a liver biopsy specimen was obtained either by a biopsy needle or as a wedge removal at laparotomy if operation was carried out. Alterations of liver function were seldom observed, but in the 49 patients from whom biopsy material was taken hepatic histological abnormalities were found in 94%, and these were more than minor in 71%. The commonest change was increased hepatic fibrosis—the so-called pericholangitis—as in ulcerative colitis, but generally less severe than in colitis. No patient had serious liver disease, such as cirrhosis. The amount of hepatic fibrosis was greater the more extensive the disease in the bowel, and particularly if the large intestine was involved. Cohen et al. (1971) and Perrett et al. (1971) reported incidences of pericholangitis on liver biopsy in patients with Crohn's disease of 75% and 50% respectively. The cause of these hepatic changes in Crohn's disease is just as debatable as in ulcerative colitis (see p. 729).

Disease of the Biliary Tract. Loss of functioning ileum due to disease or surgical excision is now known to have an adverse effect on the enterohepatic circulation of bile acids, with a consequent predisposition to the development of gall-stones (Heaton and Read 1969; Cohen et al. 1971; Dowling et al. 1972). In this connection it may be mentioned that in a special survey of 33 of my patients who had had proctocolectomy with resection of a variable amount of lower ileum gall-stones were found to have developed in no less than 12 (Hill et al. 1975). Of 22 cases in which the amount of ileum excised was less than 10 cm seven subsequently produced gall-stones, whilst of 11 cases in which a greater amount of ileum had been removed five were later found to have developed gall-stones. Clearly cholelithiasis is a major complication of sacrifice of lower small bowel.

Sclerosing cholangitis has been described as occurring in association with Crohn's disease by Atkinson (1965).

PEPTIC ULCER

Fielding and Cooke (1970a) report an incidence of peptic ulcer of 8% in their series of some 300 cases of Crohn's disease and quote several comparable frequencies of ulcer formation in other published series. They speculate as to whether this is a higher incidence than in the general population and also whether some of the ulcers might be secondary to gastric hypersecretion following extensive small bowel resection (see p. 793). But unfortunately representative figures for the frequency of peptic ulcer in the population at large are not available. It is noteworthy, too, that more than half of Fielding and Cooke's (1970a) patients with Crohn's disease and peptic ulceration first manifested their ulcers before resection of their Crohn's lesions was undertaken.

OBSTRUCTIVE UROPATHY AND LITHIASIS

Schofield et al. (1968), Enker and Block (1973), Mooney and Sant (1973) and Fasth et al. (1976) have drawn attention to the occasional occurrence in patients with Crohn's disease of periureteric fibrosis implicating the right ureter at or below the pelvic brim and causing hydronephrosis which necessitated ureterolysis. Schofield (1974) also alleges an increased incidence of urolithiasis in cases with Crohn's disease.

AMYLOID DISEASE

Amyloidosis is a rare complication of Crohn's disease. According to Fausa et al. (1977), who observed amyloid disease as a complication in seven of 85 patients with Crohn's disease, only 20 examples of this complication of the condition have been recorded in the literature. Renal involvement is the serious development in these cases and renal function is apt to deteriorate rapidly after operation. However, Fausa et al. (1977) feel that in some cases progression of the amyloidosis may be delayed or halted by timely surgical treatment of the Crohn's disease.

RADIOLOGICAL EXAMINATION

The radiological findings have been well described by Wolf and Marshak (1962), Lindner et al. (1963) and Simpkins (1972).

BARIUM ENEMA STUDIES

Distribution of Lesions. One way in which the radiological examination may be helpful in diagnosis is by defining the pattern of involvement of the large intestine. The finding of a short segmental lesion or stricture (Fig. 606), 'skipping' (Fig. 607) or non-involvement of the rectum should be regarded as strong presumptive evidence in favour of Crohn's disease.

Detailed Radiographic Appearances. In Crohn's disease the radiological appearances are usually less uniform than in ulcerative colitis. The contour of the bowel is generally more irregular, with greater rigidity of the wall and more contraction of the lumen, but sometimes areas of apparently normal mucosa and haustration may be evident in the midst of grossly diseased bowel. A 'cobblestone' mucosa may be recognizable radiologically as a shaggy nodular outline to the bowel (Fig. 608), and deep linear ulceration or fissuring of the mucosa can sometimes be shown in the form of fine radiating spikes (Fig. 609). The demonstration of a leak of barium outside the bowel lumen into an abscess cavity or skin surface is virtually diagnostic of Crohn's disease, for internal fistulas, other than rectovaginal communications, do not occur in ulcerative colitis.

But it must be admitted that the radiological findings are sometimes equivocal as between Crohn's disease and ulcerative colitis or the radiological diagnosis does not agree with the pathological findings.

BARIUM PROGRESS MEAL OR SMALL BOWEL ENEMA

Though the lower ileum may be outlined by reflux of opaque medium from the colon during a barium enema examination, a full study of the small bowel is also indicated in these cases to exclude an independent focus of Crohn's disease higher up in the ileum or jejunum.

SELECTIVE MESENTERIC ARTERIOGRAPHY

Though selective mesenteric arteriography has been advocated by some workers as a means of distinguishing between Crohn's disease and ulcerative colitis, it is doubtful if it has anything to offer over and above examination by conventional methods (see p. 706).

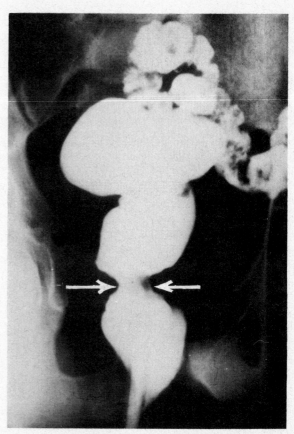

Fig. 606. Barium enema plate showing rectal stricture (indicated by arrows) due to Crohn's disease as proved by biopsy.

FURTHER INVESTIGATIONS

BIOPSY OF ANAL AND RECTAL LESIONS

As Lockhart-Mummery and Morson (1964) have shown, biopsy of anal ulcers or sigmoidoscopy of diseased rectal mucosa may be of great diagnostic value in revealing the presence of a focus of sarcoid reaction. However, a negative result is not significant. It may be due, for instance, to faulty technique in taking a rectal biopsy, so that the tissue is secured not from one of the patches of disease but from an area of normal mucosa. It may also be due to the sarcoid foci being very few in number so that they have been missed in the sections. In this connection a great deal depends on the skill and perseverance of the pathologist. Likewise, in the interpretation of the giant cell follicle, confusion may arise with foreign body giant cells and with tuberculosis. Morson (1971) stresses that, even when the rectal mucosa appears normal on sigmoidoscopy, histological evidence of Crohn's disease may sometimes be obtained on rectal biopsy.

As will be gathered, conventional histological examination of rectal biopsies sometimes fails to distinguish between ordinary ulcerative colitis and Crohn's disease. It remains to be seen whether the differences observed by Aluwihare (1971) and Cook and Turnbull (1975) on *electron microscopical* study of rectal biopsies from cases of Crohn's disease and ulcerative colitis may be of value in the future in making this differentiation in doubtful cases. It seems possible from the work of Filipe and Dawson (1970) that *histochemical examination* of rectal biopsies for mucins may be more helpful in this respect, in that acid non-sulphated mucins are present in Crohn's disease but are reduced in amount or absent in active ulcerative colitis.

FIBREOPTIC COLONOSCOPY

Since 1971–2 colonoscopy and colonoscopic biopsy have proved helpful in the diagnosis of certain cases of Crohn's disease of the colon and terminal ileum (see p. 70).

ESTIMATION OF SERUM LYSOZYME

Falchuk et al. (1975) suggested that the levels of serum lysozyme (muramidase) were elevated in patients with inflammatory bowel disease compared with normal individuals, and that usually much higher levels were found in Crohn's disease than in ulcerative colitis. It seemed, therefore, that this test might provide a useful aid in diagnosis and in differentiation of ulcerative from Crohn's colitis. Several other workers have also studied the levels of serum lysozyme in patients with inflammatory bowel disease and in normal individuals (Dronfield and

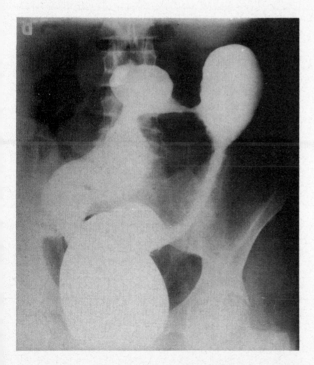

Fig. 607. Barium enema film of a female patient aged 60 with extensive Crohn's lesion of the colon producing considerable shortening and segmental stenosis. Pathological examination of the colectomy specimen showed the gross and microscopic appearances of a regional enteritis of Crohn's type.

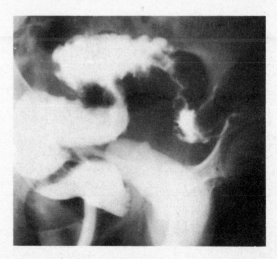

Fig. 608. Lateral view of rectum and sigmoid on barium enema examination in a case with granulomatous colitis, showing coarse nodularity of the bowel outline and also a marked stricture at the rectosigmoid junction.

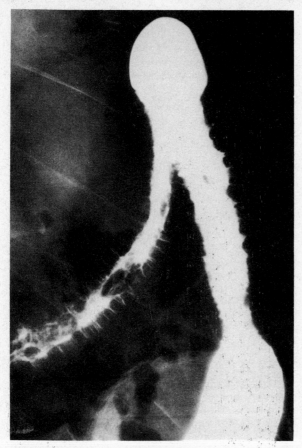

Fig. 609. Barium enema plate in a case of Crohn's disease showing radiating spicules of barium very characteristic of this condition. (*From Lockhart-Mummery and Morson 1964*)

Langman 1975; Nugent et al. 1976; Peeters et al. 1976; Hylander et al. 1976), and, whilst for the most part they agree that there are differences such as Falchuk et al. (1975) indicated, they feel that there is unfortunately too much overlap in the values for different categories of patients for the test to be of much practical assistance.

MANTOUX TEST

The Mantoux test has been found to be negative in 70% (Phear 1958) and 64% (Williams 1965) of cases of Crohn's disease, so that this reaction may be useful in helping to exclude a tuberculous lesion of the anal region.

KVEIM TEST

This test has long been regarded as highly specific for sarcoidosis, but the close similarity of the histological appearances in sarcoidosis and in Crohn's disease would certainly arouse interest as to the response to the test in this latter condition. However, Williams (1965) found consistently negative results with the Kveim test in patients with Crohn's disease. Then in 1969 Mitchell et al. reported positive responses in 50% of a series

of such cases. More recently, Siltzbach et al. (1971) have reaffirmed that in their experience the Kveim test is negative in Crohn's disease, and Williams (1971) in an extension of his series of tests found only one equivocally positive response in 32 cases. It appears from an annotation in *The Lancet* (1972, *1*, 188) that those who reported positive responses probably used a faulty batch of serum.

FAT BALANCE AND OTHER TESTS OF SMALL BOWEL ABSORPTION

In defining the extent of involvement of the small intestine, it may occasionally be advisable to supplement radiological examination after a small bowel meal by tests for malabsorption, preferably by a fat balance (see p. 77). The finding of gross malabsorption is evidence of extensive disease of the small intestine, and may have a considerable bearing on the treatment and prognosis of the case.

DIAGNOSIS

In most cases of Crohn's disease of the large bowel a careful review of the clinical and radiological features will leave little doubt as to the probable diagnosis. The points of particular diagnostic importance are: the occurrence of anal ulceration; the sigmoidoscopic findings, with either a normal rectum or a diseased rectal mucosa showing patchy lesions or a 'cobblestone' mucosa; and the radiological appearances. If a positive biopsy is obtained from an anal or rectal lesion, this is conclusive evidence, but even without this confirmation the clinician can often feel pretty certain of the diagnosis.

The diagnosis of Crohn's disease of the small bowel is often a good deal more elusive, because of the greater uncertainty of radiological findings in the small intestine compared with the large. As Dyer and Dawson (1970) have emphasized, patients may often languish under a diagnosis of psychoneurosis for a long time before the true nature of the condition is appreciated.

MEDICAL MANAGEMENT

CONVENTIONAL MEDICAL MEASURES

The medical treatment of Crohn's disease is in general unsatisfactory, in so far as there are no specific therapeutic agents available which can be relied upon to influence the course of the disease. In this respect medical therapy suffers the same limitations as in ulcerative colitis, and the physician has to depend on a varying use, as required, of the same non-specific measures employed in the treatment of the latter condition (Bárány 1971)—namely bed rest; high-protein, high-calorie, low-residue diet; blood transfusions or iron (or vitamin B_{12}) therapy; plasma or electrolyte infusions; antidiarrhoeal drugs, such as hydrophilic mucilloids or hemicelluloses, codeine phosphate up to 60 mg thrice daily, or, if impaired absorption of bile salts due to involvement or previous resection of the lower ileum, with their consequent leakage into the irritation of the colon, is deemed to be a factor in the production of the diarrhoea, the ion exchange resin cholestyramine, which has an affinity for bile salts, may be tried in a dose of 4 g four to five times daily (two hours after meals so as not to mix with the post-cibal chyme in the small intestine); sulphasalazine; and systemic or topical steroid therapy (see p. 730).

It is a common clinical experience that patients suffering from exacerbations of Crohn's disease of the large or small intestine sometimes seem to undergo a remission of their symptoms when placed on a medical regimen of the kind used in ulcerative colitis and including steroid therapy with or without sulpha-salazine (Jones and Lennard-Jones 1966). I can certainly recall many patients, particularly with Crohn's disease of the large bowel, who have made good immediate symptomatic responses to such medical measures, like patients with ulcerative colitis, and remained well subsequently for many months or sometimes longer (de Dombal et al. 1974). Not only has there been a complete resolution of symptoms and a return to very good general health, but abnormal sigmoidoscopic appearances have often reverted to normal and radiological abnormalities have likewise frequently improved. Small anal fissures have sometimes healed and small anal fistulas have become relatively quiescent, whilst systemic manifestations such as skin lesions may also have remitted temporarily. But the precise value of sulphasalazine and steroids in the treatment of Crohn's disease has only very recently been subjected to controlled clinical trial. Summers et al. (1978) found in the U.S. National Cooperative Crohn's Disease Study (NCCDS) that in the management of active disease, in the small bowel or ileocaecal region, steroids did better than a placebo, sulphasalazine not; if the condition affected mainly the large bowel, sulphasalazine was significantly better than placebo and steroids were not. As regards the treatment of quiescent disease by maintenance therapy, no advantage was shown in the NCCDS from the use of either steroids or sulphasalazine (Summers et al. 1978). This observation accords well with the frequent clinical finding that patients who have responded to medical treatment often relapse and operation often becomes necessary, as Jones and Lennard-Jones (1966), Jones et al. (1966), Sparberg and Kirsner (1966), Cooke and Fielding (1970) and de Dombal et al. (1974), have emphasized.

NUTRITIONAL SUPPORT BY INTRAVENOUS FEEDING OR ELEMENTAL DIET

A very topical subject is the use of total parenteral nutrition to improve nutrition and to afford bowel rest in the medical treatment of Crohn's disease and as a preparation for possible operation, or, as a less drastic move in the same direction, the administration of an elemental diet. The comments made on p. 732 in regard to the treatment of ulcerative colitis apply equally here.

RADIOTHERAPY

Radiation therapy for Crohn's disease was strongly advocated by Bargen (1957), but on critical analysis has not been found to be beneficial (Fruin et al. 1967).

IMMUNOSUPPRESSIVE THERAPY

The first reports of immunosuppressive therapy in Crohn's disease was from Winkelman and Brown (1965), who used *mechlorethamine* (nitrogen mustard) intravenously and claimed improvement in 9 of 13 patients treated. Since then several other favourable reports with immunosuppressive treatment have been published and also a number of complications noted, such as leucopenia and septicaemia, sometimes fatal. More recently *azathioprine* has been the drug of choice, because of its slow steady action, which makes it possible to adjust the dosage to a level giving a satisfactory therapeutic effect without producing serious toxicity, and also because it can be administered by the oral route. Brooke et al. (1969, 1970) have given an enthusiastic report of their results using this drug in a dose of 4 mg/kg body weight for 10 days and 2 mg/kg thereafter. They have treated 24 patients with various forms of Crohn's disease, some of whom were seriously ill and failed to respond to corticosteroid therapy. They reckon that there was an improvement in all but two patients and the criteria of improvement included the closing of fistulas, the healing of skin lesions and rectal ulcers, considerable gain in weight and restored capacity for work. Jones et al. (1969) have also used azathioprine in the treatment of Crohn's disease but in a small dose of 2 mg/kg and combined with a small dose of corticosteroids. Of 10 patients treated, four showed remarkable improvement but in the remainder there was no obvious benefit. My own experience, using azathioprine alone at an initial dosage of 4 mg/kg, has been similar to that of Lennard-Jones (1971), with no less than four of nine cases coming eventually to operation.

What has been badly needed to evaluate immunosuppressive therapy in this disease is the institution of controlled thera-peutic trials. Fortunately four of these have now been conducted and the outcomes recorded. In one trial by Rhodes et al. (1971) azathioprine was compared with a placebo in the treatment of active Crohn's disease and no significant advantage was obser-ved. Of eight patients with fistulas (six abdominal, one colo-vesical and one anal) treated by azathioprine in the trial, only one healed completely and another showed some improvement. In another trial by Willoughby et al. (1971) azathioprine was compared with a placebo in the maintenance of a remission of Crohn's disease secured by preliminary corticosteroid therapy. By somewhat sophisticated statistical methods they succeed in showing that the patients treated by azathioprine enjoyed some benefit over those treated by the placebo. In a further trial of azathioprine as maintenance therapy, O'Donoghue et al. (1978a) confirmed its value at St Bartholomew's and St Mark's Hospitals, London. In addition they emphasized that, in over 300 cases treated with this drug for inflammatory bowel disease at their hospitals, it has proved safe, with only one death attributed to immunosuppression (O'Donoghue et al. 1978b). Most recent of all is the trial of the NCCDS which has not shown any benefit for azathioprine over placebo in securing remission or in its subsequent maintenance (see Singleton, in Martin and Malchow 1979).

The evidence on the value of immunosuppressive therapy is thus contradictory. It has to be borne in mind, too, that this form of treatment is potentially dangerous and its continued use carries, amongst other hazards, the risk of stimulating the formation of malignant growths (Penn and Starzl 1970).

CROHN'S DISEASE AND PREGNANCY

The mutual interaction of Crohn's disease and pregnancy has been studied specially by Crohn et al. (1956), Fielding and Cooke (1970b) and ourselves (de Dombal et al. 1972). Our enquiry concerned 86 women who developed Crohn's disease whilst they were of child-bearing age. It showed that such patients, conservatively managed, were less fertile than normal, but that after surgical treatment for Crohn's disease the chances of a patient becoming pregnant were only marginally less than that of other members of the general population. The Crohn's disease had very little effect on the course of the pregnancy as a rule. As for the effect of the pregnancy on the intestinal lesion, it was found that, if anything, it exercised a beneficial effect. But after the delivery relapse of bowel symptoms was very common. There is thus considerable similarity between the effects of pregnancy on Crohn's disease and on ulcerative colitis (see p. 711).

On these findings it would not be reasonable to regard Crohn's disease as an indication for termination of pregnancy. But patients with Crohn's enteritis should be carefully supervised for three months after their confinement and might be well to be on steroid therapy during this time. It could, however, be argued that, as the long-term prognosis of Crohn's disease is apt to be poor, patients suffering from this condition would be well advised not to increase the number of persons dependent on them by having further children.

SURGICAL MANAGEMENT

The distinction that has been drawn earlier (p. 828) between Crohn's disease restricted mainly or completely to the small bowel and that confined chiefly or entirely to the large bowel is admittedly somewhat arbitrary and there are occasions when it is difficult to decide into which category to place a patient. But in discussing surgical treatment it is convenient to consider these two patterns of disease separately.

Disease Mainly or Entirely of Small Bowel (Classical Crohn's Ileitis or Ileocolitis)

INDICATIONS FOR SURGICAL TREATMENT

In the earlier years following the initial description of regional enteritis by Crohn et al. (1932) surgery was freely invoked in the treatment of this condition. But the not infrequent development of recurrence after operation led to a certain amount of disillusionment, which reached its climax following the publication by van Patter et al. in 1954 of their important paper on the late results of surgical treatment in a large series of patients suffering from this condition at the Mayo Clinic. They found a very high incidence of recurrence amounting to 80% after 15 years of follow-up. This melancholy report, and equally depressing ones from Cooke (1955) and Crohn and Yarnis (1958), had the effect of convincing many physicians and surgeons of the advisability of avoiding surgical intervention in this disease as far as possible and of reserving it essentially for cases in which it was specially indicated by the occurrence of abdominal or anal abscess formation or fistulation, of intestinal obstruction or of severe abdominal pain (Edwards 1964). For all other patients the

trend was towards conservative management in the first instance. But the fact has had to be faced that medical therapy has had very little to offer and that many of the medically treated patients have failed to progress satisfactorily on such a regimen and have subsequently developed complications, providing an indication for operation; consequently even conservatively minded physicians have had to resort to surgical treatment for the majority of their patients. For example Crohn and Yarnis (1958) reported that, of a personal series of 542 cases of regional enteritis, 385 (71%) needed operation. In my own experience of 165 cases of Crohn's disease mainly or entirely of the small bowel, no less than 133 or approximately 81% sooner or later came to surgery.

As regards the frequency of the different indications for surgical treatment, Farmer et al. (1976), in an analysis of 355 surgically treated cases of Crohn's disease mainly or entirely of the small bowel at the Cleveland Clinic, listed the indications for operation as abdominal abscess or fistula in 39%, intestinal obstruction in 42% and perianal disease in 8%. Unfortunately I cannot give precise figures for the specific indications in my own cases of mainly small bowel disease, but I am sure that intraabdominal abscess and fistula were not nearly as common as at the Cleveland Clinic and have no doubt that the severity of the alimentary symptoms and their intractability to conserative management was the most frequent indication, as it was in the experience of Glotzer and Silen (1975) and Young et al. (1975). The special problems presented by so-called 'acute ileitis' and its management at emergency operation are discussed on p. 850, as is also the tactical approach to acute intraabdominal or perianal abscess (pp. 850, 851), acute obstruction (p. 850) and perforation (p. 850).

SURGICAL METHODS AVAILABLE

For many years there was great controversy as to the relative merits of two methods of treating this form of Crohn's disease—*by-pass with unilateral exclusion* (i.e. division of the small bowel proximal to the lesion in the ileum, closure of the distal open end and anastomosis of the proximal open end to the side of the transverse colon beyond any disease) and *resection with anastomosis* (i.e. terminal ile-ectomy with or without some amount of right colectomy as well). It should be added that a simple by-pass without exclusion has generally been held to be of little curative value (Brill et al. 1969), though it proved very successful in the case of the late President Eisenhower of the USA (Heaton et al. 1964). It was the surgeons of the Mount Sinai Hospital, New York City (Garlock et al. 1951), who in the mid-1930s first advocated the by-pass exclusion procedure on the score that it was simpler and safer than resection and gave as good results. For a time it enjoyed a vogue, but, with the gradually increasing safety of surgery, the great majority of surgeons have preferred to use resection (Glotzer and Silen 1971; J. A. Williams 1971). There are, however, no good data establishing the superiority of one or other method, for, though the by-pass operation has given poorer results in many reported series (Atwell et al. 1965; Goligher et al. 1971a; J. A. Williams 1971; Koudahl et al. 1974; Young et al. 1975), it has often been reserved for technically difficult and possibly unfavourable cases and not always been combined with exclusion. Young et al.'s (1975) small series seems to emphasize the importance of including exclusion with by-pass. One clear indication for the use of a by-pass operation alone is Crohn's disease of the duodenum, which, if surgery is indicated, is best treated by gastroenterostomy (Fielding et al. 1970; Burgess et al. 1971; Paget et al. 1972; Farmer et al. 1972; Tootla et al. 1976).

As regards the now fashionable resection procedure, it can take several forms depending on the location and extent of the disease. If the lesion is entirely in the small bowel and with a good margin of normal ileum between it and the caecum, a simple small bowel resection with end-to-end anastomosis is what is required. But in many patients with a lesion in the lower ileum, the disease either extends a variable distance into the right colon or terminates so close to the ileocaecal valve that it is necessary to perform a certain amount of right colectomy as well as a terminal ile-ectomy to remove it adequately. Occasionally, depending on the extent of the original disease or of a recurrence or due to technical misjudgements regarding blood supply to the bowel at operation, considerably more of the small or large bowel may have to be removed. In some cases, it may be preferable to complete the operation, not with an anastomosis, but by bringing the proximal end of the bowel out as a temporary ileostomy and closing the distal end by suture (or exteriorizing it as an inactive opening). This step is particularly indicated in patients who have a very septic state of affairs in the peritoneal cavity due to a chronic abdominal abscess or fistula, and in cases with severe perianal disease but a normal left colon and rectum. Some idea of the frequency with which the various operative methods may be required is given in Table 68, which records the elective operations used by me in the treatment of 133 patients with Crohn's disease mainly or entirely in the small bowel. It will be ntoed that there were 98 primary operations and another 48 operations for recurrent disease.

FURTHER POINTS IN SURGICAL MANAGEMENT

CHOICE OF INCISION IN ELECTIVE OPERATIONS

Because of the way in which Crohn's disease may spread or recur in the intestinal tract, it is well to bear in mind that a patient who starts with resection of the terminal ileum may finish eventually with a proctocolectomy and ileostomy or for some other reason may need an ileostomy instead of an anastomosis. It is a good plan, therefore, to *keep the right lower quadrant of the anterior abdominal wall free from incisions* in case it is ever needed for an ileostomy, and to perform all resections—even right hemi-colectomies—through a left paramedian or median incision. Re-operations are best done through the scar of this wound. However, if another surgeon has previously used a right paramedian approach on the patient, it will probably be better to perform all further explorations and resections through this old wound and to keep the left half of the abdominal wall unscarred for any subsequent ileostomy (see p. 786), that is unless many years have elapsed and the scar of the old wound is soft, flat and pliable and not likely to make it difficult to fix an ileostomy appliance over it.

HOW MUCH BOWEL AND MESENTERY TO EXCISE?

Surgical opinion is divided as to how great a margin of clearance beyond ostensibly diseased bowel should be sought proximally and distally in resecting lesions of Crohn's enteritis (Glotzer and Silen 1971; J. A. Williams 1971; Goligher et al. 1971*b*). Some surgeons are satisfied to keep relatively close to the lesion, others such as Garlock and Crohn (1945), Wenckert (1971) and Krause et al. (1971) believe that a generous segment of, say, 10–

30 cm should be excised above and below the affected area. An additional argument for wide removal of apparently normal bowel proximal to the lesion is that recurrence most commonly develops immediately above the anastomosis (see p. 842), which might suggest that it originated in residual disease that had not been eliminated at the original operation. Equally debatable is the question as to how much mesentery should be removed along with the bowel and, in particular, how energetically the surgeon should aim to take away enlarged lymph nodes. Vigorous pursuit of enlarged nodes will often mean sacrificing a very much larger segment of bowel than would otherwise be necessary. It has to be remembered, too, that nodes may be considerably swollen for simple reactive changes without exhibiting the typical histological picture of Crohn's disease (see p. 830).

Unfortunately, until recently there was no good comparative information to show whether the choice of a more 'radical' or more conservative type of resection as regards excision of bowel and lymph nodes made any significant difference to the risk of recurrence. But in a very recent study Bergman and Krause (1977) were able to point to a recurrence rate of 29% after 'radical' operations as contrasted with 84% after 'non-radical' both in a follow-up period of $7\frac{1}{2}$ to $19\frac{1}{2}$ years. It is not clear, however, whether the two series of cases in this study were strictly comparable, for it was certainly not a controlled trial. My own practice has been to aim for removal of 12–20 cm of apparently normal bowel proximal and distal to the lesion but, on completing the excision and before carrying out the anastomosis, to open up the specimen to make sure that the disease has not extended more widely on the mucosal aspect than on the serosal surface and especially to exclude satellite ulcers beyond the main lesion. This naked-eye study is simpler and, I think, probably more valuable than frozen section examination of the bowel at the line of division, as advocated by Edwards (1964). If necessary, further bowel may then be excised. As for enlarged mesenteric nodes, I have usually removed these as widely as can be accomplished by a deep excision of mesentery not necessitating any major extension of the bowel resection.

TREATMENT OF VERY EXTENSIVE DISEASE OR MULTIPLE 'SKIP' LESIONS

A closely related question is what policy should be adopted in dealing with very long primary lesions or multiple 'skip' lesions or with recurrent lesions after a previous resection. Clearly patients with diffuse jejunoileitis are unsuitable for excisional surgery and are better left without any form of surgical treatment unless severe obstructive symptoms are present and there remains above and below the long diseased segment a small portion of normal jejunum and ileum respectively, when a simple side-to-side anastomosis may be performed between these parts of the gut, or between jejunum and colon or stomach and ileum. In patients with numerous skip lesions—I have had several with up to 24 skip lesions—it has to be decided whether it is possible or necessary to excise or by-pass some or all of the lesions. If the lesions are concentrated within one or two limited stretches of bowel it may be possible to remove them all with a single or double segmental resection comprising a total of, say, 1 m or so of intestine. Alternatively, if the lesions are more widely scattered, it may be wiser to leave them entirely untreated, or, if one or more of them in particular seem to be causing some degree of obstruction, to resect or by-pass these lesions and leave the rest *in situ*. As for patients who have already lost perhaps a third or more of their small intestine from one or two previous resections and develop a further recurrence, the surgeon should consider very carefully before advising further surgical intervention. If, however, his hand is forced from the development of obstruction or septic complications, he can take courage from the fact that it is possible for patients to survive in reasonably good health with only 1·75–2 m of upper small bowel, particularly if the deprivation of gut took place in stages and if the small bowel remnant has been joined to a normal transverse and left colon. In this connection a very interesting recent development has been maintenance on long-term domiciliary total parenteral nutrition of several patients who underwent total or subtotal removal of their small bowel for a variety of conditions (Broviac and Scribner 1974; Bordos and Cameron 1975; Jeejeebhoy et al. 1976).

OPERATIVE MORTALITY

The main risk of these various operations for mainly small bowel Crohn's disease, which usually involve an anastomosis, is of leakage with resulting peritonitis and possibly septicaemia. All the operative deaths listed in Table 68 were due to this cause. The mortality rates there shown of 4·4% for primary operations and 8·3% for subsequent ones are very similar to those reported in several other large series of surgically treated cases of Crohn's disease, in most of which the small bowel was the part chiefly affected: van Patter et al. (1954) 3·9%; Barbour et al. (1962) 2·4%, J. A. Williams (1971) 3·9% and Krause et al. (1971) 3·6%.

LATER RESULTS

RECURRENCE

The issue that has dominated consideration of the later results is the all too frequent development of recurrence of the disease, which has been fully documented in many publications including two previous ones of our own (Atwell et al. 1965; de Dombal et al. 1971b). Of my personal series of 98 patients undergoing primary surgery for Crohn's disease mainly or entirely of the small bowel (Table 68), 89 had had resection procedures. After exclusion of the three cases who died in the postoperative period

after such operations, three cases that died subsequent to discharge from hospital of unrelated causes, and five cases lost to follow-up, there are 81 patients who have been traced. Recurrence developed in 18 of these, an overall incidence of 22·3%. In 13 cases the recurrence was sited, as in the majority of other published recurrences, in the small bowel proximal to the anastomosis, in four it was both above and below the anastomosis and in one it was confined to the colon distal to the anastomotic site.

Factors Influencing the Incidence of Recurrence

Age and Sex of the Patient. In this series it was not possible to demonstrate a significant effect of the age of the patient on the frequency of recurrence, but in our previous studies (Atwell et al. 1965; de Dombal et al. 1971b) we were able to show, as Stahlgren and Ferguson (1961) had earlier done, that the risk of recurrence was greater in young patients. There was no significant difference in the incidence of recurrence according to the sex of the patients in the present series, though one of our previous studies (Atwell et al. 1965) suggested a slightly higher incidence in men.

Siting and Extent of Original Disease. Farmer et al. (1975) have reported a lower incidence of recurrence (21%) in patients whose lesion had been confined entirely to the small bowel than in those who had had ileocolic disease (27%). Bergman and Krause (1977) had no recurrences in 10 patients whose disease was restricted to the small bowel and left the lower ileum free, but 24 recurrences in 64 patients with the disease extending from the ileum into the caecum or right colon. In my personal series of 81 traced cases, the original disease was located solely in the small bowel in 41 with six recurrences (14·6%), and involved also the caecum or right colon in 40 with 12 recurrences (30%).

It would be reasonable to expect that the greater the extent of the original disease, the greater might be the risk of subsequent recurrence, and in fact van Patter et al. (1954), Schofield (1965), and we ourselves in one of our studies (Atwell et al. 1965) noted an increased incidence of recurrence in patients with an extensive segment of bowel involved. But in a latter study (de Dombal et al. 1971a) and in the present series it was not possible to confirm this

TABLE 68. *Primary and Subsequent Operations Used in the Treatment of 133 Patients with Crohn's Disease Mainly or Entirely of Small Bowel*

Operations employed	Primary		Subsequent	
	No. of cases	Operative deaths	No. of cases	Operative deaths
Small bowel resection (SBR)	5	0	3	0
SBR and right colectomy (RC)	75	2	34	3
SBR and RC with ileostomy	3	0	5	0
SBR and RC and separation of sigmoid	2	1	0	0
SBR, RC and sigmoid colectomy	4	0	0	0
SBR and subtotal colectomy with anastomosis	0	0	1	0
Complete proctocolectomy with ileostomy	0	0	1	1
Small bowel bypass	5	1	1	0
Ileotransverse anastomosis	2	0	1	0
Gastroenterostomy	1	0	1	0
Laparotomy alone	1	0	1	0
All operations	98	4 (4·1%)	48	4 (8·3%)

trend, partly because the pathological data were in many cases inadequate for adjudicating on this point. A related issue is whether the frequency of recurrence was affected by the size of the margins of clearance of the disease in the original operative specimen. Regrettably this was a point on which documentation was inadequate in all our studies and in most reported series, a notable exception being that of Bergman and Krause (1977), in which, as already mentioned (see p. 841), the incidence of recurrence was 29% in cases with a wide margin of clearance and 84% in those with a much narrower margin.

The Length of Time since Resection. It is generally agreed that the most important factor in determining the frequency of recurrence is the length of time that has elapsed since the original operation. Thus in the present series, if all 81 cases followed up 1–18 years are considered, the recurrence rate is 18 of 81 (22·2%); if only 48 cases followed up at least five years are considered, the rate is 14 of 48 (29·2%); whilst, if the study is confined to 26 patients followed up at least 10 years, the rate is 12 of 26 (46·2%). In Bergman and Krause's (1977) survey, which includes a few cases with what has been termed above (see p. 828) mainly large bowel Crohn's disease, on a 7·5 to 19·5 year follow-up the incidence of recurrence was 72 of 141 (51%). The general impression is that the predisposition to recurrence is a continuing factor predisposing to a steadily increasing accumulation of recurrences the longer the follow-up (de Dombal et al. 1971b), but most studies contain inadequate data on the outcome at longer terms of follow-up than 15 and 20 years.

Treatment of Recurrent Disease by Re-Resection

It would be not unreasonable to surmise that the risk of recurrence after a re-resection for a previous recurrence might prove greater than that after a primary resection of Crohn's disease. Indeed Lennard-Jones and Stalder (1967) have produced information to this effect and Bergman and Krause (1977), who had a recurrence rate of 51% after 141 primary resections, report 60% of re-recurrences after 56 second resections for recurrences, and 76% of re-recurrences after 34 third resections for recurrence. On the other hand, our previous study (de Dombal et al. 1971a) did not find any increased tendency to recurrence after second and third operations. The subject is a difficult one on which to adjudicate, as Grogono and Parks (1972) have pointed out, because of possible differences in the length of follow-up after these various operations which could profoundly affect the chance of recurrence and also because of the lack of uniformity of the criteria for diagnosis of recurrence.

In this context the findings in the re-operation cases listed in Table 68 are of interest. They comprise second and sometimes third operations on cases that recurred after the primary operations recorded in Table 68, and also a number of re-operations on 35 patients who had had previous resections in other hospitals. Of these 48 re-operations, 44 involved further resection. After excluding the four patients who died during the postoperative period, four who died of related or unrelated causes after discharge from hospital and four who were lost to follow-up, 32 patients remained for assessment of the risk of recurrence. Seven developed recurrent disease, an overall incidence of seven of 32 (21·8%). But if only the 22 patients followed up for at least five years are considered, the incidence is six of 22 (27·3%). These figures, when compared with the recurrence rates at different times after primary resections (see above), are encouraging, but they are not the only factor to be considered when contemplating operation for recurrence. Others are the amount of healthy small bowel that remains as

well as the extent of the recurrence and the nutritional state of the patient (see below).

GENERAL AND SYMPTOMATIC STATE OF PATIENT

As has already been emphasized by us (de Dombal et al. 1971a) and Bergman and Krause (1977), as important an aspect of the outcome of surgery for Crohn's disease as the development of recurrence is the state of the patient's general health and the presence or absence of troublesome side-effects of operation, such as diarrhoea, anaemia, malnutrition and gall-stones. Fortunately the tendency to diarrhoea after resection of small bowel with or without the ileocaecal valve and right colon, can usually be largely corrected with codeine phosphate, loperamide, Lomotil or cholestyramine. Similarly the impairment of vitamin B12 after ileal resection can be compensated for by monthly injections of this vitamin. Unfortunately the interference with the enterohepatic circulation of bile acids after ileal resection cannot be corrected by any medical means and these patients are exposed to an increased risk of developing cholesterol gall-stones (Hill et al. 1975). Depending on the extent of the resection nutrition may be grossly impaired, but even with the loss of a third, a half or even more of the small intestine the nutritional state may be quite good. For example in a recent review of 43 patients after small bowel resection, mostly for Crohn's disease and in some with residual disease present, Compston and Creamer (1977) found that half of them were at or above their 'ideal' weight, and only five were prevented from working because of their condition. In another study of 28 patients who had been subjected to much more extensive small bowel resections (75–270 cm) Kristensen et al. (1974) reported that only three cases were incapacitated by diarrhoea, and half the patients were fit for full work, another quarter for somewhat reduced work, and the remaining quarter completely unfit.

Bergman and Krause (1977) placed their patients in three categories according to their general health and functional state: (A) perfect, (B) some restriction of capacity for work or leisure activities because of tiredness or diarrhoea and (C) patients severely incapacitated by debility diarrhoea or complications; 87% of their cases fell into Category A, 9% into Category B, and 4% into Category C.

Disease Mainly or Entirely of Large Bowel

INDICATIONS FOR SURGICAL TREATMENT

The indications for surgical intervention are essentially the same as in ulcerative colitis, but the clinician has to bear in mind one most important distinction. It is that, by contrast with ulcerative colitis, for which removal of the entire large bowel, though possibly followed by a stormy convalescence and many complications, affords a certain guarantee that there will never be any reassertion of the primary disease, in Crohn's colitis no such assurance can be given. Recurrence of the Crohn's disease can occur in other parts of the alimentary tract and, even if there is considerable dispute as to the precise frequency of such recurrences (see p. 846), the fact that there is a significant risk of reappearance of the disease naturally enjoins some caution on the clinician in his resort to surgery. Depending on how highly he rates the risk, his attitude towards surgical treatment may vary from somewhat discriminating to ultra-conservative.

FAILURE OF MEDICAL TREATMENT

Crohn's colitis is distinguished from ordinary ulcerative colitis by several characteristic features (see p. 832), but there are many points of similarity between these two conditions. Certainly the Crohn's form often pursues a relapsing course like ulcerative colitis, and the more acute episodes seem not infrequently to respond well to the sort of medical treatment that is used for acute exacerbations of ordinary colitis with sulphasalazine and intensive steroid therapy (see p. 730). I have been impressed by the response of many of my Crohn's patients, with complete remission of symptoms and reversion of a grossly inflamed rectal mucosa on sig-moidoscopy to complete normality. This happy outcome has been secured even in some initially most unpromising cases. I am sure, therefore, that medical treatment as for ordinary colitis should be vigorously pursued in the first instance as a rule for Crohn's colitis. Patients thus treated successfully may remain well for periods of months or weeks or indefinitely, but further more severe attacks in due course are common. These in turn may respond equally well to an intensive medical regimen, but eventually the frequency, severity or inconvenience of these recurring episodes, or the fact that the patient remains in a chronically ill and debilitated state, may constitute an indication for resorting to surgery. In this context a rare additional factor to be considered is the fear of retardation of the physical development of young pre-pubertal patients. On the other hand, though there is some evidence to suggest that Crohn's disease of the small bowel may predispose to the occurrence of car-cinoma, there are no convincing data to incriminate Crohn's disease of the large bowel in such pre-disposition, and certainly the risk of malignant change in Crohn's disease of large or small bowel has not so far been considered sufficiently genuine to be taken into account when framing indications for surgery or indeed planning the actual operative programme.

SYSTEMIC OR LOCAL COMPLICATIONS

The indication for surgery may be strengthened by the presence of troublesome systemic complications, such as arthritis, or of gross local complications such as, rarely, stricture formation or the occurrence of an abdominal abscess or fistula, or, commonly, the development of severe anal complications. The latter are so important that their relation to surgical intervention will be specially discussed on p. 851.

SEVERE ACUTE EXACERBATIONS THAT FAIL TO RESPOND TO MEDICAL TREATMENT

Increasing experience of Crohn's disease of the large bowel has shown that a not infrequent indication for surgical treatment is the failure of one of the more severe attacks to remit on medical treatment, so that an urgent or emergency operation may be required exactly as in certain similar acute episodes of ordinary ulcerative colitis. I reckon that just under 15% of the operations done by me for Crohn's disease of the large bowel have been performed under these circumstances. The cases dealt with included some with toxic megacolon, even perforation and massive haemorrhage.

PROPORTION OF PATIENTS COMING TO OPERATION

Obviously the proportion of patients submitted to operation in any series of cases of Crohn's disease of the large bowel will be considerably influenced by the composition of the original series. If it is made up largely of patients referred to physicians for medical or surgical treatment there is quite a good chance that quite a number of cases will be managed satisfactorily along medical lines. For example at the Nutritional and Intestinal Unit at the General Hospital, Birmingham, England, of 204 patients seen with Crohn's disease of the large bowel between 1950 and 1972, 73 or roughly 36% proceeded to operation (Steinberg et al. 1974). In my practice most patients are sent for a surgical opinion and with operative treatment very much in the mind of the referring physician or surgeon. Of the 353 patients with Crohn's colitis so referred between 1958 and 1977, 250 (71%) were actually treated surgically by me, a total of 326 operations and re-operations being employed in the process.

SURGICAL METHODS AVAILABLE

TEMPORARY DEFUNCTIONING ILEOSTOMY FOLLOWED BY LATER RESTORATION OF CONTINUITY

As pointed out on pp. 733–4, though ileostomy alone sometimes led to the subsidence of the inflammation in the large bowel in ulcerative colitis, this step was rarely followed by complete resolution of the disease and it was seldom if ever that intestinal continuity could subsequently be restored. However, Truelove et al. (1965) and Oberhelman et al. (1968) suggested that Crohn's colitis might respond more favourably, particularly if a double-barrelled technique of ileostomy were used to allow topical steroid therapy to be administered to the colon through the distal opening. Unfortunately a further report from Oberhelman and Kohatsu (1971) indicated that the earlier optimistic expectations for this method of treatment had not been anything like fully realized. Of 21 patients with Crohn's colitis submitted to this regimen by Oberhelman et al. (1968) only six had proceeded to closure of their ileostomies; three of these remained well, but three had had further relapses or inflammation. Jones et al. (1966), Burman et al. (1971b) and McIlrath (1971) have recorded similarly disappointing results with exclusion by ileostomy (or colostomy) in the treatment of Crohn's disease of the colon and rectum.

RESECTION

It is not generally agreed that excisional surgery offers the best prospects. It may take several forms. A short segment of disease may be easily and satisfactorily removed by a very localized *segmental colectomy with colocolonic anastomoses*, but such cases are rare. Much more commonly the disease is widespread in the large bowel and its excision requires more extensive operations like those used for ordinary ulcerative colitis, but with some additions and possibly with a slight difference of emphasis due to two special features of Crohn's disease of the large bowel.

One feature is the involvement of more or less of the lower ileum in nearly half the patients with primary Crohn's disease of the large bowel coming to operation. It means that in that proportion of cases a *variable amount of ile-ectomy* has to be combined with the colectomy, with the sort of implications in regard to the functional and nutritional state of the patients indicated in connection

with resection for Crohn's disease of the small bowel on p. 843, but compounded by the fact that these large bowel cases usually have an ileostomy as well.

The other feature is that in nearly a quarter of the patients with Crohn's disease mainly or entirely confined to the large bowel, the rectum and possibly some of the distal sigmoid colon are apparently normal (see Fig. 603). This state of affairs naturally provides the surgeon with a strong incentive to consider keeping this ostensibly normal distal large bowel and treating the condition by a *total or subtotal colectomy (possibly with some ile-ectomy) and an ileorectal or ileosigmoid anastomosis* using a similar technique to that described for this operation for familial polyposis (see p. 365). But, when employed for inflammatory bowel disease, ileorectal or ileosigmoid anastomosis seems to carry increased risks of anastomotic dehiscence according to several reports (see p. 847), due either to the disease being more extensive than was originally imagined and involving some of the remaining rectal or ileal wall, or to the poor nutritional state of the patient. To lessen this immediate hazard of the operation it has been advocated by Lefton et al. (1975), Turnbull (1975) and Flint et al. (1977) that a covering loop ileostomy (see p. 759 for technique) should be established a short distance proximal to the anastomosis, but Burman et al. (1971a) and Weterman and Peña (1976) found that dehiscence still occurred despite such a covering ileostomy, though possibly there was less chance of serious leakage. Another method that may diminish the risks of dehiscence is to do the actual anastomosis at a second stage operation after a previous ileostomy and subtotal colectomy, leaving at least three to six months between the two stages in order to secure a full return to normal health before the second stage and also to verify as far as possible by repeat sigmoidoscopies in the interval that the rectum is indeed normal. The other serious disadvantage of colectomy and ileorectal anastomosis for Crohn's disease is that it is unquestionably followed by a high recurrence rate, not less than 50% in most published series (see p. 847).

My own experience confirms these drawbacks of ileorectal anastomosis and I feel that the operation should therefore be used with the utmost caution in Crohn's colitis, perhaps preferably as a two-stage procedure. It is to be noted, too, that, though Turnbull (1975) and his colleagues at the Cleveland Clinic (Lefton et al. 1975) warmly recommend this procedure, it has in fact been reserved for but 4% of the patients coming to surgery for Crohn's disease at that clinic.

The operations that have been mainly used for the treatment of Crohn's colitis are *ileostomy (possibly with some ileal resection) and complete proctocolectomy or subtotal colectomy* (for technical details see pp. 748–59). At one stage hopes were high that these procedures, unlike an anastomotic operation, would seldom be followed by recurrence (Cornes and Stecher 1961; Jones et al. 1966; Glotzer et al. 1970; Nugent et al. 1973) but more recent reports have shown that there is a progressive risk of recurrence, though there are differences of opinion as to the magnitude of the danger (de Dombal et al. 1971*b*; Goligher 1972; Korelitz et al. 1972; Ritchie and Lockhart-Mummery 1973; Steinberg et al. 1974). The chief objection to these operations from the patient's point of view is the ileostomy, which because of the not infrequent sacrifice of some lower ileum may act more profusely than that after ileostomy for ordinary ulcerative colitis and prove more difficult to manage. The other problem is the frequent delay in the healing of the perineal wound and the occasional need for re-operations for a persistent perineal sinus, not always with success. As between complete proctocolectomy and subtotal colectomy, the latter operation has the advantage of avoiding the problems of a perineal wound and, if the disease in the rectum or anal region is relatively slight (or the anorectum is questionably normal), little inconvenience may result from it and it may in fact largely subside. If the rectum should turn out to be normal or become so, a second stage ileorectal anastomosis can be considered after 6–12 months or longer, though many patients by then have become quite happy with their ileostomy and prefer not to proceed to a further major operation for an anastomosis, the success of which cannot be guaranteed in advance. Alternatively if the disease in the anorectum should become more severe and troublesome rectal excision may have to be advised as a second procedure.

If the disease is confined entirely to the rectum and possibly the distal sigmoid colon and surgical treatment becomes necessary, it may be quite adequately dealt with by *an abdominoperineal excision with terminal iliac colostomy.* Such a localized distal distribution of disease is relatively uncommon in most surgeons' experience and I have only used abdominoperineal rectal excision alone in a very few cases (Table 69) but at St Mark's Hospital, London, where this type of patient with purely rectal involvement is a good deal more common (Ritchie and Lennard-Jones 1976) presumably because of the more specialized clientèle there, very many more purely rectal excision have been performed. It is tempting in such cases with purely rectal disease to try the effect of a divided iliac colostomy alone in the first instance, being prepared to proceed to rectal excision later if the defunctioning provided by the colostomy does not secure an

TABLE 69. *Operations Employed and Immediate Mortality in Treatment of 225 Patients with Primary and 79 Patients with Recurrent Crohn's Disease of the Large Bowel (1958–77 Inclusive)*

Operations employed	For primary disease		For recurrent disease	
	Times used	Op. deaths	Times used	Op. deaths
Ileostomy and proctocolectomy*	124	11	10	0
Ileostomy and subtotal colectomy*	57	3	4	0
Rectal excision				
Complementing previous ileostomy and subtotal colectomy	10	0	0	0
Primary operation with iliac colostomy	8	1	0	0
Ileorectal, ileosigmoid or colocolonic anastomosis				
With primary total, subtotal or segmental colectomy*	36	1	0	0
After previous ileostomy and subtotal colectomy	12	0	0	0
Excision of recurrence following previous excisional surgery				
with abdominal stoma and establishment of new				
ileostomy	0	0	38	2
Excision of recurrence following previous colectomy and				
ileorectal or ileosigmoid anastomosis				
and establishment of new ileostomy	0	0	23	1
and construction of ileorectal anastomosis	0	0	4	0
All operations	247	16 = 6·5%	79	3 = 3·8%

* Including often resection of variable amount of ileum depending on the extent of the disease.

improvement in the condition of the rectum. I have to admit, however, that in the three cases in which I tried colostomy alone, the result was disappointing, my experience thus confirming that earlier recorded by Jones et al. (1966).

Whilst on the subject of more restricted distal disease the question of disease confined to the rectum and distal left colon, which in my experience is a good deal commoner than purely rectal lesions, should be raised. Disease of this extent could be removed by a *rectal excision and left colectomy* leaving the right colon and part of the transverse colon in position *and finishing with a transverse colostomy.* Unlike the situation in ulcerative colitis (see p. 736) removal of the normal right colon to give the patient a complete proctocolectomy and ileostomy has no special virtue in protecting the patient from recurrence of his Crohn's disease. The only argument for it is that an ileostomy may be more manageable than a transverse colostomy. I personally have not hitherto practised rectal excisions with left colectomy and transverse colostomy for Crohn's colitis, but Hughes (1977) has shown that the functional result of this operation can be very satisfactory. My feeling is therefore to use this method in the future in suitable cases.

Lastly a few words may be appropriate on the form of operation for recurrence after excision of Crohn's colitis either by resection with ileosigmoid or ileorectal anastomosis or excisional methods leaving an abdominal stoma (ileostomy or colostomy). After the former type of operation what is usually required is *excision of the terminal ileum, the anastomosis and the rectum or rectosigmoid, with establishment of an ileostomy.* Because of adhesions to adjacent loops of small gut and to structures at the brim of the pelvis, this may be quite a difficult undertaking with some additional risk of damage to small intestine or ureters. After previous proctocolectomy or subtotal colectomy and ileostomy, operation for recurrence in the ileum entails a laparotomy through the previous laparotomy wound, freeing of the ileostomy from the abdominal wall, with *resection of the diseased segment of bowel and mesentery* with a suitable margin of clearance, and *establishment of a new ileostomy* at the same site or, if there has been much peristomal sepsis or weakness of the abdominal wall, at a fresh site on the other side of the abdomen. Reassertion of disease in a retained rectal stump after subtotal colectomy simply requires *an abdominoperineal excision of this remnant.*

The extent to which I have used these various operative methods for primary Crohn's disease of the large bowel and its recurrences is indicated in Table 69.

OPERATIVE MORTALITY AND MORBIDITY

As Table 69 shows there were 16 operative deaths in my 247 operations for primary Crohn's colitis, an immediate mortality rate of 6·5% which is a little higher than in some other reported series (e.g. Ritchie and Lockhart-Mummery 1973: 2·5%; Steinberg et al. 1974: 4·1%), but my series includes no less than 34 patients undergoing urgent or emergency ileostomy and colectomy or proctocolectomy and 10 of the deaths occurred in this group of specially ill patients. In neither of the other two papers quoted is there any mention of such more acute cases being included. The causes of death were peritonitis and septicaemia in 11 cases and cardiopulmonary complications in five. One of the patients who died of peritonitis developed this complication as a result of an anastomotic dehiscence following ileorectal anastomosis. Two other patients from the group of 48 who had such anastomoses also developed leakages and had emergency operations for conversion to ileostomy with survival. Attention is also drawn to the risk of leakage after ileorectal anastomosis for Crohn's disease by Burman et al. (1971), Baker (1971), Adson et al. (1972), Weterman and Peña (1976) and Flint et al. (1977).

LATER RESULTS

RECURRENCE

After Resection with Anastomosis (Mostly Ileorectal or Ileosigmoid)
There were 44 patients available for assessment of the late results and no less than 27 (or approximately 61%) of these developed recurrence, 15 of the recurrences being in the terminal ileum, eight in the rectum and four in both ileum and rectum. Most of the ileal recurrences appeared in patients who had had involvement of the ileum at the time of the original operation, but in a few the ileum had not been implicated (Goligher 1979). Twenty of our patients with recurrence have proceeded to excision of the recurrent disease usually with rectal excision and ileostomy, but seven have been treated conservatively for their recurrence, with good to fair results in four or five.

These results are in keeping with those of other authors for this operation in Crohn's disease. Thus the recurrence rate is reported as 50% in 26 cases by Baker (1971), 60% in 25 cases by Burman et al. (1971a), 50% in 25 patients by Adson et al. (1972), 66% in 18 cases by Nugent et al. (1973), 53% in 65 cases by Lefton et al. (1975), 75% in 20 cases by Weterman and Peña (1976), and 32% in 37 cases by Flint et al. (1977). Several of these writers (Adson et al. 1972; Baker 1971; Weterman and Peña 1976) comment on the fact that recurrence could develop even when there had been no obvious original ileal involvement. Adson et al. (1972), Lepton et al. (1975) and Weterman and Peña (1976) make the point that, though surgical excision was usually required for recurrence, some patients seemed to be reasonably comfortable on conservative management. It is a sad commentary on the vagaries of clinical judgement that with such similar results some of the authors should recommend the operation more or less warmly, others condemn it!

After Primary Excision with Ileostomy (or Colostomy)

Of the 144 patients available for follow-up (for periods ranging from one year to 18 years) 19 (13·2%) developed recurrence in the bowel proximal to the stoma, most of them, as described previously (Goligher 1962), above the stoma but three more extensively in the remaining bowel (Goligher 1979). In seven cases the recurrence was detected within one year of the operation, in six between two and four years, in four between six and nine years, and in two between 10 and 12 years. There was no significant difference in the frequency of recurrence as between men and women, but younger patients had a higher incidence. Surprisingly, recurrence was not more common in patients whose original disease had extended into the terminal ileum than in those with the condition confined initially to the large bowel. But, as with Crohn's disease of the small bowel, the factor that has exercised most influence on the incidence of recurrence is the length of time elapsing since operation (Table 70). Clearly the incidence rises the longer the minimum period of follow-up for the group of cases studied, but, because of the much smaller numbers of patients available at the longer periods of follow-up, caution must be exercised in drawing conclusions as to the incidence of recurrence at 15–18 years or forecasting what the incidence is likely to be beyond that period.

There has been a wide variation in the estimates of the frequency of recurrence after excisional

TABLE 70. *Influence of Length of Follow-up on Frequency of Recurrence after Excisional Surgery with Ileostomy (or Colostomy) for Primary or Recurrent Crohn's Colitis*

Length of follow-up (years)	Primary colitis		Recurrent colitis	
	No. of cases	Recurrences	No. of cases	Recurrences
1–18	144	19 (13·2%)	70	12 (17·1%)
5–18	96	17 (17·7%)	46	12 (26·1%)
10–18	35	13 (37%)	27	9 (33·3%)
15–18	14	6 (43%)	8	3 (37·5%)

surgery with an abdominal stoma for Crohn's colitis in different series that have been published in the last few years. Glotzer et al. (1967, 1970) of Boston maintain that there is no tendency to prestomal recurrent Crohn's disease in these cases and that any stomal problems requiring re-operation are of the same nature as those encountered after similar operations for ulcerative colitis and no more frequent. It is hard to reconcile this view with the clear and unequivocal pathological evidence of recurrent disease in our Crohn's cases (Goligher 1972, 1979) and with Steinberg et al.'s (1974) careful comparative study of two groups of patients who had had ileostomy for Crohn's disease and ordinary ulcerative colitis respectively. At the other extreme are Korelitz et al. (1972) of the Mount Sinai Hospital, New York City, and Steinberg et al. (1974) of Birmingham, England, who report overall incidences of recurrence of 46% in 67 cases and 33% in 70 cases respectively and offer very sombre predictions as to the prospects of increasing incidence with more prolonged follow-up. Thus Steinberg et al. (1974) state that all six of the patients in their series who had been followed-up for more than 15 years had developed recurrence, which contrasts with our 43% incidence in 14 patients followed for that length of time (Table 70).

In between these extremes but closer to Glotzer et al.'s (1970) estimate are the incidences reported by Nugent et al. (1973) of the Lahey Clinic, Boston (3% in 28 cases), and Ritchie and Lockhart-Mummery (1973) of St Mark's Hospital, London (5% in 80 cases). It is particularly significant that Nugent et al.'s (1973) small series had all been followed-up for 10–15 years and yet only one recurrence developed. The follow-up period for Ritchie and Lockhart-Mummery's (1973) larger series ranged from two to 20 years and no recurrences were encountered at any shorter period than 10 years. Our own previous estimate of recurrence (de Dombal et al.

1971*b*; Goligher 1976) and the current one (Table 69) are admittedly higher than those of Nugent et al. (1973) and Ritchie and Lockhart-Mummery (1973), but they are certainly not as depressing as those of Korelitz et al. (1973) and Steinberg et al. (1974). What is particularly frustrating is our inability to explain why the frequency of recurrence should vary so dramatically in different centres.

Treatment of Prestomal Ileal and Colonic Recurrences. All but three of the patients who developed such recurrences were subjected to further surgical excision, the results of which are given in Table 70 along with the results of operations for recurrence in other cases. One of the three non-surgically treated patients has very extensive disease in the small bowel and is in a poor state of health. The other two have extensive lower ileal disease with periodically discharging enterocutaneous peristomal fistulas, but both adamantly refuse further operation; they remain in remarkably good general health considering their local condition.

It should be added that of 37 traced patients who were initially treated by us by ileostomy and sub-total colectomy and did not proceed to a secondary ileorectal anastomosis, no less than 27 showed evidence of *residual disease in the rectal stump on follow-up*. In many of them the existence of mild rectal inflammation had been recognized on pre-operative sigmoidoscopy. In most of these patients with persistent proctitis the general health has been good and the symptoms of rectal discharge and bleeding have been relatively slight and quite tolerable but in nine cases the discharge was much more profuse and rectal excision was necessary.

After Further Excision with Ileostomy for Recurrent Disease
Of 75 patients who developed recurrences after previous proctocolectomy, colectomy or rectal excision with ileostomy or colostomy or after colectomy and ileorectal or ileosigmoid anastomosis and were subjected to a further excision with ileostomy 70 were available for follow-up (Goligher 1979). Recurrence proximal to the stoma developed in 12 (14·7%), the interval between the re-operation and the appearance of the further recurrence was two to three years in five cases, four to five years in six cases and eight years in one. The influence of the length of follow-up on the frequency of recurrence is shown in Table 70. Unfortunately the number of patients followed-up for a very long time is small, but so far as the data go, they indicate a steady increase in the incidence of

recurrent disease the longer the follow-up but not at a very different level from that after primary operations.

As mentioned in dealing with recurrence after classical ileal or ileocolic Crohn's disease (see p. 843), there has been controversy as to whether the risk of recurrence is higher after re-resection than after primary resections (Lennard-Jones and Stalder 1967; de Dombal et al. 1971*a*; Grogono and Parks 1972; Bergman and Krause 1977). It would certainly seem from our analysis (Table 70) that re-operation for recurrence in cases of Crohn's colitis has a good deal to offer, and that is my personal clinical impression from dealing with many of these patients. But the full evaluation of re-resection and the decision about advising it in an individual patient involves consideration of its possible effects on his general and functional condition (see below).

GENERAL AND FUNCTIONAL STATE OF
PATIENTS

Three aspects of the overall results of excisional surgery with ileostomy for Crohn's colitis and its recurrences are particularly relevant:

Difficulties with Ileostomy Management
The not infrequent necessity when operating for Crohn's colitis of sacrificing some of the lower ileum exposes the patients concerned to the potential ill-effects of ileal resection mentioned on pp. 42, 843, and in addition means that the ileostomy resulting from proctocolectomy or subtotal colectomy is apt to act more profusely than that made for ordinary ulcerative colitis. Obviously the larger the amount of ileum resected, as in patients who have undergone one or more re-resection for ileal recurrence, the greater the tendency to an excessively loose output from the ileostomy and increased difficulties in stomal care due to leakage and soreness of the peristomal skin. Fortunately the latter can be obviated or substantially lessened in

TABLE 71. *Patient's Verdict on Inconvenience Caused by Ileostomy after Resection and Re-resection for Crohn's Colitis*

Inconvenience	Primary resection ($n = 119$)	Subsequent resection ($n = 62$)
Absolutely no trouble	68%	49%
Occasional skin soreness but easily manageable	24%	33%
Many problems with leakage and profuse output	8%	17%

many cases by the prescription of antidiarrhoeal agents and the use of specially bland sticking agents for the appliance such as Stomahesive.

A rough measure of how much residual inconvenience referable to the stoma was being experienced by my patients is provided by Table 71, from which it will be seen that the great majority—certainly after primary resection—have adapted well to their stoma and suffer little trouble on account of it.

Delay in Healing of the Perineal Wound

It is well recognized that healing of the perineal wound resulting from excision of the rectum for inflammatory bowel disease is often considerably delayed and this seems to apply more to cases of Crohn's disease than of ulcerative colitis (Watts et al. 1966a, b; de Dombal et al. 1971a; Ritchie and Lockhart-Mummery 1973). It is not uncommon for patients to require further operation for a persistent perineal sinus, not always successfully. Unquestionably these difficulties with perineal healing represent one source of partial dissatisfaction with the results of surgical treatment.

It is not always easy from ordinary clinical notes to determine retrospectively exactly how long it took for a perineal wound to heal. Accordingly, in our survey of the 117 patients who were followed up after rectal excision for primary Crohn's disease, no attempt was made to gauge the length of time required for final healing. Instead we have simply ascertained the current status of the perineum—whether soundly healed or the seat of persistent or recurring fistulas—and whether repeat operations had been necessary to secure complete healing. Sound healing was noted in 85% and persistent or recurring fistulation in 15%. Reoperations had been necessary in 18% of the cases.

TABLE 72. *Clinical Impression of General Health and Fitness after Resection and Re-resection for Crohn's Colitis*

Clinical impression	Primary resection (n = 119)	Subsequent resection (n = 62)
Very good. Patient fit for full work or ordinary activities	81%	73%
Fair. Patient managing most but not all ordinary activities	15%	19%
Poor. Patient considerably restricted or complete invalid	4%	8%

Overall Fitness and Capacity for Work and Recreation

On the basis of simple clinical assessment supplemented by information from the patient as to his workaday life and occasionally by haematological and biochemical investigations, the patients were grouped into three categories as shown in Table 72, from which it will be seen that after both primary and subsequent operations the great majority of patients managed to return to a reasonable state of general health and activity, but the proportion totally or partially incapacitated was greater after re-resection (27%) than after primary resections (19%).

Other Problems in the Surgery of Crohn's Disease

ACUTE MANIFESTATIONS OF CROHN'S DISEASE

Crohn's disease may present as an abdominal emergency in several ways.

Terminal Ileitis Mimicking Acute Appendicitis. Some patients present with pain of sudden onset in the right lower quadrant of the abdomen simulating that due to acute appendicitis, so that emergency operation is undertaken, at which the appendix is found to be normal but the lower ileum appears thickened and congested. Whether these cases are a form of Crohn's disease or a *Yersinia* infestation is debatable (Gump et al. 1967; Sjöström 1971; Goligher et al. 1971a; Kewenter et al. 1974). As the orthodox surgical management is to eschew any direct attack on the ostensibly inflamed small bowel (and not even remove the appendix because of the fear of a subsequent faecal fistula—though we have performed 35 appendicectomies in such a situation without development of any fistulas, and Kewenter et al. (1974) have had a very similar experience), histopathological information is lacking in most instances. Most of these patients do very well on this conservative regimen and have no further trouble, but about 30% subsequently develop typical chronic Crohn's enteritis (Goligher et al. 1971a). It would seen sensible in cases of acute terminal ileitis to request serological studies for *Yersinia enterocolitica* agglutinins, or indeed to try to isolate this organism by culture of the stool found in the appendix in such cases submitted to appendicectomy, as suggested by Winblad et al. (1966) and Gurry (1974). A very good account of *Yersinia* enteritis and enterocolitis is given by Vantrappen et al. (1977).

Acute Intestinal Obstruction. Acute intestinal obstruction may arise as the first manifestation of Crohn's disease or may occur as an emergency complication in a patient known to be suffering from chronic Crohn's disease, usually in the small intestine. If the obstruction does not respond to conservative measures, exploration will be required. The choice of operation will naturally depend on the precise findings at laparotomy. It may, for example, take the form of a simple by-pass or of a resection with anastomosis, but a very good safe procedure if the lesion is in the lower ileum is a resection finished by bringing both ends of bowel to the surface, the proximal one as a formal end-ileostomy (Goligher 1971). Restoration of continuity can be achieved at a second intervention some months later.

Free Perforation of the Lesion. Free perforation into the peritoneal cavity is a rare complication of Crohn's disease of the ileum, most usually occurring during an acute exacerbation of chronic disease associated with some degree of distal obstruction due to stenosis (J. A. Williams 1971). Treatment by simple suture with drainage has usually proved disastrous (J. A. Williams 1971; Menguy 1972). Primary excision of the perforated segment and all the distal diseased intestine is preferable and is better followed, not by an immediate anastomosis, but by exteriorization of the two ends of bowel, the active one being fashioned as an ileostomy to take an adherent bag. Menguy (1972) advocates a somewhat similar operation.

Abdominal Abscess. It is difficult to define the precise incidence of abdominal abscess formation in relation to Crohn's disease, but in several of the published series (Barbour et al. 1962; Colcock and Vansant 1960; Edwards 1969) it seems that 15–25% of the patients had complicating abdominal abscesses. Abscesses may arise spontaneously, probably as a result of slow penetration of the gut wall in Crohn's lesions that are being treated conservatively, or may occur as a complication of operative treatment. If the condition is managed expectantly with antibiotic therapy, the acute inflammation may subside—this process probably being assisted in many instances by spontaneous rupture into a neighbouring viscus such as a loop of intestine or the urinary bladder, with establishment of an internal fistula. Alternatively, the inflammation may persist and the tender mass may become larger and apparently closer to the surface, so that it is eventually possible to drain it surgically by a small incision without opening the general peritoneal cavity. Usually such drainage is followed by the development of an external abdominal faecal fistula. Occasionally in the course of an elective operation for Crohn's disease, an abscess is encountered in relation to the intestinal lesion; this may change the operative plan, but usually it is possible to proceed with resection, though it may be advisable after excising the diseased segment not to restore intestinal continuity but to establish a temporary terminal ileostomy.

Massive Haemorrhage. As J. A. Williams (1971) points out, massive bleeding is very rarely an indication for emergency resection in Crohn's disease. It should be borne in mind that haemorrhage in these cases may come not from the intestinal lesion, but from an associated peptic ulcer or from a steroid-induced ulcer.

ABDOMINAL FISTULAS

As pointed out on p. 834, abdominal fistulas, external or internal, are fairly common, especially with Crohn's disease involving the small intestine. They may arise spontaneously or may follow operation. Simple drainage of an intra-abdominal abscess in connection with Crohn's enteritis nearly always results in the development of an external faecal fistula. Resection operations may also be followed by faecal fistulation due to anastomotic dehiscence. Such dehiscence often indicates that the lesion has been incompletely removed and that the line of resection has inadvertently traversed diseased tissue.

Abdominal fistulas usually continue discharging, though perhaps with occasional intermissions, till any remaining diseased segment of bowel has been completely excised. With an external fistula it is not necessary additionally to excise the track

in the abdominal wall. Similarly internal fistulation (e.g. ileum to bladder or to sigmoid) does not usually spread the enteritis into the adherent viscus, so that it generally suffices to 'pinch' or dissect the ileum (or other part of gut) off it. When this is done, the resulting hole in the other organ is as a rule minute and the wall itself is soft and uninvolved. Under these circumstances it is adequate to close the perforation with a few sutures—or in the case of bladder, to leave it unsutured and rely on catheter drainage. Rarely, when the neighbouring viscus appears to be infiltrated with the disease, it is wiser to excise part of it.

In patients with external fistulas, particularly those situated high in the small intestine, there may be very gross malnutrition, which may add considerably to the risks of surgical treatment. The great advance in the management of such cases in recent years has been the introduction of efficient intravenous feeding which enables an adequate supply of calories to be administered in addition to replacement of fluid and electrolyte losses from the fistula (MacFadyen et al. 1973; Himal et al. 1974; Blackett and Hill 1978). With this regimen it may be possible to induce some fistulas to heal spontaneously over a period of several weeks, and even if this happy result is not achieved—and it was not in 70% of the series of 38 fistula cases treated along these lines by Aguirre et al. (1974)—the great improvement in the patient's nutritional state makes him a much better risk for surgical treatment. Aguirre et al. (1974) recommend that, as soon as the patient's general condition has been sufficiently improved, good radiological studies of the bowel with Gastrografin meals and sinography should be carried out to show the precise nature of the fistula. If a large abscess, distal obstruction or intestinal discontinuity is discovered, surgical intervention should be undertaken as soon as the patient's general condition makes it reasonably safe. If no such adverse findings are revealed, the conservative regimen, with intravenous feeding and either sump suction drainage from the fistulous tract or the application of an ileostomy appliance with the aid of broad sheets of Stomahesive, should be continued for four to six weeks if necessary, provided that there is a steady diminution in the discharge (Irving 1977; Monod-Broca 1977; Blackett and Hill 1978; Reber et al. 1978). Elemental diets have also been recommended for the treatment of intestinal fistulas (Voitk et al. 1973), but their role is not in the immediate management of very ill, severely undernourished patients with high fistulas. They are probably better reserved for use in the later stages when the fistula has largely closed.

Another matter that should be considered in these patients with intestinal fistulas who come to operation is whether, after excision of the affected bowel by segmental resection, continuity should be restored by an immediate anastomosis, or alternatively the proximal stump of bowel should be brought to the surface as an active stoma and the distal one closed or exteriorized as an inactive stoma (Goligher 1971). In my experience this is a very safe method, applicable to lesions in the lower half of the small intestine. The integrity of the intestinal tract is re-established some four to six months later when the patient has been restored to normal general health.

The prospects of inducing abdominal fistulas to heal by means of a by-pass with unilateral exclusion are uncertain (Enker and Block 1969) and, in my limited experience of this method, very poor. Strong claims have been made for the effectiveness of azathioprine therapy in inducing such fistulas to close, but I have been bitterly disappointed in my own practice and the report of Rhodes et al. (1971) is not encouraging.

ANAL LESIONS

Anal Fissures and Skin Tags. Fissures in the anal canal itself may sometimes heal spontaneously—even if they had yielded a positive biopsy for Crohn's disease—if the underlying intestinal lesion is dealt with surgically or can be got into a quiescent state on medical treatment. Coincidentally with this regression of the fissure the oedema of the associated skin tags gradually resolves. Clearly, therefore, a conservative attitude can often usefully be adopted towards these minor anal lesions, depending on the site and nature of the related intestinal component of the disease.

Extensive Perianal Ulceration. In my experience these ulcers extending out into the perianal region are invariably associated with Crohn's disease of the rectum and always necessitate radical surgical treatment to remove the rectum and any other diseased part of the intestine. At this operation it may or may not be feasible to excise all the perianal ulceration, but, even if some of the ulcerated area is left, it usually heals after the intestinal disease has been eradicated, though it may take an inordinately long time to do so (see below). Lockhart-Mummery's (1972) experience has been similar and in addition he has found that diversion of the faecal stream alone by establishing an ileostomy or colostomy has not usually produced any significant improvement in the perianal ulceration.

Anal Abscesses and Fistulas. In treating *acute abscesses*, drainage will be required as a matter of urgency to relieve the patient's discomfort. If a low fistulous opening into the anal canal is found, it may reasonably be laid open at the same time, but no extensive procedure involving considerable division of the sphincter musculature should be contemplated at this stage. Biopsy of the granulation tissue should certainly be performed.

As for *anal fistulas*, their surgical management should be postponed till the related intestinal condition has been assessed and treated, usually surgically. It may be—as, for example, when the rectum and distal colon are severely implicated and require excision—that the fistula will be removed as part of the treatment of the enteritis. In other cases—as when the small bowel or right colon are involved and a right hemicolectomy is required—the anal fistula may subsequently improve to a considerable extent, so that only a quite restricted operation on it is eventually needed. A useful recent article on anorectal Crohn's disease, which is relevant to the management of these anal abscesses and fistulas is that of Hughes (1978).

CHOLELITHIASIS AFTER ILEAL RESECTION FOR CROHN'S DISEASE

It is now well established that there is an increased tendency to gall-stones when the re-absorption of bile salts from the intestinal tract is impaired by resection or disease of the lower ileum (Heaton and Read 1960; Hill et al. 1975; see also p. 835). Consequently gall-stones are common in sufferers from Crohn's disease after surgical treatment.

PROPHYLACTIC USE OF SYSTEMIC STEROID OR SULPHASALAZINE MEDICATION AFTER RESECTION IN THE HOPE OF LESSENING THE FREQUENCY OF RECURRENCE

Turnbull (1975) advocated prolonged administration of systemic steroids after resection for Crohn's disease to try to reduce the incidence of recurrence, but this regimen was not found to be effective by Lefton et al. (1975). More recently two controlled trials of low-dosage steroid therapy after surgical excision (Smith et al. 1978; Summers et al. 1978) failed to show any significant lessening of recurrence. Wenckert et al. (1978), in a controlled trial of sulphasalazine as a prophylactic agent to prevent recurrence after intestinal resection for Crohn's disease, found a slight advantage in the treated cases but the difference was not statistically significant. It seems unlikely that much help is going to be derived from drug therapy in lessening the frequency of recurrence after surgery.

Conclusion

I would be the last to pretend that the results of surgery for Crohn's disease of the large bowel are anything like entirely satisfactory, but the picture is certainly not uniformly black. Due to the great inadequacies of medical treatment I believe that the surgeon has still a considerable part to play in the management of this condition.

REFERENCES

ACHESON, E. (1960a) The distribution of ulcerative colitis and regional enteritis in United States veterans, with particular reference to the Jewish religion. *Gut, 1,* 291.

—— (1960b) An association between ulcerative colitis, regional enteritis and ankylosing spondylitis. *Q. Jl. Med., 29,* 489.

ADSON, M. A., COOPERMAN, A. M. and FARROW, G. M. (1971) Ileorectostomy for ulcerative disease of the colon. *Archs Surg., Chicago, 104.* 424.

AGUIRRE, A., FISCHER, J. E. and WELCH, C. E. (1974) The role of surgery and hyperalimentation in therapy of gastrointestinal-cutaneous fistulae. *Ann. Surg., 180,* 393.

ALMY, T. P. and SHERLOCK, P. (1966) Genetic aspects of ulcerative colitis and regional enteritis. *Gastroenterology, 51,* 757.

ALUWIHARE, A. P. R. (1971) Electronmicroscopy in Crohn's disease. *Gut, 12,* 509.

ANSELL, B. and WIGLEY, R. (1964) Arthritic manifestations in regional enteritis. *Ann. rheum. Dis., 23,* 64.

ATKINSON, A. (1965) Sclerosing cholangitis. Association with regional enteritis. Report of two cases. *Gastroenterology, 49,* 548.

ATHERTON, D. J., MASSAM, M., WELLS, R. S., HARRIES, J. T. and PINCOTT, J. R. (1978) Congenital Crohn's disease in a 6-year-old boy. *Br. med. J., 1,* 552.

ATWELL, J. D., DUTHIE, H. L. and GOLIGHER, J. C. (1965) The outcome of Crohn's disease. *Br. J. Surg., 52,* 996.

BAKER, W. N. W. (1971) Ileorectal anastomosis for Crohn's disease of the colon. *Gut, 12*, 427.

BÁRÁNY, F. (1971) Medical management of Crohn's disease. In *Skandia Symposium on Regional Enteritis (Crohn's Disease)*. Stockholm: Nordiska Bokhandelns Förlag.

BARBOUR, K. W., Jr., WAUGH, J. M., BEAHRS, O. H. and SAUER, W. G. (1962) Indication for and results of surgical treatment of regional enteritis. *Ann. Surg., 156*, 472.

BARGEN, J. A. (1957) Regional enteritis: an evaluation of the present-day therapeutic management. *Ann. intern. Med., 47*, 875.

BERGMAN, L. and KRAUSE, U. (1977) Crohn's disease: a long-term study of the clinical course in 186 patients. *Scand. J. Gastroent., 12*, 937.

BISHOP, R. P., BREWSTER, A. C. and ANTONIOLI, D. A. (1972) Crohn's disease of the mouth. *Gastroenterology, 62*, 302.

BLACKETT, R. L. and HILL, G. L. (1978) Postoperative external small bowel fistulas: a study of a consecutive series of patients treated with intravenous alimentation. *Br. J. Surg., 65*, 775.

BOCHUS, H. L. (1965) In panel discussion on regional entero-colitis. *Dis. Colon Rect., 8*, 1.

BORDOS, D. U. and CAMERON, J. L. (1975) Successful long-term intravenous alimentation in the hospital and at home. *Archs Surg., Chicago, 10*, 439.

BRILL, C. B., KLEIN, S. F. and KARK, A. E. (1969) Regional enteritis and entero-colitis. A study of 74 patients over 15 years. *Ann. Surg., 170*, 766.

BROOKE, B. N. (1959) Granulomatous disease of the intestine. *Lancet, 2*, 745.

—— HOFFMANN, D. C. and SWARBRICK, E. T. (1969) Azathioprine for Crohn's disease. *Lancet, 2*, 612.

—— JAVETT, S. L. and DAVIDSON, O. W. (1970) Further experiences with azathioprine for Crohn's disease. *Lancet, 2*, 1050.

BROVIAC, J. W. and SCRIBNER, B. H. (1974) Prolonged parenteral nutrition in the home. *Surgery Gynec. Obstet., 139*, 28.

BURGESS, J. N., LEGGE, D. A. and JUDD, E. S. (1971) Surgical treatment of regional enteritis of the stomach and duodenum. *Surgery Gynec. Obstet., 132*, 628.

BURMAN, J. H., COOKE, W. T. and WILLIAMS, J. A. (1971a) The fate of ileo-rectal anastomosis in Crohn's disease. *Gut, 12*, 432.

—— WILLIAMS, J. A., THOMPSON, H. and COOKE, W. T. (1971b) The effect of diversion of intestinal contents on the progress of Crohn's disease of the large bowel. *Gut, 12*, 11.

CAVE, D. R., MITCHELL, D. N. and BROOKE, B. N. (1975) Experimental animal studies of the etiology and pathogenesis of Crohn's disease. *Gastroenterology, 69*, 618.

CLARK, R. L. and DIXON, C. F. (1939) Regional enteritis. *Surgery, St Louis, 5*, 277.

COHEN, S., KAPLAN, M., GOTTLIED, L. and PATTERSON, J. (1971) Liver disease and gall stones in regional enteritis. *Gastroneterology, 60*, 237.

COLCOCK, B. P. and VANSANT, J. H. (1960) Surgical treatment of regional enteritis. *New Engl. J. Med., 262*, 435.

—— —— and CONTRERAS, O. (1961) Surgical treatment of co-existing regional enteritis and ulcerative colitis. *Surgery Gynec. Obstet., 112*, 96.

COLP, R. (1934) Case of non-specific granuloma of the terminal ileum and cecum. *Surg. Clins N. Am., 14*, 443.

COMPSTON, J. E. and CREAMER, B. (1977) The consequences of small intestinal resection. *Q. Jl Med., 46*, 485.

COOK, M. (1972) The size and histological appearances of mesenteric lymph nodes in Crohn's disease. *Gut, 13*, 970.

—— and DIXON, M. F. (1973) An analysis of the reliability of detection and diagnostic value of various pathological features in Crohn's disease and ulcerative colitis. *Gut, 14*, 255.

—— and TURNBULL, G. J. (1975) A hypothesis for the pathogenesis of Crohn's disease based on ultrastructural study. *Virchows Arch. path. Anat. Physiol., 365*, 327.

COOKE, W. T. (1955) Nutritional and metabolic factors in the aetiology and treatment of regional ileitis. *Ann. R. Coll. Surg. Engl., 17*, 137.

—— and FIELDING, J. F. (1970) Corticosteroid or corticotrophin therapy in Crohn's disease (regional enteritis). *Gut, 11*, 921.

CORNES, J. S. and STECHER, M. (1961) Primary Crohn's disease of colon and rectum. *Gut, 2*, 189.

CROFT, C. B. and WILKINSON, A. R. (1972) Ulceration of the mouth, pharynx and larynx in Crohn's disease of the intestine. *Br. J. Surg., 59*, 249.

CROHN, B. B. (1965) In panel discussion on enterocolitis. *Dis. Colon Rect., 8*, 3.

—— GARLOCK, J. H. and YARNIS, H. (1947) Right sided (regional) colitis. *J. Am. med. Ass., 134*, 324.

—— GINZBURG, L. and OPPENHEIMER, G. D. (1932) Regional ileitis: a pathologic and clinical entity. *J. Am. med. Ass., 99*, 1323.

—— and ROSENAK, B. D. (1936) A combined form of ileitis and colitis. *J. Am. med. Ass., 106*, 1.

—— and YARNIS, H. (1958) *Regional Ileitis*, 2nd ed. New York: Grune & Stratton.

—— —— and KORELITZ, B. I. (1956) Regional ileitis complicating pregnancy. *Gastroenterology, 31*, 615.

DALZIEL, T. K. (1913) Chronic interstitial enteritis. *Br. med. J., 2*, 1068.

DARKE, S. G., PARKS, A. G., GROGONO, J. C. and POLLOCK, D. J. (1973) Adenocarcinoma and Crohn's disease: a report of 2 cases and an analysis of the literature. *Br. J. Surg., 60*, 169.

DE DOMBAL, F. T. (1971) Symposium on Crohn's disease: epidemiology and natural history. *Proc. R. Soc. Med., 64*, 161.

—— BURTON, I. and GOLIGHER, J. C. (1971a) The early and late results of surgical treatment for Crohn's disease. *Br. J. Surg., 58*, 807.

—— —— —— (1971b) Recurrence of Crohn's disease after primary excisional surgery. *Gut, 12*, 519.

—— —— —— (1972) Crohn's disease and pregnancy. *Br. med. J., 3*, 550.

—— —— —— (1974) Short term course and prognosis of Crohn's disease. *Gut, 15*, 435.

—— WATTS, J. McK., WATKINSON, G. and GOLIGHER, J. C. (1966) The incidence and management of anorectal abscesses, fistulae and fissure, occurring in patients with ulcerative colitis. *Dis Colon Rect., 9*, 201.

DOWLING, R. H., BELL, G. D. and WHITE, J. (1972) Lithogenic bile in patients with ileal dysfunction. *Gut, 13*, 415.

DRONFIELD, M. W. and LONGMAN, M. J. S. (1975) Serum lysozyme in inflammatory bowel disease. *Gut, 16*, 985.

DYER, N. and DAWSON, A. M. (1970) Diagnosis of Crohn's disease: a continuing source of error. *Br. med. J., 1*, 735.

EADE, M. N., COOKE, W. T. and WILLIAMS, J. A. (1970) Liver disease in Crohn's disease. A study of 100 consecutive patients. *Scand. J. Gastroent., 6*, 199.

EDWARDS, H. C. (1964) Crohn's disease. *J. R. Coll. Surg. Edinb.*, *9*, 115.

—— (1969) Crohn's disease: an enquiry into the nature and consequences. *Ann. R. Coll. Surg. Engl.*, *44*, 121.

ENGEL, A. and LARSSON, T. (1971) *Skandia Symposium on Regional Enteritis (Crohn's Disease)*. Stockholm: Nordiska Bokhandelns Forlag.

ENKER, W. E. and BLOCK, G. E. (1969) The operative treatment of Crohn's disease complicated by fistulae, a personal consecutive series. *Archs Surg., Chicago*, *98*, 493.

—— —— (1973) Occult obstructive uropathy complicating Crohn's disease. *Archs Surg., Chicago*, *110*, 319.

EVANS, J. G. (1972) The epidemiology of Crohn's disease. *Clinics Gastroent.* *1*, 335.

FARMER, R. G., HAWK, W. A. and TURNBULL, R. B., Jr. (1972) Crohn's disease of the duedenum (transmural duodenitis): clinical manifestations. Report of 11 cases. *Am. J. dig. Dis.*, *17*, 191.

—— —— —— (1975) Clinical patterns in Crohn's disease: a statistical study of 615 cases. *Gastroenterology*, *68*, 627.

—— —— (1976) Indications for surgery in Crohn's disease: analyses of 500 cases. *Gastroenterology*, *71*, 245.

FALCHUK, K. R., PERROTTO, J. L. and ISSELBACHER, K. J. (1975) Serum lysozyme in Crohn's disease and ulcerative colitis. *New Engl. J. Med.*, *299*, 395.

FASTH, S., FILIPSSON, S., HULTÉN, L. and LINDHAGER, J. (1976) Ureteric obstruction complicating Crohn's disease in the terminal ileum. *Acta chir. scand.*, *142*, 275.

FAUSA, O., NYGAARD, K. and ELGJO, K. (1977) Amyloidosis and Crohn's disease. *Scand. J. Gastroent.*, *12*, 657.

FIELDING, J. F. (1972) Perianal lesions in Crohn's disease. *J. R. Coll. Surg. Edinb.*, *17*, 32.

—— and COOKE, W. T. (1970a) Peptic ulceration in Crohn's disease (regional enteritis). *Gut*, *11*, 998.

—— —— (1970b) Pregnancy and Crohn's disease. *Br. med. J.*, *2*, 76.

—— —— (1971a) Finger clubbing and regional enteritis. *Gut*, *12*, 422.

—— —— (1971b) Treatment of Crohn's disease. *Lancet*, *2*, 771, 930.

—— TOYE, D. K. M., BETON, D. C. and COOKE, W. T. (1970) Crohn's disease of the stomach and duodenum, *Gut*, *11*, 1001.

FILIPE, M. I. and DAWSON, I. M. P. (1970) The diagnostic value of mucosubstances in rectal biopsies from patients with ulcerative colitis and Crohn's disease. *Gut*, *11*, 229.

FLINT, G., STRAUSS, R., PLATT, N. and WISE, L. (1977) Ileorectal anastomosis in patients with Crohn's disease of the colon. *Gut*, *18*, 236.

FRUIN, R. C., MIREE, J., Jr. and LITTMAN, A. (1967) Roentgen therapy for regional enteritis. *Gastroenterology*, *52*, 134.

GARLOCK, J. H. and CROHN, B. B. (1945) An appraisal of the results of surgery in the treatment of regional ileitis. *J. Am. med. Ass.*, *127*, 205.

—— —— and KLEIN, S. H. (1951) An appraisal of the long term results of surgical treatment of regional enteritis. *Gastroenterology*, *19*, 414.

GLOTZER, D. J., GARDNER, R. C., GOLDMAN, H., HINRICHS, H. R., ROSEN, H. and ZETZEL, L. (1970) Comparative features and course of ulcerative and granulomatous colitis. *New Engl. J. Med.*, *282*, 582.

—— and SILEN, W. (1975) Indications for surgical treatment in chronic ulcerative colitis and Crohn's disease of the colon. In *Inflammatory Bowel Disease*, ed. J. B. Kirsner and R. G. Shorter, p. 323. Philadelphia: Lea and Febiger.

—— STONE, P. A. and PATERSON, J. F. (1967) Prognosis after surgical treatment of granulomatous colitis. *New Engl. J. Med.*, *277*, 273.

GOLIGHER, J. C. (1971) Resection with exteriorization in the management of faecal fistulas originating in the small intestine. *Br. J. Surg.*, *58*, 163.

—— (1972) Ileal recurrence after ileostomy and excision of the large bowel for Crohn's disease. *Br. J. Surg.*, *59*, 253.

—— (1979) The immediate and long term results of surgery for Crohn's disease of the large bowel. *Surgery Gynec. Obstet.*, *148*, 1.

—— DE DOMBAL, F. T. and BURTON, I. (1971a) Surgical treatment and its results. In *Skandia Symposium on Regional Enteritis (Crohn's Disease)*. Stockholm: Nordiska Bokhandelns Förlag.

—— —— —— (1971b) Crohn's disease, with special reference to surgical management. In *Progress in Surgery*. Basle: Karger.

—— HOFFMANN, D. C. and DE DOMBAL, F. T. (1970) The surgical treatment of severe attacks of ulcerative colitis, with special reference to advantages of early operation. *Br. med. J.*, *2*, 703.

GRAY, B. K., LOCKHART-MUMMERY, H. E. and MORSON, B. C. (1965) Crohn's disease of the anal region. *Gut*, *6*, 515.

GREENSTEIN, A. J., SACHAR, D. and PUCILLO, A. (1978) Cancer in Crohn's disease after diversionary surgery: a report of seven carcinomas occurring in excluded bowel. *Am. J. Surg.*, *135*, 86.

GROGONO, J. L. and PARKS, A. G. (1972) Surgical resection of recurrent Crohn's disease. *Br. J. Surg.*, *59*, 892.

GUMP, F. E., LEPORE, M. and BARKER, H. G. (1967) A revised concept of acute regional enteritis. *Ann. Surg.*, *166*, 942.

GURRY, J. F. (1974) Acute terminal ileitis and *Yersinia* infection. *Br. med. J.*, *2*, 264.

HADFIELD, G. (1939) The primary histological lesion of regional enteritis. *Lancet*, *2*, 773.

HAMMER, B., ASHURST, P. and NAISH, J. (1968) Diseases associated with ulcerative colitis and Crohn's disease. *Gut*, *9*, 17.

HAWK, W. A. and TURNBULL, R. B., Jr. (1966) Primary ulcerative disease of the colon. *Gastroenterology*, *51*, 802.

—— —— and FARMER, R. G. (1967) Regional enteritis of the colon. Distinctive features of the entity. *J. Am. med. Ass.*, *201*, 738.

HEATLEY, R. V., BOLTON, P. M., OWEN, B. E., WILLIAMS, W. J. and HUGHES, L. E. (1975) A search for a transmissable agent in Crohn's disease. *Gut*, *16*, 528.

HEATON, K. W. and READ, A. E. (1969) Gallstones in patients with disorders of the terminal ileum and disturbed bile salt metabolism. *Br. med. J.*, *3*, 494.

HEATON, L. D., RAVDIN, I. S. and BLADES, B. (1964) President Eisenhower's operation for regional enteritis. A footnote to history. *Ann. Surg.*, *159*, 661.

HILL, G. L., MAIR, W. S. J. and GOLIGHER, J. C. (1975) Gallstones after ileostomy and ileal resection. *Gut*, *16*, 932.

HIMAL, H. S., ALLARD, J. R., NADEAU, J. E., FREEMAN, J. B. and MACLEAN, L. D. (1974) Importance of adequate nutrition in closure of small intestinal fistulas. *Br. J. Surg.*, *16*, 724.

HUGHES, L. E. (1977) Personal communication.

—— (1978) Surgical pathology and management of anorectal Crohn's disease. *J. R. Soc. Med.*, *71*, 644.

HYLANDER, E., HANSEN, N. E., KARLE, H. and JANRUM, S. (1976) Serum lysozyme in Crohn's disease and ulcerative colitis. *Scand. J. Gastroent.*, *11*, 213.

IRVING, M. (1977) Local and surgical management of enterocutaneous fistulas. *Br. J. Surg.*, *64*, 690.

JAVETT, S. L. and BROOKE, B. N. (1970) Acute dilatation of colon in Crohn's disease. *Lancet*, *2*, 126.

JEEJEEBHOY, K. N., LANGER, B. and TSALLAS, G. (1976) Total parenteral nutrition at home: studies in patients surviving 4 months to 5 years. *Gastroenterology*, *71*, 943.

JONES, F. AVERY, BROWN, P., LENNARD-JONES, J. E., JONES, J. H. and MILTON-THOMPSON, G. J. (1969) Azothiaprine for Crohn's disease. *Lancet*, *2*, 795.

JONES, J. H. (1969) Colonic cancer and Crohn's disease. *Gut*, *10*, 651.

—— and LENNARD-JONES, J. E. (1966) Corticosteroids and corticotrophin in the treatment of Crohn's disease. *Gut*, *7*, 181.

—— —— and LOCKHART-MUMMERY, H. E. (1966) Experience in the treatment of Crohn's disease of the large intestine. *Gut*, *7*, 448.

KEWENTER, J., HULTÉN, L. and KOCK, N. G. (1974) The relationship and epidemiology of acute terminal ileitis and Crohn's disease. *Gut*, *15*, 801.

KIRSNER, J. B. (1970) Ulcerative colitis 1970—recent developments. *Scand. J. Gastroent.*, Suppl., *6*, 63.

—— SPENCER, J. A. (1963) Family occurrence of ulcerative colitis, regional enteritis and ileocolitis. *Ann. intern. Med.*, *59*, 133.

KORELITZ, B. I. (1967) Clinical course, late results and pathological nature of inflammatory disease of the colon initially sparing the rectum. *Gut*, *8*, 281.

—— PRESENT, D. H., ALPERT, L. I., MARSHAK, R. H. and JANOWITZ, H. D. (1972) Recurrent regional ileitis after ileostomy and colectomy for granulomatous colitis. *New Engl. J. Med.*, *287*, 110.

KOUDAHL, G., KRISTENSEN, M. and LENZ, K. (1974) By-pass compared with resection for ileal Crohn's disease. *Scand. J. Gastroent.*, *9*, 203.

KRISTENSEN, M., LENZ, K., NIELSON, O. S. and JARNUM, S. (1974) Short bowel syndrome following resection for Crohn's disease. *Scand. J. Gastroent.*, *9*, 559.

KRAUSE, U. (1971) Epidemiology in Sweden. In *Skandia Symposium on Regional Enteritis (Crohn's Disease)*. Stockholm: Nordiska Bokhandelns For̈lag.

—— BERGMAN, L. and NORLÉN, B. J. (1971) Crohn's disease. A clinical study based on 186 patients. *Scand. J. Gastroent.*, *6*, 97.

KYLE, J. (1971a) An epidemiological study of Crohn's disease in North East Scotland. *Gastroenterology*, *61*, 826.

—— (1971b) Psoas abscess in Crohn's disease. *Gastroenterology*, *61*, 149.

LEFTON, H. B., FARMER, R. G. and FAZIO, V. (1975) Ileorectal anastomosis for Crohn's disease of the colon. *Gastroenterology*, *69*, 612.

LENNARD-JONES, J. E. (1968) Natural history and characteristics of Crohn's disease. *Postgrad. med. J.*, *44*, 674.

—— (1971) In discussion of BÁRÁNY, F. (1971).

—— and STALDER, G. A. (1967) Prognosis after resection of chronic regional ileitis. *Gut*, *8*, 332.

LEWIN, K. and SWALES, J. D. (1966) Granulomatous colitis and atypical ulcerative colitis. Histological features, behaviour and prognosis. *Gastroenterology*, *50*, 211.

LINDNER, A. E., MARSHAK, R. H., WOLF, B. S. and JANOWITZ, H. D. (1963) Granulomatous colitis: a clinical study. *New Engl. J. Med.*, *269*, 379.

LOCKHART-MUMMERY, H. E. (1972) Anal lesions of Crohn's disease. *Clinics Gastroent.* *1*, 377.

—— and MORSON, B. C. (1960) Crohn's disease (regional enteritis) of the large intestine and its distinction from ulcerative colitis. *Gut*, *1*, 87.

—— —— (1964) Crohn's disease of the large intestine. *Gut*, *5*, 493.

LONDON, D. and FITTON, J. M. (1970) Acute septic arthritis complicating Crohn's disease. *Br. J. Surg.*, *57*, 536.

MCCALLUM, D. I. and KINMONT, P. D. C. (1968) Dermatological manifestations of Crohn's disease. *Br. J. Derm.*, *80*, 1.

MCCONNELL, R. B. (1971) Genetic factors in Crohn's disease. In *Skandia Symposium on Regional Enteritis (Crohn's Disease)*. Stockholm: Nordiska Bokhandelns Förlag.

MACFADYEN, B. V., Jr., DUDRICK, S. J. and RUBERG, R. L. (1973) Management of gastrointestinal fistulas with parenteral hyperalimentation. *Surgery, St Louis*, *74*, 100.

MCILRATH, D. C. (1971) Diverting ileostomy or colostomy in the management of Crohn's disease of the colon. *Archs Surg., Chicago*, *103*, 308.

MACPHERSON, R. R., ALBERTINI, R. J. and BEEKEN, W. L. (1976) Immunological studies in patients with Crohn's disease. *Gut*, *17*, 100.

MADDEN, J. L., RAVID, J. M. and HADDAD, J. R. (1969) Regional oesophagitis. A specific entity and simulating Crohn's disease. *Ann. Surg.*, *170*, 370.

MANNING, J. H., WARREN, R. and ADI, A. S. (1955) Segmental colitis. Results of surgery. *New Engl. J. Med.*, *252*, 850.

MARSHAK, R. H., WOLF, B. S. and ELIASOPH, J. (1959) Segmental colitis. *Radiology*, *73*, 707.

MARTINI, G. A. and MALCHOW, H. (1979) Symposium on Crohn's Disease in Hemmenhofen. *Z. Gastroent.*, Supplement, in the press.

MAYO-ROBSON, A. W. (1908) Some abdominal tumours simulating malignant disease and their treatment. *Br. med. J.*, *1*, 425.

MENGUY, R. (1972) Surgical management of free perforation of the small intestine complicating regional enteritis. *Ann. Surg.*, *175*, 178.

MITCHELL, D. N., CANNON, P., DYER, N., HINSON, K. F. W. and WILLOUGHBY, J. M. T. (1969) The Kveim test in Crohn's disease. *Lancet*, *2*, 571.

—— and REES, R. J. W. (1970) Agent transmissible from Crohn's disease tissue. *Lancet*, *3*, 168.

MIXTER, C. G. (1935) Regional ileitis. *Ann. Surg.*, *102*, 674.

MONK, M., MENDELOFF, A. I., SIEGEL, C. I. and LILIENFIELD, A. (1967) An epidemiological study of ulcerative colitis and regional enteritis among adults in Baltimore. I. Hospital incidence and prevalence. *Gastroenterology*, *53*, 198.

—— —— —— —— (1969) An epidemiological study of ulcerative colitis and regional enteritis among adults in Baltimore. II. Social and demographical factors. *Gastroenterology*, *56*, 847.

MONOD-BROCA, P. (1977) Treatment of intestinal fistulas. *Br. J. Surg.*, *64*, 685.

MOONEY, R. A. H. and SANT, G. R. (1973) Obstructive uropathy in granulomatous bowel disease. *Br. J. Surg.*, *60*, 525.

MOROWITZ, D. A., BLOCK, G. E. and KIRSNER, J. B. (1968) Adenocarcinoma of the ileum complicating chronic regional enteritis. *Gastroenterology*, *55*, 397.

MORSON, B. C. (1971) Histopathology of Crohn's disease. In *Skandia Symposium on Regional Enteritis (Crohn's Disease)*. Stockholm: Nordiska Bokhandelns Förlag.

—— and LOCKHART-MUMMERY, H. E. (1959a) Crohn's disease of the colon. *Gastroenterologia, 92*, 168.

—— (1959b) Anal lesions in Crohn's disease. *Lancet, 2*, 1122.

MOUNTAIN, J. C. (1970) Cutaneous ulceration in Crohn's disease. *Gut, 11*, 18.

MOYNIHAN, B. G. A. (1907) The mimicry of malignant disease in the large intestine. *Edinb. med. J., 21*, 228.

NEALE, G., KELSALL, A. R. and DOYLE, F. H. (1968) Crohn's disease and diffuse symmetrical periostitis. *Gut, 9*, 383.

NEUMAN, H. W., BARGEN, J. A. and JUDD, E. S., Jr. (1954) Clinical study of 201 cases of regional (segmental) colitis. *Surgery Gynec. Obstet., 99*, 563.

NUGENT, F. W., MALLARI, R., GEORGE, H. and RIDLEY, N. (1976) Serum lysozyme in inflammatory bowel disease. *Gastroenterology, 70*, 1014.

—— VEIDENHEIMER, M. C., MEISSNER, W. A. and HAGGITT, R. C. (1973) Prognosis after colonic resection for Crohn's disease of the colon. *Gastroenterology, 65*, 398.

OBERHELMAN, H. A., Jr. and KOHATSU, S. (1971) Diversion by ileostomy for Crohn's disease of the colon. In *Skandia Symposium on Regional Enteritis (Crohn's Disease)*. Stockholm: Nordiska Bokhandelns Förlag.

—— —— TAYLOR, K. B. and KIVEL, R. M. (1968) Diverting ileostomy in the surgical management of Crohn's disease of the colon. *Am. J. Surg., 115*, 231.

O'DONOGHUE, D. P., DAWSON, A. M., POWELL-TUCK, J., POOWN, R. L. and LENNARD-JONES, J. E. (1978a) Double-blind withdrawal trial of azathioprine as maintenance treatment for Crohn's disease. *Lancet, 4*, 955.

—— —— —— —— —— (1978b) Maintenance azathioprine in Crohn's disease (letter). *Lancet, 4*, 1306.

PAGET, E. T., OWENS, M. P. PENISTON, W. O. and MATHEWSON, C. (1972) Massive upper gastrointestinal track haemorrhage from Crohn's disease of duodenum. *Archs Surg., Chicago, 104*, 397.

PARRISH, R. A., KARSTEN, M. B., MCRAE, A. T. and MORETZ, W. H. (1968) Segmental Crohn's colitis associated with adenocarcinoma. *Am. J. Surg., 115*, 371.

PEETERS, T. L., VANTRAPPEN, G. and GEBOES, K. (1976) Serum lysozyme levels in Crohn's disease and ulcerative colitis. *Gut, 17*, 300.

PENN, I. and STARZL, T. E. (1970) Incidence of malignant disease in patients on azathioprine for transplant. *Int. J. clin. Pharmac., 3*, 49.

PERRETT, A. D., HIGGINS, G., JOHNSTON, H. H., MASSARELLA, G. R., TRUELOVE, S. C. and WRIGHT, R. (1971) The liver in Crohn's disease. *Q. Jl Med., 40*, 187.

—— TRUELOVE, S. C. and MASSARELLA, G. R. (1968) Crohn's disease and carcinoma of the colon. *Br. med. J., 2*, 468.

PHEAR, D. N. (1958) The relation between regional ileitis and sarcoidosis. *Lancet, 2*, 1250.

PUGH, H. L. (1945) Regional enteritis. *Ann. Surg., 132*, 845.

RAMUS, N. I. and SHOREY, B. A. (1975) Crohn's disease and psoas abscess. *Br. med. J., 3*, 574.

REBER, H. A., ROBERTS, C., WAY, L. W. and DUNPHY, J. E. (1978) Management of external gastrointestinal fistulas. *Ann. Surg., 188*, 460.

RHA, C-K., KLEIN, N. C. and WILSON, T. M. (1971) Adenocarcinoma of the ileum with co-existing regional enteritis. *Archs Surg., Chicago, 102*, 630.

RHODES, J., BAINTON, B. and BECK, P. (1971) Azathioprine in Crohn's disease: a controlled trial. *Lancet, 2*, 1273.

RITCHIE, J. K. and LENNARD-JONES, J. E. (1976) Crohn's disease of the distal large bowel. *Scand. J. Gastroent., 11*, 433.

—— and LOCKHART-MUMMERY, H. E. (1973) Non-restorative surgery in the treatment of Crohn's disease of the large bowel. *Gut, 14*, 263.

ROSS, S. T. (1965) Granulomatous colitis. *Surgery, St Louis, 58*, 357.

SCHOFIELD, P. F. (1965) The natural history and treatment of Crohn's disease. *Ann. R. Coll. Surg., 36*, 258.

—— (1974) Personal communication.

—— STAFF, W. G. and MOORE, T. (1968) Ureteral involvement in regional ileitis (Crohn's disease). *J. Urol., 99*, 412.

SHIEL, F. O'M., CLARK, C. G. and GOLIGHER, J. C. (1968) Adenocarcinoma associated with Crohn's disease. *Br. J. Surg., 55*, 53.

SILTZBACH, L. E., VIEIRA, L. O. P. D., TOPILSKY, M. and JANOWITZ, H. D. (1971) Is there Kveim responsiveness in Crohn's disease? *Lancet, 2*, 634.

SIMONOWITZ, D., BLOCK, G. E., RIDDELL, R. N., KRAFT, S. C. and KIRSNER, J. B. (1977) The production of an unusual tissue reaction in rabbit bowel injected with Crohn's disease homogenates. *Surgery, St Louis, 82*, 211.

SIMPKINS, K. C. (1972) Some aspects of the radiology of Crohn's disease. *Br. J. Surg., 59*, 810.

SJÖSTRÖM, B. (1971) Acute terminal ileitis and its relation to Crohn's disease. In *Skandia Symposium on Regional Enteritis (Crohn's Disease)*. Stockholm: Nordiska Bokhandelns Förlag.

SMITH, R. C., RHODES, J. and HEATLEY, R. V. (1978) Low-dose steroids and clinical relapse in Crohn's disease: a controlled trial. *Gut, 19*, 606.

SPARBERG, M. and KIRSNER, J. B. (1966) Long-term corticosteroid therapy for regional enteritis: an analysis of 58 courses in 54 patients. *Am. J. dig. Dis., 11*, 865.

STAHLGREN, L. H. and FERGUSON, L. K. (1961) The results of surgical treatment of chronic regional enteritis. *J. Am. med. Ass., 175*, 986.

STEINBERG, D. M., ALLAN, R. N., THOMPSON, H., BROOKE, B. N., ALEXANDER-WILLIAMS, J. and COOKE, W. T. (1974) Excisional surgery with ileostomy for Crohn's colitis with particular reference to factors affecting recurrence. *Gut, 15*, 845.

SUMMERS, R. W., SESSIONS, J. T., SWITZ, D. M. and SINGLETON, J. W. (1978) National Cooperative Crohn's Disease Study (NCCDS): response of subgroups to drug treatment. *Gastroenterology, 74*, 1100.

THAYER, W. R. (1970) Crohn's disease (regional enteritis). A look at the last four years. *Scand. J. Gastroent.*, Suppl. 6, 165.

TOOTLA, F., LUCAS, R. J., BERNACKI, E. G. and TABOR, H. (1976) Gastroduodenal Crohn's disease. *Archs Surg., Chicago, 111*, 855.

TRUELOVE, S. C., ELLIS, H. and WEBSTER, C. D. (1965) The place of a double-barrelled ileostomy in ulcerative colitis and Crohn's disease of the colon: a preliminary report. *Br. med. J., 1*, 150.

—— and REYNELL, P. C. (1963) *Diseases of the Digestive System*. Oxford: Blackwell Scientific.

PLATE V

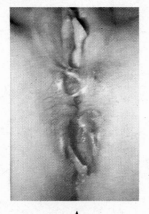 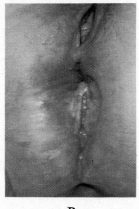 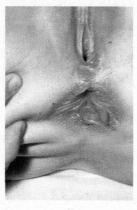

A   B   C

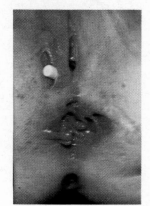

D

Anal Ulcers in Crohn's Disease

A,   From Lockhart-Mummery and Morson (1965)
D,   Mr H. R. Thompson's case

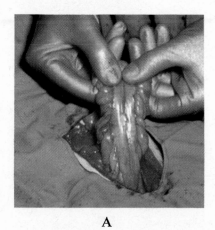

A   B

Diverticular Disease of the Sigmoid

Reilly incision for sigmoid myotomy. A, Exposure of sigmoid colon. B, Muscle coat divided through longitudinal incision in one of the antimesenteric teniae. The incision is continued into apparently normal bowel above and below for 1–2 cm. (*From Reilly 1966*)

TURNBULL, R. B., Jr. (1975) The surgical approach to the treatment of inflammatory bowel disease: a personal view of techniques and prognosis. In *Inflammatory Bowel Disease*, ed. J. B. Kirsner and R. G. Shorter. p. 338. Philadelphia: Lea and Febiger.

—— SCHOFIELD, P. F. and HAWK, W. A. (1968) Non-specific ulcerative colitis. *Advanc. Surg. 3*, 161.

VALDES-DAPENA, A. and VILARDELL, F. (1962) Granulomatous lesions in ileocolitis. *Gastroenterologia, 97*, 191.

VAN PATTER, W. N., BARGEN, J. A., DOCKERTY, M. B., FIELDMAN, W. H., MAYO, C. W. and WAUGH, J. M. (1954) Regional enteritis. *Gastroenterology, 26*, 347.

VANTRAPPEN, G., AGG, H. D. and PONETTE, E. (1977) *Yersinia* enteritis and enterocolitis: gastroenterological aspects. *Gastroenterology, 72*, 220.

VOITK, A. J., ECHAVE, V., BROWN, R. A., McARDLE, A. H. and GURD, F. N. (1973) Elemental diet in treatment of fistulas of the alimentary tract. *Surgery Gynec. Obstet., 137*, 68.

WARREN, S. and SOMMERS, S. C. (1954) Pathology of regional ileitis and ulcerative colitis. *J. Am. med. Ass., 154*, 189.

WATKINSON, G., THOMPSON, H. and GOLIGHER, J. C. (1960) Right-sided or segmental ulcerative colitis. *Br. J. Surg., 47*, 22.

WATTS, J. McK., DE DOMBAL, F. T. and GOLIGHER, J. C. (1966a) The early results of surgery for ulcerative colitis. *Br. J. Surg., 53*, 1005.

—— —— —— (1966b) Long-term complications and prognosis following major surgery for ulcerative colitis. *Br. J. Surg., 53*, 1014.

WELLS, C. A. (1952) Ulcerative colitis and Crohn's disease. *Ann. Rev. Coll. Surg. Engl., 11*, 105.

WENCKERT, A. (1971) Results of surgical treatment of Crohn's disease in Sweden. In *Skandia Symposium on Regional Enteritis (Crohn's Disease)*. Stockholm: Nordiska Bokhandelns Förlag.

—— KRISTENSEN, M. and EKLUND, A. E. (1978) The long term prophylactic effect of salazopyrin in primarily resected patients with Crohn's disease—the controlled double-blind trial. *Scand. J. Gastroent., 13*, 161.

WETERMAN, I. T. and PEÑA, A. S. (1976) The long term prognosis of ileorectal anastomosis and proctocolectomy in Crohn's disease. *Scand. J. Gastroent., 11*, 185.

WILLIAMS, J. A. (1971) The place of surgery in Crohn's disease. *Gut, 12*, 739.

WILLIAMS, R. J. (1954) Vesico-intestinal fistula and Crohn's disease. *Br. J. Surg., 42*, 179.

WILLIAMS, W. J. (1964) Histology of Crohn's syndrome. *Gut, 5*, 510.

—— (1965) A study of Crohn's syndrome using tissue extracts and the Kveim-Mantoux tests. *Gut, 6*, 503.

—— (1971) The Kveim controversy. *Lancet, 2*, 926.

WILLOUGHBY, J. M. T., KUMAR, P. J., BECKETT, J. and DAWSON, A. M. (1971) Controlled trial of azathioprine in Crohn's disease. *Lancet, 2*, 944.

WINBLAD, S., NILÉHN, B. and STERNBY, N. H. (1966) Yersinia enterocolitica (Pasteurella X) in human enteric infections. *Br. med. J., 3*, 1363.

WINKELMAN, E. I. and BROWN, C. H. (1965) Nitrogen mustard in the treatment of chronic ulcerative colitis and regional enteritis: a preliminary report. *Cleveland clin. Quart., 32*, 165.

WOLF, B. S., and MARSHAK, R. H. (1962) Granulomatous colitis (Crohn's disease of the colon): roentgen features. *Am. J. Roentg., 88*, 662.

WYATT, A. P. (1969) Regional enteritis leading to carcinoma of the small bowel. *Gut, 10.* 924.

YOUNG, S., SMITH, I. S., O'CONNOR, J., BELL, J. R. and GILLESPIE, G. (1975) Results of surgery for Crohn's disease in the Glasgow region, 1961–70. *Br. J. Surg., 62*, 528.

ZETZEL, L. (1970) Medical progress: Granulomatous (ileo) colitis. *New Engl. J. Med., 282*, 600.

23

Other Forms of Colitis, Proctitis and Ulceration

ISCHAEMIC COLITIS

During the past few years there has been a growing awareness of the fact that lesions of the colon may sometimes result from sudden deprivation of its blood supply. These have arisen in two ways:

FOLLOWING OPERATIVE OCCLUSION OF THE INFERIOR MESENTERIC ARTERY DURING RESECTION OF ABDOMINAL AORTIC ANEURYSMS

Usually division of the inferior mesenteric artery during this operation is not attended by any ill-effects, owing to the adequacy of the collateral blood supply to the left colon through the marginal artery from above and from below, but in a number of recorded cases changes have occurred in the sigmoid and descending colon (McKain and Shumacker 1958; Bernatz 1960; Smith and Szilagyi 1960; Ochsner et al. 1960; MacVaugh and Roberts 1961; Bernstein and Bernstein 1963; Young et al. 1963; Miller and Knox 1966). The colonic lesions have varied from frank necrosis of the full thickness of the bowel wall over a considerable segment, to 'inflammatory' and ulcerative changes confined largely to the mucosa and mimicking a mild or severe ulcerative colitis, and as a sequel to the latter a certain number of patients have subsequently developed strictures, most often apparently in the lower sigmoid.

The frequency of these colonic complications of aortic surgery has varied markedly in different reported series, ranging from 0·25% to nearly 4% for frank necrosis, but the variations may be partly related to differences in operative technique. Beall et al. (1965) claim that, if the inferior mesenteric artery is divided close to its origin above where it bifurcates, the collateral circulation to the left colon is much less likely to be impaired than if the vessel is taken at a lower level dividing the main branches. Yet in the radical treatment of rectal carcinoma by abdominoperineal excision or anterior resection I have in the last 17 years frequently tied the inferior mesenteric artery at its origin, and have then divided the ascending and descending branches of the left colic, as shown in Fig. 19B, leaving the iliac colon stump dependent for its blood supply on the marginal artery descending from the middle colic. But, in several hundreds of cases treated in this way, including many elderly subjects suffering also from advanced arteriosclerosis, I have never encountered any suggestion of an ischaemic lesion in the left colon proximal to the iliac colostomy or colorectal anastomosis. The vascular deprivation of the left colon in these operations would seem to be identical with that in cases undergoing aortic resection. To account for the difference in the outcome one must postulate an additional factor in the latter cases, such as that the more distal vessels closer to the bowel wall have had their efficiency impaired by arterial disease, particularly if the pressure in the mesenteric vessels has been lowered by general hypotension resulting from shock.

However, whatever the explanation, the occurrence of gross changes in the colon after aortic surgery would seem to provide virtually experimental proof in the human subject that such lesions can be produced by ischaemia. It is also known from experiments in animals that a variety of changes can be caused in the colon wall by acute occlusion of a major artery (Boley et al. 1963; Marston 1964). The brunt of the ischaemia seems to fall on the mucosa, which is the layer most sensitive to hypoxia, so that it undergoes extensive necrosis and ulceration while the outer layers usually remain intact. If complete necrosis does not occur, a remarkable degree of recovery may be possible with a return almost to complete normality. Alternatively, widespread mucosal destruction may result in a fibrous stricture varying in length from a few centimetres to a metre or more.

OCCURRING SPONTANEOUSLY

Quite a few cases have now been reported where a lesion has been produced in the colon apparently by the spontaneous occurrence of intestinal ischaemia in *older* patients with arterial disease (Boley et al. 1963; Marston 1964; Marshak et al. 1965; Roberts 1965; McGovern and Goulston 1965; Marston et al. 1966; Williams et al. 1968; Brown 1972). The cause of the ischaemia in some of these cases has been clearly established to be a block of the inferior mesenteric artery by a thrombosis or embolism, often with an associated lesion of the superior mesenteric trunk; in others the major vessels, though arteriosclerotic, were not actually occluded, and the impairment of blood supply was attributed to disease of the distal intestinal vessels aggravated by hypotension due to cardiac failure, which was often present in these cases (Marrash et al. 1962; Roberts 1965; McGovern and Goulston 1965), but, as Williams and Wittenberg (1975) have emphasized, in many patients with so-called ischaemic colitis mesenteric arteriography has shown no evidence of occlusion or spasm of the distal vessels. The effects of the ischaemia on the bowel have varied, as in the aortic resection cases and in experimental animals, from full necrosis of the colon wall to mainly mucosal changes, and from the latter there might be a complete recovery or a short or long stricture might develop.

More recently a few cases have been reported of apparent 'ischaemic' colitis in *young* patients, some of them whilst on contraceptive pills (Cotton and Thomas 1971; Clark et al. 1972).

CLINICAL FEATURES

The clinical manifestations accord with the pathological changes and, following Marston et al. (1966), it is convenient to describe three main types of presentation, though some cases may be atypical:

Cases with Gangrene of the Colon Wall. These patients, who often have advanced cardiac disease, present as abdominal catastrophes with overwhelming shock and are likely to die very soon if they cannot be sufficiently resuscitated for laparotomy. For this reason there may or may not be an indication from the occurrence of diarrhoea with passage of altered blood that necrosis of the bowel may be the cause. Marston et al. (1966) would regard the necrotizing or *Clostridium welchii* type of colitis, described by Killingback and Williams (1961) and Tate et al. (1965), as essentially an ischaemic lesion with superadded anaerobic infection, but this is debatable (see p. 861 for further discussion).

Cases Showing Transient Ischaemic Changes. The cardinal symptoms in this group are lower abdominal pain, often of a colicky nature, diarrhoea, and the passage of blood and mucus. But the incidence and timing of these symptoms has varied in different reports. Thus, all of Marston et al.'s (1966) patients started with sudden abdominal pain, which was soon followed by diarrhoea and the occurrence of rectal bleeding. But in Roberts' (1965) cases severe diarrhoea was the more usual presenting symptom, though abdominal pain sometimes occurred simultaneously or later. As for bleeding per anum, this was usually a later development not evident for several days or as long as two weeks; the passage of mucus was evident earlier as a rule. Nausea and vomiting were also frequent symptoms in both series. One of Roberts' (1965) cases complained also of a pyoderma gangrenosum of the fingers. Several patients gave a history of a previous similar episode or of occasional abdominal pain suggestive of 'intestinal angina'.

On examination the patients are often pyrexial and there is a moderate leucocytosis. There may be signs of cardiac disease or arteriosclerosis. Abdominal examination will usually elicit some abdominal tenderness and guarding in the lower abdomen particularly in the left iliac fossa. Sigmoidoscopy may show a normal rectum throughout, but blood, mucus or pus may be observed descending from above. Alternatively, a common sigmoidoscopic finding is that the mucosa is normal up to 12–15 cm, above which level it becomes oedematous, granular, friable and often extensively ulcerated. Barium enema examination confirms that an inflammatory process is present in the colon, usually of a limited or segmental distribution, and may show certain distinctive features of an ischaemic lesion (see below).

In the further course of these cases two outcomes are possible. One is that over a period of several weeks the condition may gradually subside and eventually undergo a complete restoration to normal, as has been demonstrated by Boley et al. (1963), Schwartz et al. (1963), Marshak et al. (1965), Roberts (1965), Irwin (1965) and Marston et al. (1966). The other is that a progressively increasing fibrous stenosis of the affected segment of bowel ensues with the ultimate production of a long or short stricture.

Cases with Stricture Formation. As already explained, these cases may have been followed through from the earliest stage of an episode of transient ischaemic colitis. Alternatively, they may present for the first time after the acute attack has subsided, but with some residual bowel symptoms leading to investigation, at which the presence of a stricture of the colon is demonstrated. This may be long or short and in Marston et al.'s. (1966) experience was usually centred on the region of the splenic flexure, but it may occur also in the sigmoid or rectosigmoid (Roberts 1965). It may present a very difficult problem of differential diagnosis, for it has to be distinguished from so-called segmental ulcerative colitis, from Crohn's disease and, if very short, from carcinoma or diverticulitis. There are some clinical and radiological points of difference from these lesions which may be helpful, and, if the stricture can be reached by the sigmoidoscope or colonoscope, a biopsy should be of great assistance. But the final decision will often depend on laparotomy, resection and histological examination.

RADIOLOGICAL FEATURES

Boley et al. (1963), Schwartz et al. (1963), Marshak et al. (1965) and Irwin (1965) have described the radiological appearances of ischaemic colitis on barium enema examination. The lesion is seen as a long or short segment in which there is loss of haustration, a smooth or irregular contour and a variable amount of encroachment on the lumen ranging up to almost complete obstruction. Usually the affected part of bowel is clearly demarcated from the adjoining normal colon. Four radiological features are considered to be particularly characteristic of ischaemic colitis—'thumb-printing' (Boley et al. 1963), ragged 'saw-tooth' irregularity of the bowel contour, tubular narrowing and sacculation.

'Thumb-printing', which is probably the most valuable diagnostically, is due to polypoid change

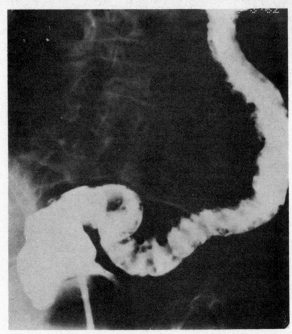

Fig. 610. Barium enema plate showing typical 'thumb printing' appearance of ischaemic colitis. (*From Marston 1966*)

in the mucosa, which produces a series of crescentic irregularities along the margin of the bowel and possibly also a number of rounded filling defects in the lumen (Fig. 610). Sacculation is due to wide-mouthed pseudo-diverticula of the colon wall, and is considered by Marston et al. (1966) to be the second most suggestive radiological sign of ischaemic colitis.

PATHOLOGICAL FEATURES

Gross. Though in ischaemic colitis produced experimentally in animals Marston (1964) observed appearances such as 'cobble-stoning' of the mucosa, resembling those of human Crohn's disease, in a series of operative specimens of ischaemic colitis removed from patients Marston et al. (1966) were unable to point to any such abnormalities. What they did find was a varying mixture of thickening of the colon wall, stenosis and mucosal ulceration. Ulceration was patchy, serpiginous, mainly longitudinal and often situated chiefly on the mesenteric aspect. Peritoneal adhesions and fibrosis were also frequently evident. Enlargement of the regional lymph nodes was not a feature.

Microscopic. In the areas of ulceration the mucosa is lost and its place taken by vascular granulation tissue. The submucosa is greatly widened with oedema and with infiltration by granulation tissue consisting of fibroblasts and a few lymphocytes, and eosinophil and plasma cells. There is also an increase in the amount of collagen. Usually *many macrophages laden with haemosiderin* are present, and Marston et al. (1966) consider this the most characteristic histopathological feature of ischaemic colitis.

DIAGNOSIS

The diagnosis of ischaemic colitis is greatly aided by a high degree of suspicion of a possible vascular origin in older patients, particularly in those with established cardiovascular disease. A characteristic feature is the abruptness of onset of the bowel symptoms. The segmental distribution of the lesion, sparing the rectum, should distinguish it from ordinary diffuse ulcerative colitis, but leaves it to be differentiated from other forms of segmental colitis including Crohn's disease. The radiological appearances may be helpful or equivocal in this respect. The absence of anal ulceration or fistulation is a point against a Crohn's lesion. If a biopsy of the affected colon wall is possible through the sigmoidoscope, the pathologist may be able to contribute to the clinical diagnosis.

TREATMENT

Cases with Frank Gangrene. It would seem that the mortality of this state of affairs will always be very high, but clearly the only prospect of survival lies with immediate operation and excision of the affected segment by an extraperitoneal type of resection. In addition to systemic antibiotic cover it would be reasonable to administer polyvalent anti-gas-gangrene serum in case there is a clostridial infection.

Cases with Mild Symptoms Unassociated with Severe Shock or Evidence of Perforation or Major Peritonitis. In these patients, in whom there is a good chance that the 'colitis' will resolve spontaneously, an expectant attitude is indicated. During the acute phase close supervision is essential, as in the conservative management of an acute attack of ordinary ulcerative colitis. Frequent re-examinations are required to detect any aggravation or extension of abdominal tenderness or deterioration of the general condition which might suggest that leakage or a spread of local peritonitis had occurred and call for operative intervention to resect the lesion and exteriorize the ends of bowel or anastomose them

depending on circumstances. After cessation of more urgent symptoms and discharge from hospital, the subsequent progress of the lesion should be followed by a regular barium enema examination every two or three months to detect any permanent stricture formation or show a restoration to normal.

Cases with Strictures. Surgical treatment will be required for these patients if they have persistent troublesome symptoms from a strictured chronically inflamed segment of large bowel or if there is uncertainty in the diagnosis from carcinoma. The operation will consist of excision of the affected part of bowel, followed usually by anastomosis. As Marston (1964) points out, it is well at this laparotomy to examine the state of the superior mesenteric system in case any form of arterial reconstruction may be advisable. To this end, too, a preoperative aortogram might give helpful information about the patency of the mesenteric arteries, and it would be well to arrange for the collaboration of a colleague interested in vascular surgery at the actual operation.

NECROTIZING OR CLOSTRIDIUM WELCHII COLITIS

Killingback and Williams (1961) report six cases of a hitherto unrecognized gangrenous process affecting the colon, in which there is extensive necrosis of the mucosa with patches of full-thickness gangrene of the bowel wall, and which they have designated 'necrotizing colitis'. A further example of the same condition has been described by Tate et al. (1965).

CLINICAL FEATURES

The condition is characterized by a fulminant course beginning with sudden severe abdominal pain, usually accompanied by bilious vomiting, but not diarrhoea or passage of blood. On examination, the patients were found to be collapsed and cyanotic with cold extremities and the abdomen was generally tender, guarded, and sometimes distended. The tentative clinical diagnosis was usually generalized peritonitis, intestinal obstruction, or an intra-abdominal vascular catastrophe, and urgent laparotomy was advised in all cases.

OPERATIVE AND PATHOLOGICAL FINDINGS

On opening the abdomen within a few hours of the onset of symptoms large amounts of putrid-smelling, non-haemorrhagic fluid were found within the peritoneal cavity. Areas of gangrene were evident on the serosal aspect of the colon, the distribution varying in different cases but being always confined to the large bowel. Examination of the affected colon from the inner aspect after removal showed a swollen, gelatinous blackish-brown mucosa without ulceration or blood-stained exudate. The mucosal changes were continuous, not patchy, and usually extended for a considerable distance beyond the limits of the necrotic areas seen on the serosal surface. *No significant arterial or venous occlusion could be demonstrated.*

AETIOLOGY

The sudden onset, profound shock, and eventual gangrene suggested that the condition might be due to *infarction*, but against this explanation is the absence of demonstrable vascular occlusion on pathological examination, and the fact that gangrene was restricted to the large bowel, which is a most unusual finding in intestinal infarction. In Tate et al.'s (1965) case the distribution of the gangrene was even more bizarre for an infarction, for the caecum was necrotic but the appendix not. The possibility that this might be some form of *acute ulcerative colitis* seemed to be excluded because of the dramatically rapid course and the absence of any ulceration of the mucosa or bloody diarrhoea. *Staphylococcal or pseudomembranous enterocolitides* were rejected because in these conditions the small bowel is also extensively affected and there is often a highly characteristic yellowish-white pseudomembrane. Ulceration of the mucosa is also present and diarrhoea is usual, though it may be delayed. Killingback and Williams (1961) stress that enormous numbers of Gram-positive organisms showing morphological features of *Clostridium welchii* were present in the wall of the bowel in all their operative specimens and, though these were unfortunately not cultured, they incline to the opinion that the condition is one of *gas gangrene of the colon wall*. In the case reported by Tate et al. (1965) clostridial infection seems to have been established. Marston et al. (1966) incline to the view that necrotizing colitis is initiated by ischaemic changes in the colon, which facilitate the entrance of clostridia into the bowel wall (see p. 859).

TREATMENT

What is needed is immediate resection of the affected segment of bowel as soon as the patient can be made fit for this operation. Because of the greater extent of the gangrenous process on the mucosal than the serosal aspect, and the occurrence of isolated outlying patches of the disease, it is important to make the excision sufficiently wide to avoid incomplete removal. Killingback and Williams (1961) advise against primary anastomosis because of the risk of breakdown and leakage and instead recommend the establishment of proximal and distal colostomies. It would be reasonable to administer not only broad-spectrum antibiotics, but also gas-gangrene antitoxin.

NON-SPECIFIC ULCERATION OF THE LARGE INTESTINE

The occurrence of 'simple ulcers' of the intestine, small or large, was first described by Baillie (1795) and Cruveilhier (1829). In 1925 Grassmann gave a very lucid account of this lesion as found in the small gut, defining it as a sharp-bordered, solitary ulceration with no surrounding inflammation, of unknown cause, indefinite pathogenesis and an acute or chronic course. Comprehensive surveys of the literature on simple ulcers of the large intestine have been provided by Barlow (1941) and Friedman and MacKenzie (1959), and a good review of the whole subject of non-specific ulceration of the intestine is that of Guest (1963).

PATHOLOGY

The majority of simple ulcers are described by Guest (1963) as punched out in appearance with no gross surrounding inflammation, but in several of the cases reported by Russell (1961) with ulcers in the caecum there was considerable induration of the adjacent bowel wall and stenosis. Usually the ulcers are single but occasionally they occur in small groups from two to six in number (Guest 1963; Russell 1961). When multiple they usually occur within 10–20 cm of one another. Many authors have noted a tendency for the ulceration to be on the antimesenteric border of the bowel. The site distribution of the ulcers in the different segments of the large intestine in 78 cases analysed by Barlow (1941) was: caecum 50%; sigmoid colon 16%; ascending colon 9%; and hepatic flexure, transverse colon, splenic flexure, descending colon and rectum, each 5%.

Microscopically, simple ulcers closely resemble peptic ulcers. There is a central area of necrosis surrounded by varying amounts of fibrous tissue interspersed with relatively small numbers of inflammatory cells, the character of which is determined by the acuteness of the process. By comparison the ulcerations found in bacterial dysentery, ulcerative colitis or Crohn's disease are shallower, more irregular lesions surrounded by considerably more acute diffuse inflammation.

NATURAL HISTORY

It seems possible that many simple ulcers of the large intestine heal spontaneously. Others progress to perforation and some cases undergo repeated perforation at the same site. Another complication that may occur is haemorrhage.

AETIOLOGY

There has been much speculation as to the cause of simple ulcers of the intestine but no convincing explanation of their aetiology has been forthcoming. A *vascular insufficiency* to the wall of the caecum was postulated by Wilkie (1937), Cameron (1939) and Barlow (1941) as a factor in the production of ulcers in this region. *Trauma* to the colon wall by hard objects in the faeces, such as fish bones, with resulting *infection* has been suggested by Barron (1928) and Bearse (1929). A similar suggestion was that *dietary factors* might be important (Wilkie 1937; Harrison 1940; Cromar 1946)—either that a diet containing much cereal might predispose to simple ulcer by the traumatic effect of the roughage on the mucosa or that the inclusion of much protein might in some inexplicable way be responsible. Needless to say, *habitual constipation* has also been incriminated (Kerr 1935). In the caecal region a solitary diverticulum may become inflamed, leading to an appearance very like that of a non-specific ulcer, and this has led to the suggestion that all simple ulcers of the caecum are *due to an underlying diverticulum* (Lipton and Riesman 1951). But on this theory it would be necessary to assume that the mucous membrane of the entire diverticulum had always been so destroyed by inflammation that it could not be identified, which seems unlikely. Furthermore this suggestion does not provide an explanation for the occurrence of simple ulcers in other parts of the large bowel.

DIAGNOSIS AND TREATMENT

The correct diagnosis of non-specific ulcer has seldom been made before laparotomy or autopsy, except in cases with rectal ulceration accessible to sigmoidoscopy (see below). More usually the patient comes to operation (or necropsy) on a diagnosis of perforated peptic ulcer, appendicitis or carcinoma of the caecum and the surgeon finds himself faced with three possible situations:

1. A Chronic Inflammatory Mass or Pericaecal Abscess. A mass, which may have been apparent clinically, may be found in the ileocaecal region and will probably be misdiagnosed as an appendix mass or abscess or a carcinoma of the caecum or ascending colon. This will lead to the performance of simple drainage or to a right hemicolectomy, the correct diagnosis being made at subsequent laparotomy or on examination of the resected piece of bowel.

2. General Peritonitis. Exploration will reveal the actual perforation, the difficulty being probably to determine whether this has arisen from a simple ulcer, a carcinoma or diverticular disease, or is a spontaneous perforation of normal bowel. Depending partly on the decision as to cause and partly on the patient's general condition, the perforation will be oversewn or a resection carried out.

3. An Unperforated Ulcer. Opinions vary as to how a simple unperforated ulcer should be managed. Most surgeons, feeling perhaps unsure as to whether they may not be dealing with an early carcinoma, or fearing progression to perforation or haemorrhage, have performed a segmental resection or at least have oversewn the ulcer (Eagleson 1952). But Russell (1961) has suggested that no direct attack of any kind should be made on the ulcer and that the abdomen should be closed without doing anything.

SOLITARY ULCER OF THE RECTUM

The term solitary ulcer of the rectum was introduced by O. V. Lloyd-Davies of St Mark's Hospital, London, 30 years ago to denote a peculiar idiopathic form of rectal ulceration. Since then 68 cases of this condition have been seen at that hospital, and Madigan and Morson (1969) give a very helpful account of the salient clinical and pathological features on the basis of a review of these patients. It is largely a complaint of young adults, males and females being equally affected. The outstanding symptoms are frequent calls to stool to pass mucus and blood (rarely profuse). Somewhat less commonly there is also a pain or discomfort in the rectum.

On sigmoidoscopy the ulcer, which is usually single, is seen to lie on the anterior rectal wall in its middle third. It is shallow, generally 2–3 cm in diameter with a sloughy washleather base and often considerable heaping-up of the surrounding mucosa. In about a third of the cases more than one ulcer is present. Biopsies taken from the adjacent mucosa characteristically show obliteration of the lamina propria by fibroblasts and muscle fibres derived from the muscularis mucosae. Sometimes the overlying epithelium exhibits a brisk reactive hyperplasia with a tendency to goblet cell depletion. In about 10% of cases misplaced mucosa is seen in the submucosa at the margins of the ulcer and has often undergone cystic dilatation (see also Colitis cystica profunda, p. 877).

Clinically, solitary ulcer is most often confused with carcinoma of the rectum or Crohn's disease, but biopsy should confidently exclude these conditions. It appears that there is a non-ulcerative stage of the disease characterized by a localized thickening of the mucosa, similar to that seen around frank ulcers; a biopsy may be required to differentiate this form of the condition from other types of proctitis.

The cause of solitary ulcer is obscure. Madigan and Morson (1969) could not adduce any good evidence in favour of self-inflicted trauma as a causal factor. They postulate a hamartomatous origin mainly because of the presence on section of submucosal epithelial cysts. Schweiger and Alexander-Williams (1977) believe that an associated, often undetected, complete rectal prolapse is a frequent and important aetiological factor. It was present in all 12 of a series of solitary rectal ulcers reported by them. Moreover, following a transabdominal rectopexy in 10 of these cases, the rectal ulcer has healed in 9. I must add, however, that in eight cases of solitary rectal ulcer recently surveyed in my practice, no evidence of overt or concealed rectal prolapse could be evinced. Morgan (1978), of the Royal Prince Henry Hospital, Sydney, was similarly unable to demonstrate rectal prolapse in a larger series of cases of solitary ulcer.

Solitary ulcer of the rectum is a benign condition, which may rarely undergo complete healing, but more often persists for many years or indefinitely. Its treatment is most unsatisfactory. Medical therapy that has been employed includes suppositories, cortisone enemas and other local applications, but it is uncertain whether any of these measures have been of the slightest value. Conservative forms of surgical treatment, which have included diathermy, cauterization of the ulcer, proximal colostomy or even local excision of the bowel by anterior resection, have all failed significantly to alter the chronic course of the disease. Schweiger and Alexander-Williams (1977) have reported very successful results in curing these ulcers by treating associated rectal prolapse by rectopexy. Complete removal of the rectum by abdominoperineal excision with permanent iliac colostomy is, of course, a certain cure, but rarely has the severity of the patient's symptoms justified this extreme measure (but I have four times had to take this step with very satisfactory results).

TUBERCULOSIS

Hyperplastic Tuberculous Enteritis

Since the emergence of Crohn's disease as a well-recognized and frequently encountered patho-

TABLE 73. *Numbers of Patients with Ileocaecal Tuberculosis and Crohn's Disease Respectively, Treated at the Leeds General Infirmary from 1925 to 1969 Inclusive*

Year	Ileocaecal tuberculosis	Crohn's disease
1925–9	20	—
1930–4	18	—
1935–9	19	3
1940–4	12	13
1945–9	3	25
1950–4	2	38
1955–9	2	72
1960–4	1	98
1965–9	4	110

After Goligher et al. (1971).

logical entity, hyperplastic ileocaecal tuberculosis has largely disappeared from clinical experience in Western countries (Table 73). Some authorities, indeed, such as Warren and Sommers (1948) and Boyd (1955), have taken the view that most of the lesions in the ileocaecal region and colon previously diagnosed and demonstrated as tuberculous were in fact examples of Crohn's disease. Whilst this contention may be largely correct, it is equally certain that the total rejection of hyperplastic tuberculous enteritis is unwarranted. Cases are still occasionally seen where the tubercle bacillus can be demonstrated in the affected bowel wall or related lymph glands, or where a guinea-pig inoculation test is positive. For example, Hoon et al. (1950) report on 58 proven cases of hyperplastic tuberculous enteritis of the colon encountered at the Mayo Clinic between 1921 and 1946; and Howell and Knapton (1964), Anscombe et al. (1967) and Byrom and Mann (1969) have published smaller groups of cases in this country, some but not all the patients being immigrants from India or Pakistan. The condition is well known to be extremely common in India and other tropical countries, as Misra and Pathak (1954), Anand (1956), Hancock (1958), Stock and Li (1964) and Tandon and Prakash (1972) have emphasized. The diagnosis of tubercle in most of these Indian cases has rested on the histological appearances, with the occurrence of caseation and sometimes the demonstration of acid-fast bacilli on tissue staining or culture, and only rarely on the results of guinea-pig inoculation, but I think there can be no doubt that many of them were in fact tuberculous. Certainly a study of 69 cases of ileocaecal tuberculosis in Amritsar, India, by Wig et al. (1961) included guinea-pig and rabbit inoculations of material from several of the cases, with positive results in a number of them.

Though this form of tuberculous enteritis is commonest in the ileocaecal region it may involve any part of the large intestine, as Hoon et al. (1950), Hancock (1958) and Tandon and Prakash (1972), who point out that multiple or 'skip' lesions may occur, have shown. The incidence of an associated pulmonary tuberculous lesion has been variously estimated by different authors, but in as many as 50% of the recorded cases it appears to have been absent, so that the enteritis may sometimes be the primary focus of tuberculosis. The wall of the affected part of the colon becomes greatly thickened due to granulomatous infiltration, fibrosis and caseation in the submucosa and other layers so that a large mass is formed and the lumen is con-

siderably reduced. Usually the mucosa becomes 'cobblestoned', due to irregularly disposed furrows, though rarely more definite ulceration occurs.

The disease is two or three times as common in females as in males; it may occur at any age but is most frequent from 20 to 39 years (Tandon and Prakash 1972).

CLINICAL FEATURES AND DIAGNOSIS

As Byron and Mann (1969) point out, the most prominent symptom in the majority of cases is abdominal pain, either central or in the right lower quadrant. Diarrhoea occurs in nearly half the patients and constipation or alternating constipation and diarrhoea in most of the remainder. Blood or mucus is passed in a few cases. A certain amount of weight loss is common. A mass is palpable in the right iliac region in the majority and, taken in conjunction with the other features, usually leads to a provisional diagnosis of Crohn's disease or carcinoma of the caecum, an impression which usually survives through the barium enema examination. Admittedly Anscombe et al. (1967) have described characteristic radiological appearances, in which the caecum disappears, the ascending colon shortens and the ileum retains its normal calibre but passes vertically upwards into the colon; but Byrom and Mann (1969) emphasize that these findings do not always reliably exclude Crohn's enteritis. A positive radiograph of the chest for a pulmonary tuberculous lesion would obviously be a strong point in favour of the abdominal condition being tuberculous as would the fact of the patient being of Indian or Pakistani origin. The diagnosis would be clinched if tubercle bacilli can be demonstrated in the stools, as was possible in three of eight patients tested in this way in Byrom and Mann's (1969) series. But, as Shukla and Hughes (1978) have pointed out, misdiagnosis of abdominal tuberculous lesions is all too common.

TREATMENT

If a certain clinical diagnosis can be reached, it would be theoretically possible to treat the condition simply by antituberculous chemotherapy and streptomycin. But the results of such treatment *per se* have not been impressive (Byrom and Mann 1969). In actual practice most patients in this country are likely to proceed to surgical exploration on a tentative diagnosis of Crohn's disease or new growth, and on the same basis it will be advisable at laparotomy to eradicate the lesion by resection. The results of this procedure in the short and long term seem to be very good (Anscombe et al. 1967; Byrom and Mann 1969). A debatable point is whether postoperative chemotherapy should be given or not. Some patients seem to have done very well without such treatment, but it would appear a wise precaution to give it in case any infected glands remain beyond the scope of the resection. A common schedule of dosage is streptomycin 1 g and isonicotinic acid hydrazide (INH) 300 mg daily for 90 days, followed by *para*-aminosalicylic acid (PAS) 9 g and INH 300 mg daily for four to five months (Tandon and Prakash 1972).

ACTINOMYCOSIS

This unusual infection may affect the large intestine anywhere from the ileocaecal region to the anus (Cope 1949).

ILEOCAECAL ACTINOMYCOSIS

The least uncommon site for actinomycosis in the abdomen is the ileocaecal region. The infection usually arises after an attack of acute perforating appendicitis, which presumably allows the organism to escape from the lumen of the appendix. Nothing exceptional is noted at the time of operation but within two or three weeks a hard lump develops in the right iliac fossa and around the drainage track if the wound was drained. The mass is painless and steadily increases in size extending towards the liver and kidney. If a sinus has persisted it may be possible to diagnose the condition from the nature of the pus with its 'sulphur granules' and contained actinomyces. Otherwise the swelling will continue to enlarge and gradually come closer to the surface as an abscess which will be incised, the nature of the lesion then being revealed by examination of the pus.

Till suppuration occurs and discharges it will be difficult to diagnose the condition from Crohn's disease, carcinoma of the caecum or colon, or a simple appendix abscess.

COLONIC ACTINOMYCOSIS

This is invariably mistaken for carcinoma of the colon till late in the course of the disease. It is diagnosed either on pathological and bacteriological examination of the lesion after surgical excision as a growth, or by finding actinomyces in the pus of an abscess which has formed and pointed on the surface.

RECTAL ACTINOMYCOSIS

This may occur primarily in the rectum (Morson 1961; Fry et al. 1965) or may be found as a chronic anorectal abscess secondary to actinomycotic lesions elsewhere in the alimentary tract. The condition may obviously be confused with other forms of chronic abscess and fistula in this region, notably tuberculosis, Crohn's disease or a secondarily infected carcinoma, and the diagnosis again depends on bacteriological examination of the pus.

TREATMENT AND PROGNOSIS

Formerly the prognosis with abdominal actinomycosis was gloomy, but now with large doses of penicillin, or ordinary dosage of oral tetracycline (Martin et al. 1956; Fry et al. 1965) most cases recover satisfactorily. The drug should be continued for some weeks after all symptoms have disappeared.

DYSENTERY

It is important to remember the specific dysenteries as a cause of acute diarrhoea with passage of blood and slime even in temperate climates, for an occasional case of apparent ulcerative colitis is found on examination of the stools to have an amoebic or bacillary dysentery. Alternatively, some patients sent to an isolation hospital with suspected dysentery—or enteric fever—subsequently turn out to have no specific infection but to be examples of ulcerative colitis. Amoebic dysentery is, of course, almost unknown in Britain, except in people who have been resident for a time in certain tropical or subtropical zones, but bacillary dysentery may occur in those who have never left these shores. The important thing is to bear in mind the possibility of dysentery and in any suspicious case to have repeated fresh stool samples examined for amoebae or stool cultures done for dysentery bacilli. Agglutination tests with specific sera which become positive within a few days of the onset of the disease may also be helpful in diagnosis of the bacillary form of the disease.

The sigmoidoscopic appearances of *bacillary* dysentery are not in any way specific, but resemble those seen at various stages of ordinary ulcerative colitis. In *amoebic* dysentery the sigmoidoscopic features may be more valuable in diagnosis. In the acute stage numerous small pinpoint or buttonhole ulcers occur with hyperaemic undermined edges but with a normal mucosa intervening between individual ulcers, except for occasional submucous telangiectatic haemorrhages. Scrapings taken by means of a small sharp spoon with a suitably long handle, such as Manson-Bahr's, and consisting of actual slough or secretion from the floor of an ulcer, may often be found on examination of the microscopic slide to contain numerous *Entamoeba histolytica*. Manson-Bahr and Muggleton (1957) have emphasized the need for the utmost speed in the execution of this manoeuvre; a delay of even 5–10 minutes may be fatal to success. It is not necessary to mix the biopsy material with normal saline or other diluent. The scraping is simply removed from the scoop with the aid of a matchstick on to the slide, and a 'squash preparation' is made by pressing on to it a 2 × 2 cm cover-glass.

For detailed advice on the clinical features and management of cases of acute dysentery reference should be made to standard medical texts. Though the great majority of patients will respond to specific therapy with emetine or metronidazole, an occasional patient fails to respond and may be salvaged by emergency ileostomy and colectomy, as advocated by Stein and Bank (1970). Sometimes perforation of the colon occurs, too, requiring surgical intervention (Chen et al. 1971; Eggleston et al. 1978). It is recommended by Eggleston et al. (1978) that, if the perforation is in the more proximal colon, it should be bypassed by an end-to-side ileocolostomy and the perforation site drained; if, however, it is in the sigmoid colon, a simple ileostomy should be performed, together with drainage of the region of the perforated colon through a separate incision. These authors counsel strongly against immediate resection because the friable state of the inflamed large bowel makes it a specially difficult and dangerous form of treatment. I myself have no practical experience of treating this condition, but on theoretical grounds would start with a bias in favour of ileostomy and subtotal colectomy for such colonic perforation, wherever situated.

Chronic or Latent Amoebiasis and Amoebic Granuloma ('Amoeboma')

Of greater significance to the surgeon practising in a temperate climate is the so-called chronic or latent form of amoebic infection of the intestine, which may be encountered in those who were formerly resident in a tropical or subtropical country. This type of amoebiasis is well described by Nevin (1947) and Archampong and Clark (1973). In some cases the patient may give a clear history of a previous acute attack of dysentery which was treated and apparently completely cured; in others the infection is acquired quite insidiously without any definite initial symptoms, sometimes without even residence abroad. The interval between the original infection and the later manifestations may vary from months to as long as several years. The main incidence of chronic amoebiasis in the intestinal tract is usually in the caecal region; more rarely other parts of the colon or rectum are affected.

Manifestations of Chronic Intestinal Amoebiasis

CHRONIC DIARRHOEA

A persistent or recurrent diarrhoea may be due to a smouldering amoebic infection and in any case of chronic diarrhoea, where the patient has ever been exposed to the risk of acquiring an amoebic infection in the past, the possibility of a chronic amoebiasis as the cause of the symptoms must always be borne in mind. The most important investigation to exclude such an infection is repeated examination of the stools for *Entamoeba histolytica*. On sigmoidoscopy the rectal and lower colonic mucosa may appear normal or may show a very fine superficial type of ulceration that is very easily missed. This consists of numerous tiny ulcers, which give the mucosa a 'pock-marked' or 'pig-skin' appearance (Manson-Bahr and Muggleton 1957), which has also been likened to that of multiple bomb-craters seen in an aerial photograph (Cropper 1945, 1951). Scrapings should be taken of any suspicious lesion for examination for amoebae. Barium enema and barium meal examination may reveal a deformity or irregularity of the caecum.

CAECAL MANIFESTATIONS MIMICKING ACUTE OR SUBACUTE APPENDICITIS

Exacerbation of a chronic amoebic infection of the caecum may give rise to acute symptoms and signs closely resembling those of an acute or subacute appendicitis. Patients with chronic amoebiasis may, of course, also develop an ordinary acute appendicular inflammation, so that even if entamoebae have been isolated from the stools a difficult diagnostic problem may present itself to the surgeon, with grave implications in regard to treatment. Appendicectomy in the presence of active amoebic infection of the caecal region carries serious risks of tearing the bowel wall, with leakage and infection, as James (1946) and Nevin (1947) have pointed out. On the other hand, there are obviously very considerable hazards in leaving an acute obstructive appendicitis without operation.

Sometimes a careful appraisal of the history may enable a fairly confident decision to be made. Thus in acute appendicitis the pain generally starts in the epigastrium or centre of the abdomen, whilst the pain in amoebiasis of the caecal region usually commences in the lower abdomen or right iliac fossa. Acute appendicitis tends to occur in a patient who was previously fit, though he may have had previous attacks of a similar nature, whilst the symptoms of amoebiasis often present in a person who has been below par for some considerable time.

If the surgeon feels compelled to operate despite the presence of a proven or suspected amoebiasis, because of the serious possibility of ordinary appendicitis, he should institute immediate treatment with emetine, the first injection of 60 mg being given before operation, and further injections continued post-operatively. When the abdomen is opened, if the caecum and appendix are found to be involved in the same process and the condition is deemed to be one of amoebic infection, the appendix should not be removed, the tissues should be most gently handled and, at most, a soft corrugated rubber drain should be inserted for 72 hours (James 1946).

THE DEVELOPMENT OF A MASS IN THE CAECUM, COLON OR RECTUM

The occurrence of an amoebic granuloma producing a large mass is actually very rare, but when it is encountered it may cause considerable difficulty in diagnosis. The usual sites are the caecal and rectosigmoid regions. The mass may be associated with partial or complete obstruction or with chronic bowel symptoms, so that it may closely simulate a carcinoma, a Crohn's lesion or an appendix abscess. The difficulty is accentuated by the fact that these conditions may occur as intercurrent diseases in a patient with established chronic intestinal amoebiasis. If the granuloma is in the rectosigmoid within reach of the sigmoidoscope, great assistance may be obtained by biopsy, which if repeatedly negative excludes a neoplasm. With the more common caecal amoebomas this aid is not available and reliance has to be placed on a therapeutic test, the effect of a course of emetine injections (60 mg intramuscularly per day for seven days) or of oral metronidazole (Flagyl) (200 mg four times daily for five to ten days) being carefully noted on the size of the mass and other signs and symptoms. In cases of 'amoeboma' the response is usually dramatic. Unless a complete resolution is obtained the diagnosis of amoebic granuloma cannot be considered to be established, for Morgan (1944) has recorded cases where a partial response occurred in patients with coexistent chronic amoebiasis and carcinoma. Under these circumstances laparotomy should be carried out under emetine cover.

ULCERATIVE PROCESSES AFFECTING OPERATION WOUNDS IN THE ANAL CANAL AND ABDOMINAL WALL

Nevin (1947) has drawn attention to the liability of patients with chronic intestinal amoebiasis to develop spreading infections in haemorrhoidectomy and other wounds in the anal canal, or in abdominal wounds, particularly around a colostomy. The characteristic appearance of these lesions is of a progressive irregular ulcer with overhanging gangrenous edges. Surrounding these edges is a pigmented zone which has been described as a 'halo' of a dusky, reddish colour. The floor of the ulcer consists of adherent greyish necrotic material and the discharge is fetid and offensive. Amoebae are not usually present in the exudate but can be demonstrated in the tissues beneath the undermined edges of the ulcer. The condition resembles closely the progressive postoperative gangrene of the skin described by Meleney (1948), and now believed to be due to a micro-aerophilic streptococcus. The response to emetine treatment, however, is striking and provides an immediate confirmation of the diagnosis.

In conclusion, then, it may be said that chronic intestinal amoebiasis may present the surgeon with a number of diagnostic problems. If, however, *the possibility of this condition is remembered* most of these difficulties can be quickly resolved.

BILHARZIASIS OF THE RECTUM AND COLON

Bilharzial dysentery occurs in tropical and subtropical countries, such as Egypt, Japan and certain parts of Africa and South America. In the acute stage it gives rise to symptoms similar to those of any other acute dysentery. At a later stage adenopapillomas occur which resemble ordinary adenomas, and fibrous induration of the rectal or colon wall may be encountered leading to stricture formation. Perianal fistulas may be present extending into the buttocks. For a full account of the disease standard texts on tropical diseases, such as Manson-Bahr (1943), should be consulted. It suffices for the surgeon to remember bilharzial infection of the rectum and colon as a cause of proctocolitis, polyps, strictures, anorectal fistulas and occasionally granulomas in the colon (Stock and Li 1964) and to think of it particularly in patients who have lived in Egypt. The diagnosis is established by demonstrating the ova of the bilharzia (usually *Schistosoma mansoni*) in the stools or in sections of the adenomas removed by biopsy forceps. In patients with long-standing disease who have developed a tight stricture, operative treatment may be required to remove the strictured area, which may sometimes be possible by a sphincter-saving technique and at others may require an abdominoperineal excision depending on the height of the lesion. These operations may be technically very difficult because of adhesions between the affected bowel and neighbouring structures. Bilharzial infection of the large bowel, unlike the corresponding condition in the bladder, does not predispose to carcinoma, though obviously a supposed bilharzial stricture or granuloma must be distinguished from an ordinary idiopathic malignant tumour of the bowel.

GONORRHOEAL PROCTITIS

This form of proctitis is much commoner in male patients, in whom it is almost always due to passive rectal coitus with an infected partner. Sometimes it assumes the proportions of a small epidemic in boys' schools or penal institutions due to adolescent homosexual practices, but usually it occurs more sporadically in overt adult homosexuals. The recent increase in this country in venereal infections transmitted by homosexuals lends additional importance to this variety of proctitis.

Gonorrhoeal proctitis may also affect women and does so much more commonly than is often realized. Thus Nicol (1948) and Jensen (1953) found gonococcal proctitis in 35% and 31%, respectively, of female patients with gonorrhoea who were submitted to proctoscopic examination. In most of these cases anorectal involvement is only detected if search is made for it. It gives rise to neither symptoms nor external signs. Opinions differ as to how many of these infections result from anorectal intercourse and how many are due to spread of infective material to the anus from a gonorrhoeal lesion of the vulva. The latter probably occurs during defaecation when increased intrapelvic pressure causes menstrual blood and vaginal discharge to flow over the everted anal mucous membrane. Patients with uncomplicated genital gonorrhoea seldom have much discharge and it seems likely that spread to the anorectum will occur more often in patients whose genital gonorrhoea is complicated by trichomonal vaginitis, giving rise to a profuse vaginal discharge (King 1962). Infants with gonorrhoeal vulvovaginitis may similarly acquire a proctitis from backward spread.

Clinical Features

A good account of the clinical features of the condition is given by Harkness (1948) in his report on 168 males with established gonorrhoeal proctitis acquired by admitted sodomy. He emphasizes that acute symptoms consisting of tenesmus, a burning sensation and painful defaecation were infrequent. More commonly the condition caused only minimal discomfort: just a slight amount of anal moisture and pruritus, and sometimes warts of the anal region. The largest proportion of the patients were in fact entirely symptom-free, the diagnosis in these cases having been made during examinations carried out in search of venereal contacts.

On proctoscopy and sigmoidoscopy in the more acute cases the rectal mucosa is seen to be congested, oedematous and friable, the changes being most marked in the lower part of the rectum and in the region of the anal valves where pus is generally present. The diagnosis is readily established by demonstrating gonococci in a smear of the material obtained through the proctoscope.

Treatment

Since the introduction of penicillin the treatment of gonorrhoeal proctitis, as of other manifestations of gonococcal infection, has presented no problem—at least not till a few years ago, when resistant strains were for the first time encountered, and have occasionally required the use of other antibiotics.

LYMPHOGRANULOMA VENEREUM

This condition, also known as lymphogranuloma inguinale, is a disease of world-wide distribution but with a specially high incidence in coloured peoples. It has hitherto been rare in Britain, and most of the patients seen with it have come from abroad and are usually coloured. With the great influx of negro immigrants in the last few years from the West Indies, where lymphogranuloma is rife, it seemed likely that the number of patients encountered with the disease in this country would increase markedly, but this has fortunately not happened. A most helpful account of lymphogranuloma as seen in West Indian natives is that of Miles (1957).

Aetiology and Pathology

Lymphogranuloma is due to infection with a virus of the psittacosis group, which is introduced into the body by sexual intercourse. Three forms of the disease may result:

The Inguinal Variety

In this form, after a transient primary sore on the penis, an inguinal lymphadenitis develops. This eventually softens to produce inguinal abscesses or buboes which burst or subside.

The Genital Variety

In this type the primary lesion on the genitals assumes a massive form and there is extensive oedema, abscess formation, fistulation and destruction of tissue.

The Anorectal Variety

It was Bensaude and Lambling (1936), who, with the aid of the Frei (1925) test, first established that many inflammatory strictures of the rectum, which were previously regarded as being due to syphilis or gonorrhoea, were in fact caused by lymphogranuloma venereum. They believed that in men the stricture was the consequence of a proctitis produced by direct infection of the rectal mucosa with the virus, but that in women the initial lesion was a primary sore high on the posterior vaginal wall or cervix. This was followed by backward spread along the lymphatics to the perirectal tissues with subsequent inflammation and fibrosis in the rectal wall proceeding from without inwards, the mucosa being the last layer affected. In support of this idea of the pathogenesis of the rectal lesion in the two sexes, Bensaude and Lambling (1936) claimed that most male patients showed a stricture with proctitis, but female cases usually a stricture without proctitis.

There are, however, several arguments against their theory of the mechanism of involvement of the rectum in the female. First, no direct evidence is available as to the existence of a high vaginal or cervical primary sore and, even if such a lesion were present, it is odd that lymphatic spread from it should implicate the rectal lymphatic system, for the usual lymph drainage from this site is to the obturator or medial external iliac glands. Admittedly primary lesions have been seen occasionally at the vaginal orifice or on the fourchette, but these sites normally drain to the inguinal and iliac glands and not to the rectal lymphatics.

Secondly, other workers do not agree with Bensaude and Lambling's (1936) finding that in the female stricture is usually unassociated with evidence of proctitis. Grace (1941) reported that proctitis was present in 92% of his female patients, and Miles' (1957) experience was similar. It seems likely therefore that a stage of proctitis precedes stricture formation in the majority of female cases, as it does in males. In other words rectal lymphogranuloma in both sexes is due to a primary infection of the anorectal mucosa with the virus, following sodomy or backward seepage of infective material after normal intercourse.

As a result of the infection, an acute proctitis ensues which may extend proximally into the lower sigmoid colon. In the absence of treatment the inflammation persists in a subacute or chronic form and after months or years fibrosis of the rectal wall takes place; this is the 'prestricture phase' of Spiesman et al. (1937). Finally a definite stricture forms. Rectal lymphogranuloma is *much more common in women than men*.

Clinical Features

The earliest symptoms are usually those caused by the proctitis, with passage of blood and mucopus and the occurrence of spurious diarrhoea. This state of affairs is usually attributed by the patient to piles and may be allowed to continue for a considerable time before medical advice is sought. At a later stage stricture formation may cause a partial obstruction with colicky abdominal pains, distension, difficulty in securing proper motions and sometimes the passage of narrow ribbon-like stools. Rarely a complete obstruction may be produced. Finally it should be mentioned that recurrent perianal or ischiorectal abscesses are common in this condition with resulting fistula formation. In female patients the fistula is often of rectovaginal type being almost invariably situated at the level of the anorectal ring, and the passage of faeces per vaginam may be the presenting symptom.

Findings on Rectal Examination and Barium Enema Studies

Three types of lesion may be found on examination: proctitis alone, proctitis and stricture, and stricture alone.

PROCTITIS

This is mainly a granular proctitis which differs in no essential respect from an idiopathic granular proctocolitis. The mucosa is said by Miles (1957) to have a characteristic coarsely granular feel resembling morocco leather to the examining finger; sometimes larger polypoid swellings can be palpated.

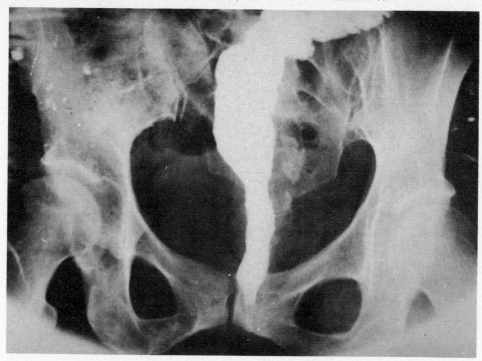

Fig. 611. Tubular stricture of lymphogranuloma venereum involving rectum and lower part of pelvic colon. (*From Miles 1957*)

THE STRICTURE

The stricture varies greatly in its density and length. In some cases it amounts to only a slight constriction gripping the finger; in others it is a tight stenosis which will not admit the smallest probe. The lower limit of the stricture usually lies 3–5 cm from the anal verge, and even below this the mucosa shows evidence of proctitis. The 'face' of the stricture is covered with intact, smooth, atrophic mucosa, which may be split by attempts at passage of the finger.

The upper limit and extent of the stricture are displayed by barium enema examination (Fig. 611). This shows that the stricture is usually long and tubular and involves the whole rectum and often the terminal part of the sigmoid colon as well. Only rarely is it of shorter extent, when it may be conical or diaphragmatic. Sometimes two or three separate strictures are present in the rectum and distal sigmoid.

In a few patients a 'dry' stricture alone is present without any active proctitis, but in many of these cases the mucosa shows scarring indicative of an inflammatory condition in the past.

LESIONS ABOVE THE RECTUM

As Miles (1957) has pointed out, the barium enema examination in cases of rectal lymphogranuloma reveals that the disease is not confined to the anus and rectum, but as a rule involves the left side of the colon as well, sometimes as far proximally as the splenic flexure. A variety of radiological appearances may be encountered in the affected distal colon. In some cases the sigmoid loop, which is normally redundant in the Negro, becomes short, thickened and inelastic; in others the whole left colon shows an absence of haustration and a tubular appearance as in ulcerative colitis, whilst in yet others there may be one or more strictures in the sigmoid and descending colon separated by apparently normal bowel.

Diagnosis

In cases with a definite rectal stricture the diagnosis is usually easy, though other causes of stricture have to be borne in mind and differentiated as mentioned on p. 913. However, a dense, non-neoplastic stricture in a negroid patient is almost certainly the result of rectal lymphogranuloma venereum. Confirmation can be obtained by the Frei test or the complement-fixation test. When a proctocolitis alone is present, the diagnosis is much more difficult. There is nothing in the objective findings to distinguish the conditions from a non-specific proctocolitis. The type of patient and the clinical history will possibly suggest lymphogranuloma, but the final diagnosis will depend on a positive Frei test or complement-fixation test.

Treatment

ANTIBIOTIC TREATMENT

At the stage of proctitis without stricture formation, only medical treatment is required, the essential item of which is the administration of broad-spectrum antibiotics. According to Miles (1957), chloromycetin, erythromycin and aureomycin are all equally effective and can all be relied upon to arrest rectal lymphogranuloma at the proctitis or pre-stricture phase. They are best given in doses of 2 g daily for 14 days and generally produce rapid and complete symptomatic and sigmoidoscopic improvement. Occasionally a relapse of symptoms follows the cessation of treatment, but this usually responds to a further course of therapy with a different antibiotic.

In cases with actual stricturing antibiotic treatment may also produce a considerable amelioration of symptoms, as Miles (1957) and Annamunthodo (1961) have claimed, due to the elimination of residual proctitis and in some cases even to 'widening' of early strictures, presumably from subsidence of inflammatory oedema. In cases with slighter degrees of stricture formation the effect of a full course of antibiotic therapy should therefore be tried before resorting to surgery, and indeed this may be a useful preliminary to operation even when the latter seems inevitable.

SURGICAL TREATMENT

This is indicated in cases with severe strictures causing some degree of obstruction, with rectovaginal fistulas, with gross damage to the anal sphincters, or very rarely because of acute obstruction. It may take several forms.

PERIODIC DILATATION

This traditional form of palliative treatment is condemned by Miles (1957) as likely to aggravate rather than arrest the tendency to stenosis, for in the Negro particularly, attempts at stretching of fibrous tissue are apt to produce a violent tissue reaction so that still more fibrosis may result. The danger of perforation during dilatation is also stressed by Annamunthodo (1961), who considers that this manoeuvre should be reserved for soft annular strictures.

COLOSTOMY

A colostomy may be required as an emergency procedure for acute intestinal obstruction. If it appears likely that an abdominoperineal excision of the rectum will be necessary in the final treatment of the condition, the emergency colostomy should be established in the iliac colon provided this is not actually diseased. But if there are hopes of being able to resect the lesions subsequently by some form of sphincter-saving excision, a transverse colostomy will be better emergency treatment for acute obstruction.

Hawe (1951) and Miles (1957) emphasize that a colostomy alone, without later removal of the diseased bowel, exposes the patient with rectal lymphogranuloma to the danger of the lesion extending gradually proximally to implicate the stoma. But Annamunthodo (1961) reports seven cases treated by permanent colostomy, placed well above the lesion, without later spread of the disease to the stoma.

EXCISIONAL SURGERY

Removal of the diseased rectum and colon is best carried out either by a straightforward abdominoperineal excision or by some form of sphincter-saving resection. The decision in favour of the latter type of operation will obviously depend on the presence of good functioning sphincters and an adequate margin of essentially normal bowel between the stricture and the sphincters, and it is probably unwise to consider a sphincter-preserving operation with lesions the lower margin of which lies less than 5 cm from the anal verge. As for the choice of technique for conservative excision, a purely anterior resection is usually out of the question, and an abdominoanal or abdominosacral method has to be employed. Most surgeons with considerable experience in the treatment of these lesions, such as Wright et al. (1946), Breidenbach and Slattery (1949) and Miles (1957), prefer a pull-through abdominoanal excision rather similar to the Bacon operation (see p. 510) used for rectal cancer, but actually modelled on the operation employed by Hartmann (1922) of Paris in the management of his large series of cases of rectal strictures. Though the functional result is often very imperfect after this operation, the type of patient who acquires rectal lymphogranuloma is frequently tolerant of a degree of incontinence that would be quite unacceptable to more fastidious individuals. Annamunthodo (1961) states that in the treatment of lymphogranulomatous rectal strictures at the University College Hospital of the West Indies, Jamaica, during 1952–8, 39 rectal excisions were performed—10 abdominoperineal excisions with colostomy, and 29 sphincter-saving resections. The functional result after the latter operations is described as good in six and satisfactory in 10. Provided the stricture is low and does not extend far proximally in the long axis of the rectum, it may be amenable to simple segmental resection though the posterior transsphincteric approach of Mason (1970), as suggested by Miles (1972) (see p. 355).

ANORECTAL SYPHILIS

PERIANAL CONDYLOMAS

These are a well known manifestation of secondary syphilis and are mentioned on p. 370; they will not be further described here.

PRIMARY SYPHILIS OF THE ANORECTAL REGION

This used to be relatively rare, but in the last decade has become almost the commonest form of primary syphilis in Britain. Thus, according to Jefferiss (1962) and Nicol (1962), no less than 76% and 31·6%, respectively, of the patients attending their venereal disease clinics in London with early syphilis admitted homosexual exposure and were believed to have acquired the disease in this way. King (1962) aptly commented that homosexual practices seem to be keeping syphilis alive in this country. As homosexual patients are often unaware of the risk of contracting a venereal infection in this way, they tend to report any complaint to the proctologist, and therefore the responsibility of making a correct diagnosis usually rests with him. As with rectal gonorrhoea, the initial symptoms may be very mild, so that the patient may not seek medical advice at all at this stage. The primary chancre may then heal and the disease is missed till secondary or tertiary manifestations appear.

The most common *primary lesion of anorectal syphilis* is a single painless circular indurated ulcer at the anal margin or in the anal canal, but multiple or contact lesions are not uncommon (Nicol 1962). There is often a characteristic, rather offensive discharge, which causes the entire perianal skin to become sodden. The inguinal glands are often enlarged and have a 'rubbery' feel on palpation. Occasionally a primary chancre occurs in the lower rectum and causes a localized ulcer with surrounding proctitis as described by Lieberman (1951). If the diagnosis is suspected it is readily established by examination of a sample of the serous discharge from the lesion by dark ground illumination for the spirochaetes (see p. 77). The patient may already be in the secondary stage and show lesions in the skin, mucous membranes, mucocutaneous junctions, as well as a generalized lymphadenopathy (and possibly iritis, hepatitis or periostitis). The blood Wassermann reaction only becomes positive three or four weeks after the appearance of the primary lesion.

TERTIARY SYPHILIS OF THE RECTUM

This used to be diagnosed fairly frequently as a cause of strictures, but the work of Bensaude and Lambling (1936) referred to on p. 868 has shown that most such strictures are due to lymphogranuloma venereum. Gumma of the rectum, however, is occasionally encountered, and I have seen one case with this condition, which was wrongly diagnosed in the first instance as a malignant tumour, probably a sarcoma because of its intact mucosa. However, a negative biopsy and a positive Wassermann reaction suggested a gumma. It responded well to penicillin therapy, as do lesions of anal and rectal syphilis in general.

IRRADIATION PROCTITIS AND ENTERITIS

Füth and Ebeler (1915) were apparently the first to draw attention to the occurrence of a rectal lesion following irradiation of an extrarectal structure. Buie and Malmgren (1930) focused attention on this condition by describing 65 cases with irradiation proctitis after radium treatment of cancer of the cervix uteri. Todd (1938) gave a most detailed account of the effects on the rectum of radium treatment for cervical cancer. He found that an acute proctitis with a hyperaemic granular mucosa was a fairly common *early* complication, occurring whilst the irradiation was in progress, but usually clearing up completely soon after the termination

of treatment. The *late* radium reactions were much more serious, though fortunately less frequent, and occurred in about 5% of cases; the average time of onset was about six months after the irradiation, but might be as soon as one month or as late as six years afterwards. (I have seen such a late radium reaction first manifesting itself 22 years after treatment, as have Localio et al. (1969).) The form the late reactions might take varied and included a mixture of changes—granular proctitis, ulceration, stricture formation and fistulation into the vagina. Except for stricturing, the changes were confined largely to the anterior rectal wall.

More recent accounts of irradiation injuries to the bowel have come from Localio et al. (1969) and DeCosse et al. (1969). They have emphasized that these injuries may be produced by conventional or supervoltage radiotherapy as well as by radium treatment, and that they may occur not only in the rectum but in other parts of the alimentary tract, such as the sigmoid, the small bowel, and even the duodenum and stomach. Thus, of the 100 cases reported by DeCosse et al. (1969), 81 had irradiation injuries to the rectum (including 29 rectovaginal fistulas), and 34 sustained similar damage to the intestine apart from the rectum (17 to the small bowel, nine to the colon and eight to both small intestine and colon). It must also be remembered that the urinary tract may be injured by the same forms of irradiation, especially for carcinoma of the uterine cervix, with the production of ureteric stenosis or vesicovaginal fistulation, so that a patient may present with simultaneous rectovaginal and vesicovaginal fistulas arising as a sequel to such treatment.

Clinical Features and Diagnosis

IRRADIATION PROCTITIS

The symptoms are like those of an ordinary idiopathic proctitis, with frequent calls to stool to pass blood and mucus, sometimes alone, sometimes along with faeces. Tenesmus is quite often a symptom and there may be some rectal discomfort or pain. Patients may become quite anaemic if the bleeding is severe and they may also lose weight. The development of a rectovaginal fistula is indicated by the complaint that faeces and flatus are being lost per vaginam as well as per rectum.

If the history of previous radium or X-ray treatment is elicited, it will immediately suggest the diagnosis, but, if this was administered many years previously, the patient may forget to mention it and mistakes in diagnosis are then more liable to occur. Todd (1938) records cases where the rectum was actually excised under the mistaken impression that the rectal condition was a carcinoma. However, the peculiar situation of the lesion at the level of the cervix uteri with any ulcer present situated on the anterior wall, and the features of the ulcer on sigmoidoscopy, with clear-cut edges without eversion, and with surrounding proctitis, should make the surgeon suspicious that it is not a carcinoma. If no ulceration has taken place and the changes are simply those of proctitis, it is characterized by its more localized nature and the fact that it usually spares the lower third of the rectum, unlike ordinary forms of distal proctitis or proctocolitis. Craig and Buie (1949) emphasize the finding of telangiectases in the mucosa on sigmoidoscopy as an important diagnostic sign, but I have not encountered this myself.

Even if the history of previous radium treatment or radiotherapy has been elicited and the connection between this treatment and the proctitis, rectal ulceration or stricture established, there may still be doubt as to whether the rectal lesion is due to irradiation or represents a recurrence of the cervical carcinoma. The upper vagina has usually been so obliterated by the radiation that it would conceivably be possible for the growth to reassert itself and show as a rectal ulcer without producing any frank ulceration in the vaginal vault. A *biopsy* is essential to resolve doubts of this kind and to establish whether or not active residual cancer is present. This decision is crucial not only because tumour will prevent successful closure of the fistula, but also because prolongation of life in the presence of active cancer may be a positive disservice. The biopsy specimens should be generous in order to penetrate the surface necrosis. In addition to biopsy the patient should be examined generally and by X-ray films of the chest to exclude metastases.

IRRADIATION ENTERITIS

Irradiation injuries of the small or large intestine apart from the rectum more usually cause obstructive symptoms with constipation, abdominal colic, distension, and eventually nausea and vomiting. It is on radiological examination of the small or large bowel that the precise diagnosis generally rests at this stage. As DeCosse et al. (1969) have pointed out, there is a considerable risk of eventual necrosis of bowel with perforation and peritonitis in these cases or the development of an external faecal fistula. Occasionally an area of irradiation enteritis may be the source of intestinal bleeding, which may be difficult to diagnose.

Prevention

Following Todd's (1938) important paper radiotherapists and gynaecologists have been alive to the danger of irradiation of the rectum and have adopted various prophylactic measures to lessen this hazard. These have comprised the use of locking devices to hold the vaginal applicators of radium in position, and frequent radiographs to confirm that their position is being maintained. Vaginal packing or screens of platinum, gold and tungsten have also been employed to protect the rectum to some extent from irradiation. It is also possible by means of a rectal probe counter to determine how much irradiation is getting through to the rectum. It seems likely that the use of cobalt instead of radium may be followed by less risk of irradiation extending to the bowel (Cochrane and Yarnold 1979).

Treatment and Prognosis

CONSERVATIVE MEASURES

In the majority of cases of irradiation proctitis no active treatment is required. Any tendency to anaemia from bleeding should be countered by giving an iron preparation and by periodic haemoglobin estimations, or by blood transfusion if necessary. It is reasonable to try topical steroid therapy in the form of retention enemas, as for idiopathic distal proctocolitis (see p. 731) but the results in my cases have been very inconclusive. It probably is a good plan to prescribe a mild aperient such as liquid paraffin if there is any tendency to constipation, to keep the stools soft and minimize the amount of trauma to the ulcerated or inflamed area of bowel.

It is important to emphasize to the patient that she may continue to have occasional bleeding and other symptoms for a considerable time, and that she should report to hospital if there are any fresh developments, such as more severe haemorrhage or a discharge from the vagina, suggesting that the ulcer has deepened.

SURGICAL MEASURES

Operative treatment may become necessary on account of really severe symptoms of proctitis, the occurrence of fistulation, or the development of obstruction.

FOR SEVERE TENESMUS, PASSAGE OF BLOOD AND PUS, DIARRHOEA AND PAIN

For patients with really severe symptoms of proctitis, which have not improved under conservative management, but in whom fistulation has not occurred, a temporary proximal colostomy may be tried. It is probably best established in the iliac colon, and may have to be maintained for quite a long time—say 6 or 12 months or longer, depending on the state of the mucosa on sigmoidoscopy—before it is safe to close it. Simple colostomy may, however, be disappointing in the relief of tenesmus and discharge and in the arrest of haemorrhage. Of four of my patients who had colostomies performed because of very severe haemorrhage, two continued to bleed alarmingly and came to emergency removal of the rectum to save life. If the tenesmus, discharge and other symptoms of proctitis continue indefinitely to be a major discomfort to the patient, the question of rectal excision will arise, either as abdominoperineal operation with permanent colostomy, or as some form of sphincter-saving resection, depending on the extent of the proctitis and the surgeon's personal experience, but probably safest and best as a complete rectal excision with colostomy.

FOR RECTOVAGINAL FISTULA

An immediate colostomy is essential in every case with a fistula, because it is always easier to care for a colostomy than to endure the discomforts of an uncontrolled fistula discharging faeces and flatus per vaginam. Eventual spontaneous closure of the fistula under cover of the colostomy is most unlikely, however long the faecal diversion is maintained. Unless therefore the patient is to have a permanent colostomy, some form of direct surgical attack on the fistula itself will have to be undertaken. Apart from the inconvenience of the colostomy there is the added discomfort that a certain amount of discharge of mucus and blood from the rectum may continue to escape through the fistula and the vagina. On the other hand reconstructive operations on the fistula are quite difficult and may fail. If the patient is elderly and frail or averse to further operative treatment it would be well to settle for a permanent colostomy, which is best sited in the iliac colon and made with a divided loop, the proximal end being brought out as a terminal iliac colostomy, the distal closed and

dropped back into the abdomen. But if an attempt is to be made subsequently to deal with the fistula, it is better to use a right transverse colostomy for the preliminary defunctioning, as being less likely to interfere with the course of the second operation. It is also essential to maintain this colostomy for at least 9–12 months to allow necrosis to disappear and the inflammatory reaction to subside so that the tissues of the rectum and vagina have regained their normal pliability before embarking on any conservative operation, though this restriction need not apply if a radical rectal excision is being contemplated. Three main forms of direct attack on a post-irradiation fistula are possible:

Local Repair of the Fistula. As a result of the irradiation of the adjacent tissues their healing capacity is impaired, so that attempts at local repair by the conventional methods for a rectovaginal fistula (see p. 191) are likely to result in necrosis and breakdown. What is needed to give a reasonable chance of success to such manoeuvres is, as Graham (1965) has emphasized, to bring to the area of the repair some tissue with a normal potentiality for healing. This may be voluntary muscle—the gracilis or rectus (Ingleman-Sundberg 1960)—or omentum (Bastiaanse 1960). Graham (1965) gives an excellent account of his technique for repairing fistulas *from below* using a pedicle flap of *gracilis*. He has had outstanding success with this method, for of 18 cases treated by it—five with associated vesicovaginal fistulas—16 were completely successful, though in one of these patients the operation had to be repeated after an initial failure, using the opposite gracilis muscle on the second occasion.

I have no experience of this technique but have recently used the method of repair *from above* employing a tail of *omentum* as an insertion between the separated rectum and vagina with a successful outcome. In this operation the abdomen is opened in the usual way and a plane of dissection is struck between the rectum and the posterior vaginal wall. This is followed down to the fistula, which is divided. In my case no attempt was made to close the holes in the rectum and vagina by suture for fear of causing necrosis. Instead the end of the omentum, which was long, was tucked between these two organs and fixed in position with a few sutures to the surrounding tissues to hold it as a barrier between the fistulous openings. (In many cases I am sure that in order to secure a long enough tail of omentum to fit between the rectum and vagina the preparation of a pedicle graft as described on p. 438 would be necessary.) A covering colostomy had been established some months previously and was maintained for four months subsequently.

Sphincter-saving Resection of the Rectum. In the application of this operation it is essential to excise not merely the segment of rectum bearing the fistula but also sufficient bowel wall above and below to leave for anastomosis stumps with healthy tissue at their cut ends undevitalized by irradiation. There is no problem about satisfying this requirement proximally; the difficulty relates entirely to the distal stump. If the fistula happens to be relatively high—say in the rectum 9–10 cm or more above the anal verge, or in the rectosigmoid—an adequate distal stump can be retained to permit of a low anterior resection with a sutured anastomosis, as in some of the cases reported by Craig and Buie (1949) and by Brintall (1953), and in several of my cases. But most post-irradiation fistulas lie at a lower level, so that the distal stump remaining after segmental resection is usually very short and amounts to little more than the anal canal with a tiny fringe of rectum at its top. For technical reasons completion of the operation as an anterior resection is impossible and other techniques have to be used instead. A purely sacral or abdominosacral technique would appear feasible, but the more popular method has been abdominoanal resection. This was used by Brintall (1953) in four cases, in two of which he performed a Maunsell–Weir type of operation (see p. 510) with excellent functional results, and in two a Bacon–Babcock operation (see p. 510) with indifferent function; by myself in five cases, using the Turnbull–Cutait pull-through technique (see p. 512), with good results in three and fair in two; and by Parks et al. (1978) using an abdominotransanal technique preserving the muscle coat of the rectum from just below the level of the fistula downwards, with good results in four cases. All these operations were performed after a preliminary colostomy. The disadvantages of abdominoanal or transanal resection are that it may be quite difficult to perform, it is a major undertaking and may be followed by troublesome complications, and it sacrifices the greater part of the rectum so that function may be impaired. At the present time my preference is for the more conservative procedure of local repair with interposition of a pedicle graph of omentum.

Abdominoperineal Excision with Permanent Iliac Colostomy. For fistulas deemed too low for anterior or abdominoanal resection, and for which a local repair is considered unsuitable because there is severe associated stricturing or the surgeon lacks familiarity with the technique, the only operation available, if continued discharge and discomfort despite colostomy call for direct operative treatment, is abdominoperineal excision. During this operation (or subsequently) the temporary loop transverse colostomy is closed and the patient is converted to a terminal iliac colostomy. This is the procedure that has probably most often been used in the past for post-irradiation rectovaginal fistulas that required further intervention, and for the average surgeon without special experience in this field it is the wisest choice.

FOR RECTAL STRICTURE FORMATION

Some degree of fibrous narrowing is common with post-irradiation proctitis and often occurs in association with fistulation, but a complete obstruction in my experience and that of Craig and Buie (1969) is rare. In most cases the amount of stenosis present is insufficient to cause symptoms or call for any treatment *per se*, but the development of complete or nearly complete obstruction may demand relief by proximal colostomy, followed later possibly by resection of the narrowed segment if its situation lends itself to this treatment.

FOR IRRADIATION ENTERITIS

In DeCosse et al.'s (1969) experience the majority of patients with irradiation enteritis in the small or large intestine apart from the rectum eventually come to surgical treatment on account of obstructive symptoms, faecal fistulation or haemorrhage. For lesions of the *small bowel* a resection is the best plan. Because of the fact that a lesser degree of irradiation injury may extend far beyond the obviously diseased zone and may seriously impair healing, a very wide excision is desirable, otherwise dehiscence of the anastomosis may be frequent. For lesions of the *colon* expectant management may sometimes be of value, but more usually surgical intervention in the form of a proximal colostomy or a resection is required.

MUCOUS COLITIS

This form of colitis is characterized by the discharge from the rectum of large quantities of mucus and usually also pieces of the mucous membrane in the form of casts. It is described in all the older textbooks and apparently used to be fairly common, occurring particularly in middle-aged, neurotic females, less frequently in children (Cawadias 1927). Usually such patients suffered from habitual constipation with abdominal discomfort. An attack of the disease was accompanied by severe griping pains, which were followed by discharge of mucus or casts. The casts might be several centimetres long, and were quite thin and semi-transparent, looking like skins; embedded in them were epithelial cells, eosinophil leucocytes, cholesterin and ammonium magnesium phosphate. Sigmoidoscopy does not seem to have been regularly practised in these patients and I have been unable to discover from the literature whether the mucous membrane regularly showed any abnormality. The radiological appearances after a barium enema have apparently been those of a rather spastic colon.

So-called mucous colitis seems to have almost completely disappeared in modern times, and though I have seen hundreds of patients with colitis or alleged colitis I have only met two who might conceivably have been diagnosed as suffering from mucous colitis. They were both seen in the intervals between attacks and, though they gave a history of passing casts from the rectum, these were never available for examination. Sigmoidoscopy showed no objective changes in the rectal or distal sigmoid mucosa, and a barium enema was negative. The predominant feature of both cases was their neurotic temperament, so that it was tempting to believe that the alleged casts were figments of their imagination; however, in one case they had been seen by the family practitioner.

(See also Irritable Colon Syndrome, p. 932.)

PSEUDOMEMBRANOUS OR NECROTIZING ENTEROCOLITIS

Aetiology and Pathology

This fulminating form of enteritis, which usually involves the small intestine and a variable amount of the large gut, is associated with necrosis of the mucous membrane and profound circulatory collapse. The condition first attracted serious attention as a complication of abdominal operations, particularly gastric or colonic resections, in the late 1950s (see Bruce 1955; Pullan 1955), but it is clear from the report of Pettet et al. (1954) that it had been recognized as a rare but definite entity two decades earlier. It is now known that it can occur also after operations other than those implicating the abdominal cavity, or even apart from any form of surgical treatment. For example, Goulston and McGovern (1965) reported a group of 14 patients who developed pseudomembranous enteritis whilst in a medical ward, the process being entirely confined to the large bowel; five of the patients had obstructive lesions of the colon such as carcinoma, the other nine had medical conditions such as chronic cardiac or renal disease. The greatly increased incidence of this form of enterocolitis 15–20 years ago—which has now largely subsided so that this is currently a rare disease—was attributed mainly to the widespread use in hospital practice of antibiotics, particularly the tetracyclines and neomycin (Dearing and Needham 1960; Altemeier et al. 1963). The effect of these agents had often been to alter the flora of the intestinal tract by killing off most of the contained organisms but allowing certain resistant stains to survive and become dominant. In many cases of pseudomembranous enterocolitis an antibiotic-resistant *Staphylococcus aureus*, often of UC_{18}-phage type (Dearing and Needham 1960; Altemeier et al. 1963) could be recovered from the stools. But in some cases with this complication stool cultures did not contain such organisms, and there may indeed have been no history of previous oral or parenteral administration of antibiotics.

This form of enterocolitis was never as common in Great Britain as in America and fortunately in the last decade it has become relatively rare in both countries, certainly in its more extreme forms. Recent work by Larson et al. (1978), Bartlett et al. (1978) and Keighley et al. (1978), on what appear to be mainly milder examples of the condition, seems to have incriminated the toxin-producing *Clostridium difficile* as the causative organism.

Clinical Picture

In the grossest form of the disease the clinical picture is one of severe circulatory collapse which precedes or follows the occurrence of profuse diarrhoea with green, foul-smelling stools, which often have an oily appearance. The patient looks ill and toxic and rapidly becomes very grossly dehydrated and depleted in electrolytes. The temperature and pulse rate normally show a sharp elevation coinciding with, or preceding, the onset of symptoms. The abdomen is moderately or considerably distended, diffusely tender—though not exquisitely so—and tympanitic. Bowel sounds may be heard in the earliest stages, but later the abdomen becomes silent on auscultation.

Diagnosis

Any patient who develops severe diarrhoea with some degree of collapse after rectal or colonic resection, particularly if oral antibiotics were used preoperatively, should be suspected of having a pseudomembranous enterocolitis. The offensive character of the stools will strengthen this suspicion, and, if they are collected in a large Winchester, the appearance of deposit of pseudomembrane in the bottom of the jar, looking like seaweed, makes a striking and characteristic picture. The diagnosis may be confirmed by observing large numbers of staphylococci in a direct smear of the faeces stained by Gram's method, and by stool culture with the growth of staphylococci resistant to all the commonly-used antibiotics. Perhaps more pertinent now is the demonstration of the presence of *Clostridium difficile* in the stools. However, negative bacteriological examination does not exclude the possibility of a pseudomembraneous enterocolitis, and in any case effective treatment cannot be withheld till the results of stool culture are available.

The difficult cases to diagnose are those in which the development of pyrexia, tachycardia, profound collapse and abdominal tenderness and distension *precede* by a considerable interval the onset of diarrhoea. The similarity in the clinical appearances to those of peritonitis, due to leakage from an intestinal suture line or to other causes, may be very close. Another condition that may be mimicked is an acute small bowel obstruction. Not a few of these patients have in fact been re-explored on either of these latter two diagnoses. At operation the absence of evidence of peritonitis or mechanical obstruction and the purple or bluish discoloration of the distended loops of small intestine should suggest the existence of an enterocolitis.

TREATMENT

An urgent necessity is to *replace lost fluid by intravenous infusion*, and in the severer cases very large quantities may have to be given for this purpose. Plasma or dextran is perhaps the best initial infusate to combat shock. Thereafter normal or half normal saline should be used, the amount to be given being gauged from the volume of the collected stools. In severe cases amounts of up to 10 or 15 litres may be required in the course of 36–48 hours. As soon as the urinary output is adequate (say 600–1000 ml/day) potassium chloride should be added to the intravenous infusion, 120–180 mg to each litre of saline. If the blood pressure remains low despite adequate replacement, vasopressor agents such as hydrocortisone and noradrenaline may be required intravenously.

The other important item of treatment is the administration of *specific antibiotic therapy*. It is customary to employ 'blindly' in the first instance one of the several antibiotics now available which are known to be specially effective against resistant staphylococci. These have included: erythromycin 300–600 mg eight-hourly, intravenously or orally; kanamycin 1 g daily in divided doses, intramuscularly; methicillin 1 g four- or six-hourly intramuscularly or intravenously; cloxacillin 0·5 g six-hourly, orally, intramuscularly or intravenously; and cephaloridine, 0·5–1 g six-hourly, intramuscularly or intravenously. In the light of Keighley et al.'s (1978) investigation an additional, probably more relevant, antibiotic that might be considered is vancomycin, which is effective against *Clostridium difficile* and also against most staphylococci. It has the virtue, too, that it is not absorbed in the small intestine and is therefore available for action in the colon. It is administered in a dose of 125 mg orally every six hours for five days. At the earliest possible moment, however, and preferably before commencing this therapy if possible, a sample of stool should be obtained for culture, so that the sensitivity of any organism present to various antibiotics may be determined, and more specific treatment given.

Isolation of Patients Suffering from Pseudomembranous Enterocolitis. An important aspect of the management of a case of staphylococcal enterocolitis is the prevention of infection of other patients. Ideally the case should be isolated in a separate ward or cubicle, and the most stringent care should be taken with the segregation and sterilization of utensils, bed clothes, night attire, etc.

PROGNOSIS

Postoperative enterocolitis varies greatly in severity from patient to patient, but one can perhaps recognize two main types: a very severe fulminating form which usually proceeds to a fatal termination despite all therapy within 48–72 hours; and a milder form in which the diarrhoea may be quite severe but toxicity is much less marked, and recovery normally occurs with appropriate treatment (see Kay et al. 1958). Some idea of the frequency and gravity of enterocolitis in some centres is conveyed by the report of Altemeier et al. (1963) on 155 patients who developed this condition in the Surgical Services of the University of Cincinnati during the years 1958–62. All had had antibiotic therapy. No less than 48 died, the commonest cause of death being septicaemia.

PROPHYLAXIS

As mentioned on p. 426, at one stage the high incidence of postoperative staphylococcal enterocolitis had led to the abandonment in some centres of oral antibiotics in the preparation of patients for colon operations in favour of non-absorbable sulphonamides. However, in the last few years there has been a considerable revival of interest in both oral antibiotic preparation and prophylactic systemic antibiotic cover in colorectal surgery, so far without any apparent increase in the incidence of enterocolitis. As previously emphasized staphylococcal enterocolitis is a highly infective condition, and the utmost care should be taken to avoid cross-infection in hospital wards to other patients.

PROCTOCOLITIS DUE TO ANTIBIOTICS AND OTHER MEDICAMENTS

ANTIBIOTICS

The role of antibiotics in the causation of some cases of *staphylococcal or pseudomembranous enterocolitis* has been referred to above. But apart from producing this clearly defined and serious condition, certain antibiotics given orally are irritating to the alimentary tract and may be responsible for *a simple irritative enteritis and colitis*, as also *pruritus ani*. It has been said that sigmoidoscopic examination in such cases may show the typical changes of a mild proctitis, but in a few cases in which I had the opportunity to perform sigmoidoscopy no definite abnormality could be observed. Usually the mild diarrhoea clears up fairly rapidly on cessation of the antibiotic therapy.

Lincomycin–Clindamycin Colitis. In recent years several authors (Kaplan and Weinstein 1968; Benner and Tellman 1970; Scott et al. 1973; Viteri et al. 1974) have drawn attention to the tendency of clindamycin and its parent compound lincomycin to produce diarrhoea. There has been a good deal of controversy as to the frequency of this complication but one estimate is a 20% incidence after oral lincomycin and a 2% incidence after oral clindamycin (Geddes et al. 1970). At first the diarrhoea was considered to be of little consequence until the publication of instances of pseudomembranous colitis, which could be fatal on occasion (Scott et al. 1973).

The clinical features have varied greatly, ranging from a mild bloodless, watery diarrhoea to an overwhelming illness comparable to severe ulcerative colitis. Sigmoidoscopy in the milder cases may show some oedema and friability of the mucosa, but according to Condon and Anderson (1978) may reveal an absolutely normal appearance. However, in more severe cases diffuse ulceration and extensive creamy-white plaque-like lesions are seen (Tedesco et al. 1974). The radiographic findings have also varied according to the severity of the clinical manifestations, in that mild cases have usually exhibited no obvious changes on barium enema examination, whilst severe cases have shown evidence of extensive mucosal ulceration and polyp formation.

As for treatment, in mild cases, apart from stopping the lincomycin–clindamycin and possibly administering simple antidiarrhoeal agents, no particular therapy is required. The diarrhoea often takes several weeks to subside. In more severe cases full supportive measures including steroids as for florid idiopathic ulcerative colitis are indicated. Some cases in the literature have come to emergency colectomy and ileostomy.

RECTAL INJECTIONS

The ordinary soap and water enema and a glycerine enema or suppository are irritating to the rectal and colonic mucosa and lead to a considerable outpouring of mucus which may be confusing to the surgeon during rectal examination and sigmoidoscopy. Even more irritating to the mucosa are retention enemas of avertin, ether in olive oil, or paraldehyde, which used to be favoured by anaesthetists in certain cases.

APERIENTS

It was claimed by Gabriel (1948) that mild proctitis is often attributable to the habitual use of aperients such as aloes, phenolphthalein or saline purgatives, but I very much doubt if this is so.

PROCTITIS AUTOPHYTICA

A localized area of proctitis or ulceration in the lower rectum may be due to self-inflicted trauma. This may be produced by the fingernail during repeated digital examination by the patient herself, or by the frequent introduction of an implement such as a pencil or poker for erotic or other reasons. I have encountered four such cases, and Hughes (1957) has also met this form of proctitis.

EOSINOPHILIC COLITIS

Dunstone (1959) describes a patient who presented acutely with pain and distension in the right abdomen, for which an emergency laparotomy was performed. This revealed a normal appendix but showed the caecum and ascending colon to be grossly oedematous and the lymph nodes draining these parts greatly enlarged. A right hemicolectomy was carried out with uninterrupted recovery. The pathological examination of the operative specimen confirmed the oedematous state of the bowel and showed on section large numbers of eosinophil cells in the submucosal, muscular and subserosal layers. There was no evidence of arteritis and the eosinophil cells were not grouped around blood vessels. The histological picture was very similar to that in 'eosinophilic gastritis'.

Salmon and Paulley (1967) have presented a comprehensive review of eosinophilic granuloma of the alimentary tract.

COLITIS CYSTICA PROFUNDA

Interest in this extremely rare form of 'colitis' was revived by Goodall and Sinclair in 1957, and a good description of it is given by Howard et al. (1971). It is characterized by the occurrence of cysts lined by intestinal epithelium situated deep to the muscularis mucosae, the overlying mucosa being normal. These changes may be found *diffusely* throughout the colon, often in association with ulcerative colitis, or *in a localized form* in the lower or mid-rectum, exceptionally in the sigmoid or descending colon. The localized lesion is an elevated plaque-like or nodular polypoid area up to 3 cm in diameter; rarely the centre is ulcerated. On digital and sigmoidoscopic examination it may resemble a carcinoma, and the symptoms, which include passage of mucus and blood, diarrhoea and tenesmus, may also suggest this condition. Some patients, indeed, have been subjected to rectal excision on a mistaken diagnosis of neoplasm. But though the pathogenesis of the disease is uncertain, it is benign. If the symptoms are bad enough to warrant surgical treatment, it is reasonable to consider in the first instance local excision per anum (see p. 350) by a posterior transsphincteric incision (see p. 355) or by a Kraske approach (see p. 503). But complete rectal excision may be technically the simplest way of dealing with the condition, as well as the most effective, provided the patient is prepared to accept a permanent colostomy.

REFERENCES

ALTEMEIER, W. A., HUMMEL, R. P. and HILL, E. O. (1963) Staphylococcal enterocolitis following antibiotic therapy. *Ann. Surg., 157*, 847.

ANAND, S. S. (1956) Hypertrophic ileocaecal tuberculosis in India with a record of fifty hemicolectomies. *Ann. R. Coll. Surg. Engl., 19*, 205.

ANNAMUNTHODO, H. (1961) Rectal lymphogranuloma venereum in Jamaica. *Dis. Colon Rect., 41*, 17.

ANSCOMBE, A. R., KEDDIE, N. C. and SCHOFIELD, P. F. (1967) Caecal tuberculosis. *Gut, 8*, 337.

ARCHAMPONG, E. Q. and CLARK, C. G. (1973) Surgical problems in amoebiasis. *Proc. R. Coll. Surg. Engl., 52*, 36.

BAILLIE, M. (1795) *The Morbid Anatomy of Some of the Most Important Parts of the Human Body.* 1st Am. ed. Albany: printed by Barber and Smithwick for Thomas Spencer, Bookseller. London: Johnson & Nicol.

BARLOW, D. (1941) 'Simple' ulcers of the caecum, colon and rectum. *Br. J. Surg., 28*, 575.

BARRON, M. E. (1928) Simple, non-specific ulcer of the colon. *Archs Surg., Chicago, 17*, 355.

BARTLETT, J. G., TE WEN CHANG, GURWITH, M., GARDACH, S. L. and ONDERDONK, A. B. (1978) Antibiotic-associated pseudomembranous colitis due to toxin-producing clostridia. *New Engl. J. Med., 298*, 531.

BASTIAANSE, M. A. VAN B. (1960) Bastiaanse's method for surgical closure of very large irradiation fistulae of the bladder and rectum. In *Gynaecological Urology,* ed. A. F. Youssef, Springfield, Ill.: Charles C. Thomas.

BEALL, A. C., CROSTHWAIT, R. W. and DEBAKEY, M. E. (1965) Injuries of the colon, including surgery upon the aorta. *Surg. Clins N. Am., 45*, 1273.

BEARSE, C. (1929) Fishbones as a cause of intestinal perforation. *New Engl. J. Med., 201*, 885.

BENNER, E. and TELLMAN, W. (1970) Pseudomembraneous colitis as a sequel to oral lincomycin therapy. *Am. J. Gastroent., 54*, 55.

BENSAUDE, R. and LAMBLING, A. (1936) Discussion on the aetiology and treatment of fibrous stricture of the rectum (including lymphogranuloma inguinale). *Proc. R. Soc. Med., 29*, 1441.

BERNATZ, P. E. (1960) Necrosis of the colon following resection for abdominal aortic aneursysms. *Archs Surg., Chicago, 81*, 373.

BERNSTEIN, W. C. and BERNSTEIN, E. F. (1963) Ischaemic ulcerative colitis following inferior mesenteric arterial ligation. *Dis. Colon Rect., 6*, 54.

BOLEY, S. J., SCHWARTZ, S., LASH, J. and STERNHILL, V. (1963) Reversible vascular occlusion of the colon. *Surgery Gynec. Obstet., 116*, 53.

BOYD, W. (1955) *Pathology for the Surgeon,* 7th ed. Philadelphia and London: Saunders.

BREIDENBACH, L. and SLATTERY, L. R. (1949) Rectal stricture of lymphogranuloma venereum. *Ann. Surg., 128*, 1079.

BRINTALL, E. S. (1953) Surgical treatment of post-irradiation rectal stricture and rectovaginal fistula. *Archs Surg., Chicago, 67*, 346.

BROWN, A. R. (1972) Non-gangrenous ischaemic colitis. *Br. J. Surg., 59*, 463.

BRUCE, J. (1955) In discussion on toxic and nutritional disturbances in the small intestine associated with surgery of the gastro-intestinal tract. *Proc. R. Soc. Med., 48*, 245.

BUIE, L. A. and MALMGREN, G. E. (1930) Factitial proctitis. *Int. Clin., 3*, 68.

BYROM, H. B. and MANN, C. V. (1969) Clinical features and surgical management of ileocaecal tuberculosis. *Proc. R. Soc. Med., 62*, 38.

CAMERON, J. R. (1939) Simple non-specific ulcer of the caecum. *Br. J. Surg., 26*, 526.

CAWADIAS, A. P. (1927) *Diseases of the Intestines.* London: Baillière.

CHEN, W. J., CHEN, K.-M. and LIN, M. (1971) Colon perforation in amoebiasis. *Archs Surg., Chicago, 103*, 676.

CLARK, A. W., LLOYD-MOSTYN, R. H. and SADLER, M. R. de C. (1972) 'Ischaemic' colitis in young adults. *Br. med. J., 4*, 70.

COCHRANE, J. P. S. and YARNOLD, J. R. (1979) Management of radiation injuries to the bowel associated with treatment of uterine carcinoma by radiotherapy: preliminary communication. *J. R. Soc. Med., 72*, 195.

CONDON, R. E. and ANDERSON, M. J. (1978) Diarrhoea and colitis in clindamycin-treated surgical patients. *Archs Surg., Chicago, 113*, 794.

COPE, SIR Z. (1949) Actinomycosis involving the colon and rectum. *J. int. Coll. Surg., 12*, 401.

COTTON, P. B. and THOMAS, M. L. (1971) Ischaemic colitis and the contraceptive pill. *Br. med. J., 3*, 27.

CRAIG, M. S., Jr. and BUIE, L. A. (1949) Factitial (irradiation) proctitis. *Surgery, St Louis, 25*, 472.

CROMAR, C. D. L. (1946) Benign ulcer of the caecum. *Am. J. dig. Dis., 13*, 230.

CROPPER, C. F. J. (1945) Sigmoidoscopy in amoebic dysentery. *Lancet, 2*, 460.

—— (1951) Histopathology of amoebic pin-point craters. *J. trop. Med., 54*, 71.

CRUVEILHIER, J. (1829) *Anatomie Pathologique du Corps Humain.* Paris: J. B. Baillière.

DEARING, W. H. and NEEDHAM, G. M. (1960) Hospitalized patients with Staphylococcus aureus in the intestine. *J. Am. med. Ass., 174*, 1597.

DeCosse, J. J., Rhodes, R. S., Wentz, W. B. Reagen, J. W., Dworken, H. J. and Holden, W. D. (1969) The natural history and management of radiation induced injury of the gastrointestinal tract. *Ann. Surg., 170*, 369.

Dunstone, G. H. (1959) A case of eosinophilic colitis. *Br. J. Surg., 46*, 474.

Eagleson, W. M. (1952) Non-specific ulcer of the large bowel. *Can. med. Ass. J., 67*, 563.

Eggleston, F. C., Verghese, M. and Handa, A. K. (1978) Amoebic perforation of the bowel: experiences with 26 cases. *Br. J. Surg., 65*, 748.

Frei, W. (1925) Eine neue Hautreaktion bei 'Lymphogranuloma inguinale'. *Klin. Wschr., 4*, 2148.

Friedman, M. H. and Mackenzie, W. C. (1959) Simple ulcer of the colon: report of four cases. *Can. J. Surg., 2*, 279.

Fry, G. A., Martin, W. J., Dearing, W. H. and Culp, C. E. (1965) Primary actinomycosis of the rectum with multiple peri-anal and perineal fistulae. *Proc. Mayo Clin., 40*, 296.

Füth, H. and Ebeler, F. (1915) Röntgen- und Radiumtherapie des Uteruskarzinoms. *Zbl. Gynaek., 39*, 217.

Gabriel, W. B. (1948) *The Principles and Practice of Rectal Surgery*, 4th ed. London: H. K. Lewis.

Geddes, A. M., Bridgewater, F. A. J. and Williams, D. N. (1970) Clinical and bacterial studies with clindamycin. *Br. med. J., 2*, 703.

Goligher, J. C., de Dombal, F. T. and Burton, I. (1971) Crohn's disease with special reference to surgical treatment. *Progress in Surgery*. Basle: Karger.

Goodall, H. B. and Sinclair, I. S. R. (1957) Colitis cystica profunda. *J. Path. Bact., 73*, 33.

Goulston, S. J. M. and McGovern, V. J. (1965) Pseudo-membranous colitis. *Gut, 6*, 207.

Grace, A. W. (1941) Lymphogranuloma venereum. *Bull. N. Y. Acad. Med., 17*, 627.

Graham, J. B. (1965) Vaginal fistulas following radiotherapy. *Surgery Gynec. Obstet., 120*, 1019.

Grassmann, M. (1925) Zur Frage des Ulcus Simplex des Dünndarmes. *Arch. klin. Chir., 136*, 449.

Guest, J. L. (1963) Non-specific ulceration of the intestine. *Surgery Gynec. Obstet. int. Abstr. Series, 117*, 409.

Hancock, D. M. (1958) Hyperplastic tuberculosis of the distal colon. *Br. J. Surg., 46*, 63.

Harkness, A. H. (1948) Anorectal gonorrhoea. *Proc. R. Soc. Med., 41*, 476.

Harrison, H. (1940) Importance of simple ulcer of the right side of the colon in diagnosis of abdominal disease. *Archs Surg., Chicago, 40*, 959.

Hartmann, H. (1922) An address on inflammatory strictures of the rectum. *Lancet, 1*, 307.

Hawe, P. (1951) Fibrous stricture of the rectum due to lymphogranuloma venereum. *Proc. R. Soc. Med., 44*, 426.

Hoon, J. R., Dockerty, M. B. and Pemberton, J. de J. (1950) ileorectal tuberculosis including a comparison of this disease with non-specific regional enterocolitis and noncaseous tuberculated enterocolitis. *Surgery Gynec. int. Abstr. Surg., 91*, 417.

Howard, R. J., Mannax, S. J., Eusebio, E. B., Shea, M. A. and Goldberg, S. M. (1971) Colitis cystica profunda. *Surgery, St Louis, 69*, 306.

Howell, J. S. and Knapton, P. J. (1964) Ileorectal tuberculosis. *Gut, 5*, 524.

Hughes, E. S. R. (1957) *Surgery of Anus, Anal Canal and Rectum*. Edinburgh: Livingstone.

Ingelman-Sundberg, A. (1960) Pathogenesis and operative treatment of urinary fistulae in irradiated tissue. In *Gynaecological Urology*, ed. A. F. Youssef. Springfield, Ill.: Charles C. Thomas.

Irwin, A. (1965) Partial infarction of the colon due to reversible vascular occlusion. *Clin. Radiol. 16*, 261.

James, K. L. (1946) The surgical complications of amoebic dysentery. *Proc. R. Soc. Med., 39*, 766.

Jerreriss, F. J. (1962) Personal communication to King.

Jensen, T. (1953) Rectal gonorrhoea in women. *Br. J. vener. Dis., 29*, 222.

Kaplan, K. and Weinstein, L. (1968) Lincomycin. *Pediat. Clins N. Am., 15*, 131.

Kay, A. W., Richards, R. L. and Watson, A. J. (1958) Acute necrotizing (pseudo-membranous) enterocolitis. *Br. J. Surg., 46*, 45.

Keighley, M. R. B., Burden, D. W. and Arabi, Y. (1978) Randomized controlled trial of vancomycin for pseudomembraneous colitis and postoperative diarrhoea. *Br. med. J., 4*, 1167.

Kerr, R. A. (1935) Simple ulcer of the large bowel. *Lancet, 2*, 550.

Killingback, M. J. and Williams, K. L. (1961) Necrotizing colitis. *Br. J. Surg., 49*, 175.

King, A. J. (1962) The complications of homosexuality. *Proc. R. Soc. Med., 55*, 869.

Larson, H. E., Price, A. B., Honour, P. and Borriello, S. P. (1978) *Clostridium difficile* and the aetiology of pseudomembraneous colitis. *Lancet, 1*, 1063.

Lieberman, W. (1951) Syphilis of the rectum. *Rev. Gastroent., 18*, 67.

Lipton, S. and Riesman, E. D. (1951) Simple ulcer of the cecum. *Ann. Surg., 134*, 279.

Localio, S. A., Stone, A. and Friedman, M. (1969) Surgical aspects of radiation enteritis. *Surgery Gynec. Obstet., 129*, 1163.

McGovern, V. J. and Goulston, S. J. M. (1965) Ischaemic enterocolitis. *Gut, 6*, 213.

McKain, J. and Shumacker, H. B. Jr. (1958) Ischaemia of the left colon associated with abdominal aortic aneurysms and their treatment. *Archs Surg., Chicago, 76*, 355.

MacVaugh, H. and Roberts, B. (1961) Results of resection of abdominal aortic aneurysm. *Surgery Gynec. Obstet., 113*, 17.

Madigan, M. R. and Morson, B. C. (1969) Solitary ulcer of the rectum. *Gut, 10*, 871.

Manson-Bahr, Sir P. (1943) *The Dysenteric Disorders*, 2nd ed. London: Cassell.

—— and Muggleton, W. J. (1957) Rectal biopsy as an aid to the diagnosis of amoebic dysentery and allied diseases of the colon. *Lancet, 1*, 763.

Marrash, S. E., Gibson, J. B. and Simeone, F. A. (1962) A clinicopathologic study of intestinal infarction. *Surgery Gynec. Obstet., 114*, 323.

Marshak, R. H., Maklansky, D. and Calem, S. H. (1965) Segmental infarction of the colon. *Am. J. dig. Dis., 10*, 86.

Marston, A. (1964) Patterns of intestinal ischaemia. *Ann. R. Coll. Surg. Engl., 35*, 151.

—— Pheils, M. T., Thomas, M. L. and Morson, B. C. (1966) Ischaemic colitis. *Gut, 7*, 1.

Martin, W. J., Nichols, D. R., Wellman, W. E. and Weed, I. A. (1956) Disseminated actinomycosis treated with tetracycline. *Archs intern. Med., 97*, 252.

MASON, A. Y. (1970) Surgical access to the rectum—a trans-sphincteric exposure. *Proc. R. Soc. Med.,* Suppl. *63,* 1.

MELENEY, F. L. (1948) *Treatise on Surgical Infections.* London: Oxford University Press.

MILES, R. P. M. (1957) Rectal lymphogranuloma venereum. *Br. J. Surg., 45,* 180.

—— (1972) Benign strictures of the rectum. *Ann. R. Coll. Surg. Engl., 50,* 310.

MILLER, R. E. and KNOX, W. G. (1966) Colon ischaemia following infrarenal aortic surgery: Report of four cases. *Ann. Surg., 163,* 639.

MISRA, S. C. and PATHAK, S. S. (1954) Surgery in treatment of abdominal tuberculosis. *J. Indian med. Ass., 23,* 240.

MORGAN, B. (1978) Personal communication.

MORGAN, C. N. (1944) Amoebiasis: some difficulties of diagnosis. *Br. med. J., 2,* 7121.

MORSON, B. C. (1961) Primary actinomycosis of the rectum. *Proc. R. Soc. Med., 54,* 723.

NEVIN, R. W. (1947) The surgical aspects of intestinal amoebiasis. *Ann. R. Coll. Surg. Engl., 1,* 69.

NICOL, C. S. (1948) Some aspects of gonorrhoea in the female—with special reference to infection of the rectum. *Br. J. vener. Dis., 24,* 26.

—— (1962) Anal syphilis. *Proc. R. Soc. Med., 55,* 870.

OCHSNER, J. L., COOLEY, D. A. and DE BAKEY, M. E. (1960) Associated intra-abdominal lesions encountered during resection of aortic aneurysms: Surgical considerations. *Dis. Colon Rect., 3,* 485.

PARKS, A. G., ALLEN, C. L. O., FRANK, J. D. and McPARTLIN, J. F. (1978) A method of treating post-irradiation rectovaginal fistulae. *Br. J. Surg., 65,* 417.

PETTET, J. D., BEGGENSTOSS, A. H., DEARING, W. H. and JUDD, E. S. (1954) Postoperative pseudo-membranous enterocolitis. *Surgery Gynec. Obstet., 98,* 546.

PULLAN, J. M. (1955) Necrotizing enteritis. *British Surgical Practice: Surgical Progress,* ed. Carling, Sir E. R. and Ross, Sir J. Paterson, p. 104. London: Butterworth.

ROBERTS, W. M. (1965) Ischaemic lesions of the colon and rectum. *S. Afr. J. Surg., 3,* 141.

RUSSELL, I. S. (1961) Non-specific ulceration of the caecum. *Br. J. Surg., 49,* 54.

SALMON, P. R. and PAULLEY, J. W. (1967) Eosinophilic granuloma of the gastrointestinal tract. *Gut, 8,* 8.

SCHWARTZ, S., BOLEY, S., LASH, J. and STERNHILL, V. (1963) Roentgenologic aspects of reversible vascular occlusion of the colon and its relationship to ulcerative colitis. *Radiology, 80,* 625.

SCHWEIGER, M. and ALEXANDER-WILLIAMS, J. (1977) Solitary ulcer syndrome of the rectum: its association with occult rectal prolapse. *Lancet, 1,* 170.

SCOTT, A. J., NICHOLSON, G. L. and KERR, A. R. (1973) Lincomycin as a cause of pseudomembranous colitis. *Lancet, 2,* 1232.

SHUKLA, H. S. and HUGHES, L. E. (1978) Abdominal tuberculosis in the 1970s: a continuing problem. *Br. J. Surg., 65,* 403.

SMITH, R. F. and SZILAGY, D. E. (1960) Ischaemia of the colon as a complication in the surgery of the abdominal aorta. *Archs Surg., Chicago, 80,* 806.

SPIESMAN, M. G., LEVY, R. C. and BROTMAN, D. M. (1937) Lymphogranuloma inguinale, rectal stricture, and pre-stricture. *Am. J. dig. Dis., 3,* 931.

STEIN, D. and BANK, S. (1970) Surgery in amoebic colitis. *Gut, 11,* 941.

STOCK, F. E. and LI, F. W. P. (1964) Granulomas of the large bowel simulating malignant disease. *Br. J. Surg., 51,* 898.

TANDON, H. D. and PRAKASH, A. (1972) Pathology of intestinal tuberculosis and its distinction from Crohn's disease. *Gut, 13,* 260.

TATE, G. T., THOMPSON, H. and WILLIS, A. T. (1965) *Clostridium welchii* colitis. *Br. J. Surg., 52,* 194.

TEDESCO, F. T., BARTON, R. W. and ALPERS, D. H. (1974) Clindamycin-associated colitis: a prospective study. *Ann. int. Med., 81,* 429.

TODD, T. F. (1938) Rectal ulceration following irradiation treatment of carcinoma of the cervix uteri. Pseudo-carcinoma of the rectum. *Surgery Gynec. Obstet., 67,* 617.

VITERI, A. L., HOWARD, P. H. and DYCK, W. P. (1974) The spectrum of lincomycin-clindamycin colitis. *Gastroenterology, 66,* 1137.

WARREN, S. and SOMMERS, S. C. (1948) Cicatrizing enteritis (regional ileitis) as a pathologic entity: analysis of 120 cases. *Am. J. Path., 24,* 475.

WIG, K. L., CHITAKARA, N. L., GUPTA, S. P., KISHORE, K. and MANCHANDA, R. L. (1961) Ileocaecal tuberculosis with particular reference to isolation of Mycobacterium tuberculosis. With a note on its relation to regional ileitis (Crohn's disease). *Am. Rev. resp. Dis., 84,* 169.

WILKIE, SIR DAVID. (1937) Simple ulcer of the ascending colon and its complications. *Surgery, St Louis, 1,* 655.

WILLIAMS, L. F. and WITTENBERG, J. (1975) Ischemic colitis: a useful clinical diagnosis, but is it ischemic? *Ann. Surg., 182,* 439.

—— BOSNIAK, M. A., WITTENBERG, J., MANUEL, B., GRIMES, E. T. and BYRNE, J. J. (1968) Ischaemic colitis. *Am. J. Surg., 117,* 254.

WRIGHT, L. T., BERG, B. N., BOLDEN, J. V. and FREEMAN, W. A. (1946) Rectal strictures due to lymphogranuloma venereum; with especial reference to Pauchet's excision operation. *Surgery Gynec. Obstet., 82,* 449.

YOUNG, J. R., HUMPHRIES, A. W., DE WOLFE, V. G. and LEFEVRE, F. A. (1963) Complications of abdominal aortic surgery. II. Intestinal ischaemia. *Archs Surg., Chicago, 86,* 51.

24

Diverticulosis and Diverticulitis of the Colon

The colon is the commonest site in the alimentary tract for the formation of diverticula. These are usually multiple. When the diverticula are un-inflamed the condition is known as 'diverticulosis'; when superadded inflammation has occurred, the term 'diverticulitis' is used. It has been fairly generally assumed in the past that diverticulosis *per se* is a symptomless condition and that the occurrence of any clinical complaint indicates the development of diverticulitis or some other complication, but often in cases with quite pronounced symptoms the pathologist has great difficulty in finding any clear evidence of inflammation in the excised specimen of colon. For this reason it is becoming popular clinically to use the less committal expression 'diverticular disease' in referring to any stage of this condition. The considerable tendency to complications renders the term diverticulum for the initial condition very appropriate; in Latin the word *diverticulum* means a wayside inn—presumably often a place of ill repute!

HISTORICAL

As with so many other diseases, the first clear pathological description of diverticula of the colon was apparently that of Cruveilhier, who wrote in 1849: 'we not infrequently find between the bands of longitudinal muscle fibres in the sigmoid a series of small, dark, pear-shaped tumours, which are formed by herniae of the mucous membrane through the gaps in the muscle coat.' Habershon also gave a good account of diverticulosis in 1857, but it was not until Graser's paper in 1899 that interest was aroused. He pointed out that diverticulosis of the colon was far from uncommon, and described the changes resulting from inflammation in and around the diverticula, a condition which he termed 'peridiverticulitis' and which we now know as 'diverticulitis'. Graser also emphasized the resemblance of diverticulitis to new growths. His work, and that of subsequent authors, such as Moynihan (1907), Keith (1910), Maxwell-Telling and Gruner (1916), Drummond (1917), Mailer (1928), Lockhart-Mummery (1930), Lockhart-Mummery and Hodgson (1931) and Edwards (1939), established diverticulosis and its complications as a definite disease entity.

An important factor, too, in shaping our present-day conception of diverticulosis and diverticulitis of the colon has been the radiological study of the gastrointestinal tract. De Quervain (1914) and Case (1914, 1929) were the first to demonstrate colonic diverticula by means of X-rays. To denote the state of affairs when diverticula were present without evidence of inflammatory changes the term 'diverticulosis' was suggested by the former. No historical account of the radiological elucidation of diverticulosis and diverticulitis would be complete without reference to the work of Spriggs and Marxer (1925, 1927, 1937), who claimed to be able to recognize a 'prediverticular stage' of the disease and thereby stimulated a controversy that has persisted to the present day (see p. 887).

INCIDENCE

An accurate estimate of the incidence of diverticulosis and diverticulitis in the general population is not possible, but useful information as to their frequency in certain groups of hospital patients has been obtained by study of the findings in large series of barium enema examinations and of autopsies. Some of the more weighty data of this kind have been based on the vast clinical material of the Mayo Clinic. Thus Rankin and Brown (1930) reported that diverticula were noted in 5·67% of 24 620 patients undergoing barium enema and 5·2% of 1925 cases coming to autopsy at the Clinic. All but one of the autopsy cases with diverticula were over the age of 40, and 70% were males. Of the patients found on X-ray examination to have diverticulosis 17% were considered also to have diverticulitis; of the autopsy cases showing diverticula, 14% had associated inflammatory changes. Later reports from the Mayo Clinic by Pemberton et al. (1947), from Philadelphia by Willard and Bochus (1936) and from Sheffield by Grout (1949), on the incidence of diverticular disease in large numbers of patients having barium enema examinations, yielded very similar figures. On the other hand Welch et al. (1953), who reviewed the results of barium enema studies at the Massachusetts General Hospital, found a rather higher incidence—approximately one-third of the patients had diverticulosis and nearly a tenth had diverticulitis. Though the ages of the affected patients ranged from 29 to 87, the incidence of diverticular disease was infinitesimal below the age of 35. Above 35 years the incidence increased steadily so that by the sixth decade nearly 30% of all patients had diverticula and 10% had evidence of diverticulosis. 57% of all the patients with diverticulosis in this Boston series were females.

Parks (1968) of Belfast, in a study comprising 300 unselected autopsy examinations (171 in men and 129 in women), found a higher incidence of diverticular disease than has hitherto been recorded. 33% of the men and 42% of the women showed diverticula. The youngest male patient with it was 44, the youngest female 29, the incidence rising steadily with increasing age and reaching a figure of 50% in the ninth decade. Of a smaller group of the patients with diverticular disease submitted to special dissection, 31% showed definite thickening of the muscle coat of the bowel and 15% gross evidence of previous inflammation. Hughes (1969) of Brisbane had slightly different findings as regards the incidence of diverticula in 200 unselec-ted autopsy examinations, with 45% in men and 40% in women.

In a series of 521 clinical cases of diverticular disease surveyed by Parks (1969), the male : female ratio was 2 : 3, virtually all the patients were over 30 years of age and the maximal incidence was in the sixth, seventh and eighth decades. Barium enema examination was performed on 461 of the cases on first presentation at hospital, so that the distribution of the colonic diverticula at this stage is known in these patients. The sigmoid was involved alone in 65·5% and in combination with other regions in 96%; 6·7% had total colonic involvement. But patients with many diverticula or total colonic involvement were on average younger and had a shorter history than those with less extensive disease, which does not support the idea, frequently entertained, that there is a relentless tendency for diverticula to become progressively more extensive with the passage of time. On the contrary, it seems that, if a segment of colon is to be affected by the disease, this is usually determined early in its course.

PATHOLOGY

To the clinician fresh from contemplation of the X-ray plates in a case of diverticulosis the appearances of the affected bowel at laparotomy or on pathological examination are often bitterly disappointing. A piece of colon that was shown radiologically to be studded with large diverticula may on first inspection from the serosal aspect reveal no abnormality whatsoever. The reason for this apparent inconsistency is that the diverticula usually project into appendices epiploicae, which frequently contain more fat than usual, so that the lesions are often completely blurred. When the fat is less abundant the diverticula may sometimes be observed as bluish-black discolorations in the bases of the appendices, this appearance being due to the contained pellets of faeces. Indeed because of the frequent presence of faecoliths in this way diverticulosis is often more easily recognized at laparotomy by palpation of the colon than by inspection, the faecal pellets being felt like hard peas on the surface of the bowel.

When the appendices epiploicae are few and the amount of surrounding fat is minimal the diverticula may show clearly on the surface of the colon. In such cases, and in others after the fat has been dissected away, it is found that the position of the

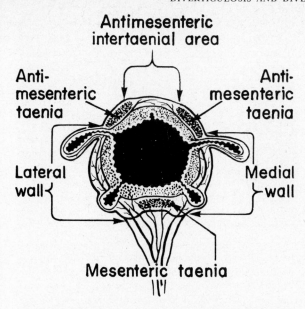

Fig. 612. Transverse section of the sigmoid colon and meso-colon, to illustrate the relation of diverticula to the taeniae, to the blood vessels penetrating the bowel wall and to the appendices epiploicae (based on the findings of Slack (1962) and Marcus and Watt (1964)).

diverticula on the bowel circumference relative to the longitudinal taeniae is remarkably constant (Fig. 612): (*a*) They never penetrate a taenia; (*b*) Most of them occur *on the side-walls* between the mesenteric taenia and the two antimesenteric taeniae, and, as Slack (1962) has shown, they may emerge at *two points on either side*, rather than one as used to be thought; (*c*) Occasionally, as Marcus and Watt (1964) in particular have demonstrated, smaller

mucosal protrusions may be situated in the anti-mesenteric intertaenial area (Figs 612, 613). These are often so slight that they do not reach the serosa (*intramural* diverticula), sometimes they do involve the serosa to the extent of producing faint trans-verse ridges on this coat in the antimesenteric inter-taenial area (*ridge* diverticula), and rarely they are developed into full-blown saccular diverticula in this sector of the bowel. All three types of diverticula may be present together in the same cases. The *relationship of diverticula to the intramural blood vessels* has been studied by Drummond (1917), Spriggs and Marxer (1925), Edwards (1939), Lloyd-Davies (1953) and Slack (1962), who point out that diverticula occur at the sites of entry of blood vessels (Fig. 612). Though the main circumferential arteries pass round the bowel to meet in the antimesenteric inter-taenial area, they send numerous small branches at right-angles to penetrate the muscle coat and supply the mucosa, and the mucosal protrusions, at any rate on the side-walls, are closely related to such vessels.

Histological section of an individual *lateral* diverticulum shows that it possesses in the main only two coats: an inner mucosa and an outer serosal (Fig. 614). There is sometimes an attenuated muscle layer at the neck of the diverticulum, but as the pouch is traced towards its fundus this coat rapidly disappears. Section of *antimesenteric inter-taenial diverticula* of intramural and ridge type (Fig. 615) reveals that the mucosal projection extends between circular muscle bundles. By contrast with these diverticula and with lateral diverticula, sac-cular diverticula in the antimesenteric intertaenial area do not herniate between the circular muscle fibres, but have a thinned-out layer of circular muscle in their walls (Fig. 616).

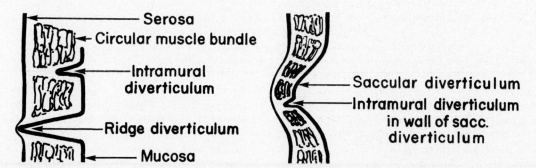

Fig. 613. Intramural, ridge and saccular diverticula of the antimesenteric intertaenial area, showing their relationship to the circular muscle bundles; saccular diverticula in this area do not herniate between the bundles but may show intramural diverticula in their wall. (*After Marcus and Watt 1964*)

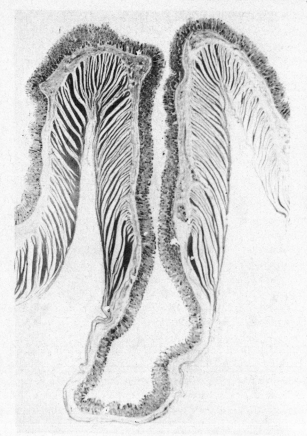

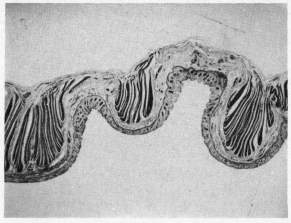

Fig. 615. Longitudinal section through the antimesenteric intertaenial area showing an intramural diverticulum on the left and a ridge diverticulum on the right (×10). (*From Marcus and Watt 1964*)

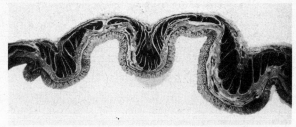

Fig. 614. Histological section of a *lateral* diverticulum of the colon showing that a muscle coat is present only at its neck. (*From Lloyd-Davies 1953*)

Fig. 616. Longitudinal section through the antimesenteric intertaenial area showing two saccular diverticula associated with thinning of the circular muscle (×10). (*From Marcus and Watt 1964*)

When the affected segment of colon is viewed as a whole, the diverticula on the sidewalls are seen to form one or two longitudinal rows of projections on either side behind each antimesenteric taenia (Fig. 617). As for the antimesenteric intertaenial area, it may be quite smooth, or may show transverse linear striae (Fig. 618) due to ridge diverticula, or be studded with a series of rounded projections (Fig. 619) due to saccular diverticula. When the bowel is sectioned longitudinally and the interior inspected the mouths of the diverticula may sometimes be seen as rounded or slit-like openings, but often they are relatively inconspicuous and can only be detected when faecal matter is expressed from them. What is striking as a rule is the way in which the circular muscle and mucosa are thrown up into transverse folds which project into the lumen like series of interdigitating valves (Fig. 620). Equally noticeable—and causally related to this

effect—is *thickening of the muscle coat*. Such thickening was observed by Keith (1910), Edwards (1939) and Celio (1952), and its occurrence has been strongly confirmed by Slack (1962), Morson (1963), Arfwidsson (1964) and Ming and Fleischner (1965), who found it to be consistantly present in operative specimens of diverticular disease, *even when no signs of inflammation could be detected*. The thickening affects both longitudinal and circular muscle fibres, and the thickening and contraction of the taeniae have been considered by Keith (1910), Morson (1963), Williams (1963) and Arfwidsson (1964) to be responsible for shortening and pleating the sigmoid, with the production of the folds of mucosa and thickened circular muscle coat which in some specimens seem partly to obstruct the lumen.

Arfwidsson (1964) has investigated whether the muscle thickening is due to hyperplasia or hypertrophy and concludes from his studies that there is a

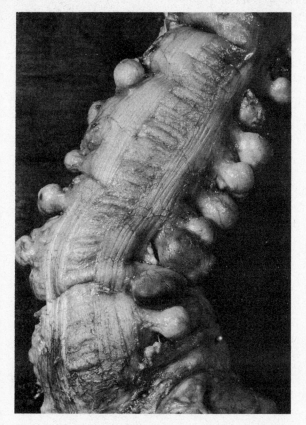

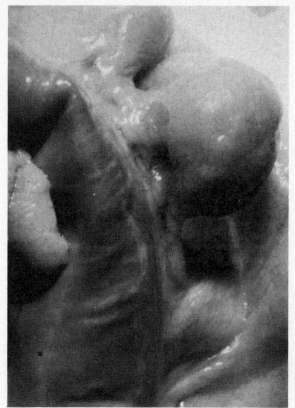

Fig. 617. Diverticula of colon seen as a row of projections along the side of the colon just behind the lateral longitudinal muscle band. Usually a second row situated more posteriorly is present on either side as well. (*From Lloyd-Davies 1953*)

Fig. 618. Transverse linear striae in the antimesenteric inter-taenial area. (*From Marcus and Watt 1964*)

genuine hypertrophy of both circular and long-itudinal muscle bundles at all stages of diverti-cular disease, both with and without inflammation. In a few cases reported by Arfwidsson (1964) the operative specimens of colon showing shortening and pleating contained no grossly visible diverticula (Fig. 620), but on careful histological examination they were found to exhibit minute mucosal pro-trusions between the muscle bundles, indicating an incipient state of diverticulosis. He regards this as supporting evidence for his belief, and that of Keith (1910), Edwards (1939), Morson (1963), Almy (1965) and others, that the muscle thickening precedes the development of diverticula. But it is to be noted that Slack (1962), who also found muscle hypertrophy in *operative* specimens, was able to demonstrate such muscle thickening in only two of 26 specimens of sigmoid colon containing diverti-cula, *obtained at routine autopsies*. However, Parks (1968) observed such thickening in 14 of 15

autopsy-room bodies with diverticular disease. Celio (1952) suggested that the muscle hypertrophy in diverticular disease might be secondary to changes in the intrinsic nerve plexuses, but Morson (1963) found Auerbach and Meissner's plexuses to be normal in all his specimens.

Though practically all cases of diverticular disease treated by operation are considered clinically to be suffering from diverticulitis, in about a third of the colon specimens thus obtained there is no evidence of inflammation, past or present (Morson 1963; Arfwidsson 1964; Ming and Fleischner 1965). When inflammation does occur, though it may originate in the diverticula its main effects are experienced in the extramural pericolonic tissues, which is not un-natural, for the diverticula project entirely into these tissues. Ming and Fleischner (1965) claim that the pericolitis is the result not of inflammation in the diverticular wall but of macro- or micro-perforations, which they were able to demonstrate frequently in their operative specimens, specially

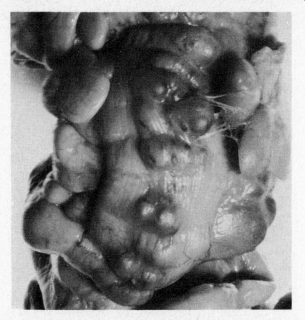

feature is the deposition of fibrofatty tissue in the subserosa, in the appendices epiploicae, and in the mesocolon, though Morson (1963) believes that much of the apparent increase of fat around the sigmoid colon in these cases is due to shortening of the bowel. As a consequence of these changes, as well as the associated muscle hypertrophy, the affected segment becomes thickened, rigid and irregularly contracted. Contraction of the meso-colon may lead to angulation or abnormal fixation, as may adhesions to other structures, which are very common. A most important point is that, however diseased the bowel may be, the mucosa lining the lumen *never shows gross ulceration* as found in carcinoma.

RADIOLOGICAL APPEARANCES

Diverticulosis

The Diverticula

A much better impression of the extent and severity of diverticulosis is as a rule obtained by radiological examination after barium enemas than by morbid anatomical studies. Diverticula may very occasionally be found distributed throughout the entire colon, even implicating the caecum and ascending colon (Fig. 621), but, in the main, it is the left colon, and particularly the sigmoid loop, that is

examined from this point of view. The pericolitis or peridiverticulitis shows itself in the form of localized peritonitis and abscess formation. Extension of the abscess to neighbouring viscera or the abdominal wall may lead to fistula formation. In cases with long-standing inflammation another prominent

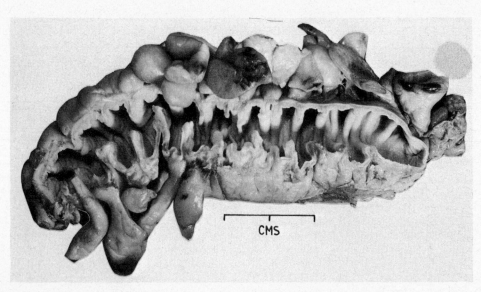

Fig. 620. Longitudinal section of a segment of colon, the seat of diverticulosis. Note the prominent transverse folds of mucosa and thickened circular muscle coat. (*From Lloyd-Davies 1953*)

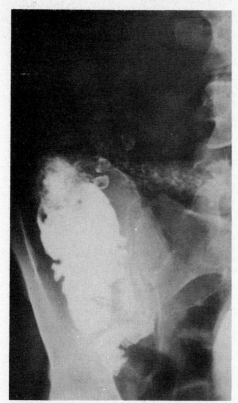

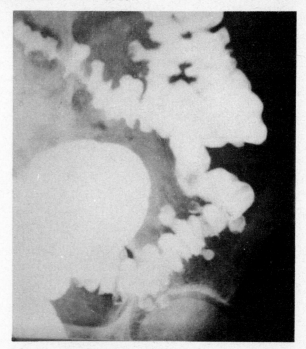

Fig. 622. Barium enema plate showing gross diverticulosis of the sigmoid and descending colon.

Fig. 621. Barium enema plate showing multiple diverticula of the caecum and right colon. Diverticula were also present in the left colon.

affected, as has already been pointed out on p. 882 (Figs 622 and 623). The most revealing X-ray film is often that made after evacuation of the enema (Fig. 624). The diverticula are then very clearly depicted and, in cases with gross diverticulosis, they may be clustered like a bunch of grapes in the pelvis or sigmoid region. The size and shape of the individual diverticula vary greatly. In the early stages they are small and globular in outline and their necks are relatively wide, almost as broad as the widest part of the diverticulum. Later the pouches are larger and more flask-shaped with narrow necks. Sometimes a diverticulum is completely filled with barium or with air; at other times the filling is incomplete due to the presence of a faecolith in the diverticulum.

The Colon Itself

A common finding on radiological examination of colon the seat of diverticula is that the affected segment is in a contracted state usually taken to indicate some degree of colon spasm. In its grossest form this produces the characteristic 'zig-zag' ap-

pearance shown in Fig. 625. In the past an element of inflammation has frequently been indicted in the genesis of such appearances, but from the combined radiological and pathological studies by Morson (1963), Williams (1963), Arfwidsson (1964) and Ming and Fleischner (1965) (see p. 885) it seems that they may be produced entirely by associated hypertrophy of the circular and longitudinal muscle fibres in the colon wall without any inflammatory changes. Arfwidsson (1964) has shown, moreover, that these appearances of spasm may be present without any radiological evidence of diverticula in certain cases in which intracolonic tension is known to be raised as in diverticular disease, or in which subsequent histopathological examination of the affected segment of bowel after surgical excision revealed very small incipient diverticula (Figs 626, 627).

The 'Prediverticular State'

Though the appearances of the colon spasm already mentioned (Figs 626, 627) might be regarded as a prediverticular state, this term is generally reserved for a particular radiological appearance originally described by Spriggs and Marxer (1925) (Fig. 628). As defined by them it referred to a 'ragged outline of the wall of the bowel, which does not dilate even in the most

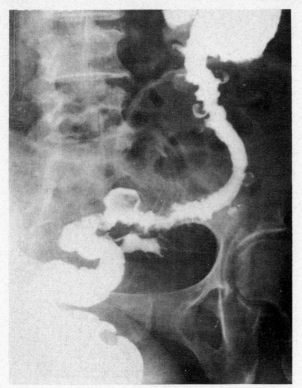

Fig. 623. Barium enema plate showing large diverticula in the sigmoid colon.

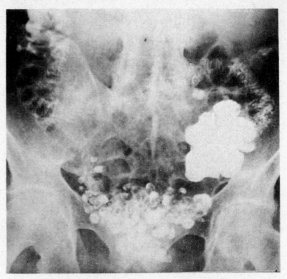

Fig. 624. Post-evacuation film after barium enema; numerous large diverticula of the sigmoid are outlined by the retained barium.

favourable position. If one aspect only of the wall is involved, the contraction is less. The appearance is not the result of irritation from the small herniae, but precedes their formation'. The sigmoid colon was the part most often involved but rarely the appearance extended into the descending colon as well. The 'prediverticular state' was observed in 20 or 100 cases of diverticulosis examined radiologically by Spriggs and Marxer (1925); in 16 of these 20 cases small diverticula were recognized in or close to the affected areas.

In subsequent writings on the subject Spriggs and Marxer (1927, 1937) modified their original description to include two stages of prediverticulosis—an early one characterized by a 'finely serrated' edge, and a later one with coarser irregularity to which they applied the term 'concertina-like' appearance (Fig. 628). In nearly all their illustrations they depicted a unilateral change. They claimed that if a case is examined at intervals, diverticula will be found to develop in an area which had previously shown the radiological appearances of the 'prediverticular state'.

As regards the aetiology of the 'prediverticular state' Spriggs and Marxer (1925, 1927, 1937) believed that the irregularity of the bowel outline was due to irritation of the circular muscle, which in turn they attributed to bacterial infection. They seemed prepared to concede, however, in their later writings that the coarse 'concertina-like' appearance might be due partly to early established diverticulosis.

As Marcus and Watt (1964) have pointed out many subsequent authors on the subject, such as Moynihan (1927), Mailer (1928), Case (1929), Lockhart-Mummery (1930), Lockhart-Mummery and Hodgson (1931), Edwards (1934, 1939), Barclay (1933), Henderson (1944), Grout (1949), Schinz et al. (1954), Todd

(1955), Shanks et al. (1958), have commented on the 'prediverticular state', using a variety of terms to describe the appearances, e.g. 'ripple border', 'palisade', 'saw-edge', 'saw-tooth' and 'spastic notches'. Though these radiological findings have been readily recognized and accepted, the significance attributed to them has varied greatly. Perhaps the majority of radiologists, following the lead of Barclay (1933), have doubted whether the 'prediverticular state' was really a precursor to overt diverticulosis and would not diagnose it unless there was at least one diverticulum elsewhere in the colon (Grout 1949).

As for Spriggs and Marxer's (1925) conception of the aetiology of the 'prediverticular state', though this gained the support of Henderson (1944) and Todd (1955) it was rejected by most other authors. Spriggs and Marxer (1927, 1938) had provided virtually no clear pathological evidence for their belief that the colon wall was the seat of inflammatory changes in these cases. Mailer's (1928) careful histopathological studies failed to reveal any inflammatory process preceding the development of diverticula, and the more recent researches of Morson (1963) and Arfwidsson (1964) have also shown that inflammation is often completely absent from the colon wall in cases of diverticulosis. Lockhart-Mummery (1930) and Lockhart-Mummery and Hodgson (1931) were early to suggest that the appearances in the 'prediverticular state' were due to the presence of very small diverticular buds in the wall of the colon. Edwards (1934, 1939) believed that the finer irregularity of the colon wall in the 'prediverticular state' was due to irregular spasm of the circular muscle fibres, but the coarser appearances resembling a 'saw-edge' (and corresponding to Spriggs and Marxer's (1927) 'concertina-like' appearance) was caused by established small diverticula.

The histopathological basis of the radiological 'prediverticular state' was re-examined by Arfwidsson (1964) and Marcus and Watt (1964). Arfwidsson (1964) suggested that the 'saw-tooth' appearance may be due to hypertrophy of the circular and longitudinal muscle coats of the colon wall drawing the bowel together lengthwise and pleating it. Marcus and Watt (1964) have emphasized that the 'prediverticular state' has usually been described as a unilateral change. They believe that it is due to the radiologist securing a profile view of the antimesenteric intertaenial area in which numerous intramural or ridge diverticula

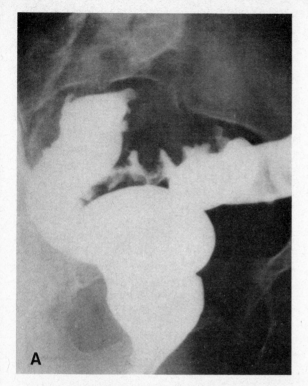
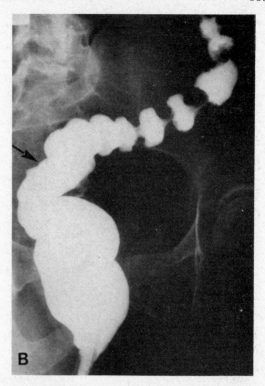

Fig. 625. (A) Barium enema plate of a patient with diverticular disease of the sigmoid, showing typical zig-zag appearance due to spasm and muscle hypertrophy with shortening. (B) Same case after sigmoidectomy, showing distal limit of the resection (marked by arrow at level of anastomosis).

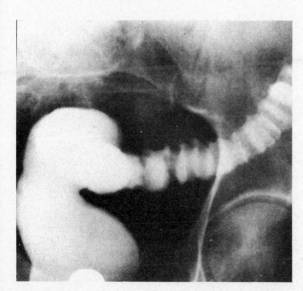

Fig. 626. Barium enema plate of a patient without diverticula who was demonstrated to have high intrasigmoid pressure, showing the spastic state of the colon which seems to be drawn together in the long axis and corrugated. The haustra are small and the indentations separating them broad and circular. (*From Arfwidsson 1964*)

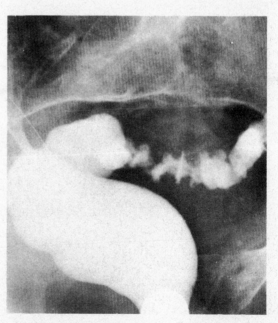

Fig. 627. Barium enema plate from a patient without radiologically overt diverticula, showing the typical spastic, almost zig-zag, appearance found in diverticular disease. Histopathological examination of the sigmoid after resection revealed that it contained incipient diverticula. (*From Arfwidsson 1964*)

are present giving a jagged irregular 'saw-tooth' edge to the outline of the colon on this aspect. They have put this theory to the test by X-raying excised specimens of colon filled with opaque medium to show the antimesenteric area in profile and have obtained an appearance (Fig. 629) very similar to that observed clinically as the 'prediverticular state' (Fig. 628).

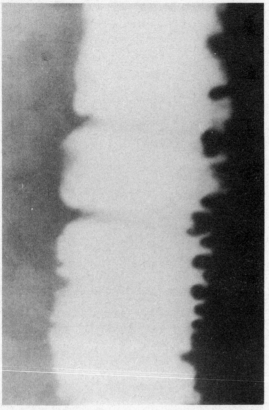

Fig. 628. 'Ripple border' or 'palisading' appearance of the alleged 'prediverticular stage' of diverticulosis. (*From Arfwidsson 1964*)

Diverticulitis

The radiological signs of diverticulitis depend mainly on encroachment on the lumen of the colon in the affected segment from thickening and contracture of the bowel wall. But it is now known (see p. 884) that considerable thickening of the colon wall and narrowing of the lumen may occur due to hypertrophy and spasm of the muscle coat in simple diverticulosis quite apart from any associated inflammatory changes. Consequently it can be very difficult to decide on radiological examination whether an element of inflammation is present or not. A grossly irregular narrowing of the outline of the colon on the barium enema plates as shown in Figs 630 and 631 would suggest that one is dealing with diverticulitis rather than diverticulosis with associated thickening and spasm of the muscle coats. The stricture is usually longer and less definite than that found with a carcinoma. In the colon proximal or distal to the area of diverticulitis uninflamed diverticula are often evident radiologically. Even more certain evidence of the existence of inflammatory changes superimposed on diverticulosis is provided by the finding of very gross distortion of the colonic outline on radiological examination with some barium lying outside the bowel lumen in an extracolonic abscess cavity (Fig. 632).

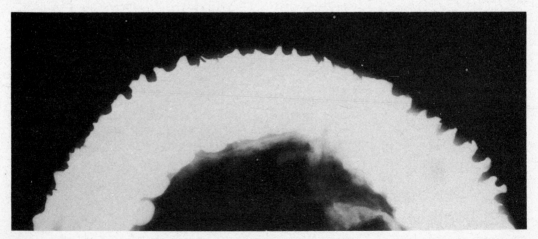

Fig. 629. Lateral radiograph of excised sigmoid colon filled with contrast medium, showing diverticulosis of the antimesenteric intertaenial area. The unilateral spiky irregularity closely resembles the so-called 'prediverticular state'. (*From Marcus and Watt 1965*)

AETIOLOGY

It is generally agreed that diverticula of the colon are as a rule *acquired* and not congenital (but solitary diverticulum of the caecum is an exception, see p. 907). This seems to be established beyond doubt by the findings of barium enema examinations and autopsies referred to on p. 882, which indicate the extreme rarity of diverticula in young patients and the progressively increasing incidence with advancing age.

It seems reasonable to suppose that colonic diverticula are of the nature of *pulsion diverticula* or *mucosal herniations*, which develop at weak points in the bowel wall under the influence of increased intraluminal pressure. Drummond (1917), Spriggs and Marxer (1925), Edwards (1939), Lloyd-Davies (1953) and Slack (1962) have emphasized that the diverticula consistently occur at the sites of entry of blood vessels into the colon wall on either side between the mesenteric taenia and the anti-mesenteric taeniae, and to a lesser extent in the antimesenteric intertaenial area. They have argued that the circular muscle coat is weakened by the penetration of the vessels and that this determines the localization of the diverticula at these points.

The other main site of entry of vessels into the colon wall is at the mesenteric border itself, but here the strong taenia probably provides additional support and counteracts any tendency to herniation. Another source of weakness that is often mentioned is fatty infiltration of the colon wall, for patients with diverticulosis are often obese. This may be a factor in some cases, but not all sufferers from diverticula of the colon are excessively stout (Hughes 1969). Spriggs and Marxer (1925) held that the initial abnormality in diverticular disease was infection of the bowel wall, which, in addition to producing the radiological appearances of the 'prediverticular state', weakened the wall and predisposed to the development of diverticula, but this theory has been rendered quite untenable by the pathological studies made by several workers (Mailer 1928; Morson 1963; Arfwidsson 1964), which show that in its earlier stages diverticulosis is a non-inflammatory condition (see p. 885).

The explanation of the raised intracolonic tension, which the theory of a pulsion diverticulum postulates, is more debatable. Constipation has often been cited as an important factor in this connection, but it is present in less than half the cases. A more plausible hypothesis is that, originally

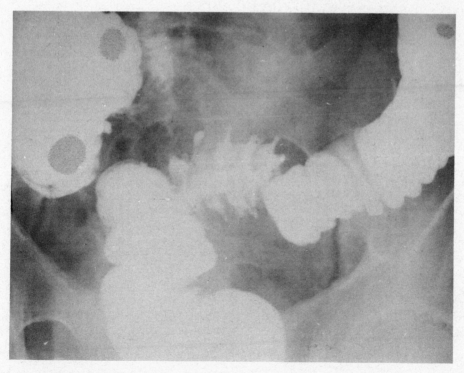

Fig. 630. Diverticulitis of sigmoid producing an irregularly narrowed segment.

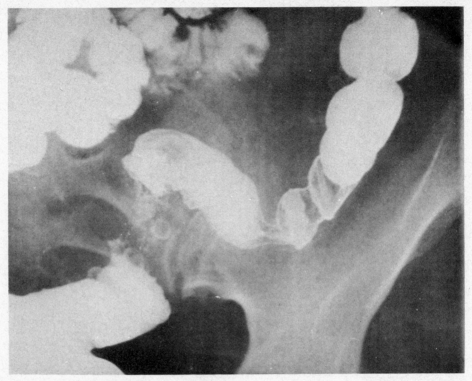

Fig. 631. Diverticulitis of sigmoid producing a long filling defect.

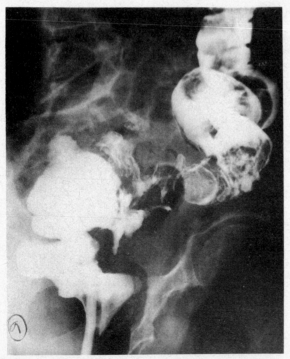

Fig. 632. Barium enema plate showing gross irregularity of the sigmoid loop due to gross diverticulitis. At operation a pericolonic abscess was found to be present, as can be surmised from the radiograph (Professor A. S. Johnstone's case).

advanced by Keith (1910) and strongly supported by Edwards (1934), Arfwidsson (1964), Painter (1964) and Painter and Truelove (1964), of muscular spasm and irregular incoordinated contraction of the affected part of the colon; it is supported by the radiographic appearances of spasm in many cases (see p. 887), by the finding of gross hypertrophy of the circular and longitudinal muscle fibres of the colon wall in the affected segment (Morson 1963; Arfwidsson 1964; Ming and Fleischner 1965), and to some extent by recordings of intracolonic tension in patients with diverticular disease (Painter and Truelove 1964; Arfwidsson 1964; Parks and Connell 1969). In Painter and Truelove's (1964) study no difference was found in the resting pressure patterns produced by the sigmoid colon in health and in diverticulosis. But *morphine*, which given intravenously or intramuscularly in therapeutic dosage caused the normal colon to generate an increased number of pressure waves compared with the number produced under resting condition, evoked an even greater response in segments of colon containing diverticula. *Prostigmine* also elicited somewhat exaggerated activity in diverticular segments of colon compared with its effect on normal segments. By contrast Arfwidsson (1964) noted a significantly *higher mean resting total pressure* and more numerous strong waves in patients suffering from diverticulosis than in normal individuals. He also demonstrated that *intake of food* induced a marked increase of the total intraluminal pressure in the sigmoid colon and in the number of strong waves recorded in both normal subjects and patients with diverticula disease. *Prostigmine* given intravenously in a dose of 0·5 mg produced a striking increase in colonic activity and pressure in normal subjects and even more so in those suffering from diverticulosis. Parks and Connell (1969) were able to confirm Arfwidsson's (1964) finding of increased basal and postprandial activity in diverticular disease compared with normal *only if they used open-ended tubes* to record the pressure, as had been done by Arfwidsson (1964) and Painter and Truelove (1964). But, using miniature balloons to record activity, no difference was observed by them in diverticular disease and in health under basal conditions and after the physiological stimulus of eating food. Parks and Connell (1969) felt, as did Painter and Truelove (1964) and Painter et al. (1965), that an important factor in the genesis of unusually high pressure in localized areas of the colon in cases of diverticular disease might be the tendency for the prominent arc-like folds of pleated mucosa and circular muscle coat (see Fig. 620) to be forced close together during contractions of the bowel, producing a series of bladders.

Emotion has been shown to increase the motility of the colon (Almy et al. 1949a, b, 1950; Chaudhary and Truelove 1961) and Painter and Truelove (1964) have postulated, without producing any direct evidence, however, that emotional stress might generate sufficiently high pressures to initiate herniation of the mucosa through weaknesses in the colonic wall. But an even more important factor in the production of high pressures within the colon is believed by Painter and Burkitt (1971) and Painter et al. (1972) to be the highly refined diet of modern Western nations. As these authors point out, diverticular disease is virtually unknown in primitive communities, as in many parts of contemporary Africa, in which a coarse diet including much fibre is eaten. The disease seems to become gradually more common as traditional eating habits of this kind are abandoned in favour of more refined foods, which are deficient in fibre and which produce much less bulky and frequent stools. (Segal et al. 1977), but Archampong et al. (1978) record examples of diverticular disease of an extensive kind occurring in African patients who have not departed from their traditional high-residue diet. Also, according to Antia and Desai (1974), diverticular disease is seen quite frequently in India, despite the high fibre content of the diet of unrefined cereals and vegetables eaten by most Indian patients. Painter et al. (1972) postulate that the colon, and particularly the sigmoid part, has to segment more vigorously to propel the more viscous faeces resulting from this diet and thereby generates higher intracolonic tension which causes the mucosal herniations that are diverticulosis. Hodgson (1972) reports some experimental work on the production of colonic diverticula in rabbits fed on a low residue diet. The whole concept of diverticular disease in contemporary civilized society as being due to lack of cereal fibre in the diet is strenuously challenged by Eastwood et al. (1974).

SYMPTOMS

Diverticulosis

Uncomplicated diverticulosis is generally believed to be asymptomatic and is often discovered incidentally during barium enema examination. However, some of these patients have vague symptoms, which were the reason for requesting the radiological examination. These comprise occasional ill-defined discomfort or pain in the central abdomen or left iliac fossa, flatulent distension and slight alteration of bowel habit. It is difficult to know whether they should be attributed to the diverticulosis, to the colonic spasm (Arfwidsson 1964; Almy 1965) which is alleged to be important in the production of the diverticula or to a mild degree of diverticulitis not severe enough to produce radiological signs. They may also originate outside the intestinal tract (Hughes 1970b), and, rightly or wrongly, have often been dismissed as manifestations of a psychoneurosis.

Diverticulitis

The symptoms of diverticulitis include abdominal pain, disturbance of bowel habits, abdominal distension, nausea, vomiting, rectal bleeding (and other symptoms such as dysuria, pneumaturia, and faecal fistula, depending on the occurrence of complications).

Abdominal pain is the cardinal symptom. Characteristically it is referred to the left iliac or suprapubic region. It may be severe, mild or absent depending on fluctuations in the local inflammatory state of the lesion. Commonly it persists for several days and then subsides or disappears completely till a further exacerbation of the diverticulitis occurs. In addition to this more typical diverticulitis pain there may be a more central colicky abdominal pain due to some degree of organic obstruction.

Alteration of bowel habit. Intermittent diarrhoea, or alternating periods of diarrhoea and constipation, are common in diverticulitis. As increasing stenosis of the colon develops, constipation becomes a more prominent symptom and may be associated with some degree of abdominal distension.

Nausea and vomiting are rare but may occur during more acute attacks or when organic obstruction is far advanced.

Rectal bleeding. Though rectal bleeding has in the past generally been regarded as an excessively rare manifestation of diverticulitis, a number of surgeons have now recorded a fairly high incidence of haemorrhage with both diverticulosis and diverticulitis. The bleeding may be slight and continuous as in carcinoma of the colon but on occasions is massive and exsanguinating. As Stone (1944), Hoar and Bernard (1954) and Fraenkel (1954) point out, this profuse type of haemorrhage, occurring in an older patient, is highly suggestive of diverticular disease (see also p. 897).

EXAMINATION

In cases of diverticulosis alone there are no abnormal physical signs on abdominal examination. But in patients with diverticulitis tenderness in the left lower quadrant of the abdomen or in the suprapubic region is a frequent finding. Its acuteness depends on the stage of the inflammatory process and it may vary from a slight discomfort on deep palpation in a relatively quiescent case to exquisite tenderness at a more florid phase of the disease. The tender thickened sigmoid colon itself can be palpated in many cases. Some abdominal distension may be noted secondary to local peritonitis in the left iliac region or to organic obstruction of the sigmoid.

Digital examination of the rectum may reveal some tenderness in the pelvis or an actual mass may be palpable. Sigmoidoscopy is frequently unsatisfactory, for distortion of the colon often prevents a full instrumentation being effected. Usually the actual lesion is not reached and an inconclusive verdict has to be returned. It is only very rarely that the openings of diverticula of the sigmoid can be seen with the sigmoidoscope. Even if they are observed, this does not prove that the lesion at a higher level is a diverticulitis and not a carcinoma.

X-ray examination. The radiological appearances at different stages of the disease have already been described on p. 886.

DIAGNOSIS

The paramount importance of radiological examination in diagnosis needs no emphasis. The detection of simple diverticulosis depends virtually entirely on this means, and, whilst diverticulitis may be strongly suspected from the symptomatology and findings on clinical examination, radiological investigation plays an important part in establishing the diagnosis. The one over-riding consideration for the radiologist is the differentiation of an area of apparent diverticulitis from a carcinoma, and in this connection he will take into account the following points, as summarized by Schatzki (1940) in a classical paper:

1. In diverticulitis a long segment of bowel is usually affected, whilst in carcinoma the lesion is often short, but there are many exceptions to this generalization.
2. In carcinoma the transition from normal to diseased bowel is usually abrupt, whilst in diverticulitis it is more gradual.
3. A bizarre, fringed contour is more often associated with diverticulitis.
4. In diverticulitis the mucosa is intact but in carcinoma it is destroyed.
5. The presence of diverticula in the bowel above or below the area of narrowing is slightly in favour of a diagnosis of diverticulitis. However, too much weight must not be attached to this point, for diverticulosis and carcinoma are both common conditions and they not infrequently coincide in the same patient. The fact that a patient has diverticula does not confer on him immunity to carcinoma of the colon.
6. Spasm of the colon is more constant in diverticulitis than in carcinoma. Lloyd-Davies (1953) has stressed the value of the antispasmodic, propantheline bromide, 100 mg one hour before the examination, in relaxing the spasm in these cases and aiding the interpretation of the radiological appearances.

It must be recognized that despite the most expert radiological examination accurate differentiation between diverticulitis and carcinoma is sometimes impossible. Thus it was found impossible to exclude carcinoma in 25% of a series of patients with diverticulitis surveyed by Pemberton et al. (1947) and in 18% of a group reported by Welch et al. (1953). Actually at laparotomy in such cases the surgeon frequently finds himself in the same quandary as the radiologist—for example in 21% of the cases published by Waugh and Walt (1957)—and is unable to say with confidence whether the lesion is carcinoma or diverticulitis. There are many cases on record where a laparotomy decision in favour of diverticulitis, and followed by a simple proximal colostomy as a palliative measure, was shown by subsequent events to be wrong. Likewise some patients, treated in the past by palliative colostomy for alleged inoperable carcinoma of the distal sigmoid, have lived in excellent health for many years afterwards, indicating that the condition was almost certainly one of diverticulitis rather than growth. I have indeed had the opportunity to resect three or four such 'irremovable tumours', the subsequent pathological examination demonstrating that they were in fact diverticulitis masses. The procedure to be adopted at laparotomy when there is doubt as to whether the lesion found is diverticulitis or carcinoma is detailed on p. 901.

The problem of diagnosis as between diverticular disease and carcinoma is further confused by the occasional simultaneous occurrence of carcinoma or adenoma with diverticulosis and diverticulitis. Thus in 197 cases of carcinoma of the sigmoid Ponka et al. (1959) found closely associated diverticulosis or diverticulitis in 35 (18%). Morton and Goldman (1962) in a survey of 141 patients with diverticular disease of the sigmoid found that 11% had also benign polyps, 3% malignant polyps and 5% carcinoma, whilst of 180 patients with carcinoma of the sigmoid 19% had diverticular disease.

Colonoscopy is now proving useful in differentiating diverticular disease from carcinoma, though diverticular cases may be technically difficult for this examination.

COMPLICATIONS

Perforation

Rupture of an individual diverticulum may occur either in pure diverticulosis or in diverticulitis. Usually it develops quite spontaneously, but oc-

casionally the perforation is produced by the administration of an enema or colonic lavage. I have seen three patients who sustained rupture of a diverticulum of the colon in this way with fatal results in two. Clinically the condition presents as an acute diffuse peritonitis with maximal signs in the lower abdomen, possibly on the left side, which may suggest the diagnosis. Often, however, the source of the peritonitis is unsuspected till the abdomen is opened.

Acute Diverticulitis (Acute Peridiverticulitis or Pericolitis, Acute Perforated Diverticulitis) with Localized or Diffuse Peritonitis or Pericolic Abscess

In a sense every exacerbation of symptoms in a case of chronic diverticulitis is due to a superimposed acute diverticulitis which usually subsides spontaneously in the course of time. But what is implied by the above heading is a much more severe attack, which, as emphasized by Dawson et al. (1965), is nearly always in fact the first clinical manifestation of diverticular disease. There is severe pain in the lower abdomen, maximal on the right as often as on the left, and accompanied by acute tenderness and guarding in that region; an ill-defined mass may sometimes be palpable, though the muscle rigidity often masks its presence. Constitutional disturbance usually occurs with an elevated temperature and pulse, and with nausea and vomiting; some patients may be gravely ill in a state of severe shock. Occasionally the patient has diarrhoea and passes blood and mucus.

It will be apparent from the foregoing account of the clinical manifestations that in some cases a clinical diagnosis of an acute inflammatory process originating in the sigmoid colon may be reached with reasonable confidence, but that in other cases

TABLE 74. *Preoperative Diagnosis in 93 Cases of Acute Diverticulitis*

Diagnosis	No. of patients
Perforated diverticulitis	33
Appendicitis	31
Peritonitis (cause unknown)	9
Perforated viscus	7
Perforated peptic ulcer	5
Mesenteric vascular occlusion	2
Strangulated umbilical hernia	1
Not diagnosed during life	5

After Dawson et al. (1965).

TABLE 75. *Causes of* Mild *or* Moderate *Rectal Bleeding in 221 Patients admitted to Louisville General Hospital and Louisville V.A. Hospital 1955–60*

Causes	No. of cases
Carcinoma of left colon	73
Diverticulosis	45 ⎱ 61
Diverticulitis	16 ⎰
Ulcerative colitis	39
Polyps	23
Carcinoma of right colon	13
Miscellaneous	12

After Noer et al. (1962).

TABLE 76. *Causes of* Severe *Rectal Bleeding in 24 Patients admitted to Louisville General Hospital and Louisville V.A. Hospital 1955–60*

Causes	No. of cases
Diverticulosis	17
Carcinoma of left colon	3
Polyps	1
Carcinoma of right colon	1
Sarcoma of rectum	1
Undetermined	1

After Noer et al. (1962).

diverticular disease, but has sometimes come from other lesions. Thus, in 12 such patients reported by Eisenberg et al. (1973) an origin for the haemorrhage was found in diverticular disease in four, other sources were demonstrated in four (a caecal ulcer, a small bowel lymphoma, an area of small bowel ischaemia, and an arteriovenous abnormality of the small bowel), and no definite site of bleeding could be discovered in four. Afidi et al. (1971), Whitehouse (1973) and Boley et al. (1977) have particularly stressed the diagnostic problem presented by *minute abnormalities of the vasculature of the colon wall, which may be difficult to detect on naked-eye examination of the bowel at laparotomy or even on subsequent pathological examination of an operative specimen.* Fortunately they can sometimes be demonstrated on selective mesenteric arteriography, especially when bleeding acutely. They appear to be at least as common on the right side as on the left side of the colon. Mesenteric arteriography is clearly important in the diagnosis of alleged bleeding diverticular disease. It may also be helpful in permitting conservative treatment of this source of bleeding as

well as some others by intra-arterial injection of vasoconstrictors or embolizing agents (see p. 907).

Mechanism of Bleeding

As Rigg and Ewing (1966) have emphasized, the precise cause of the bleeding in diverticular disease has been established in only a handful of cases, because relatively few patients have come to operation during the acute phase of haemorrhage. Smith (1951), Maynard and Voorhees (1956), Weingarten et al. (1959) and Quinn (1961) have observed blood emerging from an individual diverticulum in the lower sigmoid on sigmoidoscopy or in the transverse colon, at the hepatic flexure or the splenic flexure on colotomy. Salgado et al. (1961), Slack (1962) and Rosenberg and Rosenberg (1964) were able to demonstrate ulcers in the wall of a diverticulum in operative specimens, which were presumed to be the source of the bleeding. Bleeding is *more often found with diverticulosis than with diverticulitis* (Rosser 1955; Rives 1955; Noer et al. 1962; Eisenberg et al. 1973).

(For treatment see pp. 906–7).

TREATMENT

Simple Diverticulosis

It has been customary in the past to consider uncomplicated diverticulosis as a condition requiring only expectant or medical management. A common practice used to be to prescribe a *low-residue diet* and particularly one avoiding fruit pips and coarse vegetable fibres, but I have always been doubtful of the value of this dietetic restriction. Arfwidsson (1964), Truelove and Reynell (1963) and Almy (1965) suggested that the traditional low-residue foods might with advantage in such cases be replaced by a *high-residue* diet supplemented by *hydrophilic colloids* (e.g. Isogel, Normacol, Metamucil, one teaspoonful in a little water once to thrice daily) to provide a bigger faecal mass in the sigmoid which might make more difficult the close approximation of its walls and the creation of high intracolonic pressures in very short localized segments. Years ago Carlson and Hoelzel (1949) showed that a high-residue diet was successful in retarding the development of diverticula in the experimental animal. With the same object in mind Painter et al. (1972) have championed the advantage of adding unprocessed bran to the diet, two teaspoonfuls thrice daily, in patients with diverticular disease. Taylor and Duthie (1976) suggest as a substitute for ordinary bran, which many patients find singularly unpalatable, bran compressed in the form of tablets, nine of which are taken per day (18 g bran). In a controlled cross-over trial, comparing them with a high-roughage diet and with Normacol plus an antispasmodic respectively, Taylor and Duthie (1976) found the bran tablets to be significantly more effective not only in improving symptoms but also in returning to normal the abnormal myoelectrical tracings from the colon wall. *Mild aperients*, especially liquid paraffin and other stool softeners, are often ordered with the object of keeping the faeces soft and preventing faecal stasis with the formation of hard stercoliths in the diverticula, but it is rather dubious whether the latter development can be avoided by such means. With the same object in mind *frequent enemas or colonic lavage* are sometimes recommended, but I am sure that this is thoroughly bad advice. Apart from the danger of perforation, which I know from personal experience (see p. 895) that this treatment carries in cases of diverticulosis, it seems to me ill suited psychologically to the average patient with diverticulosis and likely to encourage still further any pre-existent tendency to introspection. The use of *antispasmodics* such as propantheline bromide, 15 mg four times daily, might seem logical in view of the part believed to be played by colon spasm in causation, and is particularly indicated when pronounced contraction of the colon has been demonstrated on X-ray examination. The continuous administration of non-absorbable sulphonamides or antibiotic preparations as *intestinal antiseptics* to sterilize the faeces and prevent infective complications had been recommended, but raises the possibility of undesirable side-effects from alteration of the bacterial flora of the gut.

The extent to which I myself have employed medical therapy has been influenced by the manner of presentation of the diverticulosis. If the condition has been detected by routine barium studies as part of the investigation to exclude neoplasm of the alimentary tract and there are no symptoms that could reasonably be attributed to the diverticular lesion, my own personal practice has been to advise the patient that the findings are of no significance and to recommend no treatment. If, on the other hand, the condition is accompanied by a complaint of pain that might be due to associated colon spasm and there is radiological evidence to this effect, I have usually prescribed antispasmodics, but have not as a rule invoked any other item of medical therapy, such as dietetic restriction. Clearly oral administration of bran, bran tablets or an hydrophilic colliod agent would be a fashionable and possibly useful addition.

As pointed out on pp. 881, 882 and 886, there has latterly been considerably blurring of the distinction between diverticulosis and diverticulitis, and it seems in retrospect (see p. 885) that a proportion of patients with simple diverticulosis and gross structural deformity due to muscle hypertrophy, but with no superadded inflammatory changes, have been submitted to radical surgical treatment because of the severity of the symptoms and on a mistaken diagnosis of diverticulitis. Indeed, Arfwidsson (1964) and Almy (1965) have advocated the cautious trial of radical surgery in certain patients with pronounced symptoms at an early stage of diverticulosis, before gross diverticula have become radiologically evident, but I must say I would disapprove of any such trend (see Indications for elective resection, p. 900, and Sigmoid myotomy, p. 902).

Diverticulitis

EXPECTANT TREATMENT

There is unfortunately no really effective medical treatment for diverticulitis, any more than there is for, say, cholecystitis. The same measures are available as for uncomplicated diverticulosis (see p. 898), but antispasmodics may be particularly important in view of the pronounced muscle hypertrophy known to be present in many of these cases. In addition for more acute episodes bed rest and analgesics may be necessary, and in the use of the latter it is clearly advisable from the work of Painter and Truelove (1964) to avoid morphine and employ instead drugs such as pethidine which do not generate raised intracolonic tension. At such times systemic antibiotic therapy may also be indicated, but the frequent use of antibiotics in this way is apt to lead to the development of resistant strains of organism. If there is any tendency to stenosis, mild aperients will be needed. Despite the unsatisfactory nature of conservative treatment, most cases of diverticulitis are in fact managed more or less adequately along expectant lines, and this is well brought out by the reports of Bolt and Hughes (1966), Kyle (1968), Parks (1969) and McGregor et al. (1970). For example, Parks (1969) found that, of 297 patients admitted to the Royal Victoria Hospital, Belfast, for medical treatment only and followed up for 2 to 16 years thereafter, 28% died of intercurrent conditions, 2% died of their diverticular disease, 4% were alive with severe symptoms of this condition, 26% were alive with mild symptoms of diverticulitis, and 40% were alive and entirely free of complaints referable to the bowel. Of the original 297 patients, 78 (25%) had to re-enter hospital for a second admission (half of them within one year), another 12 (4%) for a third time, and five (under 2%) for a fourth time. Of the patients who were re-admitted, 20 (6·7%) of the original 297 patients underwent surgical treatment, and six (2%) died.

SURGICAL TREATMENT

The rational surgical treatment of diverticulitis would seem to be resection of the affected segment of bowel followed by axial anastomosis. Actually W. J. Mayo applied this principle with very satisfactory results to five cases in 1907, but for many years most surgeons were deterred by the anticipated difficulties and dangers of such an operation. Instead they preferred indirect surgery consisting of a proximal colostomy as a temporary or permanent measure. By this means it was hoped that the inflammation in the diseased sigmoid would subside, and that it might eventually be possible to close the colostomy. Unfortunately, when this was done, there was usually a return of symptoms. Indeed, in many cases the diverticulitis remained active *even whilst the colostomy was in position*, and I have known patients develop a pericolic abscess or colovesical fistula despite the complete diversion of faeces provided by this regimen. Smithwick (1942) and Pemberton et al. (1947) have had similar experiences testifying to the inadequacy of simple proximal colostomy in the treatment of diverticulitis.

However, in the period since World War II the surgery of diverticulitis has undergone a complete transformation and now assumes the direct form hitherto generally thought to be unattainable. The main reason for this change of attitude has undoubtedly been the extensive experience which surgeons have had in recent years of anterior resection with anastomosis for carcinoma of the upper rectum and rectosigmoid, as a consequence of which they have felt better able to tackle the technical difficulties—more anticipated than real—associated with resection of adherent diverticulitis segments. Such operations can now be carried out with relatively little risk and have the great attraction over lesser operations, in the eyes of the patient, that they obviate the necessity for a permanent colostomy.

The effect of these changes in surgical policy are well shown in the statistics that have emanated from the Massachusetts General Hospital during the last 20 years. Smithwick (1942), analysing the experience of that hospital in the management of diverticulitis of the colon from 1927 to 1942, found that of 333 cases admitted with this condition 64 (19%) proceeded to operation, and only 33 (10%) of the entire series had resection of the lesion, most of these resections being by a staged method and the mortality being 6%. Rodkey and Welch (1959) carried out a similar study of the cases admitted from 1942 to 1956 and found that the number having operation of some kind had risen to 234, whilst the proportion having ultimate resection was 218, 100 of which had primary resection and anastomosis. The overall mortality in resected cases was 2·7%. During the period 1960–4, 200 patients with diverticulitis were admitted to the Massachusetts General Hospital for surgical treatment (Rodkey and Welch 1965). Of these 61 were operated on for acute complications of the disease with a mortality of 14·7%, whilst 139 had elective resection with a mortality of only 1·4%.

Waugh and Walt (1957) have similarly demonstrated from the experience of the Mayo Clinic the great safety of resection for diverticulitis in recent years. Of 320 patients admitted with this condition to the Clinic between 1945 and 1954 inclusive 291 came to elective resection with an overall mortality of 2·1%; in 93 cases treated by one-stage primary resection with anastomosis there was only one death. My own personal experience of resection for diverticular disease over ten years comprises 102 cases, mostly treated by one-stage operations, with three deaths.

INDICATIONS FOR ELECTIVE RESECTION

As a result of these improvements in surgical methods there has been a considerable broadening of the indications for operation for diverticulitis in recent years. Previously surgical treatment was reserved essentially for the complications of the disease—namely perforation, abscess, fistula formation, obstruction and rarely bleeding. The operation employed consisted of the emergency measures necessary to deal with these various situations—suture, drainage, colostomy—and seldom included resection of the lesion. Now, in addition to the complicated cases (see pp. 895–8), many patients with 'uncomplicated' diverticulitis (or even simple diverticulosis, see p. 898) associated with repeated attacks of pain and tenderness, and disturbances of bowel habit and flatulence, are also accepted for operation. In considering elective resection in this latter type of case, it is important to bear in mind the quite good long-term results that may be expected from expectant management of many patients (see p. 899), and also the fact that after operation, though the immediate mortality may be quite low in good hands, a proportion of the patients—rated as high as 18·5% by Leigh et al. (1962), 30% by Bolt and Hughes (1966) and 48% by Charnock et al. (1977)—continue with mild symptoms similar to those often experienced by conservatively treated patients with diverticular disease. Needless to say, any case in which there is the slightest doubt as to the existence of a carcinoma should certainly proceed to laparotomy and resection. Other indications for elective operation are the development of recurrent abscesses or fistulas, the occurrence of a frank colovesical fistula or the complaint of severe urinary symptoms suggesting that this development is imminent, or the occurrence of repeated massive haemorrhages.

TECHNIQUE OF ELECTIVE RESECTION

Preliminary or Simultaneous Colostomy

As with resection of the distal colon for carcinoma, the question arises whether the main operation should be preceded by a proximal transverse colostomy or not. In some cases such a diversionary opening has already been established as part of the emergency treatment of a perforation, an acute obstruction or a fistula in connection with the diverticulitis. But in uncomplicated cases coming to elective operation the necessity for a preliminary colostomy is debatable. Hitherto most resections have been performed as second-stage operations but there has been a decided trend in recent years towards one-stage resection, and Judd and Mears (1955), Waugh and Walt (1957), Rodkey and Welch (1959), Waugh (1961) and Ponka and Shaalan (1964) have strongly recommended this plan, though Rodkey and Welch (1965) have expressed some reservations regarding the use of this technique.

My own practice is to avoid a preliminary colostomy as far as possible, and this applies even to cases with colovesical fistula. However, in any case treated by primary resection, in which there is reason to feel at all dissatisfied with the quality of the anastomosis, I have invariably established a concomitant transverse colostomy at the conclusion of the operation. The detailed techniques for making—and subsequently closing—a preliminary or simultaneous transverse colostomy are described on pp. 479–87. If a primary resection is planned, the preparation for operation is similar to that employed in carcinoma cases except that enemas and wash-outs should be used with caution or completely avoided.

The Actual Resection

This follows the general lines of an anterior resection for carcinoma of the rectosigmoid as described on p. 563, but certain points of difference in procedure arise. On opening the abdomen through the usual long left paramedian incision the sigmoid colon may be found adherent to small bowel, uterus, uterine appendages or front of rectum, or to the peritoneum on the top of the bladder, left iliac fossa or pelvic brim, and at first sight its removal may appear a very difficult proposition. Depending on the preoperative radiological evidence available, one of the first decisions that may have to be made is whether the lesion is to be regarded as a diverticulitis or a carcinoma. If there is a reasonably good chance on clinical grounds that the condition may be entirely diverticular, and if no unequivocal signs of malignant disease, such as metastases in liver or peritoneum, are found at laparotomy, I think the best plan so far as the adhesions to adjoining structures are concerned is to proceed in the first instance on the basis that the lesion is benign and to separate the colon from the adherent organs and tissues. In the process a pericolic abscess may be encountered—which perhaps strengthens, but does not establish beyond doubt, the belief that the condition is purely inflammatory—so that a sucker should be connected and ready for immediate use and a bacteriological swab should also be available. It is also a wise precaution to define both ureters, especially the left one, at an early stage of the dissection to avoid the risk of injury. (Preoperative intravenous pyelography is a sensible precaution in all cases of diverticulitis coming to operation.) When the adhesions have all been divided, and the sigmoid loop has been restored to its natural state of mobility, attention is directed to planning the resection.

As regards the *distal extent*, however complex the adhesions may have seemed initially, an agreeable finding after thorough mobilization is that the diverticular disease as a rule never extends from the sigmoid into the rectum, so that it is usually possible to preserve a supraperitoneal rectal stump below for anastomosis and to complete the operation as a *high* anterior resection, which has significant advantages (see p. 573). To make sure that no vestige of disease, and particularly no element of hypertrophied muscle coat, is allowed to remain distally I usually take the distal line of section through the rectum 12–25 mm below its upper end (see Fig. 625).

Proximally, though the diverticulosis may extend upwards into the descending, transverse or right colon, symptoms and complications of the disease seem to originate chiefly in its sigmoid section, so that most surgeons consider that more proximal diverticula unassociated with any obvious signs of inflammation can safely be left and the excision confined to the sigmoid loop. Leigh et al. (1962) investigated the adequacy of such a resection in 65 patients at the Mayo Clinic who had had an average length of 14·6 cm of colon excised 5–17 years previously for diverticular disease, and in whom it was specifically noted at operation that uninflamed diverticula were present in the remaining left colon. they found that 10·8% of these patients subsequently suffered symptoms suggestive but not definitely diagnostic of diverticulitis, while only 7·7% presented definite signs and symptoms indicating recurrence (but only 3·1% of these required further operation). Rodkey and Welch (1965), reporting on the Massachusetts General Hospital series of cases, state that of 418 patients treated by resection for diverticulitis between 1942 and 1964 nine cases are known to have developed recurrent diverticulitis, an incidence of 2·1%. The average length of sigmoid removed in this series has apparently increased from 13·6 cm in 1942 to 23·8 cm in 1964. My own practice has been to confine the resection to the sigmoid unless there is obvious gross inflammatory involvement in the descending or other parts of the colon or if the operation is being performed as an elective procedure in cases with recurrent massive haemorrhage and the diverticula are found to extend farther proximally. Under these circumstances I extend the resection upwards to include the left colon, the left end or middle third of the transverse colon being swung down into the pelvis for union with the rectal stump.

It has been suggested by Rodkey and Welch (1959) that in carrying out a resection for diverticular disease of the sigmoid it is not necessary to sacrifice the main inferior mesenteric and superior haemorrhoidal vessels, but instead the sigmoidal and left colic branches may be divided in the mesocolon close to the main trunks. Clearly this method is only legitimate when there is absolutely no doubt about the benign nature of the bowel lesion, but even then I cannot see any particular advantage in it over the method of taking the main vessels above and below as in a carcinoma case.

A most important point in the conduct of a resection for diverticulitis, when the slightest dubiety exists as to whether the condition may not be a carcinoma, is *to have the operative specimen opened up for macroscopic inspection before the anastomosis is undertaken.* The absence of an obvious malignant ulcer on the mucosal surface is satisfactory proof that the disease is not malignant, and the anastomosis may be commenced forthwith. If, however, a typical carcinomatous lesion is revealed, it will be necessary to review the operative field and decide whether any extension to the excision is required in the form of removal of previously adherent tissues by resection of a loop of small bowel, hysterectomy, partial cystectomy or diathermization of raw areas.

SIGMOID MYOTOMY

As pointed out on pp. 884–6, a striking abnormality evident in many specimens of sigmoid colon containing diverticular disease is hypertrophy and thickening of the muscle coats, and there is a fair amount of evidence to suggest that increased intracolonic tension resulting from spasm of the colon wall may be an important factor in the genesis of the diverticula. Impressed by these facts, Reilly (1964, 1966a, b, 1969) proposed a new operation for the treatment of sigmoid diverticulosis comparable to Ramstedt's pyloromyotomy for hypertrophic pyloric stenosis, and consisting of incising the circular muscle coat down to the mucosa in the mainly affected part of the sigmoid colon. The division is effected through a longitudinal incision in the line of one of the antimesenteric taeniae (Plate V), care being taken to prolong it on to apparently normal bowel above and below for 12–25 mm. The initial cut is made with a scalpel, any remaining strands of circular fibre being snipped with scissors till the mucosa bulges throughout the length of the incision. In the process of dividing these strands there is a real danger of snicking the mucosa. This happened in three of Reilly's (1969) 50 cases and in no less than 18 of Daniel's (1969a) 30 cases. Though the perforation may be closed by fine catgut sutures, subsequent peritonitis and faecal fistulation have been not uncommon—in four of Daniel's (1969a) 30 cases and in four or five of Smith et al.'s (1969) 29 cases. Daniel (1969a) was so impressed by the risk of damaging the mucosa, either by cutting it inadvertently or by diathermy coagulation in the course of haemostasis, that he found it preferable to carry out the myotomy with the colon distended by inflation per anum to reveal any minute perforations, and to complete the operation by applying a free graft of peritoneum to the myotomy wound. He believes that these precautions have been valuable in lessening the risk of colonic perforation and of resultant leakage and fistula formation.

In considering the outcome of sigmoid myotomy, particular interest attaches to the effect of the operation on the pressure activity of the colon. Attisha and Smith (1969) found that the exaggerated pressure noted by them in the colon in diverticular disease, especially in response to stimulation by prostigmine, was considerably reduced in cases after sigmoid myotomy. Daniel's (1969a) findings were similar, but he emphasized that the fall in bowel pressure only lasts for 18–24 months (Daniel 1969b). As regards clinical results, Reilly (1969) and Daniel (1969a), who between them have treated a total of 80 patients by sigmoid myotomy, had four operative deaths, none directly related to the myotomy itself, and 96% of the patients are said to be completely free of symptoms on a one to five year follow-up. Smith et al. (1969) reported major abdominal sepsis in the immediate postoperative period in three of 14 cases treated by sigmoid myotomy by them, with two operative deaths. The results on follow-up of the survivors for one to three years, however, were excellent, with complete relief of the pains in the left iliac region that were these patients' main complaint before operation. My own experience of sigmoid myotomy for diverticular disease is quite limited and comprises only nine cases. There were no technical difficulties or mucosal perforations at operation and no serious complications or immediate deaths afterwards. But, though all the patients were deemed to have the disease in a relatively early stage (but with some diverticula evident in all cases), three have continued to complain of the same sort of pains as they had before operation.

This is an interesting innovation in the therapy of diverticular disease. It must be admitted that myotomy would seem to be more logically indicated for the treatment of *early* diverticulosis, or of colon spasm without diverticula or with only incipient mucosal herniations (see Fig. 627), than for an established state of gross diverticulosis or diverticulitis. But the clinical distinction between spastic colon and psychoneurosis is so difficult and the two conditions are often so intermixed that any attempt to apply the operation to this group of patients seems likely to result in a certain number of unsuitable subjects being subjected to surgical treatment. As regards the more advanced cases of diverticular

disease it is, indeed, difficult to discern a clear rationale for the use of myotomy, for it presumably is not going to cause established diverticula to reduce themselves. It was originally argued by Reilly (1964) that it was a less severe operation than a colon resection, but it is clear from the published results that myotomy carries its own particular risks, and I doubt if there would be much difference in the operative morbidity and mortality of the two operations if applied to strictly comparable series of patients. Admittedly the relief of symptoms claimed for sigmoid myotomy by Reilly (1969), Daniel (1969a) and Smith et al. (1969) is greater than that achieved in several reported series of cases after resection (see p. 900); but it is very difficult to understand why this should be so, because a resection removes the entire segment of sigmoid whilst a myotomy merely incises it. However, comparisons of the results of operations in different centres are notoriously unreliable.

TRANSVERSE TAENIAMYOTOMY

Impressed by the shortening of the taeniae coli often found in diverticular disease, which is responsible as Keith (1910) pointed out for the shortening of the bowel in this condition, Hodgson (1974) suggested that a more logical form of sigmoid myotomy than a longitudinal division of the circular muscle fibres would be a transverse division of the taeniae. Theoretically this should allow the sigmoid colon to lengthen itself. As practised by Hodgson (1974) the operation consists in making a series of transverse cuts in the *two antimesenteric taeniae* at intervals of 2 cm, starting on the anterior rectal wall just above the anterior peritoneal reflection with a long transverse incision to divide the fused taeniae at that level and extending to just above the upper limit of the disease in the upper sigmoid or lower descending colon. The cuts do not divide any circular muscle and thus do not reach the submucous coat.

The great theoretical weakness of this technique is that it does nothing to the presumably equally shortened mesenteric taenia, and so it is hard to see how the ideal of allowing the colon to lengthen and lose much of its puckering can be achieved. At a practical level there is a dearth of clinical experience with the operation which prevents a proper attempt at assessing its usefulness in the management of patients. Hodgson (1974) himself has used transverse taeniamyotomy in 17 patients with diverticular disease, but unfortunately in five of them other conditions, such as carcinoma or polyp of the colon, were also present and in these five cases as well as in another three cases additional surgical procedures such as partial colectomy were performed at the time of the taeniamyotomy. Obviously this series provides a very unsatisfactory basis for trying to assess the value of this new surgical method. Until more clinical experience with the operation becomes available no worthwhile appraisal is possible.

TREATMENT OF COMPLICATIONS OF DIVERTICULAR DISEASE

ACUTE DIVERTICULITIS WITH PERITONITIS

There has been much recent writing in the literature on this subject (MacLaren 1957; Ryan 1958, 1964; Brown and Toomey 1960; Bevan 1961; Madden and Tan 1961; Beard and Gazet 1961; Staunton 1962; Hughes et al. 1963; Large 1964; Madden 1965; Dawson et al. 1965; Muir 1966; Roxburg et al. 1968), and a wide range of opinion has been expressed as to the correct management of acute diverticulitis. Thus, some authors have advocated an extremely conservative approach in most cases; others have favoured the frequent use of immediate radical surgery. The truth of the matter, however, is that several different clinical and morbid anatomical states seem to be included under this diagnosis, and that these probably carry different prognoses and require different forms of treatment.

Medical Treatment

In my experience and that of Ryan (1964) and Muir (1966), about half the patients with acute diverticulitis have relatively restricted physical signs and little constitutional disturbance, allowing a fairly confident diagnosis of acute diverticulitis with localized peritonitis. These patients, who are indeed often admitted primarily to the medical wards or sometimes treated by their general practitioners at home, are suitable for conservative management in the first instance. This consists essentially of bedrest, systemic broad-spectrum antibiotic therapy and close observation of the clinical course. Usually intravenous fluids are not necessary unless exceptionally there has been some nausea and vomiting. Under this regimen three terminations are possible:

1. In the majority of patients symptoms and signs gradually diminish over a period of a few days or a week or so.

2. In some cases, however, they persist and become slowly more marked, and, where there was previously doubt about the existence of a palpable mass in the left iliac or suprapubic region or in the pelvis, none now remains. The swelling gradually enlarges and this finding together with the occurrence of a persistent pyrexia will indicate that a pericolic abscess has developed. If conservative treatment is continued, the overlying skin in the left lower quadrant of the abdomen may become reddened and fluctuation may be elicited. At this stage, if not sooner, surgical drainage should be undertaken (see p. 905). The occurrence of urinary symptoms in a patient with symptoms and signs of acute diverticulitis with a possible developing abscess should always arouse suspicion that the collection of pus is about to rupture into the bladder with the production of a colovesical fistula. It is an indication for more urgent intervention to effect external drainage.

3. In a certain proportion of patients there is a more rapid and pronounced deterioration of the patient's general condition and an extension of the abdominal tenderness and guarding, indicating the development of a more diffuse peritonitis. In such cases laparotomy should be undertaken without further delay (see below).

Surgical Treatment

In many cases, however, urgent laparotomy is clearly indicated. These include patients admitted with features of severe diffuse peritonitis—often insufficiently localized to permit of a diagnosis of acute diverticulitis and calling for exploration in any event—and patients who were initially treated along expectant lines and whose condition has deteriorated. The first requirement is to correct fluid and electrolyte depletion, institute gastric suction and combat shock as necessary. Unfortunately a proportion of these patients—estimated at 15% by Dawson et al. (1965), 21%, by Muir (1966) and 22·8% by Bevan (1961)—are in such a state of severe collapse that they are unable to be sufficiently resuscitated to stand any form of surgery and rapidly succumb. These cases are frequently found at autopsy to have a faecal peritonitis (MacLaren 1957; Dawson et al. 1965).

The abdomen is opened by a vertical incision and, if it seems likely that the peritonitis has originated in the lower abdomen and that acute diverticulitis is a possible cause, a left paramedian approach is to be preferred. In some cases the site of leakage and peritoneal contamination is seen to be a hole in the sigmoid, which is the seat of diverticular disease, but in the majority of instances—for example in 50 of MacLaren's (1957) 75 cases and 55 of Dawson et al.'s (1965) 93 cases—an actual perforation cannot be demonstrated and it has to be inferred from the thickening of the colon and the concentration of the signs of peritonitis around it that the infection originated in this part of the alimentary tract. In some cases the cause of the diffuse peritonitis is rupture of a previously localized pericolic abscess, as stressed by Lockhart-Mummery (1930), Hughes et al. (1963), Ryan (1964), Large (1964) and Dawson et al. (1965). Occasionally there may be difficulty in deciding whether the lesion, in or proximal to which the perforation has arisen, is not a carcinoma. Thus, in a group of 18 patients treated by operation for what appeared at laparotomy to be perforated diverticulitis, the bowel condition was subsequently shown to be a carcinoma in five (Large 1964). The nature and the extent of the peritonitis varies, being frankly faeculent in some cases—actually in 19 of MacLaren's (1957) 75 cases and 11 of Dawson et al.'s (1965) 79 patients coming to laparotomy—and purulent in others. Faecal peritonitis is always associated with a gross perforation of the bowel, purulent peritonitis more usually not (Dawson et al. 1965).

Several surgical procedures are available for the treatment of acute diverticulitis with diffuse peritonitis: simple drainage of the site; attempted suture of the perforation or covering it over with appendices epiploicae or greater omentum, together with drainage; either of the preceding combined with a defunctioning transverse colostomy; exteriorization of the affected segment of colon; a Paul–Mikulicz or Hartmann type of resection; or a primary resection with anastomosis, with or without a temporary transverse colostomy. Till recently the most commonly used method has been to *drain the site and establish a right transverse colostomy* as near as possible to the hepatic flexure, it being hoped by this manoeuvre to rest the sigmoid colon and induce the inflammation to subside. However, the left colon beyond the colostomy at the time of operation often contains a fair amount of faeces, so that contamination may persist indefinitely. This may explain the disappointingly high mortality usually following the use of this procedure: given as 48% in 33 cases by MacLaren (1957), 24% in 21 cases by Hughes et al. (1963), 31% in 61 cases by Dawson et al. (1965) and 10%, in 20 cases by Muir (1966). Actually *simple drainage with or without attempted suture (if a perforation were present), but without proximal colostomy*, has in some series given no worse results. Thus, MacLaren (1957) reported 31 patients treated

in this way with a mortality of 32% and Hughes et al. (1963) 27 with a mortality of 11%. But it seems highly probable that in these various collective series of cases patients with less serious lesions were selected for treatment without colostomy.

In the last few years a number of surgeons have turned to more radical initial surgical treatment for acture diverticulitis with diffuse peritonitis with encouraging results. Staunton (1962) practised *exteriorization of the affected segment of bowel* as an iliac colostomy in five patients with no deaths. He pointed out that, despite initial appearances, the lesion can usually be readily mobilized for the performance of this procedure. Previously Shepherd (1960) had reported six cases treated by *Paul–Mikulicz resection* with only one death. He also has been impressed by the frequency with which the procedure is found to be technically feasible (Shepherd 1966). More daring has been the use of *primary resection with anastomosis* as reported by several authors. Ryan (1958) treated four cases in this way without fatality, Large (1964) 18 with two deaths, and Madden (1965) 25 also with only two deaths. Madden (1965) emphasizes, however, that there was a high postoperative morbidity rate with a high incidence of temporary faecal fistulation, and wound infection and dehiscence. None of these authors used a defunctioning proximal colostomy as a routine in conjunction with primary resection, but Madden (1965) did employ it in two cases with particularly low anastomoses. Another very encouraging report on the feasibility of using immediate resection in these cases has been that of Roxburgh et al. (1968), who employed this method in 24 consecutive cases (end-to-end anastomosis in eight, Mikulicz technique in eight and Hartmann's operation in eight) with only three deaths, all in patients with faecal peritonitis. Eng et al. (1977) describe 46 cases of diverticular disease with general peritonitis, abscess or fistula treated by primary resection, usually Hartmann's operation, with no deaths.

One of the problems in comparing the modern more radical surgical approach to acute diverticulitis with the more conservative type of operation used in the past is that cases treated at the present day enjoy the benefits of more efficient supporting antibiotic therapy than was available 10 or 20 years ago. This factor may exercise a considerable influence on the results of contemporary treatment. Whatever surgical technique is employed, it is certainly important to use systemic and local antibiotic therapy and peritoneal irrigation with noxythiolin, as indicated on p. 441. As regards the

the so-called *simple solitary ulcers of the caecum*, described by Cameron (1939), are usually examples of acute caecal diverticulitis; this opinion is also shared by Williams (1960) (see p. 862).

Miangolarra (1961) emphasized that *diverticulosis* of the right colon and caecum is a much commoner condition than has usually been imagined. In a series of 758 patients with confirmed colonic diverticulosis no less than 231 (30%) had diverticula in the right colon, and in 109 (14%) these were *not* associated with diverticulosis of the left colon. It is not made clear how many of these cases had solitary diverticula and how many had multiple diverticula of the caecum and ascending colon of the same acquired kind as are found in the left colon.

CLINICAL FEATURES

In the great majority of cases the presence of diverticula in the right colon is not attended by any symptoms and the condition passes entirely unrecognized or the diagnosis is a purely coincidental radiological one. In a very few patients, where the radiological changes of the diverticulosis have been gross and other conditions such as cholecystitis and subacute appendicitis have been excluded, the persistence of vague right-sided abdominal pain has led to a diagnosis of 'chronic diverticulitis' (Miangolarra 1961). But usually the only clinical manifestations of diverticula, single or multiple, of the caecum or ascending colon are due to the development of acute diverticulitis or haemorrhage.

Acute Diverticulitis
This was noted in 31 (13.4%) of Miangollarra's (1961) 231 patients with right-sided diverticulosis. In no case was it correctly diagnosed preoperatively, being invariably mistaken for acute appendicitis or cholecystitis. Similarly Anderson (1947) found that in a collective series of 99 cases of acute caecal diverticulitis a preoperative diagnosis of acute appendicitis was made in 84, and all of Laimon and Cohn's (1962) eight patients with caecal diverticulitis were thus erroneously diagnosed before operation. Rarely a palpable mass is present and has to be differentiated from masses produced by an appendix abscess, a carcinoma of the caecum, Crohn's disease, or other rarer conditions.

Haemorrhage
In the form of melaena, this was a prominent sign in 47% of the patients with diverticulosis limited to the right colon reported by Miangolarra (1961).

TREATMENT

Usually cases of caecal diverticulitis come to operation on a mistaken diagnosis of acute appendicitis, and even at laparotomy it may be difficult to make a precise diagnosis if there is much surrounding inflammation or a large mass. If an abscess is present it should be drained and that is probably all that is required in the first instance. If the inflammatory reaction in the caecal wall is fairly circumscribed a local excision extending to normal bowel wall all round should be performed followed by suture; or alternatively the diverticulum should be invaginated by inverting stitches. If a large mass is present suggestive of the presence of a carcinoma a right hemicolectomy will be required, as was necessary in nine of Miangolarra's (1961) 31 patients with acute diverticulitis and in two of Laimon and Cohn's (1962) eight cases with this complication.

If the case is less acute and presents with a mass in the right iliac region, radiological examination may suggest the correct diagnosis, and conservative treatment with antibiotics, parenteral fluids and nasogastric suction may be instituted. If a solitary diverticulum of the caecum is encountered incidentally in the course of another abdominal operation, it is best invaginated into the caecum with a purse-string suture.

In most cases with massive haemorrhage from right-sided diverticula the bleeding ceases on conservative treatment, but in no less than eight of the 51 patients with diverticulosis of the right colon associated with haemorrhage reported by Miangolarra (1961) emergency operation was required, and in five others elective operation was performed some time after cessation of the bleeding. Right hemicolectomy was the usual elective or emergency procedure; there were two operative deaths.

REFERENCES

AFIDI, R. J., ESSELSTYN, C. D. and TARAR, R. (1971) Recognition and angiosurgical detection of arteriovenous malformations of the bowel. *Ann. Surg., 174*, 573.
ALMY, T. P. (1965) Diverticular disease of the colon—the new look. *Gastroenterology, 49*, 109.

ALMY, T. P., ABBOT, F. K. and HINKLE, L. E. Jr. (1950) Alterations in colonic function in man under stress. IV. Hypomotility of the sigmoid colon, and its relationship to the mechanism of functional diarrhoea. *Gastroenterology, 15*, 95.

—— —— BERLE, B. and KERN, F., Jr. (1949a) Alterations in colonic functions in man under stress. III. Experimental production of sigmoid spasm in patients with spastic constipation. *Gastroenterology, 12*, 437.

—— KERN, F., Jr. and TULIN, M. (1949b) Alterations in colonic function in man under stress. II. Experimental production of sigmoid spasm in healthy persons. *Gastroenterology, 12*, 425.

ANDERSON, L. (1947) Acute diverticulitis of the caecum. *Surgery, St Louis, 22*, 479.

ANSCOMBE, A. R., KEDDIE, N. C. and SCHOFIELD, P. F. (1967) Solitary ulcers and diverticulitis of the caecum. *Br. J. Surg., 54*, 553.

ANTIA, F. P. and DESAI, H. G. (1974) Colonic diverticula and dietary fibre. *Lancet, 1*, 814.

ARCHAMPONG, E. Q., CHRISTIAN, F. and BADOE, E. A. (1978) Diverticular disease in an indigenous African community. *Ann. R. Coll. Surg. Edin., 60*, 464.

ARFWIDSSON, S. (1964) Pathogenesis of multiple diverticula of the sigmoid colon in diverticular disease. *Acta chir. scand.*, Suppl. *342*.

ATHANASOULIS, C. A., BAUM, S. and RÖSCH, J. (1975) Mesenteric arterial infusions of vasopressin for haemorrhage from colonic diverticulosis. *Am. J. Surg., 129*, 212.

ATTISHA, R. P. and SMITH, A. N. (1969) Pressure activity of the colon and rectum in diverticular disease before and after sigmoid myotomy, *Br. J. Surg., 56*, 891.

BARCLAY, A. E. (1933) *The Digestive Tract*, p. 281. London: Cambridge University Press.

BEARD, R. G. and GAZET, J.-C. (1961) Perforated diverticulitis of the colon with generalized peritonitis. *Guy's Hosp. Rep., 110*, 263.

BEVAN, P. G. (1961) Acute diverticulitis. A review of emergency admissions. *Br. med. J., 1*, 400.

BOLEY, S. J., SAMARTANO, R. and ADAMS, A. (1977) On the nature and etiology of vascular ectaseas of the colon. Degenerative lesions of aging. *Gastroenterology, 72*, 650.

BOLT, D. E. and HUGHES, L. E. (1966) Diverticulitis: a follow-up of 100 cases. *Br. med. J., 1*, 1205.

BRANT, B., RÖSCH, J. and KRIPPAEHNE, W. W. (1972) Experiences with angiography in diagnosis and treatment of acute gastro-intestinal bleeding of various etiologies. *Ann. Surg., 176*, 419.

BROWN, D. B. and TOOMEY, W. F. (1960) Diverticular disease of the colon. *Br. J. Surg., 47*, 485.

CAMERON, J. R. (1939) Simple or non-specific ulcer of caecum. *Br. J. Surg., 26*, 526.

CARLSON, A. J. and HOELZEL, F. (1949) Relation of diet to diverticulosis of the colon in rats. *Gastroenterology, 12*, 108.

CASE, J. T. (1914–15) The roentgen demonstration of multiple diverticula of the colon *Am. J. Roentg., 2*, 654.

—— (1929) The roentgen study of colonic diverticula. *Am. J. Roentg., 21*, 207.

CELIO, A. (1952) Zur Pathologie der chronischen stenosierenden Diverticulitis coli (sog. Diverticulitistumor). *Helv. chir. Acta, 19*, 93.

CHARNOCK, F. M. L., RENNIE, J. R., WELLWOOD, J. M. and TODD, I. P. (1977) Results of colectomy for diverticular disease of the colon. *Br. J. Surg., 64*, 417.

CHAUDHARY, N. A. and TRUELOVE, S. C. (1961) Human colonic motility: A comparative study of normal subjects, patients with ulcerative colitis, and patients with the irritable colon syndrome. III. Effects of emotions. *Gastroenterology, 40*, 27.

COLCOCK, B. P. and SASS, R. E. (1949) Diverticulitis and carcinoma of the colon: differential diagnosis. *Surgery Gynec. Obstet., 99*, 627.

CRIPPS, H. (1888) *The Passage of Air and Faeces from the Urethra*. London: Churchill.

CRUVEILHIER, J. (1849) *Traité d'Anatomie Pathologique*, vol. 1, p. 593. Paris: Baillière.

DANIEL, O. (1969a) Sigmoid myotomy with peritoneal graft. *Proc. R. Soc. Med., 62*, 39.

—— (1969b) Personal communication.

DAWSON, J. L., HANON, I. and ROXBURGH, R. A. (1965) Diverticulitis coli complicated by diffuse peritonitis. *Br. J. Surg., 52*, 354.

DE QUERVAIN, F. (1914) Zur Diagnose der erworbenen Dickdarmdivertikel und der Sigmoiditis diverticularis. *Dt. Z. Chir., 128*, 67.

DRAPANAS, T., PENNINGTON, D. G., KAPPELMAN, M. and LINDSEY, E. S. (1973) Emergency subtotal colectomy: preferred approach to management of massively bleeding diverticular disease. *Ann. Surg., 177*, 519.

DRUMMOND, H. (1917) Sacculi of the large intestine. *Br. J. Surg., 4*, 407.

DUNNING, M. W. F. (1963) The clinical features of haemorrhage from diverticular disease of the colon. *Surgery Gynec. Obstet., 108*, 49.

EASTWOOD, M. A., FISHER, N., GREENWOOD, C. T. and HUTCHINSON, J. B. (1974) Perspectives on the bran hypothesis. *Lancet, 1*, 1029.

EDWARDS, H. C. (1934) Diverticula of the colon and vermiform appendix. *Lancet, 1*, 221.

—— (1939) *Diverticula and Diverticulitis of the Intestine*. Bristol: John Wright.

EISENBERG, H., LAUFER, I. and SKILLMAN, J. J. (1973) Arteriographic diagnosis and management of suspected colonic diverticular hemorrhage. *Gastroenterology, 64*, 1091.

ENG, K., RANSON, J. H. C. and LOCALIO, S. A. (1977) Resection of the perforated segment: a significant advance in treatment of diverticulitis with free perforation or abscess. *Am. J. Surg., 133*, 67.

FAIRBANK, T. J. and ROB, C. G. (1947) Solitary diverticulitis of caecum and ascending colon. *Br. J. Surg., 26*, 526.

FOSTER, R. L. and FISHER, R. F. (1954) Colostomy as emergency treatment for massive melena secondary to diverticulitis: case report. *Am. Surg., 20*, 734.

FRAENKEL, G. L. (1954) rectal bleeding and diverticulitis. *Br. J. Surg., 41*, 643.

GOLDBERGER, E. and BOOKSTEIN, J. J. (1977) Transcatheter embolization for the treatment of diverticular haemorrhage. *Radiology, 122*, 613.

GRASER, E. (1899) Über multiple falsche Darmdivertikel in der Flexura sigmoidea. *Münch. med. Wschr., 46*, 74.

GROUT, J. L. (1949) Diverticulosis and diverticulitis of the large intestine. *Br. J. Radiol., 22*, 442.

HABERSHON, S. O. (1857) *On Diseases of the Alimentary Canal*, p. 296. London: Churchill.

HENDERSON, N. P. (1944) Diverticulitis and diverticulosis. *Br. J. Radiol., 17*, 197.

HOAR, C. S. and BERNARD, W. F. (1954) Colonic bleeding and diverticular disease of the colon. *Surgery Gynec. Obstet., 99*, 101.

HODGSON, J. (1974) Transverse taenia myotomy: a new surgical approach for diverticular disease. *Ann. R. Coll. Surg. Engl., 55*, 80.

HODGSON, W. J. B. (1972) An interim report on the production of colonic diverticula in the rabbit. *Gut, 13*, 802.

HUGHES, E. S. R. (1965) Diverticulitis with vesico-colitis fistula. *Aust. N. Z. J. Surg., 34*, 188.

—— CUTHBERTSON, A. M. and CARDEN, A. B. G. (1963) The surgical management of acute diverticulitis. *Med. J. Aust., 1*, 780.

HUGHES, L. E. (1969) Postmortem survey of diverticular disease of the colon. *Gut, 10*, 336.

—— (1970*a*) A study of abnormal muscular patterns in diverticular disease of the colon using the polysiloxane foam enema. *Gut, 11*, 111.

—— (1970*b*) Diverticular disease of colon. *Br. med. J., 1*, 496.

JUDD, E. S. and MEARS, T. W. (1955) Diverticulitis. Progress toward wider application of single stage resection. *Archs Surg., Chicago, 70*, 818.

—— and POLLOCK, L. W. (1924) Diverticulitis of the colon. *Ann. Surg., 80*, 425.

KEITH, Sir A. (1910) Diverticula of the alimentary tract of congenital or of obscure origin. *Br. med. J., 1*, 376.

KNIGHT, C. D. (1957) Massive haemorrhage from diverticular disease of the colon. *Surgery, St Louis, 42*, 853.

KUNATH, C. A. (1956) Massive bleeding from diverticulosis of the colon. *Am. J. Surg., 91*, 911.

KYLE, J. (1968) Prognosis in diverticulitis. *J. R. Coll. Surg. Edinb., 13*, 136.

LAIMON, H. and COHN, P. (1962) Diverticulitis of the cecum: A report of eight cases. *Am. J. Surg., 103*, 146.

LARGE, J. M. (1964) Treatment of perforated diverticulitis. *Lancet, 1*, 413.

LAURIDSEN, J. and ROSS, F. P. (1952) Acute diverticulitis of the caecum. *Archs Surg., Chicago, 64*, 320.

LEIGH, J. E., JUDD, E. S. and WAUGH, J. M. (1962) Diverticulitis of the colon. Recurrence after apparently adequate segmental resection. *Am. J. Surg., 103*, 51.

LETT, Sir H. (1932) In Discussion of urinary complications of diseases of large intestine. *Proc. R. Soc. Med., 25*, 1811.

LEWIS, E. E. and SNAG, G. E. (1972) Importance of angiography in the management of haemorrhage from colonic diverticula. *Am. J. Surg., 124*, 573.

LLOYD-DAVIES, O. V. (1953) Diverticulitis. *Proc. R. Soc. Med., 46*, 407.

LOCKHART-MUMMERY, H. E. (1958) Vesico-intestinal fistula. *Proc. R. Soc. Med., 51*, 1032.

LOCKHART-MUMMERY, J. P. (1923) *Diseases of the Rectum and Colon and Their Surgical Treatment*, p. 448. London: Baillière, Tindall and Cox.

—— (1930) The aetiology of diverticulitis. *Lancet, 1*,231.

—— and HODGSON, H. G. (1931) Diverticula of the colon and their sequelae. *Br. med. J., 1*, 525.

McGREGOR, A. B., ABERNETHY, B. C. and THOMSON, J. W. W. (1970) The role of surgery in diverticular disease of the colon. *J. R. Coll. Surg. Edinb., 15*, 137.

McGUIRE, H. H. and HAYNES, B. W. (1972) Massive bleeding from diverticulosis of the colon: guidelines for therapy based on bleeding patterns observed in fifty cases. *Ann. Surg., 175*, 847.

MacLAREN, I. F. (1957) Perforated diverticulitis. A survey of 75 cases. *J. R. Coll. Surg. Edinb., 3*, 129.

MADDEN, J. L. (1965) Primary resection and anastomosis in the treatment of perforated lesions of the colon. *Am. Surg., 31*, 781.

—— and TAN, P. Y. (1961) Primary resection and anastomosis in the treatment of perforated lesions of the colon, with abscess or diffusing peritonitis. *Surgery Gynec. Obstet., 113*, 646.

MAILER, R. (1928) Observations on diverticula of the colon: a pathological and clinical study. *Lancet, 2*, 51.

MARCUS, R. and WATT, J. (1964) The 'pre-diverticular state'. Its relationship to diverticula in the anti-mesenteric intertaenia area of the pelvic colon. *Br. J. Surg., 51*, 676.

—— —— (1965) The radiological appearances of diverticula in the antimesenteric intertaenia areas of the pelvic colon. *Clin. Radiol., 16*, 87.

MAXWELL-TELLING, W. H. and GRUNER, O. C. (1916–17) Acquired diverticula, diverticulitis and peridiverticulitis of the large intestine. *Br. J. Surg., 4*, 468.

MAYNARD, E. P., III and VOORHEES, A. B., Jr. (1956) Arterial hemorrhage from a large bowel diverticulum. *Gastroenterology, 31*, 210.

MAYO, C. W. and BLUNT, C. P. (1950) Vesicosigmoidal fistulas complicating diverticulitis. *Surgery Gynec. Obstet., 91*, 612.

MIANGOLARRA, C. J. (1961) Diverticulitis of the right colon: an important surgical problem. *Ann. Surg., 153*, 861.

MING, SI-CHUN and FLEISCHNER, F. G. (1965) Diverticulitis of the sigmoid colon: reappraisal of the pathology and pathogenesis. *Surgery, St Louis, 58*, 627.

MORSON, B. C. (1963) The muscle abnormality in diverticular disease of the sigmoid colon. *Br. J. Radiol., 36*, 385.

MORTON, D. L. and GOLDMAN, L. (1962) Differential diagnosis of diverticulitis and carcinoma of the sigmoid colon. *Am. J. Surg., 103*, 55.

MORTON, J. J., Jr. (1946) Diverticulitis of the colon. *Ann. Surg., 124*, 725.

MOYNIHAN, B. G. A. (1907) The mimicry of malignant disease in the large intestine. *Edinb. med. J., 21*, 228.

—— (1927) Diverticula of the alimentary canal. *Lancet, 1*, 1061.

MUIR, E. G. (1966) Diverticulitis. *Lancet, 1*, 195.

NOER, R. J. (1955) Haemorrhage as a complication of diverticulitis. *Ann. Surg., 141*, 674.

—— HAMILTON, J. E., WILLIAMS, D. J. and BROUGHTON, D. S. (1962) Rectal haemorrhage: moderate and severe. *Ann. Surg., 155*, 794.

NUSBAUM, M., BAUM, S. and BLAKEMORE, W. S. (1969) Clinical experience with the diagnosis and management of gastrointestinal hemorrhage by selective mesenteric cathererization. *Ann. Surg., 170*, 506.

—— —— —— and TUMEN, H. (1972) Clinical experience with selective intraarterial infusion of vasopressin in the control of gastrointestinal bleeding from arterial sources. *Am. J. Surg., 123*, 165.

PAINTER, N. S. (1964) The aetiology of diverticulosis of the colon with special reference to the action of certain drugs on the behaviour of the colon. *Ann. R. Coll. Surg. Engl., 34*, 98.

—— ALMEIDA, A. Z. and COLEBOURNE, K. W. (1972) Unprocessed bran in the treatment of diverticular disease of the colon. *Br. med. J., 1*, 137.

—— and BURKITT, D. P. (1971) Diverticular disease of the colon: a deficiency disease of Western civilization. *Br. med. J., 2*, 450.

—— and TRUELOVE, S. C. (1964) The intraluminal pressure patterns in diverticulosis of the colon. *Gut, 5*, 201, 365.

—— —— ARDRAN, G. M. and TUCKEY, M. (1965) Effect of morphine, prostigmine, pethidine, and probanthine on the human colon in diverticulosis studies by intraluminal pressure recording and cineradiography. *Gut, 6*, 57.

PARKS, T. G. (1968) Post-mortem studies on the colon with special reference to diverticular disease. *Proc. R. Soc. Med., 61*, 932.

—— (1969) Natural history of diverticular disease of the colon. A review of 521 cases. *Br. med. J., 4*, 639.

—— and CONNELL, A. M. (1969) Motility studies in diverticular disease of the colon. Part I. Basal activity and response to food assessed by open-ended tube and miniature balloon techniques. *Gut, 10*, 534.

PEELING, W. B. and AUBREY, D. A. (1969) Diverticulum of caecum. *Br. J. Surg., 56*, 145.

PEMBERTON, J. DE J., BLACK, B. M. and MAINO, C. R. (1947) Progress in the surgical management of diverticulitis of the sigmoid colon. *Surgery Gynec. Obstet., 85*, 523.

PONKA, J. L., FOX, J. DE W. and BRUSH, B. E. (1959) Co-existing carcinoma and diverticula of the colon. *Archs Surg., Chicago, 79*, 373.

—— and SHAALAN, K. (1964) Changing aspects of diverticulitis. *Archs Surg., Chicago, 89*, 31.

PUGH, J. I. (1964) On the pathology and behaviour of acquired non-traumatic vesico-intestinal fistula. *Br. J. Surg., 51*, 644.

QUINN, W. C. (1961) Gross haemorrhage from presumed diverticular disease of the colon: results of treatment in 103 patients. *Ann. Surg., 153*, 851.

RANKIN, F. W. and BROWN, P. W. (1930) Diverticulitis of the colon. *Surgery Gynec. Obstet., 50*, 836.

—— and GRIMES, A. E. (1938) The surgical treatment of diverticulitis. *Sth. Surg., 7*, 1.

REILLY, M. (1964) Sigmoid myotomy. *Proc. R. Soc. Med., 57*, 556.

—— (1966a) In correspondence. *Lancet, 1*, 261.

—— (1966b) Sigmoid myotomy. *Br. J. Surg., 53*, 859.

—— (1969) Sigmoid myotomy—interim report. *Proc. R. Soc. Med., 62*, 715.

RIGG, B. M. and EWING, M. R. (1966) Current attitudes on diverticulitis with particular reference to colonic bleeding. *Archs Surg., Chicago, 92*, 321.

RIVES, J. D. (1955) Discussion of Noer (1955).

—— and EMMETT, R. O. (1954) Melena: survey of 206 cases. *Am. Surg., 20*, 458.

RODKEY, G. V. and WELCH, C. E. (1959) Diverticulitis and diverticulosis of the colon. In *Diseases of the Colon and Anorectum*, ed. R. Turrell, vol. 2. Philadelphia and London: W. B. Saunders.

—— —— (1965) Diverticulitis of the colon: evolution in concept and therapy. *Surg. Clins N. Am., 45*, 1231.

RÖSCH, J., DOTTER, C. T. and ROSE, R. W. (1971) Selective arterial infusions of vasocontrictors in acute gastrointestinal bleeding. *Radiology, 99*, 27.

—— GRAY, R. K., GROLLMAN, J. H., Jr., ROSS, G., STECKEL, R. J. and WEINTER, M. (1970) Selective arterial drug infusions in the treatment of acute gastrointestinal bleeding. *Gastroenterology, 59*, 341.

ROSENBERG, I. K. and ROSENBERG, B. F. (1964) Massive haemorrhage from diverticula of the colon, with demonstration of the source of bleeding. *Ann. Surg., 159*, 570.

ROSSER, C. (1955) Discussion of Noer (1955).

ROXBURGH, R. A., DAWSON, J. L. and YEO, R. (1968) Emergency resection in treatment of diverticular disease of colon complicated by peritonitis. *Br. med. J., 3*, 465.

RUSHFORD, A. J. (1956) The significance of bleeding as a symptom in diverticulitis. *Proc. R. Soc. Med., 49*, 577.

RYAN, P. (1958) Emergency resection and anastomosis for perforated sigmoid diverticulitis. *Br. J. Surg., 45*, 611.

—— (1964) Acute diverticulitis and diverticulitis with perforation. *Med. J. Aust., 2*, 51.

SALGADO, I., WLODEK, G. K., MATHEWS, W. H. and ROBERTSON, H. R. (1961) Massive haemorrhage due to diverticular disease of the colon: a case illustrating the bleeding point. *Can. J. Surg., 4*, 473.

SCARBOROUGH, R. A. (1958) The significance of rectal bleeding in diverticulosis and diverticulitis of the colon. *Dis. Colon Rect., 1*, 49.

—— and KLEIN, R. R. (1948) Polypoid lesions of the colon and rectum. *Am. J. Surg., 76*, 723.

SCHATZKI, R. (1940) The roentgenologic differential diagnosis between carcinoma and diverticulitis of the colon. *Radiology, 34*, 651.

SCHINZ, H. R., BAENSCH, W. E., FRIEDL, E. and UEHLINGER, E. (1954) *Roentgen-Diagnostics*, trans. J. T. Case, vol. 4, p. 3561. New York: Grune and Stratton.

SEGAL, I., SOLOMON, A. and HUNT, J. A. (1977) Emergence of diverticular disease in the urban Soth African blacks. *Gastroenterology, 72,*, 215.

SHANKS, S. C., KERLEY, P. and TWINING, E. W. (1958) *A Textbook of X-ray Diagnosis*, 3rd. ed., vol. 3, p. 429. London: H. K. Lewis.

SHEPHERD, J. A. (1960) *Surgery of the Acute Abdomen*. Edinburgh: Livingstone.

—— (1966) Personal communication.

SLACK, W. W. (1962) The anatomy, pathology and some clinical features of diverticulitis of the colon, *Br. J. Surg., 50*, 185.

SMITH, A. N., ATTISHA, R. P. and BALFOUR, T. (1969) Clinical and manometric results one year after sigmoid myotomy for diverticular disease. *Br. J. Surg., 56*, 895.

SMITH, N. D. (1951) Diverticulosis and diverticulitis: General consideration and sigmoidoscopic diagnosis. *Am. J. Surg., 82*, 583.

SMITHWICK, R. H. (1942) Experiences with the surgical management of diverticulitis of the sigmoid. *Ann. Surg., 115*, 969.

SPRIGGS, E. I. and MARXER, O. A. (1925) Intestinal diverticula. *Q. Jl Med., 19*, 1.

—— —— (1927) Multiple diverticula of the colon. *Lancet, 1*, 1067.

—— —— (1937) *The British Encyclopaedia of Medical Practice*, vol. 4, p. 207. London: Butterworth

STAUNTON, M. D. M. (1962) Treatment of perforated diverticulitis coli. *Br. med. J., 1*, 916.

STONE, H. B. (1944) Large melena of obscure origin. *Ann. Surg., 120*, 582.

TAGART, R. E. B. (1953) Acute phlegmonous caecitis. *Br. J. Surg., 40*, 437.

TAYLOR, I. and DUTHIE, H. L. (1976) Bran tablets and diverticular disease. *Br. med. J., 1*, 988.

TODD, I. P. (1955) The role of elective surgery in diverticulitis of the colon. *Ann. R. Coll. Surg. Engl., 16*, 118.

TRUELOVE, S. C. and REYNELL, P. C. (1963) *Diseases of the Digestive System*. Oxford: Blackwell Scientific.

WAGNER, D. E. and ZOLLINGER, R. W. (1961) Diverticulitis of the cecum and ascending colon. *Archs Surg., Chicago, 83*, 436.

WAUGH, J. M. (1961) Surgical management of diverticulitis of the colon. *Proc. Mayo Clin., 36*, 489.

—— and WALT, A. J. (1957) An appraisal of one stage anterior resection in diverticultis of the sigmoid colon. *Surgery Gynec. Obstet., 104*, 690.

WEINGARTEN, M., VENET, L. and VICTOR, M. B. (1959) Direct observations of massive arterial hemorrhage from a diverticulum of the hepatic flexure. *Gastroenterology, 36*, 642.

WELCH, C. E., ALLEN, A. W. and DONALDSON, G. A. (1953) An appraisal of resection of the colon for diverticulitis of the sigmoid. *Ann. Surg., 138*, 332.

WHITEHOUSE, G. H. (1973) Solitary angiodysplastic lesions in the ileocaecal region diagnosed by angiography. *Gut, 14*, 977.

WILLARD, J. H. and BOCHUS, H. L. (1936) Clinical and therapeutic status of colonic diverticulosis seen in office practice. *Am. J. digest. Dis., 3*, 580.

WILLIAMS, I. (1963) Changing emphasis in diverticular disease of the colon. *Br. J. Radiol., 36*, 393.

WILLIAMS, K. L. (1960) Acute solitary ulcers and acute diverticulitis of the caecum and ascending colon. *Br. J. Surg., 47*, 351.

WILLIAMS, R. J. (1954) Vesico-intestinal fistula. *Br. J. Surg., 42*, 179.

YOUNG, E. L. and YOUNG, E. L., III (1944) Diverticulitis of the colon. A review of the literature and an analysis of 91 cases. *New Engl. J. Med., 230*, 33.

25

Stricture of the Rectum

AETIOLOGY

By far the commonest cause of a rectal stricture is carcinoma, but as ordinarily used the term is taken to mean a non-malignant stricture. In the past many strictures were thought to carry a venereal taint and to be due to syphilis or gonorrhoea, but it was usually impossible to substantiate this impression on a bacteriological basis. Then in 1936, as explained on p. 868, Bensaude and Lambling clarified the situation by showing with the aid of the Frei test that these strictures were due to lymphogranuloma venereum. It is now extremely doubtful whether such a thing as a gummatous stricture of the rectum exists, and a gonorrhoeal stricture is probably very rare.

Actually stricture of the rectum in contemporary clinical practice in this country is hardly ever due to lymphogranuloma. Usually it is a sequel to a non-specific proctitis or proctocolitis, to a previous operation or to irradiation (Table 77).

DIAGNOSIS

This history or other salient clinical features may strongly suggest the cause of the stricture. Thus in a young child it is probably congenital. If there has been a previous operation on the rectum or anus or radium treatment to the uterine cervix, it has to be considered whether the stricture could be attributable to it. Most *strictures of the anal region* can be satisfactorily explained on the basis of spasm and fibrosis due to an anal fissure or addiction to liquid paraffin, or to scarring following previous anal operations. The difficult cases are those with a

TABLE 77. *Causes of Stricture of the Rectum and Anus*

Congenital	Congenital deformities of the anorectum
Spasmodic	Tight spasm of the anus may occur with a chronic anal fissure. In the long run a *fibrous stenosis of the internal sphincter* may develop. A similar anal stenosis may be found in patients who habitually take paraffin or saline purgatives
Inflammatory	Non-specific ulcerative or granular proctitis or proctocolitis Crohn's disease of the rectum Rarely other forms of proctitis, for example, gonorrhoea, lymphogranuloma, dysentery or bilharzial infections
Traumatic	PREVIOUS OPERATIONS *Anal operations* for fistula, fissure, haemorrhoids or anal warts may rarely be followed by stricture of anus. Whitehead's operation was notorious in this respect. Injections for haemorrhoids may rarely produce a stricture. Operations for imperforate anus or rectum may be complicated by stenosis *Sphincter-saving resections of the rectum* especially abdominoanal excisions, less commonly anterior resections; rectosigmoidectomy for prolapse *Ligature and excision of benign tumours of the rectum* may be followed by stricture *Diathermy treatment for benign tumours of the rectum* is an important cause of stricture, especially in cases of familial polyposis ACCIDENTAL INJURIES Gunshot wounds of the rectum, and rectal injuries by enema syringes may be followed by stricture IRRADIATION Radium treatment for carcinoma of the cervix uteri may cause a severe stricture through the medium of an irradiation proctitis. Radium implantation for carcinoma of the anus was frequently followed by stricturing.

spontaneously occurring *stricture of the rectum proper*. Here the diagnosis usually lies between the following:

1. Rectal carcinoma with much extrarectal spread inferiorly so that its lower end presents to the examining finger or sigmoidoscope as a stricture with an intact mucosal covering.
2. Stricture in association with ulcerative colitis or other form of proctitis or colitis—which may be 'fibrous' or carcinomatous.
3. Stricture due to rectal lymphogranuloma.
4. Irradiation proctitis and stricture.
5. Rarely carcinoma of the prostate encircling the rectum, as described by Jackman and Anderson (1952).

Sigmoidoscopy will be helpful in showing if the rectal mucosa below or covering the stricture is normal or displays the characteristic changes of proctocolitis. In rectal lymphogranuloma the mucosa may be normal or may show similar changes, often with coarse granularity. With the sigmoidoscope a careful search is made for any sign of ulceration within the stricture itself, and a biopsy is taken of any ulcerated area, several snippets being obtained. Even if no ulcer is present a biopsy should still be taken of the overlying mucosa and as much of the tissue of the stricture itself underneath it as possible. To do so, considerable force must be used and a general anaesthetic is usually necessary. Unless the findings on the rectal and sigmoidoscopic examination strongly suggest that the condition is one of rectal carcinoma or ordinary ulcerative colitis or proctitis, it is wise to have a Frei test or complement fixation test done to exclude lymphogranuloma. In cases of suspected carcinoma of the prostate, urological examination—including transperineal biopsy, X-ray examination of the spine and pelvis, and estimation of the serum phosphate levels—is indicated, and the effect of stilboestrol therapy is sometimes instructive.

TREATMENT

The treatment of the various forms of stricture is described in detail in the appropriate sections of this book and will not be further discussed in this chapter.

REFERENCES

BENSAUDE, R. and LAMBLING, A. (1936) Discussion on the aetiology and treatment of fibrous stricture of the rectum (including lymphogranuloma inguinale). *Proc. R. Soc. Med., 24*, 1441.

JACKMAN, R. J. and ANDERSON, J. R. (1952) Proctologic manifestations of carcinoma of the prostate. *Am. J. Surg., 83*, 491.

26

Injuries of the Rectum and Colon

RECTAL INJURIES

Injuries from Particles in the Faeces

The possibility of laceration of the anorectal mucosa by sharp particles in the faeces has already been referred to on p. 154. Fish bones, rabbit bones and fragments of egg shell, enamel or glass are the principal offenders, but rarely gall-stone or other form of enterolith in the intestinal tract may make its way to the rectum. In psychiatric patients a bizarre selection of foreign bodies—needles, nails, screws, hairpins, etc.—may be swallowed and may eventually reach the rectum. They may lodge there or they may be passed, causing trauma to the anal canal in the process. Swallowed toothpicks may also cause perforation or laceration of the small or large intestine (Schwartz and Graham 1977). Needless to say the passage of a large hard faecal mass alone without any particular foreign body in it may provoke injury to the anal canal, especially in individuals who from addiction to liquid paraffin or saline purgatives have been accustomed for many years to passing only soft stools.

The initial effect of such an injury may be to produce severe pain due to impaction of the foreign body in the wall of the anal canal, usually in one of the anal crypts. This may lead the patient to seek immediate medical advice. The complaint is apt to be dismissed as due to an acute anal fissure, but if a careful rectal examination is carried out the foreign particle may be felt or seen on proctoscopy and removed. A short general anaesthetic or an inferior haemorrhoidal nerve block may be necessary to do justice to this examination.

Alternatively the initial discomfort may subside spontaneously, especially if the fragment causing the injury is passed. The laceration may heal spontaneously or may be followed by the development of a submucous, perianal, or ischiorectal abscess (see p. 154).

Injuries From Foreign Bodies Introduced per Anum

Foreign bodies may rarely be introduced into the rectum through the anus, and the literature contains records of a most remarkable series of objects that have thus found their way into the bowel (see particularly Tuttle 1903; Lockhart-Mummery 1934). These include bottles of different sizes and shapes, electric light bulbs, door handles, various forms of fruit, and candles and other phallic-like objects. In some instances apparently the foreign bodies have slipped accidentally into the rectum whilst being used to control a rectal prolapse or prolapsing haemorrhoids, but more commonly they have been inserted deliberately as an erotic manoeuvre or during a drunken orgy. Rarely they have been forced by sadists into the rectum of their victims. The most recently described bizarre object to be introduced into the rectum is the human fist in what Sohn et al. (1977) term 'fist fornication'. They encountered a number of rectal lacerations (and also perforation of the sigmoid) due to this practice. The dramatic features associated with many of the reported cases have secured a prominence for this condition in standard tests quite out of proportion to its frequency. Actually foreign bodies in the rectum are excessively rare, and more common than the sensational items that have been listed above are objects such as clinical thermometers and rubber enema tips which have accidentally sliped into the rectum during nursing attentions.

Such foreign bodies, if irregular and sharp, may cause laceration or perforation of the anorectal wall during introduction but once in position in the rectum are often surprisingly well tolerated. Injury is more likely to occur indeed during unskilful attempts at removal. Depending on the size and nature of the body it may be possible to withdraw it endoscopically or digitally through the anal canal under a general anaesthetic, but large globular objects will probably have to be extracted from above by laparotomy and incision of the anterior wall of the rectum in its intraperitoneal part.

Injuries During Parturition

One of the commonest causes of injury to the anorectum is tearing of the perineum during parturition. It is not proposed to discuss this common obstetrical complication further, except to say that, if the injury is subjected to immediate repair with accurate suture of the sphincters and puborectales as well as the anorectal and vaginal mucosae, healing *per primam* is often obtained. If this is not done or if sepsis complicates repair and union *per primam* fails, the resulting defect of the sphincter mechanism will probably lead to incontinence.

Episiotomy is often practised to avoid tearing of the perineum into the rectum during parturition; if inexpertly done, however, this operation may occasionally injure the bowel.

Surgical Injuries

GYNAECOLOGICAL OPERATIONS

The rectum is exposed to the risk of injury on its anterior aspect during the operations of posterior colporrhaphy and perineorrhaphy from below, or of Wertheim's hysterectomy from above. Such an injury may be detected at the time and suitably repaired by an inverting suture, possibly supplemented by a proximal colostomy. If overlooked by the gynaecologist, its presence will become apparent later from the development of wound infection or pelvic peritonitis. At this stage the

correct procedure will be to re-operate. In the case of an intraperitoneal injury the abdomen will require to be reopened, the site of the injury being repaired or drained, and a proximal colostomy established, preferably in the transverse colon. With an extraperitoneal laceration the perineal wound will be opened and a proximal colostomy provided.

Another gynaecological manoeuvre that may lead to a more gradual form of rectal injury is the intravaginal application of radium to carcinoma of the cervix uteri (see p. 871).

UROLOGICAL OPERATIONS

Similarly, in the male, the rectum on its anterior aspect is exposed to hazard during a number of operations on the urethra, prostate and bladder. During *instrumentation of the urethra* a false passage may be created and may implicate the anal canal or rectum. Injury to the front of the rectum is one of the recognized dangers of *perineal prostatectomy* or *open operations on the male urethra*. Even during *suprapubic or retropubic prostatectomy or total cystoprostatectomy* a faulty plane may be struck posteriorly with resulting laceration of the anterior rectal wall, or the latter may be damaged by deep diathermy coagulation employed to control bleeding. If these complications are detected at the time of operation they should be treated by immediate repair supplemented by a transverse colostomy. Even with a proximal colostomy a temporary communication may take place between the rectum and the urinary tract. For treatment of an established rectoprostatic fistula after prostatectomy see p. 193.

ANORECTAL PROCEDURES

Apart from the deliberate trauma of operations on the anus and rectum, unintentional injury may occur during a number of surgical or nursing procedures.

SIGMOIDOSCOPIC INJURIES

The rectum or sigmoid colon may be perforated during sigmoidoscopy, but considering the great frequency with which this examination is performed, such injuries are exceedingly rare. In many thousands of sigmoidoscopies performed by me only once has the bowel been perforated. However, a collective enquiry concerning 94 cases of sigmoidoscopic perforations has been published by

Andreson (1974). The injury may occur when the bowel wall has been weakened by disease such as colitis or dysentery, but most perforations have taken place in patients whose rectum and colon is normal. The usual site of injury is the front wall at or just below the rectosigmoid flexure due to difficulty in negotiating this bend. In most instances the perforation is immediately recognized because the end of the sigmoidoscope enters the peritoneal cavity through it and the examiner is suddenly confronted by the serosal aspect of the small intestine and possibly of the colon with its appendices epiploicae and tortuous intramural vessels. The patient may or may not experience instant abdominal pain at this occurrence. For example in my single case of perforation no discomfort was felt at first and it was for that reason difficult to induce the patient to submit to operation. The correct management is immediate laparotomy. Any free blood or intestinal contents are aspirated out of the pelvis and the rent exposed and closed by two rows of inverting stitches. A proximal iliac or transverse colostomy has frequently been established at the conclusion of the operation to relieve tension on the suture line, but it is doubtful whether this is really necessary. A corrugated rubber drain should be laid down to the site of injury.

In some instances the perforation is overlooked at the time of the sigmoidoscopy; the examination is then followed in due course by the development of symptoms and signs of pelvic peritonitis. These will eventually demand the exploration of the abdomen, but the inevitable delay may have a very adverse effect on the prognosis.

INJURY DURING DILATATION OF A HIGH RECTAL STRICTURE

As pointed out on p. 606, splitting of the rectum into the peritoneal cavity is one of the hazards of dilatation of a high rectal stricture such as sometimes forms after anterior resection.

PERFORATION FROM RECTAL BIOPSY OR FROM DIATHERMY DESTRUCTION OR LOCAL EXCISION OF A BENIGN RECTAL TUMOUR

The possibility of perforation of the rectal or colonic wall during treatment of benign tumours of the intraperitoneal part of the bowel by the diathermy electrode or snare or other forms of local excision has already been referred to on p. 343. Injury may also occur during a simple rectal biopsy of a sessile tumour or of an area of ulceration that has thinned the rectal wall, as pointed out by Thorbjarnarson (1962).

INJURY BY ENEMA NOZZLES, AND CLINICAL THERMOMETERS

Injuries of the rectum, anus or perianal region may be *produced by hard enema nozzles* of bone, vulcanite or glass as in the cases reported by King (1930), Rayner (1932), Pinnock (1937), Galbraith (1937), Murray (1937), Gabriel (1948) and Large and Mukheiber (1956). There seems to be a special predisposition to these accidents in obstetrical patients who have undergone the repair of perineal tears during childbirth. The injury is caused by the unskilful or clumsy introduction of the nozzle, by a sudden movement on the part of the patient, by bad lighting or by the presence of skin tags or prolapsed piles which obscure the actual anus. The result is that the nozzle may be thrust not into the anal canal but into the perianal tissues lateral or anterior to the anus, or if correctly introduced into the canal, is passed too far and too forcibly, impinging on and perforating the lower part of the anterior rectal wall. The introduction of the soapy enema fluid, which is irritating, increases the damage, especially if considerable pressure is used as with a Higginson syringe, and the result is usually a perianal or pelvic cellulitis, often with a variable amount of sloughing of the rectal wall.

These injuries can be prevented by avoiding any form of hard enema nozzle. The safest plan is to use a rubber rectal catheter and a funnel, the latter being raised not more than 50 cm above the level of the anus. If for any reason it is considered necessary to employ a Higginson syringe, a short rectal tube should invariably be attached to the tip in place of any more rigid type of introducer.

In treating enema injuries, each case must be judged according to the extent of the injury and to the time that has elapsed since it was inflicted. Incision to facilitate drainage of pus and separation of necrotic material will probably be necessary in most cases with perianal injuries, and in cases with perforation of the rectal wall and pelvic cellulitis or peritonitis laparotomy is urgently required, at which the peritoneal cavity is sucked out, the perforation exposed and sutured, a drain left down to it, and possibly a temporary loop iliac colostomy established. The serious nature of these injuries may be judged from the fact that in 31 cases collected by Large and Mukheiber (1956) from the literature, eight died, four had permanent colostomies and all had long and severe illnesses.

Injuries to the anterior rectal wall have also been reported by Siebner (1931) as having been *caused by clinical thermometers* inserted into the anal canal. It should be impressed on nursing staff that in taking the rectal temperature it is never necessary to insert the thermometer for more than 2–3 cm into the anal canal.

PERFORATION AS A COMPLICATION OF A
BARIUM ENEMA EXAMINATION

Perforation of rectum or sigmoid has been recorded as occurring during the administration of a barium enema by several authors (Isaacs 1952; Spiro 1958; Lorinc and Brahame 1959; Roland and Rogers 1959; Hemley and Kanick 1963). The clinical features and management are similar to those of ordinary enema injuries, except that the diagnosis is often expedited by the radiologist observing opaque medium or air in the peritoneal cavity.

Impalement Injuries

Impalement injuries of the rectum may be caused by a variety of accidents such as falls from windows on to railings, falls off haystacks or hay-carts on to the handles or spikes of pitch-forks, the breaking of shooting-sticks, or games involving climbing or jumping over objects which are liable to collapse leaving sharp spikes which may penetrate the rectum (see Habhegger 1912; Powers and O'Meara 1939; Gabriel 1939, 1940). Such injuries are liable to involve other organs as well, particularly the urethra, bladder, vagina and, if the wound penetrates to the pelvic peritoneum, the small intestine or sigmoid colon. The gravity of the lesion depends largely on the occurrence of associated visceral injuries and especially of peritoneal involvement.

Clinically impalement injuries can be very deceptive and in cases with a suggestive history the possibility of rectal or other visceral damage should always be borne in mind. There may be a penetrating wound in the perianal region, which will obviously call for exploration, but if the impaling object has entered the rectum through the anal canal no external signs of injury may be evident. Bleeding per anum or per urethram may indicate that the rectum, urethra or bladder has been damaged. Visceral injury may also be suggested by signs of pelvic peritonitis or the existence of a severe degree of shock.

It is difficult to particularize regarding the treatment of impalement injuries, for so much depends on the precise nature of the injury and on the length of time that elapsed since its infliction. It is important to determine whether the urinary tract has been implicated; if a catheter can be passed without difficulty and clear urine is withdrawn, it may be assumed that the bladder and urethra have escaped injury. If in addition there are no clinical signs of peritoneal involvement and if on gentle probing it seems that the perianal penetrating wound or the perforating wound of the rectal wall extends too short a distance upwards to endanger the peritoneum, a simple local operation to remove foreign material and damaged tissue and improve drainage will suffice. Rarely a completely expectant attitude with the exhibition of systemic antibiotics may be permissible. In cases seen very soon after injury, particularly where the sphincters have been torn, it may be feasible after excision of devitalized tissue to carry out a primary suture. Probably in most cases of this kind a proximal colostomy will not be necessary, and the wound will be sufficiently protected by systemic antibiotic therapy.

If, on the other hand, there is the slightest doubt about the peritoneum having been penetrated, laparotomy should be performed without delay. The perforation of the rectal wall is then sutured and any associated intra-abdominal injuries appropriately treated. Repair of any injury to the bladder or urethra will also require operative attention, either through the abdominal approach or by means of a suprapubic cystotomy or perineal incision. Finally the advisability of a temporary colostomy in the iliac or transverse colon remains to be considered. Where there has been a simple penetrating wound of the anterior or lateral wall of the intraperitoneal rectum, it should not be necessary to protect this after suture by a colostomy, though a drain should be placed down to the site of repair. Where a more complicated injury has been found involving the urinary tract, it is wise to establish a defunctioning colostomy for a time to diminish the risk of fistulation developing between the rectum and the bladder or urethra.

Gunshot Wounds

Owing to the very oblique course which missiles may pursue in the body, the rectum may be injured in association with wounds situated anywhere between the levels of the costal margin and the lower thigh, particularly on the posterior aspect. Gunshot wounds of the buttocks, hips, sacral region and back of the thighs are moderately common in warfare because of the prone position usually assumed by soldiers whilst under fire. Fortunately the rectum usually escapes injury unless the projectile has crossed, or lodged near, the midline; for example, only 6% of the buttock wounds observed by Laufmann (1946) involved the rectum.

It is customary to classify gunshot injuries of the rectum into *extraperitoneal* and *intraperitoneal* wounds, of which the former are much the commoner; thus 26 of Morgan's (1945*b*) 32 cases with wounds of the rectum had extraperitoneal injuries. It is also possible for a combination of these two types of injury to be present in the same patient, for, if the missile track is very oblique, the rectum may be perforated in its extraperitoneal part on one side and in its intraperitoneal portion on the other. Similarly very severe injuries with much destruction of the bowel wall may implicate both extraperitoneal and intraperitoneal compartments. The rectal lesion may be the only injury apart from the wound of the adjacent soft tissues, but there are usually associated skeletal and visceral injuries, such as extensive comminuted fractures of the sacrum or hip bone, or wounds of the bladder, urethra, small intestine, colon, stomach or almost any abdominal or indeed thoracic viscus. The rectal injury may be a simple clean-cut perforation or there may be extensive destruction of the rectal wall, especially in the cases with complicating fractures of the pelvis. Dunn and Drummond (1917) pointed out that widespread damage to the rectal or colon wall could result from a 'near miss', the projectile passing close to the bowel but not actually striking it. Subsequently areas of necrosis were liable to occur with the development of faecal fistulation and virulent infection of the retrorectal or retrocolonic soft tissues.

Another unusual type of gunshot wound of the rectum is that described by Gordon-Watson (1919) in which a bullet traversing the perineum immediately deep to the surface exercises a bursting effect whereby the perianal skin becomes completely detached at the anal verge from the lower end of the anal canal, which then retracts upwards together with the sphincter muscles. The resulting wound has an appearance as if the lower part of the canal had been destroyed. Gabriel (1948) has recorded a similar effect due to blast.

DIAGNOSIS

The diagnosis of *intraperitoneal injuries* of the rectum is usually fairly easy and depends on the development of lower abdominal tenderness, rigidity and other signs of an abdominal wound with visceral perforation. Laparotomy is thus soon clearly indicated and the precise nature of the rectal and other lesions is exposed at operation. The risk of injury to the abdominal viscera by penetrating wounds of the buttock is well recognized and a careful examination of the abdomen is essential in such cases. A careful review of the circumstances of the wounding—the position of the soldier at the time, the type and trajectory of the missile—will help the surgeon to decide in doubtful cases whether the rectum or peritoneal cavity could have been implicated. With a lodging wound a radiological examination to show the position of the retained missile may also be of considerable assistance in visualizing the course of the track. If there is no external abdominal wound, further help in the decision as to whether visceral (possibly including rectal) injury is present may be obtained from peritoneal lavage (see p. 932).

The much commoner *extraperitoneal* injuries of the rectum are more easily overlooked, for the clinical evidence of involvement may at first be very slight. Thus, in Morgan's (1945*b*) series of 21 cases with extraperitoneal wounds of the rectum the diagnosis had been completely missed in seven till faeces and flatus escaped from the wound of entry. Of course wounds of the extreme lower end of the rectum involving the anal and perianal region would be obvious on simple inspection, though it may not be possible to determine the extent of the injury till the patient has been examined under an anaesthetic and the urinary tract has been investigated by catheterization. Injuries of the rectal ampulla, however, in association with penetrating wounds of the buttock and without external anal wounds, may present no obvious signs and often have to be carefully sought to be detected. Extensive comminution of the sacrum strongly suggests the possibility of rectal damage in such cases, and a steady stream of blood from entry or exit wounds usually indicates a serious injury which may well implicate the rectum, as does profound shock in association with such a wound. Proof of the existence of a rectal injury is afforded by the escape of blood per anum or of faeces through the wound.

Digital examination of the rectum is very helpful in most cases. It may be possible to feel the actual defect in the rectal wall, or, on withdrawal, blood may be observed on the fingertip (needless to say it is important not to be misled by allowing blood from the perianal skin on the gloved finger to be interpreted as coming from within the bowel). But not all perforations can be palpated, either because they may be beyond reach of the finger or because they are small and have been sealed off by contraction of the mucosa. In such cases, also, the examining finger may come away without revealing blood. A foreign body may be palpable through the rectal wall, and it is most important to determine whether the mucosa overlying it is intact or breached.

When palpation fails to reveal the presence of a rectal perforation, direct inspection of the interior of the rectum by means of the sigmoidoscope should be performed. This can be easily and quickly done either at the time of the initial assessment or whilst the patient is on the operating table immediately prior to operation. The reason for advocating a painstaking search for rectal perforations in these cases is that their discovery has a profound influence on the treatment of the wound.

A catheter should be passed in all cases with gunshot wounds of the pelvis and perineum to exclude the possibility of injury to the urethra or bladder.

TREATMENT

Intraperitoneal Wounds
The treatment of these injuries follows that of any other gunshot wounds of the abdomen with suspected visceral perforation and consists of laparotomy as soon as the general condition has been sufficiently restored by transfusion, if necessary. The abdomen is explored and the extent of the intra-abdominal injuries determined. Their operative treatment may involve a variety of procedures which need not be detailed here. So far as the rectal injury is concerned it is usually possible to suture an intraperitoneal tear, or to shut it off from the general peritoneal cavity by stitching the pelvic peritoneum to the rectal wall above it. A rubber drain is inserted down to the site of the injury. In the 1939–45 war it was the invariable practice of surgeons in the British and American armies to supplement the repair of intraperitoneal wounds of the rectum by establishment of a loop iliac colostomy, preferably at a separate gridiron incision in the left iliac region (Ogilvie 1944; Morgan 1945b; Laufmann 1946). This policy was based on the distrust of any form of intraperitoneal suture of the left colon that was prevalent at that time, particularly when applied to war wounds with their well-known tendency to be associated with extensive devitalization of the surrounding bowel wall leading to subsequent necrosis. With the great experience that has been obtained of sutured anastomoses in the colon since those days and the present availability of potent antibiotics for systemic use it is permissible to question whether a proximal colostomy should still be regarded as essential in

the treatment of all intraperitoneal wounds of the rectum. I imagine that for some of these injuries with particularly clear-cut perforations in a readily accessible part of the intraperitoneal rectum allowing of easy suture and with no other serious pelvic injuries, it should now be possible to omit proximal colostomy. But for larger and more difficult lacerations of the rectum, particularly if associated with an injury to the bladder or urethra, or an extensive skeletal or soft tissue wound of the pelvis or buttock, an iliac colostomy is a wise precaution, and in any case in which the surgeon is in doubt, it is better to establish a colostomy.

The operation for an intraperitoneal wound of the rectum is completed by carrying out a débridement of the associated wound of the buttock, thigh etc. as required.

Extraperitoneal Wounds
In cases in which the findings on examination do not suggest that the peritoneal cavity has been entered the surgical treatment should be directed primarily to exploration of the causal wound of the buttock or perineum, with excision of damaged tissues and the provision of free external drainage. The entrance and exit wounds are first enlarged, foreign material such as dirt and clothing removed, all devitalized tissues, especially damaged buttock muscles being freely excised, and the wound tracks traced towards the rectum. To afford freer access to the bowel in these cases Drummond (1919) recommended removal of the coccyx, but in the Second World War Hurt (1945) and Laufmann (1946) found that this was sometimes followed by troublesome osteomyelitis in the end of the sacrum and, instead, they favoured a vertical incision along the lateral edge of the coccyx and sacrum. In the Vietnam war Lung et al. (1970) became convinced of the value of coccygectomy not only for access at operation but for good subsequent drainage. The fascia of Waldeyer is then incised, all foreign material such as fragments of clothing, shell fragments or bone is removed and the extraperitoneal surface of the rectum is stripped bare till the perforation is exposed. In some cases conditions may be such that the hole in the rectal wall can be closed with inverting fine chromic catgut stitches, but in other cases this is not possible. Under either circumstances the wound is then lightly packed with petroleum jelly gauze which extends to the site of the perforation.

Wounds of the anorectal region involving the sphincter musculature merit special comment. The utmost conservatism in the excision of sphincter muscle is indicated in so far as this is compatible with the requirements of efficient débridement. Through in the past suture of the sphincters in the initial operative treatment of war wounds has been condemned, at the present time with efficient antibiotic 'cover' it seems that primary suture of these important structures ought to be seriously considered in all early cases where the sphincters have been completely or nearly completely divided. Lung et al. (1970) are strongly in favour of this step wherever possible, for, if primary suture of the sphincter muscles does succeed, the functional results are much more satisfactory than those likely to be obtained by any form of secondary suture of these muscles. Probably the most appropriate material for sphincteric suture is polyglycolic acid, 2/0.

The next step is the establishment of an iliac colostomy. It is probably best to explore the abdomen and pelvis through a left paramedian incision to exclude any other abdominal injury, particularly if the perforation of the rectum is high. Any such associated visceral injuries are appropriately dealt with and the iliac colostomy is established at a separate gridiron incision in the left lower quadrant of the abdomen. Lung et al. (1970) make a plea for a divided rather than a loop colostomy, in order to secure better faecal diversion, but my experience is that, if the glass rod or subsequent supporting rubber tube (see p. 653) is retained in position for several weeks to establish a good spur, a simple loop colostomy may be adequately diverting. Lung et al. (1970) also suggest that the segment of bowel beyond the colostomy should be washed out from colostomy to anus at the time of the primary operation to clear it of any residual faeces and lessen the risk of subsequent persisting infection, and Lavenson and Cohen (1971) make a similar plea. (It may also be a good plan to irrigate the perineal wound with noxythiolin or other antiseptic solution or at any rate with abundant quantities of normal saline (see p. 441).)

Because of the considerable risk of clostridial infection of buttock wounds associated with rectal injury, it is important to give a full prophylactic dose of polyvalent gas gangrene antitoxin and tetanus antitoxin or toxoid, and to institute prophylactic systemic antibiotic therapy with penicillin and streptomycin or other appropriate antibiotics, in addition to the surgical treatment outlined above.

Postoperative Care

The subsequent management of patients after operation for rectal wounds follows the lines of military surgery developed during the latter part of the 1939–45 war. On the fourth or fifth postoperative day a review of the perineal sacral or buttock wounds is carried out in the operating theatre under a general anaesthetic. If infection has not occurred delayed primary suture of the skin edges of these wounds should be carried out, a long rubber drain being inserted up to the site of the perforation in the rectum if it is an extraperitoneal lesion; this drain is retained for four or five days. In many instances healing *per primam* is obtained but there may be a temporary fistula from the rectum along the drain track. This will usually close spontaneously in time provided that the defunctioning colostomy is maintained with a good spur or separation between proximal and distal limbs. In certain cases, however, a secondary operation may be necessary to open the fistulous track and expose and suture the internal opening. Preparatory to attempting closure of the perforation it is essential to mobilize the rectal wall sufficiently all round to allow of suture with inversion and without tension. This is often extremely difficult to do because the opening may lie high up under cover of the sacrum, and the rectum may be firmly adherent to the bone. Often a non-absorbable suture material such as silk or fine stainless steel wire has been used for the stitches, but a fine grade of polyglycolic acid might be a satisfactory alternative.

In cases where the buttock wound, on review at the fourth or fifth postoperative day, shows some degree of infection delayed primary suture should be avoided and reliance placed on healing by granulation. Rectal perforations may close spontaneously in due course or a persistent fistula may develop requiring attempts at operative closure eventually.

Results of Surgical Treatment

The mortality of rectal wounds in the First World War according to Gordon-Taylor (1942) was approximately 66%. The Second World War saw a very remarkable reduction in this figure. Thus Laufmann (1946), in a series of 35 penetrating wounds of the rectum, had a mortality of only 8·5%. The improvement in the results was probably attributable in large measure to the routine use of proximal colostomy, as well as to other more general factors making surgery much safer in the second war. A report by Vannix et al. (1963) of civilian gunshot wounds of the rectum, in the treatment of which the same principles of management were adopted as outlined above for military injuries, quotes an operative mortality of 31% in 25 cases. As Lung et al. (1970) have emphasized, if these patients survive, they generally have a pro-

longed period in hospital with several subsequent operations.

Pneumatic Injuries

These injuries result from practical joking in which
a powerful current of compressed air is applied
through a nozzle to the unfortunate victim's anus.
The classical paper on the subject is that of Andrews
(1911) of Chicago. As he points out, the usual effect
of the sudden increase of intrarectal and intracolonic pressure is to rupture the bowel, usually in
the anterior wall of the intraperitoneal portion of
the rectum or in the sigmoid. The patient experiences sudden severe abdominal pain and shock.
Vomiting soon follows. On examination a striking
physical sign is the great distension of the abdomen
due to air in the peritoneal cavity.

A consideration of the history and findings on
examination leave no doubt as a rule as to the
diagnosis and the need for laparotomy as soon as
the patient can be made fit for it. Tears of the
intraperitoneal rectum will call for the same
operative management as sigmoidoscopic perforation (see p. 916).

Miscellaneous Other Injuries

The rectum may be punctured by bony spicules *in
association with fractures of the pelvis*, though this is a
much rarer complication of pelvic fracture than is
rupture of the urethra or bladder, and is usually
associated with the latter injuries. This combined
lesion represents a very serious injury causing severe
shock from which the patient may never rally
sufficiently even with vigorous resuscitation to
warrant active treatment.

COLONIC INJURIES

Injury to the colon may occur in several ways:

1. Due to violence applied from within the
   lumen of the bowel as in sigmoidoscopic,
   colonoscopic or 'pneumatic' injuries to the
   upper rectum or lower sigmoid (see above).
2. 'Closed' lesions resulting from external violence, as in crushing injuries without external
   wound, or injuries due to blast in air or water
   (Goligher et al. 1943).

3. 'Open' injuries from penetrating wounds, as
   in gunshot or stab injuries.

The diagnosis and treatment of the lesions
referred to in (2) and (3) are inseparably bound up
with the possibility of similar injuries occurring in
the other abdominal viscera, and it is quite unrealistic to discuss their clinical features apart from
those of injuries of the small gut, stomach, etc. A
detailed consideration of the latter, however, lies
outside the scope of this work. In regard to 'open'
abdominal injuries from penetrating wounds, the
presence of perforating lesions of the abdominal
viscera will always be suspected and will be particularly suggested by signs of peritoneal irritation
with tenderness and muscular rigidity of the abdominal wall. However, the diagnosis may be
difficult, confusion arising with more superficial
wounds implicating only the abdominal parietes
but associated with tenderness and guarding on that
account, or with thoracic wounds producing similar
abdominal signs. In doubtful cases it was considered safer in wartime to follow the dictum of Sir
Cuthbert Wallace (1917) to 'look and see' than to
'wait and see'. But in comtemporary civilian life,
when the surgeon has had a good deal of experience in evaluating these patients, a more
selective approach is apparently often safely possible, some doubtful cases being kept under close
supervision for a limited period to see how their
physical signs progress (Shafton 1960; Mason 1964;
Ryzoff et al. 1966; Steichen 1967; Richter and
Mahfouz 1967; Stein and Lissoos 1968). In this way
operation may be avoided in a proportion of
patients who would otherwise be submitted to an
unnecessary laparotomy. The diagnosis of the
presence of traumatic visceral lesions in cases of
blunt abdominal injury is much more difficult, but
the decision can be aided by special investigative
measures (see below).

The management of open or closed abdominal
injuries has been much influenced by the extensive
experience of them available in recent years in
major American cities. A policy of treatment in
civilian practice that would probably be accepted by
most surgeons is as follows (Shires 1978):

Gunshot Wounds. These should all be explored
unless the wound obviously does not penetrate the
abdominal cavity.

Stab Wounds. Many cases with these injuries are
suitable for expectant management in the first
instance. Obvious exceptions are patients with

frank evisceration or very gross abdominal signs, as also those with otherwise unexplained shock.

Blunt Injuries. These will involve the spleen, liver or kidney in nearly 70%. Though the clinical signs on abdominal examination may be suggestive of intraperitoneal injury, they may be misleading, and a much more reliable assessment is provided by *peritoneal lavage* (Root et al. 1965), which is 90–95% accurate and gives very few false negative results (Shires 1978). It should be a routine investigation in all cases of blunt injury except patients who have had previous abdominal operations or are pregnant; care must also be taken to ensure that the bladder is empty. Under local anaesthesia a small cut is made transversely or vertically in the midline of the anterior abdominal wall 6–10 cm below the umbilicus. The linea alba is exposed and incised to display the peritoneum. A plastic catheter, size No. 18F, with side holes as in a peritoneal dialysis set, is inserted into the peritoneal cavity through a needle or cannula and 1 litre of Ringer's lactate solution is injected fairly rapidly into the abdominal cavity with a syringe. If the patient's condition permits he is shifted from side to side before the fluid is sucked back. The fluid is examined with regard to blood-staining, a rough-and-ready test of normality in that regard being that it should be possible to read the small print of a newspaper through it. If a greater amount of blood than that is present laparotomy should be performed on the assumption that a significant visceral injury is present.

Mesenteric ateriography, ultrasonography (and possibly *CAT scanning*) may be helpful in cases of suspected solid visceral injury.

OPERATIVE TREATMENT

In cases to be explored, as soon as the patient has been sufficiently resuscitated by blood transfusion, the abdomen is opened by a right or left para-median incision. The presence of blood, gas or intestinal contents in the peritoneal cavity is observed and a careful systematic exploration carried out to determine the extent of the injuries. Of the hollow viscera the jejunum and ileum are from their extent the ones most likely to be injured with gunshot wounds, the chances of the large gut being perforated being only about half that of the small gut. The actual lesions in the colon are much the same as those in the small gut but are less often multiple, or if multiple, less numerous. The larger size of the colon makes it less liable to complete transection than in gunshot wounds of the small

intestine. One of the most important and dangerous forms of colon injury is perforation or laceration of the posterior bare surface of the ascending or descending colon, which is liable to result from wounds of the loin. Whenever the signs on clinical examination and the probable track of the missile focus suspicion on the vertical parts of the colon, these posterior perforations should be sought for by dividing the peritoneum in the paracolic gutter and mobilizing the colon so as to bring its bare surface into view. The lethal character of spreading cellulitis, expecially by gas gangrene infection, of the retroperitoneal tissues in association with missed perforations of the ascending or descending colon was abundantly demonstrated in both world wars (Fraser and Drummond 1917; Gordon-Taylor 1942).

The management of the injuries revealed may involve a variety of procedures depending on the precise nature of the lesions—suture or resection of small gut, nephrectomy or splenectomy, suture or packing of the liver, suture of the stomach, and repair, exteriorization or excision of injured segments of colon. Only the treatment of injuries of the large intestine will be considered in this chapter. Contrary to the usual policy in the care of small gut injuries where suture of the lesions, even if multiple, is to be preferred where possible, resection being reserved for injuries which damage the mesenteric attachment or blood supply of the bowel, in the treatment of injuries of the colon simple suture has been regarded with disfavour. This disapproval is based on the fact that perforations or lacerations of the large intestine often seem to involve more extensive devitalization of the colon wall than may at first be apparent to the naked eye (Gordon-Taylor 1942). This may result in subsequent necrosis, and there are indeed cases on record where such necrosis has been produced by a missile passing close to the colon or rectum without actually striking it (Dunn and Drummond 1917). Apart from this danger of widespread tissue damage, there is presumably a greater risk of sepsis and leakage from sutured wounds of the unprepared large intestine with its high bacterial content, than from similar repaired wounds of the small gut.

As a result of these apprehensions about simple intraperitoneal repair of injuries of the colon the policy was developed in the Second World War by Ogilvie (1944) of exteriorization or extraperitoneal resection of the affected portion of colon wherever possible, and it usually was possible anywhere down to the midsigmoid. For injuries in the lower sigmoid or upper rectum which could not be sufficiently mobilized to come to the surface the treatment adopted was simple suture, drainage to the site of repair, and a proximal colostomy. For all other large bowel perforations, lacerations or contusions exteriorization was practised, the fixed ascending and descending portions of the colon being, if necessary, mobilized to make this possible. If there was a single or simple through-and-through wound of the colon, it was usually effectively exteriorized by making an ordinary loop colostomy at this site. If the colon injury was more extensive, the affected segment was resected between clamps and the two ends brought to the surface as a double-barrelled colostomy as in the Paul–Mikulicz type of colonic resection.

However, it is debatable whether this policy of exteriorization is necessary at the present time in dealing with civilian injuries of the colon. I feel sure that there must be many small solitary perforations of the large bowel without significant soiling that could now be safely treated by simple suture or, if more extensive, by a straightforward resection with intraperitoneal anastomosis. Without putting these opinions to the test of extensive war experience it is difficult to reach a firm conclusion, but reports on the treatment of quite large series of civilian injuries in America from Woodhall and Ochsner (1951), Pontius et al. (1957), Roof et al. (1960), Vannix et al. (1963), Beall et al. (1965), Josen et al. (1972) and Schrock and Christiansen (1972), and in South Africa from Stein and Lissoos (1968), suggest that primary suture is indeed the treatment of choice when circumstances permit, though, when colon wounds are accompanied by extensive local tissue injury or massive faecal peritonitis, exteriorization methods are probably still preferable. Beall et al. (1965) had an operative mortality of only 5% in 256 cases of colon injury treated by primary repair. In 32 cases treated by exteriorization the mortality was 31% and in 30 cases managed by primary repair supplemented by a proximal colostomy it was 27%. These uncontrolled clinical impressions are confirmed by a recent controlled trial randomizing patients with injuries suitable for primary suture to either suture or exteriorization (Stone and Fabian 1979). Suture was followed by less sepsis and a shorter period in hospital but no lower mortality.

A compromise plan that has been tried by some surgeons in the management of colonic injuries is that of 'exteriorized primary repair' (Okies et al. 1972). In this technique the injured segment of colon is repaired by primary suture but then exteriorized as a loop over a glass rod or other supporting device. If the repair holds and the loop remains viable by the fourteenth postoperative day, the rod is removed and the exteriorized loop of bowel freed from the abdominal wall and returned to the peritoneal cavity. If, on the other hand, the repair breaks down, all that happens is that the patient has a colostomy. Though Okies et al. (1972) have been much impressed with the value of this method, Shrock (1975) is much less enthusiastic.

Probably very important items in the care of patients with penetrating wounds of the hollow abdominal viscera are the antibiotic and antiseptic measures outlined on p. 921.

SEATBELT INJURIES TO THE COLON

It is now well established that in car accidents injuries may occasionally be sustained by the occupants due to the seatbelts or lap-straps which they are wearing. These injuries take three forms: abdominal, thoracic and those affecting the spinal cord (Garrett and Braunstein 1962). All three types of injury may occur in an individual case or single injuries may be found. Of the abdominal injuries, most have been to the solid viscera in the upper abdomen or to the small gut or its mesentery. But the colon may be damaged and rarely it may be the only organ injured (Towne and Coe 1971). The clinical features, diagnosis and management of abdominal seatbelt injuries are similar to those of blunt abdominal injuries in general (see p. 923), though associated vertebral and thoracic injuries may introduce special problems.

SPONTANEOUS PERFORATION OF THE NORMAL LARGE BOWEL

Usually perforation of the colon or rectum arises as a complication of pathological states, such as diverticular disease, carcinoma, colitis or simple ulcer, or as a result of trauma in the form of external violence to the abdomen or intraluminal injury from faulty instrumentation, etc. But, rarely, rupture of the large bowel may occur spontaneously, as was first pointed out by Sir Benjamin Brodie in 1827. In 1961 Dickinson and Gilmour were able to collect 19 such cases from the literature and to add six of their own. Since them further cases have been reported by Kirkham (1960), Jokinen and Stuckey (1962), Kessing (1962), Sanan (1962), Lewis (1963) and no doubt others more recently. From the 31 cases described by these authors the following account has been compiled.

SITE OF PERFORATION

In 30 cases perforation lay in *the distal large bowel*: 10 in the anterior wall of the rectum above the peritoneal reflection; 11 in the sigmoid colon (six on the antimesenteric border, one on the mesocolic aspect, and in four the position not clearly defined); and nine at the rectosigmoid junction on its antimesenteric aspect. Thus in 26 of 31 cases the rupture was on the anterior wall of the bowel. It is interesting to note that in two cases (Kirkham 1960; Kessing 1962) there was a *re-perforation at the same site* some years later.

In one case the perforation was situated elsewhere than in the distal colon, namely in the *ascending colon anteriorly* just above the level of the ileocaecal junction (Sanan 1962).

APPEARANCE OF PERFORATION

Precise data regarding the gross appearance of the rupture were often lacking, but, where they were available, the lesion was usually described as 'clear-cut' or 'slit-like', rarely with a ragged edge, and running usually longitudinally, sometimes transversely.

AGE AND SEX INCIDENCE

The ages of the patients varied from 16 to 76 years, 17 being male and 14 female.

CLINICAL FEATURES AND DIAGNOSIS

The presenting symptom was usually sudden lower abdominal pain, which later spread to the rest of the abdomen and sometimes to the shoulder tips. Sometimes it came on dramatically during defaecation, but in others there was no history of any form of strain. Indeed, in one patient it occurred during sleep. Rectal bleeding was recorded in only one case. The findings on examination were those of a perforation or peritonitis and the tentative clinical diagnosis was usually a perforated appendix, peptic ulcer or colonic diverticulum, the correct diagnosis depending on laparotomy.

AETIOLOGY

Nothing definite can be said about the causation of these lesions. It is important to emphasize that in none of the cases quoted was there any underlying pathological lesion such as a diverticulum, solitary ulcer or infarction to account for the bowel perforating. It has been suggested that the bowel wall ruptures at a site where the muscle coat is abnormally thin but, as Kirkham (1960) points out, the perforation has on occasion taken place not at the point where the bowel wall is obviously exceptionally thin but elsewhere. Brearley (1954), Birbis (1955) and Kirkham (1960) have commented on the frequency with which a large faecal mass was present in the pelvis or plugged the gap in the bowel wall, and believe that impaction of such a scybalous mass on the antimesenteric wall of the bowel where the blood supply is poorest, aided by repeated straining at stool, leads eventually to perforation. Obviously, unusually sited perforations are even more difficult to explain.

TREATMENT

In the 31 cases referred to, treatment consisted usually of laparotomy with evacuation of pus or faeces from the peritoneal cavity and usually suture of the perforation with or without proximal colostomy or caecostomy. In four cases in which the perforation was in the sigmoid loop this segment was exteriorized.

MORTALITY

Eleven of the 31 patients died. Of the seven patients recorded in the literature up to 1928, only one survived; but of the 24 reported since 1944 only five have died, reflecting the improvement in modern methods of colonic surgery and the assistance of antibiotics and other antiseptic agents.

REFERENCES

ANDRESON, A. F. R. (1947) Perforations from proctoscopy. *Gastroenterology, 9*, 32.
ANDREWS, E. W. (1911) Pneumatic ruptures of the intestine, or new type of industrial accident. *Surgery Gynec. Obstet., 12*, 63.
BEALL, A. C., CROSTHWAIT, R. W. and DEBAKEY, M. E. (1965) Injuries of the colon including surgery upon the aorta. *Surg. Clins N. Am., 45*, 1273.
BIRBIS, P. (1955) Les perforations par effort du colon rectosigmoidien. *Bordeaux Chir.*, Jan., 17.
BREARLEY, R. (1954) Spontaneous perforation of colon due to alkaline medication. *Br. med. J., 1*, 743.
BRODIE, B. C. (1827) Case of a singular variety of hernia treated at St George's Hospital. *Lond. med. phys. J., 57* (2), 529.
DICKINSON, P. H. and GILMOUR, J. (1961) 'Spontaneous' rupture of the distal large bowel. *Br. J. Surg., 49*, 157.
DRUMMOND, H. (1919) Gunshot wounds of the large intestine and rectum, with special reference to surgical treatment. *Proc. R. Soc. Med., 13*, 24.
DUNN, J. S. and DRUMMOND, H. (1917) Ulceration of the colon in the neighbourhood of gunshot wounds. *Br. J. Surg., 5*, 59.
FRASER, J. and DRUMMOND, H. (1917) Three hundred perforating wounds of the abdomen. *Br. med. J., 1*, 321.
GABRIEL, W. B. (1939) In: Rectum. *Med. Ann.*, 251.
—— (1940) In: Rectum. *Med. Ann.*, 395.
—— (1948) *Principles and Practice of Rectal Surgery*, 4th ed. London: H. K. Lewis.
GALBRAITH, W. W. (1937) Severe rectal injuries caused by an enema given through a rigid nozzle. *Br. med. J., 1*, 859.
GARRETT, J. W. and BRAUNSTEIN, P. W. (1962) The seatbelt syndrome. *J. Trauma, 2*, 220.
GOLIGHER, J. C., KING, D. P. and SIMMONS, H. T. (1943) Injuries produced by blast in water. *Lancet, 2*, 119.
GORDON,-TAYLOR, Sir G. (1942) The abdominal surgery of 'total war'. *Br. J. Surg., 30*, 89.
GORDON-WATSON, Sir C. (1919) Discussion on gunshot wounds of great bowel and rectum. *Proc. R. Soc. Med., 12*, 47.
HABHEGGER, C. J. (1912) Impaling injuries of the pelvis: report of a case with some of the literature. *Wisconsin med. J., 10*, 449.
HEMLEY, S. D. and KANICK, V. (1963) Perforation of the rectum: a complication of barium enema following rectal biopsy. *Am. J. dig. Dis., 8*, t882.
HURT, L. A. (1945) The surgical management of colon and rectal injuries in the forward areas. *Ann. Surg., 122*, 398.
ISAACS, I. (1952) Intraperitoneal escape of barium enema fluid in perforation of the sigmoid colon. *J. Am. med. Ass., 150*, 645.
JOKINEN, T. I. T. and STUCKEY, W. H. (1962) Spontaneous rupture of the sigmoid colon. Report of a case. *Acta chir. scand., 123*, 155.
JOSEN, A. S., FERRER, J. M., Jr., FORDE, K. A. and ZIKRIA, B. A. (1972) Primary closure of civilian colorectal wounds. *Ann. Surg., 176*, 782.

KESSING, S. V. (1962) Spontaneous perforation of the normal sigmoid colon. *Acta chir. scand., 123,* 149.

KING, W. W. (1930) Rectal injury caused by simple enema. *Br. med. J., 1,* 113.

KIRKHAM, C. S. (1960) Spontaneous perforation of the normal pelvic colon. *Br. J. Surg., 48,* 126.

LARGE, P. G. and MUKHEIBER, W. J. (1956) Injury to rectum and anal canal by enema syringes. *Lancet, 2,* 596.

LAUFMANN, H. (1946) Initial surgical treatment of penetrating wounds of the rectum. *Surgery Gynec. Obstet., 82,* 219.

LAVENSON, G. S. and COHEN, A. (1971) Management of rectal injuries. *Am. J. Surg., 122,* 226.

LEWIS, E. C. (1963) Spontaneous perforation of the colon associated with gross surgical emphysema. *Br. J. Surg., 50,* 548.

LOCKHART-MUMMERY, J. P. (1934) *Diseases of the Rectum and Colon and their Surgical Treatment.* London: Baillière.

LORINC, P. and BRAHAME, F. (1959) Perforation of the colon during examination by the double contrast method. *Gastroenterology, 37,* 770.

LUNG, J. A. TURK, R. P., MILLER, R. E. and EISEMAN, B. (1970) Wounds of the rectum. *Ann. Surg., 172,* 985.

MASON, T. H. (1964) The expectant management of abdominal stab wounds. *J. Trauma, 4,* 210.

MORGAN, C. N. (1945a) Wounds of the colon. *Br. J. Surg., 32,* 337.

—— (1945b) Wounds of the rectum. *Surgery Gynec. Obstet., 81,* 56.

MURRAY, F. (1937) Rectal injuries from an enema nozzle. *Br. med. J., 1,* 1044.

OGILVIE, W. H. (1944) Abdominal wounds in the Western Desert. *Surgery Gynec. Obstet., 78,* 225.

OKIES, J. E., BRICKER, D. L. and JORDAN, G. L. (1972) Exteriorized repair of colon injuries. *Am. J. Surg., 124,* 807.

PINNOCK, D. (1937) Dangerous rectal trauma due to a rigid nozzle. *Lancet, 1,* 205.

PONTIUS, R. G., CREECH, O. and DEBAKEY, M. E. (1957) Management of large bowel injuries in civilian practice. *Ann. Surg., 146,* 291.

POWERS, J. N. and O'MEARA, E. S. (1939) Perforated wounds of the rectum into the Pouch of Douglas. *Ann. Surg., 109,* 468.

RAYNER, H. H. (1932) Injury of the rectum caused by the faulty administration of an enema. *Br. med. J., 1,* 419.

RICHTER, R. M. and MAHFOUZ, H. Z. (1967) Selective conservative management of penetrating abdominal wounds. *Ann. Surg., 166,* 238.

ROLAND, C. G. and ROGERS, A. G. (1959) Rectal perforation after enema administration. *Can. med. Ass. J., 81,* 815.

ROOF, W. R., MORRIS, G. C. and DEBAKEY, M. E. (1960) Management of perforating injuries to the colon in civilian practice. *Am. J. Surg., 99,* 641.

ROOT, H. D., HAUSER, C. W. and MCKINLEY, C. R. (1965) Diagnostic peritoneal lavage. *Surgery, St Louis, 57,* 633.

RYZOFF, R. T., SHAFTON, G. W. and HERBSMAN, H. (1966) Selective conservatism in penetrating abdominal trauma. *Surgery, St Louis, 59,* 650.

SANAN, D. P. (1962) Spontaneous rupture of the ascending colon. *Br. J. Surg., 50,* 199.

SCHWARTZ, J. T. and GRAHAM, D. Y. (1977) Toothpick perforation of the intestines. *Am. Surg., 185,* 64.

SHAFTON, G. W. (1960) Indications for operation in abdominal trauma. *Am. J. Surg., 99,* 657.

SHIRES, G. T. (1978) Personal communication.

SHROCK, T. R. (1975) Personal communication.

—— and CHRISTIANSEN, N. (1972) Management of perforating injuries of the colon. *Surgery Gynec. Obstet., 135,* 65.

SIEBNER, M. (1931) Instrumentelle Verletzungen des Mastdarms, insbesonders durch Fieber-thermometer. *Chirurg, 3,* 208.

SOHN, N., WEINSTEIN, M. A. and GONCHAR, J. (1977) Social injuries of the rectum. *Am. J. Surg., 134,* 611.

SPIRO, R. K. (1958) Perforation of the rectum following barium enema. *Am. J. Gastroent., 30,* 540.

STEICHEN, F. M. (1967) Penetrating wounds of the chest as well as the abdomen. *Curr. Probl. Surg., 1,* 73.

STEIN, A. and LISSOOS, I. (1968) Selective management of penetrating wounds of the abdomen. *J. Trauma, 8,* 1015.

STONE, H. H. and FABIAN, T. C. (1979) Management of perforating colon trauma: randomization between primary closure and exteriorization. *Ann. Surg.,* in the press.

THORBJARNARSON, B. (1962) Iatrogenic and related perforations of the large bowel. *Archs Surg., Chicago, 84,* 28.

TOWNE, J. B. and COE, J. D. (1971) Seatbelt trauma of the colon. *Am. J. Surg., 122,* 683.

TUTTLE, J. P. (1903) *A Treatise on Diseases of the Anus, Rectum and Pelvic Colon.* London: Appleton.

VANNIX, R. S., CARTER, R., HINSHAW, D. B. and JOERGENSON, E. J. (1963) Surgical management of colon trauma in civilian practice. *Am. J. Surg., 106,* 364.

WALLACE, Sir C. (1971) A study of 1200 cases of gunshot wounds of the abdomen. *Br. J. Surg., 4,* 679.

WOODHALL, J. P. and OCHSNER, A. (1951) Management of perforating injuries of the colon and rectum in civilian practice. *Surgery, St Louis, 29,* 305.

27

Miscellany

VOLVULUS

The colon is the commonest part of the alimentary tract to be affected by volvulus, in which the gut becomes twisted on its mesenteric axis, with resulting partial or complete obstruction to its lumen and a varying degree of impairment of its circulation. The most usual site in the large intestine for volvulus to occur is the sigmoid colon, and sigmoid volvulus is a well recognized, if rather rare, form of acute closed-loop obstruction in older individuals. Very much less frequent is volvulus of the caecum, ascending colon and terminal ileum. This may be encountered as a cause of obstruction in neonates in whom the normal fixation of the right colon to the posterior abdominal wall has failed to take place. It may also rarely occur in adults in whom there has likewise been some persisting imperfection of peritoneal fusion so that the right colon has remained unduly mobile. Exceptionally volvulus can occur in the transverse colon (Kerry and Ransom 1969), but I have never personally met with an example of it in this situation.

Volvulus accounts for only a small proportion of the cases of acute obstruction of the large bowel in Britain, America and most Western European countries, but is generally held to be much more frequent in Eastern Europe, Scandinavia, parts of Africa and India (Bruusgaard 1947; Shepherd 1968; Sinha 1969).

Volvulus of the Sigmoid

Clinical Features
The symptoms of volvulus of the sigmoid as a rule closely resemble those of an acute obstruction due to carcinoma of the distal colon, with cramp-like abdominal pains, abdominal distension and complete constipation with non-passage of flatus. Nausea and vomiting are at first absent and the symptoms increase in severity gradually over a period of two or three days or longer, by which time the abdomen may be very considerably distended, to such an extent indeed as to interfere with respiration and even impede cardiac action.

Diagnosis
There is usually no difficulty in reaching a diagnosis of large bowel obstruction, and the gross abdominal distension may suggest the possibility of a sigmoid volvulus. A plain X-ray examination of the abdomen is usually very helpful for not only does it show gaseous distension of the colon with fluid levels, but it usually also reveals the outline of the enormously dilated sigmoid loop, which often extends almost up to the diaphragm.

Treatment
It has been customary in Britain and America till a few years ago to consider that there is no satisfactory non-operative treatment for the condition, but practice in Scandinavia has been very different. There operation is only rarely employed and the usual initial treatment for all cases is an attempt at deflation and untwisting of the sigmoid loop by the passage of rubber rectal tube, 7 mm in diameter and 60 cm long, through a sigmoidoscope. It might be feared that, if this manoeuvre were successful in relieving the obstruction, it would leave the patient exposed to the risk of gangrene and perforation of the bowel, but apparently this is a rare complication. Thus Bruusgaard (1947) reported on the use of this method in the treatment of 136 episodes of sigmoid

volvulus in 91 patients with satisfactory decompression in 123 (90%). Emergency laparotomy was
performed in 18 patients who showed clinical signs
of peritonitis or on whom conservative treatment
failed. The overall mortality was 14·2%. More
recently British and American surgeons have turned
to this method also (Bolt 1956; Drapanas and
Stewart 1961; Prather and Bowers 1962; Nayman
1962; Wilson and Dunavant 1965; Wuepper et al.
1966; Shepherd 1968; Kerry and Ransom 1969),
and have mostly had a fair amount of success with
it—for example, Drapanas and Stewart (1961),
Wuepper et al. (1966) and Shepherd (1968) report
respectively 84%, 80% and 88% of successful de-
rotations with it.

In the performance of sigmoidoscopic decompression the patient is placed on the left side or in a
prone position. The sigmoidoscope is passed till the
site of narrowing is encountered, which is usually
within 25 cm of the anal margin. Sometimes the
scope itself can be induced to go through the point
of torsion, but it is probably safer to pass a well-
lubricated rectal rubber catheter through the
twisted bowel with a gentle rotating movement. The
immediate escape of flatus and liquid faeces
through the sigmoidoscope or catheter indicates
that the obstruction has been negotiated. The tube
is left *in situ* and fixed to the perianal skin by
adhesive strapping after the sigmoidoscope has
been withdrawn. It is retained for 48 hours and
irrigated frequently during that time. Attempts at
sigmoidoscopic decompression are abandoned if
mucosa of dubious viability is seen, if efforts to
pass the tube through the twisted colon fail, or if the
twist is too high to be reached.

Ghazi et al. (1976) have more recently advocated
the use of the colonoscope to effect de-rotation of
sigmoid volvulus, but whether this has any real
advantage over ordinary tubal de-rotation through
a rigid sigmoidoscope remains to be established.

If sigmoidoscopic decompression fails or if
necrosis of the bowel is feared, laparotomy is
carried out. The abdomen is opened by a long left
paramedian incision. The diagnosis is confirmed by
finding the enormously distended sigmoid loop
which may have almost the calibre of a Rugby football. As the twist that produces the obstruction is
usually in an anticlockwise direction, an attempt is
made to undo the volvulus by rotating it first in a
clockwise direction. The rotation may have to be
carried through 180° to 360° or more to complete
the untwisting, and it may be that the reverse
direction will have to be tried. It is useful to have
had a stout stomach tube passed into the rectum per

anum before the start of the operation, so that it
can at this stage be further advanced by an assistant
from below, its point being guided by the surgeon's
fingers into the dilated but now untwisted loop.
Immediate deflation is thus achieved. The sigmoid
loop is now collapsed and flaccid but still very
redundant. Examination of the base of the loop
may show that the two limbs of colon are bound
closer together than usual by fibrous adhesions in
the peritoneum. This, and the dependency of the
loop, are presumably the factors that predispose
these patients to volvulus.

If the *colon shows evidence of necrosis*, it will be
necessary to resect it right away. As the bowel wall is
oedematous and friable, making a sutured
anastomosis probably hazardous, it is safer to
employ either a Paul–Mikulicz type of resection, or,
if there is difficulty in getting the distal colon stump
to reach to the surface, as there frequently is
(Shepherd 1968; Neely 1970), to do a sort of
Hartmann's operation suturing the top of the lower
end and placing a drain down to it, and then
bringing the upper end out as a terminal iliac
colostomy. On a subsequent occasion the continuity of the large intestine can be restored by
suture. If the *sigmoid is found to be quite viable*, it may
likewise be resected by either of these two techniques, for there is a 40% risk of recurrence of the
volvulus if the collapsed decompressed loop is
simply returned to the abdomen and chances of
recurrence are almost as great if an attempt is made
to fix the sigmoid by sutures (Shepherd 1968). It can
be argued that it is more comfortable for the patient
to undergo a second laparotomy a few weeks later
and have a formal resection with anastomosis
performed then than to be subjected to a staged
extraperitoneal type of sigmoid colectomy, but an
immediate Paul-Mikulicz or Hartmann operation
has proved very satisfactory in my hands. Sinha
(1969) of Patna, India, who has personally treated
over 211 cases of sigmoid volvulus, has used
primary resection with immediate anastomosis in
70% of these patients with a 5% incidence of
anastomotic leakage. But most surgeons would be
reluctant to embark on immediate restoration of
continuity by primary suture in these patients with
an unprepared grossly distended and oedematous
bowel, and this is the view of Shepherd (1968).
Naturally patients whose volvulus has been successfully decompressed by sigmoidoscopic intubation
should subsequently proceed to elective resection
after suitable bowel preparation, unless there are
strong medical contraindications to this plan. The
operative mortality of resection at this stage can be

very low—it was under 2% in Shepherd's (1968) series of 74 elective operations.

Recurrent Sigmoid Volvulus

Apart from recurrence of sigmoid volvulus after previous operation, at which the loop of colon was simply untwisted but not resected, another form of recurrent or chronic volvulus may occur. In this variety the volvulus is less acute and undergoes spontaneous reduction, but is liable to recur, so that the patient may experience several attacks before finally coming to surgical treatment (Sturzaker et al. 1976). The attack commences with colicky central abdominal pain, which is followed by the development of considerable abdominal distension and an inability to pass faeces or flatus. The cessation of symptoms usually occurs suddenly, immediately after the patient succeeds in getting rid of wind or motion per anum. A plain X-ray examination during the attack will show the distended sigmoid loop and may lead to a correct diagnosis. But even during the symptom-free intervals barium enema studies may reveal that the sigmoid colon is grossly redundant with close juxtaposition of its afferent and efferent limbs at its base. In turn this state of affairs is also disclosed at laparotomy, and, in addition, binding adhesions are usually found between the basal parts of the two limbs of the sigmoid loop. The treatment required is excision of the affected portion of colon, which in the intervals between attacks of acute volvulus may safely take the form of a segmental resection with anastomosis. If, however, the patient is operated on during an actual attack, it is probably wiser to be content with untwisting the volvulus and emptying the bowel through a rectal tube, resection being deferred for a subsequent occasion. Alternatively, if conditions for a sutured anastomosis are not too unfavourable, an immediate resection with anastomosis may be practised, preferably with a covering transverse colostomy.

Volvulus of the Caecum and Ascending Colon

Clinical Features

There are no characteristic clinical features to distinguish volvulus of the right colon from other forms of intestinal obstruction; a plain radiograph of the abdomen may be informative, but the diagnosis is often made only at laparotomy.

Treatment

There is considerable controversy as to the correct surgical treatment for this form of closed loop obstruction. The simplest plan is just to untwist the volvulus and fix the caecum and right colon to the peritoneum of the right paracaecal and paracolic gutter, either by simple suture or by raising a peritoneal flap and stitching it to the front of the bowel, so that the latter fits into a sort of retroperitoneal pocket. Because of a high incidence of recurrence after this operation, an alternative or additional method of anchoring the right colon, much favoured by Hinshaw et al. (1959), Hjelmstedt (1960), Chamberlain (1960) and Smith and Goodwin (1973), is the establishment of a caecostomy, which also has the advantage of decompressing the dilated bowel. Smith and Goodwin (1973) claimed very good results with this combination in the treatment of 17 cases. The alternative, favoured by Bagley et al. (1961) and Sawyer et al. (1962)—which probably carries a higher initial mortality—is to excise the mobile bowel by a formal right hemicolectomy, and this will usually be essential if gangrene has occurred, though a very small patch of omentum, if suitably located, might simply be excised and a caecostomy established at this site or elsewhere. It may be possible to complete the operation by a sutured anastomosis between the ileum and transverse colon, Muir's method of ileotransverse colostomy with drainage of the terminal ileum being specially suitable (see p. 455), but, if the small gut is grossly distended, it may be safer to exteriorize both ends of bowel, or to close the distal relatively collapsed end by suture and to bring the proximal end out as a temporary terminal ileostomy.

PNEUMATOSIS CYSTOIDES INTESTINALIS

Intestinal pneumatosis is a very rare condition, first described by Duvernoy in 1738 and more comprehensively by Bang in 1876, in which multiple cysts are present in the wall of the intestine. The cysts range in size from one to several centimetres in diameter. They contain mainly hydrogen (Forgacs et al. 1973) and have a lining of flattened or cubical cells often some giant cells. They occur either in the subserosa, or in the submucosa, or in both layers. In nearly all of the 213 published cases collected by Koss (1952) the disease affected the small bowel, but in only 13 did it involve the colon, and in none was the rectum implicated. More recently cases have been reported by Mathews (1954), Griffiths (1955), McGee et al. (1956), Shoesmith and Crone (1959) and Williams (1961) in which the condition occurred also in the sigmoid colon and rectum (Figs 633, 634). Though examples of pneumatosis intestinalis have been recorded in children and infants, the vast majority of the

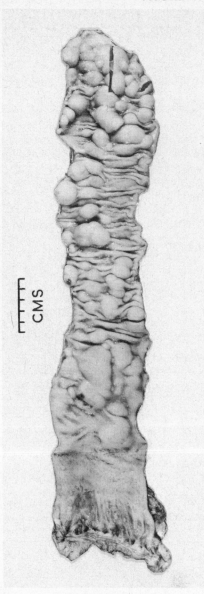

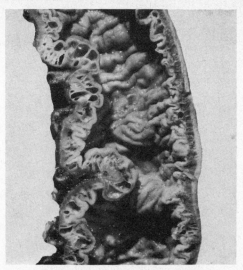

Fig. 634. Section of the colon in a case of pneumatosis cystoides intestinalis. (*From Shoesmith and Crone 1959*)

Fig. 633. View of the sigmoid colon and rectum from the mucosal aspect in a case of pneumatosis cystoides intestinalis, showing numerous grape-like swellings due to cysts in the submucosa. (*From Shoesmith and Crone 1959*)

published cases have been adults, particularly men, between the ages of 30 and 50. A frequent concomitant in these patients was a stenosing peptic ulcer of the pylorus, less commonly an associated gastric carcinoma or intestinal tuberculous ulceration. Underwood et al. (1978) have described the occurrence of pneumatosis in a woman and her son.

The various theories of aetiology of the disease have been well reviewed by Mathews (1954), Forgacs et al. (1973), Yale et al. (1973) and Underwood et al. (1978). The most generally accepted explanation is that of Masson (1925) who studied the condition

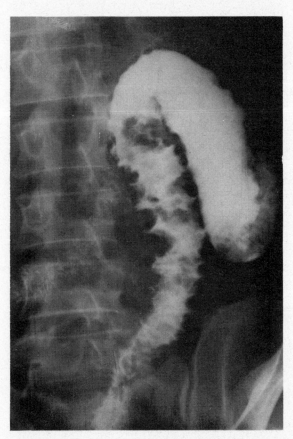

Fig. 635. The striking appearance of the sigmoid colon on barium enema examination in a case of pneumatosis cystoides involving the large intestine. (*From Shoesmith and Crone 1959*)

in swine in which it is very much more common than in man. He believed that the cysts were due to dilatation of lymphatics following lymph statis in tortuous and obstructed channels. He postulated that carbon dioxide and lactic acid were absorbed from the bowel into the blocked lymphatics and that this was followed by liberation of carbon dioxide and by diffusion of nitrogen, oxygen, and occasionally methane and hydrogen from the capillaries. Forgacs et al. (1973) found on sampling one of the rectal cysts in pneumatosis that it contained mainly hydrogen.

The presence of intestinal pneumatosis is not associated with any characteristic clinical picture and in most cases the condition has been brought to light in a fortuitous manner. Symptoms of concurrent gastrointestinal disease may lead to radiological investigation or operation at which the cystic condition of the intestine is revealed. The gas in the cysts may be evident on a plain X-ray examination of the abdomen, and in addition a very striking appearance may be obtained on barium enema studies in cases with pneumatosis of the colon (Fig. 635). Rarely intestinal obstruction may be caused by a mass of cysts blocking the lumen of the bowel or serving as the starting point of an intussusception. Rupture of cysts into the peritoneal cavity may lead to a persistent or recurrent pneumoperitoneum.

Intestinal pneumatosis has been confused with other conditions, such as a tumour of the rectum, and operation undertaken on that account (Thomson et al. 1977). However, a careful sigmoidoscopic and radiological examination combined with biopsy should avoid such errors of diagnosis and procedure. In the ordinary way no active surgical treatment is required for pneumatosis, and until recently there was no effective medical management. But in 1973 treatment by breathing oxygen was suggested by Forgacs et al. Their patient was given 70% oxygen *continuously* in an oxygen tent for six days and a repeat X-ray examination at the end of this period showed that the cysts had disappeared. They had not re-appeared on a further examination six months later. Further reports testifying to the efficacy of this form of treatment in dispersing the cysts of pneumatosis cystoides intestinalis have come from Höflin and van der Linden (1974), and Gruenberg et al. (1977). But, as van der Linden and Marsell (1979) point out, there is an insidious tendency for the cysts to reform. These authors found an elemental diet successful in causing regression of the cysts.

SOLITARY ANGIODYSPLASTIC LESIONS OF THE COLON WALL AS A CAUSE OF INTESTINAL BLEEDING

This rare but immensely important condition, which should always be thought of in the differential diagnosis of a case of obscure intestinal haemorrhage, is discussed on p. 897.

DISEASES OF THE APPENDICES EPIPLOICAE

It may be useful to summarize briefly some of the ways in which the appendices epiploicae may be affected by, or cause, disease:

Involvement in Diverticulosis and Diverticulitis of the Colon. As explained on p. 882 the diverticula in this condition often project into the appendices epiploicae so that the latter may be largely occupied by diverticula with their contained faecoliths. When chronic diverticulitis supervenes, one of the characteristic changes that occurs in the affected segment of colon is an increased deposition of subserous and pericolonic fat. In this process the appendices epiploicae share so that they may become considerably enlarged and hang like festoons from the bowel.

Tumours of the Appendices Epiploicae. Though primary connective tissue tumours such as lipomas may occur in the appendices, as reported by Godenne et al. (1957), these are excessively rare. Much more common is secondary involvement of the appendices epiploicae by direct spread of a carcinoma of the colon into them, or by adhesion and direct extension or transcolonic implantation from a carcinoma elsewhere in the abdomen.

Acute Inflammation, Torsion and Infarction. The appendices epiploicae may become acutely inflamed in association with an acute inflammatory condition of a neighbouring organ such as acute appendicitis and salpingitis. But there is a form of primary acute epiploic appendagitis in which the inflammatory changes originate in an appendage itself. Lynn et al. (1956) have described this condition in detail. The cause of the appendagitis is not always clear but in the majority of cases it would seem that the initial factor is an interference with the blood supply either by torsion of the appendage or by some kind of vascular thrombosis of its vessels.

Acute appendagitis causes acute abdominal pain and tenderness, and occasionally some nausea and vomiting. Though it is usually a sigmoid appendage that is affected, the pain is commonly experienced in the right lower quadrant. Consequently the clinical diagnosis is generally that of ordinary acute appendicitis and operation is usually undertaken with removal of the appendage (and appendix). If the condition were treated expectantly because the symptoms were mild, it would presumably end in spontaneous resolution or separation of the appendage, and spontaneous separation as a result of a previous torsion is the probable explanation of some fibrous or calcified free bodies occasionally found in the peritoneal cavity (Ross and McQueen 1948).

Incarceration in a Hernia Sac. Appendices epiploicae may be incarcerated in a hernia either along with the related portion of colon or, rarely, alone without involvement of the bowel.

As a Cause of Acute Intestinal Obstruction. Occasionally an appendage causes acute intestinal obstruction by becoming adherent to another viscus or the parietal peritoneum and kinking or compressing a loop of small gut.

MELANOSIS COLI

In patients who have been in the habit of taking a daily laxative of the anthracene group (cascara, aloes, senna and rhubarb) over a period of years, a peculiar brown or black pigmentation of the mucosa of the rectum and colon is often observed on sigmoidoscopy. At first it may be thought that the mucosa is uniformly affected, but closer inspection, especially after a slight degree of inflation, shows that the pigmentation is confined to closely packed, irregular, small areas, each of them a few square millimetres in size, separated by thin lines of normal mucosa, the appearance resembling that of a crazy pavement. If the condition is studied in autopsy-room bodies, it is seen that it affects the whole large intestine uniformly, but benign and malignant tumours of the colon and rectum are not stained and are rendered more conspicuous by their contrasting bright pink or red colour. Speare (1951) claims that if the administration of the causal aperient is stopped, the pigmentation gradually fades or disappears completely in the course of a year or so.

Histological examination reveals that the granules of pigment are contained in the cytoplasm of large mono-nuclear—presumably phagocytic—cells situated in the sub-mucosa between the epithelium and the muscularis mucosae. The exact nature of the pigment is unknown but its chemical composition resembles that of melanin. In an electron microscopy study Schrodt (1963) suggests that the pigment originates in degenerating mitochondria.

Melanosis coli is encountered fairly commonly in clinical practice; thus Bochus et al. (1933) found it in 4·7% of their patients examined sigmoidoscopically. So far as is known, the condition is quite symptomless and has no special significance. It may be of some slight value in rendering small adenomas more evident against the blackish background of the surrounding mucosa on sigmoidoscopy. (A good general review of the subject of melanosis coli is provided by Wittoesch et al. 1958.)

IRRITABLE COLON SYNDROME

For years the diagnosis of 'irritable' or 'spastic colon'—or in an earlier era 'mucous colitis' (see p. 874)—has frequently been applied to patients with persistent symptoms referable to the bowel, but with no objective abnormality demonstrable in the intestine except possibly a rather contracted colon on barium enema examination. It has been freely recognized that there is a very considerable psychological factor in the genesis of this complaint. Chaudhary and Truelove (1962) have attempted to define the characteristics of this syndrome. They distinguish two main clinical types: one has a spastic colon, the chief manifestation of which is pain of colicky, aching, continuous or stabbing kind and occurring almost anywhere in the abdomen or occasionally in the back, sometimes accompanied by con-stipation or diarrhoea; and the other has painless diarrhoea. 106 of their cases fell into the former category, 24 into the latter. In both groups women predominated in the ratio of two to one; they also tended to develop the syndrome fairly evenly from 20 to 60 years of age, whilst with men the highest incidence was in the forties. Previous abdominal operations, usually appendicec-tomy or gynaecological procedures, were common in these patients.

As regards aetiology, about a quarter of the patients dated their symptoms to an attack of proven or suspected infective dysentery. Abuse of purgatives was admitted in only a sixth of the cases. But about half the patients had been impressed by the fact that certain items of diet, particularly fruits such as apples, oranges or pears, aggravated their symptoms. In over three-quarters of the cases psychological factors could be identified. the underlying disorder of motor function in the colon in this condition has been recently elucidated by Chaudhary and True-love (1961) by motility studies. They found evidence of motor hyperactivity in a number of their patients in response to emotional stimuli or to parasympatheticomimetic drugs.

The diagnosis of this syndrome is reached largely by a process of exclusion of serious organic disease by a scrupulous physical examination including sigmoidoscopy and barium studies. The latter may be additionally valuable by showing a characteristic set of appearances, well described by Lumsden et al. (1963) and illustrated to some extent in Figs 626 and 627. The lumen of the colon is usually reduced in size. Haustral markings are promi-nent and very numerous. Sometimes a segment of bowel may close down completely and refuse to fill with barium, and this is

often accompanied by the pain of which the patient ordinarily complains. The intravenous injection of propantheline bromide immediately abolishes the spasm, allowing the bowel to dilate normally; it also relieves any pain.

An important item of treatment is reassurance to the patient that no growth or other serious lesion is present. The use of anti-spasmodics (e.g. propantheline bromide 15 mg four times a day) is logical. Sedation with barbiturates may also be helpful. Colloid hydrophilic agents such as Isogel or Normacol may be useful in providing bulk to the colon contents. Codeine phosphate can sometimes be of assistance in controlling intract-able diarrhoea. But the overall results of such medical treatment leave a great deal to be desired for only about a third of the patients are relieved of their symptoms and relapse is common.

For the surgeon the important thing is to regard a diagnosis of spastic colon with grave mistrust and to accept it only after the most searching physical examination including if necessary repeat sigmoidoscopic and radiological investigations. Like many other surgical colleagues I have seen several patients with colon carcinoma, colitis or Crohn's disease who had initially been misdiagnosed elsewhere as cases of irritable colon.

CATHARTIC COLON

A condition known as 'purge colon' or 'cathartic colon' has been described by radiologists in which there are characteristic radiological appearances apparently due to prolonged ad-ministration of purgatives. Plum et al. (1960) have reported on cases of this kind seen at the Mayo Clinic. The changes were first seen on the right side of the colon, and later extended to involve

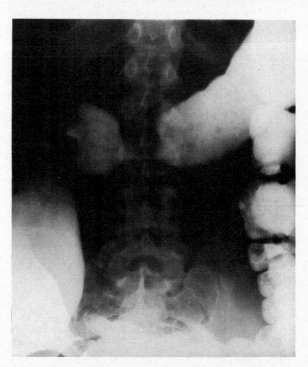

Fig. 636. Radiological appearances of 'cathartic colon', the outline of the colon being smooth and free from haustral mark-ings or irregularities and 'pseudostrictures' being present. (*From Rawson 1966*)

the entire colon, sometimes also the terminal ileum. There is an absence of the normal haustral markings with a smooth outline showing no irregularity. Yet there is no stiffening or thickening of the bowel wall, which on the contrary is easily distendable. Smooth tapering contractions are often noted and might be interpreted as strictures, but when observed they slowly disappear and reappear in another part of the colon. These pseudo-strictures seem to be absolutely typical of this condition and have great diagnostic value (Fig. 636).

Associated with such X-ray changes and a long history of regular purgation, various metabolic disturbances may be found—hypokalaemia with gross muscle weakness (Schwartz and Relman 1953; Houghton and Pears 1958; Rawson 1966), steatorrhoea (French et al. 1956) and hypocalcaemia (Meulengracht 1939; Rawson 1966).

Clearly the radiological appearances are open to misinterpretation as due to colitis, but the pseudo-strictures, the negative sigmoidoscopic findings, and history of addiction to aperients should be helpful in leading to a correct diagnosis, as they were in two cases of this kind that have come under my care and were reported by Rawson (1966). Once the cause of the condition has been appreciated, treatment consists in providing suitable electrolyte supplements and stopping the purgation. Unfortunately many of the patients relapse in their addiction. No doubt administration of bran would now be an approved measure for this condition.

PROCTALGIA FUGAX

The first recorded clinical description of this severe, intermittent, idiopathic, rectal pain was apparently given by MacLennan of Glasgow in 1917 when he reported two cases of 'rectal crises of non-tabetic origin'. The term 'proctalgia fugax' was introduced by Thaysen in 1935.

The pain in proctalgia is of considerable severity, but of short duration as a rule. It most often occurs at night and wakens the patient. It at first feels like a cramp or spasm situated in the rectum 5–10 cm above the anus; it gradually increases in intensity till it becomes well nigh unbearable and sometimes causes fainting. After reaching a peak it gradually subsides. The attacks occur irregularly, usually at long intervals of several months. They vary in duration from a few minutes to half an hour. They are always referred to the same situation in the bowel. Many, but not all, patients complaining of proctalgia are of tense excitable nature. Ewing (1953) and Ibrahim (1961) give good clinical descriptions of the condition.

The cause of proctalgia is quite unknown, though several theories have been advanced (Karras and Angelo 1951). It has often been suggested that it is due to spasm of the levator muscles (Douthwaite 1962). Again it has been attributed to a sigmoidorectal intussusception. The opportunity for examining these patients during an attack seldom presents itself, but certainly during the intervals between attacks no consistent physical abnormality is evident, though other, propably unrelated, conditions such as piles may be observed. The absence of any objective abnormality and the temperament of many of these patients suggest that in a considerably proportion of the cases, if not in all, the condition is a psychogenic disorder (Granet 1954).

The treatment of proctalgia fugax is thoroughly unsatisfactory. Measures that have been employed with varying degrees of success to terminate an attack of pain are inhalation of amyl nitrate or sublingual dissolution of a tablet of nitroglycerine, taking a hot sitz bath, passing flatus or a motion, or inserting a finger into the anus.

REFERENCES

BAGLEY, E. C., CRABTREE, H., FISH, J. C., MILLER, E. B., MORRIS, W. R. and WILLIAMS, G. H. (1961) Volvulus of the right colon. *Ann. Surg., 154*, 268.

BANG, B. L. F. (1876) Luftholdiger Kyster i Vöggen af ileum og i nydannet bindevav på sammes serosa. *Nord. med. Ark., 8*, 1.

BOCHUS, H. L., WILLARD, J. H. and BANK, J. (1933) Melanosis coli. *J. Am. med. Ass., 101*, 1.

BOLT, D. E. (1956) The management of volvulus of the sigmoid colon. *Br. J. Surg., 44*, 1.

BRUUSGAARD, C. (1947) Volvulus of the sigmoid colon and its treatment. *Surgery, St Louis, 22*, 466.

CHAMBERLAIN, G. (1960) Volvulus of the caecum. *Gut, 1*, 106.

CHAUDHARY, N. A. and TRUELOVE, C. (1961) Human colonic motility: a comparative study of normal subjects, patients with ulcerative colitis, and patients with the irritable colon syndrome. *Gastroenterology, 40*, 1.

—— —— (1962) The irritable colon syndrome. *Q. Jl Med., 31*, 307.

DOUTHWAITE, A. H. (1962) Proctalgia fugax. *Br. med. J., 2*, 164.

DRAPANAS, T. and STEWART, J. D. (1961) Acute sigmoid volvulus. Concepts in surgical treatment. *Am. J. Surg., 101*, 70.

DUVERNOY, J. G. (1738) Quoted by Koss (1952).

EWING, M. R. (1953) Proctalgia fugax. *Br. med. J., 1*, 1083.

FORGACS, P., WRIGHT, P. H. and WYATT, A. P. (1973) Treatment of intestinal cysts with oxygen breathing. *Lancet, 1*, 579.

FRENCH, J. M., GADDIE, R. and SMITH, N. (1956) Diarrhoea due to phenolphthalein. *Lancet, 1*, 551.

GHAZI, A., SHINYA, H. and WOLFF, W. (1976) Treatment of volvulus of the colon by colonoscopy. *Am. Surg., 182*, 263.

GODENNE, G. D., BURKE, E. C. and HALLENBECK, G. A. (1957) Epiploic lipomatosis; report of a case. *Proc. Mayo Clin., 32*, 370.

GRANET, E. (1954) In *Manual of Proctology*. Chicago: Yearbook Publishers.

GRIFFITHS, G. J. (1955) Pneumatosis cystoides intestinalis. *Lancet, 2*, 905.

GRUENBERG, J. C., BATRA, S. K. and PRIEST, R. J. (1977) Treatment of pneumatosis cystoides with oxygen. *Archs Surg., Chicago, 112*, 62.

HINSHAW, D. B., CARTER, R. and JOERGENSON, E. J. (1959) Volvulus of the caecum and right colon. *Am. J. Surg., 98*, 175.

HJELMSTEDT, A. (1960) Volvulus of the right colon. *Acta chir. scand., 118*, 455.

HÖFLIN, F. and VAN DER LINDEN, W. (1974) Pneumatosis cystoides intestinalis treated by oxygen breathing. *Scand. J. Gastroent., 9*, 427.

HOUGHTON, B. J. and PEARS, M. A. (1958) Chronic potassium depletion due to purgation with cascara. *Br. med. J., 1*, 1328.

IBRAHIM, H. (1961) Proctalgia fugax. *Gut, 2*, 137.

KARRAS, J. D. and ANGELO, G. (1951) Proctalgia fugax. *Am. J. Surg., 82*, 616.

KERRY, R. L. and RANSOM, H. K. (1969) Volvulus of the colon. *Archs Surg., Chicago, 99*, 215.

KOSS, L. G. (1952) Abdominal gas cysts (pneumatosis cystoides intestinorum hominis). *Archs Path., 53*, 523.

LUMSDEN, K., CHAUDHARY, N. A. and TRUELOVE, S. C. (1963) The irritable colon syndrome. *Clin. Radiol., 14*, 54.

LYNN, T. E., DOCKERTY, M. B. and WAUGH, J. M. (1956) A clinico-pathologic study of the epiploic appendages. *Surgery Gynec. Obstet.,* *103*, 423.

McGEE, A. R., PENNY, S. F. and WILLIAMSON, N. L. (1956) Pneumatosis cystoides intestinalis. *Radiology, 66*, 88.

MacLENNAN, A. (1917) Rectal crises of non-tabetic origin. *Glasgow med. J., 88*, 129.

MASSON, P. (1925) La lymphopneumatose kystique. *Ann. Anat. path. méd.-chir., 2*, 541.

MATHEWS, F. J. C. (1954) Enteric pneumatosis. *Br. med. J., 1*, 851.

MEULENGRACHT, E. (1939) Osteomalacia of the spinal column from deficient diet or from disease of the digestive tract. *Acta med. scand., 101*, 187.

NAYMAN, J. (1962) Treatment of sigmoid volvulus. *Aust. N.Z. J. Surg., 32*, 111.

NEELY, J. (1970) Treatment of gangrenous sigmoid volvulus. *Br. J. Surg., 57*, 670.

PLUM, G. E., WEBER, H. M. and SAUER, W. G. (1960) Prolonged cathartic abuse resulting in roentgen evidence suggestive of entero-colitis. *Am. J. Roentg., 83*, 919.

PRATHER, J. R. and BOWERS, R. F. (1962) Surgical management of volvulus of the sigmoid. *Archs Surg., Chicago, 85*, 869.

RAWSON, M. D. (1966) Cathartic colon. *Lancet, 1*, 1121.

ROSS, J. A. and McQUEEN, A. (1948) Peritoneal loose bodies. *Br. J. Surg., 35*, 313.

SAWYER, R. B., SAWYER, K. C. and SAWYER, K. C. (1962) Volvulus of the colon. *Am. J. Surg., 194*, 468.

SCHRODT, G. R. (1963) Melanosis coli: a study with the electron microscope. *Dis. Colon Rect., 6*, 277.

SCHWARTZ, W. B. and RELMAN, A. S. (1953) Metabolic and renal studies in chronic potassium depletion resulting from overuse of laxatives. *J. clin. Invest., 32*, 258.

SHEPHERD, J. J. (1968) Treatment of volvulus of sigmoid colon: a review of 425 cases. *Br. med. J., 1*, 280.

SHOESMITH, J. H. and CRONE, W. P. (1959) Pneumatosis cystoides intestinalis. *Br. J. Surg., 46*, 601.

SINHA, R. S. (1969) A clinical appraisal of volvulus of the pelvic colon with special reference to aetiology and treatment. *Br. J. Surg., 56*, 838.

SMITH, W. R. and GOODWIN, J. N. (1973) Caecal volvulus. *Am. J. Surg., 126*, 215.

SPEARE, G. S. (1951) Melanosis coli. *Am. J. Surg., 82*, 63.

STURZAKER, H. G., LAWRIE, R. S. and JOINER, C. L. (1976) Recurrent sigmoid volvulus in young people: a missed diagnosis. *Br. med. J., 4*, 338.

THAYSEN, E. H. (1935) Proctalgia fugax. *Lancet, 2*, 243.

THOMSON, W. O., GILLESPIE, G. and BLUMGART, L. H. (1977) The clinical significance of pneumatosis cystoides intestinalis: a report of 5 cases. *Br. J. Surg., 64*, 590.

UNDERWOOD, J. W., FINNIS, D. and SCOTT, W. (1978) Pneumatosis coli: a familial association. *Br. J. Surg., 65*, 64.

VAN DER LINDEN, W. and MARSELL, R. (1979) Pneumatosis cystoides associated with high H_2 excretion: treatment with an elemental diet. *Scand. J. Gastroent., 14*, 173.

WILLIAMS, J. L. (1961) Pneumatosis cystoides intestinalis involving the left half of the colon and rectum. *Br. J. Surg., 49*, 67.

WILSON, H. and DUNAVANT, W. D. (1965) Volvulus of the sigmoid colon. *Surg. Clins N. Am., 45*, 1245.

WITTOESCH, J. H., JACKMAN, R. J. and McDONALD, J. R. (1958) Melanosis coli: general review and a study of 887 cases. *Dis. Colon Rect., 1*, 172.

WUEPPER, K. D., OTTEMAN, M. G. and STAHLGREN, L. H. (1966) An appraisal of the operative and non-operative treatment of sigmoid volvulus. *Surgery Gynec. Obstet., 122*, 84.

YALE, C. E., BALISH, E. and WU, J. P. (1974) The bacterial etiology of pneumatosis cystoides intestinalis. *Archs Surg., Chicago, 109*, 89.

Appendix A

Combined Proctoscope and Rubber Band Ligation

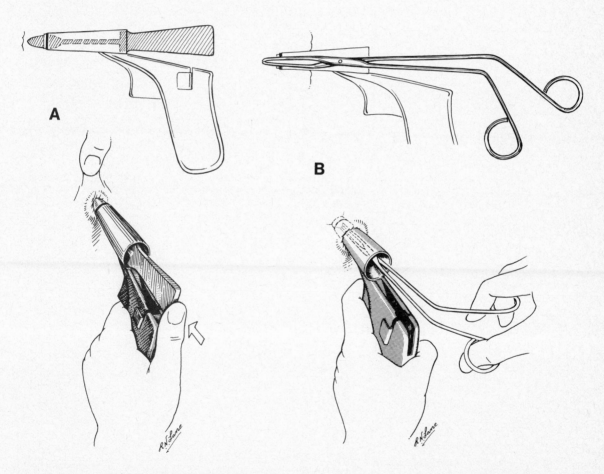

Fig. 637. The van Hoorn ligating proctoscope. (A) The instrument with obturator in place ready for introduction into anus. Note the rubber band surrounding the terminal part of the tube of the instrument. (B) When the proctoscope is in position in the anal canal and the obturator has been withdrawn, illumination can be provided by a fibreoptic cable from a distant light source or quite adequately by a properly positioned Anglepoise lamp. The end of the proctoscopic tube is pressed against the haemorrhoid being treated, care being taken that the lower edge is at least 0·5 cm above the pectinate line. The pile is then grasped by a special forceps and drawn further into the lumen of the proctoscope whilst the rubber band is pushed off the end by pulling the trigger handle.

The subject of rubber band ligation for haemorrhoids is discussed on p. 133, but an innovation in the technique of this procedure, which has only recently become available in Great Britain, seems worth mentioning. It is the development of a special proctoscope* which is itself capable of applying the rubber band to the haemorrhoid without the need to introduce a separate ligator (van Hoorn 1967). This proctoscope functions as the drum of a ligator and carries a rubber band around its distal end (Fig. 637). When the haemorrhoid is drawn into the proctoscope by a grasping forceps the band can be slipped off the tip of the proctoscope on to the neck of the pile. As the diameter of the distal end of the proctoscope is 1·8 cm, compared with a diameter of 1·1 cm for most conventional haemorrhoid

* Marketed by: 3C PMBA, Karmelietenstraat 118, B-2600 Berchem-Antwerp, Belgium.

ligators, the use of the ligating proctoscope means that a larger amount of haemorrhoidal tissue is included in the grip of the rubber band.

The great advantage claimed for this new instrument is that it enables a surgeon to perform rubber band ligation without an assistant, which is certainly a considerable convenience in office or consulting-room practice. In addition, as already mentioned, it may allow a more radical removal of haemorrhoids than is possible with ordinary ligators. My personal experience of the device is only just commencing, but it would tend to support both these claims. However, I have the firm impression that the combined proctoscope and ligator is a little rougher and more uncomfortable for the patient than are the smaller conventional ligators used in conjunction with an ordinary proctoscope. But further trial of the method appears justified.

REFERENCE

van Hoorn, M. (1972) The haemorrhoidal ligating proctoscope. In *Urgent Endoscopy of Digestive and Abdominal Diseases*, ed. Z. Maratka and J. Setka. Basel: Karger.

Appendix B

Use of Fascial Sling to Retain Mesentery to Nipple-valve in Position in Reservoir Ileostomy

---

As mentioned on p. 796 the outstanding problem in regard to the reservoir ileostomy has been the inability to devise a technique that ensures the stability of the nipple-valve, on which continence so much depends. Certainly the method of splitting the mesentery to the valve and separating the two halves of it during the suturing process (see p. 797) does not, contrary to earlier expectations, provide a

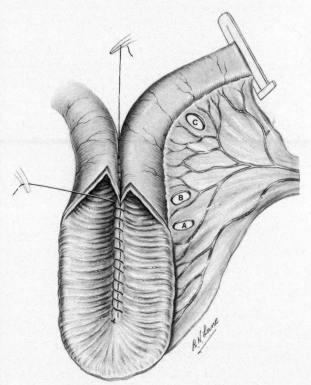

Fig. 638. Fascial sling technique for making nipple-valve. The three slits in relevant ileal mesentery are marked A, B and C. (*After Bokey and Fazio 1979*)

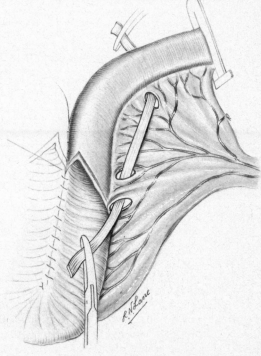

Fig. 639. Fascial sling technique for making nipple-valve. The strip of anterior rectum sheath has been threaded through the mesenteric slits and the ends are held with forceps pending invagination of the ileum into the reservoir. (*After Bokey and Fazio 1979*).

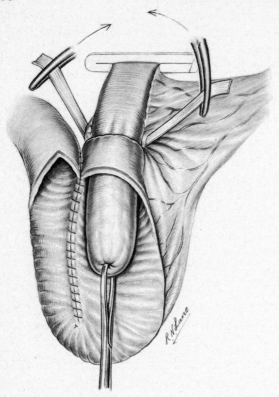

Fig. 640. Fascial sling technique for making nipple-valve. The ileum has now been drawn into the reservoir and the fascial strip has been pulled taut preparatory to wrapping its tails round the ileum for suture to it and the wall of the reservoir. (*After Bokey and Fazio 1979*)

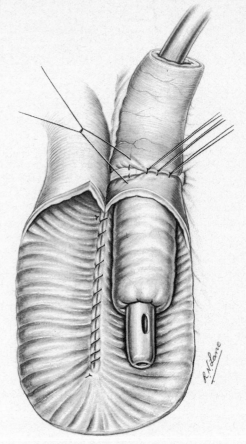

Fig. 641. Fascial sling technique for making nipple-valve. The strip of fascia has been wrapped round the ileum and fixed to the ileum and reservoir by a circumferential row of interrupted fine silk sutures, which takes bites of all three structures. The sutures commence at the edge of the ileal mesentery on one side of the bowel and extend round to the corresponding point on the other side. Here the series is not quite complete. Note that the tails of the knotted sutures are left long, and with the needles retained, for subsequent attachment of the reservoir to the abdominal wall at the end of the operation. (*After Bokey and Fazio 1979*)

guarantee against subsequent extrusion. Experience with the use of metal stapling in making the valve (see p. 803) is too recent for a reliable assessment to be made as yet of the value of this method. But a recent suggestion by Bokey and Fazio (1979), to introduce a fascial sling to hold in place the piece of mesentery attached to the valve, seems promising. The fascial band is most conveniently taken as a strip of the posterior or anterior rectus sheath 1·0–1·5 cm wide and 7·5 cm long, either through the main laparotomy wound or by making a separate longitudinal incision over the upper rectus muscle on one or other side of the abdomen. The part of the ileal mesentery connected to the segment of the ileal exit conduit that will be used for the construction of the valve is now spread out and its vascular arrangement examined by transillumination. Two small snicks are made in avascular areas of the mesentery close to the ileum (Fig. 638) about 1·5 cm apart in the mesentery close to the reservoir (A and

B) and one in the most distant part of the mesentery that will be used in the construction of the nipple-valve (C). The strip of sheath is threaded through these mesenteric holes as shown in Fig. 639. Then the ileum is drawn into the reservoir and, when it is fully in position and producing a 4 cm projection, the ends of the aponeurotic strip are wrapped round the exit ileal conduit just where it makes contact with the wall of the reservoir (Fig. 640) and drawn sufficiently taut to hold the mesentery firmly against the bowel without constricting the contained blood vessels or producing significant narrowing of the ileal lumen. To make sure that the intestinal lumen is adequate a Medena plastic tube, size 28 Charrière, is passed through the ileum and valve. Usually the tails of the fascial strip meet and slightly overlap on the antimesenteric border. They are now fixed to one another and to the ileum and wall of the reservoir by a close series of interrupted sutures of 3/0 silk or other non-absorbable material, which take bites of all three structures (Fig. 641). The tails of each suture are left long after tying and with the needle still attached, so that they can be used at the end of the operation to attach the reservoir at the base of the nipple-valve to the edges of the opening in the abdominal wall for transmission of the exit conduit. But, first of all, consideration has to be given to the use of other measures to reinforce the fixation of the valve, such as the application of three longitudinal rows of staples with the modified GIA stapler—one on either side of the mesentery and one on the antimesenteric border of the valve. The reservoir is then closed with two rows of continuous 3/0 Dexon or chromic catgut and fixed as already indicated to the anterior abdominal wall at the site of the separate ileostomy wound.

My own personal experience of this technique combined with stapling is confined to four cases done in the last few weeks. Obviously it does not give any indication of the long-term efficacy of the method in avoiding valve extrusion, but it confirms that it is an eminently practicable procedure.

REFERENCE

Bokey, L. and Fazio, V. W. (1979) A new method of constructing an intestinal nipple-valve for the continent ileostomy. *Ann. Surg.*, in the press.

Appendix C

Further Practical Considerations in Regard to Ileoanal Anastomosis With or Without Proximal Ileal Reservoir in Treatment of Ulcerative Colitis

RESULTS AND INDICATIONS FOR USE

This is indeed an awkward time (May 1979) to be writing about this procedure, because, though there has been a great revival of interest in ileoanal pull-through anastomosis in the last couple of years (Martin et al. 1977; Ferrari and Fonkalsrud 1978; Goligher 1978; Parks and Nicholls 1978; Fonkalsrud 1979), the plain fact is that insufficient experience is yet available to permit of other than tentative answers to several of the questions that arise in regard to its use in practice.

There is no doubt that, contrary to earlier short-term impressions (Goligher 1951), ileoanal anastomosis without a proximal ileal pouch can in many cases be followed by complete continence (Martin et al. 1977; Goligher 1979), but it may take many weeks or months for this state of control to be achieved and initially there is often a good deal of incontinence, especially at night, which may be very distressing to the patient. An additional cause of inconvenience, even when the patient is fully continent, is the greatly increased frequency of defaecation, sometimes amounting to 10–12 times a day or more. It is indeed hard to resist the conclusion that some of the patients would be much more comfortable with a well managed ileostomy (Goligher 1979; Fonkalsrud 1979), but there are obvious attractions, particularly to young persons, to be without any form of abdominal stoma.

Similarly it seems clear that most patients after an ileoanal anastomosis with proximal ileal pouch achieve continence, but some suffer leakage particularly at night (Parks 1978; Parks and Nicholls 1978; Goligher 1979). Nearly all these patients with an associated pelvic ileal pouch do not at first secure spontaneous defaecation, but instead have to rely on emptying the pouch three or four times a day by intubation per anum whilst they sit on the toilet. Later, some patients have achieved a normal defaecation without the use of a tube (Fonkalsrud 1979; Goligher 1979).

Though there has been no operative mortality in Martin et al.'s (1978) 17 cases of ileoanal anastomosis, in Parks' (1978) nine or Fonkalsrud's (1979) five cases of ileoanal anastomosis with ileal reservoir and in my own seven cases of ileoanal anastomosis (three with ileal reservoir), some septic complications occurred in all four groups of patients. Pull-through operations are notoriously prone to be followed by complications of this kind. Certainly it would take much larger series of cases to indicate reliably the operative morbidity and mortality of ileoanal pull-through anastomosis and to allow of a more accurate assessment of the functional results. Until we have such information it is difficult to decide on the part which this procedure, with or without associated ileal reservoir, should play in the overall plan of surgical management of ulcerative colitis. Meanwhile it would probably be wise to reserve it mainly for those patients who have found life with an ileostomy intolerable and who still retain their rectum. But in such cases the choice of ileoanal pull-through anastomosis after mucosal proctectomy has to be considered in competition with a straightforward ileorectal anastomosis (see p. 736) or with an abdominal reservoir ileostomy (see p. 796) (and, if the patient had already been submitted to a complete proctolectomy, the third of those possibilities would be the only one open to her in this situation). In this connexion it would seem reasonable, whilst awaiting the accumulation of more information about the value of ileoanal pull-through anastomosis, to urge surgeons not to sacrifice the rectum during their initial surgical treatment of colitis (unless it is very badly diseased with associated anal fistulae), so that the patient may be eligible for consideration of an anastomotic procedure of some kind at a later date.

A debatable issue is whether the construction of the ileoanal anastomosis (with or without ileal pouch) should always be reserved for a second stage, whilst a conventional ileostomy and subtotal colectomy, retaining an inactive rectal or rectosigmoid stump, is performed in the first instance. This plan has the attraction that it makes it possible to restore the patient to a fully normal state of general health and nutrition before embarking on an operation that involves the healing of an intricate and delicate anastomosis and possibly the occurrence of troublesome septic complications. Staging also has the advantage that it spares the patient a fairly lengthy combined operation, and by securing some subsidence of the inflammation in the rectal mucosa may make the subsequent mucosal proctectomy technically a good deal easier. Certainly it would be foolhardy to contemplate a single-stage combined total colectomy, partial proctectomy and ileoanal pull-through anastomosis in a patient suffering from an acute exacerbation of colitis, but if the colitis is in a phase of remission and the patient's general condition is good, there is no reason why a one-stage plan should not be adopted, as has in fact been done by Martin et al. (1977) in most of their cases. There seems to be general agreement that, whenever the ileoanal anastomosis is established, it should be 'covered' by a temporary loop ileostomy, the closure of which after eight weeks or so adds yet another stage to the programme. It is thus attractive to reduce the number of stages from three to two by amalgamating the first two when it seems possible to do so without obviously increasing the risks.

OPERATIVE TECHNIQUE

The performance of a mucosal proctectomy with ileoanal pull-through anastomosis, with or without a proximal ileal reservoir involves three or four integrated manoeuvres:

MUCOSAL PROCTECTOMY

It is customary to preserve the lower half of the rectum—that is from the level of the anterior peritoneal reflection—and to excise the mucosa from it down to the level of the pectinate line in the anal canal. This may be done in two or three ways. In one of them the rectum is bared all round just above the reflection and divided at this level, bleeding from the cut edge of the rectal stump being controlled by diathermy coagulation. A trivalve anal speculum is then inserted into the anal canal and opened up to expose the posterior wall of the anorectal remnant. The submucosa is then infiltrated with a weak adrenaline solution and the mucosa is dissected off the underlying circular muscle coat of that wall exactly as in abdominotransanal resection (see Figs 463–5). Subsequently by rotating the speculum the same procedure is employed to remove the mucosa from the other walls of the anorectal remnant in turn.

Alternatively the mucosal dissection may be performed mainly or entirely from above, as favoured by Martin et al. (1977). Again the rectum is bared of its mesorectum just above the anterior peritoneal reflection (Fig. 642), but instead of dividing the bowel across at this level its wall is infiltrated with an adrenaline solution to 'blow up' the submucosa (Fig. 643). A circular incision is then made through the muscle coat and a circumferential plane of dissection is struck between the mucosa and muscle coat (Fig. 644). By a mixture of sharp scissor dissection and blunt dissection with small gauze 'pushers' the tube of mucosa is freed from the muscle coat, which tends to collapse unless it is held up with three or four tissue forceps (Figs 644, 645). It is quite difficult to avoid some breaches of the mucosal tube during dissection and the freeing of the mucosa from the lower part of the rectum from above is certainly far from easy, especially in male patients. For this reason I prefer a combination of dissection from above and from below. Bleeding during the mucosal separation can be troublesome and requires careful haemostasis by diathermy coagulation.

Actually, so far as subsequent rectal sensation is concerned the preservation of the muscle coat of the wall of the rectum is probably unnecessary, for there is reason to believe that such sensation is at any rate partly mediated by nerve endings in the levator muscles (see p. 35), but avoiding a dissec-

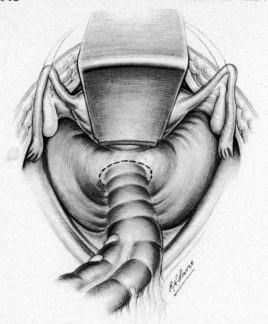

Fig. 642. Mucosal proctectomy from above. Mesorectun divided posteriorly and peritoneal coat incised on anterior and lateral walls of rectum just above the anterior reflection.

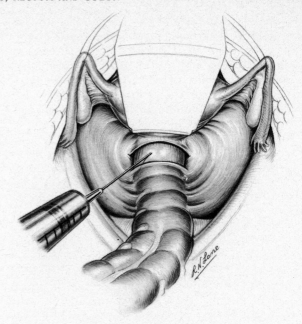

Fig. 643. Mucosal proctectomy from above. Infiltration of rectal wall with weak adrenaline solution.

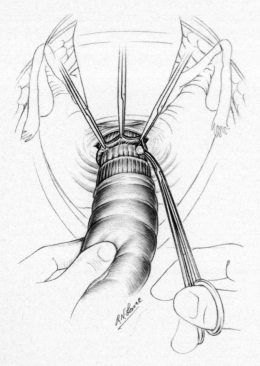

Fig. 644. Mucosal proctectomy from above. Circumferential incision of muscle coat of rectal wall down to submucosa. Whilst cut edge of muscle coat is held up with tissue forceps a plane of dissection is developed between the mucosa and muscle layers with a mixture of sharp scissor and blunt dissection.

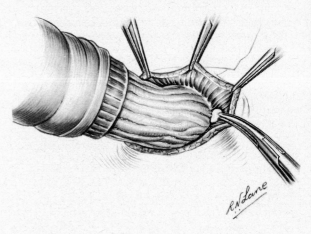

Fig. 645. Mucosal proctectomy from above. The mucosal tube is being separated from the muscle coat.

tion outside the rectum probably lessens the risks of injury to the pelvic autonomic nerves and the retention of the muscle tube may make the ileoanal anastomosis more secure.

PREPARATION OF ILEAL STUMP AND RESERVOIR

If it is intended to do a simple ileoanal pull-through anastomosis without any accompanying

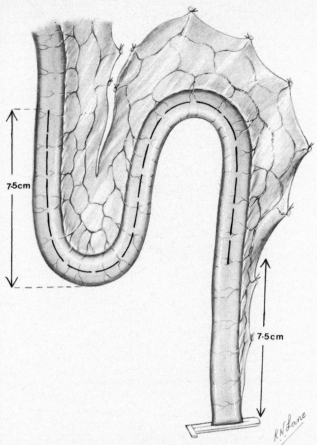

7·5cm

7·5cm

Fig. 646. Making the ileal reservoir. Sigmoid disposition of ileal segment and outline of incision used to make the reservoir. Note that each of the three limbs of bowel incised is 7·5 cm long and another 7·5 cm of ileum extends beyond to be pulled through to the anal canal.

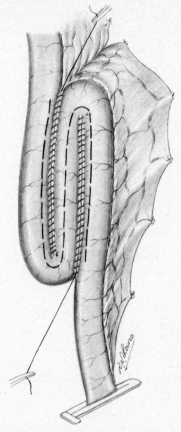

Fig. 647. Making the ileal reservoir. Two running sutures of 3/0 Dexon or chromic catgut placed to approximate the three limbs of ileum.

ileal reservoir, it is just a matter of making sure that the ileal stump that is available after separating the previous ileostomy from the abdominal wall (or dividing the ileum from the caecum in a primary operation or from the rectum or sigmoid in a case previously treated by colectomy and ileorectal anastomosis) is able to extend without tension to the anal orifice. If necessary, suitable division of vessels in the mesentery may be required to make this possible.

If on the other hand an ileal pouch is going to be prepared in the stump, even greater care is required to ensure that there is sufficient slack bowel to extend to the anus and yet allow for the duplication and suturing necessary to make the pouch. As for the method of manufacturing the reservoir, it is

important to emphasize that what is intended is a *reservoir without a valve* and that the actual technique of reservoir construction used by Kock (see p. 798) is unsuitable in this situation, for it produces a very broad pouch which does not fit easily into the tube of rectal muscle coat. A method which provides an ovoid-shaped reservoir better suited to a subsequent ileoanal pull-through anastomosis is that of Ferrari and Fonkalsrud (1978) and Parks and Nicholls (1978), in which a segment of ileum is cast in the form of a sigmoid loop and then opened and anastomosed, as shown in Figs 646–9.

PULL-THROUGH ILEOANAL ANASTOMOSIS

The technique for the anastomosis is essentially that used in abdominotransanal resection (see Figs 466, 467), except that the smaller lumen of the ileum makes the instrumentation with the bivalve specu-

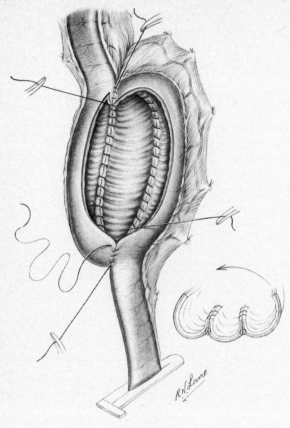

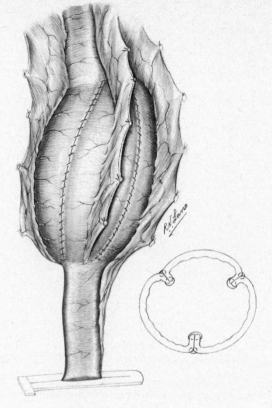

Fig. 648. Making the ileal reservoir. The bowel has now been incised and contiguous cut edges of ileum have been sutured with 3/0 running Dexon or chromic catgut.

Fig. 649. Making ileal reservoir. Completed reservoir.

lum a little more difficult. For the final state see Fig. 541B. If an ileal pouch has been provided an indwelling Medena plastic tube, size 28 F, is passed through the anus and ileum into the reservoir for continuous drainage, and fixed with a stitch to the perianal skin. Two or three sump suction drains are placed in the deep pelvis and brought out in the suprapubic region.

COVERING LOOP ILEOSTOMY

At a comfortable distance proximal to the top of the ileal reservoir—usually about 25–30 cm—a loop ileostomy with protruding active opening and receding inactive opening is fashioned in the right or left lower quadrant of the anterior abdominal wall, using the technique described on p. 759.

POSTOPERATIVE CARE

The sump drains are retained as long as they continue producing fluid, usually for four to five days at least. The plastic peranal tube in the reservoir is maintained constantly in position for two and a half weeks and thereafter passed intermittently two or three times a day to withdraw any seromucous fluid accumulating in the pouch. Vigilance is required regarding the possible development of pelvic sepsis or some degree of anastomotic dehiscence. However smooth the convalescence it is usually much easier to close the loop ileostomy after an interval of two months or so to allow all oedema to settle. After the ileostomy has been closed and the patient is experiencing the initially very frequent motions after an ileoanal anastomosis without associated ileal reservoir, a most important item of treatment is *the generous administration of antidiarrhoeal agents, such as Lomotil or loperamide.*

REFERENCES

FERRARI, B. T. and FONKALSRUD, E. W. (1978) Endorectal ileal pull-through operation with ileal reservoir after total colectomy. *Am. J. Surg.*, *136*, 113.

FONKALSRUD, E. W. (1979) Personal communication.

GOLIGHER, J. C. (1951) The functional results after sphincter-saving resections of the rectum. *Ann. R. Coll. Surg. Engl.*, *8*, 421.

—— (1978) The surgical treatment of colitis: past, present and future. *Ann. R. Coll. Surg. Engl.*, *60,* 258.

—— (1979) Unpublished data.

MARTIN, L., LE COULTRE, C. and SCHUBERT, W. K. (1977) Total colectomy and mucosal proctectomy with preservation of continence in ulcerative colitis. *Ann. Surg.*, *186*, 477.

PARKS, A. G. (1978) Personal communication.

—— and NICHOLLS, J. (1978) Proctocolectomy without ileostomy for ulcerative colitis. *Br. med. J.*, *2*, 85.